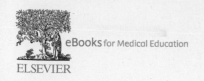

ELSEVIER

eBooks for Medical Education

T0195185

Any screen.
Any time.
Anywhere.

Activate the eBook version
of this title at no additional charge.

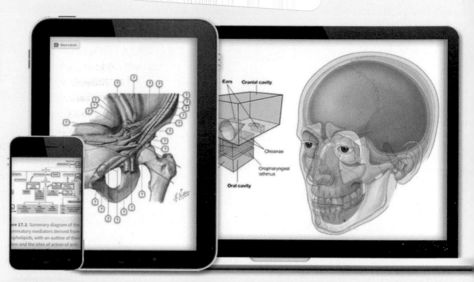

Elsevier eBooks for Medical Education gives you the power to browse and search content, view enhanced images, highlight and take notes—both online and offline.

Unlock your eBook today.

1. Visit **studentconsult.inkling.com/redeem**
2. Scratch box below to reveal your code
3. Type code into "Enter Code" box
4. Click "Redeem"
5. Log in or Sign up
6. Go to "My Library"

It's that easy!

HEICK
Scratch Gently
to Reveal Code

For technical assistance:
email studentconsult.help@elsevier.com
call 1-800-401-9962 (inside the US)
call +1-314-447-8300 (outside the US)

2020_ME

GOODMAN AND SNYDER'S
DIFFERENTIAL DIAGNOSIS
FOR PHYSICAL THERAPISTS
SCREENING FOR REFERRAL

7th
EDITION

GOODMAN AND SNYDER'S
DIFFERENTIAL DIAGNOSIS
FOR PHYSICAL THERAPISTS

SCREENING FOR REFERRAL

John D. Heick, PT, DPT, PhD, OCS, NCS, SCS

Associate Professor
Department of Physical Therapy and Athletic Training
Northern Arizona University
Flagstaff, Arizona

Rolando Lazaro, PT, PhD, DPT

Professor
Department of Physical Therapy
California State University Sacramento
Sacramento, California

ELSEVIER

3251 Riverport Lane
St. Louis, Missouri 63043

GOODMAN AND SNYDER'S DIFFERENTIAL DIAGNOSIS   ISBN: 978-0-323-72204-9
FOR PHYSICAL THERAPISTS, SEVENTH EDITION

Notice

Practitioners and researchers must always rely on their own experience and knowledge in evaluating
and using any information, methods, compounds or experiments described herein. Because of rapid
advances in the medical sciences, in particular, independent verification of diagnoses and drug dosages
should be made. To the fullest extent of the law, no responsibility is assumed by Elsevier, authors,
editors or contributors for any injury and/or damage to persons or property as a matter of products
liability, negligence or otherwise, or from any use or operation of any methods, products, instructions,
or ideas contained in the material herein.

Previous editions copyrighted 2018, 2013, 2007, 2000, 1995, and 1990.

Senior Content Strategist: Lauren Willis
Senior Content Development Manager: Luke Held
Senior Content Development Specialist: Maria Broeker
Publishing Services Manager: Deepthi Unni
Project Manager: Aparna Venkatachalam
Design Direction: Ryan Cook

Printed in Canada

Last digit is the print number: 9 8 7 6 5 4 3 2

The profession of physical therapy was founded by women. One hundred years ago, women worked as reconstruction aides to serve injured soldiers during World War I. They may not have realized what was ahead, but they did what they felt was right and always with the patient in mind.
The concept of this textbook on Differential Diagnosis was also started by a woman, Catherine Goodman. Catherine's vision for unrestricted direct access continues to advance. This edition of this textbook is dedicated to the women who started this great profession that much like Catherine have advanced our profession beyond our expectations.

JH and RTL

Annie Burke-Doe, PT, MPT, PhD
Dean
Department of Physical Therapy
West Coast University
Los Angeles, California

Marty Fontenot, PT, DPT, OCS, SCS
Assistant Professor
Physical Therapy Program
Murphy Deming College of Health Sciences at Mary
    Baldwin University
Fishersville, Virginia

William Garcia, PT, DPT, OCS, FAAOMPT
Associate Professor
Department of Physical Therapy
California State University, Sacramento
Sacramento, California

Erin Green, PT, DPT, OCS, FAAOMPT
Associate Professor
Department of Physical Therapy
California State University, Sacramento
Sacramento, California

John D. Heick, PT, DPT, PhD, OCS, NCS, SCS
Associate Professor
Department of Physical Therapy and Athletic Training
Northern Arizona University
Flagstaff, Arizona

Rolando Lazaro, PT, PhD, DPT
Professor
Department of Physical Therapy
California State University Sacramento
Sacramento, California

Jeannette Lee, PT, PhD
Associate Professor
UCSF/SFSU Graduate Program in Physical Therapy
San Francisco State University
San Francisco, California

Filippo Maselli, PT BSc, MSc, PhD, OMPT, Cert. SMT, Cert. VRS, Cert. HN
Orthopaedic Manipulative Physical Therapist, Physiotherapy,
Ph.D. in Neuroscience, DINOGMI Department, University
    of Genova

Lecturer and Skills Coordinator in Musculoskeletal &
    Rheumatological Physiotherapy Master, Sapienza
    University of Rome
Lecturer in the Musculoskeletal & Rheumatological
    Physiotherapy Master, University of Molise
President of Gruppo di Terapia Manuale e Fisioterapia
    Muscoloscheletrica Italiano (IFOMPT MO) - AIFI
Sovrintendenza Sanitaria Regionale Puglia INAIL
Bari, Italy

Seth Peterson, PT, DPT, OCS, CSCS, FAAOMPT
Founder
Physical Therapy
The Motive
Oro Valley, Arizona
Adjunct Professor
Physical Therapy
Arizona School of Health Sciences, A.T. Still University
Mesa, Arizona

Michael Ross, PT, DHSc, OCS, FAAOMPT
Associate Professor
Physical Therapy Department
Daemen College
Amherst, New York

Richard Severin, PT, DPT, PhD, CCS
Clinical Assistant Professor
Baylor University
Waco, Texas

Elizabeth Shelly, PT, DPT, WCS, BCB PMD
Physical Therapy
Beth Shelly Physical Therapist
Moline, Illinois

Brian A. Young, MS, PT, DSc, OCS, FAAOMPT
Clinical Associate Professor
Assistant Program Director &
Graduate Program Director, Physical Therapy Department
Robbins College of Health and Human Sciences
Baylor University
Waco, Texas

Author's Vision for the Future: *Cloudy with a Chance of Meatballs*

The associate editors of *DDPT* (to whom I have entrusted the future of this text) asked me (Catherine) to provide a vision of our future as a profession. When I think about our future, the title of a children's book *Cloudy With a Chance of Meatballs* (Judi and Ron Barrett, Atheneum Books for Young Readers, 1978) comes to mind, as uncertainty with unexpected outcomes may be the most apt description.

As we prepare this text for its seventh edition, the American Physical Therapy Association is celebrating its Centennial Year. One hundred years have passed and our profession is in need of clarity more than ever before. Centered around these Centennial celebrations, articles and editorials with a wide range of "visions for our future" abound. There has been much discussion as to how we will interact with artificial intelligence, how we will integrate with digital health care, how physical therapy education will evolve, how the profession will be impacted by the growth of telehealth, how research will provide data to direct treatment protocols, and more as the digital revolution comes to healthcare. As questions and predictions continue to circulate, all that is currently clear is that the crystal ball is cloudy… with a chance of meatballs.

Our (Catherine and Ellen) vision is informed by the past as much as by our hope for the future. What can we learn from looking back that will help us move successfully forward? Our history is rich and ripe with good advice for us today. Physical therapy was born of a need as Reconstruction Aides stepped up to care for our injured soldiers during the first World War. Decades of subsequent war and a polio epidemic further developed our rehabilitation skills and expanded our toolkits as wound care, splinting, and electrical stimulation entered our repertoire in answer to the calls of injured soldiers, military veterans, and children. Cardiac rehabilitation and more advanced neurorehabilitation skills were added to the toolbox during a mid-century spike in heart attacks and strokes, another example of physical therapy finding a way to meet crisis with action. Time and again we have adapted the old ways and developed new ways to rise up and meet the challenges of the day.

As physical therapists, we pride ourselves on our "can-do" attitude and have a long track record of putting that attitude to work in the world. The first edition of this text was born from both a passion as a clinician and a clear need within the profession — we were at the doorstep of Direct Access without adequate training in medical screening and I (Catherine) was ready to put my "can-do" attitude to work. The absence of this training was potentially dangerous; the first edition aimed to fill in the gap for the modern physical therapist.

It was only 30 years ago we dared to publish a physical therapy text with the word "diagnosis" as part of the title. Today, the word "diagnosis" has become an accepted word in our lexicon. Diagnosis evolved to differential diagnosis, then further parsed out to include *screening for medical disease*, and finally *screening for referral*. The next logical step now is to create differential diagnoses of neuromuscular and musculoskeletal conditions within the scope of a physical therapist's practice from which to create a best practice plan of care.

With some form of Direct Access currently available in all 50 states, the heat I (Catherine) took for that decision seems unimaginable now. But that was when Direct Access was still just a "vision of the future." The future always seems further away than it actually is. So, we can dream, can't we? And those dreams of the future can absolutely become our present.

We are in a similar place today, standing in the doorway of a transition to primary care without a clear understanding of the links between medical pathology and what we see as neuromusculoskeletal impairments. The aging Baby Boom generation and more complex health conditions are becoming new challenges for our profession. It is my hope (Catherine) that texts such as *Differential Diagnosis for Physical Therapists: Screening for Referral* and Ellen Helinski's forthcoming text, *A Physical Therapy Approach to the Modern Pain Patient*, will lead the way into the future of physical therapy care.

In the not-so-distant future, healthcare may look more like the science fiction of the not-so-distant past. Physical therapy evaluations could be performed via artificial intelligence with no physical visit even necessary as machines do the bulk of our work for us. Imagine handheld devices or automated kiosks where a person need only place a hand on the screen to get an immediate read out of biologic age and telomere length, Body Mass Index, blood type, and indicators of health and/or disease such as blood values, inflammatory markers, condition of the gut microbiome, and body/organ frequencies and functions. Practical suggestions to improve health or address disease would then be offered based on these findings.

Today this new vision may seem far away. Standing at the precipice of our future yet mired in the messy trenches of patient/client care, it has been (and continues to be) a difficult time for the physical therapy profession. Declining referrals, plummeting reimbursement rates, soaring educational costs, and the inexhaustible pain epidemic — each of these variables is taking a toll, contributing to both burnout and what many have called an identity crisis at a time when we (and our history of can-do) are needed more than ever. How will the profession get back on its feet and meet the challenges of the day? Call us biased, but we feel the answer is in the evolution of differential diagnosis.

We see a more immediate future where the physical therapist is the gatekeeper and primary practitioner for all neuromusculoskeletal conditions, including pain. Established standards like differential diagnosis and screening for referral will be the foundation from which we build new skills in pharmacology, diagnostic imaging, functional medicine, indirect manual therapy, and wellness education and practice. A standardized emphasis on integration will mean no one is viewed in terms of separate pieces and parts, but rather as a whole being—a multifaceted summation of all parts.

We see a future where what once was called "alternative" is finally seen as *advanced* and where all students of physical therapy hit the field with the tools they need to contribute and thrive. To get there, we will need to take on our new role as a doctor in healthcare by leading a shift from standardization to individualization, exclusion to inclusion, specialization to holism, and compartmentalization to integration. The task is big, the need immense. We must bring the lessons of the past to carve the way to this new future.

With rising incidences of diabetes, cancer, immunocompromise, and neurologic disorders, all healthcare professionals need to step back and embrace a more integrated view of the body. Patient/client presentations are no longer as straightforward as they once were. Individual medical conditions do not exist in isolation from the neuromusculoskeletal conditions we target. Specialization plays out like a game of pass-the-buck as patients/clients are sent from one professional to the next, with no one tracking the big picture (i.e., the individual person). We see a vision of the future in which the physical therapist takes the helm for complex patients, such as the aging adult and those struggling with pain.

Pain is the new battlefield in America for the physical therapist. The knowledge, skills, and tools needed to fight this battle will push us out of our comfort zone as movement experts into uncharted waters. If we have any hope of truly winning the war against pain, we will need to step up and take on our new role as a doctor in healthcare as we discover how thin the line has become between neuromuscular/musculoskeletal pain and dysfunction and medical pathology.

Now more than ever, we must conduct careful and thorough interviews (whether in person or via telehealth visits),

identify associated signs and symptoms, note risk factors for specific diseases, and screen for yellow and red flags. We need to overcome our outdated beliefs, learn new tools to meet the needs of each individual, and embrace new methods for addressing variables we have only begun to consider, such as epigenetics and the microbiome. The decision to treat, refer, or treat and refer remains the question of the day, only now with many more layers to peel back, more variables to consider, and a bigger role for the physical therapist to play.

As the role of the physical therapist continues to expand toward a more holistic, advanced approach, the basics will remain the same. We will still be responsible for evaluating each individual to make sure a differential diagnosis is made in order to be as specific as possible when creating the most appropriate plan of care. As always, screening begins the process and continues throughout the evaluation and subsequent treatment to determine the need for direct referral and/or interprofessional collaboration.

Like death and taxes, healthcare will remain a certainty, front and center in all our lives, but change is 100% guaranteed. In this moment, will we choose to be the profession that steps up and helps define the future of healthcare, or will we let that future define us?

So, with our history at our backs, let us move forward together with bravery, curiosity, anticipation, and joy as we craft and make manifest what we want for our profession, for patients and clients, and for all our futures. Here's to blue skies ahead…sans meatballs.

Catherine Cavallaro Goodman, MBA, PT
Ellen Hope Helinski, MS, PT, IMT.C

It is my pleasure and honor to write the foreword for the seventh edition of *Differential Diagnosis for Physical Therapists: Screening for Referral*. This textbook has been a staple in physical therapy programs for over 30 years and has stood the test of time. If you are in graduate school learning to become a physical therapist, this book is a requirement. I will go one step further. If you are a practicing clinician who treats patients, this book is a requirement. Since its inception in 1990, this text has documented the changes in our profession from one dominated by referral from physicians to that of direct access. Differential diagnosis and screening for referral continues to be increasingly important as more physical therapists, in a greater number of states, have increased autonomy due to direct access. Patients are coming into our clinics with more co-morbidities, more complex medical issues than ever before. As a physical therapist, we need to know how to navigate this tide of change which has opened our practices to the ability to see more varied and unique cases. As a professor who has been teaching orthopedics for over 20 years, and a practicing orthopedic and sports clinician for almost 30 years, I understand the importance of clearly knowing what pathologies may be masquerading as something benign. Differential diagnosis and screening for referral is foundational to our present practice of physical therapy.

Differential Diagnosis for Physical Therapists: Screening for Referral helps us navigate these changes by presenting a screening model that is rooted in standard clinical practice and reflects the patient management process in the *Guide to Physical Therapists Practice*. This text, like previous versions, is divided into three main sections. Section I: Introduction to the Screening Process; Section II: Viscerogenic Causes of Neuromusculoskeletal Pain and Dysfunction; and Section III: Systemic Origins of Neuromusculoskeletal Pain and Dysfunction. Each chapter has been edited and updated with relevant references that have become available since the last edition. These updates within each chapter clearly describe new and evolving methods of medical screening. One clear example of the latest updated edition of the text is the chapter on neurologic screening. This chapter is updated with new relevant references and concisely describes the screening process for a patient with neurological issues.

I congratulate John Heick and Rolando Lazaro for their efforts to continue Catherine Goodman's tradition of educating physical therapists through the seventh edition of the foundational textbook. Any physical therapist entrusted in examining and treating patients will benefit from this textbook.

Robert C. Manske, PT, DPT, MPT, MEd, SCS, ATC, CSCS
Professor
Department of Physical Therapy
College of Health Professions
Wichita State University

The vision of the American Physical Therapy Association (APTA) is to "Transform society by optimizing movement to improve the human experience."[1] To reach this vision, the APTA goal is to "Drive demand and access to physical therapy as a proven pathway to improve the human experience."[2] The expected outcome that APTA hopes to achieve is "Use of and access to physical therapist services as a primary entry point of care for consumers will increase."[2] This textbook supports this outcome as physical therapists are ideal health care providers to work in a primary care setting. This movement towards primary care makes sense as physical therapists work across a wide range of clinical settings, are doctorate trained musculoskeletal experts, and an important profession that contributes to the health of society by screening all systems of the body. This overarching theme is present within this updated edition of this textbook. The focus on this seventh edition is to continue to look forward and improve the abilities of physical therapy students and physical therapist clinicians to consider the three options when the therapist evaluates a patient/client, that is: 1) treat, 2) treat and refer, or 3) refer the patient.

This process is done on an ongoing basis throughout the episode of care for the patient/client and follows the standards of competency established by the APTA related to conducting a screening examination. Throughout this text, we present a screening model that allows for an efficient examination that includes the critical parts of the screening process. This screening model is an accepted part of standard clinical practice and reflects the patient/client management process in the updated edition of the *Guide to Physical Therapist Practice*. This screening process has also contributed to the movement towards a diagnostic classification scheme for our profession.

Differential diagnosis has been an area of concentration that has vastly increased over the past decade in physical therapy and is well represented on the physical therapist licensure examination. In addition, screening for medical referral continues to be an increasingly important component of physical therapist practice in all clinical practice settings, due to physical therapy direct access, medical complexity of individuals being seen by physical therapists, and limitations in health care reimbursement. As we updated the literature in this edition of the text, we have found even stronger documented evidence on the role of the physical therapist in the screening process, showing the skill and capability of the therapist to identify the need for referral to other health professionals, therefore saving lives as well as optimizing the quality of lives of individuals under their care. Information contained in this text is therefore immensely important in all clinical practice settings in the contemporary and future practice of physical therapy.

This text is divided into three sections. Section I introduces the screening process as well as a focus on interviewing the client with clarity. Chapters 3 and 4 dive deeper into pain presentations and physical assessment of the patient/client.

Section II follows a systems approach that focuses on the nine viscerogenic causes that may masquerade as a neuromusculoskeletal presentation. Each system is presented and the common conditions that occur within this system as well as red flags, risk factors, clinical presentations, and signs and symptoms are reviewed for the system. Clinical practice guidelines and helpful screening clues supported by evidence of all levels are presented for each system.

Section III covers the axial and appendicular regions of the body and reviews the systemic origins to consider when treating a patient/client with a condition in these regions.

At the end of each chapter, the reader is presented with practice questions to check for understanding and further facilitate learning. In this edition, we updated the practice questions and added several more items for review.

A comprehensive index can be found at the end of the text to allow the reader to more easily find content in the text.

The Appendices can be found in the accompanying eBook. It is important to note that part of the Appendices is a list of specific questions to consider asking when screening specific problems (e.g., headache, depression, substance use/abuse, bladder function, joint pain) (Appendix B). This list is provided alphabetically and is a special feature of the appendix.

We also encourage the reader to access additional resources related to this text in the accompanying eBook to provide you with a complete learning experience. The resources include forms that can be used in clinical practice, practice questions, weblinks, and references. For instructors, we also provide additional resources to support the use of this text in your courses, including selected images, PowerPoint slides, and a test bank.

It is our intention to provide the physical therapist clinician and physical therapist student with evidence-based approaches to screen for systemic conditions that mimic neuromusculoskeletal conditions and assist the physical therapist in optimal decision-making to benefit the patient/client. We feel that this textbook moves the profession one step closer to realizing our vision of transforming society by optimizing movement to improve the human experience.

[1]Vision Statement for the Physical Therapy Profession. American Physical Therapy Association. Available at: https://www.apta.org/apta-and-you/leadership-and-governance/vision-mission-and-strategic-plan Accessed February 15, 2022.

[2]APTA Strategic Plan 2022-2025. American Physical Therapy Association. Available at: https://www.apta.org/apta-and-you/leadership-and-governance/vision-mission-and-strategic-plan/strategic-plan Accessed February 15, 2022.

ACKNOWLEDGMENTS

As we started editing the seventh edition of this book, we realized how much has changed in such a short period of time! We were able to include a new chapter on screening for the neurologic system in this edition and we feel that this chapter will add to the understanding of the physical therapist. We are fortunate to have had the expertise and support of several individuals who made the task easier and more enjoyable. Your immense contribution to the text is very much appreciated.

To the following content experts who provided support and/or edited chapters:
Annie Burke-Doe
Marty Fontenot
Bill Garcia
Erin Green
Jeanette Lee
Seth Peterson
Filippo Maselli

Michael Ross
Richard Severin
Beth Shelly
Brian Young

To our partners at Elsevier, thank you for the help and support behind the scenes:
Lauren Willis, Senior Content Strategist
Maria Broeker, Senior Content Development Specialist
Aparna Venkatachalam, Project Manager

To Sherrill Brown at the University of Montana Skaggs School of Pharmacy: thank you for helping us update several tables related to drug information in the text.

To our research assistants: Sherene Thompson and Gita Mariel L. Manuel, thank you for assisting us with numerous research and editing tasks.

John Heick
Rolando T. Lazaro

CONTENTS

APPENDICES*

All appendixes are included in the accompanying eBook

CHAPTER

1

Introduction to Screening for Referral in Physical Therapy

In this ever changing health care system, physical therapists must screen our patients/clients* to make sure that they are appropriate candidates for physical therapy. The term *screening* denotes a methodical examination which is aimed to separate into various diagnostic groups. In this textbook, the focus is to screen for referral. The authors make this distinction because the term *differential diagnosis* invokes two different ideas. One is to differentiate between one condition versus another condition. A simplistic example of this would be a patient complaining of knee pain who potentially has patellofemoral pain syndrome or has peripatellar bursitis. The second idea of differential diagnosis is that a physical therapist needs to rule out diseases and conditions that masquerade as musculoskeletal conditions. The latter of these two approaches is the direction that the authors of this textbook take, that is screening for referral. In both scenarios, physical therapists perform within their scope of practice to provide optimal health care. By doing so we determine what biomechanical or neuromusculoskeletal problem is present that affects the client's activity and participation, and then treat the problem as specifically as possible.

As part of this process of practicing within our scope, it is the therapist's responsibility to screen for medical disease. As a health care provider, the physical therapist must be able to identify signs and symptoms of systemic disease that can mimic neuromuscular or musculoskeletal (herein referred to as neuromusculoskeletal, or NMS) dysfunction. Peptic ulcers, gallbladder disease, liver disease, and myocardial ischemia are only a few examples of systemic diseases that can cause shoulder or back pain. Other diseases can present as primary neck, upper back, hip, sacroiliac (SI), or low back pain and/or symptoms.

The purpose and the scope of this text are not to teach therapists to be medical diagnosticians. The purpose of this text is twofold. The first is to help therapists recognize the areas that are beyond the scope of a physical therapist's practice or expertise. The second is to provide a step-by-step method for therapists to identify clients who need a referral or consultation to a physician or other health professionals who can then best manage the patient.

As more states move toward unrestricted direct access, physical therapists are increasingly becoming the practitioner of choice and thereby the first contact that patients/clients seek particularly for the care of musculoskeletal dysfunction. This makes it critical for physical therapists to be well versed in determining when and how referral to a physician, nurse practitioner, physician assistant, nutritionist, psychologist, another health professional, or even another physical therapist who is a certified specialist in an area that the patient/client needs. Each patient/client case must be reviewed carefully (see Fig. 1.1).

Even without unrestricted direct access, screening is an essential skill because any client can present with red flags, or warning signs, requiring reevaluation by a medical specialist. The methods and clinical decision-making model for screening presented in this text remain the same with or without direct access and in all practice settings.

THE USE OF YELLOW OR RED FLAGS

A large part of the screening process is identifying yellow (caution) or red (warning) flag histories and identifying signs and symptoms during the examination (Box 1.1). A

---

*The *Guide to Physical Therapist Practice*1 defines *patients* as "individuals who are the recipients of physical therapy care and direct intervention" and *clients* as "individuals who are not necessarily sick or injured but who can benefit from a physical therapist's consultation, professional advice, or prevention services." In this introductory chapter, the term *patient/client* is used in accordance with the patient/client management model as presented in the *Guide*. In all other chapters, the term *client* is used except when referring to hospital inpatients/clients or outpatients/clients.

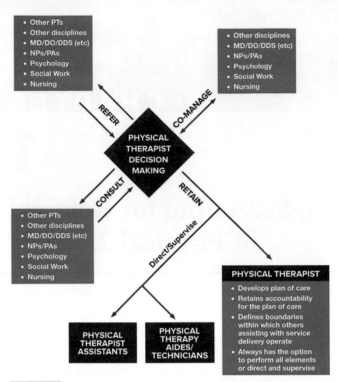

Fig. 1.1 Physical therapist referrals to other providers. PT = physical therapist, MD = doctor of medicine, DO = doctor of osteopathy, DDS = doctor of dental surgery, NP = nurse practitioner, PA = physician assistant. (From *APTA Guide to Physical Therapist Practice*, American Physical Therapy Association.)

yellow flag is a cautionary or warning symptom that signals "slow down" and is used specifically to assess pain-associated psychological distress. A useful screening tool to identify yellow flags is the Optimal Screening for Prediction of Referral and Outcome for Yellow Flags (OSPRO-YF)[1]. The OSPRO-YF asks the patient questions to identify negative coping, negative mood, and positive affect/coping domains via a multidimensional questionnaire. This tool assists clinicians in recognizing the need for referral to other health care providers to benefit the patient/client.

Red flags are features of the individual's medical history and clinical examination thought to be associated with a high risk of serious disorders, such as infection, inflammation, cancer, or fracture.[2] Think of a red flag as a means to stop and consider the information gathered in history-taking or within the examination of a patient/client. When a pattern emerges to reveal a cluster of red-flags, the clinician should stop and evaluate if the patient/client requires immediate attention, or to pursue further screening questions and/or tests, or to make an appropriate referral. A useful screening tool to identify red flags is the Optimal Screening for Prediction of Referral and Outcome-Review of Systems (OSPRO-ROS).[3] The OSPRO-ROS is a 10-item review of systems questionnaire completed by the patient that helps the clinician identify symptoms that suggest the need for referral to another health care provider (see Appendix at the end of this chapter, p. 30).

The presence of a single yellow or red flag is not usually a cause for immediate medical attention. Each cautionary or

---

BOX 1.1   RED FLAGS

The presence of any one of these symptoms is not usually cause for extreme concern but should raise a red flag for the alert therapist. The therapist is looking for a pattern that suggests a viscerogenic or systemic origin of pain and/or symptoms. The therapist will proceed with the screening process, depending on which symptoms are grouped together. Often the next step is to conduct a risk factor assessment and look for associated signs and symptoms.

Past Medical History (Personal or Family)

- Personal or family history of cancer
- Recent (last 6 weeks) infection (e.g., mononucleosis, upper respiratory infection [URI], urinary tract infection [UTI]; bacterial such as streptococcal or staphylococcal; viral such as measles, hepatitis), especially when followed by neurologic symptoms 1 to 3 weeks later (Guillain-Barré syndrome), joint pain, or back pain
- Recurrent colds or flu with a cyclical pattern (i.e., the client reports that he or she just cannot shake this cold or the flu—it keeps coming back over and over)
- Recent history of trauma, such as motor vehicle accident or fall (fracture, any age), or minor trauma in older adult with osteopenia/osteoporosis
- History of immunosuppression (e.g., steroids, organ transplant, human immunodeficiency virus [HIV])
- History of injection drug use (infection)

Risk Factors

Risk factors vary, depending on family history, previous personal history, and disease, illness, or condition present. For example, risk factors for heart disease will be different from risk factors for osteoporosis or vestibular or balance problems. As with all decision-making variables, a single risk factor may or may not be significant and must be viewed in context of the whole patient/client presentation. This represents only a partial list of all the possible health risk factors.

Substance use/abuse	Alcohol use/abuse
Tobacco use	Sedentary lifestyle
Age	Race/ethnicity
Gender	Domestic violence
Body mass index (BMI)	Hysterectomy/oophorectomy
Exposure to radiation	Occupation

Clinical Presentation

No known cause, unknown etiology, insidious onset
Symptoms that are not improved or relieved by physical therapy intervention are a red flag.
Physical therapy intervention does not change the clinical picture; client may get worse!
Symptoms that get better after physical therapy, but then get worse again is also a red flag identifying the need to screen further

Continued

BOX 1.1   RED FLAGS—cont'd

Significant weight loss or gain without effort (more than 10% of the client's body weight in 10 to 21 days)

Gradual, progressive, or cyclical presentation of symptoms (worse/better/worse)

Unrelieved by rest or change in position; no position is comfortable

If relieved by rest, positional change, or application of heat, in time, these relieving factors no longer reduce symptoms

Symptoms seem out of proportion to the injury

Symptoms persist beyond the expected time for that condition

Unable to alter (provoke, reproduce, alleviate, eliminate, aggravate) the symptoms during examination

Does not fit the expected mechanical or neuromusculoskeletal pattern

No discernible pattern of symptoms

A growing mass (painless or painful) is a tumor until proved otherwise; a hematoma should decrease (not increase) in size with time

Postmenopausal vaginal bleeding (bleeding that occurs a year or more after the last period [significance depends on whether the woman is taking a hormone replacement therapy and which regimen is used])

Bilateral symptoms:

Edema	Clubbing
Numbness, tingling	Nail-bed changes
Skin-pigmentation changes	Skin rash

Change in muscle tone or range of motion (ROM) for individuals with neurologic conditions (e.g., cerebral palsy, spinal cord injury, traumatic brain injury, multiple sclerosis)

Pain Pattern

Back or shoulder pain (most common location of referred pain; other areas can be affected as well, but these two areas signal a particular need to take a second look)

Pain accompanied by full and painless range of motion (see Table 3.1)

Pain that is not consistent with emotional or psychologic overlay (e.g., Waddell's test is negative or insignificant; ways to measure this are discussed in Chapter 3); screening tests for emotional overlay are negative

Night pain (constant and intense; see complete description in Chapter 3)

Symptoms (especially pain) are constant and intense (Remember to ask anyone with "constant" pain: Are you having this pain right now?)

Pain made worse by activity and relieved by rest (e.g., intermittent claudication; cardiac: upper quadrant pain with the use of the lower extremities when upper extremities are inactive)

Pain described as throbbing (vascular) knife-like, boring, or deep aching

Pain that is poorly localized

Pattern of coming and going like spasms, colicky

Pain accompanied by signs and symptoms associated with a specific viscera or system (e.g., GI, GU, GYN, cardiac, pulmonary, endocrine)

Change in musculoskeletal symptoms with food intake or medication use (immediately or up to several hours later)

Associated Signs and Symptoms

Recent report of confusion (or increased confusion); this could be a neurologic sign; it could be drug-induced (e.g., NSAIDs) or a sign of infection; usually it is a family member who takes the therapist aside to report this concern

Presence of constitutional symptoms (see Box 1.3) or unusual vital signs (see Discussion, Chapter 4); body temperature of 100° F (37.8° C) usually indicates a serious illness

Proximal muscle weakness, especially if accompanied by change in DTRs (see Fig. 14.3)

Joint pain with skin rashes, nodules (see discussion of systemic causes of joint pain, Chapter 3; see Table 3.6)

Any cluster of signs and symptoms observed during the Review of Systems that are characteristic of a particular organ system (see Box 4.15; Table 14.5)

Unusual menstrual cycle/symptoms; association between menses and symptoms

It is imperative, at the end of each interview, that the therapist ask the client a question like the following:

- Are there any other symptoms or problems anywhere else in your body that may not seem related to your current problem?

---

warning flag must be viewed in the context of the whole person given the age, gender, past medical history, known risk factors, medication use, and current clinical presentation of that patient/client. For example, in the examination of a patient that has had a stroke, the presence of clonus is not a red flag sign because it is expected in this patient's condition.

Clusters of yellow and/or red flags do not always warrant medical referral. Each case is evaluated on its own. Clusters of flags suggest it is time to take a closer look when risk factors for specific diseases are present, or both risk factors and red flags are present at the same time. Even as we say this, the heavy emphasis on red flags in screening has been called into question.[4,5]

It has been reported that in the primary care (medical) setting, some red flags have high false-positive rates and have very little diagnostic value when used by themselves.[6] Efforts are being made to identify reliable red flags that are valid based on patient-centered clinical research. Whenever possible, those yellow/red flags are reported in this text.[7,8]

EVIDENCE-BASED PRACTICE

All components of evidence-based practice are incorporated in the practice of physical therapy. Clinical decisions must be a product of the integration of the therapist's clinical expertise, the client's values and preferences, and the best available research evidence.[9]

Each therapist must develop the skills necessary to assimilate, evaluate, and make the best use of evidence when screening patients/clients for possible medical diseases. Clinical practice guidelines (CPG) are ideal evidence-based tools to consider as they facilitate this process of using the evidence available to facilitate screening. At the current time, the profession of physical therapy has developed 25 CPGs that are open-access available electronically, free and easy to download. At the time of publication of this book, a differential diagnosis-specific CPG is being conducted.

In the latest edition of this text, every effort has been made to consider pertinent literature, but it remains up to the reader to keep up with peer-reviewed literature reporting on the likelihood ratios; predictive values; measurement properties such as reliability, sensitivity, and specificity; and validity of yellow (cautionary) and red (warning) flags and the confidence level/predictive value behind screening questions and tests. Therapists will want to build their set of specific screening tools based on their practice setting by using the best evidence screening strategies available. These strategies are rapidly changing and require careful attention to current patient-centered peer-reviewed research/literature. One suggestion by the editors is to consider using Pubmed as it allows for *push evidence* as opposed to *pull evidence*. These terms refer to the work that the physical therapist has to do to receive literature, i.e., push evidence is evidence that is sent to the therapist via email, and pull evidence involves the therapist searching for the evidence. Push evidence such as MY NCBI from Pubmed enables the therapist who works in outpatient, and treats specific populations such as those with spinal conditions, to have literature specific to spinal conditions sent to them on a weekly or daily basis, thus allowing the therapist to stay up-to-date in their focused musculoskeletal area.

Evidence-based clinical decision-making consistent with the patient/client management model as presented in the *Guide to Physical Therapist Practice*[9] will be the foundation upon which a physical therapist's differential diagnosis is made. Screening for systemic disease or viscerogenic causes of NMS symptoms begins with a well-developed client history and interview.

The foundation for these skills is presented in Chapter 2. In addition, the therapist will rely heavily on clinical presentation and the presence of any associated signs and symptoms to alert him or her to the need for more specific screening questions and tests.

Under evidence-based practice, relying on a red-flag checklist such as the OSPRO-ROS is a more evidence-based approach that allows for consideration of serious disorders. Efforts are being made to validate red flags currently in use (see further discussion in Chapter 2). When serious conditions have not been identified, it is not for a lack of special investigation, but for a lack of adequate and thorough attention to clues usually found during a thorough history.[10,11]

Some conditions will not be identified with screening because the condition may be early in its presentation and has not progressed enough to be recognizable. In some cases, early recognition makes no difference to the outcome, either because nothing can be done to prevent progression of the condition or there is no adequate treatment available.[10]

STATISTICS

How often does it happen that a systemic or viscerogenic problem masquerades as a neuromuscular or musculoskeletal problem? There are very limited statistics to quantify how often an organic disease masquerades or presents as NMS problems. Osteopathic physicians suggest this happens in approximately 1% of cases seen by physical therapists, but little data exist to confirm this estimate.[12,13] At the present time, the screening concept remains a consensus-based approach patterned after the traditional medical model and research derived from military medicine (primarily case reports/studies).

Efforts are underway to develop a physical therapists' national database to collect patient/client data that can assist us in this effort. It is up to each of us to look for evidence in peer-reviewed journals to guide us in this process.

Personal experience suggests the 1% figure would be higher if therapists were screening routinely. In support of this hypothesis, a systematic review of 78 published case reports and case series reported that physical therapists involved in the care referred 20 patients (25.6%) to a physician because they either had worsening of symptoms or were not meeting the original prognosis. Out of the 20 who were referred, 8 cases or 10% had new symptoms that were unrelated to the initial primary symptoms.[14] Physical therapists involved in the cases were therefore routinely performing screening examinations, regardless of whether or not the client was initially referred to the physical therapist by a physician. These results demonstrate the importance of a therapist screening beyond the chief presenting complaint (i.e., for this group the red flags were not related to the reason physical therapy was started), or when new presenting signs and symptoms appear to not be related to the primary condition. For example, it is important to listen to our clients when they are not improving in our care, either postoperatively[15] or if the presentation does not match the referring diagnosis.[16] In these cases, red flags may lead the therapist to further evaluate systems that are not included in the original referring diagnosis by the health care professional. This approach benefits our clients/patients by using our knowledge and providing the best care!

KEY FACTORS TO CONSIDER

Three key factors that create a need for screening are:
- Side effects of medications
- Comorbidities
- Visceral pain mechanisms

If the medical diagnosis is delayed, then the correct diagnosis is eventually made when:

1. The patient/client does not get better with physical therapy intervention.
2. The patient/client gets better then worse.
3. Other associated signs and symptoms eventually develop.

There are times when a patient/client with NMS complaints is really experiencing the side effects of medications. This may be the most common source of associated signs and symptoms observed depending on the clinical setting. Side effects of medication as a cause of associated signs and symptoms, including joint and muscle pain, will be discussed more completely in Chapter 2. Visceral pain mechanisms may be found in Chapter 3.

As for comorbidities, many patients/clients are affected by other conditions such as depression, diabetes, incontinence, obesity, chemical dependency, hypertension, osteoporosis, and deconditioning. These conditions can contribute to significant morbidity and mortality and must be documented as a part of the problem list. Physical therapy intervention is often appropriate in affecting outcomes, and/or referral to a more appropriate health care professional or to another physical therapist with advanced skills or certifications may be needed.

Movement, physical activity, and moderate exercise aid the body and boost the immune system,[17,18] but sometimes such measures are unable to prevail, especially if other factors are present, such as inadequate hydration, poor nutrition, fatigue, depression, immunosuppression, and stress. In such cases the condition will progress to the point that warning signs and symptoms will be observed or reported and/or the patient's/client's condition will deteriorate. For these types of patients, the need for medical referral or consultation becomes evident over the episode of care.

REASONS TO SCREEN

There are many reasons why the therapist needs to screen for medical disease. Direct access (see definition and discussion later in this chapter) is only one of those reasons (Box 1.2).

Early detection and referral is the key to prevention of further significant comorbidities or complications. In all practice settings, therapists must know how to recognize systemic disease mimicking the clinical presentation of a neuromusculoskeletal condition. This includes practice by physician referral, practitioner of choice via the direct access model, or as a primary practitioner.

The practice of physical therapy has evolved over time since the profession began as Reconstruction Aides. Clinical practice, as it was shaped by World War I and then World War II, was eclipsed by the polio epidemic in the 1940s and 1950s. With the widespread use of the live, oral polio vaccine in 1963, polio was eradicated in the United States and clinical practice changed again (Fig. 1.2).

Today most clients seen by therapists have impairments, activity limitations, and participation restrictions that are clearly NMS-related. Frequently the client history and

> ### BOX 1.2   REASONS FOR SCREENING
>
> - Direct access: Therapist has primary responsibility or first contact.
> - Quicker and sicker patient/client base.
> - Signed prescription: Clients may obtain a signed prescription for physical/occupational therapy based on similar past complaints of musculoskeletal symptoms without direct physician contact.
> - Medical specialization: Medical specialists may fail to recognize underlying systemic disease.
> - Disease progression: Early signs and symptoms are difficult to recognize, or symptoms may not be present at the time of medical examination.
> - Patient/client disclosure: Client discloses information previously unknown or undisclosed to the physician.
> - Client does not report symptoms or concerns to the physician because of forgetfulness, fear, or embarrassment.
> - Presence of one or more yellow (caution) or red (warning) flags.

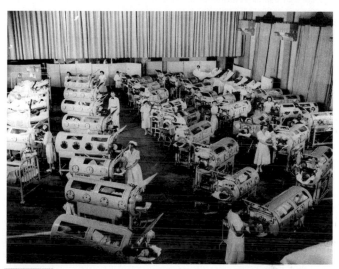

Fig. 1.2 Patients in iron lungs receive treatment at Rancho Los Amigos during the polio epidemic of the 1940s and 1950s. (Courtesy Rancho Los Amigos, 2005).

mechanism of injury point to a known cause of movement dysfunction.

However, therapists practicing in all settings must be able to evaluate a patient's/client's complaint knowledgeably and determine whether there are signs and symptoms of a systemic disease or a medical condition that should be evaluated by a more appropriate health care provider. This text endeavors to provide the necessary information that will assist the therapist in making these decisions.

Quicker and Sicker

The aging of America has affected general health in significant ways. "Quicker and sicker" is a term used to describe patients/clients in the current health care arena (Fig. 1.3).[19,20]

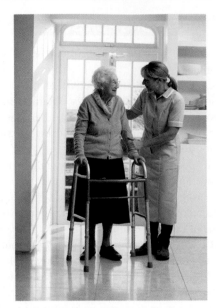

Fig. 1.3   The aging of America from the "traditionalists" (born before 1946) and the Baby Boom generation ("boomer" born 1946–1964) will result in older adults with multiple comorbidities in the care of the physical therapist. Even with a known orthopedic and/or neurologic impairment, these clients will require a careful screening for the possibility of other problems, side effects from medications, and primary/secondary prevention programs. (From monkeybusinessimages).

"Quicker" refers to how health care delivery has changed in the last 10 years to combat the rising costs of health care. In the acute care setting, the focus is on rapid recovery protocols. As a result, earlier mobility is emphasized and more complex patients are being discharged much faster than in the past.[21] Better pharmacologic management of agitation has allowed earlier and safer mobility. Hospital inpatients/clients are discharged much faster today than they were even 10 years ago. Patients are discharged from the intensive care unit (ICU) to rehab or even home. Patients/clients on the medical-surgical wards of most hospitals today would have been in the ICU 20 years ago. Same-day discharge for selected orthopedic procedures, that would have required a much longer hospitalization in the past, is also now more common. Physical therapy may or may not be ordered by the physician after discharge from an outpatient/client surgery.

Today's health care environment is complex, rapidly changing, and highly demanding. The therapist must be alert to red flags of systemic disease at all times and in all practice settings, but especially in those clients who have been given early release from the hospital or transitional units. Warning flags may come in the form of reported symptoms or observed signs. It may be a clinical presentation that does not match the recent history. Red warning and yellow caution flags will be discussed throughout this text to emphasize the importance relevant to each content area.

"Sicker" refers to patients/clients in acute care, rehabilitation, or in the outpatient/client setting with any orthopedic or neurologic problem who may have a past medical history of cancer or a current personal history of diabetes, liver disease, thyroid condition, peptic ulcer, and/or other conditions or diseases.

Our society is faced with challenges in terms of managing chronic conditions. It is estimated that two out of three older Americans have multiple chronic conditions. This accounts for 25% of the entire U.S. population, and 66% of the U.S. health care expenditure.[22] The presence of multiple comorbidities emphasizes the need to view the whole patient/client and not just the body part in question.

Natural History

Improvements in treatment for neurologic, cardiovascular and pulmonary conditions previously considered fatal (e.g., cancer, cystic fibrosis) are now extending the life expectancy for many individuals. Improved interventions bring new areas of focus such as issues related to quality of life. The artificial dichotomy of pediatric versus adult care is gradually being replaced by a continuum of care lifestyle approach that takes into consideration what is known about the natural history of the condition.

Many individuals with childhood-onset diseases now live well into adulthood, and age with chronic disabilities. Their original pathology or disease process has given way to secondary impairments, creating further activity and participation restrictions as the person ages. For example, a 30-year-old with cerebral palsy may experience chronic pain, changes or limitations in ambulation and endurance, and increased fatigue that prevents the client from performing functional activities and participating in events that they enjoy.

These symptoms result from the atypical compensatory movement patterns and musculoskeletal strains caused by chronic increase in tone and muscle imbalances that were originally caused by cerebral palsy. In this case the screening process may be identifying signs and symptoms that have developed as a natural result of the primary condition (e.g., cerebral palsy) or long-term effects of treatment (e.g., chemotherapy, biotherapy, or radiotherapy for cancer).

Signed Prescription

Under direct access, the physical therapist may have primary responsibility or become the first contact for some clients in the health care delivery system. On the other hand, clients may obtain a signed prescription for physical therapy from their primary care physician or other health care provider, based on similar past complaints of musculoskeletal symptoms, without actually seeing the physician or being examined by the physician (Case Example 1.1).

? FOLLOW-UP QUESTIONS

Always ask a client who provides a signed prescription:
- Did you actually see the physician (chiropractor, dentist, nurse practitioner, physician assistant)?
- Did the doctor (dentist) examine you and how did this occur?

CASE EXAMPLE 1.1

Physician Visit Without Examination

A 60-year-old man retired from his job as the president of a large vocational technical school and called his physician the next day for a long-put-off referral to physical therapy. He arrived at an outpatient orthopedic physical therapy clinic with a signed physician's prescription that said, "Evaluate and Treat."

His primary complaint was left anterior hip and groin pain. This client had a history of three previous total hip replacements (THRs) (anterior approach, lateral approach, posterior approach) on the right side, performed over the last 10 years.

Based on previous rehabilitation experience, he felt certain that his current symptoms of hip and groin pain could be alleviated by physical therapy.

- Social history: Recently retired as the director of a large vocational rehabilitation agency, married, three grown children
- Past medical history (PMHx): Three THRs to the left hip (anterior, posterior, and lateral approaches) over the last 10 years
  - Open heart surgery 10 years ago
  - Congestive heart failure (CHF) 3 years ago
  - Medications: Lotonsin daily, 1 baby aspirin per day, Zocor (20 mg) once a day
- Clinical presentation:
  - Extensive scar tissue around the left hip area with centralized core of round, hard tissue (4 × 6 cm) over the greater trochanter on the left
  - Bilateral pitting edema of the feet and ankles (right greater than left)
  - Positive Thomas (30-degree hip flexion contracture) test for left hip
  - Neurologic screen: Negative but general deconditioning and global decline observed in lower extremity strength
  - Vital signs:*
  Blood pressure (sitting, right arm) 92/58 mm Hg
  Heart rate 86 bpm
  Respirations 22/min
  Oxygen saturation (at rest) 89%
  Body temperature 97.8° F

The client arrived at the physical therapy clinic with a signed prescription in hand, but when asked if he had actually seen the physician, he explained that he received this prescription after a telephone conversation with his physician.

How Do You Communicate Your Findings and Concerns to the Physician? It is always a good idea to call and ask for a copy of the physician's dictation or notes. It may be that the doctor is well aware of the client's clinical presentation. Health Insurance Portability and Accountability Act (HIPAA) regulations require the client to sign a disclosure statement before the therapist can gain access to the medical records. To facilitate this process, it is best to have the paperwork requirements completed by the first appointment before the therapist sees the client.

Sometimes a conversation with the physician's office staff is all that is needed. They may be able to look at the client's chart and advise you accordingly. At the same time, in our litigious culture, outlining your concerns or questions almost always obligates the medical office to make a follow-up appointment with the client.

It may be best to provide the client with your written report that he or she can hand carry to the physician's office. Sending a fax, email, or mailed written report may place the information in the chart but not in the physician's hands at the appropriate time. It is always advised to either fax or mail and provide a hand-carried copy.

Make your documentation complete, but your communication brief. Thank the physician for the referral. Outline the problem areas (human movement system diagnosis, impairment classification, and planned intervention). Be brief! The physician is only going to have time to scan what you sent.

Any associated signs and symptoms or red flags can be pointed out as follows:

During my examination, I noted the following:
Bilateral pitting edema of lower extremities
Vital signs:
Blood pressure (sitting, right arm) 92/58 mm Hg
Heart rate 86 bpm
Respirations 22/min
Oxygen saturation (at rest) 89%
Body temperature 97.8 F
Some of these findings seem outside the expected range. Please advise.

Note to the Reader: If possible, highlight this last statement in order to draw the physician's eye to your primary concern.

It is outside the scope of our practice to suggest possible reasons for the client's symptoms (e.g., congestive failure, side effect of medication). Just make note of the findings and let the physician make the medical diagnosis. An open-ended comment such as "Please advise" or a question such as "What do you think?" may be all that is required.

Of course, in any collaborative relationship you may find that some physicians ask for your opinion. It is quite permissible to offer the evidence and draw some possible conclusions.

Result: An appropriate physical therapy program of soft tissue mobilization, stretching, and home exercise was initiated. However, the client was returned to his physician for an immediate follow-up appointment. A brief report from the therapist stated the key objective findings and outlined the proposed physical therapy plan. The letter included a short paragraph with the following remarks:

> *Given the client's sedentary lifestyle, previous history of heart disease, and blood pressure reading today, I would like to recommend a physical conditioning program. Would you please let me know if he is medically stable? Based on your findings, we will begin with a preaerobic training program here and progress to a home-based or fitness center program for him.*

---

*The blood pressure and pulse measurements are difficult to evaluate given the fact that this client is taking antihypertensive medications. ACE inhibitors and beta-blockers, for example, reduce the heart rate so that the body's normal compensatory mechanisms (e.g., increased stroke volume and therefore increased heart rate) are unable to function in response to the onset of congestive heart failure. Low blood pressure and high pulse rate with higher respiratory rate and mildly diminished oxygen saturation (especially on exertion) must be considered red flags. Auscultation would be in order here. Light crackles in the lung bases might be heard in this case.

Medical Specialization

Additionally, with the increasing specialization of medicine, clients may be evaluated by a medical specialist who does not immediately recognize the underlying systemic disease, or the specialist may assume that the referring primary care physician has ruled out other causes (Case Example 1.2).

Progression of Time and Disease

In some cases, early signs and symptoms of systemic disease may be difficult or impossible to recognize until the disease has progressed enough to create distressing or noticeable signs or symptoms (Case Example 1.3). In some cases, the patient's/client's clinical presentation in the physician's office may be very different from what the therapist observes when days or weeks separate the two appointments.

CASE EXAMPLE 1.2
Medical Specialization

A 45-year-old long-haul truck driver with bilateral carpal tunnel syndrome was referred for physical therapy by an orthopedic surgeon specializing in hand injuries. During the course of treatment the client mentioned that he was also seeing an acupuncturist for wrist and hand pain. The acupuncturist told the client that, based on his assessment, acupuncture treatment was indicated for liver disease.

Comment: Protein (from food sources or from a GI bleed) is normally taken up and detoxified by the liver. Ammonia is produced as a by-product of protein breakdown and then transformed by the liver to urea, glutamine, and asparagine before being excreted by the renal system. When liver dysfunction results in increased serum ammonia and urea levels, peripheral nerve function can be impaired. (See detailed explanation on neurologic symptoms in Chapter 10.)

Result: The therapist continued to treat this client, but knowing that the referring specialist did not routinely screen for systemic causes of carpal tunnel syndrome (or even screen for cervical involvement) combined with the acupuncturist's information, raised a red flag for possible systemic origin of symptoms. A phone call was made to the physician with the following approach:

> Say, Mr. Y was in for therapy today. He happened to mention that he is seeing an acupuncturist who told him that his wrist and hand pain is from a liver problem. I recalled seeing some information here at the office about the effect of liver disease on the peripheral nervous system. Because Mr. Y has not improved with our carpal tunnel protocol, would you like to have him come back in for a reevaluation?

Comment: How to respond to each situation will require a certain amount of diplomacy, with consideration given to the individual therapist's relationship with the physician and the physician's openness to direct communication.

It is the physical therapist's responsibility to recognize when a client's presentation falls outside the parameters of a true neuromusculoskeletal condition. Unless prompted by the physician, it is not the therapist's role to suggest a specific medical diagnosis or medical testing procedures.

Given enough time, a disease process may eventually progress and get worse. Symptoms may become more readily apparent or more easily clustered. In such cases, the alert therapist may be the first to ask the patient/client pertinent

CASE EXAMPLE 1.3
Progression of Disease

A 44-year-old woman was referred to the physical therapist with a complaint of right paraspinal/low thoracic back pain. There was no reported history of trauma or assault and no history of repetitive movement. The past medical history was significant for a kidney infection treated 3 weeks ago with antibiotics. The client stated that her follow-up urinalysis was "clear" and the infection resolved.

The physical therapy examination revealed true paraspinal muscle spasm with an acute presentation of limited movement and exquisite pain in the posterior right middle to low back. Spinal accessory motions were tested following application of a cold modality and were found to be mildly restricted in right sidebending and left rotation of the T8–T12 segments. It was the therapist's assessment that this joint motion deficit was still the result of muscle spasm and guarding and not true joint involvement.

Result: After three sessions with the physical therapist in which modalities were used for the acute symptoms, the client was not making observable, reportable, or measurable improvement. Her fourth scheduled appointment was cancelled because of the "flu."

Given the recent history of kidney infection, the lack of expected improvement, and the onset of constitutional symptoms (see Box 1.3), the therapist contacted the client by telephone and suggested that she make a follow-up appointment with her doctor as soon as possible.

As it turned out, this woman's kidney infection had recurred. She recovered from her back sequelae within 24 hours of initiating a second antibiotic treatment. This is not the typical medical picture of a urologically compromised person. Sometimes it is not until the disease progresses that the systemic disorder (masquerading as a musculoskeletal problem) can be clearly differentiated.

Last, sometimes clients do not relay all the necessary or pertinent medical information to their physicians but will confide in the physical therapist. They may feel intimidated, forget, become unwilling or embarrassed, or fail to recognize the significance of the symptoms and neglect to mention important medical details (see Box 1.1).

Knowing that systemic diseases can mimic neuromusculoskeletal dysfunction, the therapist is responsible for identifying as closely as possible what neuromusculoskeletal pathologic condition is present.

The final result should be to treat as specifically as possible. This is done by closely identifying the underlying neuromusculoskeletal pathologic condition and the accompanying movement dysfunction, while simultaneously investigating the possibility of systemic disease.

This text will help the clinician quickly recognize problems that are beyond the expertise of the physical therapist. The therapist who recognizes hallmark signs and symptoms of systemic disease will know when to refer clients to the appropriate health care practitioner.

CASE EXAMPLE 1.4
Bilateral Hand Pain

A 69-year-old man presented with pain in both hands that was worse in the left. He described the pain as "deep aching" and reported that it interfered with his ability to write. The pain got worse as the day went on.

There was no report of fever, chills, previous infection, new medications, or cancer. The client was unaware that joint pain could be caused by sexually transmitted infections but said that he was widowed after 50 years of marriage to the same woman and did not think this was a problem.

There was no history of occupational or accidental trauma. The client viewed himself as being in "excellent health." He was not taking any medications or herbal supplements.

Wrist range of motion was limited by stiffness at end ranges in flexion and extension. There was no obvious soft tissue swelling, warmth, or tenderness over or around the joint. A neurologic screening examination was negative for sensory, motor, or reflex changes.

There were no other significant findings from various tests and measures performed. There were no other joints involved. There were no reported signs and symptoms of any kind anywhere else in the muscles, limbs, or general body.

What Are the Red-Flag Signs and Symptoms Here? Should a Medical Referral Be Made? Why or Why Not?
Red Flags
Age
Bilateral symptoms
Lack of other definitive findings

It is difficult to treat as specifically as possible without a clear differential diagnosis. You can treat the symptoms and assess the results before making a medical referral. Improvement in symptoms and motion should be seen within one to three sessions.

However, in light of the red flags, best practice suggests a medical referral to rule out a systemic disorder before initiating treatment. This could be rheumatoid arthritis, osteoarthritis, osteoporosis, the result of a thyroid dysfunction, gout, or other arthritic condition.

How Do You Make This Suggestion to the Client, Especially if He Was Coming to You to Avoid a Doctor's Visit/Fee? Perhaps something like this would be appropriate:

Mr. J,

You have very few symptoms to base treatment on. When pain or other symptoms are present on both sides, it can be a sign that something more systemic is going on. For anyone over the age of 40 years with bilateral symptoms and a lack of other findings, we recommend a medical examination.

Do you have a regular family doctor or primary care physician? It may be helpful to have some x-rays and laboratory work done before we begin treatment here. Who can I call or send my report to?

Result: Radiographs showed significant joint space loss in the radiocarpal joint, as well as sclerosis and cystic changes in the carpal bones. Calcium deposits in the wrist fibrocartilage pointed to a diagnosis of calcium pyrophosphate dihydrate (CPPD) crystal deposition disease (pseudogout).

There was no osteoporosis and no bone erosion present.

Treatment was with oral NSAIDs for symptomatic pain relief. There is no evidence that physical therapy intervention can change the course of this disease or even effectively treat the symptoms.

The client opted to return to physical therapy for short-term palliative care during the acute phase.

To read more about this condition, consult the *Primer on the Rheumatic Diseases*, ed 13, Atlanta, 2008, Arthritis Foundation.

Data from Raman S, Resnick D: Chronic and increasing bilateral hand pain, *J Musculoskeletal Med* 13(6):58–61, 1996.

questions to determine the presence of underlying symptoms requiring medical referral.

The therapist must know what questions to ask clients in order to identify the need for medical referral. Knowing what medical conditions can cause shoulder, back, thorax, pelvic, hip, SI, and groin pain is essential. Familiarity with risk factors for various diseases, illnesses, and conditions is an important tool for early recognition in the screening process.

Patient/Client Disclosure

Sometimes patients/clients tell the therapist things about their current health and social history unknown or unreported to the physician. The content of these conversations can hold important screening clues to point out a systemic illness or viscerogenic cause of musculoskeletal or neuromuscular impairment.

The patient's/client's history, presenting pain pattern, and possible associated signs and symptoms must be reviewed along with results from the objective evaluation in making a treatment-versus-referral decision.

Medical conditions can cause pain, dysfunction, and impairment of the:
- Back/neck
- Shoulder
- Chest/breast/rib
- Hip/groin
- SI/sacrum/pelvis

For the most part, the organs are located in the central portion of the body and refer symptoms to the nearby major muscles and joints. In general, the back and shoulder represent the primary areas of referred viscerogenic pain patterns. Cases of isolated symptoms will be presented in this text as they occur in clinical practice. Symptoms of any kind that present bilaterally should raise a red flag for concern and further investigation (Case Example 1.4).

Monitoring vital signs is a quick and easy way to screen for medical conditions. Vital signs are discussed more completely in Chapter 4. Asking about the presence of constitutional symptoms is important, especially when there is no known cause. Constitutional symptoms refer to a constellation of signs and symptoms present whenever the patient/client is

---

BOX 1.3   CONSTITUTIONAL SYMPTOMS

Fever
Diaphoresis (unexplained perspiration)
Sweats (can occur anytime night or day)
Nausea
Vomiting
Diarrhea
Pallor
Dizziness/syncope (fainting)
Fatigue
Weight loss

BOX 1.4   PHYSICAL THERAPIST ROLE IN DISEASE PREVENTION

Primary Prevention: Stopping the process(es) that lead to the development of disease(s), illness(es), and other pathologic health conditions through education, risk factor reduction, and general health promotion.

Secondary Prevention: Early detection of disease(es), illness(es), and other pathologic health conditions through regular screening; this does not prevent the condition but may decrease duration and/or severity of disease and thereby improve the outcome, including improved quality of life.

Tertiary Prevention: Providing ways to limit the degree of disability while improving function in patients/clients with chronic and/or irreversible diseases.

Health Promotion and Wellness: Providing education and support to help patients/clients make choices that will promote health or improve health. The goal of wellness is to give people greater awareness and control in making choices about their own health.

---

experiencing a systemic illness. No matter what system is involved, these core signs and symptoms are often present (Box 1.3).

MEDICAL SCREENING VERSUS SCREENING FOR REFERRAL

Therapists can have an active role in both primary and secondary prevention through screening and education. Primary prevention involves stopping the process(es) that lead to the development of diseases such as diabetes, coronary artery disease, or cancer in the first place (Box 1.4).

According to the *Guide*,[9] physical therapists are involved in primary prevention because they identify "risk factors and implement services to reduce risk in individuals and populations." Risk factor assessment and risk reduction fall under this category.

Secondary prevention involves the regular screening for early detection of disease or other health-threatening conditions such as hypertension, osteoporosis, incontinence,

diabetes, or cancer. This does not prevent any of these problems but improves the outcome and the efficiency of getting the client to the appropriate healthcare provider. Physical therapists "prevent or slow the progression of functional decline and disability and enhance activity and participation in chosen life roles and situations in individuals and populations with an identified condition."[9] Although the terms *screening for medical referral* and *medical screening* are often used interchangeably, these are two separate activities. Medical screening is a method for detecting disease or body dysfunction before an individual would normally seek medical care. Medical screening tests are usually administered to individuals who do not have current symptoms, but who may be at high risk for certain adverse health outcomes (e.g., colonoscopy, fasting blood glucose, blood pressure monitoring, assessing body mass index, thyroid screening panel, cholesterol screening panel, prostate-specific antigen, mammography).

In the context of a human movement system diagnosis, the term *medical screening* has come to refer to the process of screening for referral. The process involves determining whether the individual has a condition that can be addressed by the physical therapist's intervention, and if not, whether the condition requires evaluation by a physician or another healthcare professional.

Both terms (*medical screening* and *screening for referral*) will probably continue to be used interchangeably to describe the screening process. It may be important to keep the distinction in mind, especially when conversing/consulting with physicians whose concept of medical screening differs from the physical therapist's use of the term to describe screening for referral.

DIAGNOSIS BY THE PHYSICAL THERAPIST

The term "diagnosis by the physical therapist" is language used by the American Physical Therapy Association (APTA). It is the policy of the APTA that physical therapists shall establish a diagnosis for each patient/client. Before making a patient/client management decision, physical therapists shall utilize the diagnostic process in order to establish a diagnosis for the specific conditions in need of the physical therapist's attention.[23]

In keeping with advancing physical therapy practice, *Diagnosis by Physical Therapists* (HOD P06-12-10-09), has been updated to include ordering of tests that are performed and interpreted by other health professionals (e.g., radiographic imaging, laboratory blood work). The position now states that it is the physical therapist's responsibility in the diagnostic process to organize and interpret all relevant data.[23]

The diagnostic process requires evaluation of information obtained from the patient/client examination, including the history, systems review, administration of tests, and interpretation of data. Physical therapists use diagnostic labels that identify the effect of a condition on function at the level of the system (especially the human movement system) and the level of the whole person.[24]

In 2013 the APTA adopted a bold vision statement that the profession will move towards "Transforming society by optimizing movement to improve the human experience."[25] The APTA continues to work towards developing the concept of human movement as a physiologic system and to advance physical therapists recognition as experts in human movement.[25,26] The Movement System is therefore the core of who physical therapists are and what physical therapists do.[27] The Movement System is defined as "the anatomic structures and physiologic functions that interact to move the body or its component parts."[28]

Further Defining Diagnosis

To arrive at a physical therapy diagnosis, the clinician collects and sorts data gathered in the examination based on a classification scheme that is relevant to the clinician.[29] This process may result in the generation of diagnostic labels to describe the impact of a condition on function at the level of the system (especially the movement system) and at the level of the whole person.[29]

The approach taken by a physical therapist for diagnosis is in contrast to the physician's approach to medical diagnosis. The physician makes a medical diagnosis based on the pathologic or pathophysiologic state at the cellular level. In a diagnosis-based physical therapist's practice, the therapist places an emphasis on the identification of specific human movement impairments, activity limitations, and participation restrictions, and then matches established effective interventions and considers the prognosis of the patient based on a biopsychosocial model of the patient.[30,31]

Others have supported a revised definition of the physical therapy diagnosis as: a process centered on the evaluation of multiple levels of movement dysfunction whose purpose is to inform treatment decisions related to functional restoration.[32] According to the *Guide*, the diagnostic-based practice requires the physical therapist to integrate the elements of patient/client management (Box 1.5) in a manner designed to maximize outcomes (Fig. 1.4).

Within the Elements of the Patient/Client Management Model from the Guide to Physical Therapist Practice "Referral/Consultation" as a potential pathway for the therapist during the evaluation process. The referral pathway was previously described and detailed by Boissonnault to show three alternative decisions[33,34] (Fig. 1.5), including:

- Referral/consultation (no treatment; referral may be a nonurgent consult or an immediate/urgent referral)
- Diagnose and treat
- Both (treat and refer)

The decision to refer or consult with the physician can also apply to referral to other appropriate health care professionals and/or practitioners (e.g., dentist, chiropractor, nurse practitioner, psychologist, or even a physical therapist that specializes in an area that the patient needs).

In summary, there has been considerable discussion that evaluation is a process with diagnosis as the end result.[35] The concepts around the "diagnostic process" remain part of an

---

BOX 1.5   ELEMENTS OF PATIENT/CLIENT MANAGEMENT

Examination: History, systems review, and tests and measures
Evaluation: Assessment or judgment of the data
Diagnosis: Determined within the scope of practice
Prognosis: Optimal level of improvement within a time frame
Intervention: Coordination, communication, and documentation of an appropriate treatment plan for the diagnosis based on the previous four elements
Outcomes: Actual result of the implementation of the plan of care

Data from *Guide to physical therapist practice*, ed 3, Alexandria, VA, 2014, American Physical Therapy Association (APTA).

The process of physical therapist patient and client management.

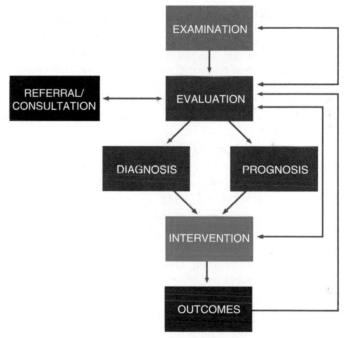

© 2014 by American Physical Therapy Association

Fig. 1.4   The elements of patient/client management leading to optimal outcomes. (Reprinted from *Guide to Physical Therapist Practice 3.0*, [http://www.apta.org/Guide/], with permission from the American Physical Therapy Association. © 2014 American Physical Therapy Association.)

---

evolving definition that will continue to be discussed and clarified by physical therapists.

When communicating with physicians, it is helpful to understand the definition of a medical diagnosis and how it differs from a physical therapist's diagnosis. The medical diagnosis is traditionally defined as the recognition of disease. It is the determination of the cause and nature of pathologic conditions. Medical differential diagnosis is the comparison of symptoms of similar diseases and medical diagnostics (laboratory and test procedures performed) so

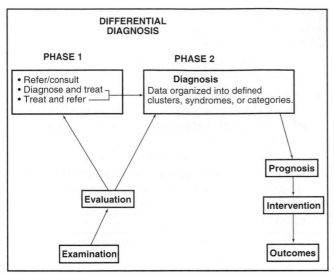

Fig. 1.5   Modification to the patient/client management model. On the left side of this figure, the therapist starts by collecting data during the examination. Based on the data collected, the evaluation leads to clinical judgments. In this adapted model, a fork in the decision-making pathway provides the therapist with the opportunity to make one of three alternative decisions as described in the text. This model is more in keeping with recommended clinical practice. (From Boissonault WG: Differential Diagnosis Phase I. In: Umphred DA, Lazaro RT, Roller ML, Burton GU: *Umphred's Neurological Rehabilitation*, ed 6, 2012, St. Louis, Elsevier.)

that a correct assessment of the patient's/client's actual problem can be made.

A differential diagnosis by the physical therapist is the comparison of NMS signs and symptoms to identify the underlying human movement dysfunction so that treatment can be planned as specifically as possible. If there is evidence of a pathologic condition, referral is made to the appropriate health care professional. This step requires the therapist to consider the possible pathologic conditions, even if unable to verify the presence or absence of said condition.[36]

One of the APTA goals is that physical therapists will be universally recognized and promoted as the practitioners of choice for persons with conditions that affect human movement, function, health, and wellness.[37]

Purpose of the Diagnosis

In the context of screening for referral, the purpose of the diagnosis is to:

- Treat as specifically as possible by determining the most appropriate plan of care and intervention strategy for each patient/client
- Recognize the need for a medical referral

More broadly stated, the purpose of the human movement system diagnosis is to guide the physical therapist in determining the most appropriate intervention strategy for each patient/client with a goal of decreasing disability and increasing function. In the event the diagnostic process does not yield an identifiable cluster, disorder, syndrome, or category,

Verify Medical Diagnosis

A 31-year-old man was referred to physical therapy by an orthopedic physician. The diagnosis was "shoulder-hand syndrome." This client had been evaluated for this same problem by three other physicians and two physical therapists before arriving at our clinic. Treatment to date had been unsuccessful in alleviating symptoms.

The medical diagnosis itself provided some useful information about the referring physician. "Shoulder-hand syndrome" is outdated nomenclature previously used to describe reflex sympathetic dystrophy syndrome (RSDS or RSD), now known more accurately as complex regional pain syndrome (CRPS).[38,78]

Shoulder-hand syndrome was a condition that occurred following a myocardial infarct, or MI (heart attack), usually after prolonged bed rest. This condition has been significantly reduced in incidence by more up-to-date and aggressive cardiac rehabilitation programs. Today CRPS, primarily affecting the limbs, develops after injury or surgery, but it can still occur as a result of a cerebrovascular accident (CVA) or heart attack.

This client's clinical presentation included none of the typical signs and symptoms expected with CRPS such as skin changes (smooth, shiny, red skin), hair growth pattern (increased dark hair patches or loss of hair), temperature changes (increased or decreased), hyperhidrosis (excessive perspiration), restricted joint motion, and severe pain. The clinical picture appeared consistent with a trigger point of the latissimus dorsi muscle, and in fact, treatment of the trigger point completely eliminated all symptoms.

Conducting a thorough physical therapy examination to identify the specific underlying cause of symptomatic presentation was essential to the treatment of this case. Treatment approaches for a trigger point differ greatly from intervention protocols for CRPS.

Accepting the medical diagnosis without performing a physical therapy diagnostic evaluation would have resulted in wasted time and unnecessary charges for this client.

The International Association for the Study of Pain replaced the term *RSDS* with *CRPS I* in 1995.[38] Other names given to RSD included neurovascular dystrophy, sympathetic neurovascular dystrophy, algodystrophy, "red-hand disease," Sudeck's atrophy, and causalgia.

intervention may be directed toward the alleviation of symptoms and remediation of impairment, activity limitation, and participation restrictions.[29]

Sometimes the patient/client is too acute to examine fully during the first visit. At other times, physical therapists evaluate nonspecific referral diagnoses such as problems medically diagnosed as "shoulder pain" or "back pain." When the patient/client is referred with a previously established diagnosis, the physical therapist determines that the clinical findings are consistent with that diagnosis[29] (Case Example 1.5).

Sometimes the screening and diagnostic process identifies a systemic problem as the underlying cause of NMS symptoms. At other times, it confirms that the patient/client has a human movement system syndrome or problem (see Case Examples 1.5[38] and 1.6).

CASE EXAMPLE 1.6

Identify Mechanical Problems: Cervical Spine Arthrosis Presenting as Chest Pain

A 42-year-old woman presented with primary chest pain of unknown cause. She was employed as an independent pediatric occupational therapist. She has been seen by numerous medical doctors who have ruled out cardiac, pulmonary, esophageal, upper GI, and breast pathology as underlying etiologies.

Because her symptoms continued to persist, she was sent to physical therapy for an evaluation.

She reported symptoms of chest pain/discomfort across the upper chest rated as a 5 or 6 and sometimes an 8 on a scale of 0 to 10. The pain does not radiate down her arms or up her neck. She cannot bring the symptoms on or make them go away. She cannot point to the pain but reports it as being more diffuse than localized.

She denies any shortness of breath but admits to being "out of shape" and has not been able to exercise because of a failed bladder neck suspension surgery 2 years ago. She reports fatigue but states this is not unusual for her with her busy work schedule and home responsibilities.

She has not had any recent infections, no history of cancer or heart disease, and her mammogram and clinical breast examination are up-to-date and normal. She does not smoke or drink but by her own admission has a "poor diet" as a result of time pressure, stress, and fatigue.

Final Result: After completing the evaluation with appropriate questions, tests, and measures, a Review of Systems pointed to the cervical spine as the most likely source of this client's symptoms. The jaw and shoulder joint were cleared, although there were signs of shoulder movement dysfunction.

After relaying these findings to the client's primary care physician, radiographs of the cervical spine were ordered. Interestingly, despite the thousands of dollars spent on repeated diagnostic workups for this client, a simple x-ray had never been taken.

Results showed significant spurring and lipping throughout the cervical spine from early osteoarthritic changes of unknown cause. Cervical spine fusion was recommended and performed for instability in the midcervical region.

The client's chest pain was eliminated and did not return even up to 2 years after the cervical spine fusion. The physical therapist's contribution in pinpointing the location of referred symptoms brought this case to a successful conclusion.

Historical Perspective

The idea of "physical therapy diagnosis" is not a new concept. It was first described in the literature by Shirley Sahrmann[39] as the name given to a collection of relevant signs and symptoms associated with the primary dysfunction toward which the physical therapist directs treatment. The dysfunction is identified by the physical therapist based on the information obtained from the history, signs, symptoms, examination, and tests the therapist performs or requests.

In 1984, the APTA House of Delegates (HOD), similar to the Congress of the United States but for the physical therapy profession, presented and passed a motion that "the physical therapist may establish a diagnosis within the scope of their knowledge, experience, and expertise." This was further qualified in 1990 when the Education Standards for Accreditation described "Diagnosis" for the first time.

In 1990, teaching and learning content and the skills necessary to determine a diagnosis became a required part of the curriculum standards established then by the Standards for Accreditation for Physical Therapist Educational Program. At that time the therapist's role in developing a diagnosis was described as:

- Engage in the diagnostic process in an efficient manner consistent with the policies and procedures of the practice setting.
- Engage in the diagnostic process to establish differential diagnoses for patients/clients across the lifespan based on evaluation of results of examinations and medical and psychosocial information.
- Take responsibility for communication or discussion of diagnoses or clinical impressions with other practitioners.

In 1995, the HOD amended the 1984 policy to make the definition of diagnosis consistent with the then upcoming *Guide to Physical Therapist Practice*. The first edition of the *Guide* was published in 1997. The second edition was published in 2001 and revised in 2003. The third edition was published in 2014 and revised in 2016.

The APTA HOD adopted a position on diagnosis titled "Management of the Movement System" (HOD P06-15-25-24).[40] In this position statement, the "APTA endorses the development of diagnostic labels and/or classification systems that reflect and contribute to the physical therapist's ability to properly and effectively manage disorders of the movement system."

Earlier in this chapter, we attempted to summarize various opinions and thoughts presented in our literature defining diagnosis. A "working" definition of diagnosis is:

Diagnosis is both a process and a descriptor. The diagnostic process includes integrating and evaluating the data that are obtained during the examination for the purpose of guiding the prognosis, the plan of care, and intervention strategies. Physical therapists assign diagnostic descriptors that identify a condition or syndrome at the level of the system, especially the human movement system, and at the level of the whole person.[41]

The human movement system has become the focus of the physical therapist's "diagnosis." The suggested template for this diagnosis under discussion and development is currently as follows:

- Use recognized anatomic, physiologic, or movement-related terms to describe the condition or syndrome of the human movement system.
- Include, if deemed necessary for clarity, the name of the pathology, disease, disorder, or symptom that is associated with the diagnosis.
- Be efficient to improve clinical usefulness.

Classification System

According to Rothstein,[42] in many fields of medicine when a medical diagnosis is made, the pathologic condition is determined and stages and classifications that guide treatment are also named. Although we recognize that the term diagnosis relates to a pathologic process, we know that pathologic evidence alone is inadequate to guide the physical therapist.

Physical therapists do not diagnose disease in the sense of identifying a specific organic or visceral pathologic condition. However, identified clusters of signs, symptoms, symptom-related behavior, and other data from the patient/client history and other testing can be used to confirm or rule out the presence of a problem within the scope of the physical therapist's practice. These diagnostic clusters can be labeled as *impairment classifications* or *human movement dysfunctions* by physical therapists and can guide efficient and effective management of the client.[43]

Diagnostic classification systems that direct treatment interventions are being developed based on client prognosis and definable outcomes demonstrated in the literature.[9,44] At the same time, efforts continue to define diagnostic categories or diagnostic descriptors for the physical therapist.[39-43] There is also a trend toward identification of subgroups within a particular group of individuals based on diagnostic characteristics (e.g., low back pain, carpal tunnel syndrome, shoulder dysfunction) and predictive factors (positive and negative) for treatment and prognosis.

DIFFERENTIAL DIAGNOSIS VERSUS SCREENING

If you are already familiar with the term *differential diagnosis*, you may be wondering about the change in title for this text. Previous editions were entitled *Differential Diagnosis in Physical Therapy*.

The name *Differential Diagnosis for Physical Therapists: Screening for Referral*, first established for the fourth edition of this text, does not reflect a change in the content of the text as much as it reflects a better understanding of the screening process and a more appropriate use of the term "differential diagnosis" to identify and describe the specific movement impairment present (if there is one).

When the first edition of this text was published, the term *physical therapy diagnosis* was not common. Diagnostic labels were primarily within the domain of the physician. Over the years, as our profession has changed and progressed, the concept of diagnosis has evolved.

A *diagnosis by the physical therapist* as outlined in the *Guide* describes the patient's/client's primary dysfunction(s). The diagnostic process begins with the collection of data (examination), proceeds through the organization and interpretation of data (evaluation), and ends in the application of a label (i.e., the diagnosis).[9]

As part of the examination process, the therapist should conduct a screening examination. This is especially true if the diagnostic process does not yield an identifiable movement dysfunction. Throughout the evaluation process, the therapist must ask himself or herself:

- Is this an appropriate physical referral?
- Is there a history or cluster of signs and/or symptoms that raises a yellow (cautionary) or red (warning) flag?

The presence of risk factors and yellow or red flags alerts the therapist to the need for a screening examination. Once the screening process is complete and the therapist has confirmed the client is appropriate for physical therapy intervention, then the objective examination continues.

Sometimes in the early presentation, there are no red flags or associated signs and symptoms to suggest an underlying systemic or viscerogenic cause of the client's NMS symptoms or movement dysfunction.

It is not until the disease progresses that the clinical picture changes enough to raise a red flag. This is why the screening process is not necessarily a one-time evaluation. Screening can and should take place anywhere along the continuum represented in Fig. 1.4.

The most likely place screening occurs is during the examination when the therapist obtains the history, performs a systems review, and carries out specific tests and measures. It is at this point that the client presents with indicators of systemic disease. Hence in the revised figure in the third edition of the *Guide*, the pathway for Consultation/Referral is presented after Examination.

As the therapist works with the patient throughout the episode of care, the client may relate a new onset of symptoms that were not present during the examination. If the patient/client does not progress in physical therapy, or presents with a new onset of symptoms previously unreported, the screening process should be repeated.

Red-flag signs and symptoms may appear for the first time or develop more fully during the course of physical therapy intervention. In some patients, having the patient exercise stresses the physiology and the previously unnoticed, unrecognized, or silent symptoms suddenly present more clearly.

A lack of progress signals the need to conduct a reexamination or to modify/redirect intervention. The process of reexamination may identify the need for consultation with or referral to another health care provider. The physician is the most likely referral recommendation, but referral to a nurse practitioner, physician assistant, chiropractor, dentist, psychologist, counselor, a certified physical therapist specialist or fellow, or other appropriate health care professional may be more appropriate at times.

Scope of Practice

A key phrase in the APTA standards of practice is "within the scope of physical therapist practice." Establishing a diagnosis is a professional standard within the scope of a physical therapist's practice, but may not be permitted in the state that the physical therapist practices (Case Example 1.7).

Throughout the text, we will point out that a systemic condition can masquerade as a mechanical or movement

CASE EXAMPLE 1.7
Scope of Practice

A licensed physical therapist volunteered at a high school athletic event and screened an ankle injury. After performing a heel strike test (negative), the physical therapist recommended RICE (Rest, Ice, Compression, and Elevation) and follow-up with a medical doctor if the pain persisted.

A complaint was filed 2 years later claiming that the physical therapist violated the state practice act by "... engaging in the practice of physical therapy in excess of the scope of physical therapy practice by undertaking to diagnose and prescribe appropriate treatment for an acute athletic injury."

The therapist was placed on probation for 2 years. The case was appealed and amended as it was clearly shown that the therapist was practicing within the legal bounds of the state's practice act. Imagine the effect this had on the individual in the community and as a private practitioner.

Know your state practice act and make sure it allows physical therapists to draw conclusions and make statements about findings of evaluations (i.e., diagnosis).

dysfunction. Identification of causative factors or etiology by the physical therapist is an important step in the screening process. By remaining within the scope of our practice the diagnosis is limited primarily to those pathokinesiologic problems associated with faulty biomechanical or neuromuscular action.

When no apparent movement dysfunction, causative factors, or syndrome can be identified, the therapist may treat symptoms as part of an ongoing diagnostic process. Sometimes even physicians use physical therapy as a diagnostic tool, observing the client's response during the episode of care to confirm or rule out medical suspicions.

If, however, the findings remain inconsistent with what is expected for the human movement system and/or the patient/client does not improve with intervention,[4,45] then referral to an appropriate medical professional may be required. Always keep in mind that the screening process may confirm the presence of a musculoskeletal or neuromuscular problem.

The flip side of this concept is that client complaints that cannot be associated with a medical problem should be referred to a physical therapist to identify mechanical problems (see Case Example 1.6). Physical therapists have a responsibility to educate the medical community as to the scope of our practice and our role in identifying mechanical problems and movement disorders.

Staying within the scope of physical therapist practice, the therapist communicates with physicians and other health care practitioners to request or recommend further medical evaluation. Whether in a private practice, school or home health setting, acute care hospital, or rehabilitation setting, physical therapists may observe and report important findings outside the realm of NMS disorders that require additional medical evaluation and treatment.

DIRECT ACCESS AND SELF-REFERRAL

Direct access and self-referral is the legal right of the public to obtain examination, evaluation, and intervention from a licensed physical therapist without previous examination by, or referral from, a physician, gatekeeper, or other practitioner. In the civilian sector, the need to screen for medical disease was first raised as an issue in response to direct-access legislation. Until direct access, the only therapists screening for referral were physical therapists in the military.

Before 1957 a physician referral was necessary in all 50 states for a client to be treated by a physical therapist. Direct access was first obtained in Nebraska in 1957, when that state passed a licensure and scope-of-practice law that did not mandate a physician referral for a physical therapist to initiate care.[46]

At the present time, all 50 states, the District of Columbia, and the US Virgin Islands permit some form of direct access and self-referral to allow patients/clients to consult a physical therapist without first being referred by a physician.[47,48] Direct access is relevant in all practice settings and is not limited just to private practice or outpatient services.

Following changes in the Medicare Benefit Policy Manual in 2005 (Publication 100-02), clients under Medicare can see physical therapists directly without consultation or referral from a physician. A patient, however must be "under the care of a physician," indicated by the physician's certification of the physical therapy plan of care. The physician or nonphysician practitioner (NPP) must certify this physical therapy plan of care within 30 days of the initial PT visit, and the physical therapist must comply with applicable laws in their state related to direct access. Additional information can be obtained from "Direct Access and Medicare" page in the APTA website.[49]

Full, unrestricted direct access is not available in all states with a direct-access law. Various forms of direct access are available on a state-by-state basis. Many direct-access laws are permissive, as opposed to mandatory. This means that consumers are permitted to see therapists without a physician's referral; however, a payer can still require a referral before providing reimbursement for services. Each therapist MUST be familiar with the practice act and direct-access legislation for the state in which he or she is practicing.

Sometimes states enact a two- or three-tiered restricted or provisional direct-access system. For example, some states' direct access law only allows evaluation and treatment for therapists who have practiced for 3 years. Some direct-access laws only allow physical therapists to provide services for up to 14 days without physician referral. Other states list up to 30 days as the standard.

There may be additional criteria in place, such as the patient/client must have been referred to physical therapy by a physician within the past 2 years or the therapist must notify the patient's/client's identified primary care practitioner no later than 3 days after intervention begins.

Some states require a minimum level of liability insurance coverage by each therapist. In a three-tiered–direct access state, three or more requirements must be met before practicing without a physician referral. For example, licensed physical therapists must practice for a specified number of years, complete continuing education courses, and obtain references from two or more physicians before treating clients without a physician referral.

There are other factors that prevent therapists from practicing under full direct-access rights even when granted by state law. For example, Boissonnault[50] presents regulatory barriers and internal institutional policies that interfere with the direct access practice model.

In the private sector, some therapists think that the way to avoid malpractice lawsuits is to continue operating under a system of physician referral. Therapists in a private practice driven by physician referral may not want to be placed in a position as competitors of the physicians who serve as a referral source.

Internationally, direct access has become a reality in some, but not all, countries. It has been established in Australia, New Zealand, Canada, the United Kingdom, and the Netherlands. In a study of member countries of the World Confederation of Physical Therapy, of the 72 member organizations who responded, 40 (58%) reported availability of direct access or self-referral in their countries.[51]

Primary Care

Primary care is the coordinated, comprehensive, and personal care provided on a first-contact and continuous basis. It incorporates primary and secondary prevention of chronic disease states, wellness, personal support, education (including providing information about illness, prevention, and health maintenance), and addresses the personal health care needs of patients/clients within the context of family and community.[32] Primary care is not defined by who provides it but rather it is a set of functions as described. It is person- (not disease- or diagnosis-) focused care over time.[52]

In the primary care delivery model, the therapist is responsible as a patient/client advocate to see that the patient's/client's NMS and other health care needs are identified and prioritized, and a plan of care is established. The primary care model provides the consumer with first point-of-entry access to the physical therapist as the most skilled practitioner for human movement system dysfunction. The physical therapist may also serve as a key member of an interdisciplinary primary care team that works together to assist the patient/client in maintaining his or her overall health and fitness.

Through a process of screening, triage, examination, evaluation, referral, intervention, coordination of care, education, and prevention, the therapist prevents, reduces, slows, or remediates impairments, functional limitations, and disabilities while achieving cost-effective clinical outcomes.[9,53]

Expanded privileges beyond the traditional scope of the physical therapist practice may become part of the standard future physical therapist primary care practice. In addition to the usual privileges included in the scope of the physical therapist practice, the primary care therapist may eventually refer patients/clients to radiology for diagnostic imaging and other diagnostic evaluations. For example, U.S. military physical therapists refer patients/clients to radiology for imaging, laboratory tests and are credentialed to prescribe analgesic and nonsteroidal antiinflammatory medications.[54]

Direct Access and Primary Care

Direct access is the vehicle by which the patient/client comes directly to the physical therapist without first seeing a physician, dentist, chiropractor, or other health care professional. Direct access does not describe the type of practice the therapist is engaging in.

Primary care physical therapy is not a setting but rather describes a philosophy of whole-person care. The therapist is the first point-of-entry into the health care system. After screening and triage, patients/clients who do not have NMS conditions are referred to the appropriate health care specialist for further evaluation.

The primary care therapist is not expected to diagnose conditions that are not neuromuscular or musculoskeletal. However, risk factor assessment and screening for a broad range of medical conditions (e.g., high blood pressure, incontinence, diabetes, vestibular dysfunction, peripheral vascular disease) is possible and an important part of primary and secondary prevention. Thus the primary care therapist should have sufficient experience to be able to recognize a broad range of medical conditions and to ask the specific questions about the client during the history portion of the exam, to identify the specific system involvement of the client. The primary care therapist is more likely to treat patients/clients across the continuum of care whereas the direct access therapist could be more likely to see patients/clients that fit the setting the therapist works at.

Autonomous Practice

Autonomous physical therapist practice is defined as "self-governing;" "capable of existing independently"; "not controlled (or owned) by others."[55] Autonomous practice is described as "independent, self-determining professional judgment and action."[56] Autonomous practice for the physical therapist does not mean practice independent of collaborative and collegial communication with other health care team members (Box 1.6) but rather, interdependent evidence-based practice that is patient- (client-) centered. Professional autonomy meets the health needs of people who are experiencing disablement by providing a service that supports the autonomy of that individual.[57]

Five key objectives set forth by the APTA in achieving an autonomous physical therapist practice include (1) demonstrating professionalism, (2) achieving direct access to physical therapist services, (3) basing practice on the most up-to-date evidence, (4) providing an entry-level education at the level of Doctor of Physical Therapy, and (5) becoming the practitioner of choice.[56]

BOX 1.6   ATTRIBUTES OF AUTONOMOUS PRACTICE

Direct and unrestricted access: The physical therapist has the professional capacity and ability to provide to all individuals with the physical therapy services they choose without legal, regulatory, or payer restrictions

Professional ability to refer to other health care providers: The physical therapist has the professional capability and ability to refer to others in the health care system for identified or possible medical needs beyond the scope of physical therapy practice

Professional ability to refer to other professionals: The physical therapist has the professional capability and ability to refer to other professionals for identified or patient/client needs beyond the scope of physical therapy services

Professional ability to refer for diagnostic tests: The physical therapist has the professional capability and ability to refer for diagnostic tests that would clarify the patient/client situation and enhance the provision of physical therapy services

From Diagnosis by Physical Therapists HOD P06-12-10-09. Last updated 08/22/12. Available online at: https://www.apta.org/apta-and-you/leadership-and-governance/policies/diagnosis-by-physical-therapist Accessed February 18, 2021.

BOX 1.7   GOODMAN SCREENING FOR REFERRAL MODEL

- Past medical history
- Personal and family history
- Risk factor assessment
- Clinical presentation
- Associated signs and symptoms of systemic diseases
- Review of systems

Reimbursement Trends

A systematic review in 2014 confirmed that physical therapy direct access is associated with decreased health care costs while providing quality care.[58] Despite this, many payers, hospitals, and other institutions still require physician referral.[50,59]

Direct access laws give consumers the legal right to seek physical therapy services without a medical referral. These laws do not always make it mandatory that insurance companies, third-party payers (including Medicare/Medicaid), self-insured, or other insurers reimburse the physical therapist without a physician's prescription.

Some state home-health agency license laws require referral for all client care regardless of the payer source. In the future, we hope to see all insurance companies reimburse for direct access without restriction. Further legislation and regulation are needed in many states to amend the insurance statutes and state agency policies to assure statutory compliance.

This policy, along with large deductibles, poor reimbursement, and failure to authorize needed services has resulted in a trend toward a cash-based, private-pay business. This trend in reimbursement is also referred to as direct contracting, first-party payment, direct consumer services, or direct fee-for-service.[60] In such an environment, decisions can be made based on the good of the clients rather than on cost or volume.

In such circumstances, consumers are willing to pay out-of-pocket for physical therapy services, by-passing the need for a medical evaluation unless requested by the physical therapist. A therapist can use a cash-based practice only where direct access has been passed and within the legal parameters of the state practice act.

Also in relation to new models of reimbursement, companies are giving their employees an annual stipend to spend on health care services either not covered or for which they have not met their deductible. The Flex Plan and Health Savings Plan also provides for this approach. This gives more people the opportunity to receive/choose physical therapy beyond the number of visits covered, and/or for visits billed before the deductible is met. Other services such as acupuncture, massage, BodyTalk, etc. can also be utilized through the stipend and/or Health Savings Plan.

In any situation where authorization for further intervention by a therapist is not obtained despite the therapist's assessment that further skilled services are needed, the therapist can notify the client and/or the family of their right to an appeal with the agency providing health care coverage.

The client has the right to make informed decisions regarding pursuit of insurance coverage or to make private-pay arrangements. Too many times the insurance coverage ends, but the client's needs have not been met. Creative planning and alternate financial arrangements should be made available.

DECISION-MAKING PROCESS

This text is designed to help students, physical therapist assistants, and physical therapy clinicians screen for medical disease when it is appropriate to do so. But just exactly how is this done? The proposed Goodman screening model can be used in conducting a screening evaluation for any client (Box 1.7).

By using these decision-making tools, the therapist will be able to identify chief and secondary problems, identify information that is inconsistent with the presenting complaint, identify noncontributory information, generate a working hypothesis regarding possible causes of complaints, and determine whether referral or consultation is indicated.

The screening process is carried out through the client interview and verified during the physical examination. Therapists compare the subjective information (what the client tells us) with the objective findings (what we find during the examination) to identify movement impairment or other neuromuscular or musculoskeletal dysfunction (that which is within the scope of our practice) and to rule out systemic involvement (requiring medical referral). This is the basis for the evaluation process.

Given today's time constraints in the clinic, a fast and efficient method of screening is essential. Checklists (see Appendix A-1 available in the accompanying enhanced eBook version included with print purchase of this textbook), special questions to ask (Appendix B available in the accompanying enhanced eBook version included with print purchase of this textbook), and the screening model outlined in Box 1.7 can guide and streamline the screening process. Once the clinician is familiar with the use of this model, it is possible to conduct the initial screening examination in 3 to 5 minutes when necessary. This can include (but is not limited to):

- Take vital signs
- Use the word "symptom(s)" rather than "pain" during the screening interview
- Watch for red flag histories, signs, and symptoms
- Review medications; observe for signs and symptoms that could be a result of drug combinations (polypharmacy), dual drug dosage; consult with the pharmacist
- Ask a final open-ended question such as:
  1. Are you having any other symptoms of any kind anywhere else in your body we have not talked about yet?
  2. Is there anything else you think is important about your condition that we have not discussed yet?

If a young, healthy athlete comes in with a sprained ankle and no other associated signs and symptoms, there may be no need to screen further. But if that same athlete has an eating disorder, uses anabolic steroids illegally, or is taking antidepressants, the clinical picture (and possibly the intervention) changes. Risk factor assessment and a screening physical examination are the most likely ways to screen more thoroughly.

Or take, for example, an older adult who presents with hip pain of unknown cause. There are two red flags already present (age and insidious onset). As clients age, the past medical history and risk factor assessment become more important assessment tools. After investigating the clinical presentation, screening would focus on these two elements next.

Or, if after ending the interview by asking, "Are there any symptoms of any kind anywhere else in your body that we have not talked about yet?" the client responds with a list of additional symptoms, it may be best to step back and conduct a Review of Systems.

Past Medical History

Most of history taking is accomplished through the client interview and includes both family and personal history. The client/patient interview is very important because it helps the physical therapist distinguish between problems that he or she can treat and problems that should be referred to a physician (or other appropriate health care professional) for medical diagnosis and intervention.

In fact, the importance of history taking cannot be emphasized enough. Physicians cite a shortage of time as the most common reason to skip the client history, yet history taking is the essential key to a correct diagnosis by the physician (or physical therapist).[61,62] At least one source recommends performing a *history and differential diagnosis* followed by *relevant examination.*[63]

In Chapter 2, an interviewing process is described that includes concrete and structured tools and techniques for conducting a thorough and informative interview. The use of follow-up questions (FUPs) helps complete the interview. This information establishes a solid basis for the therapist's objective evaluation, assessment, and therefore intervention.

During the screening interview it is always a good idea to use a standard form to complete the personal/family history (see Fig. 2.2). Any form of checklist assures a thorough and consistent approach and spares the therapist from relying on his or her memory.

The types of data generated from a client history are presented in Fig. 2.1. Most often, age, race/ethnicity, gender, and occupation (general demographics) are noted. Information about social history, living environment, health status, functional status, and activity level is often important to the patient's/client's clinical presentation and outcomes. Details about the current condition, medical (or other) intervention for the condition, and use of medications is also gathered and considered in the overall evaluation process.

The presence of any yellow or red flags elicited during the screening interview or observed during the physical examination should prompt the therapist to consider the need for further tests and questions. Many of these signs and symptoms are listed in Appendix A-2 available in the accompanying enhanced eBook version included with print purchase of this textbook.

Psychosocial history may provide insight into the client's clinical presentation and overall needs. Age, gender, race/ethnicity, education, occupation, family system, health habits, living environment, medication use, and medical/surgical history are all a part of the client history evaluated in the screening process.

Risk Factor Assessment

Greater emphasis has been placed on risk factor assessment in the health care industry. Risk factor assessment is an important part of disease prevention. Knowing the various risk factors for different kinds of diseases, illnesses, and conditions is an important part of the screening process.

Therapists can have an active role in both primary and secondary prevention through screening and education. According to the *Guide,*[9] physical therapists are involved in primary prevention by preventing a target condition in a susceptible or potentially susceptible population through such specific measures as general health promotion efforts.

Educating clients about their risk factors is a key element in risk factor reduction. Identifying risk factors may guide the therapist in making a medical referral sooner than would otherwise seem necessary.

In primary care, the therapist assesses risk factors, performs screening examinations, and establishes interventions to prevent impairment, dysfunction, and disability. For example, does the client have risk factors for osteoporosis, urinary incontinence, cancer, vestibular or balance problems, obesity, cardiovascular disease, and so on? The physical therapist practice can include routine screening for any of these, as well as other problems.

More and more evidence-based clinical decision rules for specific conditions (e.g., deep venous thrombosis) are available and included in this text; research is needed to catch up in the area of clinical decision rules and identification of specificity and sensitivity of specific red flags and screening tests currently being presented in this text and used in clinical practice. Prediction models based on risk that would improve outcomes may eventually be developed for many diseases, illnesses, and conditions currently screened by red flags and clinical findings.[64,65]

Genetic screening may augment or even replace risk factor assessment. Virtually every human illness is believed to have a hereditary component. The most common problems seen in a physical therapist practice (outside of traumatic injuries) are now thought to have a genetic component, even though the specific gene may not yet be discovered for all conditions, diseases, or illnesses.[66,67]

Exercise is a successful intervention for many diseases, illnesses, and conditions will become prescriptive as research shows how much, and what specific type of, exercise can prevent or mediate each problem. There is already a great deal of information on this topic published, and an accompanying need to change the way people think about exercise.[68]

Convincing people to establish lifelong patterns of exercise and physical activity will continue to be a major focus of the health care industry. Therapists can advocate disease prevention, wellness, and promotion of healthy lifestyle by delivering health care services intended to prevent health problems or maintain health and by offering annual wellness screening as a part of primary prevention.

Clinical Presentation

Clinical presentation, including pain patterns and pain types, is the next part of the decision-making process. To assist the physical therapist in making a treatment-versus-referral decision, specific pain patterns corresponding to systemic diseases are provided in Chapter 3. Drawings of primary and referred pain patterns are provided in each chapter for quick reference. A summary of key findings associated with systemic illness is listed in Box 1.1.

The presence of any one of these variables is not cause for extreme concern but should raise a yellow or red flag for the therapist. The therapist is looking for a pattern that suggests a viscerogenic or systemic origin of pain and/or symptoms. This pattern will not be consistent with what we might expect to see with the neuromuscular or musculoskeletal systems.

The therapist will proceed with the screening process, depending on all findings. Often the next step is to look for associated signs and symptoms. Special FUPs are listed in the subjective examination to help the physical therapist

determine when these pain patterns are accompanied by associated signs and symptoms that indicate visceral involvement.

Associated Signs and Symptoms of Systemic Diseases

One focus of this text is the recognition of yellow- or red-flag signs and symptoms, either reported by the client subjectively or observed objectively by the physical therapist.

Signs are observable findings detected by the therapist in an objective examination (e.g., unusual skin color, clubbing of the fingers [swelling of the terminal phalanges of the fingers or toes], hematoma [local collection of blood], effusion [fluid]). Signs can be seen, heard, smelled, measured, photographed, shown to someone else, or documented in some other way.

Symptoms are reported indications of disease that are perceived by the client but cannot be observed by someone else. Pain, discomfort, or other complaints, such as numbness, tingling, or "creeping" sensations, are symptoms that are difficult to quantify but are most often reported as the chief complaint. As signs are observable by the therapist, they provide objective data, and this differentiation between signs and symptoms is important. Symptoms are what the client perceives and may not always be as reliable, however they are definitely important because the therapist does not know what the patient is feeling and therefore the patient may not know to tell the therapist what they are feeling somewhere else in their body than where they think the problem is presenting.

Because physical therapists spend a considerable amount of time investigating pain, it is easy to remain focused exclusively on this symptom when clients might otherwise bring to the forefront other important problems.

Thus the physical therapist is encouraged to become accustomed to using the word *symptoms* instead of *pain* when interviewing the client. It is likewise prudent for the physical therapist to refer to symptoms when talking to clients with chronic pain in order to move the focus away from pain.

Instead of asking the client, "How are you today?" try asking:

❓ FOLLOW-UP QUESTIONS

- Are you better, the same, or worse today?
- What can you do today that you could not do yesterday? (Or last week/last month?)

This approach to questioning progress (or lack of progress) may help you see a systemic pattern sooner rather than later.

The therapist can identify the presence of associated signs and symptoms by asking the client:

❓ FOLLOW-UP QUESTIONS

- Are there any symptoms of any kind anywhere else in your body that we have not yet talked about?
- *Alternately:* Are there any symptoms or problems anywhere else in your body that may not be related to your current problem?

The patient/client may not see a connection between shoulder pain and blood in the urine from kidney impairment or blood in the stools from chronic nonsteroidal anti-inflammatory drug (NSAID) use. Likewise, the patient/client may not think the diarrhea present is associated with the back pain (gastrointestinal [GI] dysfunction).

The client with temporomandibular joint pain from a cardiac source usually has some other associated symptoms, and in most cases, the client does not see the link. If the therapist does not ask, the client does not offer the information.

Each visceral system has a typical set of core signs and symptoms associated with impairment of that system (see Box 4.15). Systemic signs and symptoms that are listed for each condition should serve as a warning to alert the informed physical therapist of the need for further questioning and possible medical referral.

For example, the most common symptoms present with pulmonary pathology are cough, shortness of breath, and pleural pain. Liver impairment is marked by abdominal ascites, right upper quadrant tenderness, jaundice, and skin and nailbed changes. Signs and symptoms associated with *endocrine* pathology may include changes in body or skin temperature, dry mouth, dizziness, weight change, or excessive sweating.

Being aware of signs and symptoms associated with each individual system may help the therapist make an early connection between viscerogenic and/or systemic presentation of NMS problems. The presence of constitutional symptoms is always a red flag that must be evaluated carefully (see Box 1.3).

Systems Review Versus Review of Systems

The components of the physical therapy examination include the patient history, systems review, and tests and measures. The Systems Review is defined in the *Guide* as a brief or limited examination of the anatomic and physiologic status of the cardiovascular/pulmonary, integumentary, musculoskeletal, and neuromuscular systems. The Systems Review also includes assessment of the client's communication ability, affect, cognition, language, and learning style.[69]

The Systems Review looks beyond the primary problem that brought the client to the therapist in the first place. It gives an overview of the "whole person," and guides the therapist in choosing appropriate tests and measures. The Systems Review helps the therapist answer the questions, "What should I do next?" and "What do I need to examine in depth?" It also answers the question, "What do I not need to do?"[70]

In the screening process, a slightly different approach may be needed, perhaps best referred to as a Review of Systems. In the new version of the *Guide*, Review of Systems is now a part of the history.[9] After conducting an interview, performing an assessment of the pain type and/or pain patterns, and reviewing the clinical presentation, the therapist looks for any characteristics of systemic disease. Any identified clusters of associated signs and symptoms are reviewed to search for a potential pattern that will identify the underlying system involved.

The Review of Systems as part of the screening process (see discussion, Chapter 4) is a useful tool in recognizing clusters of associated signs and symptoms and the possible need for medical referral. Using this tool, the therapist steps back and looks at the big picture, taking into consideration all of the presenting factors, and looking for any indication that the client's problem is outside the scope of a physical therapist's practice.

As part of the history and interview, the therapist conducts a Review of Systems in the screening process by categorizing all of the complaints and associated signs and symptoms. Once these are listed, compare this list to Box 4.15. Are the signs and symptoms all genitourinary (GU) related? GI in nature? It may be helpful to consider this systematic process in a visual format. The therapist has lots of different buckets (systems) in front of them when evaluating a patient, and each time a system is implicated, chips are dropped into the appropriate bucket indicating involvement of that system. At the end of the examination, the therapist evaluates how many chips are in the buckets. This systematic approach provides consideration of the complex patient with multiple buckets or system involvement.

For example, a therapist observes dry skin, brittle nails, cold or heat intolerance, or excessive hair loss, and realizes these signs could be pointing to an endocrine problem. In evaluating this presentation, the therapist recognizes that the clinical presentation is not something within the musculoskeletal or neuromuscular systems.

If, for example, the client's signs and symptoms fall primarily within the GU group, turn to Chapter 11 and use the additional, pertinent screening questions at the end of the chapter. The client's answers to these questions will guide the therapist in making a decision about referral to a physician or other health care professional.

The physical therapist is not responsible for identifying the specific systemic or visceral disease underlying the clinical signs and symptoms present. However, the therapist who classifies groups of signs and symptoms in a Review of Systems will be more likely to recognize a problem outside the scope of physical therapy practice and make a timely referral. Use of the OSPRO-ROS should be considered in outpatient physical therapy practice as a tool to consider additional healthcare provided referral. This allows our patients to receive the best care possible and the care that they need to improve the human experience!

CASE EXAMPLES AND CASE STUDIES

Case examples and case studies are provided with each chapter to give the therapist a working understanding of how to recognize the need for additional questions. In addition, information is given concerning the type of questions to ask and how to correlate the results with the objective findings.

Cases will be used to integrate screening information in making a physical therapy differential diagnosis and deciding when and how to refer to the physician or other health care professional. Whenever possible, information about when and how to refer a client to the physician is presented.

Each case study is based on actual clinical experiences in a variety of inpatient/client and outpatient/client physical therapy practices to provide reasonable examples of what to expect when the physical therapist is functioning under any of the circumstances listed in Box 1.2.

PHYSICIAN REFERRAL

As previously mentioned, the therapist may treat symptoms as a part of an ongoing medical diagnostic process. In other words, sometimes the physician sends a patient/client to physical therapy "to see if it will help." This may be part of the medical differential diagnosis. Medical consultation or referral is required when no apparent movement dysfunction, causative factors, or syndrome can be identified and/or the findings are not consistent with an NMS dysfunction.

Communication with the physician is a key component in the referral process. Phone and email make this process faster and easier than ever before. Persistence may be required in obtaining enough information to glean what the doctor knows or thinks to avoid sending the very same problem back for his/her consideration. This is especially important when the physician is using physical therapy intervention as a part of the medical differential diagnostic process.

The hallmark of professionalism in any health care practitioner is the ability to understand the limits of their professional knowledge. The physical therapist, either on reaching the limit of their knowledge or on reaching the limits prescribed by the client's condition, should refer the patient/client to the appropriate provider. In this way, the physical therapist will work within the scope of their level of skill, knowledge, and practical experience.

Knowing when and how to refer a client to another health care professional is just as important as the initial screening process. Once the therapist recognizes red flag histories, risk factors, signs and symptoms, and/or a clinical presentation that do not fit the expected picture for NMS dysfunction, then this information must be communicated effectively to the appropriate referral source.

Knowing how to refer the client or how to notify the physician of important findings is not always clear. In a direct access or primary care setting, the client may not have a personal or family physician. In an orthopedic setting, the client in rehab for a total hip or total knee replacement may be reporting signs and symptoms of a nonorthopedic condition. Do you send the client back to the referring (orthopedic) physician or refer him or her to the primary care physician?

Suggested Guidelines

When the client has come to physical therapy without a medical referral (i.e., self-referred) and the physical therapist recommends medical follow-up, the patient/client should be referred to the primary care physician if the patient/client has one.

Occasionally, the patient/client indicates that he or she has not contacted a physician, or was treated by a physician (whose name cannot be recalled) a long time ago, or that he or she has just moved to the area and does not have a physician.

In these situations, the client can be provided with a list of recommended physicians. It is not necessary to list every physician in the area, but the physical therapist can provide several appropriate choices. Whether the client makes or does not make an appointment with a medical practitioner, the physical therapist is urged to document subjective and objective findings carefully, as well as the recommendation made for medical follow-up. The therapist should make every effort to get the physical therapy records to the consulting physician.

Before sending a client back to his or her doctor, have someone else (e.g., case manager, physical therapy colleague or mentor, nursing staff if available) double-check your findings and discuss your reasons for referral. The therapist may consider to review your own findings at a second appointment. Are they consistent?

Consider checking with the medical doctor by telephone. Perhaps the physician is aware of the problem, but the therapist does not have the patient/client records and is unaware of this information. As previously mentioned, it is not uncommon for physicians to send a client to physical therapy as a part of their own differential diagnostic process. For example, they may have tried medications without success and the client does not want surgery or medications. The doctor may suggest, "I think you should see a physical therapist. If physical therapy does not improve your symptoms, the next step is …"

As a general rule, try to send the client back to the referring physician. If this does not seem appropriate, call and ask the physician how he or she wants to handle the situation. Describe the problem and ask:

 ## FOLLOW-UP QUESTIONS

- Do you want Mr. X/Mrs. Y to check with his/her family doctor … or do you prefer to see him/her yourself?

Perhaps an orthopedic client is demonstrating signs and symptoms of depression. This may be a side effect from medications prescribed by another physician (e.g., gynecologist, gastroenterologist). Provide the physician with a list of the observed cluster of signs and symptoms and an open-ended question such as:

FOLLOW-UP QUESTIONS

- How do you want to handle this? or How do you want me to handle this?

Do not suggest a medical diagnosis. When providing written documentation, a short paragraph of physical therapy findings and intervention is followed by a list of concerns, perhaps with the following remarks, "These do not seem consistent with a neuromuscular or musculoskeletal problem (choose the most appropriate description of the human movement system syndrome/problem or name the medical diagnosis [e.g., S/P THR])." Then followup with one of two questions/comments:

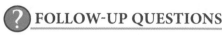

FOLLOW-UP QUESTIONS

- What do you think? or Please advise.

Special Considerations

What if the physician refuses to see the client or finds nothing wrong? We recommend being patiently persistent. Sometimes it is necessary to wait until the disease progresses to a point that medical testing can provide a diagnosis. This is unfortunate for the client but a reality in some cases.

Sometimes it may seem like a good idea to suggest a second opinion. You may want to ask your client:

FOLLOW-UP QUESTIONS

- Have you ever thought about getting a second opinion?

It is best not to tell the client what to do. If the client asks you what he or she should do, consider asking this question:

FOLLOW-UP QUESTIONS

- What do you think your options are? or What are your options?

It is perfectly acceptable to provide a list of names (more than one) where the client can get a second opinion. If the client asks which one to see, suggest whoever is closest geographically or with whom he or she can get an appointment as soon as possible.

What do you do if the client's follow-up appointment is scheduled 2 weeks away and you think immediate medical attention is needed? Call the physician's office and see what is advised: Does the physician want to see the client in the office or send him/her to the emergency department?

For example, what if a patient/client with a recent total hip replacement develops chest pain and shortness of breath during exercise? The client also reports a skin rash around the surgical site. This will not wait for 2 weeks. Take the client's vital signs (especially body temperature in case of infection), report these to the physician, and document your results. In some cases, the need for medical care will be obvious such as in the case of acute myocardial infarct or if the client collapses.

Documentation and Liability

Documentation is any entry into the patient/client record. Documentation may include consultation reports, initial examination reports, progress notes, recap of discussions with physicians or other health care professionals, flow sheets,

checklists, reexamination reports, discharge summaries, and so on.[9] Various forms are available for use in the *Guide* to aid in collecting data in a standardized fashion. Remember, in all circumstances, in a court of law, if you did not document it, you did not do it (a common catch phrase is "not documented, not done").

Documentation is required at the onset of each episode of physical therapy care and includes the elements described in Box 1.5. Documentation of the initial episode of physical therapy care includes examination, comprehensive screening, and specific testing leading to a diagnostic classification and/or referral to another practitioner.[9]

Clients with complex medical histories and multiple comorbidities are increasingly common in a physical therapist's practice. Risk management has become an important consideration for many clients. Documentation and communication must reflect this practice.

Sometimes the therapist will have to be more proactive and assertive in communicating with the client's physician. It may not be enough to suggest or advise the client to make a follow-up appointment with his or her doctor. Leaving the decision up to the client is a passive and indirect approach. It does encourage client/consumer responsibility but may not be in their best interest.

In the APTA *Standards of Practice for Physical Therapy* it states, "The physical therapy service collaborates with all disciplines as appropriate" [Administration of the Physical Therapy Service, Section II, Item J].[71] In the APTA *Referral Relationships*, it states, "The physical therapist must refer patients/clients to the referring practitioner or other health care practitioners if symptoms are present for which physical therapy is contraindicated or are indicative of conditions for which treatment is outside the scope of his/her knowledge."[72]

In cases where the seriousness of the condition can affect the client's outcome, the therapist may need to contact the physician directly and describe the problem. If the therapist's assessment is that the client needs medical attention, advising the client to see a medical doctor as soon as possible may not be enough.

Good risk management is a proactive process that includes taking action to minimize negative outcomes. If a client is advised to contact his or her physician and fails to do so, the therapist should call the doctor.[73]

Failure on the part of the therapist to properly report on a client's condition or important changes in condition reflects a lack of professional judgment in the management of the client's case. A number of positions and standards of the APTA Board of Directors emphasize the importance of physical therapist communication and collaboration with other health care providers. This is a key to providing the best possible client care (Case Example 1.8).[74]

In the APTA Policy on *Diagnosis by Physical Therapists*, it is stated that, "as the diagnostic process continues, physical therapists may identify findings that should be shared with other health professionals, including referral sources, to ensure optimal patient/client care."[75] Part of this process may require appropriate follow-up or referral.

CASE EXAMPLE 1.8

Failure to Collaborate and Communicate with the Physician

A 43-year-old woman was riding a bicycle when she was struck from behind and thrown to the ground. She was seen at the local walk-in clinic and released with a prescription for painkillers and muscle relaxants. X-ray imaging of her head and neck was unremarkable for obvious injury.

She came to the physical therapy clinic 3 days later with complaints of left shoulder, rib, and wrist pain. There was obvious bruising along the left chest wall and upper abdomen. In fact, the ecchymosis was quite extensive and black in color, indicating a large area of blood extravasation into the subcutaneous tissues.

She had no other complaints or problems. Shoulder range of motion was full in all planes, although painful and stiff. Ribs 9, 10, and 11 were painful to palpation but without obvious deformity or derangement.

A neurologic screening examination was negative. The therapist scheduled her for three visits over the next 4 days and started her on a program of pendulum exercises, progressing to active shoulder motion. The client experienced progress over the next 5 days and then reported severe back muscle spasms.

The client called the therapist and cancelled her next appointment because she had the flu with fever and vomiting. When she returned, the therapist continued to treat her with active exercise progressing to resistive strengthening. The client's painful shoulder and back symptoms remained the same, but the client reported that she was "less stiff."

Three weeks after the initial accident, the client collapsed at work and had to be transported to the hospital for emergency surgery. Her spleen had been damaged by the initial trauma with a slow bleed that eventually ruptured.

The client filed a lawsuit in which the therapist was named. The complaint against the therapist was that she failed to properly assess the client's condition and failed to refer her to a medical doctor for a condition outside the scope of physical therapy practice.

Did the physical therapist show questionable professional judgment in the evaluation and management of this case?

There are some obvious red-flag signs and symptoms in this case that went unreported to a medical doctor. There was no contact with the physician at any time throughout this client's physical therapy episode of care. The physician on-call at the walk-in clinic did not refer the client to physical therapy—she referred herself.

However, the physical therapist did not send the physician any information about the client's self-referral, physical therapy evaluation, or planned treatment.

Subcutaneous blood extravasation is not uncommon after a significant accident or traumatic effect such as this client experienced. The fact that the physician did not know about this and the physical therapist did not report it demonstrates questionable judgment. Left shoulder pain after trauma may be Kehr's sign, indicating blood in the peritoneum (see the discussion in Chapter 18).

The new onset of muscle spasm and unchanging pain levels with treatment are potential red-flag symptoms. Concomitant constitutional symptoms of fever and vomiting are also red flags, even if the client thought it was the flu.

The therapist left herself open to legal action by failing to report symptoms unknown to the physician and failing to report the client's changing condition. At no time did the therapist suggest the client go back to the clinic or see a primary care physician. She did not share her findings with the physician either by phone or in writing.

The therapist exercised questionable professional judgment by failing to communicate and collaborate with the attending physician. She did not screen the client for systemic involvement, based on the erroneous thinking that this was a traumatic event with a clear etiology.

She assumed in a case like this, where the client was a self-referral and the physician was a "doc-in-a-box," that she was "on her own." She failed to properly report on the client's condition, failed to follow the APTA's policies governing a physical therapist's interaction with other health care providers, and was legally liable for mismanagement in this case.

Failure to share findings and concerns with the physician or other appropriate health care provider is a failure to enter into a collaborative team approach. Best-practice standards of optimal patient/client care that support and encourage interactive exchange.

Prior negative experiences with difficult medical personnel do not exempt the therapist from best practice, which means making every attempt to communicate and document clinical findings and concerns.

The therapist must describe his or her concerns to the health care provider that the patient is being referred to in a succinct approach. Using the key phrase "scope of practice" may be helpful. It may be necessary to explain that the symptoms do not match the expected pattern for a musculoskeletal or neuromuscular problem. The problem appears to be outside the scope of a physical therapist's practice, or the problem requires a greater collaborative effort between health care disciplines.

It may be appropriate to make a summary statement regarding key objective findings with a follow-up question for the physician. This should be documented in the client's chart or electronic medical record in the hospital or sent in a letter to the outpatient's/client's physician (or other health care provider).

For example, after treatment of a person who has not responded to physical therapy, a report to the physician may include additional information: "Miss Jones reported a skin rash over the backs of her knees 2 weeks before the onset of joint pain and experiences recurrent bouts of sore throat and fever when her knees flare up. These features are not consistent with an athletic injury. Would you please examine her?" (For an additional sample letter, see Fig. 1.6.)

Other useful wording may include "Please advise" or "What do you think?" The therapist does not suggest a medical cause or attempt to diagnose the findings medically. Providing a report and stating that the clinical presentation

Referral. A 32-year-old female university student was referred for physical therapy through the student health service 2 weeks ago. The physician's referral reads: "Possible right oblique abdominis tear/possible right iliopsoas tear." A faculty member screened this woman initially, and the diagnosis was confirmed as being a right oblique abdominal strain.

History. Two months ago, while the client was running her third mile, she felt "severe pain" in the right side of her stomach, which caused her to double over. She felt immediate nausea and had abdominal distention. She cannot relieve the pain by changing the position of her leg. Currently, she still cannot run without pain.

Presenting Symptoms. Pain increases during sit-ups, walking fast, reaching, turning, and bending. Pain is eased by heat and is reduced by activity. Pain in the morning versus in the evening depends on body position. Once the pain starts, it is intermittent and aches. The client describes the pain as being severe, depending on her body position. She is currently taking aspirin when necessary.

SAMPLE LETTER

Date

John Smith, M.D.
University of Montana Health Service
Eddy Street
Missoula, MT 59812

Re: Jane Doe

Dear Dr. Smith,

Your client, Jane Doe, was evaluated in our clinic on 5/2/11 with the following pertinent findings:

She has severe pain in the right lower abdominal quadrant associated with nausea and abdominal distention. Although the onset of symptoms started while the client was running, she denies any precipitating trauma. She describes the course of symptoms as having begun 2 months ago with temporary resolution and now with exacerbation of earlier symptoms. Additionally, she reports chronic fatigue and frequent night sweats.

Presenting pain is reproduced by resisted hip or trunk flexion with accompanying tenderness/tightness on palpation of the right iliopsoas muscle (compared with the left iliopsoas muscle). There are no implicating neurologic signs or symptoms.

Evaluation. A musculoskeletal screening examination is consistent with the proposed medical diagnosis of a possible iliopsoas or abdominal oblique tear. Jane does appear to have a combination of musculoskeletal and systemic symptoms, such as those outlined earlier. Of particular concern are the symptoms of fatigue, night sweats, abdominal distention, nausea, repeated episodes of exacerbation and remission, and severe quality of pain and location (right lower abdominal quadrant). These symptoms appear to be of a systemic nature rather than caused by a primary musculoskeletal lesion.

Recommendations. The client has been advised to return to you for further medical follow-up to rule out any systemic involvement before the initiation of physical therapy services. I am concerned that my proposed plan of care, including soft tissue mobilization and stretching may aggravate an underlying infectious or disease process.

I will contact you directly by telephone by the end of the week to discuss these findings and to answer any questions that you may have. Thank you for this interesting referral.

Sincerely,

Catherine C. Goodman, M.B.A., P.T.

Result. This client returned to the physician, who then ordered laboratory tests. After an acute recurrence of the symptoms described earlier, she had exploratory surgery. A diagnosis of a ruptured appendix and peritonitis was determined at surgery. In retrospect, the proposed plan of care would have been contraindicated in this situation.

Fig. 1.6 Sample letter of the physical therapist's findings that is sent to the referring physician.

does not follow a typical neuromuscular or musculoskeletal pattern may be all that is needed.

Guidelines for Immediate Medical Attention

After each chapter in this text, there is a section on Guidelines for Physician Referral. Guidelines for immediate medical attention are provided whenever possible. An overall summary is provided here, but specifics for each viscerogenic system and NMS situation should be reviewed in each chapter as well.

Keep in mind that prompt referral is based on the physical therapist's overall evaluation of client history and clinical presentation, including red/yellow flag findings and associated signs and symptoms. The recent focus on validity, reliability, specificity, and sensitivity of individual red flags has shown that there is little evidence on the diagnostic accuracy of red flags in the primary care medical (physician) practice.[76]

Experts agree that red flags are important and ignoring them can result in morbidity and even mortality for some individuals. On the other hand, accepting them uncritically can result in unnecessary referrals.[77] Until the evidence supporting or refuting red flags is complete, the therapist is advised to consider all findings in context of the total picture.

For now, immediate medical attention is still advised when:
- Client has anginal pain not relieved in 20 minutes with reduced activity and/or administration of nitroglycerin; has angina at rest
- Client with angina has nausea, vomiting, profuse sweating
- Client presents with bowel/bladder incontinence and/or saddle anesthesia secondary to cauda equina lesion or cervical spine pain concomitant with urinary incontinence
- Client is in anaphylactic shock (see Chapter 13)
- Client has symptoms of inadequate ventilation or CO_2 retention (see the section on Respiratory Acidosis in Chapter 8)
- Client with diabetes appears confused or lethargic or exhibits changes in mental function (perform finger stick glucose testing and report findings)
- Client has positive McBurney's point (appendicitis) or rebound tenderness (inflamed peritoneum) (see Chapter 9)
- Sudden worsening of intermittent claudication may be caused by thromboembolism and must be reported to the physician immediately
- Throbbing chest, back, or abdominal pain that increases with exertion accompanied by a sensation of a heartbeat when lying down and a palpable pulsating abdominal mass may indicate an aneurysm
- Changes in size, shape, tenderness, and consistency of lymph nodes; detection of palpable, fixed, irregular mass in the breast, axilla, or elsewhere, especially in the presence of a previous history of cancer

Guidelines for Physician Referral

Medical attention must be considered when any of the following are present. This list represents a general overview of warning flags or conditions presented throughout this text. More specific recommendations are made in each chapter based on impairment of each individual visceral system.

General Systemic
- Unknown cause
- Lack of significant objective NMS signs and symptoms
- Lack of expected progress with physical therapy intervention
- Development of constitutional symptoms or associated signs and symptoms any time during the episode of care
- Discovery of significant past medical history unknown to physician
- Changes in health status that persist 7 to 10 days beyond expected time period
- Client who is jaundiced and has not been diagnosed or treated

For Women
- Low back, hip, pelvic, groin, or SI symptoms without known etiologic basis and in the presence of constitutional symptoms
- Symptoms correlated with menses
- Any spontaneous uterine bleeding after menopause
- For pregnant women:
  - Vaginal bleeding
  - Elevated blood pressure
  - Increased Braxton-Hicks (uterine) contractions in a pregnant woman during exercise

Vital Signs (Report These Findings)
- Persistent rise or fall of blood pressure
- Blood pressure elevation in any woman taking birth control pills (should be closely monitored by her physician)
- Pulse amplitude that fades with inspiration and strengthens with expiration
- Pulse increase over 20 breaths per minute (bpm) lasting more than 3 minutes after rest or changing position
- Difference in pulse pressure (between systolic and diastolic measurements) of more than 40 mm Hg
- Persistent low-grade (or higher) fever, especially associated with constitutional symptoms, most commonly sweats
- Any unexplained fever without other systemic symptoms, especially in the person taking corticosteroids
- See also yellow cautionary signs presented in Box 4.7 and the section on Physician Referral: Vital Signs in Chapter 4

Cardiac
- More than three sublingual nitroglycerin tablets required to gain relief from angina
- Angina continues to increase in intensity after stimulus (e.g., cold, stress, exertion) has been eliminated
- Changes in pattern of angina
- Abnormally severe chest pain
- Anginal pain radiates to jaw/left arm
- Upper back feels abnormally cool, sweaty, or moist to touch

- Client has any doubts about his or her condition
- Palpitation in any person with a history of unexplained sudden death in the family requires medical evaluation; more than six episodes of palpitation in 1 minute or palpitations lasting for hours or occurring in association with pain, shortness of breath, fainting, or severe light-headedness requires medical evaluation.
- Clients who are neurologically unstable as a result of a recent cerebrovascular accident (CVA), head trauma, spinal cord injury, or other central nervous system insult often exhibit new arrhythmias during the period of instability; when the client's pulse is monitored, any new arrhythmias noted should be reported to the nursing staff or physician.
- Anyone who cannot climb a single flight of stairs without feeling moderately to severely winded or who awakens at night or experiences shortness of breath when lying down should be evaluated by a physician.
- Anyone with known cardiac involvement who develops progressively worse dyspnea should notify the physician of these findings.
- Fainting (syncope) without any warning period of light-headedness, dizziness, or nausea may be a sign of heart valve or arrhythmia problems; unexplained syncope in the presence of heart or circulatory problems (or risk factors for heart attack or stroke) should be evaluated by a physician.

Cancer

Early warning sign(s) of cancer:
- The CAUTION mnemonic for early warning signs is pertinent to the physical therapy examination (see Box 14.2)
- All soft tissue lumps that persist or grow, whether painful or painless
- Any woman presenting with chest, breast, axillary, or shoulder pain of unknown etiologic basis, especially in the presence of a positive medical history (self or family) of cancer
- Any man with pelvic, groin, SI, or low back pain accompanied by sciatica and a history of prostate cancer
- New onset of acute back pain in anyone with a previous history of cancer
- Bone pain, especially on weight-bearing, that persists more than 1 week and is worse at night
- Any unexplained bleeding from any area

Pulmonary

- Shoulder pain aggravated by respiratory movements; have the client hold his or her breath and reassess symptoms; any reduction or elimination of symptoms with breath holding or the Valsalva maneuver suggests pulmonary or cardiac source of symptoms.
- Shoulder pain that is aggravated by supine positioning; pain that is worse when lying down and improves when sitting up or leaning forward is often pleuritic in origin (abdominal contents push up against diaphragm and in turn against parietal pleura; see Figs. 3.4 and 3.5).

- Shoulder or chest (thorax) pain that subsides with auto-splinting (lying on painful side)
- For the client with asthma: signs of asthma or abnormal bronchial activity during exercise
- Weak and rapid pulse accompanied by fall in blood pressure (pneumothorax)
- Presence of associated signs and symptoms, such as persistent cough, dyspnea (rest or exertional), or constitutional symptoms (see Box 1.3)

Genitourinary

- Abnormal urinary constituents, for example, change in color, odor, amount, flow of urine
- Any amount of blood in urine
- Cervical spine pain accompanied by urinary incontinence (unless cervical disk protrusion has already been medically diagnosed)

Gastrointestinal

- Back pain and abdominal pain at the same level, especially when accompanied by constitutional symptoms
- Back pain of unknown cause in a person with a history of cancer
- Back pain or shoulder pain in a person taking NSAIDs, especially when accompanied by GI upset or blood in the stools
- Back or shoulder pain associated with meals or back pain relieved by a bowel movement

Musculoskeletal

- Symptoms that seem out of proportion to the injury or symptoms persisting beyond the expected time for the nature of the injury
- Severe or progressive back pain accompanied by constitutional symptoms, especially fever
- New onset of joint pain following surgery with inflammatory signs (warmth, redness, tenderness, swelling)

Precautions/Contraindications to Therapy

- Uncontrolled chronic heart failure or pulmonary edema
- Active myocarditis
- Resting heart rate 120 or 130 bpm*
- Resting systolic rate 180 to 200 mm Hg
- Resting diastolic rate 105 to 110 mm Hg
- Moderate dizziness, near-syncope
- Marked dyspnea
- Unusual fatigue
- Unsteadiness
- Irregular pulse with symptoms of dizziness, nausea, or shortness of breath or loss of palpable pulse
- Postoperative posterior calf pain
- For the client with diabetes: chronically unstable blood sugar levels must be stabilized (fasting target glucose range: 60 to 110 mg/dL; precaution: <70 or >250 mg/dL)

---

*Unexplained or poorly tolerated by client.

Clues to Screening for Medical Disease

Some therapists suggest a lack of time as an adequate reason to skip the screening process. A few minutes early in the evaluation process may save the client's life. Less dramatically, it may prevent delays in choosing the most appropriate intervention.

Listening for yellow- or red-flag symptoms and observing for red-flag signs can be easily incorporated into everyday practice. It is a matter of listening and looking intentionally. If you do not routinely screen clients for systemic or viscerogenic causes of NMS impairment or dysfunction, then at least pay attention to this red flag:

RED FLAG

- Client does not improve with physical therapy intervention or gets worse with treatment.[4]
- Client is not making progress consistent with the prognosis.

  If someone fails to improve with physical therapy intervention, gets better and then worse, or just gets worse, the treatment protocol may not be in error. Certainly, the first steps are to confirm your understanding of the clinical presentation, repeat appropriate examinations, and review selected intervention(s), but also consider the possibility of a systemic or viscerogenic origin of symptoms. Use the screening tools outlined in this chapter to evaluate each individual client (see Box 1.7).

■ Key Points to Remember

1. Systemic diseases can mimic NMS dysfunction.
2. It is the therapist's responsibility to identify what NMS impairment is present.
3. There are many reasons for screening of the physical therapy client (see Box 1.2).
4. Screening for medical disease is an ongoing process and does not occur just during the initial evaluation.
5. The therapist uses several parameters in making the screening decision: client history, risk factors, clinical presentation including pain patterns/pain types, associated signs and symptoms, and Review of Systems. Any red flags in the first three parameters will alert the therapist to the need for a screening examination. In the screening process, a Review of Systems includes identifying clusters of signs and symptoms that may be characteristic of a particular organ system.
6. The two body parts most commonly affected by visceral pain patterns are the back and the shoulder, although the thorax, pelvis, hip, SI, and groin can be involved.
7. The physical therapist is qualified to make a diagnosis regarding primary NMS conditions referred to as human movement system syndromes.
8. The purpose of the diagnosis, established through the subjective and objective examinations, is to identify as closely as possible the underlying NMS condition involving the human movement system. In this way

the therapist is screening for medical disease, ruling out the need for medical referral, and treating the physical therapy problem as specifically as possible.
9. Sometimes in the diagnostic process the symptoms are treated because the client's condition is too acute to evaluate thoroughly. Usually, even medically diagnosed problems (e.g., "shoulder pain" or "back pain") are evaluated.
10. Careful, objective, detailed evaluation of the client with pain is critical for accurate identification of the sources and types of pain (underlying impairment process) and for accurate assessment of treatment effectiveness.[74]
11. Painful symptoms that are out of proportion to the injury or that are not consistent with objective findings may be a red flag indicating systemic disease. The therapist must be aware of and screen for other possibilities such as physical assault (see the section on Domestic Violence in Chapter 2) and emotional overlay (see Chapter 3).
12. If the client or the therapist is in doubt, communication with the physician, dentist, family member, or referral source is indicated.
13. The therapist must be familiar with the practice act for the state in which he or she is practicing. Information can be found in the Federation of State Boards of Physical Therapy website, or by searching the respective physical therapy boards of each state.

PRACTICE QUESTIONS

1. In the context of screening for referral, the primary purpose of a diagnosis is to:
   a. Obtain reimbursement
   b. Guide the plan of care and intervention strategies
   c. Practice within the scope of physical therapy
   d. Meet the established standards for accreditation

2. Direct access is the only reason physical therapists must screen for systemic disease.
   a. True
   b. False

3. A patient/client gives you a written prescription from a physician, chiropractor, or dentist. The first screening question to ask is:
   a. What did the physician (dentist, chiropractor) say is the problem?
   b. Did the physician (dentist, chiropractor) examine you?
   c. When do you go back to see the doctor (dentist, chiropractor)?
   d. How many times per week did the doctor (dentist, chiropractor) suggest you come to therapy?

4. Screening for medical disease takes place:
   a. Only during the first interview
   b. Just before the client returns to the physician for his/her next appointment
   c. Throughout the episode of care
   d. None of the above

5. Medical referral for a problem outside the scope of the physical therapy practice occurs when:
   a. No apparent movement dysfunction exists
   b. No causative factors can be identified
   c. Findings are not consistent with neuromuscular or musculo-skeletal dysfunction
   d. Client presents with suspicious red-flag symptoms
   e. Any of the above
   f. None of the above

6. Physical therapy evaluation and intervention may be a part of the physician's differential diagnosis.
   a. True
   b. False

7. What is the difference between a yellow- and a red-flag symptom?

8. What are the major decision-making tools used in the screening process?

9. See if you can quickly name 6 to 10 red flags that suggest the need for further screening.

REFERENCES

1. Lentz TA, Beneciuk JM, Bialosky JE, Zeppieri G, Dai Y, Wu SS, George SZ. Development of a yellow flag assessment tool for orthopaedic physical therapists: results from the optimal screening for prediction of referral and outcome (OSPRO) Cohort. *Journal of Orthopaedic & Sports Physical Therapy*. 2016;46(5): 327–343. https://www.jospt.org/doi/10.2519/jospt.2016.6487.

2. Leerar PJ, Boissonnault W, Domholt E, et al. Documentation of red flags by physical therapists for patients with low back pain. *J Man Manip Ther*. 2007;15(1):42–49.

3. George SZ, Beneciuk JM, Lentz TA, et al. optimal screening for prediction of referral and outcome (OSPRO) for musculoskeletal pain conditions: results from the validation cohort. *J Orthop Sports Phys Ther*. 2018;48(6):460–475.

4. Ross MD, Boissonnault WG. Red flags: to screen or not to screen? *J Orthop Sports Phys Ther*. 2010;40(11):682–684.

5. Underwood M. Diagnosing acute nonspecific low back pain: time to lower the red flags? *Arthritis Rheum*. 2009;60:2855–2857.

6. Henschke N, Maher C, Ostelo RW, et al. Red flags to screen for malignancy in patients with low-back pain. *Cochrane Database Syst Rev (ePub)*. 2013

7. Henschke N. A systematic review identifies five "red flags" to screen for vertebral fractures in patients with low back pain. *J Clin Epidemiol*. 2008;61:110–118.

8. Henschke N. Screening for malignancy in low back pain patients: a systematic review. *Eur Spine J*. 2007;16:1673–1679.

9. American Physical Therapy Association: Guide to physical therapist practice. Available online at: https://guide.apta.org/ Accessed February 18, 2021.

10. Bogduk N: Evidence-based clinical guidelines for the management of acute low back pain, *The National Musculoskeletal Medicine Initiative, National Health and Medical Research Council*, 1999. Available online at http://www.stanleyconsulting.ns.ca/Files/pain.pdf. Accessed February 18, 2021.

11. McGuirk B, King W, Govind J, et al. Safety, efficacy, and cost effectiveness of evidence-based guidelines for the management of acute low back pain in primary care. *Spine*. 2001;26(23):2615–2622.

12. Kuchera ML. *Foundations for integrative musculoskeletal medicine*. Philadelphia: Philadelphia College of Osteopathic Medicine; 2005.

13. Henschke N. Prevalence of and screening for serious spinal pathology in patients presenting to primary care settings with acute low back pain. *Arthritis Rheum*. 2009;60(10): 3072–3080.

14. Boissonault W, Ross MDE. Physical therapists referring patients to physicians: a review of case reports and series. *J Orthop Sports Phys Ther*. 2012;42(5):447–454.

15. Heick JD, Boissoinnault WG, King PM. Physical therapist recognition of signs and symptoms of infection after shoulder reconstruction: a patient case report. *Physiother Theory Pract*. 2013;29(2):166–173.

16. Heick JD, Bustillo KL, Farris JW. Recognition of signs and symptoms of a type 1 chondrosarcoma: a case report. *Physiother Theory Pract*. 2014;30(1):49–55.

17. Goodman CC, Kapasi Z. The effect of exercise on the immune system. *Rehab Oncol*. 2002;20(1):13–26.

18. Kruijensen-Jaarsma M, Revesz D, Bierings MB, et al. Effects of exercise on immune function in patients with cancer: a systematic review. *Exer Immunol Rev*. 2013;19:120–143.

19. Qian X, Russell LB, Valiyeva E, et al. "Quicker and sicker" under Medicare's prospective payment system for hospitals: new evidence on an old issue from a national longitudinal survey. *Bull Econ Res*. 2011;63(1):1–27.

20. Deniger A, Troller P, Kennelty KA. Geriatric transitional care and readmissions review. *J Nurse Pract*. 2015;11:248–252.

21. Morris PE. Moving our critically ill patients: mobility barriers and benefits. *Crit Care Clin*. 2007;23:1–20.

22. The State of Aging and Health: National Center for Chronic Disease Prevention and Health Promotion, *Centers for Disease Control*, 2013. Available online at: https://www.cdc.gov/aging/pdf/state-aging-health-in-america-2013.pdf. Accessed February 18, 2021.

23. American Physical Therapy Association (APTA) House of Delegates (HOD): Diagnosis by physical therapists HOD 06-97-06-19 (Program 32) [Amended HOD 06-95-12-07; HOD 06-94-22-35, Initial HOD 06-84-19-78]. APTA Governance.

24. American Physical Therapy Association *A normative model of physical therapist professional education: version 2004*. Alexandria, VA: American Physical Therapy Association; 2004.

25. Vision Statement for the Physical Therapy Profession and Guiding Principles to Achieve the Vision: American Physical Therapy Association. Available online at https://www.apta.org/apta-and-you/leadership-and-governance/policies/vision-statement-for-the-physical-therapy-profession. Accessed February 18, 2021.

26. Ellis J. Paving the path to a brighter future. Sahrmann challenges colleagues to move precisely during 29th McMillan lecture at PT. *PT Bulletin*. 1998;13(29):4–10.

27. American Physical Therapy Association White Paper: Physical Therapist Practice and the Human Movement System. Available

online at http://www.apta.org, August 2015 Accessed September 2, 2016.

28. American Physical Therapy Association. Physical Therapist Practice and the Movement System. Available online at: https://www.apta.org/patient-care/interventions/movement-system-management/movement-system-white-paper. Accessed February 18, 2021.

29. Principles of Physical Therapist Patient and Client Management: *Guide to physical therapist practice*. Available at: https://guide.apta.org/patient-client-management. Accessed February 18, 2021.

30. Sahrmann S: A challenge to diagnosis in physical therapy: tradition, *American Physical Therapy Association*, CSM Opening lecture, 1997.

31. Jiandani MP, Mhatre BS. Physical therapy diagnosis: How is it different? *J Postgrad Med*. 2018;64(2):69–72. https://doi.org/10.4103/jpgm.JPGM_691_17.

32. Spoto MM, Collins J. Physiotherapy diagnosis in clinical practice: a survey of orthopaedic certified specialists in the USA. *Physiother Res Int*. 2008;13(1):31–41.

33. Boissonault WG. Differential diagnosis phase I. In: Umphred DA, Lazaro RT, Roller ML, Burton GU, eds. *Umphred's neurological rehabilitation*. ed 6: Elsevier; 2012.

34. Boissonnault WG, Ross M. Clinical factors leading to physical therapists referring patients to physicians. A systematic review paper. *J Orthop Sports Phys Ther*. 2011;41(1):A23.

35. Fosnaught M. A critical look at diagnosis. *PT Magazine*. 1996;4(6):48–54.

36. Quinn L, Gordon J. *Documentation for rehabilitation: a guide to clinical decision making*. ed 3, St Louis: Elsevier; 2015.

37. American Physical Therapy Association: *Vision 2020, annual report 2010*, American Physical Therapy Association.

38. Raj PP. *Pain medicine: A comprehensive review*. St Louis: Mosby; 1996.

39. Sahrmann S. Diagnosis by the physical therapist—a prerequisite for treatment. A special communication. *Phys Ther*. 1988;68:1703–1706.

40. The Movement System Brings it All Together: PT In Motion. Available online at https://www.apta.org/apta-magazine/2016/05/01/the-movement-system-brings-it-all-together. Accessed February 18, 2021.

41. Norton B. *Diagnosis dialog: defining the 'x' in DxPT*. New Orleans: Combined Sections Meeting; 2011.

42. Rothstein JM. Patient classification. *Phys Ther*. 1993;73(4):214–215.

43. Delitto A, Snyder-Mackler L. The diagnostic process: examples in orthopedic physical therapy. *Phys Ther*. 1995;75(3):203–211.

44. Guccione A. *Diagnosis and diagnosticians: the future in physical therapy*, Dallas, February 13–16, 1997, Combined sections meeting.

45. Desai MJ, Padmanabhan G. Spinal schwannoma in a young adult. *J Orthop Sports Phys Ther*. 2010;40(11):762.

46. Moore J. Direct access under Medicare part B: the time is now! *PT Magazine*. 2002;10(2):30–32.

47. Direct Access at the State Level: American Physical Therapy Association. Available online at http://www.apta.org/StateIssues/DirectAccess/ Accessed July 22, 2016.

48. Levels of Patient Access to Physical Therapists Services in the U.S. Available online at https://www.apta.org/advocacy/issues/direct-access-advocacy/direct-access-by-state. Accessed February 18, 2021.

49. Direct Access and Medicare: American Physical Therapy Association. Available online at https://www.apta.org/your-practice/practice-models-and-settings/direct-access/direct-access-and-medicare. Accessed February 18, 2021.

50. Boissonnault WG. Pursuit and implementation of hospital-based outpatient direct access to physical therapy services: an administrative case report. *Phys Ther*. 2010;90(1):100–109.

51. Bury TJ, Stokes EK. A global view of direct access and patient self-referral to physical therapy: implications for the profession. *Phys Ther*. 2013;93(4):449–459.

52. Roland M. The future of primary care: lessons from the UK. *N Engl J Med*. 2008;359(20):2087–2092.

53. Primary Care. American Physical Therapy Association. Available at: https://www.apta.org/your-practice/practice-models-and-settings/primary-care. Accessed February 18, 2021. 53

54. Ryan GG, Greathouse D, Matsui I, et al. Introduction to primary care medicine. In: Boissonnault WG, ed. *Primary care for the physical therapist*. ed 2 Philadelphia: WB Saunders; 2010.

55. Merriam-Webster On-line Dictionary: Available online at https://www.merriam-webster.com/dictionary/autonomous#:~:text=1a%20%3A%20having%20the%20right,existing%20independently%20an%20autonomous%20zooid. Accessed February 18, 2021.

56. Autonomous physical therapist practice. American Physical Therapy Association. Available online at https://www.apta.org/apta-and-you/leadership-and-governance/policies/autonomous-pt-practice. Accessed February 18, 2020.

57. Sandstrom RW. The meanings of autonomy for physical therapy. *Phys Ther*. 2007;87(1):98–110.

58. Ojha HA, Snyder RS, Davenport TE. Direct access compared with referred physical therapy episodes of care: a systematic review. *Phys Ther*. 2014;94:14–30.

59. Fosnaught M. Direct access: exploring new opportunities. *PT Magazine*. 2002;10(2):58–62.

60. Cash Practice: Considerations for Physical Therapists. Available online at https://www.apta.org/your-practice/payment/cash-practice/cash-practice-considerations-for-physical-therapists. Accessed February 18, 2021.

61. Gonzalez-Urzelai V, Palacio-Elua L, Lopez-de-Munain J. Routine primary care management of acute low back pain: adherence to clinical guidelines. *Eur Spine J*. 2003;12(6):589–594.

62. Sandler G. The importance of the history in the medical clinic and cost of unnecessary tests. *Amer Heart J*. 1980;100:928–931.

63. Vickers AJ. Against diagnosis. *Ann Intern Med*. 2008;149(3):200–203.

64. Enthoven WTM, Geuze J, Scheele J, et al. Prevalence and "red flags" regarding specified causes of back pain in older adults presenting in general practice. *Phys Ther*. 2016;96:305–312.

65. Cook CE, Moore TJ, Learman C, et al. Can experienced physiotherapists identify which patients are likely to succeed with physical therapy treatment? *Arch Physiother*. 2015;5.3.

66. Genetics in Physical Therapy: American Physical Therapy Association. Available online at https://www.apta.org/patient-care/interventions/genetics. Accessed February 18, 2021.

67. Poirot L. Genetic disorders and engineering: implications for physical therapists. *PT Magazine*. 2005;13(2):54–60.

68. Goodman C, Helgeson K. *Exercise prescription for medical conditions*. Philadelphia: FA Davis; 2011.

69. Principles of Physical Therapist Patient and Client Management. American Physical Therapy Association. Available online at https://guide.apta.org/patient-client-management. Accessed February 18, 2021.

70. Giallonardo L. Guide in action. *PT Magazine*. 2000;8(9):76–88.

71. Standards of Practice for Physical Therapy: American Physical Therapy Association. Available online at https://www.apta.org/apta-and-you/leadership-and-governance/policies/standards-of-practice-pt. Accessed February 18, 2021.

72. Referral to Physical Therapy. American Physical Therapy Association. Available online at https://www.apta.org/siteassets/pdfs/policies/referral-physical-therapy.pdf. Accessed February 18, 2021.

73. Arriaga R. Stories from the front, part II: complex medical history and communication. *PT Magazine*. July 2003;11(7):23–25.

74. Gersh M, Echternach JL. Management of the individual with pain—part I: physiology and evaluation. *PT Magazine.* 1996;4(11):54–63.

75. Diagnosis by Physical Therapists: American Physical Therapy Association. Available online at https://www.apta.org/apta-and-you/leadership-and-governance/policies/diagnosis-by-physical-therapist. Accessed February 18, 2021.

76. Moffett J, McLean S. The role of physiotherapy in the management of non-specific back pain and neck pain. *Rheumatol.* 2006;45(4):371–378.

77. Moffett J, McLean S. Red flags need more evaluation: reply. *Rheumatol.* 2006;45(7):921.

SCREENING TOOLS APPENDIX

Optimal Screening for Prediction of Referral and Outcome for Yellow Flags

OSPRO-YF ASSESSMENT TOOL

Negative Mood Domain
Over the last 2 weeks, how often have you been bothered by any of the following problems?

	Not at All	Several Days	More Than Half The Days	Nearly Every Day
1. Poor appetite or overeating*†	0	1	2	3

Read each statement and circle the appropriate number to the right of the statement to indicate how you generally feel.

	Almost Never	Sometimes	Often	Almost Always
2. I am content	1	2	3	4
3. Some unimportant thoughts run through my mind and bother me*†	1	2	3	4
4. I am a hotheaded person*†	1	2	3	4
5. When I get mad, I say nasty things	1	2	3	4
6. It makes me furious when I am criticized in front of others	1	2	3	4

Fear-Avoidance Domain
Circle the number next to each question that best corresponds to how you feel.

	Strongly Disagree	Somewhat Disagree	Somewhat Agree	Strongly Agree
7. I wouldn't have this much pain if there weren't something potentially dangerous going on in my body*†	1	2	3	4

Using the following scale, please indicate the degree to which you have these thoughts and feelings when you are experiencing pain.

	Not at All	To a Slight Degree	To a Moderate Degree	To a Great Degree	All the Time
8. I can't seem to keep it out of my mind*†	0	1	2	3	4

Circle the number from 0 to 6 to indicate how much physical activities affect your current pain.

	Completely Disagree						Completely agree
9. Physical activity might harm my painful body region	0	1	2	3	4	5	6
10. I cannot do physical activities which (might) make my pain worse*†	0	1	2	3	4	5	6
11. My work is too heavy for me*†	0	1	2	3	4	5	6

Continued

Use the scale rating below to indicate how often you engage in each of the following thoughts or activities.

	Never						Always
12. During painful episodes it is difficult for me to think of anything besides the pain	0	1	2	3	4	5	6

Positive Affect/Coping Domain
Please rate how confident you are that you can do the following things at present, despite the pain.

	Not at All Confident						Completely Confident
13. I can live a normal lifestyle, despite the pain	0	1	2	3	4	5	6

Please rate the truth of each statement as it applies to you.

	Never True						Always True
14. It's OK to experience pain*†	0	1	2	3	4	5	6
15. I lead a full life even though I have chronic pain*†	0	1	2	3	4	5	6
16. Before I can make any serious plans, I have to get some control over my pain	0	1	2	3	4	5	6

Please rate your degree of certainty in performing various tasks during rehabilitation based on the following statements.

	I Cannot Do It										Certain I Can Do It
17. My therapy no matter how I feel emotionally*†	0	1	2	3	4	5	6	7	8	9	10

Abbreviation: OSPRO-YF, Optimal Screening for Prediction of Referral and Outcome cohort yellow flag assessment tool.
*Items included in the 10-item version.
†Items included in the 7-item version.

From Lentz TA et al.: Development of a Yellow Flag Assessment Tool for Orthopaedic Physical Therapists: Results From the Optimal Screening for Prediction of Referral and Outcome (OSPRO) Cohort, Journal of Orthopaedic & Sports Physical Therapy, May 2016, Volume 46, Number 5, pp 327-345

Optimal Screening for Prediction of Referral and Outcome-Review of Systems

OPTIMAL SCREENING FOR PREDICTION OF REFERRAL AND OUTCOME RED FLAG SYMPTOM ITEM BANK

Items in bold font have been described as "general health," "constitional symptoms," or "general systemic" but were classified with a specific system for the purposes of this item bank.

Cardiovascular System

1. Have you recently experienced chest pain with rest?
2. Have you recently experienced chest pain with exertion?
3. Have you recently experienced chest pressure?
4. Have you recently experienced upper-quarter pressure or tightness sensations?
5. Have you recently experienced upper-quarter pain when performing lower-quarter (eg,walking)?
6. **Have you recently experienced light-headedness?**
7. **Have you recently experienced loss of consciousness?**
8. Have you recently experienced anxiety or apprehension?
9. Have you recently experienced sweating with chest pain?
10. **Have you recently experienced sweating without exercise or activity (ie, cold sweats)??**
11. **Have you recently experienced excessive sweating?**
12. Have you recently experienced decreased sweating?
13. **Have you recently experienced night sweats?**
14. **Have you recently experienced severe fatigue?**
15. **Have you recently experienced shortness of breath?**
16. Have you recently experienced rapid breathing?
17. Have you recently experienced labored or difficult breathing?
18. Have you recently experienced breathlessness?
19. Have you recently experienced shortness of breath while lying down?
20. Have you recently experienced difficulty in swallowing?
21. Have you recently experienced edema or weight gain?
22. Have you recently experienced heart palpitations?
23. Have you recently experienced a heartbeat in your abdomen when you lie down?
24. Have you recently experienced cramps in your legs when you walk for several blocks?
25. Have you recently experienced swollen calves, ankles, or feet when you wake in the morning?
26. **Have you recently experienced malaise (eg, feeling lethargic as a result of illness)?**
27. Have you recently experienced unexplained irritability?

Pulmonary System

1. Have you recently experienced wheezing?
2. Have you recently experienced a harsh, high-pitched noise on breathing?
3. Have you recently experienced the production of blood when coughing?
4. Have you recently experienced a dry, hacking cough?
5. Have you recently experienced changes in your typical cough pattern?
6. Have you recently experienced the production of abnormally colored substances upon coughing?
7. Have you recently experienced decreased tolerance for physical activity?

Continued

Gastrointestinal System

1. Have you recently experienced nausea?

2. Have you recently experienced vomiting?

3. Have you recently experienced constripation?

4. Have you recently experienced diarrhea?

5. Have you recently experienced abdominal pain?

6. Have you recently experienced change in stool color?

7. Have you recently experienced blood in your stool?

8. Have you recently experienced changes in the frequency of bowel movements?

9. Have you recently experienced excessive heartburn or indigestion?

10. Have you recently experienced specific food intolerance?

11. Have you recently experienced a change in appetite?

12. Have you recently experienced excessive belching or flatulence?

Urogenital System

1. Have you recently experienced pain or difficulty when urinating?

2. Have you recently experienced blood in the urine?

3. Have you recently experienced dark-colored urine?

4. Have you recently experienced changes in urinary frequency and/or volume?

5. Have you recently experienced an infection?

6. Have you recently experienced incontinence?

7. Have you recently experienced vaginal discharge?

8. Have you recently experienced urethral discharge?

9. Have you recently experienced abdominal bloating?

10. Have you recently experienced changes in menstruation patterns?

11. Have you recently experienced pain with sexual intercourse?

12. Have you recently experienced difficulty with sexual intercourse?

13. Have you recently experienced difficulty maintaining an erection?

14. Have you recently experienced breast tenderness?

Endocrine System

1. Have you recently experienced excessive thirst?

2. Have you recently experienced excessive hunger?

3. Have you recently experienced heat or cold intolerance?

4. Have you recently experienced an abrupt onset of cramps?

5. Have you recently experienced unexplained weight loss?

6. Have you recently experienced unexplained weight gain?

7. Have you recently experienced hoarseness of your voice?

8. Have you recently experienced easy bruising?

Continued

Nervous System

1. **Have you recently experienced abnormal sensation (eg, numbness, pins and needles)?**

2. **Have you recently experienced muscle weakness?**

3. Have you recently experienced changes in coordination?

4. Have you recently experienced gait or balance disturbances?

5. Have you recently experienced changes in vision?

6. Have you recently experienced changes in hearing?

7. Have you recently experienced changes in smelling?

8. Have you recently experienced slurred speech?

9. Have you recently experienced changes in memory?

10. Have you recently experienced unexplained confusion?

11. **Have you recently experienced frequent dizziness?**

12. Have you recently experienced headaches?

13. Have you recently experienced facial pain?

14. Have you recently experienced tremors?

15. Have you recently experienced seizures?

Integumentary System

1. **Have you recently experienced changes in skin color?**

2. Have you recently experienced changes in skin texture?

3. Have you recently experienced changes in wound healing time?

4. Have you recently experienced a skin rash?

5. Have you recently experienced changes in hair on your skin?

6. Have you recently experienced changes in the integrity of your nails?

Musculoskeletal System

1. **Have you recently experienced night pain?**

2. **Have you recently experienced pain with rest?**

3. Have you recently experienced sustained morning stffness?

4. **Have you recently experienced no symptom relief with position changes?**

5. **Have you recently experienced trauma (eg, a motor vehicle accident, a fall)?**

6. Have you recently experienced symptoms that travel to different body regions?

7. **Have you recently experienced a failure of conservative intervention?**

8. Have you recently experienced a prolonged use of corticosteroids?

From George SZ et al.: Development of a Review-of-Systems Screening Tool for Orthopaedic Phyisical Therapists: Results from the Optimal Screening for Prediction of Referral and Outcome (OSPRO) Cohort, Journal of Orthopaedic & Sports Physical Therapy, July 2015, Volume 45, Number 7, pp 512-525

Interviewing as a Screening Tool

This chapter describes the specific steps in screening for medical disease. The first step in screening for medical disease is the client interview. Interviewing should be viewed as a skill, which each physical therapist can improve upon with practice. It is generally agreed that 80% of the information needed to make a diagnosis is collected during the interview. This chapter is designed to provide the physical therapist with interviewing guidelines and important questions to ask the client.

Health care practitioners typically begin the interview by determining the client's chief complaint. The **chief complaint** is usually a symptomatic description given by the client (i.e., symptoms reported for which the person is seeking care or advice). The **present illness**, including the chief complaint and other current symptoms, gives a broad, clear account of the symptoms—how they developed and events related to them.

Questioning the client may also assist the therapist in determining whether an injury is in the acute, subacute, or chronic stage. Knowledge of this information allows the clinician to make appropriate decisions regarding the plan of care. This chapter covers the important components of the client interview process: interviewing techniques, interviewing tools, the Core Interview, and review of the inpatient hospital record. Information obtained from these components will determine the location and potential significance of any symptom, including pain.

The interview format provides detailed information regarding symptom behavior: frequency, duration, intensity, length, breadth, depth, and anatomic location as these relate to the client's chief complaint. The physical therapist will later correlate this information with objective findings from the examination to rule out a possible systemic origin of symptoms.

The subjective examination may also reveal contraindications to physical therapy intervention or indications for the kind of intervention that is most likely to be effective. The information obtained from the interview determines whether the therapist will stop the examination process and refer the client elsewhere or continue the physical therapy patient/client management process.

CONCEPTS IN COMMUNICATION

Interviewing is a skill that requires careful refinement over time. Even the most experienced health care professional should engage in continued self-assessment and improvement. Taking an accurate medical history can be a challenge.[1] It is the health care professional that guides the client during the interview process and maintains control of the interview throughout. Clients often forget details regarding their past illnesses, symptoms, or treatments.

Clients may forget, underreport, or combine separate health events into a single memory, a process called *telescoping*. Difficulty with accurate recollection of events should be seen as a human trait that is easily influenced by various factors and conditions. In a patient/client scenario, a person's personality and mental state at the time of the illness or injury may influence their recall abilities.[2]

The clinician must adopt a compassionate and caring attitude and an effective communication style that is sensitive to cultural nuances to help ensure a successful interview. Using the tools and techniques presented in this chapter will get you started or help you improve your screening abilities throughout the patient interview process.

INTERVIEWING SKILLS

Nonverbal Communication Skills

Nonverbal communication is arguably more important than verbal communication when conducting a patient interview. It is very important to notice the nonverbal communication displayed by the patient, as they often have no awareness of their body language, which can reveal information that they have not readily revealed. For example, a patient may describe having very bad shoulder pain and occasionally move or clutch their neck. Congruency and incongruency in a patient's body language can reveal numerous important messages. The physical therapist should be alert and observant to notice these signals. The physical therapist can also display welcoming nonverbal communication by sitting at an angle to the patient, matching the patient's eye contact when appropriate, and affirming their story with facial expressions and body postures that convey empathy.

Verbal Communication Skills

Some patients have an easy time with verbal communication, while others do not. It is the job of the physical therapist to maintain control of the patient interview in the case of a garrulous patient, and to elicit important information from a reticent one. If the patient does not directly answer your question or is providing unhelpful information, it is often helpful to touch the patient or raise your hand while asking a question to redirect them. There are numerous ways to do this and as mentioned, it is a skill that is developed over time.

When conducting a patient interview, the physical therapist should see themselves much like an attorney at trial, trying to gather correct information that is unbiased. In so doing, it is often helpful to keep questions brief and not to ask more than one question at a time. Some patients are also open to suggestions, so questions should be phrased in such a way as to leave the patient open to choosing. The physical therapist should particularly avoid phrasing questions in a direction toward the answer hoped for. For example, "Have you ever had difficulty initiating urination?" is less suggestive than, "You haven't had any difficulty initiating urination, have you?"

Another helpful approach is to use the patient's own words whenever possible. This will help the patient understand what the physical therapist is referring to and improve patient rapport. For example, if a patient has described their radicular symptoms as "cool water dripping down my legs," the physical therapist may ask a follow-up question such as, "when do you notice that cool water feeling?"

Interviewing Errors

One of the most common interviewing errors, as mentioned above, is letting the patient control the interview. The physical therapist has information they need to gather and must be able to politely ascertain that information in the most efficient manner possible. Another error is in misunderstanding the patient. Whether the patient miscommunicated their thoughts, the physical therapist worded the question in a confusing manner, or the physical therapist misunderstood the patient's answer, there is plenty of room for misunderstanding during repeated questioning. We use various words to convey how we feel, and some words may mean different things to different people. For example, patients commonly report feeling "numbness" when they really mean paresthesia, so this should be clarified.

Another common error is in assuming things. A common example is the patient that reports having "constant" pain, which the physical therapist takes to mean there is never a time of day or position in which the pain resolves. In reality, the patient may simply be saying that the pain is the same intensity whenever it is felt, otherwise it is absent. Information like this should be clarified, especially if it is important for the diagnostic process or planning the physical examination.

Compassion and Caring

Compassion is the desire to identify with, or sense something of, another's experience and is a precursor to caring. Caring is the concern, empathy, and consideration for the needs and values of others. Interviewing clients and communicating effectively, both verbally and nonverbally, with compassionate caring takes into consideration individual differences and the client's emotional and psychologic needs.[3,4]

Establishing a trusting relationship with the client is essential when conducting a screening interview and examination. The therapist may be asking questions no one else has asked before about body functions, assault, sexual dysfunction, and so on. A client who is comfortable physically and emotionally is more likely to offer complete information regarding personal and family history.

Be aware of your own body language and how it may affect the client. Sit down when obtaining the history and keep an appropriate social distance from the client. Take notes while maintaining adequate eye contact. Lean forward, nod, or encourage the client occasionally by saying, "Yes, go ahead. I understand." The therapist could also engage in a process called "mirroring" by reflecting similar gestures, postures, and facial expressions given by the client. These behaviors are an important way that human beings express empathy, and can assist in building rapport.[5]

Silence is also a key feature in the communication and interviewing process. Silent attentiveness gives the client time to think or organize his or her thoughts. The health care professional is often tempted to interrupt during this time, potentially disrupting the client's train of thought. According to research by Beckman and Frankel, physicians interrupt their patients an average of 18 seconds into the description of their chief complaint, and the initial concern is often never revisited.[6] Silence can give the therapist time to observe the client and plan the next question or step. Interruptions can be justified later on in the interview if done in a cooperative nature, such as when expanding on a patient's current train of thought or expressing agreement.[7]

Communication Styles

Everyone has a slightly different interviewing and communication style. The interviewer may need to adjust his or her personal interviewing style to strengthen rapport with the client. Relying on one interviewing style may not be adequate for all situations. Factors such as gender, ethnic identification, religion, beliefs, and behaviors of both the therapist and the client can have an effect on the chosen style of communication.

There are cultural differences based on family of origin or country of origin, again for both the therapist and the client. Besides spoken communication, different cultural groups may also have nonverbal, observable differences in communication style. Body language, tone of voice, eye contact, personal space, sense of time, and facial expression are only a few key components of differences in interactive style.[8]

Illiteracy

Throughout the interviewing process and even throughout the episode of care, the therapist must keep in mind that an estimated 45 million Americans are classified as "functionally illiterate."[9] These individuals may be able to read and write simple sentences with limited vocabulary, but are unable to read or write at a level sufficient to deal with everyday life. In addition, approximately half of Americans have poor reading skills and are unable to read prescription drug labels.[9] According to the Center for Immigration Studies, one in five people in the United States speak a language other than English at home, and over 40% of these individuals report that they are less proficient in speaking English.[10] Moreover, it has been found that 36% of the adult U.S. population has a Basic or Below Basic health literacy level, resulting in an economic burden between $106 to $236 billion.[11] Low health literacy means that adults with below basic skills have no more than the simplest reading skills. They cannot read a physicians (or physical therapist's) instructions or food or pharmacy labels.[12]

According to the findings of the Joint Commission, health literacy skills are not evident during most health care encounters. Clear communication and plain language should become a goal and the standard for all health care professionals.[13]

Low health literacy translates into more severe, chronic illnesses and lower quality of care when care is accessed. There is also a higher rate of health service utilization (e.g., hospitalization, emergency services) among people with limited health literacy. People with reading problems may avoid outpatient offices and clinics, and utilize emergency departments for their care because somebody else asks the questions and fills out the form.[14]

It is not just the lower socioeconomic and less-educated population that is affected. Interpreting medical jargon and diagnostic test results and understanding pharmaceuticals are challenges even for many highly educated individuals.

English as a Second Language

The therapist must keep in mind that many people in the United States speak English as a second language (ESL) or are limited English proficient (LEP), and many of those people do not read or write English.[15] More than 14 million people aged 5 years and older in the United States speak English poorly or not at all. Up to 86% of non–English speakers who are illiterate in English are also illiterate in their native language.

Although the percentages of African American and Hispanics with basic and below basic health literacy are much higher than those of whites, the actual number of whites with basic and below health literacy is twice that of African American and Hispanic nonreaders.[11]

People who have basic and below basic health literacy skills cannot read instructions on bottles of prescription medicine or over-the-counter (OTC) medications. They may not know when a medicine is past the date of safe consumption nor can they read about allergic risks, warnings to diabetics, or the potential sedative effect of medications.[12]

They cannot read about "the warning signs" of cancer or which fasting glucose levels signals a red flag for diabetes. They cannot take online surveys to assess their risk for breast cancer, colon cancer, heart disease, or any other life-threatening condition.

The Physical Therapist's Role

The therapist should be aware of the possibility of any form of illiteracy and watch for risk factors such as age (over 55 years old), education (0 to 8 years or 9 to 12 years but without a high school diploma), lower paying jobs, living below the poverty level and/or receiving government assistance, and ethnic or racial minority groups or history of immigration to the United States.

Health illiteracy can present itself in different ways. In the screening process, the therapist must be careful when having the client fill out medical history forms. The illiterate or functionally illiterate adult may not be able to understand the written details on a health insurance form, accurately complete a Family/Personal History form, or read the details of exercise programs provided by the therapist. The same is true for individuals with learning disabilities and mental impairments.

When given a choice between a "yes" or "no" answer to questions, functionally illiterate adults often circle "no" to everything. The therapist should briefly review with each client to verify the accuracy of answers given on any questionnaire or health form.

For example, you may say, "I see you circled 'no' to any health problems in the past. Has anyone in your immediate family (or have you) ever had cancer, diabetes, hypertension …" and continue to name some or all of the choices provided. Sometimes, just naming the most common conditions is enough to know the answer is really "no"—or that there may be a problem with literacy.

Watch for behavioral red flags such as misspelling words, not completing intake forms, leaving the clinic before completing the form, outbursts of anger when asked to complete paperwork, asking no questions, missing appointments, or identifying pills by looking at the pill rather than naming the medication or reading the label.[16]

The Institute of Medicine has called upon health care providers to take responsibility for providing clear communication and adequate support to facilitate health-promoting actions based on understanding. Their goal is to educate society so that people have the skills they need to obtain, interpret, and use health information appropriately and in meaningful ways.[17,18]

Therapists should minimize the use of medical terminology. Use simple but not demeaning language to communicate concepts and instructions. Encourage clients to ask questions and confirm knowledge or tactfully correct misunderstandings.[18]

Consider including the following questions:

 FOLLOW-UP QUESTIONS

- What questions do you have?
- What would you like me to go over?

Identifying individual personality style may be helpful for each therapist as a means of improving communication. Resource materials are available to help with this.[19] The Myers-Briggs Type Indicator, a widely used questionnaire designed to identify one's personality type, is also available on the Internet at www.myersbriggs.org.[20]

For the experienced clinician, it may be helpful to reevaluate individual interviewing practices. Making an audio or video recording during a client interview can help the therapist recognize interviewing patterns that may need to improve. Watch and/or listen for any of the guidelines listed in Box 2.1.

Texts are available with the complete medical interviewing process described. These resources are helpful not only to give the therapist an understanding of the training physicians receive and methods they use when interviewing clients, but also to provide helpful guidelines when conducting a physical therapy screening or examination interview.[21,22]

The therapist should be aware that under federal civil rights laws and regulative agencies, any client with LEP has the right to an interpreter free of charge if the health care provider receives federal funding. In addition, it is important to remember that that quality of care for individuals who are LEP is compromised when qualified interpreters are not used (or available). Errors of omission, false fluency, substitution, editorializing, and addition are common and can have important clinical consequences.[15] Standards for medical interpreting and translating in the United States have been published and are available online.[23]

BOX 2.1 INTERVIEWING DOS AND DON'TS

DOs

Do extend small courtesies (e.g., shaking hands if appropriate, acknowledging others in the room)

Do use a sequence of questions that begins with open-ended questions.

Do leave closed-ended questions for the end as clarifying questions.

Do select a private location where confidentiality can be maintained.

Do give your undivided attention; listen attentively and show it both in your body language and by occasionally making reassuring verbal prompts, such as "I see" or "Go on." Make appropriate eye contact.

Do ask one question at a time and allow the client to answer the question completely before continuing with the next question.

Do encourage the client to ask questions throughout the interview.

Do listen with the intention of assessing the client's current level of understanding and knowledge of his or her current medical condition.

Do eliminate unnecessary information and speak to the client at his or her level of understanding.

Do correlate signs and symptoms with medical history and objective findings to rule out systemic disease.

Do provide several choices or selections to questions that require a descriptive response.

DON'Ts

Don't jump to premature conclusions based on the answers to one or two questions. (Correlate all subjective and objective information before consulting with a physician.)

Don't interrupt or take over the conversation when the client is speaking.

Don't destroy helpful open-ended questions with closed-ended follow-up questions before the person has had a chance to respond (e.g., How do you feel this morning? Has your pain gone?).

Don't use professional or medical jargon when it is possible to use common language (e.g., don't use the term *myocardial infarct* instead of *heart attack*).

Don't overreact to information presented. Common overreactions include raised eyebrows, puzzled facial expressions, gasps, or other verbal exclamations such as "Oh, really?" or "Wow!" Less dramatic reactions may include facial expressions or gestures that indicate approval or disapproval, surprise, or sudden interest. These responses may influence what the client does or does not tell you.

Don't use leading questions. Pain is difficult to describe, and it may be easier for the client to agree with a partially correct statement than to attempt to clarify points of discrepancy between your statement and his or her pain experience.

Leading Questions	Better Presentation of Same Questions
Where is your pain?	Do you have any pain associated with your injury? If yes, tell me about it.
Does it hurt when you first get out of bed?	When does your back hurt?
Does the pain radiate down your leg?	Do you have this pain anywhere else?
Do you have pain in your lower back?	Point to the exact location of your pain.

CULTURAL COMPETENCE

Effective interviewing and communication require the clinician to possess an awareness and understanding of the uniqueness of each individual. Part of this process is the consideration of an individual's cultural background. *Culture* refers to integrated patterns of human behavior that include the language, thoughts, communications, actions, customs, beliefs, values, and institutions of racial, ethnic, religious, or social groups.[24]

Cultural competence can be defined as a set of congruent behaviors, attitudes, and policies that come together in a system, agency, or among professionals and enable that system, agency, or those professionals to work effectively in cross-cultural situations (APTA, Cultural Competence in Physical Therapy).[25] As health care professionals, we must develop a deeper sense of understanding of how factors related to culture affect the interviewing, screening, and healing process.

Minority Groups

The need for culturally competent physical therapy care has come about, in part, because of the rising number of groups in the United States. Groups other than "white" or

---

BOX 2.2 RACIAL/ETHNIC DESIGNATIONS

The categories below were used for the 2010 U.S. Census.
- American Indian/Alaska Native
- Asian Indian; Chinese; Filipino; Japanese; Korean; Vietnamese; other Asian
- Black/African American, or Negro
- Hispanic or Latino, or Spanish origins; Mexican, Mexican American, Chicano; Puerto Rican; Cuban; another Hispanic, Latino or Spanish origin
- Native Hawaiian, Guanamanian or Chamorro; Samoan; other Pacific Islander
- White
- Some other race

"Caucasian" counted as race/ethnicity by the U.S. Census are listed in Box 2.2.

Over the last five decades, the population growth of the United States has been driven by immigrants and their descendants. The Pew Research Center projects that in 2065, one in three Americans will be an immigrant or have immigrant parents; currently it is one in four. Although non-Hispanic whites will still be the largest racial and ethnic group, they will only comprise 46% of the total population, down from 62% in 2015. In 2065 Hispanics/Latinos will comprise almost a quarter of the total population, followed by Asians (14%) and African Americans (13%).[26]

Social Determinants of Health

Although cultural competence training has been embedded in health care curricula for several years, recent studies have shown that there is little evidence that it improves patient outcomes.[27] It cannot be denied that there is a need for better quality research on this topic, but it is also important to recognize other factors that contribute to widening health disparities and continued inequity in health care access. More recent literature on the social determinants of health attempts to address this topic.

Social determinants of health (SDH) is defined by the World Health Organization as "the non-medical factors that influence health outcomes. They are the conditions in which people are born, grow, work, live, and age, and the wider set of forces and systems shaping the conditions of daily life" (WHO, 2016).[28] Examples of SDH include economic policies and systems, development agendas, social norms, social policies, and political systems.[28] Although clinicians are highly encouraged to practice culturally competent delivery of health care, they must also be cognizant of the SDH to optimize patient outcomes.

Cultural Competence in the Screening Process

Clients from a racial/ethnic background may have unique health care concerns and risk factors. It is important to learn as much as possible about each group served (Case Example 2.1).

CASE EXAMPLE 2.1

Cultural Competency; Risk Factors Based On Ethnicity

A 25-year-old African American woman who is also a physical therapist came to a physical therapy clinic with severe right knee joint pain. She could not recall any traumatic injury but reported hiking 3 days ago in the Rocky Mountains with her brother. She lives in New York City and just returned yesterday.

A general screening examination revealed the following information:
- Frequent urination for the last 2 days
- Stomach pain (related to stress of visiting family and traveling)
- Fatigue (attributed to busy clinic schedule and social activities)
- Past medical history: acute pneumonia, age 11 years
- Nonsmoker, social drinker (1–3 drinks/week)

What Are the Red-Flag Signs/Symptoms?

How Do You Handle a Case Like This?
- Young age
- African American

With the combination of red flags (change in altitude, increased fatigue, increased urination, and stomach pain), there could be a possible systemic cause, not just life's stressors as attributed by the client. The physical therapist treated the symptoms locally, but not aggressively, and referred the client immediately to a medical doctor.

Result: The client was subsequently diagnosed with sickle cell anemia. Medical treatment was instituted along with client education and a rehabilitation program for local control of symptoms and a preventive strengthening program.

BOX 2.3   CULTURAL COMPETENCY IN A SCREENING INTERVIEW

- Wait until the client has finished speaking before interrupting or asking questions.
- Allow "wait time" (time gaps) for some cultures (e.g., Native Americans, English as a second language [ESL]).
- Be aware that eye contact, body-space boundaries, and even handshaking may differ from culture to culture.

When Working With an Interpreter

- Choosing an interpreter is important. A competent medical interpreter is familiar with medical terminology, cultural customs, and the policies of the health care facility in which the client is receiving care.
- There may be problems if the interpreter is younger than the client; in some cultures it is considered rude for a younger person to give instructions to an elder.
- In some cultures (e.g., Muslim), information about the client's diagnosis and condition are relayed to

the head of the household who then makes the decision to share the news with the client or other family members.
- Listen to the interpreter but direct your gaze and eye contact to the client (as appropriate; sustained direct eye contact may be considered aggressive behavior in some cultures).
- Watch the client's body language while listening to him or her speak.
- Head nodding and smiling do not necessarily mean understanding or agreement; when in doubt, always ask the interpreter to clarify any communication.
- Keep comments, instructions, and questions simple and short. Do not expect the interpreter to remember everything you said and relay it exactly as you said it to the client if you do not keep it short and simple.
- Avoid using medical terms or professional jargon.

Clients who are members of a cultural minority are more likely to be geographically isolated and/or underserved in the area of health services. Risk-factor assessment is very important, especially if there is no primary care physician involved.

Communication style may be unique from group to group; be aware of groups in your area or community and learn about their distinctive health features. For example, Native Americans may not volunteer information, requiring additional questions in the interview or screening process. Courtesy is very important in Asian cultures. Clients may act polite, smiling and nodding, but not really understand the clinician's questions. ESL may be a factor; the client may need an interpreter. The client may not understand the therapist's questions but will not show his or her confusion and may not ask the therapist to repeat the question.

Cultural factors can affect the way a person follows through on instructions, interprets questions, and participates in his or her own care. In addition to the guidelines in Box 2.1, Box 2.3 offers some "Dos" in a cultural context for the physical therapy or screening interview.

Furthermore, Kleinman and colleagues introduced the Patient's Explanatory Model[29] using a series of eight questions that are aimed at facilitating culturally competent communication. Box 2.4 includes "Kleinman's eight questions."

Although it is important to pick up on cultural cues that may explain the client's behavior and responses, the clinician must not stereotype individuals based on race and ethnicity. Treating each client as you would want to be treated will help provide the best care for that individual.

Resources

Learning about cultural preferences helps therapists become familiar with factors that could affect the screening process.

More information on cultural competency is available to help therapists develop a deeper understanding of culture and cultural differences, especially in health and health care.

The American Physical Therapy Association (APTA) maintains several resources on cultural competence in physical therapy. These resources can be found using the following link: https://www.apta.org/patient-care/public-health-population-care/cultural-competence/achieve-cultural-competence

Information on laws and legal issues affecting minority health care are also available on this website. Best practices in culturally competent health services are provided, including summary recommendations for medical interpreters, written materials, and cultural competency of health professionals.

The APTA also has a department dedicated to Minority and International Affairs with additional information available online regarding cultural competence. Information on laws and legal issues affecting minority health care are also

---

BOX 2.4   KLEINMAN'S EIGHT QUESTIONS*

1. What do you think has caused your problem?
2. Why do you think it started when it did?
3. What do you think your sickness does to you? How does it work? How severe is your sickness?
4. Will it have a short or long course?
5. What kind of treatment do you think you should receive?
6. What are the most important results you hope to receive from this treatment?
7. What are the chief problems your sickness has caused for you?
8. What do you fear most about your sickness?

*Published with Permission, Dr. Arthur Kleinman[29]

available. Best practices in culturally competent health services are provided, including summary recommendations for medical interpreters, written materials, and cultural competency of health professionals.[25]

The APTA's *Tips to Increase Cultural Competency* offers information on values and principles integral to culturally competent education and delivery systems, a Publications Corner that includes articles on cultural competence, links to resources, resources for treating patients/clients from diverse backgrounds, and more. Also, there is a *Blueprint for Teaching Cultural Competence in Physical Therapy Education* now available that was created by the Committee on Cultural Competence. This program is a guide to help physical therapists with learning core knowledge, attitudes, and skills specific to developing cultural competence as we meet the needs of diverse consumers and strive to reduce or eliminate health disparities.[25]

The U.S. Department of Health and Human Services' Office of Minority Health has published national standards for culturally and linguistically appropriate services (CLAS) in health care. These are available at the Office of Minority Health's website (http://minorityhealth.hhs.gov/omh/browse.aspx?lvl=1&lvlid=6).[30]

Resources for language and cultural needs of minorities, immigrants, refugees, and other diverse populations seeking health care are available, including strategies for overcoming language and cultural barriers to health care.[31]

THE SCREENING INTERVIEW

The therapist will use two main interviewing tools during the screening process. The first is the Family/Personal History form (see Fig. 2.2). With the client's responses on this form and/or the client's chief complaint in hand, the interview begins.

The second interviewing tool is the Core Interview (see Fig. 2.3). The Core Interview as presented in this chapter provides a guideline for the therapist when asking questions about the present illness and chief complaint. Screening questions may be interspersed throughout the Core Interview, as seems appropriate and based on each client's answers to the questions.

There may be times when additional screening questions are asked at the end of the Core Interview or even on a subsequent date at a follow-up appointment. Specific series of questions related to a single symptom (e.g., dizziness, heart palpitations, night pain) or event (e.g., assault, work history, breast examination) are included throughout the text and compiled in the general appendix in the accompanying enhanced eBook version included with print purchase of this textbook for the clinician to use easily.

Interviewing Techniques

An organized interview format assists the therapist in obtaining a complete and accurate database. Using the same outline with each client ensures that all pertinent information related to previous medical history and current medical problem(s) is included. This information is especially important when correlating the subjective data with objective findings from the physical examination.

The most basic skills required for a physical therapy interview include:

- Open-ended questions
- Closed-ended questions
- Funnel sequence or technique
- Paraphrasing technique.

Open-Ended and Closed-Ended Questions

Beginning an interview with an *open-ended question* (i.e., questions that elicit more than a one-word response) is advised, even though this gives the client the opportunity to control and direct the interview.[32,33]

People are the best source of information about their own condition. Initiating an interview with the open-ended directive, "Tell me why you are here" can potentially elicit more information in a relatively short (5- to 15-minute) period than a steady stream of *closed-ended questions* requiring a "yes" or "no" type of answer (Table 2.1).[34,35] In cognitive psychology, the term *primacy effect*[36] has been used to describe how information provided early in a conversation is more impactful. This type of interviewing style demonstrates to the client that what he or she has to say is important. Moving from the open-ended line of questions to the closed-ended questions is referred to as the *funnel technique* or *funnel sequence.*

Each question format has advantages and limitations. The use of open-ended questions to initiate the interview may allow the client to control the interview (Case Example 2.2), but it can also prevent a false-positive or false-negative response that would otherwise be elicited by starting with closed-ended (yes or no) questions.

Closed-ended questions are best used when clarifying or obtaining the answer to a very specific question. If used in the beginning of an interview before background information has been established, it is easy for closed-ended questions to become leading and yield inaccurate information.

TABLE 2.1	Interviewing Techniques	
Open-Ended Questions	**Closed-Ended Questions**
1. How does bed rest affect your back pain?	1. Do you have any pain after lying in bed all night?
2. Tell me how you cope with stress and what kinds of stressors you encounter on a daily basis.	2. Are you under any stress?
3. What makes the pain better/worse?	3. Is the pain relieved by food?
4. How did you sleep last night?	4. Did you sleep well last night?

CASE EXAMPLE 2.2

Monologue

You are interviewing a client for the first time, and she tells you, "The pain in my hip started 12 years ago, when I was a waitress standing on my feet 10 hours a day. It seems to bother me most when I am having premenstrual symptoms.

"My left leg is longer than my right leg, and my hip hurts when the scars from my bunionectomy ache. This pain occurs with any changes in the weather. I have a bleeding ulcer that bothers me, and the pain keeps me awake at night. I dislocated my shoulder 2 years ago, but I can lift weights now without any problems." She continues her monologue, and you feel out of control and unsure how to proceed.

This scenario was taken directly from a clinical experience and represents what we call "an organ recital." In this situation the client provides detailed information regarding all previously experienced illnesses and symptoms, which may or may not be related to the current problem.

How Do You Redirect This Interview? A client who takes control of the interview by telling the therapist about every ache and pain of every friend and neighbor can be rechanneled effectively by interrupting the client with a polite statement such as:

? FOLLOW-UP QUESTIONS

- I am beginning to get an idea of the nature of your problem. Let me ask you some other questions.

At this point the interviewer may begin to use closed-ended questions (i.e., questions requiring the answer to be "yes" or "no") in order to characterize the symptoms more clearly.

Use of the funnel sequence to obtain as much information as possible through the open-ended format first (before moving on to the more restrictive but clarifying "yes" or "no" type of questions at the end) can establish an effective forum for trust between the client and the therapist.

Follow-Up Questions. The funnel sequence is aided by the use of *follow-up* questions, referred to as *FUPs* in the text. Beginning with one or two open-ended questions in each section, the interviewer may follow up with a series of closed-ended questions, which are listed in the Core Interview presented later in this chapter.

For example, after an open-ended question such as: "How does rest affect the pain or symptoms?" the therapist can follow up with clarifying questions such as:

? FOLLOW-UP QUESTIONS

- Are your symptoms aggravated or relieved by any activities? If yes, what?
- How has this problem affected your daily life at work or at home?
- How has it affected your ability to care for yourself without assistance (e.g., dress, bathe, cook, drive)?

Paraphrasing Technique. A useful interviewing skill that can assist in synthesizing and integrating the information obtained during questioning is the *paraphrasing technique*. When using this technique, the interviewer repeats information presented by the client.

This technique can assist in fostering effective, accurate communication between the health care recipient and the health care provider. For example, once a client has responded to the question, "What makes you feel better?" the therapist can paraphrase the reply by saying, "You've told me that the pain is relieved by such and such, is that right? What other activities or treatments offer relief from your pain or symptoms?"

If the therapist cannot paraphrase what the client has said, or if the meaning of the client's response is unclear, then the therapist can ask for clarification by requesting an example of what the person is saying. It can also be helpful to paraphrase a client's statement in an extreme way in order to elicit greater thought by the client. For example, a client may initially say they don't have tingling in their left foot, only their right. The interviewer could reply by saying, "Have you *never had any tingling at all* in your left foot?" In this way, the interviewer can guard against new information coming up later in the interview, such as the client recalling that their left foot has also tingled on occasion.

Interviewing Tools

With the emergence of evidence-based practice, therapists are required to identify problems, to quantify symptoms (e.g., pain), and to demonstrate the effectiveness of intervention.

Documenting the effectiveness of intervention is called *outcomes management*. Using standardized tests, functional tools, or questionnaires to relate pain, strength, or range of motion to a quantifiable scale are defined as *outcome measures*. The information obtained from such measures is then compared with the functional outcomes of treatment to assess the effectiveness of those interventions.

In this way, therapists are gathering information about the most appropriate treatment progression for a specific diagnosis. Such a database shows the efficacy of physical therapy intervention and provides data for use with insurance companies in requesting reimbursement for service.

Along with impairment-based measures, therapists must use reliable and valid measures of activity and participation. No single instrument or method of assessment can be considered the best for all patient populations.

Pain assessment is often a central focus of the therapist's interview, so some way to quantify and describe pain is necessary. There are numerous pain assessment scales designed to determine the quality and location of pain or the percentage of impairment or functional levels associated with pain (see further discussion in Chapter 3).

There are a wide variety of anatomic region, function, or disease-specific assessment tools available. Each test has a specific focus—whether to assess pain levels, level of balance, risk for falls, functional status, disability, quality of life, and so on.

Some tools focus on a particular kind of problem such as activity limitations or disability in people with low back pain (e.g., Oswestry Disability Questionnaire,[37] Quebec Back Pain Disability Scale,[38] Duffy-Rath Questionnaire[39]). The Simple Shoulder Test[40] and the Disabilities of the Arm, Shoulder, and Hand Questionnaire (DASH)[41] may be used to assess physical function of the shoulder. Nurses often use the PQRST mnemonic to help identify underlying pathology or pain (see Box 3.3).

Other examples of specific tests include the:
- Visual Analog Scale (VAS; see Fig. 3.6)
- Verbal Descriptor Scale (see Box 3.1)
- McGill Pain Questionnaire (see Fig. 3.11)
- Pain Impairment Rating Scale (PAIRS).

A more complete evaluation of client function can be obtained by pairing disease- or region-specific instruments with the Short-Form Health Survey (SF-36 Version 2).[42] The SF-36 is a well-established questionnaire used to measure the client's perception of his or her health status. It is a generic measure, as opposed to one that targets a specific age, disease, or treatment group. It includes eight different subscales of functional status that are scored in two general components: physical and mental. There are now even shorter survey forms, the SF-12 Version 2, and the SF-8. All of these tools are available online at www.sf-36.org. The initial Family/Personal History form (see Fig. 2.2) gives the therapist some idea of the client's previous medical history (personal and family), medical testing, and current general health status. Make a special note of the box inside the form labeled "Therapists." This is for liability purposes. Anyone who has ever completed a deposition for a legal case will agree it is often difficult to remember the details of a case brought to trial years later.

A client may insist that a condition was (or was not) present on the first day of the examination. Without a baseline to document initial findings, this is often difficult, if not impossible to dispute. The client must sign or initial the form once it is complete. The therapist is advised to sign and date it to verify that the information was discussed with the client.

Resources

The Family/Personal History form presented in this chapter is just one example of a basic intake form. See the companion website for other useful examples with a different approach. If a client has any kind of literacy or writing problem, the therapist completes the form with him or her. If not, the therapist goes over the form with the client at the beginning of the evaluation.

Therapists may modify the information collected from these examples depending on individual differences in client base and specialty areas served. For example, hospital or institution accreditation agencies such as Commission on Accreditation of Rehabilitation Facilities (CARF) and the Joint Commission on Accreditation of Health Care Organizations (JCAHO) may require the use of their own forms.

An orthopedic-based facility or a sports-medicine center may want to include questions on the intake form concerning current level of fitness and the use of orthopedic devices used, such as orthotics, splints, or braces. Therapists working with the geriatric population may want more information regarding current medications prescribed or levels of independence in activities of daily living.

The Review of Systems (see Box 4.15 on p. 207 and Appendix D-5 in the accompanying enhanced eBook version included with print purchase of this textbook), which provides a helpful chart of signs and symptoms characteristic of each visceral system, can be used along with the Family/Personal History form.

CLIENT HISTORY AND INTERVIEW

The client history and interview are intended to provide a database of information that is important in determining the need for medical referral or the direction for physical therapy intervention. Risk factor assessment is conducted throughout the patient history and interview and the tests and measures portion of the physical therapy examination.

Key Components of the Client History and Interview

The Client History and Interview must be conducted in a complete and organized manner. These are composed of several components. The mechanisms in place for gathering the necessary information in these components may vary between therapists and clinical settings (Fig. 2.1).

The traditional medical interview begins with the family/personal history and then addresses the chief complaint. Therapists may find it works better to conduct the Core Interview and then ask additional questions after looking over the client's responses on the Family/Personal History form.

In a screening model, the therapist is advised to have the client complete the Family/Personal History form before the client-therapist interview. The therapist then quickly reviews the history form, making mental note of any red-flag histories. This information may be helpful during the Patient Interview and History and Tests and Measures portions of the examination. Information gathered will include:

Types of data that may be generated from a patient or client history.

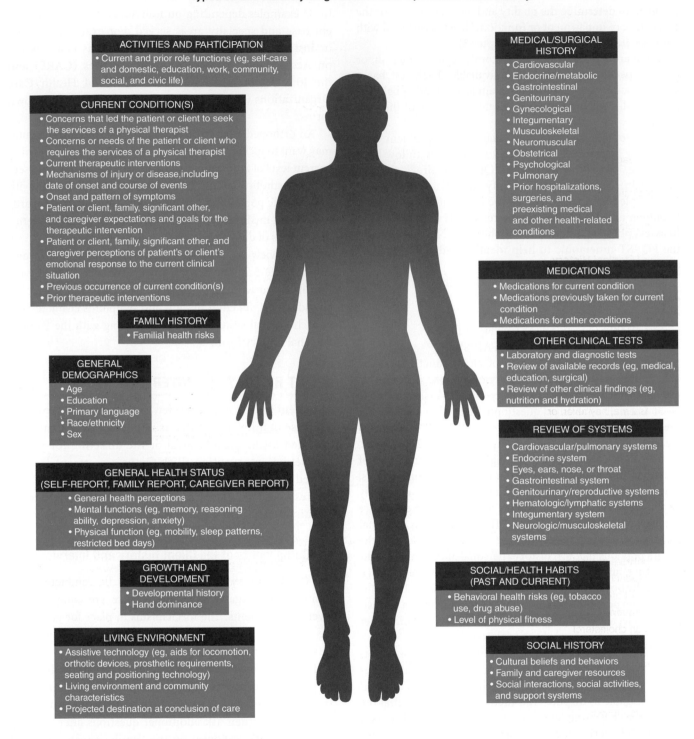

ACTIVITIES AND PARTICIPATION
- Current and prior role functions (eg, self-care and domestic, education, work, community, social, and civic life)

CURRENT CONDITION(S)
- Concerns that led the patient or client to seek the services of a physical therapist
- Concerns or needs of the patient or client who requires the services of a physical therapist
- Current therapeutic interventions
- Mechanisms of injury or disease, including date of onset and course of events
- Onset and pattern of symptoms
- Patient or client, family, significant other, and caregiver expectations and goals for the therapeutic intervention
- Patient or client, family, significant other, and caregiver perceptions of patient's or client's emotional response to the current clinical situation
- Previous occurrence of current condition(s)
- Prior therapeutic interventions

FAMILY HISTORY
- Familial health risks

GENERAL DEMOGRAPHICS
- Age
- Education
- Primary language
- Race/ethnicity
- Sex

GENERAL HEALTH STATUS (SELF-REPORT, FAMILY REPORT, CAREGIVER REPORT)
- General health perceptions
- Mental functions (eg, memory, reasoning ability, depression, anxiety)
- Physical function (eg, mobility, sleep patterns, restricted bed days)

GROWTH AND DEVELOPMENT
- Developmental history
- Hand dominance

LIVING ENVIRONMENT
- Assistive technology (eg, aids for locomotion, orthotic devices, prosthetic requirements, seating and positioning technology)
- Living environment and community characteristics
- Projected destination at conclusion of care

MEDICAL/SURGICAL HISTORY
- Cardiovascular
- Endocrine/metabolic
- Gastrointestinal
- Genitourinary
- Gynecological
- Integumentary
- Musculoskeletal
- Neuromuscular
- Obstetrical
- Psychological
- Pulmonary
- Prior hospitalizations, surgeries, and preexisting medical and other health-related conditions

MEDICATIONS
- Medications for current condition
- Medications previously taken for current condition
- Medications for other conditions

OTHER CLINICAL TESTS
- Laboratory and diagnostic tests
- Review of available records (eg, medical, education, surgical)
- Review of other clinical findings (eg, nutrition and hydration)

REVIEW OF SYSTEMS
- Cardiovascular/pulmonary systems
- Endocrine system
- Eyes, ears, nose, or throat
- Gastrointestinal system
- Genitourinary/reproductive systems
- Hematologic/lymphatic systems
- Integumentary system
- Neurologic/musculoskeletal systems

SOCIAL/HEALTH HABITS (PAST AND CURRENT)
- Behavioral health risks (eg, tobacco use, drug abuse)
- Level of physical fitness

SOCIAL HISTORY
- Cultural beliefs and behaviors
- Family and caregiver resources
- Social interactions, social activities, and support systems

Fig. 2.1 *Types of data that may be generated from a client history.* In this model, data about the visceral systems is reflected in the Medical/Surgical history. (From *Guide to physical therapist practice*, ed 3, Alexandria, VA, 2014, American Physical Therapy Association.)

- Family/Personal History (see Fig. 2.2)
  Age
  Sex
  Race and Ethnicity
  Past Medical History

General Health

Past Medical and Surgical History

Clinical Tests

Work and Living Environment

Family/Personal History

Date: _____

Client's name: _____   DOB: _____   Age: _____

Race/ethnicity:
- ☐ American Indian/Alaska Native
- ☐ Black/African American
- ☐ Hispanic/Latino
- ☐ Multiracial

- ☐ Asian
- ☐ Caucasian/white
- ☐ Native Hawaiian/Pacific Islander
- ☐ Other/unknown

Language: ☐ English understood   ☐ Interpreter needed   ☐ Primary language:

Medical diagnosis: _____   Date of onset: _____

Physician: _____   Date of surgery (if any): _____   Therapist: _____

Past Medical History

Have you or any immediate family member (parent, sibling, child) ever been told you have:

Circle one:

			(Do **NOT** complete) **For the therapist:**		
• Allergies	Yes	No	Relation to client	Date of onset	Current status
• Angina or chest pain	Yes	No			
• Anxiety/panic attacks	Yes	No			
• Arthritis	Yes	No			
• Asthma, hay fever, or other breathing problems	Yes	No			
• Cancer	Yes	No			
• Chemical dependency (alcohol/drugs)	Yes	No			
• Cirrhosis/liver disease	Yes	No			
• Depression	Yes	No			
• Diabetes	Yes	No			
• Eating disorder (bulimia, anorexia)	Yes	No			
• Headaches	Yes	No			
• Heart attack	Yes	No			
• Hemophilia/slow healing	Yes	No			
• High cholesterol	Yes	No			
• Hypertension or high blood pressure	Yes	No			
• Kidney disease/stones	Yes	No			
• Multiple sclerosis	Yes	No			
• Osteoporosis	Yes	No			
• Stroke	Yes	No			
• Tuberculosis	Yes	No			
• Other (please describe)	Yes	No			

Therapists: Use this space to record baseline information. This is important in case something changes in the client's status. You are advised to record the date and sign or initial this form for documentation and liability purposes, indicating that you have reviewed this form with the client. You may want to have the client sign and date it as well.

Fig. 2.2   Sample of a Family/Personal History Form.

Personal History

Have you ever had:

• Anemia	Yes	No		• Chronic bronchitis	Yes	No
• Epilepsy/seizures	Yes	No		• Emphysema	Yes	No
• Fibromyalgia/myofascial				• GERD	Yes	No
pain syndrome	Yes	No		• Gout	Yes	No
• Hepatitis/jaundice	Yes	No		• Guillain-Barré syndrome	Yes	No
• Joint replacement	Yes	No		• Hypoglycemia	Yes	No
• Parkinson's disease	Yes	No		• Peripheral vascular disease	Yes	No
• Polio/postpolio	Yes	No		• Pneumonia	Yes	No
• Shortness of breath	Yes	No		• Prostate problems	Yes	No
• Skin problems	Yes	No		• Rheumatic/scarlet fever	Yes	No
• Urinary incontinence				• Thyroid problems	Yes	No
(dribbling, leaking)	Yes	No		• Ulcer/stomach problems	Yes	No
• Urinary tract infection	Yes	No		• Varicose veins	Yes	No

For Women:

History of endometriosis	Yes	No
History of pelvic inflammatory disease	Yes	No
Are you/could you be pregnant?	Yes	No
Any trouble with leaking or dribbling urine?	Yes	No
Number of pregnancies _____ Number of live births _____		
Have you ever had a miscarriage/abortion?	Yes	No

General Health

1. I would rate my health as (circle one):   Excellent   Good   Fair   Poor

2. Are you taking any prescription or over-the-counter medications? If yes, please list: _____ Yes No
_____

3. Are you taking any nutritional supplements (any kind, including vitamins) Yes No

4. Have you had any illnesses within the last 3 weeks (e.g., colds, influenza, bladder or kidney infection)? Yes No
    If yes, have you had this before in the last 3 months? Yes No

5. Have you noticed any lumps or thickening of skin or muscle anywhere on your body? Yes No

6. Do you have any sores that have not healed or any changes in size, shape, or color of a wart or mole? Yes No

7. Have you had any unexplained weight gain or loss in the last month? Yes No

8. Do you smoke or chew tobacco? Yes No
    If yes, how many packs/pipes/pouches/sticks a day? _____ How many months or years? _____

9. I used to smoke/chew but I quit. Yes No
    If yes: pack or amount/day _____ Year quit _____

10. I would like to quit smoking/using tobacco. Yes No

11. How much alcohol do you drink in the course of a week? (One drink is equal to 1 beer, 1 glass of wine, or 1 shot of hard liquor) _____

12. Do you use recreational or street drugs (marijuana, cocaine, crack, meth, amphetamines, or others)? Yes No
    If yes, what, how much, how often? _____

13. How much caffeine do you consume daily (including soft drinks, coffee, tea, or chocolate)? _____
_____

14. Are you on any special diet? Yes No

Fig. 2.2, cont'd

15. Do you have (or have you recently had) any of these problems:

☐ Blood in urine, stool, vomit, mucus
☐ Dizziness, fainting, blackouts
☐ Fever, chills, sweats (day or night)
☐ Nausea, vomiting, loss of appetite
☐ Changes in bowel or bladder
☐ Throbbing sensation/pain in belly or anywhere else
☐ Skin rash or other skin changes

☐ Cough, dyspnea
☐ Dribbling or leaking urine
☐ Heart palpitations or fluttering
☐ Numbness or tingling
☐ Swelling or lumps anywhere
☐ Problems seeing or hearing
☐ Unusual fatigue, drowsiness

☐ Difficulty swallowing/speaking
☐ Memory loss
☐ Confusion
☐ Sudden weakness
☐ Trouble sleeping
☐ Other: _____
☐ None of these

Medical/Surgical History

1. Have you ever been treated with chemotherapy, radiation therapy, biotherapy, or brachytherapy (radiation implants)?   Yes   No
   If yes, please describe: _____

2. Have you had any x-rays, sonograms, computed tomography (CT) scans, or magnetic resonance imaging (MRI) or other imaging done recently?   Yes   No
   If yes, what? _____ When? _____ Results? _____

3. Have you had any laboratory work done recently (urinalysis or blood tests)?   Yes   No
   If yes, what? _____ When? _____ Results (if known)? _____

4. Any other clinical tests?   Yes   No
   Please describe: _____

5. Please list any operations that you have ever had and the date(s):
   Operation_____ Date _____

6. Do you have a pacemaker, transplanted organ, joint replacement, breast implants, or any other implants?   Yes   No
   If yes, please describe: _____

Work/Living Environment

1. What is your job or occupation? _____
2. Military service: (When and where): _____
3. Does your work involve:
   ☐ Prolonged sitting (e.g., desk, computer, driving)
   ☐ Prolonged standing (e.g., equipment operator, sales clerk)
   ☐ Prolonged walking (e.g., mill worker, delivery service)
   ☐ Use of large or small equipment (e.g., telephone, forklift, computer, drill press, cash register)
   ☐ Lifting, bending, twisting, climbing, turning
   ☐ Exposure to chemicals, pesticides, toxins, or gases
   ☐ Other: please describe
   ☐ Not applicable; none of these

4. Do you use any special supports:
   ☐ Back cushion, neck cushion
   ☐ Back brace, corset
   ☐ Other kind of brace or support for any body part
   ☐ None; not applicable

History of falls:
   ☐ In the past year, I have had no falls
   ☐ I have just started to lose my balance/fall
   ☐ I fall occasionally
   ☐ I fall frequently (more than two times during the past 6 months)
   ☐ Certain factors make me cautious (e.g., curbs, ice, stairs, getting in and out of the tub)

I live:
   ☐ Alone   ☐ With family, spouse, partner
   ☐ Nursing home   ☐ Assisted living   ☐ Other _____

For the physical therapist:

Exercise history: determine level of activity, exercise, fitness (type, frequency, intensity, duration)

Vital signs (also complete Pain Assessment Record Form, Appendix C-7 on ⓔ)

Resting pulse rate: _____ Body temperature: _____ Respirations: _____ Oxygen saturation: _____

Blood pressure: 1st reading _____ 2nd reading _____

Position: Sitting   Standing   Extremity: Right   Left

Fig. 2.2, cont'd

- The Core Interview (see Fig. 2.3)
  History of Present Illness
    Chief Complaint
    Pain and Symptom Assessment
    Medical Treatment and Medications
    Current Level of Fitness
    Sleep-related History
    Stress (Emotional/Psychologic screen)
    Final Questions
  Associated Signs and Symptoms
  Special Questions
- Review of Systems

Family/Personal History

It is unnecessary and probably impossible to complete the entire patient history and interview on the first visit. Many clinics or health care facilities use some type of initial intake form before the client's first visit with the therapist.

The Family/Personal History form presented here (Fig. 2.2) is one example of an initial intake form. Throughout the rest of this chapter, the text discussion will follow the order of items on the Family/Personal History form. The reader is encouraged to follow along in the text while referring to the form.

The therapist must keep the client's family history in perspective. Very few people have a clean and unencumbered family history. It would be unusual for a person to say that nobody in their family ever had heart disease, cancer, or some other major health issue.

A check mark in multiple boxes on the history form does not necessarily mean the person will have the same problems. Onset of disease at an early age in a first-generation family member (sibling, child, parent) can be a sign of genetic disorders and is usually considered a red flag. But an aunt who died of colon cancer at age 75 is not as predictive.

A family history brings to light not only shared genetic traits but also shared environment, shared values, shared behavior, and shared culture. Factors such as nutrition, attitudes toward exercise and physical activity, and other modifiable risk factors are usually the focus of primary and secondary prevention.

Follow-Up Questions (FUPs)

Once the client has completed the Family/Personal History intake form, the clinician can then follow up with appropriate questions based on any "yes" selections made by the client. Beware of the client who circles one column of either all "Yeses" or all "Nos." Take the time to carefully review this section with the client. The therapist may want to ask some individual questions whenever illiteracy is suspected or observed.

Each clinical situation requires slight adaptations or alterations to the interview. These modifications, in turn, affect the depth and range of questioning. For example, a client who has pain associated with a traumatic anterior shoulder dislocation and who has no history of other disease is unlikely to require in-depth questioning to rule out systemic origins of pain.

Conversely, a woman with no history of trauma but with a previous history of breast cancer who is self-referred to the therapist without a previous medical examination and who complains of shoulder pain should be interviewed more thoroughly. The simple question, "How will the answers to the questions I am asking permit me to help the client?" can serve as your guide.[43]

Continued questioning may occur both during the objective examination and during treatment. The therapist is encouraged to carry on a continuous dialogue during the objective examination, both as an educational tool (i.e., reporting findings and mentioning possible treatment alternatives) and as a method of reducing any apprehension on the part of the client. This open communication may bring to light other important information.

The client may wonder about the extensiveness of the interview, thinking, for example, "Why is the therapist asking questions about bowel function when my primary concern relates to back pain?"

The therapist may need to make a qualifying statement to the client regarding the need for such detailed information. For example, questions about bowel function to rule out stomach or intestinal involvement (which can refer pain to the back) may seem to be unrelated to the client but make sense when the therapist explains the possible connection between back pain and systemic disease.

Throughout the questioning, record both positive and negative findings from the client history and interview, and tests and measures in order to correlate information when making an initial assessment of the client's problem. Efforts should be made to quantify all information by frequency, intensity, duration, and exact location (including length, breadth, depth, and anatomic location).

Age and Aging

Age is the most common primary risk factor for disease, illness, and comorbidities. It is the number one risk factor for cancer. The age of a client is an important variable to consider when evaluating the underlying neuromusculoskeletal (NMS) pathologic condition and when screening for medical disease.

Epidemiologists report that the U.S. population is beginning to age at a rapid pace, with the first baby boomers turning 65 in 2011. Between now and the year 2030 the number of individuals aged 65 years and older will double, reaching 72 million and making up a larger proportion of the entire population (increasing from 13% in 2000 to 20% in 2030).[44] Of particular interest is the explosive growth expected among adults aged 85 and older, at particular risk of death and disability, who are expected to grow from 5.5 million in the year 2010 to at least 19 million in 2050. While growing in size, the population is also expected to get more diverse.[44]

It is helpful to be aware of NMS and systemic conditions that tend to occur during particular decades of life. Signs and symptoms associated with that condition take on greater significance when age is considered. For example, prostate problems usually occur in men after the fourth decade (age 40 +).

THE CORE INTERVIEW

HISTORY OF PRESENT ILLNESS

Chief Complaint (Onset)

- Tell me why you are here today.
- Tell me about your injury.

  Alternate question: What do you think is causing your problem/pain?

  FUPs: How did this injury or illness begin?

  ◦ Was your injury or illness associated with a fall, trauma, assault, or repetitive activity (e.g., painting, cleaning, gardening, filing papers, driving)?

  ◦ Have you been hit, kicked, or pushed? (For the therapist: See text [Assault] before asking this question.)

  ◦ When did the present problem arise and did it occur gradually or suddenly?

  Systemic disease: Gradual onset without known cause.

  ◦ Have you ever had anything like this before? If yes, when did it occur?

  ◦ Describe the situation and the circumstances.

  ◦ How many times has this illness occurred? Tell me about each occasion.

  ◦ Is there any difference this time from the last episode?

  ◦ How much time elapses between episodes?

  ◦ Do these episodes occur more or less often than at first?

  Systemic disease: May present in a gradual, progressive, cyclical onset: worse, better, worse.

PAIN AND SYMPTOM ASSESSMENT

- Do you have any pain associated with your injury or illness? If yes, tell me about it.

Location

- Show me exactly where your pain is located.

  FUPs: Do you have this same pain anywhere else?

  ◦ Do you have any other pain or symptoms anywhere else?

  ◦ If yes, what causes the pain or symptoms to occur in this other area?

Description

- What does it feel like?

  FUPS: Has the pain changed in quality, intensity, frequency, or duration (how long it lasts) since it first began?

Pattern

- Tell me about the pattern of your pain or symptoms.

  Alternate question: When does your back/shoulder (name the body part) hurt?

  Alternate question: Describe your pain/symptoms from first waking up in the morning to going to bed at night. (See special sleep-related questions that follow.)

  FUPs: Have you ever experienced anything like this before?

  ◦ If yes, do these episodes occur more or less often than at first?

  ◦ How does your pain/symptom(s) change with time?

  ◦ Are your symptoms worse in the morning or in the evening?

Frequency

- How often does the pain/symptom(s) occur?

  FUPs: Is your pain constant, or does it come and go (intermittent)?

  ◦ Are you having this pain now?

  ◦ Did you notice these symptoms this morning immediately after awakening?

Duration

- How long does the pain/symptom(s) last?

  Systemic disease: Constant.

Fig. 2.3   Core Interview.

Intensity

- On a scale from 0 to 10, with 0 being no pain and 10 being the worst pain you have experienced with this condition, what level of pain do you have right now?

  Alternate question: How strong is your pain?

  1 = Mild

  2 = Moderate

  3 = Severe

  FUPs: Which word describes your pain right now?

  ° Which word describes the pain at its worst?

  ° Which word describes the least amount of pain?

  Systemic disease: Pain tends to be intense.

Associated Symptoms

- What other symptoms have you had that you can associate with this problem?

  FUPs: Have you experienced any of the following?

  ☐ Blood in urine, stool, vomit, mucus

  ☐ Dizziness, fainting, blackouts

  ☐ Fever, chills, sweats (day or night)

  ☐ Nausea, vomiting, loss of appetite

  ☐ Changes in bowel or bladder

  ☐ Throbbing sensation/pain in belly or anywhere else

  ☐ Skin rash or other skin changes

  ☐ Headaches

  ☐ Cough, dyspnea

  ☐ Dribbling or leaking urine

  ☐ Heart palpitations or fluttering

  ☐ Numbness or tingling

  ☐ Swelling or lumps anywhere

  ☐ Problems seeing or hearing

  ☐ Unusual fatigue, drowsiness

  ☐ Joint pain

  ☐ Difficulty swallowing/speaking

  ☐ Memory loss

  ☐ Confusion

  ☐ Sudden weakness

  ☐ Trouble sleeping

Systemic disease: Presence of symptoms bilaterally (e.g., edema, nail bed changes, bilateral weakness, paresthesia, tingling, burning). Determine the frequency, duration, intensity, and pattern of symptoms. Blurred vision, double vision, scotomas (black spots before the eyes), or temporary blindness may indicate early symptoms of multiple sclerosis (MS), cerebral vascular accident (CVA), or other neurologic disorders.

Aggravating Factors

- What kinds of things affect the pain?

  FUPs: What makes your pain/symptoms worse (e.g., eating, exercise, rest, specific positions, excitement, stress)?

Relieving Factors

- What makes it better?

  Systemic disease: Unrelieved by change in position or by rest.

- How does rest affect the pain/symptoms?

  FUPs: Are your symptoms aggravated or relieved by any activities? If yes, what?

  ° How has this problem affected your daily life at work or at home?

  ° How has it affected your ability to care for yourself without assistance (e.g., dress, bathe, cook, drive)?

MEDICAL TREATMENT AND MEDICATIONS

Medical Treatment

- What medical treatment have you had for this condition?

  FUPs: Have you been treated by a physical therapist for this condition before? If yes:

  ° When?

  ° Where?

  ° How long?

  ° What helped?

  ° What didn't help?

  ° Was there any treatment that made your symptoms worse? If yes, please elaborate.

Medications

- Are you taking any prescription or over-the-counter medications?

  FUPs: If no, you may have to probe further regarding use of laxatives, aspirin, acetaminophen (Tylenol), and so forth. If yes:

  ° What medication do you take?

  ° How often?

Fig. 2.3, cont'd

- ◦ What dose do you take?
- ◦ Why are you taking these medications?
- ◦ When was the last time that you took these medications? Have you taken these drugs today?
- ◦ Do the medications relieve your pain or symptoms?
- ◦ If yes, how soon after you take the medications do you notice an improvement?
- ◦ Do you notice any increase in symptoms or perhaps the start of symptoms after taking your medication(s)? (This may occur 30 minutes to 2 hours after ingestion.)
- ◦ If prescription drugs, who prescribed them for you?
- ◦ How long have you been taking these medications?
- ◦ When did your physician last review these medications?
- ◦ Are you taking any medications that weren't prescribed for you?

If no, follow-up with: Are you taking any pills given to you by someone else besides your doctor?

CURRENT LEVEL OF FITNESS

- What is your present exercise level?
  FUPs: What type of exercise or sports do you participate in?
- ◦ How many times do you participate each week (frequency)?
- ◦ When did you start this exercise program (duration)?
- ◦ How many minutes do you exercise during each session (intensity)?
- ◦ Are there any activities that you could do before your injury or illness that you cannot do now? If yes, please describe.
  Dyspnea: Do you ever experience any shortness of breath (SOB) or lack of air during any activities (e.g., walking, climbing stairs)?
  FUPs: Are you ever short of breath without exercising?
- ◦ If yes, how often?
- ◦ When does this occur?
- ◦ Do you ever wake up at night and feel breathless? If yes, how often?
- ◦ When does this occur?

SLEEP-RELATED HISTORY

- Can you get to sleep at night? If no, try to determine whether the reason is due to the sudden decrease in activity and quiet, which causes you to focus on your symptoms.
- Are you able to lie or sleep on the painful side? If yes, the condition may be considered to be chronic, and treatment would be more vigorous than if no, indicating a more acute condition that requires more conservative treatment.
- Are you ever wakened from a deep sleep by pain?
  FUPs: If yes, do you awaken because you have rolled onto that side? Yes may indicate a subacute condition requiring a combination of treatment approaches, depending on objective findings.
- ◦ Can you get back to sleep?
  FUPs: If yes, what do you have to do (if anything) to get back to sleep? (The answer may provide clues for treatment.)
- Have you had any unexplained fevers, night sweats, or unexplained perspiration?
  Systemic disease: Fevers and night sweats are characteristic signs of systemic disease.

STRESS

- What major life changes or stresses have you encountered that you would associate with your injury/illness?
  Alternate question: What situations in your life are "stressors" for you?
- On a scale from 0 to 10, with 0 being no stress and 10 being the most extreme stress you have ever experienced, in general, what number rating would you give to your stress at this time in your life?
- What number would you assign to your level of stress today?
- Do you ever get short of breath or dizzy or lose coordination with fatigue (anxiety-produced hyperventilation)?

FINAL QUESTION

- Do you wish to tell me anything else about your injury, your health, or your present symptoms that we have not discussed yet?
  Alternate question: Is there anything else you think is important about your condition that we haven't discussed yet?

FUPs, Follow-up Questions

Fig. 2.3, cont'd

A past medical history of prostate cancer in a 55-year-old man with sciatica of unknown cause should raise the suspicions of the therapist. Table 2.2 provides some of the age-related systemic and NMS pathologic conditions.

Human aging is best characterized as the progressive constriction of each organ system's homeostatic reserve. This decline, often referred to as "homeostenosis," begins in the third decade and is gradual, linear, and variable among individuals.[45] Each organ system's decline is independent of changes in other organ systems and is influenced by diet, environment, genetics, and personal habits.

Age-related changes in metabolism increase the risk for drug accumulation in older adults. Older adults are more sensitive to both the therapeutic and toxic effects of many drugs, especially analgesics. Functional liver tissue diminishes and hepatic blood flow decreases with aging, thus impairing the liver's capacity to break down and convert drugs. Therefore aging is a risk factor for a wide range of signs and symptoms associated with drug-induced toxicities.

Memory and cognition are also important considerations with the older client. Dementia increases the risk of falls and fracture. Delirium is a common complication of hip fracture that increases the length of hospital stay and mortality. Older clients take a disproportionate number of medications, predisposing them to adverse drug events (ADEs), drug-drug interactions, poor adherence to medication regimens, and changes in pharmacokinetics and pharmacodynamics related to aging.[46,47]

The onset of a new disease in older people generally affects the most vulnerable organ system, which often is different from the newly diseased organ system and explains why disease presentation is so atypical in this population. For example, at presentation, less than one fourth of older clients with hyperthyroidism have the classic triad of goiter, tremor, and exophthalmos; more likely symptoms are atrial fibrillation, confusion, depression, syncope, and weakness.

Because the "weakest links" with aging are so often the brain, lower urinary tract, or cardiovascular or musculoskeletal system, a limited number of presenting symptoms predominate no matter what the underlying disease. These include:

- Acute confusion
- Depression
- Falling
- Incontinence
- Syncope

The corollary is equally important: The organ system usually associated with a particular symptom is less likely to be the cause of that symptom in older individuals than in younger ones. For example, acute confusion in older adults is less often caused by a new brain lesion; incontinence is less often caused by a bladder disorder; falling, to a neuropathy; or syncope, to heart disease.

Sex and Gender

In the screening process, sex (male versus female) and gender (social and cultural roles and expectations based on sex) may be important issues (Case Example 2.3). To some extent, men and

TABLE 2.2	Some Age- and Sex-Related Medical Conditions	
Diagnosis	Sex	Age (in years)
NEUROMUSCULOSKELETAL		
Guillain-Barré syndrome	Men > women	Any age; history of infection/alcoholism
Multiple sclerosis	Women > men	15–35 (peak)
Rotator cuff degeneration		30 +
Spinal stenosis	Men > women	60 +
Tietze's syndrome		Before 40, including children
Costochondritis	Women > men	40 +
Neurogenic claudication		40–60 +
Systemic		
AIDS/HIV	Men > women	20–49
Ankylosing spondylitis	Men > women	15–30
Abdominal aortic aneurysm	(hypertensive) Men > women	40–70
Buerger's disease	Men > women	20–40 (smokers)
Cancer	Men > women	Any age; incidence rises after age 50
Breast cancer	Women > men	45–70 (peak incidence)
Hodgkin's disease	Men > women	20–40, 50–60
Osteoid osteoma (benign)	Men > women	10–20
Pancreatic carcinoma	Men > women	50–70
Rheumatoid arthritis	Women > men	20–50
Skin cancer	Men=women	Rarely before puberty; increasing incidence with increasing age
Gallstones	Women > men	40 +
Gout	Men > women	40–59
Gynecologic conditions	Women	20–45 (peak incidence)
Paget's disease of bone	Men > women	60 +
Prostatitis	Men	40 +
Primary biliary cirrhosis	Women > men	40–60
Reiter's syndrome	Men > women	20–40
Renal tuberculosis	Men > women	20–40
Rheumatic fever	Girls > boys	4–9; 18–30
Shingles		60 +; increasing incidence with increasing age
Spontaneous pneumothorax	Men > women	20–40
Systemic backache		45 +
Thyroiditis	Women > Men	30–50
Vascular claudication		40–60 +

CASE EXAMPLE 2.3
Sex as a Risk Factor

Clinical Presentation: A 45-year-old woman presents with mid-thoracic pain that radiates to the interscapular area on the right. There are two red flags recognizable immediately: age and back pain. Female sex can be a red flag and should be considered during the evaluation.

Referred pain from the gallbladder is represented in Fig. 9.10 as the light pink areas. If the client had a primary pain pattern with GI symptoms, she would have gone to see a medical doctor first.

Physical therapists see clients with referred pain patterns, often before the disease has progressed enough to be accompanied by visceral signs and symptoms. They may come to us from a physician or directly.

Risk-Factor Assessment: Watch for specific risk factors. In this case look for the five Fs associated with gallstones: fat, fair, forty (or older), female, and flatulent.

Clients with gallbladder disease do not always present this way, but the risk increases with each additional risk factor. Other risk factors for gallbladder disease include:
- Age: increasing incidence with increasing age

- Obesity
- Diabetes mellitus
- Multiparity (multiple pregnancies and births)

Women are at increased risk of gallstones because of their exposure to estrogen. Estrogen increases the hepatic secretion of cholesterol and decreases the secretion of bile acids. Additionally, during pregnancy, the gallbladder empties more slowly, causing stasis and increasing the chances for cholesterol crystals to precipitate.

For any woman over 40 years of age presenting with midthoracic, scapular, or right shoulder pain, consider gallbladder disease as a possible underlying etiology. To screen for systemic disease, look for known risk factors and ask about:

Associated Signs and Symptoms: When the disease advances, GI distress may be reported. This is why it is always important to ask clients if they are having any symptoms of any kind anywhere else in the body. The report of recurrent nausea, flatulence, and food intolerances points to the GI system and a need for medical attention.

---

women experience some diseases that are different from each other. When they have the same disease, the age at onset, clinical presentation, and response to treatment is often different.

Men. It may be appropriate to ask some specific screening questions just for men. A list of these questions is provided in Chapter 14 (see also Appendices B-24 and B-37 on). Taking a sexual history (see Appendix B-32, A and B in the accompanying enhanced eBook version included with print purchase of this textbook) may be appropriate at some point during the episode of care.

For example, the presentation of joint pain accompanied by (or a recent history of) skin lesions in an otherwise healthy, young adult male or female raises the suspicion of a sexually transmitted infection (STI). Being able to recognize STIs is helpful in the clinic. The therapist who recognized the client presenting with joint pain of "unknown cause" and also demonstrating signs of an STI may help bring the correct diagnosis to light sooner than later. Chronic pelvic or low back pain of unknown cause may be linked to sexual assault.[48]

The therapist may need to ask men about prostate health (e.g., history of prostatitis, benign prostatic hypertrophy, prostate cancer) or about a history of testicular cancer. In some cases, a sexual history (see Appendix B-32, A and B in the accompanying enhanced eBook version included with print purchase of this textbook) may be helpful.

Men and Osteoporosis. Osteoporosis has been reported to be underdiagnosed in men. Normal aging results in loss of bone mineral density and one in five men over 50 years of age will sustain a fracture as a result of osteoporosis. Studies report that about a third of all hip fractures are in men. A greater proportion of men die of hip fractures compared with women.[49]

Keeping this information in mind and watching for risk factors of osteoporosis (see Fig. 12.9) can guide the therapist in recognizing the need to screen for osteoporosis in men and women.

Women. The incidence of stroke is greater in middle aged and older women compared with men. In addition, these women also have poorer outcomes following a stroke compared with men.[50] Secondary to this, the American Heart Association suggested new guidelines to lower the risk of stroke in women.[51]

The Office of Research on Women's Health of the National Institutes of Health also reported that female athletes have a higher risk of anterior cruciate ligament (ACL) tear compared with males.[52] There is now research to address risk reduction for ACL tear in this population.[53]

In addition, chronic pain disorders such as temporomandibular joint (TMJ) pain[54] and migraines[55] are more common in women than in men.

These are just a few of the many ways that being female represents a unique risk factor requiring special consideration when assessing the overall individual and when screening for medical disease.

Questions about past pregnancies, births and deliveries, past surgical procedures (including abortions), incontinence, endometriosis, history of sexually transmitted or pelvic inflammatory disease(s), and history of osteoporosis and/or compression fractures are important in the assessment of some female clients (see Appendix B-37 in the accompanying enhanced eBook version included with print purchase of this textbook). The therapist must use common sense and professional judgment in deciding what questions to ask and which follow-up questions are essential.

Life Cycles. For women, it may be pertinent to find out where each woman is in the life cycle (Box 2.5) and correlate this information with age, personal and family history, current health, and the presence of any known risk factors. It may be necessary to ask if the current symptoms occur at the same time each month in relation to the menstrual cycle (e.g., day 10 to 14 during ovulation or at the end of the cycle during the woman's period).

BOX 2.5 LIFE CYCLES OF A WOMAN

- Premenses (before the start of the monthly menstrual cycle; may include early puberty)
- Reproductive years (including birth, delivery, miscarriage, and/or abortion history; this time period may include puberty)
- Menopause Transition (time from initial reduction in estrogen until menopause)
- Menopause (12 months without menstrual cycle, may be natural or surgical menopause [i.e., hysterectomy])
- Postmenopause (time after menopause)

Each phase in the life cycle is really a process that occurs over a number of years. There are no clear distinctions most of the time as one phase blends gradually into the next one.

Menopause Transition (MT)—previously called *Perimenopause*—is a term that was first coined in the 1990s. It refers to the transitional period from physiologic ovulatory menstrual cycles to eventual ovarian shutdown. During the MT, signs and symptoms of hormonal changes may become evident. These can include fatigue, memory problems, weight gain, irritability, sleep disruptions, enteric dysfunction, painful intercourse, and change in libido. The pattern of menstrual cessation varies. It may be abrupt, but more often it occurs over 1 to 2 years. Periodic menstrual flow gradually occurs less frequently, becoming irregular and less in amount. Occasional episodes of profuse bleeding may be interspersed with episodes of scant bleeding.

Menopause is an important developmental event in a woman's life. It is the permanent cessation of menses occurring after a women has experienced one full year without of menstruation, diagnosed retrospectively.

Menopause is not a disease but rather a complex sequence of biologic aging events, during which the body makes the transition from fertility to a nonreproductive status. The usual age of menopause is between 48 and 54 years. The average age for menopause is around 51 years of age.[56,57]

Postmenopause describes the remaining years of a woman's life when the reproductive and menstrual cycles have ended. *Any spontaneous uterine bleeding after this time is abnormal and is considered a red flag.*

However, cyclic hormone therapy preparations that contain a combination of estrogen and a progestin may cause monthly bleeding that may be light or as heavy as a normal menstrual period.[58]

Hysterectomy (removal of the uterus) is the second most common surgical procedure performed in women of reproductive age.[59] The majority of these women have this operation between the ages of 25 and 44 years.

Removal of the uterus and cervix, even without removal of the ovaries, usually brings on an early menopause (surgical menopause), within 2 years of the operation. Oophorectomy (removal of the ovaries) brings on menopause immediately, regardless of the age of the woman. Surgical removal of the ovaries increases the rate of bone mineral density loss, possibly leading to osteoporosis.[60]

CLINICAL SIGNS AND SYMPTOMS

Menopause

- Fatigue and malaise
- Depression, mood swings
- Difficulty concentrating; "brain fog"
- Headache
- Altered sleep pattern (insomnia/sleep disturbance)
- Hot flashes
- Irregular menses, cessation of menses
- Vaginal dryness, pain during intercourse
- Atrophy of breasts and vaginal tissue
- Pelvic floor relaxation (cystocele/rectocele)
- Urge incontinence

Women and Hormone Therapy (HT). Hormone therapy (HT, also known as hormone replacement therapy or HRT) refers to the administration of synthetic estrogen and progesterone to alleviate symptoms related to menopause. There continues to be a debate in the medical community about the risk-benefit ratio of HT.[61] The American Cancer Society discusses how HT can affect the risk of developing certain types of cancers but "has no position or guidelines regarding menopausal hormone therapy."[62]

The American Heart Association does not recommend the use of HT to reduce the risk of coronary heart disease because several studies have shown that HT appears to not reduce that risk.[63] Both associations highly encourage women to consult their physicians to discuss their specific benefits and risks of undergoing HT.

Women and Heart Disease. When a 55-year-old woman with a significant family history of heart disease comes to the therapist with shoulder, upper back, or jaw pain it will be necessary to take the time and screen for possible cardiovascular involvement.

Heart disease is the number one cause of death in women in the United States. It is estimated that one in every five deaths in women is as a result of heart disease. Despite efforts to increase awareness, it has been reported that 54% of women do not know that heart disease is the leading cause of death in women.[64] Women die of heart disease at the same rate as men. Two thirds of women who die suddenly have no previously recognized symptoms.[64] Prodromal symptoms as much as 1 month before a myocardial infarction go unrecognized (see Table 7.4).

Therapists should recognize age combined with the female sex as a risk factor for heart disease and look for other risk factors thus contributing to heart disease prevention. See Chapter 7 for further discussion of this topic.

Women and Osteoporosis. As health care specialists, therapists have a unique opportunity and responsibility to provide screening and prevention for a variety of diseases and conditions. Osteoporosis is one of those conditions.

To put it into perspective, a woman's risk of developing a hip fracture is equal to her combined risk of developing breast, uterine, and ovarian cancer. Women have higher fracture rates than men of the same ethnicity. Caucasian women have higher rates than black women.

Assessment of osteoporosis and associated risk factors along with further discussion of osteoporosis as a condition are discussed in Chapter 12.

Transgender

Transgender is an umbrella term used to identify individuals whose gender identity or expression differs from societal norms. About 0.3% of the population identify as transgender.[65] Trans women (men-to-women) and trans men (women-to-men) both are likely to experience higher levels of depression, stigma, and to receive inadequate medical care.[65] According to one study, more than two-thirds of transgender medical students and physicians heard derogatory comments regarding transgender patients and one-third witnessed maltreatment of a transgender patient in practice.[66]

Lack of societal acceptance may be one reason for the increased rate of depression, substance abuse disorders, and STIs in this population.[67] Transgender men and women often seek to change their physical appearance by undergoing hormone therapy or surgery. The most common surgery in transgender males is breast reconstruction, while the most common surgery in transgender females is vaginoplasty or labioplasty.[68] Hormone therapy for transgender males typically involves testosterone, while hormone therapy for transgender females can involve estrogen or androgen suppression or both. Physical therapists should be aware of potential interactions and side effects that may occur from previous surgeries or medication use.

When addressing and dealing with transgender males and females, it is typically preferred to use the pronouns associated with their gender of identification. For example, addressing a transgender women as she/her/herself is preferred. If unsure how to address a transgender patient, the physical therapist can ask the patient if they have a preferred pronoun. The health care provider should also consider changing the intake forms, as this offers a more comfortable way for the patient to indicate their gender identity. The following two questions can be helpful:
1. What is your current gender identity?
2. What sex were you assigned at birth?

Race and Ethnicity

Social scientists make a distinction in that race describes membership in a group based on physical differences (e.g., color of skin, shape of eyes). Ethnicity refers to being part of a group with shared social, cultural, language, and geographic factors (e.g., Hispanic, Italian).[69]

An individual's ethnicity is defined by a unique sociocultural heritage that is passed down from generation to generation but can change as the person changes geographic locations or joins a family with different cultural practices. A child born in Korea but adopted by a Caucasian American family will most likely be raised speaking English, eating American food, and studying U.S. history. Ethnically, the child is American but will be viewed racially by others as Asian.

The Genome Project dispelled previous ideas of biologic differences based on race. It is now recognized that humans are 99.9% identical in their genetic makeup. The remaining 0.1% is thought to hold clues regarding the causes of diseases.[70] Despite tremendous advances and improved public health in America, several non-Caucasian racial/ethnic groups listed in Box 2.3 are medically underserved and suffer higher levels of illness, premature death, and disability. These include stroke, cardiovascular disease, adult diabetes, infant mortality rate, suicide, and cancer.[71,72] Examples of these health inequities according to the Centers for Disease Control (CDC) include the following:[71]

Coronary heart disease and stroke: Black men and women in the 45 to 74 age group have a much higher rate of death from the disease compared with other races.

Obesity: The prevalence of obesity in most age groups is higher among blacks and Mexican Americans than whites.

Asthma: Prevalence of asthma is higher in multiracial, Puerto Rican Hispanics, and non-Hispanic African Americans compared with non-Hispanic Caucasians.

HIV infection: Except for Asians, ethnic minorities and men who have sex with men have a higher prevalence of HIV compared with Caucasians.

Hypertension: There is a difference in prevalence of hypertension among age group, race/ethnicity, education, family income, foreign-born status, health insurance status, and diabetes, obesity and disability.

Other studies are underway to compare ethnic differences among different groups for different diseases (Case Example 2.1).

Additional information regarding incidence, prevalence, morbidity, and mortality of specific diseases according to racial/ethnic groups can be found throughout this text.

Resources. Definitions and descriptions for race and ethnicity are available through the CDC.[73] For a report on health disparities and inequities, see the CDC Health Disparities & Inequalities Report (CHDIR).[72]

Past Medical and Personal History

It is important to take time with these questions and to ensure that the client understands what is being asked. A "yes" response to any question in this section would require further questioning, correlation to objective findings, and consideration of referral to the client's physician.

For example, a "yes" response to questions on this form directed toward *allergies, asthma*, and *hay fever* should be followed up by asking the client to list the allergies and to list the symptoms that may indicate a manifestation of allergies, asthma, or hay fever. The therapist can then be alert for any signs of respiratory distress or allergic reactions during exercise or with the use of topical agents.

Likewise, clients may indicate the presence of *shortness of breath* with only mild exertion or without exertion, possibly even after waking at night. This condition of breathlessness can be associated with one of many conditions, including heart disease, bronchitis, asthma, obesity, emphysema, dietary deficiencies, pneumonia, and lung cancer.

Some "no" responses may also warrant further follow-up. The therapist can screen for diabetes, depression, liver impairment, eating disorders, osteoporosis, hypertension, substance use, incontinence, bladder or prostate problems, and so on. Special questions to ask for many of these conditions are listed in the Appendices on).

Many of the screening tools for these conditions are self-report questionnaires, which are inexpensive, require little or no formal training, and are less time-consuming than formal testing. Knowing the risk factors for various illnesses, diseases, and conditions will help guide the therapist in knowing when to screen for specific problems. Recognizing the signs and symptoms will also alert the therapist to the need for screening.

Eating Disorders and Disordered Eating. Eating disorders, such as bulimia nervosa, binge eating disorder, and anorexia nervosa, are good examples of past or current conditions that can affect the client's health and recovery. The therapist must consider the potential for a negative effect of anorexia on bone mineral density, and also keep in mind the psychologic risks of exercise (a common intervention for osteopenia) in anyone with an eating disorder. Women of reproductive age should be asked about menstrual cycle changes. Amenorrhea (lack of menstrual flow in a women of reproductive age) is a red flag for decreased bone mineral density in young female athletes with eating disorders.

The first step in screening for eating disorders is to look for common risk factors[74] associated with eating disorders, including being female, mental health disorders, a personal or family history of obesity and/or eating disorders, sports or athletic involvement, stress and history of sexual abuse or other trauma.[75]

Distorted body image and disordered eating are probably underreported, especially in male athletes. Athletes participating in sports that use weight classifications, such as wrestling and weight lifting, are at greater risk for anorexic behaviors such as fasting, fluid restriction, and vomiting.[76]

Researchers have recently described a form of body image disturbance in male bodybuilders and weight lifters referred to as *muscle dysmorphia*. This was previously referred to as "reverse anorexia," this disorder is characterized by an intense and excessive preoccupation or dissatisfaction with a perceived defect in appearance, even though the men are usually large and muscular. The goal in disordered eating for this group of men is to increase body weight and size. The use of performance-enhancing drugs and dietary supplements is common in this group of athletes.[77,78]

Gay men tend to be more dissatisfied with their body image and may be at greater risk for symptoms of eating disorders compared with heterosexual men.[79,80] Screening is advised for anyone with risk factors and/or signs and symptoms of eating disorders. Questions to ask may include:

 FOLLOW-UP QUESTIONS

- Are you satisfied with your eating patterns?
- Do you force yourself to exercise, even when you do not feel well?
- Do you exercise more when you eat more?
- Do you think you will gain weight if you stop exercising for a day or two?
- Do you exercise more than once a day?
- Do you take laxatives, diuretics (water pills), or any other pills as a way to control your weight or shape?
- Do you ever eat in secret? (Secret eating refers to individuals who do not want others to see them eat or see what they eat; they may eat alone or go into the bathroom or closet to conceal their eating.)
- Are there days when you do not eat anything?
- Do you ever make yourself throw up after eating as a way to control your weight?

CLINICAL SIGNS AND SYMPTOMS
Eating Disorders

Physical

- Weight loss or gain
- Skeletal myopathy and weakness
- Chronic fatigue
- Dehydration or rebound water retention; pitting edema
- Discoloration or staining of the teeth from contact with stomach acid
- Broken blood vessels in the eyes from induced vomiting
- Enlarged parotid (salivary) glands (facial swelling) from repeated contact with vomit
- Tooth marks, scratches, scars, or calluses on the backs of hands from inducing vomiting (Russell's sign)
- Irregular or absent menstrual periods; delay of menses onset in young adolescent girls
- Inability to tolerate cold
- Dry skin and hair; brittle nails; hair loss and growth of downy hair (lanugo) all over the body, including the face
- Reports of heartburn, abdominal bloating or gas, constipation, or diarrhea
- Vital signs: slow heart rate (bradycardia); low blood pressure
- In women/girls: irregular or absent menstrual cycles

Behavioral

- Preoccupation with weight, food, calories, fat grams, dieting, clothing size, body shape
- Mood swings, irritability
- Binging and purging (bulimia) or food restriction (anorexia); frequent visits to the bathroom after eating
- Frequent comments about being "fat" or overweight despite looking very thin
- Excessive exercise to burn off calories
- Use of diuretics, laxatives, enemas, or other drugs to induce urination, bowel movements, and vomiting (purging)

General Health

Self-assessed health is a strong and independent predictor of mortality. Research has shown that individuals who report their health as "poor" have a two-fold increase in mortality than those who reported their health as excellent.[81] Self-assessed health is also a strong predictor of functional limitation.[82] Therefore, the therapist should consider it a red flag anytime a client chooses "poor" to describe his or her overall health.

Medications. Although the Family/Personal History form includes a question about prescription or OTC medications, specific follow-up questions come later in the Core Interview under Medical Treatment and Medications. Further discussion about this topic can be found in that section of this chapter.

It may be helpful to ask the client to bring in any prescribed medications he or she may be taking. In the older adult with multiple comorbidities, it is not uncommon for the client to bring a gallon-sized plastic bag full of pill bottles. Taking the time to sort through the many prescriptions can be time-consuming.

Start by asking the client to make sure each one is a drug that is being taken as prescribed on a regular basis. Many people take "drug holidays" (skip their medications intentionally) or routinely take fewer doses than prescribed. Make a list for future investigation if the clinical presentation or presence of possible side effects suggests the need for consultation with a pharmacist.

Recent Infections. Recent infections, such as mononucleosis, hepatitis, or upper respiratory infections may precede the onset of Guillain-Barré syndrome. Recent colds, influenza, or upper respiratory infections may also be an extension of a chronic health pattern of systemic illness.

Further questioning may reveal recurrent influenza-like symptoms associated with headaches and musculoskeletal complaints. These complaints could originate with medical problems such as endocarditis (a bacterial infection of the heart), bowel obstruction, or pleuropulmonary disorders, which should be ruled out by a physician.

Knowing that the client has had a recent bladder, vaginal, uterine, or kidney infection, or that the client is likely to have such infections, may help explain back pain in the absence of any musculoskeletal findings.

The client may or may not confirm previous back pain associated with previous infections. If there is any doubt, a medical referral is recommended. On the other hand, repeated coughing after a recent upper respiratory infection may cause chest, rib, back, or sacroiliac pain.

Screening for Cancer. Any "yes" responses to early screening questions for cancer (General Health questions 5, 6, and 7) must be followed up by a physician. An in-depth discussion of screening for cancer is presented in Chapter 13.

The single most significant piece of information obtained in the patient history regarding cancer is whether the patient has had it before. Having a previous history of cancer has the largest positive predictive value of a range of "red flag" questions.[83] However, most red flag questions have high false positive rates in isolation.

Unexplained weight loss is another commonly recommended red flag question when screening for malignancy. One study showed a 10-fold increase in the odds of malignancy when the patient reported both unexplained weight loss and a history of cancer.[84] Changes in appetite and unexplained weight loss can be associated with cancer, onset of diabetes, hyperthyroidism, depression, or pathologic anorexia (loss of appetite). Weight loss significant for neoplasm would be a 10% loss of total body weight over a 4-week period unrelated to any intentional diet or fasting.[85]

A significant, unexplained weight gain can be caused by congestive heart failure, hypothyroidism, or cancer. The person with back pain who, despite reduced work levels and decreased activity, experiences unexplained weight loss demonstrates a key "red flag" symptom.

Weight gain/loss does not always correlate with appetite. For example, weight gain associated with neoplasm may be accompanied by appetite loss, whereas weight loss associated with hyperthyroidism may be accompanied by increased appetite.

Substance Abuse. Substance refers to any agent taken nonmedically that can alter mood or behavior. Addiction refers to the daily need for the substance in order to function, an inability to stop, and recurrent use when it is harmful physically, socially, and/or psychologically. *Addiction* is based on physiologic changes associated with drug use but also has psychologic and behavioral components. Individuals who are addicted will use the substance to relieve psychologic symptoms even after physical pain or discomfort is gone.

Dependence is the physiologic dependence on the substance so that withdrawal symptoms emerge when there is a rapid dose reduction or the drug is stopped abruptly. Once a medication is no longer needed, the dosage will have to be tapered down for the client to avoid withdrawal symptoms.

Tolerance refers to the individual's need for increased amounts of the substance to produce the same effect. Tolerance develops in many people who receive long-term opioid therapy for chronic pain problems. If undermedicated, drug-seeking behaviors or unauthorized increases in dosage may occur. These may seem like addictive behaviors and are sometimes referred to as "pseudoaddiction," but the behaviors disappear when adequate pain control is achieved. Referral to the prescribing physician is advised if you suspect a problem with opioid analgesics (misuse or abuse).[86,87]

Among the substances most commonly used that cause physiologic responses but are not usually thought of as drugs are alcohol, tobacco, coffee, black tea, and caffeinated carbonated beverages.

Other substances commonly abused include *depressants*, such as alcohol, barbiturates (barbs, downers, pink ladies, rainbows, reds, yellows, sleeping pills); *stimulants*, such as amphetamines and cocaine (crack, crank, coke, snow, white, lady, blow, rock); *opiates* (heroin); *cannabis derivatives* (marijuana, hashish); and *hallucinogens* (LSD or acid, mescaline, magic mushroom, PCP, angel dust).

Methylenedioxymethamphetamine (MDMA; also called ecstasy, hug, beans, and love drug), a synthetic, psychoactive drug chemically similar to the stimulant methamphetamine and the hallucinogen mescaline, has been reported to be sold in clubs around the country. It is often given to individuals without their knowledge and used in combination with alcohol and other drugs.

The National Institute of Drug Abuse maintains a website dedicated to emerging trends and alerts regarding drugs of abuse.[88]

Public health officials tell us that alcohol and other drug use/abuse is a major problem in the United States.[89] A well-known social scientist in the area of drug studies published a new report showing that overall, alcohol is the most harmful drug (to the individual and to others) with heroin and crack cocaine ranked second and third.[90]

Alcohol and other drugs are commonly used to self-medicate mental illness, pain, and the effects of posttraumatic

stress disorder (PTSD). Widespread use of alcohol has been reported to be a negative coping mechanism for stress in the workplace.[91]

Risk Factors. Many teens and adults are at risk for using and abusing various substances (Box 2.6). Often, they are self-medicating the symptoms of a variety of mental illnesses, learning disabilities, and personality disorders. The use of alcohol to self-medicate depression is very common, especially after a traumatic injury or event in one's life.

Baby boomers (born between 1946 and 1964) with a history of substance use, aging adults (or others) with sleep disturbances or sleep disorders, and anyone with an anxiety or mood disorder is at increased risk for use and abuse of substances.

Risk factors for opioid misuse in people with chronic pain have been published. These include mental disorder.[92] Physicians and clinical psychologists may use one of several tools (e.g., Current Opioid Misuse Measure, Screener and Opioid Assessment for Patients in Pain) to screen for risk of opioid misuse.

Signs and Symptoms of Substance Use/Abuse. Behavioral and physiologic responses to any of these substances depend on the characteristics of the chemical itself, the route of administration, and the adequacy of the client's circulatory system (Table 2.3).

BOX 2.6 POPULATION GROUPS AT RISK FOR SUBSTANCE ABUSE

- Teens and adults with attention deficit disorder or attention deficit disorder with hyperactivity (ADD/ADHD)
- History of posttraumatic stress disorder (PTSD)
- Baby boomers with a history of substance use
- Individuals with sleep disorders
- Individuals with depression and/or anxiety disorders
- Transgender patients

TABLE 2.3 Physiologic Effects and Adverse Reactions to Substances

Caffeine	Cannabis	Depressants	Narcotics	Stimulants	Tobacco
EXAMPLES					
Coffee, espresso Chocolate, some over-the-counter "alert aids" used to stay awake, black tea and other beverages with caffeine (e.g., Red Bull, caffeinated water)	Marijuana, hashish	Alcohol, sedatives/ sleeping pills, barbiturates, tranquilizers	Heroin, opium, morphine, codeine	Cocaine and its derivatives, amphetamines, methamphetamine, MDMA (ecstasy)	Cigarettes, cigars, pipe smoking, smokeless tobacco products (chew, snuff)
EFFECTS					
Vasoconstriction Irritability Enhances pain perception Intestinal disorders Headaches Muscle tension Fatigue Sleep disturbancesUrinary frequency Tachypnea Sensory disturbances Agitation Nervousness Heart palpitation	Short-term memory loss Sedation Tachycardia Euphoria Increased appetite Relaxed inhibitions Fatigue Paranoia Psychosis Ataxia, tremor	Agitation; mood swings; anxiety; depression Vasodilation; red eyes Fatigue Altered pain perception Excessive sleepiness or insomnia Coma (overdose) Altered behaviour Slow, shallow breathing Clammy skin Slurred speech	Euphoria Drowsiness Respiratory depression	Increased alertness Excitation Euphoria Loss of appetite Increased blood pressure Insomnia Increased pulse rate Agitation, increased body temperature, hallucinations, convulsions, death (overdose)	Increased heart rate Vasoconstriction Decreased oxygen to heart Increased risk of thrombosis Loss of appetite Poor wound healing Poor bone grafting Increased risk of pneumonia Increased risk of cataracts Disk degeneration

Adapted from Goodman CC, Fuller KS: *Pathology: implications for the physical therapist*, ed 4, Philadelphia, 2015, WB Saunders.

Behavioral red flags indicating a need to screen can include consistently missed appointments (or being chronically late to scheduled sessions), noncompliance with the home program or poor attention to self-care, shifting mood patterns (especially the presence of depression), excessive daytime sleepiness or unusually excessive energy, and/or deterioration of physical appearance and personal hygiene.

The physiologic effects and adverse reactions have the additional ability to delay wound healing or the repair of soft tissue injuries. Soft tissue infections such as abscess and cellulitis are common complications of injection drug use (IDU). Affected individuals may present with swelling and tenderness in a muscular area from intramuscular injections, as well as fever. Substance abuse in older adults often mimics many of the signs of aging: memory loss, cognitive problems, tremors, and falls. Even family members may not recognize when their loved one is an addict.

Screening for Substance Use/Abuse. Questions designed to screen for the presence of chemical substance abuse need to become part of the physical therapy assessment. Clients who depend on alcohol and/or other substances require lifestyle intervention. However, direct questions may be offensive to some people, and identifying a person as a substance abuser (i.e., alcohol or other drugs) often results in referral to professionals who treat alcoholics or drug addicts, a label that is not accepted in the early stage of this condition.

Because of the controversial nature of interviewing the alcohol- or drug-dependent client, the questions in this section of the Family/Personal History form are suggested as a guideline for interviewing.

After (or possibly instead of) asking questions about use of alcohol, tobacco, caffeine, and other chemical substances, the therapist may want to use the Trauma Scale Questionnaire[93] that makes no mention of substances but asks about previous trauma. Questions include:[93]

 ## FOLLOW-UP QUESTIONS

- Have you had any fractures or dislocations to your bones or joints?
- Have you been injured in a road traffic accident?
- Have you injured your head?
- Have you been in a fight or assaulted?

These questions are based on the established correlation between trauma and alcohol or other substance use for individuals 18 years old and older. "Yes" answers to two or more of these questions should be discussed with the physician or used to generate a referral for further evaluation of alcohol use. It may be best to record the client's answers with a simple + for "yes" or a − for "no" to avoid taking notes during the discussion of sensitive issues.

The RAFFT Questionnaire[94,95] (Relax, Alone, Friends, Family, Trouble) poses five questions that appear to tap into common themes related to adolescent substance use such as peer pressure, self-esteem, anxiety, and exposure to friends and family members who are using drugs or alcohol. Similar dynamics may still be present in adult substance users, although their use of drugs and alcohol may become independent from these psychosocial variables.

- **R:** Relax—Do you drink or take drugs to relax, feel better about yourself, or fit in?
- **A:** Alone—Do you ever drink or take drugs while you are alone?
- **F:** Friends—Do any of your closest friends drink or use drugs?
- **F:** Family—Does a close family member have a problem with alcohol or drugs?
- **T:** Trouble—Have you ever gotten into trouble from drinking or taking drugs?

Depending on how the interview has proceeded thus far, the therapist may want to conclude with one final question: "Are there any drugs or substances you take that you have not mentioned?" Other screening tools for assessing alcohol abuse are available, as are more complete guidelines for interviewing this population.[94]

Resources. Several guides on substance abuse for health care professionals are available.[96,97] These resources may help the therapist learn more about identifying, referring, and preventing substance abuse in their clients.

The University of Washington provides a Substance Abuse Screening and Assessments Instruments database to help health care providers find instruments appropriate for their work setting.[98] The database contains information on more than 980 questionnaires and interviews; many have proven clinical utility and research validity, whereas others are newer instruments that have not yet been thoroughly evaluated.

The national Institute of Drug Abuse maintains a web page containing resources regarding substance abuse.[99]

Many are in the public domain and can be freely downloaded from the Web; others are under copyright and can only be obtained from the copyright holder. The Partnership for a Drug-Free America also provides information on the effects of drugs, alcohol, and other illicit substances available online at www.drugfree.org.

Alcohol. Other than tobacco, alcohol is the most dominant addictive agent in the United States. Statistics regarding alcohol abuse were mentioned earlier in this chapter.

Alcohol use disorder (AUD) is a medical diagnosis of severe problem drinking. The Diagnostic and Statistical Manual of Mental Disorders lists several criteria to be diagnosed with AUD. The individual must meet two of the 11 criteria to have the medical diagnosis. The severity of AUD (mid, moderate, severe) can be indicated depending on the number of criteria that were met by the individual. Examples of these criteria include: times when the individual ended up drinking more than intended; tried to cut down or stop drinking more than once but could not; spent a lot of time drinking or being sick because of the after effects; and experienced a craving, strong need, or urge to drink.[100]

As the graying of America continues, the number of adults affected by alcoholism is expected to increase, especially as baby boomers, having grown up in an age of alcohol and substance abuse, carry that practice into old age.

Older adults are not the only ones affected. Alcohol consumption is a major contributor to risky behaviors and adverse health outcomes in adolescents and young adults. In addition, the use of alcohol is associated with risky sexual behavior and sexually transmitted diseases (STD),[101] and teen pregnancy.[102]

Binge drinking, defined as consuming five or more alcoholic drinks within a couple of hours, is a serious problem among adults and high-school aged youths. Binge drinking contributes to more than half of the 79,000 deaths caused by excessive drinking annually in the United States.[103]

Effects of Alcohol Use. Excessive alcohol use can cause or contribute to many medical conditions. Alcohol is a toxic drug that is harmful to all body tissues. Certain social and behavioral changes, such as heavy regular consumption, binge drinking, frequent intoxication, concern expressed by others about one's drinking, and alcohol-related accidents, may be early signs of problem drinking and unambiguous signs of dependence risk.[104]

Alcohol has both vasodilatory and depressant effects that may produce fatigue and mental depression or alter the client's perception of pain or symptoms. Alcohol has deleterious effects on the gastrointestinal (GI), hepatic, cardiovascular, hematopoietic, genitourinary (GU), and neuromuscular systems.

CLINICAL SIGNS AND SYMPTOMS
Alcohol Use Disorders in Older Adults[105]

- Memory loss, cognitive impairment
- Depression, anxiety
- Neglect of hygiene and appearance
- Poor appetite, nutritional deficits
- Disruption of sleep
- Refractory (resistant) hypertension
- Blood glucose control problems
- Refractory seizures
- Impaired gait, impaired balance, falls
- Recurrent gastritis or esophagitis
- Difficulty managing dosing of warfarin

Prolonged use of excessive alcohol may affect bone metabolism, resulting in reduced bone formation, disruption of the balance between bone formation and resorption, and incomplete mineralization.[106] Alcoholics are often malnourished, which exacerbates the direct effects of alcohol on bones. Alcohol-induced osteoporosis (the predominant bone condition in most people with cirrhosis) may progress for years without any obvious symptoms.

Alcohol may interact with prescribed medications to produce various effects, including death. Prolonged drinking changes the way the body processes some common prescription drugs, potentially increasing the adverse effects of medications or impairing or enhancing their effects.

Binge drinking commonly seen on weekends and around holidays can cause atrial fibrillation, a condition referred to as "holiday heart." The affected individual may report dyspnea, palpitations, chest pain, dizziness, fainting or near-fainting, and signs of alcohol intoxication. Strenuous physical activity is contraindicated until the cardiac rhythm converts to normal sinus rhythm. Medical evaluation is required in cases of suspected holiday heart syndrome.[107]

Of additional interest to the therapist is that alcohol diminishes the accumulation of neutrophils necessary for "cleanup" of all foreign material present in inflamed areas. This phenomenon results in delayed wound healing and recovery from inflammatory processes involving tendons, bursae, and joint structures.

Signs and Symptoms of Alcohol Withdrawal. The therapist must be alert to any signs or symptoms of alcohol withdrawal, a potentially life-threatening condition. This is especially true in the acute care setting,[108] especially for individuals who are recently hospitalized for a motor vehicle accident or other trauma or the postoperative orthopedic patient (e.g., patient with total hip or total knee replacement).[109] Alcohol withdrawal may be a factor in recovery for any patient with an orthopedic or neurologic condition (e.g., stroke, total joint, fracture), especially patients with trauma.

Early recognition can bring about medical treatment that can reduce the symptoms of withdrawal as well as identify the need for long-term intervention. Withdrawal begins 3 to 36 hours after discontinuation of heavy alcohol consumption. Symptoms of autonomic hyperactivity may include diaphoresis (excessive perspiration), insomnia, general restlessness, agitation, and loss of appetite. Mental confusion, disorientation, and acute fear and anxiety can occur.

Tremors of the hands, feet, and legs may be visible. Symptoms may progress to hyperthermia, delusions, and paranoia called *alcohol hallucinosis* lasting 1 to 5 or more days. Seizures occur in up to one third of affected individuals, usually 12 to 48 hours after the last drink or potentially sooner when the blood alcohol level returns to zero.

CLINICAL SIGNS AND SYMPTOMS
Alcohol Withdrawal

- Agitation, irritability
- Headache
- Insomnia
- Hallucinations
- Anorexia, nausea, vomiting, diarrhea
- Loss of balance, incoordination (apraxia)
- Seizures (occurs 12 to 48 hours after the last drink)
- Delirium tremens (occurs 2 to 3 days after the last drink)
- Motor hyperactivity, tachycardia
- Elevated blood pressure

The Clinical Institute Withdrawal of Alcohol Scale (CIWA)[110] is an assessment tool used to monitor alcohol withdrawal symptoms. Although it is used primarily to determine the need for medication, it can provide the therapist with an indication of stability level when determining patient safety

---

BOX 2.7   SCREENING FOR EXCESSIVE ALCOHOL

CAGE Questionnaire

C: Have you ever thought you should cut down on your drinking?

A: Have you ever been annoyed by criticism of your drinking?

G: Have you ever felt guilty about your drinking?

E: Do you ever have an eye-opener (a drink or two) in the morning?

Key

- One "yes" answer suggests a need for discussion and follow-up; taking the survey may help some people in denial to accept that a problem exists

- Two or more "yes" answers indicate a problem with alcohol; intervention likely needed

Alcohol-Related Screening Questions

- Have you had any fractures or dislocations to your bones or joints?
- Have you been injured in a road traffic accident?
- Have you ever injured your head?
- Have you been in a fight or been hit or punched in the last 6 months?

Key

- "Yes" to two or more questions is a red flag

---

before initiating physical therapy. The tool assesses 10 common withdrawal signs.

Screening for Alcohol Abuse. In the United States alcohol use/abuse is often considered a moral problem and may pose an embarrassment for the therapist and/or client when asking questions about alcohol use. Keep in mind the goal is to obtain a complete health history of factors that can affect healing and recovery as well as pose risk factors for future health risk.

There are several tools used to assess a client's history of alcohol use, including the Short Michigan Alcoholism Screening Test (SMAST),[111] the CAGE questionnaire, and a separate list of alcohol-related screening questions (Box 2.7). The CAGE questionnaire helps clients unwilling or unable to recognize a problem with alcohol, although it is possible for a person to answer "no" to all of the CAGE questions and still be drinking heavily and at risk for alcohol dependence. The test has reported good test-retest reliability (0.80-0.95) and acceptable correlations with other instruments (0.48-0.70). It is a valid test for detecting alcohol abuse.[112] After 25 years of use, the CAGE questionnaire is still widely used and considered one of the most efficient and effective screening tools for the detection of alcohol abuse.[113]

The AUDIT (Alcohol Use Disorders Identification Test) developed by the World Health Organization to identify persons whose alcohol consumption has become hazardous or harmful to their health is another popular, valid,[104,114] and easy to administer screening tool (Box 2.8).

The AUDIT is designed as a brief, structured interview or self-report survey that can easily be incorporated into a general health interview, lifestyle questionnaire, or medical history. It is a 10-item screening questionnaire with questions on the amount and frequency of drinking, alcohol dependence, and problems caused by alcohol.

When presented in this context by a concerned and interested interviewer, few clients will be offended by the questions. Results are most accurate when given in a nonthreatening, friendly environment to a client who is not intoxicated and who has not been drinking.[104]

The experience of the WHO collaborating investigators indicated that AUDIT questions were answered accurately regardless of cultural background, age, or sex. In fact, many individuals who drank heavily were pleased to find that a health worker was interested in their use of alcohol and the problems associated with it.

The best way to administer the test is to give the client a copy and have him or her fill it out (see Appendix B-1 in the accompanying enhanced eBook version included with print purchase of this textbook). This is suggested for clients who seem reliable and literate. Alternately, the therapist can interview clients by asking them the questions. Some health care workers use just two questions (one based on research in this area and one from the AUDIT) to quickly screen.

❓ FOLLOW-UP QUESTIONS

- How often do you have six or more drinks on one occasion?
  - 0=Never
  - 1=Less than monthly
  - 2=Monthly
  - 3=Weekly
  - 4=Daily or almost daily
- How many drinks containing alcohol do you have each week?
  - More than 14/week for men constitutes a problem
  - More than 7/week for women constitutes a problem

When administered during the screening interview, it may be best to use a transition statement such as:

Now I am going to ask you some questions about your use of alcoholic beverages during the past year. Because alcohol use can affect many areas of health, and may interfere with healing and certain medications, it is important for us to know how much you usually drink and whether you have experienced any problems with your drinking. Please try to be as honest and as accurate as you can be.

BOX 2.8 ALCOHOL USE DISORDERS IDENTIFICATION TEST (AUDIT)

Therapists: This form is available in Appendix B-1 in the accompanying enhanced eBook version included with print purchase of this textbook for clinical use. It is also available from the National Institute on Alcohol Abuse and Alcoholism (NIAAA) online at: www.niaaa.nih.gov. Type AUDIT in search window.

1) How often do you have a drink containing alcohol?
   NEVER (1) MONTHLY OR LESS (2) TWO TO FOUR TIMES A MONTH (3) TWO TO THREE TIMES A WEEK (4) FOUR OR MORE TIMES A WEEK

2) How many drinks containing alcohol do you have on a typical day when you are drinking?
   1 OR 2 (1) 3 OR 4 (2) 5 OR 6 (3) 7 OR 8 (4) 10 OR MORE

3) How often do you have six or more drinks on one occasion?
   NEVER (1) LESS THAN MONTHLY (2) MONTHLY (3) WEEKLY (4) DAILY OR ALMOST DAILY

4) How often during the last year have you found that you were unable to stop drinking once you had started?
   NEVER (1) LESS THAN MONTHLY (2) MONTHLY (3) WEEKLY (4) DAILY OR ALMOST DAILY

5) How often during the last year have you failed to do what was normally expected from you because of drinking?
   NEVER (1) LESS THAN MONTHLY (2) MONTHLY (3) WEEKLY (4) DAILY OR ALMOST DAILY

6) How often during the last year have you needed a first drink in the morning to get going after a heavy drinking session?
   NEVER (1) LESS THAN MONTHLY (2) MONTHLY (3) WEEKLY (4) DAILY OR ALMOST DAILY

7) How often during the last year have you had a feeling of guilt or remorse after drinking?
   NEVER (1) LESS THAN MONTHLY (2) MONTHLY (3) WEEKLY (4) DAILY OR ALMOST DAILY

8) How often during the last year have you been unable to remember the night before because you had been drinking?
   NEVER (1) LESS THAN MONTHLY (2) MONTHLY (3) WEEKLY (4) DAILY OR ALMOST DAILY

9) Have you or someone else been injured as a result of your drinking?
   NO (2) YES, BUT NOT IN THE LAST YEAR (4) YES, DURING THE LAST YEAR

10) Has a relative, friend, or health professional been concerned about your drinking or suggested you cut down?
   NO (2) YES, BUT NOT IN THE LAST YEAR (4) YES, DURING THE LAST YEAR

11) TOTAL SCORE: _____

Key

The numbers for each response are added up to give a composite score. Scores above 8 warrant an in-depth assessment and may be indicative o. an alcohol problem. See options presented to clients in Appendix B-1, AUDIT Questionnaire in the accompanying enhanced eBook version included with print purchase of this textbook.

Data from World Health Organization, 1992. Available for clinical use without permission.

Alternately, if the client's breath smells of alcohol, the therapist may want to say more directly:

? FOLLOW-UP QUESTIONS

- I can smell alcohol on your breath right now. How many drinks have you had today? As a follow-up to such direct questions, you may want to say:
- Alcohol, tobacco, and caffeine often increase our perception of pain, mask or even increase other symptoms, and delay healing. I would like to ask you to limit as much as possible your use of any such stimulants. At the very least, it would be better if you did not drink alcohol before our therapy sessions, so I can assess more clearly just what your symptoms are. You may progress and move along more quickly through our plan of care if these substances are not present in your body.

A helpful final question to ask at the end of this part of the interview may be:

? FOLLOW-UP QUESTIONS

- Are there any other drugs or substances you take that you have not mentioned?

Physical Therapist's Role. Incorporating screening questions into conversation during the interview may help to engage individual clients. Honest answers are important to guiding treatment. Reassure clients that all information will remain confidential and will be used only to ensure the safety and effectiveness of the plan of care. Specific interviewing techniques, such as normalization, symptom assumption, and transitioning may be helpful.[115,116]

Normalization involves asking a question in a way that lets the person know you find a behavior normal or at least understandable under the circumstances. The therapist might say, "Given the stress you are under, I wonder if you have been drinking more lately?"

Symptom assumption involves phrasing a question that assumes a certain behavior already occurs and that the therapist will not be shocked by it. For example, "What kinds of drugs do you use when you are drinking?" or "How much are you drinking?"

Transitioning is a way of using the client's previous answer to start a question such as, "You mentioned your family is upset by your drinking. Have your coworkers expressed similar concern?"[115]

What is the best way to approach alcohol and/or substance use/abuse? Unless the client has a chemical dependency on alcohol, appropriate education may be sufficient for the client experiencing negative effects of alcohol use during the episode of care.

It is important to recognize the distinct and negative physiologic effects each substance or addictive agent can have on the client's physical body, personality, and behavior. Some physicians advocate screening for and treating suspected or known excessive alcohol consumption no differently than diabetes, high blood pressure, or poor vision. The first step may be to ask all clients: Do you drink alcohol, including beer, wine, or other forms of liquor? If yes, ask about consumption (e.g., days per week/number of drinks). Then proceed to the CAGE questions before advising appropriate action.[117]

If the client's health is impaired by the use and abuse of substances, then physical therapy intervention may not be effective as long as the person is under the influence of chemicals.

Encourage the client to seek medical attention or let the individual know you would like to discuss this as a medical problem with the physician (Case Example 2.4).

Physical therapists are not chemical dependency counselors or experts in substance abuse, but armed with a few questions, the therapist can still make a significant difference. Hospitalization or physical therapy intervention for an injury is potentially a teachable moment. Clients with substance abuse problems have worse rehabilitation outcomes, are at increased risk for reinjury or new injuries, and additional comorbidities.

Therapists can actively look for and address substance use/abuse problems in their clients. At the very minimum, therapists can participate in the National Institute on Alcohol Abuse and Alcoholism's National Alcohol Screening Day with a program that includes the CAGE questionnaire, educational materials, and an opportunity to talk with a health care professional about alcohol.

 FOLLOW-UP QUESTIONS

- How do you feel about the role of alcohol in your life?
- Is there something you want or need to change?

Earlier referral for a physical examination may have resulted in earlier diagnosis and treatment for the cancer. Unfortunately, these clinical situations occur often and are very complex, requiring ongoing screening (as happened here).

Finally, the APTA recognizes that physical therapists and physical therapist assistants can be adversely affected by alcoholism and other drug addictions. Impaired therapists or assistants should be encouraged to enter into the recovery process. Reentry into the workforce should occur when the well-being of the physical therapy practitioner and patient/client are assured.[118]

Recreational Drug Use. As with tobacco and alcohol use, recreational or street drug use can lead to or compound already present health problems. Although the question "Do you use recreational or street drugs?" is asked on the Family/Personal History form (see Fig. 2.2), it is questionable whether the client will answer "yes" to this question.

At some point in the interview, the therapist may need to ask these questions directly:

 FOLLOW-UP QUESTIONS

- Have you ever used "street" drugs such as cocaine, crack, crank, "downers," amphetamines ("uppers"), methamphetamine, or other drugs?
- Have you ever injected drugs?
- If yes, have you been tested for HIV or hepatitis?

Cocaine and amphetamines affect the cardiovascular system in the same manner as does stress. The drugs stimulate the sympathetic nervous system to increase its production of adrenaline causing a sharp rise in blood pressure, rapid and irregular heartbeats, heart attacks, seizures and respiratory arrest, among others.[119]

CASE EXAMPLE 2.4

Substance Abuse

A 44-year-old man previously seen in the physical therapy clinic for a fractured calcaneus returns to the same therapist 3 years later because of new onset of midthoracic back pain. There was no known cause or injury associated with the presenting pain. This man had been in the construction business for 30 years and attributed his symptoms to "general wear and tear."

Although there were objective findings to support a musculoskeletal cause of pain, the client also mentioned symptoms of fatigue, stomach upset, insomnia, hand tremors, and headaches. From the previous episode of care, the therapist recalled a history of substantial use of alcohol, tobacco, and caffeine (three six-packs of beer after work each evening, 2 pack/day cigarette habit, 18+ cups of caffeinated coffee during work hours).

The therapist pointed out the potential connection between the client's symptoms and the level of substance use, and the client agreed to "pay more attention to cutting back." After 3 weeks the client returned to work with a reduction of back pain from a level of 8 to a level of 0 to 3 (intermittent symptoms), depending on the work assignment.

Six weeks later this client returned again with the same symptomatic and clinical presentation. At that time, given the client's age, the insidious onset, the cyclic nature of the symptoms, and significant substance abuse, the therapist recommended a complete physical with a primary care physician.

Medical treatment began with NSAIDs, which caused considerable GI upset. The GI symptoms persisted even after the client stopped taking the NSAIDs. Further medical diagnostic testing determined the presence of pancreatic carcinoma. The prognosis was poor, and the client died 6 months later, after extensive medical intervention.

In this case it could be argued that the therapist should have referred the client to a physician immediately because of the history of substance abuse and the presence of additional symptoms. A more thorough screening examination during the first treatment for back pain may have elicited additional red-flag GI symptoms (e.g., melena or bloody diarrhea in addition to the stomach upset).

Heart rate can accelerate by as much as 60 to 70 beats per minute (bpm). In otherwise healthy and fit people, this overload can cause death in minutes, even in first-time cocaine users. In addition, cocaine can cause the aorta to rupture, the lungs to fill with fluid, the heart muscle and its lining to become inflamed, blood clots to form in the veins, and strokes to occur as a result of cerebral hemorrhage.

Tobacco. It is reported that one in five deaths in the United States is as a result of the use of tobacco. Persons who smoke are three times at risk of dying compared with those who never smoked. There is also evidence that quitting smoking before the age of 40 decreases the risk of death from smoking-related diseases by 90%. Tobacco and tobacco products are known carcinogens.[120] This includes secondhand smoke, pipes, cigars, cigarettes, and chewing (smokeless) tobacco.

More people die of tobacco use than alcohol and all the other addictive agents combined. Cigarettes sold in the United States reportedly contain 600 chemicals and additives, ranging from chocolate to counteract tobacco's bitterness to ammonia, added to increase nicotine absorption. Cigarette smoke contains approximately 7000 chemicals, many of which are poisonous, and at least 69 are known to be carcinogenic.[121] As a health care provider, the therapist has an important obligation to screen for tobacco use and incorporate smoking cessation education into the physical therapy plan of care to improve immediate health and prevent secondary complications of chronic disease.[122] The American Cancer Society publishes a chart of the benefits of smoking cessation starting from 20 minutes since the last cigarette up to 15 years later.[123] Therapists can encourage clients to decrease (or eliminate) tobacco use during treatment.

Client education includes a review of the physiologic effects of tobacco (see Table 2.3). Nicotine in tobacco, whether in the form of chewing tobacco or from a cigar, pipe, or cigarette, smoking acts directly on the heart, blood vessels, digestive tract, kidneys, and nervous system.[124] It also has direct effects on important areas of physical therapy practice, including cardiovascular, musculoskeletal, neurologic, and integumentary health across the life span.[122] For the client with respiratory or cardiac problems, nicotine stimulates the already compensated heart to beat faster, it narrows the blood vessels, increases airflow obstruction,[124] reduces the supply of oxygen to the heart and other organs, and increases the chance of developing blood clots. Narrowing of the blood vessels is also detrimental for anyone with peripheral vascular disease, diabetes, or delayed wound healing.

Smoking markedly increases the need for vitamin C, which is poorly stored in the body.[125] One cigarette can consume 25 mg of vitamin C (one pack would consume 500 mg/day). Smoking has been linked with disc degeneration[126] and lumbar intervertebral disc herniation.[127] Nicotine interacts with cholinergic nicotinic receptors, which leads to increased blood pressure, vasoconstriction, and vascular resistance. These systemic effects of nicotine may cause a disturbance in the normal nutrition of the disc.[122]

The combination of coffee ingestion and smoking raises the blood pressure of hypertensive clients about 15/30 mm Hg for as long as 2 hours. All these effects have a direct effect on the client's ability to exercise and must be considered when the client is starting an exercise program. Careful monitoring of vital signs during exercise is advised.

The commonly used formula to estimate cigarette smoking history is done by taking the number of packs smoked per day multiplied by the number of years smoked.[128] If a person smoked 2 packs per day for 30 years, this would be a 60-pack year history (2 packs per day × 30 years=60-pack-years). A 60-pack year history could also be achieved by smoking 3 packs of cigarettes per day for 20 years, and so on (Case Example 2.5).

A significant smoking history is considered 20-pack-years and is a risk factor for lung disease, cancer, heart disease, and other medical comorbidities. Less significant smoking habits must still be assessed in light of other risk factors present, personal/family history, and other risky lifestyle behaviors.

If the client indicates a desire to quit smoking or using tobacco (see Fig. 2.2, General Health: Question 10), the therapist must be prepared to help him or her explore options for smoking cessation. Many hospitals, clinics, and community organizations, such as the local chapter of the American Lung Association, sponsor annual (or ongoing) smoking cessation programs. Pamphlets and other reading material should be available for any client interested in tobacco cessation.

CASE EXAMPLE 2.5
Recognizing Red Flags

A 60-year-old man was referred to physical therapy for weakness in the lower extremities. The client also reports dysesthesia (pain with touch).

Social/Work History: Single, factory worker, history of alcohol abuse, 60-pack year* history of tobacco use.

Clinically, the client presented with mild weakness in distal muscle groups (left more than right). Over the next 2 weeks, the weakness increased and a left foot drop developed. Now the client presents with weakness of right wrist and finger flexors and extensors.

What Are the Red Flags Presented in This Case?

Is Medical Referral Required?
- Age
- Smoking history
- Alcohol use
- Bilateral symptoms
- Progressive neurologic symptoms

Consultation with the physician is certainly advised given the number and type of red flags present, especially the progressive nature of the neurologic symptoms in combination with other key red flags.

*Pack years=# packs/day × number of years. A 60-pack year history could mean 2 packs/day for 30 years or 3 packs/day for 20 years.

Referral to medical doctors who specialize in smoking cessation may be appropriate for some clients.

Caffeine. Caffeine is a substance with specific physiologic (stimulant) effects. Caffeine ingested in toxic amounts has many effects, including nervousness, irritability, agitation, sensory disturbances, tachypnea (rapid breathing), heart palpitations (strong, fast, or irregular heartbeat), nausea, urinary frequency, diarrhea, and fatigue.

The average cup of coffee or tea in the United States is reported to contain between 40 and 150 mg of caffeine; specialty coffees (e.g., espresso) may contain much higher doses. OTC supplements used to combat fatigue typically contain 100 to 200 mg caffeine per tablet. Many prescription drugs and OTC analgesics contain between 32 and 200 mg of caffeine.

People who drink 8 to 15 cups of caffeinated beverages per day have been known to have problems with sleep, dizziness, restlessness, headaches, muscle tension, and intestinal disorders. Caffeine may enhance the client's perception of pain. Pain levels can be reduced dramatically by reducing the daily intake of caffeine.

In large doses, caffeine is a stressor, but abrupt withdrawal from caffeine can be equally stressful. Withdrawal from caffeine induces a syndrome of headaches, fatigue, anxiety, irritability, depressed mood, and difficulty concentrating.[129] Anyone seeking to break free from caffeine dependence should do so gradually over a week's time or more.

It has been noted that about 200 to 300 milligrams of coffee a day, about the equivalent of two to four cups, is safe.[130] It is not hard to exceed these safe levels. A 16-ounce energy drink can contain as much as 240 milligrams. Caffeine pills (Vivarin, EzDoz), which are widely available, can have up to 200 milligrams in each tablet. Caffeine powder is also now widely available online and is reported to be more potent.[131]

Latest evidence suggests that habitual, moderate caffeine intake from coffee and other caffeinated beverages may be associated with a neutral to potentially beneficial effect on health, specifically cardiovascular health.[132] Other sources of caffeine are tea (black and green), cocoa, chocolate, and caffeinated-carbonated beverages.

Sugar Substitutes. Sugar substitutes (also termed "high-intensity sweeteners" by the Food and Drug Administration [FDA]) are additives that sweeten foods without adding significant amounts of calories. The FDA states that based on the available scientific evidence, high-intensity sweeteners approved by FDA are safe for the general population when used in amounts specified by the agency.[133,134] Other studies still question the potential toxic effects of these substances.[135,136]

There have been anecdotal reports that some individuals who have adverse reactions to sugar substitutes complain of headaches, fatigue, myalgias and generalized joint pain. For anyone with these symptoms, connective tissue disorders, fibromyalgia, multiple sclerosis, or other autoimmune disorders such as systemic lupus erythematosus or Hashimoto thyroid disease, it may be helpful to ask about the use of products containing artificial sweeteners.

Client Checklist. Screening for medical conditions can be aided by the use of a client checklist of associated signs and symptoms. Any items checked will alert the therapist to the possible need for further questions or tests.

A brief list here of the most common systemic signs and symptoms is one option for screening. It may be preferable to use the Review of Systems checklist (see Box 4.15; see also Appendix D- in the accompanying enhanced eBook version included with print purchase of this textbook).

Medical and Surgical History. Tests contributing information to the physical therapy assessment may include radiography (x-rays, sonograms), computed tomography (CT) scans, magnetic resonance imaging (MRI), bone scans or imaging, lumbar puncture analysis, urinalysis, and blood tests. The client's medical records may contain information regarding which tests have been performed and the results of the test. It may be helpful to question the client directly by asking:

 FOLLOW-UP QUESTIONS

- What medical test have you had for this condition?
- After giving the client time to respond, the therapist may need to probe further by asking:
  - Have you had any x-ray films, sonograms, CT scans, MRI, or other imaging studies done in the last 2 years?
  - Do you recall having any blood tests or urinalyses done?

If the response is affirmative, the therapist will want to know when and where these tests were performed and the results (if known to the client). Knowledge of where the test took place provides the therapist with access to the results (with the client's written permission for disclosure).

Surgical History. Previous surgery or surgery related to the client's current symptoms may be indicated on the Family/Personal History form (see Fig. 2.2). Whenever treating a client postoperatively, the therapist should read the surgical report. Look for notes on complications, blood transfusions, and the position of the client during the surgery and the length of time in that position.

Clients in an early postoperative stage (within 3 weeks of surgery) may have stiffness, aching, and musculoskeletal pain unrelated to the diagnosis, which may be attributed to position during the surgery. Postoperative infections can lie dormant for months. Accompanying constitutional symptoms may be minimal with no sweats, fever, or chills until the infection progresses with worsening of symptoms or significant change in symptoms.

Specific follow-up questions differ from one client to another, depending on the type of surgery, age of client, accompanying medical history, and so forth, but it is always helpful to assess how quickly the client recovered from surgery to determine an appropriate pace for physical activity and exercise prescribed during an episode of care.

Clinical Tests. The therapist will want to examine the available test results as often as possible. Familiarity with the results of these tests, combined with an understanding of the clinical presentation is paramount. Knowledge of testing and test results also provides the therapist with some guidelines for suggesting or recommending additional testing for clients who have not had a radiologic workup or other potentially appropriate medical testing.

Laboratory values of interest to therapists are displayed on the inside covers of this book.

Work/Living Environment. Questions related to the client's daily work activities and work environments are included in the Family/Personal History form to assist the therapist in planning a program of client education that is consistent with the objective findings and proposed plan of care.

For example, the therapist is alerted to the need for follow-up with a client complaining of back pain who sits for prolonged periods without a back support or cushion. Likewise, a worker involved in bending and twisting who complains of lateral thoracic pain may be describing a muscular strain from repetitive overuse. These work-related questions may help the client report significant data contributing to symptoms that may otherwise have gone undetected.

Questions related to occupation and exposure to toxins such as chemicals or gases are included because well-defined physical (e.g., cumulative trauma disorder) and health problems occur in people engaging in specific occupations.[137] For example, pesticide exposure is common among agricultural workers, asthma and sick building syndrome are reported among office workers, lung disease is associated with underground mining, and silicosis is found in those who must work near silica. There is a higher prevalence of tuberculosis in health care workers compared with the general population.

Each geographic area has its own specific environmental/occupational concerns, but overall, the chronic exposure to chemically based products and pesticides has escalated the incidence of environmental allergies and cases of multiple chemical sensitivity. Exposure to cleaning products can be an unseen source of problems. Headaches, fatigue, skin lesions, joint arthralgias, myalgias, and connective tissue disorders

TABLE 2.4	Common Occupational Exposures
Occupation	Exposure
Agriculture	Pesticides, herbicides, insecticides, fertilizers
Industrial	Chemical agents or irritants, fumes, dusts, radiation, loud noises, asbestos, vibration
Health care workers	Tuberculosis, hepatitis
Office workers	Sick building syndrome
Military service	Gulf War syndrome, connective tissue disorders, amyotrophic lateral sclerosis (ALS), non-Hodgkin's lymphoma, soft tissue sarcoma, chloracne (skin blistering)

may be the first signs of a problem. The therapist may be the first person to put the pieces of the puzzle together. Clients who have seen every kind of specialist end up with a diagnosis of fibromyalgia, rheumatoid arthritis, or some other autoimmune disorder and find their way to the physical therapy clinic (Case Example 2.6).

The U.S. Department of Veterans Affairs reports of a cluster of medically unexplained symptoms that was given the term "Gulf War Syndrome." Military veterans from the Gulf War were reported to complain of chronic symptoms including fatigue, headaches, joint pain, indigestion, insomnia, dizziness, respiratory disorders, memory problems, fibromyalgia, and chronic fatigue syndromes.[139]

Survivors of the Gulf War are nearly twice as likely to develop amyotrophic lateral sclerosis (ALS; Lou Gehrig's disease) than other military personnel.[140] Classic early symptoms include irregular gait and decreased muscular coordination. Other occupationally-related illnesses and diseases have been reported (Table 2.4).

When to Screen. Taking an environmental, occupational, or military history may be appropriate when a client

---

CASE EXAMPLE 2.6

Cleaning Products

A 33-year-old dental hygienist came to physical therapy for joint pain in her hands and wrists. In the course of taking a symptom inventory, the therapist discovered that the client had noticed multiple arthralgias and myalgias over the last 6 months.

She reported being allergic to many molds, dusts, foods, and other allergens. She was on a special diet but had obtained no relief from her symptoms. The doctor, thinking the client was experiencing painful symptoms from repetitive motion, sent her to physical therapy.

A quick occupational survey will include the following questions:[138]

- What kind of work do you do?
- Do you think your health problems are related to your work?
- Are your symptoms better or worse when you are at home or at work?
- Do others at work have similar problems?

The client answered "No" to all work-related questions but later came back and reported that other dental hygienists and dental

assistants had noticed some of the same symptoms, although in a much milder form.

None of the other support staff (receptionist, bookkeeper, secretary) had noticed any health problems. The two dentists in the office were not affected either. The strongest red flag came when the client took a 10-day vacation and returned to work symptom-free. Within 24-hours of her return to work, her symptoms had flared up worse than ever.

This is not a case of emotional stress and work avoidance. The women working in the dental cubicles were using a cleaning spray after each dental client to clean and disinfect the area. The support staff was not exposed to it and the dentists only came in after the spray had dissipated. When this was replaced with an effective cleaning agent with only natural ingredients, everyone's symptoms were relieved completely.

has a history of asthma, allergies, fibromyalgia, chronic fatigue syndrome, or connective tissue or autoimmune disease or in the presence of other nonspecific disorders.

Conducting a quick survey may be helpful when a client presents with puzzling, nonspecific symptoms, including myalgias, arthralgias, headaches, back pain, sleep disturbance, loss of appetite, loss of sexual interest, or recurrent upper respiratory symptoms.

After determining the client's occupation and depending on the client's chief complaint and accompanying associated signs and symptoms, the therapist may want to ask:[141]

 FOLLOW-UP QUESTIONS

- Do you think your health problems are related to your work?
- Do you wear a mask at work?
- Are your symptoms better or worse when you are at home or at work?
- Follow-up if worse at work: Do others at work have similar problems?
- Follow-up if worse at home: Have you done any remodeling at home in the last 6 months?
- Are you now, or have you previously, been exposed to dusts, fumes, chemicals, radiation, loud noise, tools that vibrate, or a new building/office space?
- Have you ever been exposed to chemical agents or irritants such as asbestos, asphalt, aniline dyes, benzene, herbicides, fertilizers, wood dust, or others?
- Do others at work have similar problems?
- Have you ever served in any branch of the military?
  - If yes, were you ever exposed to dusts, fumes, chemicals, radiation, or other substances?

The idea in conducting a workplace/environmental screening is to look for patterns in the past medical history that might link the current clinical presentation with the reported or observed associated signs and symptoms. Further follow-up questions are listed in Appendix B-14 in the accompanying enhanced eBook version included with print purchase of this textbook.

The mnemonic CH²OPD² (Community, Home, Hobbies, Occupation, Personal habits, Diet, and Drugs) can be used as a tool to identify a client's history of exposure to potentially toxic environmental contaminants:[142]

• **C**ommunity	Live near a hazardous waste site or industrial site
• **H**ome	Home is more than 40 years old; recent renovations; pesticide(s) use in home, garden, or on pets
• **H**obbies	Work with stained glass, oil-based paints, varnishes
• **O**ccupation	Air quality at work; exposure to chemicals
• **P**ersonal habits	Tobacco use, exposure to secondhand smoke
• **D**iet	Contaminants in food and water
• **D**rugs	Prescription, OTC drugs, home remedies, illicit drug use

Resources. Further suggestions and tools to help health care professionals incorporate environmental history questions can be found online. The Children's Environmental Health Network (www.cehn.org) has an online training manual, Pediatric Environmental Health: Putting It into Practice. Download and review the chapter on environmental history taking.

The Agency for Toxic Substances and Disease Registry (ATSDR) website, (www.atsdr.cdc.gov) offers information on specific chemical exposures.

History of Falls. Falls are a serious and costly health concern in the United States. In the United States, falls are the leading cause of traumatic brain injury.[143] It is reported that the financial burden of nonfatal falls in the United States in those over 65 years to be $31 billion.[144] Of the reported 250,000 hip fractures per year, 95% were as a result of falls.[145]

One consequence of falls is fear of falling again.[143] This results in the individual severely restricting their daily activities, leading to a decreased quality of life. Ironically, this fear of falling leads to an increased risk of falling through the adoption of stiffening strategies and altered attentional processes.[147]

By assessing risk factors (prediction) and offering preventive and protective strategies, the therapist can make a significant difference in the number of fall-related injuries and fractures. There are many ways to look at falls assessment. For the screening process, there are four main categories:
- Well-adult (no falling pattern)
- Just starting to fall
- Falls frequently (more than once every 6 months)
- Fear of falling

Healthy older adults who have no falling patterns may have a fear of falling in specific instances (e.g., getting out of the bath or shower; walking on ice, curbs, or uneven terrain). Fear of falling can be considered a mobility impairment or activity limitation. It restricts the client's ability to perform specific actions, thereby preventing the client from doing the things he or she wants to do. Functionally, this may appear as an inability to take a tub bath, walk on grass unassisted, or even attempt household tasks such as getting up on a sturdy step stool to change a lightbulb (Case Example 2.7).

Risk Factors for Falls. The ability to maintain upright balance in static and dynamic conditions is a result of a complex interaction of several major body systems, including but not limited to the musculoskeletal and neuromuscular systems. The therapist is a key health care professional to make early identification of adults at increased risk for falls.

With careful questioning, any potential problems with balance may come to light. Such information will alert the therapist to the need for testing static and dynamic balance and to look for potential risk factors and systemic or medical causes of falls (Table 2.5).

All of the variables and risk factors listed in Table 2.5 for falls are important. Older adults may have impaired balance, decreased position sense, slower reaction times, and decreased strength and range of motion, leading to more frequent falls. Medications, especially polypharmacy or

CASE EXAMPLE 2.7
Fracture After a Fall

From Chanoski C: Adapted from case report presented in partial fulfillment of DPT 910, Principles of Differential Diagnosis, Institute for Physical Therapy Education, Widener University, Chester, Pennsylvania, 2005. Used with permission.

Case Description: A 67-year-old woman fell and sustained a complete transverse fracture of the left fibula and an incomplete fracture of the tibia. The client reported she lost her footing while walking down four steps at the entrance of her home.

She was immobilized in a plaster cast for 9 weeks. Extended immobilization was required after the fracture because of slow rate of healing secondary to osteopenia/osteoporosis. She was non–weight-bearing and ambulated with crutches while her foot was immobilized. Initially this client was referred to physical therapy for range of motion (ROM), strengthening, and gait training.

Client is married and lives with her husband in a single-story home. Her goals were to ambulate independently with a normal gait.

Past Medical History: Type 2 diabetes, hypertension, osteopenia, and history of alcohol use. Client used tobacco (1½ packs a day for 35 years) but has not smoked for the past 20 years. Client described herself as a "weekend alcoholic," meaning she did not drink during the week but drank six or more beers a day on weekends.

Current medications include tolbutamide, enalapril, hydrochlorothiazide, Fosamax and supplemental calcium, and a multivitamin.

Intervention: The client was seen six times before a scheduled surgery interrupted the plan of care. Progress was noted as increased ROM and increased strength through the left lower extremity, except dorsiflexion.

Seven weeks later, the client returned to physical therapy for strengthening and gait training secondary to a "limp" on the left side. She reported that she noticed the limping had increased since having both big toenails removed. She also noted increased toe dragging, stumbling, and leg cramps (especially at night). She reported she had decreased her use of alcohol since she fractured her leg because of the pain medications and recently because of a fear of falling.

Minimal progress was noted in improving balance or improving strength in the lower extremity. The client felt that her loss of strength could be attributed to inactivity following the foot surgery, even though she reported doing her home exercise program.

Neurologic screening examination was repeated with hyperreflexia observed in the lower extremities, bilaterally. There was a positive Babinski reflex on the left. The findings were reported to the primary care physician who requested that physical therapy continue.

During the next week and a half, the client reported that she fell twice. She also reported that she was "having some twitching in her [left] leg muscles." The client also reported "coughing a lot while [she] was eating; food going down the wrong pipe."

Outcome: The client presented with a referral for weakness and gait abnormality thought to be related to the left fibular fracture and fall that did not respond as expected and, in fact, resulted in further loss of function.

The physician was notified of the client's need for a cane, no improvement in strength, fasciculations in the left lower extremity, and the changes in her neurologic status. The client returned to her primary care provider who then referred her to a neurologist.

Results: Upon examination by the neurologist, the client was diagnosed with amyotrophic lateral sclerosis (ALS). A new physical therapy plan of care was developed based on the new diagnosis.

---

hyperpharmacotherapy (see definition and discussion of Medications in this chapter), can contribute to falls.[148] There are four key areas to consider when assessing falls in the older adult:[149]

Chronic health problems, such as physical impairments, function/activity limitations, medication and alcohol use, hazards in the home, coronary heart disease, peripheral vascular disease, and diabetes mellitus, are just a few of the chronic health problems that can put additional stress on the regulating function of the autonomic nervous system's ANS. The ability of the ANS to regulate blood pressure is also affected by age. A sudden drop in blood pressure can precipitate a fall.

Additional neurological conditions such as stroke, Parkinson's disease, and multiple sclerosis can cause alterations in the systems controlling balance, thereby increasing their risk for falls. Musculoskeletal conditions, such as arthritis, can cause limitations in range of motion, weakness, and skeletal and postural deformities, thereby potentially causing a fall.

Physical impairments and function/activity limitations are additional factors to consider when screening for falls. As we age, cervical spinal motion declines, as does peripheral vision.

These two factors alone contribute to changes in our vestibular system and the balance mechanism. Macular degeneration, glaucoma, cataracts, or any other visual problems can result in loss of depth perception and even greater loss of visual acuity.

Balance impairments, caused by impaired sensation and sensory integration, whether age-related or brought about by existing medical conditions, could cause falls. The clinician must check vision, somatosentation, and vestibular subsystems of the client to determine whether they are contributory to the balance dysfunction. Limitations in activity, such as functional mobility, and transfers can cause falls. The speed of ambulation may also give clues to the client's ability to maintain an upright posture in a dynamic situation.

Alcohol use in the elderly was covered earlier in this chapter. Heavy use of alcohol is a definite contributor to impairments in balance and occurrences of falls. Multiple comorbidities often mean the use of multiple medications (polypharmacy/hyperpharmacotherapy). These two variables together increase the risk of falls in older adults. Some medications (especially psychotropics such as tranquilizers and antidepressants, including amitriptyline, doxepin, Zoloft, Prozac, Paxil, Remeron, Celexa, and Wellbutrin) are red-flag

TABLE 2.5	Risk Factors for Falls			
Age Changes	Environmental/ Living Conditions	Pathologic Conditions	Medications	Other
Muscle weakness; loss of joint motion (especially lower extremities)	Poor lighting	Vestibular disorders; episodes of dizziness or vertigo from any cause	Antianxiety; benzodiazepines	History of falls
Abnormal gait	Throw rugs, loose carpet complex carpet designs	Orthostatic hypotension (especially before breakfast)	Anticonvulsants	Female sex; postmenopausal status
Impaired or abnormal balance	Cluster of electric wires or cords	Chronic pain condition	Antidepressants	Living alone
Impaired proprioception or sensation	Stairs without handrails	NeuropathiesCervical myelopathy	Antihypertensives	Elder abuse/assault
Delayed muscle response/ increased reaction time	Bathroom without grab bars	Osteoarthritis; rheumatoid arthritis	Antipsychotics	Nonambulatory status (requiring transfers)
↓Systolic blood pressure (<140 mm Hg in adults age over 65 years old)	Slippery floors (water, urine, floor surface, ice); icy sidewalks, stairs, or streets	Visual or hearing impairment; multifocal eyeglasses; change in perception of color; loss of depth perception; decreased contrast sensitivity	Diuretics	Gait changes (decreased stride length or speed)
Stooped or forward bent posture	Restraints	Cardiovascular disease	Narcotics	Postural instability; reduced postural control
	Use of alcohol or other drugs	Urinary incontinence	Sedative-hypnotics	Fear of falling; history of falls
	Footwear, especially slippers	Nocturia more than 3 times per night	Phenothiazines	Dehydration from any cause
		Central nervous system disorders (e.g., stroke, Parkinson's disease, multiple sclerosis)	Use of more than four medications (polypharmacy/ hyperpharmacotherapy)	Recent surgery (general anesthesia, epidural)
		Motor disturbance		Sleep disorder/ disturbance; sleep deprivation; daytime drowsiness; brief disorientation after waking up from a nap[146]
		Osteopenia, osteoporosis		
		Pathologic fractures		
		Any mobility impairments (e.g., amputation, neuropathy, deformity)		
		Cognitive impairment; dementia; depression		

risk factors for loss of balance and injury from falls. The clinician needs to remember that alcohol can interact with many medications, increasing the risk of falling.

The therapist should watch for clients with chronic conditions who are taking any of these medications. Anyone with fibromyalgia, depression, cluster migraine headaches, chronic pain, obsessive-compulsive disorders (OCD), panic disorder, and anxiety who is on a psychotropic medication must be monitored carefully for dizziness, drowsiness, and postural orthostatic hypotension (a sudden drop in blood pressure with an increase in pulse rate). It is not uncommon for clients taking hypertensive medication (diuretics) to become dehydrated, dizzy, and lose their balance. Postural orthostatic hypotension can (and often does) occur in the aging adult—even in someone taking blood pressure–regulating medications.

Orthostatic hypotension as a risk factor for falls may occur as a result of volume depletion (e.g., diabetes mellitus, sodium or potassium depletion), venous pooling (e.g., pregnancy, varicosities of the legs, immobility following a motor vehicle or cerebrovascular accident), side effects of medications such as antihypertensives, starvation associated with anorexia or cachexia, and sluggish normal regulatory mechanisms associated with anatomic variations or secondary to other conditions such as metabolic disorders or diseases of the central nervous system (CNS).

Lastly, hazards in the home are a significant contributor to falls in the elderly. Examples of these include poor lighting, clutter around the house, loose carpets, lack of adaptive equipment (grab bars or handrails), and lack of safety equipment in the kitchen and bathroom.[149] The clinician must make a note to consider asking clients a few questions about their home environment and offer suggestions to decrease their risk of falling at home.

Screening for Risk of Falls. Aging adults who have just started to fall or who fall frequently may be fearful of losing their independence by revealing this information, even to a therapist. If the client indicates no difficulty with falling, the therapist is encouraged to review this part of the form (see Fig. 2.2) carefully with all older clients.

Some potential screening questions may include (see Appendix B-11 in the accompanying enhanced eBook version included with print purchase of this textbook for full series of questions):

FOLLOW-UP QUESTIONS

- Do you have any episodes of dizziness?
  If yes, does turning over in bed cause (or increase) dizziness?
- Do you have trouble getting in or out of bed without losing your balance?
- Can you/do you get in and out of your bathtub or shower?
- Do you avoid walking on uneven surfaces outside, such as grass or curbs, to avoid falling?
- Have you started taking any new medications, drugs, or pills of any kind?
- Has there been any change in the dosage of your regular medications?

During the Core Interview, the therapist will have an opportunity to ask further questions about the client's Current Level of Fitness (see Current Level of Fitness section in this chapter).

Performance-based tests such as the Multidirectional Reach Test,[150,151] Five-Times-Sit-to-Stand-Test (FTSST),[152] Berg Balance Scale (BBS),[153,154] the Timed "Up and Go" Test (TUG),[155-157] and the modified Clinical Test of Sensory Integration of balance (mCTSIB), when analyzed carefully, could provide clues as to the possible contributor to the balance impairments. Some of these tests could even predict and/or quantify the risk for falls. Fear of falling can be measured using the Falls Efficacy Scale (FES)[158] and the Activities-Specific Balance Confidence Scale (ABC) can measure balance confidence.[159]

Measuring vital signs and screening for postural orthostatic hypotension is another important tool in predicting falls. Positive test results for any of the mentioned tests require further evaluation, especially in the presence of risk factors predictive of falls.

Resources. As the population of older people in the United States continues to grow, the number of falls and injuries related to it will likely grow. Therapists are in a unique position to educate people on movement and exercise to help maintain proper posture, improve balance, and prevent falls. The APTA has a Balance and Falls Kit (Item number PR-294) available to assist the therapist in this area. Related products are also available from the APTA and include: What You Need to Know about Balance and Falls: A Physical Therapist's Perspective, and Balance and Falls Awareness Event Kit Score Sheets.[160]

The American Geriatric Society (AGS) also provides excellent evidence-based guidelines for the screening and prevention of falls, including clinical algorithms, assessment materials, and intervention strategies (available online at http://www.americangeriatrics.org/health_care_professionals/clinical_practice/clinical_guidelines_recommendations/prevention_of_falls_summary_of_recommendations).

Vital Signs. Taking a client's vital signs remains the single easiest, most economic, and fastest way to screen for many systemic illnesses.

A place to record vital signs is provided at the end of the Family/Personal History form (see Fig. 2.2). The clinician must be proficient in taking vital signs, an important part of

the screening process. All vital signs are important, but the client's temperature and blood pressure have the greatest utility as early screening tools. An in-depth discussion of vital signs as a part of the screening physical assessment is presented in Chapter 4.

CORE INTERVIEW

Once the therapist reviews the results of the Family/Personal History form and reviews any available medical records for the client, the client interview (referred to as the Core Interview in this text) begins (Fig. 2.3).

Screening questions may be interspersed throughout the Core Interview and/or presented at the end. When to screen depends on the information provided by the client during the interview.

Special questions related to sensitive topics such as sexual history, assault or domestic violence (DV), and substance or alcohol use are often left to the end, or even on a separate day, after the therapist has established sufficient rapport to broach these topics.

History of Present Illness

Chief Complaint

The history of present illness (often referred to as the chief complaint and other current symptoms) may best be obtained through the use of open-ended questions. This section of the interview is designed to gather information related to the client's reason(s) for seeking clinical treatment.

The following open-ended statements may be appropriate to start an interview:

 FOLLOW-UP QUESTIONS

- Tell me how I can help you.
- Tell me why you are here today.
- Tell me about your injury.
- (Alternate) What do you think is causing your problem or pain?

During this initial phase of the interview, allow the client to carefully describe his or her current situation. Follow-up questions and paraphrasing, as shown in Fig. 2.3, can be used in conjunction with the primary open-ended questions.

Pain and Symptom Assessment

The interview naturally begins with an assessment of the chief complaint, usually (but not always) pain. Chapter 3 of this text presents an in-depth discussion of viscerogenic sources of NMS pain and pain assessment, including questions to ask to identify specific characteristics of pain.

For the reader's convenience, a summary of these questions is included in the Core Interview (see Fig. 2.3). Also, the list of questions is included in Appendices B-28 and C-7 on for use in the clinic.

Beyond a pain and symptom assessment, the therapist may conduct a screening physical examination as a part of the objective assessment (see Chapter 4). Table 4.13 and Boxes 4.15 and 4.16 are helpful tools for this portion of the examination and evaluation.

Insidious Onset

When the client describes an insidious onset or unknown cause of imbalance, it is important to ask further questions. Did the symptoms develop after a fall, trauma (including assault), or some repetitive activity (such as painting, cleaning, gardening, filing, or driving long distances)?

The client may wrongly attribute the onset of symptoms to a particular activity that is unrelated to the current symptoms. The alert therapist must seek to identify and recognize the true causative factor and avoid being unnecessarily swayed by the patient. Whenever the client presents with an unknown etiology of injury, or impairment, or with an apparent cause, always ask yourself these questions:

 FOLLOW-UP QUESTIONS

* Is it insidious?
* Is it likely to be caused by such and such (whatever the client told you)?
* Are there other likely causes that I have not considered?

Trauma

When seeking to make a diagnosis, the physical therapist should be alert for inconsistencies. When the symptoms seem out of proportion to the injury or when the symptoms persist beyond the expected time for that condition, a red flag should be raised in the therapist's mind. Emotional overlay is often the most suspected underlying cause of this clinical presentation. But trauma from assault and undiagnosed cancer can also present with these symptoms.

Even if the client has a known (or perceived) cause for his or her condition, the therapist must be alert for trauma as an etiologic factor. Trauma may be intrinsic (occurring within the body) or extrinsic (external accident or injury, especially assault or DV).

Twenty-five percent of clients with primary malignant tumors of the musculoskeletal system report a prior traumatic episode. Often the trauma or injury brings attention to a pre-existing malignant or benign tumor. Whenever a fracture occurs with minimal trauma or involves a transverse fracture line, the physician considers the possibility of a tumor.

Intrinsic Trauma. An example of intrinsic trauma is the unguarded movement that can occur during normal motion. For example, the client who describes reaching to the back of a cupboard while turning his or her head away from the extended arm to reach that last inch or two. He or she may feel a sudden "pop" or twinge in the neck with immediate pain and describe this as the cause of the injury.

Intrinsic trauma can also occur secondary to extrinsic (external) trauma. A motor vehicle accident, assault, fall, or known accident or injury may result in intrinsic trauma to another part of the musculoskeletal system or another organ system. Such intrinsic trauma may be masked by the more critical injury and may become more symptomatic as the primary injury resolves.

Take, for example, the client who experiences a cervical flexion/extension (whiplash) injury. The initial trauma causes painful head and neck symptoms. When these resolve (with treatment or on their own), the client may notice midthoracic spine pain or rib pain.

The midthoracic pain can occur when the spine fulcrums over the T4-T6 area as the head moves forcefully into the extended position during the whiplash injury. In cases like this, the primary injury to the neck is accompanied by a secondary intrinsic injury to the midthoracic spine. The symptoms may go unnoticed until the more painful cervical lesion is treated or healed.

Likewise, if an undisplaced rib fracture occurs during a motor vehicle accident, it may be asymptomatic until the client gets up the first time. Movement or additional trauma may cause the rib to displace, possibly puncturing a lung. These are all examples of intrinsic trauma.

Extrinsic Trauma. Extrinsic trauma occurs when a force or load external to the body is exerted against the body. Whenever a client presents with NMS dysfunction, the therapist must consider whether this was caused by an accident, injury, or assault.

The therapist must remain aware that some motor vehicle "accidents" may be reported as accidents but are, in fact, the result of DV in which the victim is pushed, shoved, or kicked out of the car or deliberately hit by a vehicle.

Assault. Domestic violence is a serious public health concern that often goes undetected by clinicians. Women (especially those who are pregnant or disabled), children, and older adults are at greatest risk, regardless of race, religion, or socioeconomic status. Early intervention may reduce the risk of future abuse.

Physical therapists and physical therapist assistants need to be alert to the prevalence of violence in all sectors of society. Therapists are encouraged to participate in education programs on screening, recognition, and treatment of violence and to advocate for people who may be abused or at risk for abuse. It is in the physical therapist code of ethics to "report suspected cases of abuse of children or vulnerable adults to appropriate authority, subject to law."[161]

Addressing the possibility of sexual or physical assault/abuse during the interview may not take place until the therapist has established a working relationship with the client. Each question must be presented in a sensitive, respectful manner with observation for nonverbal cues.

Although some interviewing guidelines are presented here, questioning clients about abuse is a complex issue with important effects on the outcome of rehabilitation. All therapists are encouraged to familiarize themselves with the information available for screening and intervening in this important area of clinical practice.

BOX 2.9 DEFINITIONS OF ABUSE

Abuse—Infliction of physical or mental injury, or the deprivation of food, shelter, clothing, or services needed to maintain physical or mental health

Sexual abuse—Sexual assault, sexual intercourse without consent, indecent exposure, deviate sexual conduct, or incest; adult using a child for sexual gratification without physical contact is considered sexual abuse

Neglect—Failure to provide food, shelter, clothing, or help with daily activities needed to maintain physical or mental well-being; client often displays signs of poor hygiene, hunger, or inappropriate clothing

Material exploitation—Unreasonable use of a person, power of attorney, guardianship, or personal trust to obtain control of the ownership, use, benefit, or possession of the person's money, assets, or property

by means of deception, duress, menace, fraud, undue influence, or intimidation

Mental abuse—Impairment of a person's intellectual or psychologic functioning or well-being

Emotional abuse—Anguish inflicted through threats, intimidation, humiliation, and/or isolation; belittling, embarrassing, blaming, rejecting behaviors from adult toward child; withholding love, affection, approval

Physical abuse—Physical injury resulting in pain, impairment, or bodily injury of any bodily organ or function, permanent or temporary disfigurement, or death

Self-neglect—Individual is not physically or mentally able to obtain and perform the daily activities of life to avoid physical or mental injury

Data from Smith L, Putnam DB: The abuse of vulnerable adults. Montana State Bar. *The Montana Lawyer* magazine, June/July 2001.

Generally, the term *abuse* encompasses the terms physical abuse, mental abuse, sexual abuse, neglect, self-neglect, and exploitation (Box 2.9). *Assault* is by definition any physical, sexual, or psychologic attack. This includes verbal, emotional, and economic abuse. *DV* or *intimate partner violence* (IPV) is a pattern of coercive behaviors perpetrated by a current or former intimate partner that may include physical, sexual, and/or psychologic assaults.[162,163]

Violence against women is more prevalent than violence against men,[164] but men can be in an abusive relationship with a parent or partner (male or female).[165] Intimate partner assault may be more prevalent against gay men than against heterosexual men.[166] Many men have been the victims of sexual abuse as children or teenagers.

Child abuse includes neglect and maltreatment that includes physical, sexual, and emotional abuse. Failure to provide for the child's basic physical, emotional, or educational needs is considered neglect even if it is not a willful act on the part of the parent, guardian, or caretaker.[167]

Screening for Assault or Domestic Violence. The American Medical Association (AMA) and other professional groups recommend routine screening for DV. At least one study has shown that screening does not put victims at increased risk for more violence later. Many victims who participated in the study contacted community resources for victims of DV soon after completing the study survey.[168]

As health care providers, therapists have an important role in helping to identify cases of DV and abuse. Routinely incorporating screening questions about DV into history taking only takes a few minutes and is advised in all settings. When interviewing the client, it is often best to use some other word besides *assault*.

Many people who have been physically struck, pushed, or kicked do not consider the action an assault, especially if someone they know inflicts it. The therapist may want to

preface any general screening questions with one of the following lead-ins:

 FOLLOW-UP QUESTIONS

- Abuse in the home is so common today we now ask all our clients:
  - Are you threatened or hurt at home or in a relationship with anyone?
  - Do you feel safe at home?
- Many people are in abusive relationships but are afraid to say so. We ask everyone about this now.
  - FUP: Has this ever happened to you?
- We are required to ask everyone we see about domestic violence. Many of the people I treat tell me they are in difficult, hurtful, sometimes even violent relationships. Is this your situation?

Several screening tools are available with varying levels of sensitivity and specificity. The Woman Abuse Screening Tool (WAST) has direct questions that are easy to understand (e.g., Have you been abused physically, emotionally, or sexually by an intimate partner?). It is a valid and reliable measure of abuse in the family practice setting.[169,170] There is also the Composite Abuse Scale (CAS),[171] and the Index of Spousal Abuse (ISA).

 FOLLOW-UP QUESTIONS

- Have you been kicked, hit, pushed, choked, punched, or otherwise hurt by someone in the last year?
- Do you feel safe in your current relationship?
- Is anyone from a previous relationship making you feel unsafe now?
- Alternate: Are your symptoms today caused by someone kicking, hitting, pushing, choking, throwing, or punching you?
- Alternate: I am concerned someone hurting you may have caused your symptoms. Has anyone been hurting you in any way?

- FUP: Is there anything else you would like to tell me about your situation?

Indirect Questions[167]

- I see you have a bruise here. It looks like it is healing well. How did it happen?
- Are you having problems with your partner?
- Have you ever been hurt in a fight?
- You seem concerned about your partner. Can you tell me more about that?
- Does your partner keep you from coming to therapy or seeing family and friends?

Follow-up questions will depend on the client's initial response.[167] The timing of these personal questions can be very delicate. A private area for interviewing is best at a time when the client is alone (including no children, friends, or other family members). The following may be helpful:

? FOLLOW-UP QUESTIONS

- May I ask you a few more questions?
- If yes, has anyone ever touched you against your will?
- How old were you when it started? When did it stop?
- Have you ever told anyone about this?
- *Client denies abuse*

Response: I know sometimes people are afraid or embarrassed to say they have been hit. If you are ever hurt by anyone, it is safe to tell me about it.

- *Client is offended*

Response: I am sorry to offend you. Many people need help but are afraid to ask.

- *Client says "Yes"*

Response: Listen, believe, document if possible. Take photographs if the client will allow it. If the client does not want to get help at this time, offer to give them the photos for future use or to keep them on file should the victim change their mind. See documentation guidelines. Provide information about local resources.

During the interview (and subsequent episode of care) watch out for any of the risk factors and red flags for violence (Box 2.10), or any of the clinical signs and symptoms listed in

this section. The physical therapist should not turn away from signs of physical or sexual abuse.

In attempting to address such a sensitive issue, the therapist must make sure that the client will not be endangered by intervention. Physical therapists who are not trained to be counselors should be careful about offering advice to those believed to have sustained abuse (or even those who have admitted abuse).

The best course of action may be to document all observations and, when necessary or appropriate, to communicate those documented observations to the referring or family physician.[172-174] When an abused individual asks for help or direction, the therapist must always be prepared to provide information about available community resources.

In considering the possibility of assault as the underlying cause of any trauma, the therapist should be aware of cultural differences and how these compare with behaviors that suggest excessive partner control. For example:

- Abusive partner rarely lets the client come to the appointment alone (partner control).
- Collectivist cultures (group-oriented) often come to the clinic with several family members; such behavior is a cultural norm.
- Noncompliance/missed appointments (could be either one).

Elder Abuse. Health care professionals are becoming more aware of elder abuse as a problem. It is estimated that 84% of elder abuse and neglect is never reported. The International Network for the Prevention of Elder Abuse has more information available online at www.inpea.net.

The therapist must be alert at all times for elder abuse. Skin tears, bruises, and pressure ulcers are not always predictable signs of aging or immobility. During the screening process, watch for warning signs of elder abuse (Box 2.11).

Clinical Signs and Symptoms. Physical injuries caused by battering are most likely to occur in a central pattern (i.e., head, neck, chest/breast, abdomen). Clothes, hats, and hair easily hide injuries to these areas, but they are frequently observable by the therapist in a clinical setting that requires changing into a gown or similar treatment attire.

The therapist should follow guidelines provided when documenting the nature (e.g., cut, puncture, burn, bruise,

---

BOX 2.10   RISK FACTORS AND RED FLAGS FOR DOMESTIC VIOLENCE

- Women with disabilities
- Cognitively impaired adult
- Chronically ill and dependent adult (especially adults over age 75 years)
- Chronic pain clients
- Physical and/or sexual abuse history (men and women)
- Daily headache
- Previous history of many injuries and accidents (including multiple motor vehicle accidents)
- Somatic disorders

- Injury seems inconsistent with client's explanation; injury in a child that is not consistent with the child's developmental level
- Injury takes much longer to heal than expected
- Pelvic floor problems
  - Over activity of the PFM
  - Infertility
  - Pain and dyspareunia
- Recurrent unwanted pregnancies
- History of alcohol abuse in male partner

BOX 2.11 WARNING SIGNS OF ELDER ABUSE

- Multiple trips to the emergency department
- Depression
- "Falls"/fractures
- Bruising/suspicious sores
- Malnutrition/weight loss
- Pressure ulcers
- Changing physicians/therapists often
- Confusion attributed to dementia

bite), location, and detailed description of any injuries. The therapist must be aware of Mongolian spots, which can be mistaken for bruising from child abuse in certain population groups (see Fig. 4.25).

CLINICAL SIGNS AND SYMPTOMS

Domestic Violence

Physical Cues[180]
- Bruises, black eyes, malnutrition
- Sprains, dislocations, foot injuries, fractures in various stages of healing
- Skin problems (e.g., eczema, sores that do not heal, burns); see Chapter 4
- Chronic or migraine headaches
- Diffuse pain, vague or nonspecific symptoms
- Chronic or multiple injuries in various stages of healing
- Vision and hearing loss
- Chronic low back, sacral, or pelvic pain
- Temporomandibular joint (TMJ) pain
- Dysphagia (difficulty swallowing) and easy gagging
- GI disorders
- Patchy hair loss, redness, or swelling over the scalp from violent hair pulling
- Easily startled, flinching when approached

Social Cues
- Continually missing appointments; does not return phone calls; unable to talk on the phone when you call
- Bringing all the children to a clinic appointment
- Spouse, companion, or partner always accompanying client
- Changing physicians often
- Multiple trips to the emergency department
- Multiple car accidents

Psychologic Cues
- Anorexia/bulimia
- Panic attacks, nightmares, phobias
- Hypervigilance, tendency to startle easily or be very guarded
- Substance abuse
- Depression, anxiety, insomnia
- Self-mutilation or suicide attempts
- Multiple personality disorders
- Mistrust of authority figures
- Demanding, angry, distrustful of health care provider

In the pediatric population, fractures of the ribs, tibia/fibula, radius/ulna, and clavicle are more likely to be associated with abuse than with accidental trauma, especially in children less than 18 months old. In the group older than 18 months, a rib fracture is highly suspicious of abuse.[175]

A link between a history of sexual or physical abuse and multiple somatic and other medical disorders in adults (e.g., cardiovascular,[138] GI, endocrine,[176] respiratory, gynecologic, headache and other neurologic problems) has been confirmed.[177] The Adverse Childhood Experiences, or ACE, questionnaire[178] may be a helpful tool for evaluating whether the patient experienced abuse or other psychologically harmful events as a child. Multiple positive responses is associated with multiple health conditions.[179]

Workplace Violence. Workers in the health care profession are at risk for workplace violence in the form of physical assault and aggressive acts. Threats or gestures used to intimidate or threaten are considered assault. Aggressive acts include verbal or physical actions aimed at creating fear in another person. Any unwelcome physical contact from another person is battery. Any form of workplace violence can be perpetrated by a coworker, member of a coworker's family, by a client, or a member of the client's family.

Predicting violence is very difficult, making this occupational hazard one that must be approached through preventative measures rather than relying on individual staff responses or behavior. Institutional policies must be implemented to protect health care workers and provide a safe working environment.[181]

Therapists must be alert for risk factors (e.g., dependence on drugs or alcohol, depression, signs of paranoia) and behavioral patterns that may lead to violence (e.g., aggression toward others, blaming others, threats of harm toward others) and immediately report any suspicious incidents or individuals.[182]

The Physical Therapist's Role. Providing referral to community agencies is perhaps the most important step a health care provider can offer any client who is the victim of abuse, assault, or DV of any kind. Experts report that the best approach to addressing abuse is combined law enforcement and public health effort.

Any health care professional who asks these kinds of screening questions must be prepared to respond. Having information and phone numbers available is imperative for the interested client. Each therapist must know what reporting requirements are in place in the state in which he or she is practicing (Case Example 2.8). An excellent resource for the physical therapist can be found by Schachter's article in the Journal of Physical Therapy.[183]

The therapist should avoid assuming the role of "rescuer" but rather recognize DV, offer a plan of care and intervention for injuries, assess the client's safety, and offer information regarding support services. The therapist should provide help at the pace the client can handle. Reporting a situation of DV can put the victim at risk.

The client usually knows how to stay safe and when to leave. Whether leaving or staying, it is a complex process of

CASE EXAMPLE 2.8
Elder Abuse

An 80-year-old female (Mrs. Smith) was referred to home health by her family doctor for an assessment following a mild cerebrovascular accident (CVA). She was living with her 53-year-old divorced daughter (Susan). The daughter works full-time to support herself, her mother, and three teenage children.

The CVA occurred 3 weeks ago. She was hospitalized for 10 days during which time she had daily physical and occupational therapy. She has residual left-sided weakness.

Home health nursing staff notes that she has been having short-term memory problems in the last week. When the therapist arrived at the home, the doors were open, the stove was on with the stove door open, and Mrs. Smith was in front of the television set. She was wearing a nightgown with urine and feces on it. She was not wearing her hearing aid, glasses, or false teeth.

Mrs. Smith did not respond to the therapist or seem surprised that someone was there. While helping her change into clean clothes, the therapist noticed a large bruise on her left thigh and another one on the opposite upper arm. She did not answer any of the therapist's questions but talked about her daughter constantly. She repeatedly said, "Susan is mean to me."

How Should the Therapist Respond in This Situation?
Physical therapists do have a role in prevention, assessment, and intervention in cases of abuse and neglect. Keeping a nonjudgmental attitude is helpful.

Assessment: Examination and Evaluation
1. Attempt to obtain a detailed history.
2. Conduct a thorough physical examination. Look for warning signs of pressure ulcers, burns, bruises, or other signs suggesting force. Include a cognitive and neurologic assessment. Document findings with careful notes, drawings, and photographs whenever possible.

Intervention: Focus on Providing the Client With Safety and the Family With Support and Resources
1. Contact the case manager or nurse assigned to Mrs. Smith.
2. Contact the daughter before calling the county's Adult Protective Services (APS).
3. Team up with the nurse if possible to assess the situation and help the daughter obtain help.
4. When meeting with the daughter, acknowledge the stress the family has been under. Offer the family reassurance that the home health staff's role is to help Mrs. Smith get the best care possible.
5. Let the daughter know what her options are but acknowledge the need to call APS (if required by law).
6. Educate the family and prevent abuse by counseling them to avoid isolation at home. Stay involved in other outside activities (e.g., church/synagogue, school, hobbies, friends).
7. Encourage the family to recognize their limits and seek help when and where it is available.

Result: APS referred Mrs. Smith to an adult day health care program covered by Medicaid. She receives her medications, two meals, and programming with other adults during the day while her daughter works.

The daughter received counseling to help cope with her mother's declining health and loss of mental faculties. She also joined an Alzheimer's "36-hour/day" support group. Respite care was arranged through the adult day care program once every 6 weeks.

---

decision-making influenced by shame, guilt, finances, religious beliefs, children, depression, perceptions, and realities. The therapist does not have to be an expert to help someone who is a victim of DV. Identifying the problem for the first time and listening is an important first step.

During intervention procedures, the therapist must be aware that hands-on techniques, such as pushing, pulling, stretching, compressing, touching, and rubbing, may affect a client with a history of abuse in a negative way.

Reporting Abuse. The law is clear in all U.S. states regarding abuse of a minor (under age 18 years) (Box 2.12):

> *When a professional has reasonable cause to suspect, as a result of information received in a professional capacity, that a child is abused or neglected, the matter is to be reported promptly to the department of public health and human services or its local affiliate.*[185]

Guidelines for reporting abuse in adults are not always so clear. Some states require health care professionals to notify law enforcement officials when they have treated any individual for an injury that resulted from a domestic assault. There is much debate over such laws as many DV advocate agencies fear mandated police involvement will discourage injured clients from seeking help. Fear of retaliation may prevent abused persons from seeking needed health care because of required law enforcement involvement.

BOX 2.12 REPORTING CHILD ABUSE

- The law requires professionals to report suspected child abuse and neglect.
- The therapist must know the reporting guidelines for the state in which he or she is practicing.
- Know who to contact in your local child protective service agency and police department.
- The duty to report findings only requires a reasonable suspicion that abuse has occurred, not certainty.[184]
- A professional who delays reporting until doubt is eliminated is in violation of reporting the law.
- The decision about maltreatment is left up to investigating officials, not the reporting professional.

Data from Mudd SS, Findlay JS: The cutaneous manifestations and common mimickers of physical child abuse, *J Pediatr Health Care* 18(3):123–129, 2004; Myers, JE, Berliner, L, Briere, J, Hendrix, CT, Jenny, C, Reid, TA: *The APSAC handbook on child maltreatment.* Thousand Oaks, CA: Sage Publications, 2002.

The therapist should be familiar with state laws or statutes regarding DV for the geographic area in which he or she is practicing. The National Center on Elder Abuse (NCEA) has more information online http://www.aoa.acl.gov/AoA_Programs/Elder_Rights/NCEA/index.aspx

Documentation. Most state laws also provide for the taking of photographs of visible trauma on a child without parental consent. Written permission must be obtained to photograph adults. Always offer to document the evidence of injury. The APTA publications on DV, child abuse, and elder abuse provide reproducible documentation forms and patient resources.[167,185,186]

Even if the client does not want a record of the injury on file, he or she may be persuaded to keep a personal copy for future use if a decision is made to file charges or prosecute at a later time. Polaroid and digital cameras make this easy to accomplish with certainty that the photographs clearly show the extent of the injury or injuries.

The therapist must remember to date and sign the photograph. Record the client's name and injury location on the photograph. Include the client's face in at least one photograph for identification. Include a detailed description (type, size, location, depth) and how the injury/injuries occurred.

Record the client's own words regarding the assault and the assailant. For example, "Ms. Jones states, 'My partner Doug struck me in the head and knocked me down.'" Identifying the presumed assailant in the medical record may help the client pursue legal help.[187]

Resources. Consult your local directory for information about adult and child protection services, state elder abuse hotlines, shelters for the battered, or other community services available in your area. For national information, contact:

- National Domestic Violence Hotline. Available 24 hours/day with information on shelters, legal advocacy and assistance, and social service programs. Available online at www.ndvh.org or 1-800-799-SAFE (1-800-799-7233).
- U.S. Department of Justice. Office on Violence Against Women provides lists of state hotlines, coalitions against domestic violence, and advocacy groups (https://www.justice.gov/ovw).
- Elder Care Locator. Information on senior services. The service links those who need assistance with state and local area agencies on aging and community-based organizations that serve older adults and their caregivers www.eldercare.gov/ or 1-800-677-1116.
- U.S. Department of HHS Administration for Children and Families. Provides fact sheets, laws and policies regarding minors, and phone numbers for reporting abuse. Available online at www.acf.hhs.gov/ or 1-800-4-A-CHILD (1-800-422-4453).

The APTA offers three publications related to domestic violence, available online at www.apta.org (click on Areas of Interest>Publications):

- Guidelines for Recognizing and Providing Care for Victims of Child Abuse (2005)
- Guidelines for Recognizing and Providing Care for Victims of Domestic Abuse (2005)
- Guidelines for Recognizing and Providing Care for Victims of Elder Abuse (2007)

Medical Treatment and Medications

Medical Treatment

Medical treatment includes any intervention performed by a physician (family practitioner or specialist), dentist, physician's assistant, nurse, nurse practitioner, physical therapist, or occupational therapist. The client may also include chiropractic treatment when answering the question:

 FOLLOW-UP QUESTIONS

- What medical treatment have you had for this condition?
- Alternate: What treatment have you had for this condition? (allows the client to report any and all modes of treatment including complementary and alternative medicine)

In addition to eliciting information regarding specific treatment performed by the medical community, follow-up questions related to previous physical therapy treatment include:

? FOLLOW-UP QUESTIONS

- Have you been treated by a physical therapist for this condition before?
- If yes, when, where, and for how long?
- What helped and what did not help?
- Was there any treatment that made your symptoms worse? If yes, please describe.

Knowing the client's response to previous types of treatment techniques may assist the therapist in determining an appropriate treatment protocol for the current chief complaint. For example, previously successful treatment intervention described may provide a basis for initial treatment until the therapist can fully assess the objective data and consider all potential types of treatments.

Medications

Medication use, especially with polypharmacy, is important information. Side effects of medications can present as an impairment of the integumentary, musculoskeletal, cardiovascular/pulmonary, or neuromuscular system. Medications may be the most common or most likely cause of systemically induced NMS signs and symptoms.

Hyperpharmacotherapy is a term that is relatively new in medical practice. Whereas polypharmacy is often defined as the use of multiple medications to treat health problems, the term has also been expanded to describe the use of multiple pharmacies to fill the same (or other) prescriptions, high-frequency medications, or multiple-dose medications. Hyperpharmacotherapy is the current term used to describe the excessive use of drugs to treat disease, including the use of more medications than are clinically indicated or the unnecessary use of medications.

Medications (either prescription, shared, or OTC) may or may not be listed on the Family/Personal History form at all facilities. Even when a medical history form is used, it may be necessary to probe further regarding the use of OTC preparations such as aspirin, acetaminophen (Tylenol), ibuprofen (e.g., Advil, Motrin), laxatives, antihistamines, antacids, and decongestants or other drugs that can alter the client's symptoms.

It is common for adolescents and seniors to share, borrow, or lend medications to friends, family members, and acquaintances. Medication borrowing and sharing is a behavior that has been identified in patients of all ages.[188]

Most of the sharing and borrowing is done without consulting a pharmacist or medical doctor. The risk of allergic reactions or ADEs is much higher under these circumstances than when medications are prescribed and taken as directed by the person for whom they were intended.[189]

Risk Factors for Adverse Drug Events. Pharmacokinetics (the processes that affect drug movement in the body) represents the biggest risk factor for ADEs. An ADE is any unexpected, unwanted, abnormal, dangerous, or harmful reaction or response to a medication. Most ADEs are medication reactions or side effects.

A *drug-drug* interaction occurs when medications interact unfavorably, possibly adding to the pharmacologic effects. A *drug-disease* interaction occurs when a medication causes an existing disease to worsen. Absorption, distribution, metabolism, and excretion are the main components of pharmacokinetics affected by age,[190] size, polypharmacy or hyperpharmacotherapy, and other risk factors listed in Box 2.13.

BOX 2.13   RISK FACTORS FOR ADVERSE DRUG EVENTS (ADES)

- Age (over 65 years, but especially over 75 years)
- Small physical size or stature (decrease in lean body mass)
- Sex (men and women respond differently to different drugs)
- Polypharmacy (taking several drugs at once; duplicate or dual medications) or hyperpharmacotherapy (excessive use of drugs to treat disease)
- Prescribing cascade (failure to recognize signs and symptoms as an ADE and treating it as the onset of a new illness; taking medications to counteract side effects of another medication)
- Taking medications prescribed for someone else
- Organ impairment and dysfunction (e.g., renal or hepatic insufficiency)
- Concomitant alcohol consumption
- Concomitant use of certain nutraceuticals
- Previous history of ADEs
- Mental deterioration or dementia (unintentional repeated dosage; failure to take medications as prescribed)
- Difficulty opening medication bottles, difficulty swallowing, unable to read or understand directions
- Racial/ethnic variations

Ethnic background is a risk factor to consider. Herbal and home remedies may be used by clients based on their ethnic, spiritual, or cultural orientation. Alternative healers may be consulted for all kinds of conditions from diabetes to depression to cancer. Home remedies can be harmful or interact with some medications.

Some racial groups respond differently to medications. Effectiveness and toxicity can vary among racial and ethnic groups. Differences in metabolic rate, clinical drug responses, and side effects of many medications, such as antihistamines, analgesics, cardiovascular agents, psychotropic drugs, and CNS agents, have been documented. Genetic factors also play a role.[191]

Women metabolize drugs differently throughout the month as influenced by hormonal changes associated with menses. There is conflicting data regarding differences in drug metabolism related to menopausal status.[192]

Clients receiving home health care are at increased risk for medication errors such as uncontrolled hypertension despite medication, confusion or falls while taking psychotropic medications, or improper use of medications deemed dangerous to the older adult such as muscle relaxants. Nearly one-third of home health clients are misusing their medications as well.[193]

Potential Drug Side Effects. Side effects are usually defined as predictable pharmacologic effects that occur within therapeutic dose ranges and are undesirable in the given therapeutic situation. Doctors are well aware that drugs have side effects. They may even fully expect their patients to experience some of these side effects. The goal is to obtain maximum benefit from the drug's actions with the minimum amount of side effects. These are referred to as "tolerable" side effects.

The most common side effects of medications are constipation or diarrhea, nausea, abdominal pain, and sedation. More severe reactions include confusion, drowsiness, weakness, and loss of coordination. Medications can mask signs and symptoms or produce signs and symptoms that are seemingly unrelated to the client's current medical problem. For example, long-term use of steroids resulting in side effects, such as proximal muscle weakness, tissue edema, and increased pain threshold, may alter objective findings during the examination of the client.

A detailed description of GI disturbances and other side effects caused by nonsteroidal antiinflammatory drugs (NSAIDs) resulting in back, shoulder, or scapular pain is presented in Chapter 9. Every therapist should be very familiar with these.

Physiologic or biologic differences can result in different responses and side effects to drugs. Race, age, weight, metabolism, and for women, the menstrual cycle can influence drug metabolism and effects. In the aging population, drug side effects can occur even with low doses that usually produce no side effects in younger populations. Older people, especially those who are taking multiple drugs, are two or three times more likely than young to middle-aged adults to have ADEs.

Older clients take OTC medications that may cause confusion, cause or contribute to additional symptoms, and interact with other medications. Sometimes the client is receiving the same drug under different brand names, increasing the likelihood of drug-induced confusion. Watch for the four *D*'s associated with OTC drug use:

- Dizziness
- Drowsiness
- Depression
- Disturbance in vision

Because many older people do not consider these "drugs" worth mentioning (i.e., drugs without prescription "don't count"), it is important to ask specifically about OTC drug use. Additionally, alcoholism and other drug abuse are more common in older people than is generally recognized, especially in depressed clients. Screening for substance use in conjunction with medication use and/or prescription drug abuse may be important for some clients.

Common medications in the clinic that produce other signs and symptoms include:

- Skin reactions, noninflammatory joint pain (antibiotics; see Fig. 4.12)
- Muscle weakness/cramping (diuretics)
- Muscle hyperactivity (caffeine and medications with caffeine)
- Back and/or shoulder pain (NSAIDs; retroperitoneal bleeding)
- Hip pain from femoral head necrosis (corticosteroids)
- Gait disturbances (Thorazine/tranquilizers)
- Movement disorders (anticholinergics, antipsychotics, antidepressants)
- Hormonal contraceptives (elevated blood pressure)
- GI symptoms (nausea, indigestion, abdominal pain, melena)

This is just a partial listing, but it gives an idea of why paying attention to medications and potential side effects is important in the screening process. Not all, but some, medications (e.g., antibiotics, antihypertensives, antidepressants) must be taken as prescribed to obtain pharmacologic efficacy.

Nonsteroidal Antiinflammatory Drugs. NSAIDs are a group of drugs that are useful in the symptomatic treatment of inflammation; some appear to be more useful as analgesics. OTC NSAIDs are listed in Table 9.3. NSAIDs are commonly used postoperatively to alleviate discomfort; for painful musculoskeletal conditions, especially among the older adult population; and in the treatment of inflammatory rheumatic diseases.

NSAID use is widespread. It has been reported that in the United States, 70 million prescriptions and over 30 billion OTC pills are sold every year.[194]

Side Effects of NSAIDs. In 2015, the FDA strengthened its earlier warning regarding the risk of heart attack and stroke with NSAID use. This included instructions to update warning labels and Drug Facts labels.[195] The FDA instructs clients to seek immediate medical attention if they experience symptoms consistent with a heart attack or stroke—chest pain, breathing difficulty, weakness on one side of the body, or slurred speech.[195]

This increased risk for heart attack and strokes can occur as early as the first week of taking the drug, and may increase at higher doses or longer NSAID use. The risk occurs for individuals with or without heart disease or risk factors for heart disease. Those with a history or risk factors, however, are at an increased risk; patients with a first time heart attack who were treated with NSAIDs were reported to have an increased risk of dying in the first year after the heart attack compared with those who had a first time heart attack but were not treated with NSAIDs.[195]

Older adults taking NSAIDs and antihypertensive agents must be monitored carefully. Regardless of the NSAID chosen, it is important to check blood pressure when exercise is initiated and periodically afterward.

Another major side effect of NSAID use pertains to adverse reactions affecting the GI tract. Additional information about this can be found in Chapter 9.

CLINICAL SIGNS AND SYMPTOMS
NSAID Complications

- May be asymptomatic
- May cause confusion and memory loss in the older adult

Gastrointestinal
- Indigestion, heartburn, epigastric or abdominal pain
- Esophagitis, dysphagia, odynophagia
- Nausea
- Unexplained fatigue lasting more than 1 or 2 weeks
- Ulcers (gastric, duodenal), perforations, bleeding
- Melena

Renal
- Polyuria
- Nausea, pallor
- Edema, dehydration
- Muscle weakness, restless legs syndrome

Integumentary
- Pruritus (symptom of renal impairment)
- Delayed wound healing
- Skin reaction to light (photodermatitis)

Cardiovascular/Pulmonary
- Elevated blood pressure
- Peripheral edema
- Asthma attacks in individuals with asthma

Musculoskeletal
- Increased symptoms after taking the medication
- Symptoms linked with ingestion of food (increased or decreased, depending on location of GI ulcer)
- Midthoracic back, shoulder, or scapular pain
- Neuromuscular
- Muscle weakness (sign of renal impairment)
- Restless legs syndrome (sign of renal impairment)
- Paresthesias (sign of renal impairment)

Screening for Risk Factors and Effects of NSAIDs. Screening for risk factors is as important as looking for clinical manifestations of NSAID-induced complications. High-risk individuals are older with a history of ulcers and any coexisting diseases that increase the potential for GI bleeding.

Anyone receiving treatment with multiple NSAIDs is at an increased risk, especially if the dosage is high and/or includes aspirin.

As with any risk-factor assessment, we must know what to look for before we can recognize signs of impending trouble. In the case of NSAID use, back and/or shoulder pain can be the first symptom of impairment in its clinical presentation. Look for the presence of associated GI distress such as indigestion, heartburn, nausea, unexplained chronic fatigue, and/or melena (tarry, sticky, black or dark stools from oxidized blood in the GI tract). Correlate increased musculoskeletal symptoms after taking medications. Expect to see a decrease (not an increase) in painful symptoms after taking analgesics or NSAIDs. Ask about any change in pain or symptoms (increase or decrease) after eating (anywhere from 30 minutes to 2 hours later).

Ingestion of food should not affect the musculoskeletal tissues, so any change in symptoms that can be consistently linked with food raises a red flag, especially for the client with known GI problems or taking NSAIDs.

The peak effect for NSAIDs, when used as an *analgesic* varies from product to product. For example, peak analgesic effect of aspirin is 2 hours, whereas the peak for naproxen sodium (Aleve) is 2 to 4 hours (compared with acetaminophen, which peaks in 30 to 60 minutes). Therefore the symptoms may occur at varying lengths of time after ingestion of food or drink. It is best to find out the peak time for each antiinflammatory taken by the client and note if maximal relief of symptoms occurs in association with that time.

The time to effect *underlying tissue impairment* also varies by individual and severity of impairment. There is a big difference between 220 mg (OTC) and 500 mg (by prescription) of naproxen sodium. For example, 220 mg may appear to "do nothing" in the client's subjective assessment (opinion) after a week's dosing.

What most adults do not know is that it takes more than 24 to 48 hours to build up a high enough level in the body to affect inflammatory symptoms. The person may start adding more drugs before an effective level has been reached in the body. Five hundred milligrams (500 mg) can affect tissue in a shorter time, especially with an acute event or flare-up; this is one reason why doctors sometimes dispense prescription NSAIDs instead of just using the lower dose OTC drugs.

Older adults taking NSAIDs and antihypertensive agents must be monitored carefully. Regardless of the NSAID chosen, it is important to check blood pressure when exercise is initiated and periodically afterward.

Ask about muscle weakness, unusual fatigue, restless legs syndrome, polyuria, nocturia, or pruritus (signs and symptoms of renal failure). Watch for increased blood pressure and peripheral edema (perform a visual inspection of the feet and ankles). Document and report any significant findings.

Acetaminophen. Acetaminophen, the active ingredient in Tylenol and other OTC and prescription pain relievers and cold medicines, is an analgesic (pain reliever) and antipyretic (fever reducer), but not an antiinflammatory agent.

Acetaminophen is effective in the treatment of mild-to-moderate pain and is generally well tolerated by all age groups.

It is the analgesic least likely to cause GI bleeding, but taken in large doses over time, it can cause liver toxicity, especially when used with vitamin C or alcohol. Women are more quickly affected than men at lower levels of alcohol consumption.

Individuals at increased risk for problems associated with using acetaminophen are those with a history of alcohol use/abuse, anyone with a history of liver disease (e.g., cirrhosis, hepatitis), and anyone who has attempted suicide using an overdose of this medication.[196]

Some medications (e.g., phenytoin, isoniazid) taken in conjunction with acetaminophen can trigger liver toxicity. The effects of oral anticoagulants may be potentiated by chronic ingestion of large doses of acetaminophen.[197]

Clients with acetaminophen toxicity may be asymptomatic or have anorexia, mild nausea, and vomiting. The therapist may ask about right upper abdominal quadrant tenderness, jaundice, and other signs and symptoms of liver impairment (e.g., liver palms, asterixis, carpal tunnel syndrome, spider angiomas); see discussion in Chapter 10.

Corticosteroids. Corticosteroids are often confused with the singular word "steroids." There are three types or classes of steroids:

1. Anabolic-androgenic steroids such as testosterone, estrogen, and progesterone.
2. Mineralocorticoids responsible for maintaining body electrolytes.
3. Glucocorticoids, which suppress inflammatory processes within the body.

All three types are naturally occurring hormones produced by the adrenal cortex; synthetic equivalents can be prescribed as medication. Illegal use of a synthetic derivative of testosterone is a concern with athletes and millions of men and women who use these drugs to gain muscle and lose body fat.[198]

Corticosteroids used to control pain and reduce inflammation are associated with significant side effects even when given for a short time. Administration may be by local injection (e.g., into a joint), transdermal (skin patch), or systemic (inhalers or pill form).

Side effects of *local injection* (catabolic glucocorticoids) may include soft tissue atrophy, changes in skin pigmentation, accelerated joint destruction, and tendon rupture, but it poses no problem with liver, kidney, or cardiovascular function. *Transdermal* corticosteroids have similar side effects. The incidence of skin-related changes is slightly higher than with local injection, whereas the incidence of joint problems is slightly lower.

Systemic corticosteroids are associated with GI problems, psychologic problems, and hip avascular necrosis. Physician referral is required for marked loss of hip motion and referred pain to the groin in a client taking systemic corticosteroids long-term.

Long-term use can lead to immunosuppression, osteoporosis, and other endocrine-metabolic abnormalities.

Therapists working with athletes may need to screen for non-medical (illegal) use of anabolic steroids. Visually observe for signs and symptoms associated with anabolic steroid use. Monitor behavior and blood pressure.

CLINICAL SIGNS AND SYMPTOMS
Anabolic Steroid Use

- Rapid weight gain
- Elevated blood pressure (BP)
- Peripheral edema associated with increased BP
- Acne on face and upper body
- Muscular hypertrophy
- Stretch marks around trunk
- Abdominal pain, diarrhea
- Needle marks in large muscle groups
- Personality changes (aggression, mood swings, "roid" rages)
- Bladder irritation, urinary frequency, urinary tract infections
- Sleep apnea, insomnia
- Altered ejection fraction (lower end of normal: under 55%)[198]

Opioids. Opioids, such as codeine, morphine, tramadol, hydrocodone, or oxycodone are typically prescribed to treat pain. It should be noted that there is scant evidence that supports opioids' superiority in pain management,[199,200] and that prescribing opioids for acute pain in opioid naïve patients has partially fueled long-term use patterns.[201]

They do not cause kidney, liver, or stomach impairments and have few drug interactions. Side effects can include nausea, constipation, and dry mouth. The client may also experience impaired balance and drowsiness or dizziness, which can increase the risk of falls. Most commonly, opioids cause constipation and nausea.[202]

Addiction (physical or psychologic dependence) is often a concern raised by clients and family members alike. Addiction to opioids is uncommon in individuals with no history of substance abuse, but dependence can occur after only 5 days of taking opioids.[201] The physical therapist should therefore be aware of withdrawal symptoms, such as rebound pain, in patients that stop or taper from opioids, even after taking them for a relatively short time. When compared to younger adults, older adults obtain greater pain control with lower doses and develop less tolerance than younger adults.[203] However, it does not appear that opioids are any more beneficial than nonopioids for the management of pain in patients with moderate to severe chronic low back pain, hip, or knee pain.[204]

Prescription Drug Abuse. The U.S. Drug Enforcement Administration has reported that more than 7 million Americans abuse prescription medications.[205] The CDC reports opioid drug overdose as the second leading cause of accidental death in the United States (second only to motor vehicle accidents). Opioid misuse and dependence among prescription opioid patients in the United States are likely higher than currently documented.[206] Medical and nonmedical prescription drug abuse has become an increasing problem, especially among young adolescents and teenagers.[207]

Oxycodone, hydrocodone, methadone, benzodiazepines, and muscle relaxants used to treat pain and anxiety and stimulants used to treat learning disorders are listed as the most common medications involved in nonmedical use.[208,209] Prescription opioids are monitored carefully and withdrawn or stopped gradually to avoid withdrawal symptoms.

Risk factors for prescription drug abuse and nonmedical use of prescription drugs include age under 65 years, previous history of opioid abuse, major depression, and psychotropic medication use.[206] Teen users raiding the family medicine cabinet for prescription medications (a practice referred to as "pharming") often find a wide range of mood stabilizers, painkillers, muscle relaxants, sedatives, and tranquilizers right within their own homes. Combining medications and/or combining prescription medicines with alcohol can lead to serious drug-drug interactions[210]

Hormonal Contraceptives. Some women use birth control pills to prevent pregnancy, whereas others take them to control their menstrual cycle and/or manage premenstrual and menstrual symptoms, including excessive and painful bleeding.

Originally, birth control pills contained as much as 20% more estrogen than the amount present in the low-dose, third-generation oral contraceptives available today. Women taking the newer hormonal contraceptives (whether in pill, injectable, or patch form) have a slightly increased risk of high blood pressure, and the risk is higher in women with a family history of hypertension or in those who have mild kidney disease.[211] Individuals using the injectable Depo-Provera are at risk for bone loss, which is particularly concerning in adolescents and older adults.[212] Anyone taking hormonal contraception of any kind, but especially premenopausal cardiac clients, must be monitored by taking vital signs, especially blood pressure, during physical activity and exercise. Assessing for risk factors is an important part of the plan of care for this group of individuals.

Any woman on combined oral contraceptives (estrogen and progesterone) reporting breakthrough bleeding should be advised to see her doctor.

Antibiotics. Skin reactions (see Fig. 4.12) and noninflammatory joint pain (see Box 3.4) are two of the most common side effects of antibiotics seen in a therapist's practice. Often these symptoms are delayed and occur up to 6 weeks after the client has finished taking the drug.

Fluoroquinolones, a class of antibiotics used to treat bacterial infections (e.g., urinary tract; upper respiratory tract; infectious diarrhea; gynecologic infections; and skin, soft tissue, bone and joint infections) are known to cause tendinopathies ranging from tendinitis to tendon rupture.

Commonly prescribed fluoroquinolones include ciprofloxacin (Cipro), ciprofloxacin extended-release (Cipro ER, Proquin XR), gemifloxacin (Factive), levofloxacin (Levaquin), norfloxacin (Noroxin), ofloxacin (Floxin), and moxifloxacin (Avelox). Although tendon injury has been reported with most fluoroquinolones, most of the fluoroquinolone-induced tendinopathies of the Achilles tendon are caused by ciprofloxacin.

The incidence of this adverse event has been enough that in 2008, the U.S. FDA required makers of fluoroquinolone antimicrobial drugs for systemic use to add a boxed warning to the prescribing information about the increased risk of developing tendinitis and tendon rupture. At the same time, the FDA issued a notice to health care professionals about this risk, the known risk factors, and what to advise anyone taking these medications who report tendon pain, swelling, or inflammation (i.e., stop taking the fluoroquinolone, avoid exercise and use of the affected area, promptly contact the prescribing physician).[213]

Other common side effects include depression, headache, convulsions, fatigue, GI disturbance (nausea, vomiting, diarrhea), arthralgia (joint pain, inflammation, and stiffness), yeast infections, and neck, back, or chest pain (Case Example 2.9).

Nutraceuticals. Nutraceuticals are natural products (usually made from plant substances) that do not require a prescription to purchase. They are often sold at health food

---

CASE EXAMPLE 2.9

Fluoroquinolone-Induced Tendinopathy

A 57-year-old retired army colonel (male) presented to an outpatient physical therapy clinic with a report of swelling and pain in both ankles.

Symptoms started in the left ankle 4 days ago. Then the right ankle and foot became swollen. Ankle dorsiflexion and weight-bearing made it worse. Staying off the foot made it better.

Past Medical History
- Prostatitis diagnosed and treated 2 months ago with antibiotics; placed on levofloxacin
- 11 days ago when urinary symptoms recurred
- Chronic benign prostatic hypertrophy
- Gastroesophageal reflux (GERD)
- Hypertension

Current Medications
- Omeprazole (Prilosec)
- Lisinopril (Prinivil, Zestril)
- Enteric-coated aspirin
- Tamsulosin (Flomax)
- Levofloxacin (Levaquin)

Clinical Presentation
- Moderate swelling of both ankles; malleoli diminished visually by 50%
- No lymphadenopathy (cervical, axillary, inguinal)
- Fullness of both Achilles tendons with pitting edema of the feet extending to just above the ankles, bilaterally
- No nodularity behind either Achilles tendon
- Ankle joint tender to minimal palpation; reproduced when Achilles tendons are palpated
- Range of motion (ROM): normal subtalar and plantar flexion of the ankle; dorsiflexion to neutral (limited by pain); inversion and eversion within normal limits (WNL) and pain-free; unable to squat because of painfully limited ROM
- Neuro screen: negative
- Knee screen: no apparent problems in either knee

Associated Signs and Symptoms: The client reports fever and chills the day before the ankle started swelling, but this has gone away now. Urinary symptoms have resolved. Reports no other signs or symptoms anywhere else in his body.

Vital Signs
- Blood pressure 128/74 mm Hg taken seated in the left arm
- Heart rate 78 bpm
- Respiratory rate 14 breaths per minute
- Temperature 99.0° F (client states "normal" for him is 98.6° F)

What Are the Red-Flag Signs and Symptoms Here? Should a Medical Referral Be Made? Why or Why Not?

Red Flags:
- Age
- Bilateral swelling
- Recent history of new medication (levofloxacin) known to cause tendon problems in some cases
- Constitutional symptoms × 1 day; presence of low-grade fever at the time of the initial evaluation

A cluster of red flags like this suggests medical referral would be a good idea before initiating intervention. If there is an inflammatory process going on, early diagnosis and medical treatment can minimize damage to the joint.

If there is a medical problem, it is not likely to be life-threatening, so theoretically the therapist could treat symptomatically for three to five sessions and then evaluate the results. Medical referral could be made at that time if symptoms remain unchanged by treatment. If this option is chosen, the client's vital signs must be monitored closely.

Decision: The client was referred to his primary care physician with the following request:

Date
Dr. Smith,

This client came to our clinic with a report of bilateral ankle swelling. I observed the following findings:

Moderate swelling of both ankles; malleoli diminished visually by 50%

No lymphadenopathy (cervical, axillary, inguinal)

Fullness of both Achilles tendons with pitting edema of the feet extending to just above the ankles, bilaterally

No nodularity behind either Achilles tendon

Ankle joint tender to minimal palpation; reproduced when Achilles tendons are palpated

ROM: normal subtalar and plantar flexion of the ankle; dorsiflexion to neutral (limited by pain); inversion and eversion WNL and pain-free; unable to squat due to painfully limited ROM

Neuro screen: negative

Knee screen: no apparent problems in either knee

Associated Signs and Symptoms:

The client reports fever and chills the day before the ankle started swelling, but this went away by the time he came to physical therapy. Urinary symptoms also had resolved. The client reported no other signs or symptoms anywhere else in his body.

Vital signs

Blood pressure	128/74 mm Hg taken seated in the left arm
Heart rate	78 bpm
Respiratory rate	14 breaths per minute
Temperature	99.0° F (client states "normal" for him is 98.6° F)

I'm concerned by the following cluster of red flags:
Age
Bilateral swelling
Recent history of new medication (levofloxacin)
Constitutional symptoms × 1 day; presence of low-grade fever at the time of the initial evaluation
I would like to request a medical evaluation before beginning any physical therapy intervention. I would appreciate a copy of your report and any recommendations you may have if physical therapy is appropriate.
Thank you. Best regards,

Result: The client was diagnosed (x-rays and diagnostic laboratory work) with levofloxacin-induced bilateral Achilles tendonitis. Medical treatment included NSAIDs, rest, and discontinuation of the levofloxacin.

Symptoms resolved completely within 7 days with full motion and function of both ankles and feet. There was no need for physical therapy intervention. Client was discharged from any further PT involvement for this episode of care.

Recommended Reading: Greene BL: Physical therapist management of fluoroquinolone-induced Achilles tendinopathy, **Phys Ther** 82(12):1224–1231, 2002.

Data from McKinley BT, Oglesby RJ: A 57-year-old male retired colonel with acute ankle swelling, *Mil Med* 169(3):254–256, 2004.

---

stores, nutrition or vitamin stores, through private distributors, or on the Internet. Nutraceuticals consist of herbs, vitamins, minerals, antioxidants, and other natural supplements.

The use of herbal and other supplements has increased dramatically in the last two decades. These products may be produced with all natural ingredients, but this does not mean they do not cause problems, complications, and side effects. When combined with certain food items or taken with some prescription drugs, nutraceuticals can have potentially serious complications.

Herbal and home remedies may be used by clients based on their ethnic, spiritual, or cultural orientation. Alternative healers may be consulted for all kinds of conditions from diabetes to depression to cancer. Home remedies and nutraceuticals can be harmful when combined with some medications. The therapist should ask clients about and document their use of nutraceuticals and dietary supplements.

 FOLLOW-UP QUESTIONS

- Are you taking any remedies from a naturopathic physician or homeopathic healer?
- Are you taking any other vitamins, herbs, or supplements?
- If yes, does your physician have a list of these products?
- Are you seeing anyone else for this condition (e.g., alternative practitioner, such as an acupuncturist, massage therapist, or chiropractor, or Reiki, BodyTalk, Touch for Healing, or Ayurveda practitioner)?

A pharmacist can help in comparing signs and symptoms present with possible side effects and drug-drug or drug-nutraceutical interactions. The Mayo Clinic offers information about herbal supplements.[214]

The Physical Therapist's Role. For every client, the therapist is strongly encouraged to take the time to look up indications for use and possible side effects of prescribed medications. Information regarding drugs is easily searchable online. Drug reference guidebooks that are updated and published every year are available in hospital and clinic libraries or pharmacies. Pharmacists are also invaluable sources of drug information. Websites with useful drug information are included in the next section (see Resources).

Distinguishing drug-related signs and symptoms from disease-related symptoms may require careful observation and consultation with family members or other health care professionals to see whether these signs tend to increase following each dose.[215] This information may come to light by asking the question:

 FOLLOW-UP QUESTIONS

- Do you notice any increase in symptoms, or perhaps the start of symptoms, after taking your medications? (This may occur 30 minutes to 2 hours after taking the drug.)

Because clients are more likely now than ever before to change physicians or practitioners during an episode of care, the therapist has an important role in education and screening. The therapist can alert individuals to watch for any red flags in their drug regimen. Clients with both hypertension and a condition requiring NSAID therapy should be closely monitored and advised to make sure the prescribing practitioner is aware of both conditions.

The therapist may find it necessary to reeducate the client regarding the importance of taking medications as prescribed, whether on a daily or other regular basis. In the case of antihypertensive medication, the therapist should ask whether the client has taken the medication today as prescribed.

It is not unusual to hear a client report, "I take my blood pressure pills when I feel my heart starting to pound." The same situation may occur with clients taking anti-inflammatory drugs, antibiotics, or any other medications that must be taken consistently for a specified period to be effective. Always ask the client if he or she is taking the prescription every day or just as needed. Make sure this is with the physician's knowledge and approval.

Clients may be taking medications that were not prescribed for them, taking medications inappropriately, or not taking prescribed medications without notifying the doctor. Appropriate FUPs include the following:

 FOLLOW-UP QUESTIONS

- Why are you taking these medications?
- When was the last time that you took these medications?
- Have you taken these drugs today?
- Do the medications relieve your pain or symptoms?
- If yes, how soon after you take the medications do you notice an improvement?
- If prescription drugs, who prescribed this medication for you?
- How long have you been taking these medications?
- When did your physician last review these medications?
- Are you taking any medications that were not prescribed for you?
  - If no, follow-up with: Are you taking any pills given to you by someone else other than your doctor?

Many people who take prescribed medications cannot recall the name of the drug or tell you why they are taking it. It is essential to know whether the client has taken OTC or prescription medication before the physical therapy examination or intervention because the symptomatic relief or possible side effects may alter the objective findings.

Similarly, when appropriate, treatment can be scheduled to correspond with the time of day when clients obtain maximal relief from their medications. Finally, the therapist may be the first one to recognize a problem with medication or dosage. Bringing this to the attention of the doctor is a valuable service to the client.

Resources. Many resources are available to help the therapist identify potential side effects of medications, especially in the presence of polypharmacy or hyperpharmacotherapy with the possibility of drug interactions.

Find a local pharmacist willing to answer questions about medications. The pharmacist can let the therapist know when associated signs and symptoms may be drug-related. Always bring this to the physician's attention. It may be that the "burden of tolerable side effects" is worth the benefit, but often, the dosage can be adjusted or an alternative drug can be tried.

Several resources include *Mosby's Nursing Drug Handbook*, published each year by Elsevier Science (Mosby, St. Louis), *PDR for Herbal Medicines ed 6*[216] and *Pharmacology in Rehabilitation*.[215]

A helpful general guide regarding potentially inappropriate medications for older adults called the Beers' list has been published and revised. This list along with detailed information about each class of drug is available online at: https://www.dcri.org/trial-participation/the-beers-list/.

Easy-to-use websites for helpful pharmacologic information include:

- MedicineNet (www.medicinenet.com)
- University of Montana Drug Information Service (DIS) (www.umt.edu/druginfo or by phone: 1-800-501-5491) (our personal favorite—an excellent resource)

- RxList: The Internet Drug Index (www.rxlist.com)
- DrugDigest (www.drugdigest.com)
- National Council on Patient Information and Education: BeMedWise. Advice on use of OTC medications. Available online at www.bemedwise.org.

Current Level of Fitness

An assessment of current physical activity and level of fitness (or level just before the onset of the current problem) can provide additional necessary information relating to the origin of the client's symptom complex.

The level of fitness can be a valuable indicator of potential response to treatment based on the client's motivation (i.e., those who are more physically active and healthy seem to be more motivated to return to that level of fitness through disciplined self-rehabilitation).

It is important to know what type of exercise or sports activity the client participates in, the number of times per week (frequency) that this activity is performed, the length (duration) of each exercise or sports session, how long the client has been exercising (weeks, months, years), and the level of difficulty of each exercise session (intensity). It is very important to ask:

 FOLLOW-UP QUESTIONS

- Since the onset of symptoms, are there any activities that you can no longer accomplish?

The client should describe these activities including how physical activities have been affected by the symptoms. Follow-up questions include:

 FOLLOW-UP QUESTIONS

- Do you ever experience shortness of breath or lack of air during any activities (e.g., walking, climbing stairs)?
- Are you ever short of breath without exercising?
- Are you ever awakened at night breathless?
- If yes, how often and when does this occur?

If the Family/Personal History form is not used, it may be helpful to ask some of the questions shown in Fig. 2.2: Work/Living Environment or History of Falls. For example, assessing the history of falls with older people is essential. One-third of community-dwelling older adults and a higher proportion of institutionalized older people fall annually. Aside from the serious injuries that may result, a debilitating "fear of falling" may cause many older adults to reduce their activity level and restrict their social life. This is one area that is often treatable and even preventable with physical therapy.

Older persons who are in bed for prolonged periods are at risk for secondary complications, including pressure ulcers, urinary tract infections, pulmonary infections and/or infarcts, congestive heart failure, osteoporosis, and compression fractures. See previous discussion in this chapter on History of Falls for more information.

Sleep-Related History

Sleep patterns are valuable indicators of underlying physiologic and psychologic disease processes. The primary function of sleep is believed to be the restoration of body function. When the quality of this restorative sleep is decreased, the body and mind cannot perform at optimal levels.

Physical problems that result in pain, increased urination, shortness of breath, changes in body temperature, perspiration, or side effects of medications are just a few causes of sleep disruption. Any factor precipitating sleep deprivation can contribute to an increase in the frequency, intensity, or duration of a client's symptoms.

For example, fevers and sweats are characteristic signs of systemic disease. Sweats occur as a result of a gradual increase in body temperature followed by a sudden drop in temperature; although they are most noticeable at night, sweats can occur anytime of the day or night. This change in body temperature can be related to pathologic changes in immunologic, neurologic, or endocrine function.

Be aware that many people, especially women, experience sweats associated with menopause, poor room ventilation, or too many clothes and covers used at night. Sweats can also occur in the neutropenic client after chemotherapy or as a side effect of other medications such as some antidepressants, sedatives or tranquilizers, and some analgesics.

Anyone reporting sweats of a systemic origin must be asked if the same phenomenon occurs during the waking hours. Sweats (present day and/or night) can be associated with medical problems such as tuberculosis, autoimmune disease, and malignancy.[217]

An isolated experience of sweats is not as significant as intermittent but consistent sweats in the presence of risk factors for any of these conditions or in the presence of other constitutional symptoms (see Box 1.3). Assess vital signs in the client reporting sweats, especially when other symptoms are present and/or the client reports back or shoulder pain of unknown cause.

Certain neurologic lesions may produce local changes in sweating associated with nerve distribution. For example, a client with a spinal cord tumor may report changes in skin temperature above and below the level of the tumor. At presentation, any client with a history of either sweats or fevers should be referred to the primary physician. This is especially true for clients with back pain or multiple joint pain without traumatic origin.

Pain at night is usually perceived as being more intense because of the lack of outside distraction when the person lies quietly without activity. The sudden quiet surroundings and lack of external activity create an increased perception of pain that is a major disrupter of sleep.

It is very important to ask the client about pain during the night. Is the person able to get to sleep? If not, the pain may be a primary focus and may become continuously intense so that falling asleep is a problem.

 FOLLOW-UP QUESTIONS

- Does a change in body position affect the level of pain?

If a change in position can increase or decrease the level of pain, it is likely to be a musculoskeletal problem. If, however, the client is awakened from a deep sleep by pain in any location that is unrelated to physical trauma and is unaffected by a change in position, this may be an ominous sign of serious systemic disease, particularly cancer. FUPs include:

 FOLLOW-UP QUESTIONS

- If you wake up because of pain, is it because you rolled onto that side?
- Can you get back to sleep?
- If yes, what do you have to do (if anything) to get back to sleep? (This answer may provide clues for treatment.)

Many other factors (primarily environmental and psychologic) are associated with sleep disturbance, but a good, basic assessment of the main characteristics of physically related disturbances in sleep pattern can provide valuable information related to treatment or referral decisions. The McGill Home Recording Card (see Fig. 3.7) is a helpful tool for evaluating sleep patterns.

Stress (see also Chapter 3)

By using the interviewing tools and techniques described in this chapter, the therapist can communicate a willingness to consider all aspects of illness, whether biologic or psychologic. Client self-disclosure is unlikely if there is no trust in the health professional, if there is fear of a lack of confidentiality, or if a sense of disinterest is noted.

Most symptoms (pain included) are aggravated by unresolved emotional or psychologic stress. Prolonged stress may gradually lead to physiologic changes. Stress may result in depression, anxiety disorders, and behavioral consequences (e.g., smoking, alcohol and substance abuse, accident proneness).

The effects of emotional stress may be increased by physiologic changes brought on by the use of medications or poor diet and health habits (e.g., cigarette smoking or ingestion of caffeine in any form). As part of the Core Interview, the therapist may assess the client's subjective report of stress by asking:

 FOLLOW-UP QUESTIONS

- What major life changes or stresses have you encountered that you would associate with your injury/illness?
- Alternate: What situations in your life are "stressors" for you?
- It may be helpful to quantify the stress by asking the client:
- On a scale of 0 to 10, with 0 being no stress and 10 being the most extreme stress you have ever experienced, what number rating would you give your stress in general at this time in your life?
- What number would you give your stress level today?

Emotions, such as fear and anxiety, are common reactions to illness and treatment intervention and may increase the client's awareness of pain and symptoms. These emotions may cause autonomic (branch of nervous system not subject to voluntary control) distress manifested in such symptoms as pallor, restlessness, muscular tension, perspiration, stomach pain, diarrhea or constipation, or headaches.

It may be helpful to screen for anxiety-provoked hyperventilation by asking:

 ## FOLLOW-UP QUESTIONS

- Do you ever get short of breath or dizzy or lose coordination when you are fatigued?

After the objective evaluation has been completed, the therapist can often provide some relief of emotionally amplified symptoms by explaining the cause of pain, outlining a plan of care, and providing a realistic prognosis for improvement. This may not be possible if the client demonstrates signs of hysterical symptoms or conversion symptoms (see discussion in Chapter 3).

Whether the client's symptoms are systemic or caused by an emotional/psychologic overlay, if the client does not respond to treatment, it may be necessary to notify the physician that there is not a satisfactory explanation for the client's complaints. Further medical evaluation may be indicated at that time.

Final Questions

It is always a good idea to finalize the interview by reviewing the findings and paraphrasing what the client has reported. This gives the client a chance to agree with or refute the clinician's understanding of the facts. Use the answers from the Core Interview to recall specifics about the location, frequency, intensity, and duration of the symptoms. Mention what makes it better or worse.

Recap the medical and surgical history including current illnesses, diseases, or other medical conditions; recent or past surgeries; recent or current medications; recent infections; and anything else of importance brought out by the interview process.

It is always appropriate to end the interview with a few final questions such as:

 ## FOLLOW-UP QUESTIONS

- Are there any other symptoms of any kind anywhere else in your body that we have not discussed yet?
- Is there anything else you think is important about your condition that we have not discussed yet?
- Is there anything else you think I should know?

If you have not asked any questions about assault or partner abuse, this may be the appropriate time to screen for DV.

Special Questions for Women

Gynecologic disorders can refer pain to the low back, hip, pelvis, groin, or sacroiliac joint. Any woman having pain or symptoms in any one or more of these areas should be screened for possible systemic diseases. The need to screen for systemic disease is essential when there is no known cause of pain or symptoms.

Any woman with a positive family/personal history of cancer should be screened for medical disease even if the current symptoms can be attributed to a known NMS cause.

Chapter 15 has a list of special questions to ask women (see also Appendix B-37 in the accompanying enhanced eBook version included with print purchase of this textbook). The therapist will not need to ask every woman each question listed but should take into consideration the data from the Family/Personal History form, Core Interview, and clinical presentation when choosing appropriate FUPs.

Special Questions for Men

Men describing symptoms related to the groin, low back, hip, or sacroiliac joint may have prostate or urologic involvement. A positive response to any or all of the questions in Appendix B-24 in the accompanying enhanced eBook version included with print purchase of this textbook must be evaluated further. Answers to these questions correlated with family history, the presence of risk factors, clinical presentation, and any red flags will guide the therapist in making a decision regarding treatment versus referral.

HOSPITAL INPATIENT INFORMATION

Medical Record

Treatment of hospital inpatients or residents in other facilities (e.g., step-down units, transition units, extended care facilities) requires a slightly different interview (or information-gathering) format. A careful review of the medical record for information will assist the therapist in developing a safe and effective plan of care. Watch for conflicting reports (e.g., emergency department, history and physical, consult reports). Important information to look for might include:

- Age
- Medical diagnosis
- Surgery report
- Physician's/nursing notes
- Associated or additional problems relevant to physical therapy
- Medications
- Current precautions/restrictions
- Laboratory results
- Vital signs

An evaluation of the patient's medical status in conjunction with age and diagnosis can provide valuable guidelines for the plan of care.

If the patient has had recent surgery, the physician's report should be scanned for preoperative and postoperative orders (in some cases there is a separate physician's orders book or link to click on if the medical records are in an electronic format). Read the operative report whenever available. Look for any of the following information:

- Was the patient treated preoperatively with physical therapy for gait, strength, range of motion, or other objective assessments?
- Were there any unrelated preoperative conditions?
- Was the surgery invasive, a closed procedure via arthroscopy, fluoroscopy, or other means of imaging, or virtual by means of computerized technology?
- How long was the operative procedure?
- How much fluid and/or blood products were given?
- What position was the patient placed in during the procedure?

Fluid received during surgery may affect arterial oxygenation, leaving the person breathless with minimal exertion and experiencing early muscle fatigue. Prolonged time in any one position can result in residual musculoskeletal complaints.

The surgical position for men and women during laparoscopy (examination of the peritoneal cavity) may place patients at increased risk for thrombophlebitis because of the decreased blood flow to the legs during surgery.

Other valuable information that may be contained in the physician's report may include:

- What are the current short-term and long-term medical treatment plans?
- Are there any known or listed contraindications to physical therapy intervention?
- Does the patient have any weight-bearing limitations?

Associated or additional problems to the primary diagnosis may be found within the record (e.g., diabetes, heart disease, peripheral vascular disease, respiratory involvement). The physical therapist should look for any of these conditions to modify exercise accordingly and to watch for any related signs and symptoms that might affect the exercise program:

- Are there complaints of any kind that may affect exercise (e.g., shortness of breath [dyspnea], heart palpitations, rapid heart rate [tachycardia], fatigue, fever, or anemia)?

If the patient has diabetes, the therapist should ask:

- What are the current blood glucose levels and recent A1C levels?
- When is insulin administered?

Avoiding peak insulin levels in planning exercise schedules is discussed more completely in Chapter 12. Other questions related to medications can follow the Core Interview outline with appropriate follow-up questions:

- Is the patient receiving oxygen or receiving fluids/medications through an intravenous line?
- If the patient is receiving oxygen, will he or she need increased oxygen levels before, during, or following physical therapy? What level(s)? Does the patient have chronic obstructive pulmonary disease with restrictions on oxygen use?
- Are there any dietary or fluid restrictions?

If so, check with the nursing staff to determine the full limitations. For example:

- Are ice chips or wet washcloths permissible?
- How many ounces or milliliters of fluid are allowed during therapy?
- Where should this amount be recorded?

Laboratory values and vital signs should be reviewed. For example:

- Is the patient anemic?
- Is the patient's blood pressure stable?

Anemic patients may demonstrate an increased normal resting pulse rate that should be monitored during exercise. Patients with unstable blood pressure may require initial standing with a tilt table or monitoring of the blood pressure before, during, and after treatment. Check the nursing record for pulse rate at rest and blood pressure to use as a guide when taking vital signs in the clinic or at the patient's bedside.

Nursing Assessment

After reading the patient's chart, check with the nursing staff to determine the nursing assessment of the individual patient. The essential components of the nursing assessment that are of value to the therapist may include:

- Medical status
- Pain
- Physical status
- Patient orientation
- Discharge plans

The nursing staff are usually intimately aware of the patient's current medical and physical status. If pain is a factor:

- What is the nursing assessment of this patient's pain level and pain tolerance?

Pain tolerance is relative to the medications received by the patient, the number of days after surgery or after injury, fatigue, previous history of substance abuse or chemical addiction, and the patient's personality.

To assess the patient's physical status, ask the nursing staff or check the medical record to find out:

- Has the patient been up at all yet?
- If yes, how long has the patient been sitting, standing, or walking?
- How far has the patient walked?
- How much assistance does the patient require?

Ask about the patient's orientation:

- Is the patient oriented to time, place, and person?

In other words, does the patient know the date and the approximate time, where he or she is, and who he or she is? Treatment plans may be altered by the patient's awareness; for example, a home program may be impossible without family compliance.

- Are there any known or expected discharge plans?
- If yes, what are these plans and when is the target date for discharge?

Cooperation between nurses and therapists is an important part of the multidisciplinary approach in planning the patient's plan of care. The questions to ask and factors to consider provide the therapist with the basic information needed to carry

BOX 2.14 HOSPITAL INPATIENT INFORMATION

Medical Record

- **Patient age**
- **Medical diagnosis**
- **Surgery**: Did the patient have surgery? What was the surgery for?

FUPs

- Was the patient seen by a physical therapist preoperatively?
- Were there any unrelated preoperative conditions?
- Was the surgery invasive, a closed procedure via arthroscopy, fluoroscopy, or other means of imaging, or virtual by means of computerized technology?
- How long was the procedure? Were there any surgical complications?
- How much fluid and/or blood products were given?
- What position was the patient placed in and for how long?
- **Physician's report:**
  - What are the short-term and long-term medical treatment plans?
  - Are there precautions or contraindications for treatment?
  - Are there weight-bearing limitations?
- **Associated or additional problems** such as diabetes, heart disease, peripheral vascular disease, respiratory involvement

FUPs

- Are there precautions or contraindications of any kind that may affect exercise?
- If diabetic, what are the current blood glucose levels (normal range: 70 to 100 mg/dL)?
- When is insulin administered? (Use this to avoid the peak insulin levels in planning an exercise schedule.)
- **Medications** (what, when received, what for, potential side effects)

FUPs

- Is the patient receiving oxygen or receiving fluids/medications through an intravenous line?
- **Restrictions:** Are there any dietary or fluid restrictions?

FUPs

- If yes, check with the nursing staff to determine the patient's full limitation.
- Are ice chips or a wet washcloth permissible?
- How many ounces or milliliters of fluid are allowed during therapy?
- **Laboratory values:** Hematocrit/hemoglobin level (see inside cover for normal values and significance of these tests); exercise tolerance test results if available for cardiac patient; pulmonary function test (PFT) to determine severity of pulmonary problem; arterial blood gas (ABG) levels to determine the need for supplemental oxygen during exercise
- **Vital signs:** Is their blood pressure stable?

FUPs

- If no, consider initiating standing with a tilt table or monitoring their blood pressure before, during, and after treatment.

Nursing Assessment

- **Medical status:** What is the patient's current medical status?
- **Pain:** What is the nursing assessment of this patient's pain level and pain tolerance?
- **Physical status:** Has the patient been up at all yet?

FUPs

- If yes, is the patient sitting, standing, or walking? How long and (if walking) what distance, and how much assistance is required?
- **Patient orientation:** Is the patient oriented to time, place, and person? (Does the patient know the date and the approximate time, where he or she is and who he or she is?)
- **Discharge plans:** Are there any known or expected discharge plans?

FUPs

- If yes, what are these plans and when will the patient be discharged?
- **Final question:** Is there anything else that I should know before exercising the patient?

---

out appropriate physical examination procedures and to plan the intervention. Each patient's situation may require that the therapist obtain additional pertinent information (Box 2.14).

PHYSICIAN REFERRAL

The therapist will be using the questions presented in this chapter to identify symptoms of possible systemic origin. The therapist can screen for medical disease and decide if referral to the physician (or other appropriate health care professional) is indicated by correlating the client's answers with family/personal history, vital signs, and objective findings from the physical examination.

For example, consider the client with a chief complaint of back pain who circles "yes" on the Family/Personal History form, indicating a history of ulcers or stomach problems. Obtaining further information at the first appointment by using Special Questions to Ask is necessary so that a decision regarding treatment or referral can be made immediately.

This treatment-versus-referral decision is further clarified as the interview, and other objective evaluation procedures, continue. Thus, if further questioning fails to show any association of back pain with GI symptoms and the objective findings from the back evaluation point to a true musculoskeletal lesion, medical referral is unnecessary and the physical therapy intervention can begin.

This information is not designed to make a medical diagnosis but rather to perform an accurate assessment of pain and systemic symptoms that can mimic or occur simultaneously with a musculoskeletal problem.

Guidelines for Physician Referral

As part of the Review of Systems, correlate *history* with *patterns of pain* and any *unusual findings* that may indicate systemic disease. The therapist can use the decision-making tools discussed in Chapter 1 (see Box 1.7) to decide on treatment versus referral.

Some of the specific indications for physician referral mentioned in this chapter include the following:

- Spontaneous postmenopausal bleeding
- A growing mass, whether painful or painless
- Persistent rise or fall in blood pressure
- Hip, sacroiliac, pelvic, groin, or low back pain in a woman without traumatic etiologic complex who reports fever, sweats, or an association between menses and symptoms
- Marked loss of hip motion and referred pain to the groin in a client taking long-term systemic corticosteroids
- A positive family/personal history of breast cancer in a woman with chest, back, or shoulder pain of unknown cause
- Elevated blood pressure in any woman taking birth control pills; this should be closely monitored by her physician

---

■ Key Points to Remember

1. The process of screening for medical disease before establishing a diagnosis by the physical therapist and plan of care requires a broad range of knowledge.
2. Throughout the screening process, a medical diagnosis is not the goal. The therapist is screening to make sure that the client does indeed have a primary problem that is within the scope of a physical therapist practice.
3. The screening steps begin with the client interview, but screening does not end there. Screening questions may be needed throughout the episode of care. This is especially true when progression of disease results in a changing clinical presentation, perhaps with the onset of new symptoms or new red flags after the treatment intervention has been initiated.
4. The client history is the first and most basic skill needed for screening. Most of the information needed to determine the cause of symptoms is contained within the subjective assessment (interview process).
5. The Family/Personal History form can be used as the first tool to screen clients for medical disease. Any "yes" responses should be followed up with appropriate questions. The therapist is strongly encouraged to review the form with the client, entering the date and his or her initials. This form can be used as a document of baseline information.
6. Screening examinations (interview and vital signs) should be completed for any person experiencing back, shoulder, scapular, hip, groin, or sacroiliac symptoms of unknown cause. The presence of constitutional symptoms will almost always warrant a physician's referral and further follow-up questions in making that determination.
7. It may be necessary to explain the need to ask such detailed questions about organ systems seemingly unrelated to the musculoskeletal symptoms.
8. Not every question provided in the lists offered in this text needs to be asked; the therapist can scan the lists and ask the appropriate questions based on the individual circumstances.
9. When screening for domestic violence, sexual dysfunction, incontinence, or other conditions, it is important to explain that a standard set of questions is asked and that some may not apply.
10. With the older client, a limited number of presenting symptoms often predominate—no matter what the underlying disease is—including acute confusion, depression, falling, incontinence, and syncope.
11. A recent history of any infection (bladder, uterine, kidney, vaginal, upper respiratory), mononucleosis, influenza, or colds may be an extension of a chronic health pattern or systemic illness.
12. The use of fluoroquinolones (antibiotic) has been linked with tendinopathies, especially in older adults who are also taking corticosteroids.
13. Reports of dizziness, loss of balance, or a history of falls require further screening, especially in the presence of other neurologic signs and symptoms such as headache, confusion, depression, irritability, visual changes, weakness, memory loss, and drowsiness or lethargy.
14. Special Questions for Women and Special Questions for Men are available to screen for gynecologic or urologic involvement for any woman or man with back, shoulder, hip, groin, or sacroiliac symptoms of unknown origin at presentation.
15. Consider the possibility of physical/sexual assault or abuse in anyone with an unknown cause of symptoms, clients who take much longer to heal than expected, or any combination of physical, social, or psychologic cues listed.

    In screening for systemic origin of symptoms, review the patient history and interview in light of the physical examination findings. Compare the client's history with clinical presentation and look for any associated signs and symptoms.

CASE STUDY

REFERRAL

A 28-year-old white man was referred to physical therapy with a medical diagnosis of progressive idiopathic Raynaud's syndrome of the bilateral upper extremities. He had this condition for the last 4 years.*

The client was examined by numerous physicians, including an orthopedic specialist. The client had complete numbness and cyanosis of the right second, third, fourth, and fifth digits on contact with even a mild decrease in temperature.

He reported that his symptoms had progressed to the extent that they appear within seconds if he picks up a glass of cold water. This man works almost entirely outside, often in cold weather, and uses saws and other power equipment. The numbness has created a very unsafe job situation.

The client received a gunshot wound in a hunting accident 6 years ago. The bullet entered the posterior left thoracic region, lateral to the lateral border of the scapula, and came out through the anterior lateral superior chest wall. He says that he feels as if his shoulders are constantly rolled forward. He reports no cervical, shoulder, or elbow pain or injury.

PHYSICAL THERAPY INTERVIEW

Note that not all of these questions would necessarily be presented to the client because his answers may determine the next question and may eliminate some questions.

Tell me why you are here today. (Open-ended question)

PAIN

- Do you have any pain associated with your past gunshot wound? If yes, describe your pain.

FUPs: Give the client a chance to answer and prompt only if necessary with suggested adjectives such as "Is your pain sharp, dull, boring, or burning?" or "Show me on your body where you have pain."

To pursue this line of questioning, if appropriate:

FUPs: What makes your pain better or worse?

- What is your pain like when you first get up in the morning, during the day, and in the evening?
- Is your pain constant or does it come and go?
- On a scale of 0 to 10, with zero being no pain and 10 being the worst pain you have ever experienced with this problem, what level of pain would you say that you have right now?
- Do you have any other pain or symptoms that are not related to your old injury?
- If yes, pursue as in previous questions to find out about the onset of pain, etc.
- You indicated that you have numbness in your right hand. How long does this last?

FUPs: Besides picking up a glass of cold water, what else brings it on?

How long have you had this problem?

- You told me that this numbness has progressed over time. How fast has this happened?
- Do you ever have similar symptoms in your left hand?

ASSOCIATED SYMPTOMS

Even though this client has been seen by numerous physicians, it is important to ask appropriate questions to rule out a systemic origin of current symptoms, especially if there has been a recent change in the symptoms or presentation of symptoms bilaterally. For example:

- What other symptoms have you had that you can associate with this problem?
- In addition to the numbness, have you had any of the following?

• Tingling	• Nausea
• Burning	• Dizziness
• Weakness	• Difficulty with swallowing
• Vomiting	• Heart palpitations or fluttering
• Hoarseness	• Unexplained sweating or night sweats
• Difficulty with breathing	• Problems with your vision

- How well do you sleep at night? (Open-ended question)
- Do you have trouble sleeping at night? (Closed-ended question)
- Does the pain awaken you out of a sound sleep? Can you sleep on either side comfortably?

MEDICATIONS

- Are you taking any medications? If yes, and the person does not volunteer the information, probe further:

What medications?

Why are you taking this medication?

When did you last take the medication?

Do you think the medication is easing the symptoms or helping in any way?

Have you noticed any side effects? If yes, what are these effects?

Previous Medical Treatment

- Have you had any recent medical tests, such as x-ray examination, MRI, or CT scan? If yes, find out the results.
- Tell me about your gunshot wound. Were you treated immediately?
- Did you have any surgery at that time or since then? If yes, pursue details with regard to what type of surgery and where and when it occurred.

* Adapted from Bailey W, Northwestern Physical Therapy Services, Inc., Titusville, Pennsylvania.

- Did you have physical therapy at any time after your accident? If yes, relate when, for how long, with whom, what was done, did it help?
- Have you had any other kind of treatment for this injury (e.g., acupuncture, chiropractic, osteopathic, naturopathic, and so on)?

ACTIVITIES OF DAILY LIVING (ADLs)

- Are you right-handed?
- How do your symptoms affect your ability to do your job or work around the house?

- How do your symptoms affect caring for yourself (e.g., showering, shaving, other ADLs such as eating or writing)?

FINAL QUESTION

- Is there anything else you feel that I should know concerning your injury, your health, or your present situation that I have not asked about?

Note: If this client had been a woman, the interview would have included questions about breast pain and the date when she was last screened for cancer (cervical and breast) by a physician.

PRACTICE QUESTIONS

1. What is the effect of NSAIDs (e.g., Naprosyn, Motrin, Anaprox, ibuprofen) on blood pressure?
   a. No effect
   b. Increases blood pressure
   c. Decreases blood pressure

2. Most of the information needed to determine the cause of symptoms is contained in the:
   a. Patient interview
   b. Family/Personal History Form
   c. Physical Examination
   d. All of the above
   e. a and c

3. A risk factor for NSAID-related gastropathy is the use of:
   a. Antibiotics
   b. Antidepressants
   c. Antihypertensives
   d. Antihistamines

4. After interviewing a new client, you summarize what she has told you by saying, "You told me you are here because of right neck and shoulder pain that began 5 years ago as a result of a car accident. You also have a 'pins and needles' sensation in your third and fourth fingers but no other symptoms at this time. You have noticed a considerable decrease in your grip strength, and you would like to be able to pick up a pot of coffee without fear of spilling it." This is an example of:
   a. An open-ended question
   b. A funnel technique
   c. A paraphrasing technique
   d. None of the above

5. Screening for alcohol use would be appropriate when the client reports a history of accidents.
   a. True
   b. False

6. What is the significance of sweats?
   a. A sign of systemic disease
   b. Side effect of chemotherapy or other medications
   c. Poor ventilation while sleeping
   d. All of the above

   e. None of the above

7. Spontaneous uterine bleeding after 12 consecutive months without menstrual bleeding requires medical referral.
   a. True
   b. False

8. Which of the following are red flags to consider when screening for systemic or viscerogenic causes of neuromuscular and musculoskeletal signs and symptoms:
   a. Fever, (night) sweats, dizziness
   b. Symptoms are out of proportion to the injury
   c. Insidious onset
   d. No position is comfortable
   e. All of the above

9. A 52-year-old man with low back pain and sciatica on the left side has been referred to you by his family physician. He has had a discectomy and laminectomy on two separate occasions about 5 to 7 years ago. No imaging studies have been performed (e.g., x-ray examination or MRI) since that time. What follow-up questions should you ask to screen for medical disease?

10. You should assess clients who are receiving NSAIDs for which physiologic effect associated with increased risk of hypertension?
    a. Decreased heart rate
    b. Increased diuresis
    c. Slowed peristalsis
    d. Water retention

11. Instruct clients with a history of hypertension and arthritis to:
    a. Limit physical activity and exercise
    b. Avoid OTC medications
    c. Inform their primary care provider of both conditions
    d. Drink plenty of fluids to avoid edema

12. Alcohol screening tools should be:
    a. Used with every client sometime during the episode of care
    b. Brief, easy to administer, and nonthreatening
    c. Deferred when the client has been drinking or has the smell of alcohol on their breath
    d. Conducted with one other family member present as a witness

13. With what final question should you always end your interview?

REFERENCES

1. Miranda H, Gold JE, Gore R, et al. Recall of prior musculoskeletal pain. *Scand J Work Environ Health.* 2006;32(4):294–299.

2. Barsky AJ. Forgetting, fabricating, and telescoping: the instability of the medical history. *Arch Intern Med.* 2002;162(9):981–984.

3. Wiklund GL, Wagner L. The butterfly effect of caring – clinical nursing teachers' understanding of self-compassion as a source to compassionate care. *Scand J Caring Sci.* 2013;27(1):175–183.

4. Davis CM. *Patient practitioner interaction: an experiential manual for developing the art of healthcare.* ed 5 Thorofare, NJ: Slack; 2011.

5. Chartrand TL, van Baaren R. Human mimicry. *Adv Exp Soc Psychol.* 2009;41:219–274. https://doi.org/10.1016/S0065-2601(08)00405-X.

6. Beckman HB, Frankel RM. The effect of physician behavior on the collection of data. *Annals of Internal Medicine.* 1984;101:692–696

7. Kennedy CW, Camden CT. A new look at interruption. *Western Journal of Speech Communication.* 1983;47:45–58.

8. Nonverbal communication: HelpGuide.org. Available online at. http://www.helpguide.org/articles/relationships/nonverbal-communication.htm Accessed 12.07.16.

9. Staggering Illiteracy Statistics: Literacy Project Foundation. Available online at. http://literacyprojectfoundation.org/community/statistics/ Accessed 12.07.16.

10. Dinan S: An eye-popping 20% of U.S. residents abandon English at home, *Washington Times*, Monday, October 6, 2014. Available online at http://www.washingtontimes.com/news/2014/oct/6/one-in-five-in-us-dont-speak-english-at-home-repor/. Accessed 16.07.16.

11. Vernon JA, Trujillo A, Rosenbaum M et al.: Low health literacy: implications for national health policy. Available online at. http://publichealth.gwu.edu/departments/healthpolicy/CHPR/downloads/LowHealthLiteracyReport10_4_07.pdf Accessed 16.07.16.

12. Literacy Foundation: Consequences of Illiteracy. Available online at https://www.fondationalphabetisation.org/en/foundation/causes-of-illiteracy/consequences-of-illiteracy/ Accessed 16.07.16.

13. The Joint Commission: What did the doctor say? Improving health literacy to protect patient safety. Available online at https://www.jointcommission.org/what_did_the_doctor_say/, 2007 Accessed 16.07.16.

14. Marcus EN. The silent epidemic—the health effects of illiteracy. *N Engl J Med.* 2006;355(4):339–341.

15. Nordrum J, Bonk E. Serving patients with limited English proficiency. *PT Magazine.* 2009;17(1):58–60.

16. Garcia SF, Hahn EA, Jacobs EA. Addressing low literacy and health literacy in clinical oncology practice. *J Support Oncol.* 2010;8(2):64–69.

17. Magasi S. Rehabilitation consumers' use and understanding of quality information: a health literacy perspective. *Arch Phys Med Rehabil.* 2009;90(2):206–212.

18. Nielsen-Bohlman L, Panzer AM, Kindig DA, eds. *Health literacy: a prescription to end confusion.* Washington, D.C: National Academies Press; 2004. (Available online at. http://www.nationalacademies.org/hmd/Reports/2004/Health-Literacy-A-Prescription-to-End-Confusion.aspx. (Accessed 16.07.15.

19. Cultural Competence Assessment Resources. Available online at http://iengage.multicultural.ufl.edu/resources/campus_resources/cultural_competence_resources/ Accessed 16.07.16.

20. The Myers and Briggs Foundation. Available online at http://www.myersbriggs.org/more-about-personality-type/international-use/multicultural-use-of-the-mbti.htm Accessed 16.07.16.

21. Fortin AH, Dwamena FC, Frankel RM, et al. *Smith's patient centered interviewing: an evidence-based method.* ed 3 : McGraw Hill; 2012.

22. Cole SA, Bird J. *The medical interview: the three function approach.* ed 3 St. Louis: Elsevier; 2013.

23. National Health Law Program: What's in a word: a guide to understanding interpreting and translation in health care (full guide). Available online at http://www.healthlaw.org/publications/whats-in-a-word-a-guide-to-understanding-interpreting-and-translation-in-health-care-full-guide#.V4qg-PkrKM9 Accessed 16.07.16.

24. Alexandria VA. A normative model of physical therapist professional education. *American Physical Therapy Association.* 2004

25. Cultural Competence in Physical Therapy: American Physical Therapy Association. Available online at http://www.apta.org/CulturalCompetence/ Accessed 16.07.16.

26. Cohn V: Future immigration will change the face of America by 2065. Pew Research Center. Available online at http://www.pewresearch.org/fact-tank/2015/10/05/future-immigration-will-change-the-face-of-america-by-2065/ Accessed 16.07.16.

27. Lie DA, Lee-Key E, Gomez A, et al. Does cultural competency training of health professionals improve patient outcomes? A systematic review and proposed algorithm for future research. *J Gen Intern Med.* 2011;26(3):317–325.

28. World Health Organization: Social Determinants of Health. Available online at http://www.who.int/social_determinants/en/ Accessed 16.07.16.

29. Kleinman A, Eisenberg L, Good B. Culture, illness and care: clinical lessons from anthropologic and cross-cultural research. *Ann Int Med.* 1978;88:251–258.

30. Cultural and Linguistic Competency: Office of Minority Health. US Department of Health and Human Services. Available online at http://minorityhealth.hhs.gov/omh/browse.aspx?lvl=1&lvlid=6 Accessed 16.07.16.

31. Bowen-Bailey D: Diversity Rx: multicultural best practices overview. Available online at http://healthcareinterpreting.org/diversity-rx-multicultural-health-best-practices-overview/ Accessed 16.07.16.

32. Chan Z, Fung Y, Chien W. Bracketing in phenomenology: only undertaken in the data collection and analysis process? *The Qualitative Report.* 2013;18(30):1–9.

33. Platt FW. The patient-centered interview. *Ann Intern Med.* 2001;134:1079–1085.

34. Baker LH. What else? Setting the agenda for the clinical interview. *Ann Intern Med.* 2005;143:766–770.

35. Churchill LR. Improving patient care. *Arch Intern Med.* 2008;149:720–724.

36. Asch SE. Forming impressions of personality. *Journal of Abnormal and Social Psychology.* 1946;41:258–290.

37. Fairbank JC, Couper J, Davies JB, et al. The Oswestry low back pain disability questionnaire. *Physiotherapy.* 1980;66:271–273.

38. Kopec JA, Esdaile JM, Abrahamowicz M, et al. The Quebec back pain disability scale measurement properties. *Spine.* 1995;20:341–352.

39. Ventre J, Schenk RJ. Validity of the Duffy-Rath questionnaire. *Orthopaedic Practice.* 2005;17(1):22–28.

40. Lippitt SB, Harryman DT, Matsen FA. A practical tool for evaluating function: the simple shoulder test. In: Matsen FA, Hawkins RJ, Fu FH, eds. *The shoulder: a balance of mobility and stability, Rosemont.* : American Academy of Orthopaedic Surgeons; 1993.

41. Hudak PL, Amadio PC, Bombardier C. Development of an upper extremity outcome measure: the DASH (disabilities of the arm, shoulder, and hand), the upper extremity collaborative group (UECG). *Am J Ind Med.* 1996;29:602–608. Erratum 30:372, 1996.

42. SF-36.org. Available online at http://www.sf-36.org/ Accessed 16.07.16.

43. Wolf Jr. GA. *Collecting data from patients.* Baltimore: University Park Press; 1977.

44. Older Americans: key indicators of well-being. Available online at http://www.agingstats.gov/aging-statsdotnet/Main_Site/Data/2012_Documents/Docs/EntireChartbook.pdf, 2012 Accessed 16.07.16.

45. Shega JW, Dale W, Andrew M, Paice J, Rockwood K, Weiner DK. Persistent Pain and Frailty: A case for homeostenosis. *J Am Geriatr Soc.* 2012;60(1):113–117.

46. Skinner M. A literature review: polypharmacy protocol for primary care. *Geriatr Nurs.* 2015;36(5):367–371.

47. Runganga M, Peel NM, Hubbard RE. Multiple medication use in older patients in post-acute transitional care: a prospective cohort study. *Clin Interv Aging.* 2014;9:1453–1462.

48. Ulirsch JC, Ballina LE, Soward AC, et al. Pain and somatic symptoms are sequelae of sexual assault: results of a prospective longitudinal study. *Eur J Pain.* 2014;18(4):559–566.

49. Sutton RA, Dian L, Guy P. Osteoporosis in men: an underrecognized and undertreated problem. *BCMJ.* 2011;53(10):535–540.

50. Franzén-Dahlin Å, Laska AC. Gender differences in quality of life after stroke and TIA: a cross-sectional survey of out-patients. *J Clin Nurs.* Aug 2012;21(15-16):2386–2391.

51. New guidelines for reducing stroke risks unique to women: American Heart Association/American Stroke Association Scientific Statement. Available online at http://newsroom.heart.org/news/new-guidelines-for-reducing-stroke-risks-unique-to-women?preview=378d Accessed 17.07.16.

52. National Institutes of Health: Report of the NIH Advisory Committee on Research on Women's Health | Fiscal Years 2013–2014. Available online at https://orwh.od.nih.gov/resources/pdf/3-NIH-ICs-ACRWH-Biennial-Report-FY13-14.pdf Accessed 23.10.16.

53. Sugimoto D, Myer GD, Foss KD, et al. Dosage effects of neuromuscular training intervention to reduce anterior cruciate ligament injuries in female athletes: meta- and sub-group analyses. *Sports Med.* 2014;44(4):551–562.

54. Slade GD, Fillingim RB, Sanders AE, et al. Summary of findings from the OPPERA prospective cohort study of incidence of first-onset temporomandibular disorder: implications and future directions. *J Pain.* Dec 2013;14(Suppl 12):T116–T124.

55. Prevalence of Migraine Headache in the United States: Relation to Age, Income, Race, and Other Sociodemographic Factors | JAMA | JAMA Network. https://jamanetwork.com/journals/jama/article-abstract/394233. Accessed 01.10.19.

56. Northrup C. *The wisdom of menopause, revised updated edition.* New York: Hay House; 2012.

57. Menopause: National Institute on Aging: Menopause. Available online at https://www.nia.nih.gov/health/publication/menopause Accessed 17.07.16.

58. Menopause: Mayo Clinic. Available online at http://www.mayoclinic.org/diseases-conditions/menopause/expert-answers/hormone-replacement-therapy/faq-20058499 Accessed 17.07.16.

59. 2011 Women's Health Stats and Facts: American Congress of Obstetrics and Gynecology. Available online at https://www.acog.org/-/media/NewsRoom/MediaKit.pdf Accessed 17.07.15.

60. Mucowski S, Mack WJ, Shoupe D, et al. Effect of prior oophorectomy on changes in bone mineral density and carotid artery intima-media thickness in postmenopausal women. *Fertil Steril.* 2014;101(4):1117–1122.

61. Kaur K: Menopausal hormone replacement therapy. Medscape. Available online at http://emedicine.medscape.com/article/276104-overview Updated March 17, 2016. Accessed 17.07.16.

62. Menopausal Hormone Therapy and Cancer Risk: American Cancer Society. Available online at http://www.cancer.org/cancer/cancercauses/othercarcinogens/medicaltreatments/menopausal-hormone-replacement-therapy-and-cancer-risk Accessed 17.07.16.

63. Menopause and Heart Disease: American Heart Association. Available online at http://www.heart.org/HEARTORG/Conditions/More/MyHeartandStrokeNews/Menopause-and-Heart-Disease_UCM_448432_Article.jsp#.V4wBTfkrKM8 Accessed 17.07.16.

64. Women and Heart Disease Fact Sheet: Centers for Disease Control and Prevention. Available online at http://www.cdc.gov/dhdsp/data_statistics/fact_sheets/fs_women_heart.htm Accessed 17.07.16.

65. Hafeez H, Zeshan M, Tahir MA, Jahan N, Naveed S. Health Care Disparities Among Lesbian, Gay, Bisexual,

and Transgender Youth: A Literature Review. *Cureus.* 2017;9(4):e1184. https://doi.org/10.7759/cureus.1184.

66. Dimant OE, Cook TE, Greene RE, Radix AE. Experiences of Transgender and Gender Nonbinary Medical Students and Physicians. *Transgend Health.* 2019;4(1):209–216. https://doi.org/10.1089/trgh.2019.0021.

67. Tollinche LE, Walters CB, Radix A, et al. The Perioperative Care of the Transgender Patient. *Anesth Analg.* 2018;127(2):359–366. https://doi.org/10.1213/ANE.0000000000003371.

68. James SE, Herman JL, Rankin S, Keisling M, Mottet L, Anafi M. *The Report of the 2015 Transgender Survey.* Washington, DC: National Center for Healthcare Equality; 2016.

69. LaViest T. *Minority populations and health.* San Francisco: Jossey-Boss; 2005.

70. Frequently Asked Questions About Genetic and Genomic Science: National Human Genome Institute. Available online at https://www.genome.gov/19016904/faq-about-genetic-and-genomic-science/ Accessed 17.07.16.

71. CDC Health Disparities & Inequalities Report (CHDIR): Centers for Disease Control and Prevention. Available online at http://www.cdc.gov/minorityhealth/chdireport.html Accessed 17.07.16.

72. 2015 Kelly Report on Health Disparities in America. Available online at http://www.cdc.gov/minorityhealth/chdireport.html Accessed 17.07.16.

73. Centers for Disease Control and Prevention (CDC): Race and Ethnicity Code Set. Available online at https://www.cdc.gov/phin/resources/vocabulary/documents/cdc-race-ethnicity-background-and-purpose.pdf Accessed 17.07.16.

74. Eating Disorders: Mayo Clinic. Available online at http://www.mayoclinic.org/diseases-conditions/eating-disorders/symptoms-causes/dxc-20182875 Accessed 17.07.16.

75. Trauma and Eating Disorders. National Eating Disorders Association. Available online at https://www.nationaleatingdisorders.org/sites/default/files/ResourceHandouts/TraumaandEatingDisorders.pdf Accessed 17.07.16.

76. Strother E, Lehmberg R, Stanford SC, et al. Eating Disorders. *J Treat Prevent.* 2012;20(5):346–355.

77. Pipet S, Halpern R, Woody GE, et al. Association between AAS use, muscle dysmorphia and illicit drug use among gym frequenters. *Drug Alcohol Depend.* 2014;140:e178.

78. Murray SB, Rieger E, Hildebrandt T, et al. A comparison of eating, exercise, shape, and weight related symptomatology in males with muscle dysmorphia and anorexia nervosa. *Body Image.* 2012;9(2):193–200.

79. Fussner LM, Smith AR. It's not me, it's you: perceptions of partner body image preferences associated with eating disorder symptoms in gay and heterosexual men. *J Homosex.* 2015;62(10):1329–1344.

80. Kaminski PL, Chapman BP, Haynes SD, et al. Body image, eating behaviors, and attitudes toward exercise among gay and straight men. *Eat Behav.* 2005;6(3):179–187.

81. Schnittker J, Bacak V. The increasing predictive validity of self-rated health. *PLoS ONE.* 2014;9(1):e84933.

82. Galenkamp H, Deeg DJ, Huisman M, et al. Is self-rated health still sensitive for changes in disease and functioning among nonagenarians? *J Gerontol B Psychol Sci Soc Sci.* 2013;68(5):848–858.

83. Henschke N, Maher CG, Ostelo RWJG, de Vet HCW, Macaskill P, Irwig L. Red flags to screen for malignancy in patients with low-back pain. *Cochrane Database Syst Rev.* 2013;2:CD008686. https://doi.org/10.1002/14651858.CD008686.pub2.

84. Premkumar A, Godfrey W, Gottschalk MB, Boden SD. Red flags for low back pain are not always really red: a prospective evaluation of the clinical utility of commonly used screening questions for low back pain. *J Bone Joint Surg Am.* 2018;100(5):368–374. https://doi.org/10.2106/JBJS.17.00134.

85. Stajkovic S, Aitken EM, Holroyd-Leduc J. Unintentional weight loss in older adults. *CMAJ.* 2011;183(4):443–449.

86. Ross EL, Holcomb C, Jamison RN, et al. Chronic pain update: addressing abuse and misuse of opioid analgesics. *J Musculoskel Med.* 2008;25(6):268–277. 302.

87. Greene MS, Chambers RA. Pseudoaddiction: fact or fiction? An investigation of the medical literature. *Curr Addict Rep.* 2015;2:310–317.

88. National Institute of Drug Abuse: Emerging Trends and Alerts. Available online at https://www.drugabuse.gov/drugs-abuse/emerging-trends-alerts Accessed 17.07.16.

89. National Institute of Drug Abuse: Alcohol Facts and Statistics. Available online at https://www.niaaa.nih.gov/alcohol-health/overview-alcohol-consumption/alcohol-facts-and-statistics Accessed 17.07.16.

90. Nutt D. Drug harms in the UK: a multicriteria decision analysis. *Lancet.* 2010;6736(10):61462–61466.

91. Bowen P, Edwards P, Lingard H, et al. Workplace stress, stress effects, and coping mechanisms in the construction industry. *J Constr Eng Manag.* 2014;140:3.

92. Seghal N, Manchkanti L, Smith HS. Prescription opioid abuse in chronic pain: a review of opioid abuse predictors and strategies to curb opioid abuse. *Pain Physician.* Jul 2012;15(Suppl 3):ES67–ES92.

93. Skinner HA. Identification of alcohol abuse using laboratory tests and a history of trauma. *Ann Intern Med.* 1984;101(6):847–851.

94. Pilowsky DJ, Wu LT. Screening instruments for substance use and brief interventions targeting adolescents in primary care: a literature review. *Addict Behav.* 2013;38(5):2146–2153.

95. Bastiaens L, Francis G, Lewis K. The RAFFT as a screening tool for adolescent substance use disorders. *Am J Addict.* 2000;9:10–16.

96. National Institute for Drug Addiction: Screening for drug use in general medical settings - resource guide. Available online at https://www.drugabuse.gov/sites/default/files/resource_guide.pdf Accessed 17.07.16.

97. Massachusetts Department of Public Health Bureau of Substance Abuse. Available online at http://www.masbirt.org/sites/www.masbirt.org/files/documents/toolkit.pdf Accessed 17.07.16.

98. University of Washington Alcohol and Drug Abuse Institute (ADAI): Substance Use and Screening Assessment Instruments Database. Available online at http://lib.adai.washington.edu/instruments/ Accessed 17.07.16.

99. Resources: National Institute for Drug Abuse. Available online at https://www.drugabuse.gov/publications/principles-drug-addiction-treatment-research-based-guide-third-edition/resources Accessed 17.07.16.

100. Alcohol Use Disorder: National Institute on Alcohol Abuse and Alcoholism. Available online at https://www.niaaa.nih.gov/alcohol-health/overview-alcohol-consumption/alcohol-use-disorders Accessed 17.07.16.

101. Hutton HE, McCaul ME, Santora PB, et al. The relationship between recent alcohol use and sexual behaviors: gender differences among STD clinic patients. *Alcoholism, clinical and experimental research*. 2008;32(11):2008–2015.

102. Salas-Wright CP, Vaughn MG, Ugalde J, et al. Substance use and teen pregnancy in the United States: evidence from the NSDUH 2002-2012. *Addict Behav*. 2015;45:218–225.

103. Kanny D. Vital signs: binge drinking among high school students and adults in the United States. *MMWR*. 2010;59(39):1274–1279.

104. Babor TF, de la Fuente JR, Saunders J, et al.: *AUDIT (the alcohol use disorders identification test): guidelines for use in primary health care*, ed 2. Available online at http://apps.who.int/iris/bitstream/10665/67205/1/WHO_MSD_MSB_01.6a.pdf. Accessed 17.07.16.

105. Bickley L, Szilagyi P. ,. *Bates' guide to physical examination and history-taking*. ed 11 Philadelphia: Wolters-Kluwer Health/Lippincott Williams & Wilkins; 2013:934.

106. Davis JL: Drink less for strong bones. WebMD Osteoporosis Health Center. Available online at http://www.webmd.com/osteoporosis/features/alcohol Accessed 17.07.16.

107. Budzikowski A: Holiday heart syndrome. WebMD. Available online at http://emedicine.medscape.com/article/155050-overview Accessed 17.07.16.

108. Cranston AR. Physical therapy management of a patient experiencing alcohol withdrawal. *J Acute Care Phys Ther*. 2010;1(2):56–63. Winter.

109. Vincent WR. Review of alcohol withdrawal in the hospitalized patient: diagnosis and assessment. *Orthopedics*. 2007;30(5):358–361.

110. Tompkins DA, Bigelow GE, Harrison JA, et al. Concurrent validation of the clinical opiate withdrawal scale (COWS) and single-item indices against the clinical institute narcotic assessment (CINA) opioid withdrawal instrument. *Drug and Alcohol Depend*. 2009;105(1-2):154–159.

111. Smith LA, Foxcroft D, Holloway A, et al. Brief alcohol questionnaires for identifying hazardous, harmful and dependent alcohol use in primary care (protocol). *Cochrane Database Syst Rev*. 2010;8:1–10.

112. Dhalla S, Kopec JA. The CAGE questionnaire for alcohol misuse: a review of reliability and validity studies. *Clin Invest Med*. 2007;30(1):33–41.

113. O'Brien CP. The CAGE questionnaire for detection of alcoholism: a remarkably useful but simple tool. *JAMA*. 2008;300(17):2054–2056.

114. Aalto M, Alho H, Halme JT, et al. The alcohol use disorders identification test (AUDIT) and its derivatives in screening for heavy drinking among the elderly. *Int J Geriatr Psychiatry*. 2011;26(9):881–885.

115. Henderson-Martin B. No more surprises: screening patients for alcohol abuse. *Nursing 2000*. 2000;100(9):26–32.

116. Carlat DJ. The psychiatric review of symptoms: a screening tool for family physicians. *Am Fam Physician*. 1998;58(7):1617–1624.

117. Vinson DC. Comfortably engaging: which approach to alcohol screening should we use? *Ann Fam Med*. 2004;2(5):398–404.

118. American Physical Therapy Association: SUBSTANCE ABUSE HOD P06-03-22-19. Updated 08/01/12. Available online at http://www.apta.org/uploadedFiles/APTAorg/About_Us/Policies/Health_Social_Environment/SubstanceAbuse.pdf#search=%22substance abuse%22 Accessed 18.07.16.

119. Illegal Drugs and Heart Disease: American Heart Association. Available online at http://www.heart.org/HEARTORG/Conditions/More/MyHeartandStrokeNews/Illegal-Drugs-and-Heart-Disease_UCM_428537_Article.jsp#.V4zdYPkrKM8 Accessed 18.07.16.

120. Tobacco-Related Mortality: Centers for Disease Control and Prevention. Available online at http://www.cdc.gov/tobacco/data_statistics/fact_sheets/health_effects/tobacco_related_mortality/ Accessed 18.07.16.

121. What's In a Cigarette? Smoking Facts: American Heart Association. Available online at http://www.lung.org/stop-smoking/smoking-facts/whats-in-a-cigarette.html?referrer=https://www.google.com/ Accessed 18.07.16.

122. Pignataro R, Ohtake PJ, Swisher A, et al. The role of physical therapists in smoking cessation: opportunities for improving treatment outcomes. *Phys Ther*. 2012;92(5):757–766.

123. Benefits of Quitting Smoking Over Time: American Cancer Society. Available online at http://www.cancer.org/healthy/stayawayfromtobacco/benefits-of-quitting-smoking-over-time Accessed 18.07.16.

124. Rodriguez J. The association of pipe and cigar use with cotinine levels, lung function, and airflow obstruction. The multi-ethnic study of atherosclerosis (MESA). *Ann Intern Med*. 2010;152(4):201–210.

125. Mulligan JK, Nagel W, O'Connell BP, et al. Cigarette smoke exposure is associated with vitamin D3 deficiencies in patients with chronic rhinosinusitis. *J Allergy Clin Immunol*. 2014;134(2):342–349.

126. Jackson AR, Dhawale AA, Brown MD. Association between intervertebral disc degeneration and cigarette smoking: clinical and experimental findings. *JBJS Rev*. 2015;3(3):e2.

127. Shinji M, Akio Y, Tadayoshi K, et al. Risk factors of recurrent lumbar disk herniation: a single center study and review of the literature. *J Spinal Disord Tech.* 2015;28(5):E265–E269.

128. Pack year: NCI Dictionary of Cancer Terms: National Cancer Institute. Available online at http://www.cancer.gov/publications/dictionaries/cancer-terms?CdrID=306510 Accessed 18.07.16.

129. Caffeine Myths and Facts: WebMD. Available online at http://www.webmd.com/balance/caffeine-myths-and-facts#1 Accessed 18.07.16.

130. Lyon C: Can you OD on caffeine? CNN.com. Available online at http://www.cnn.com/2013/12/03/health/upwave-caffeine-overdose/ Accessed 18.07.16.

131. National Institute of Drug Abuse: Caffeine Powder. Available online at https://www.drugabuse.gov/emerging-trends/caffeine-powder Accessed 18.07.16.

132. De Mejia EG, Ramirez-Mares MV. Impact of caffeine and coffee on our health. *TEM.* 2014;25(10):489–492.

133. How sweet it is: all about sugar substitutes. food and drug administration. Available online at http://www.fda.gov/downloads/ForConsumers/ConsumerUpdates/UCM397797.pdf Accessed 18.05.16.

134. Ain Q, Khan SA. Artificial sweeteners: safe or unsafe? *J Pak Med Assoc.* 2015;65(2):225–227.

135. Chattopadhyay S, Raychaudhuri U, Chakraborty R. Artificial sweeteners – a review. *J Food Sci Technol.* 2014;51(4):611–621.

136. Sharma A, Amarnath S, Thulasimani M, et al. Artificial sweeteners as a sugar substitute: are they really safe? *Indian J Pharmacol.* 2016;48:237–240.

137. Occupational and work-related diseases: World Health Organization. Available online at http://www.who.int/occupational_health/activities/occupational_work_diseases/en/ Accessed 18.07.16.

138. Rich-Edwards J, Mason S, Rexrode K, et al. Physical and sexual abuse in childhood as predictors of early-onset cardiovascular events in women. *Circulation.* 2012;126(8):920–927.

139. US Department of Veteran Affairs: gulf war veterans' medically unexplained illnesses. Available online at http://www.publichealth.va.gov/exposures/gulfwar/medically-unexplained-illness.asp Accessed 18.07.16.

140. Haley RW. Excess incidence of ALS in young Gulf War veterans. *Neurology.* 2003;61(6):750–756.

141. Newman LS. Occupational illness. *N Engl J Med.* 1995;333:1128–1134.

142. Kreisberg J. Preventive medicine: taking an environmental history. *Integr Med.* 2009;8(5):58–59.

143. Important Facts about Falls: Centers for Disease Control and Prevention. Available online at http://www.cdc.gov/homeandrecreationalsafety/falls/adultfalls.html Accessed 18.07.16.

144. Joo H, Wang G, Yee SL, Zhang P, Sleet D. Economic Burden of informal caregiving associated with history of stroke and falls among older adults in the US. *American Journal of Preventive Medicine.* 2017;53(6):S197–S204.

145. Slip, Trip and Fall Prevention will Keep Older Adults Safe and Independent: National Safety Council. Available online at http://www.nsc.org/learn/safety-knowledge/Pages/safety-at-home-falls.aspx Accessed 18.07.16.

146. Stone KL. Self-reported sleep and nap habits and risk of mortality in a large cohort of older women. *J Am Geriatr Soc.* 2009;57(4):604–611.

147. Young WR, Mark Williams A. How fear of falling can increase fall-risk in older adults: applying psychological theory to practical observations. *Gait Posture.* 2014;41(1):7–12. https://doi.org/10.1016/j.gaitpost.2014.09.006.

148. Woolcott JC. Meta-analysis of the impact of 9 medication classes on falls in elderly persons. *Arch Intern Med.* 2009;169:1952–1960.

149. Falls Among Older Adults: Strategies for Prevention. Washington State Department of Health. Available online at http://www.doh.wa.gov/portals/1/Documents/2900/FallsAmongOlderAdults.pdf Accessed 18.07.16.

150. Newton R. Validity of the multi-directional reach test: a practical measure for limits of stability in older adults. *J Gerontol Biol Sci Med.* 2001;56(4):M248–M252.

151. Multidirectional reach test: Rehab Measures. Available online at http://www.rehabmeasures.org/Lists/RehabMeasures/DispForm.aspx?ID=1139 Accessed 18.07.16.

152. Goldberg A, Chavis M, Watkins J, et al. The five-times-sit-to-stand test: validity, reliability and detectable change in older females. *Aging Clin Exp Res.* 2012;24(4):339–344.

153. Ross E, Purtill H, Uszynski M, et al. Cohort study comparing the Berg balance scale and the Mini-BESTest in ambulatory people with multiple sclerosis. *Physical Therapy.* 2016;96(9):1448–1455.

154. Berg K, Wood-Dauphinee S, Williams JI, et al. Measuring balance in the elderly: validation of an instrument. *Can J Pub Health.* 1992;83(Suppl 2):S7–S11.

155. Podsiadlo D, Richardson S. The timed "up & go": a test of basic functional mobility for frail elderly persons. *J Am Geriatr Soc.* 1991;39:142–148.

156. Schoene D, Wu SM, Mikolaizak AS, et al. Discriminative ability and predictive validity of the timed up and go test in identifying older people who fall: systematic review and meta-analysis. *J Am Geriatr Soc.* 2013;61(2):202–208.

157. Horn LB, Rice T, Stoskus JL, et al. Measurement characteristics and clinical utility of the clinical test of sensory interaction on balance (CTSIB) and modified CTSIB in individuals with vestibular dysfunction. *Arch Phys Med Rehabil.* 2015;96(9):1747–1748.

158. Halvarson A, Franzen E, Stahle A. Assessing the relative and absolute reliability of the falls efficacy scale-international questionnaire in elderly individuals with increased fall risk and the questionnaire's convergent validity in elderly women with osteoporosis. *Osteoporos Int.* 2013;24(6):1853–1858.

159. Scheffer AC, Schuurmans MJ, van Dijk N, et al. Fear of falling: measurement strategy, prevalence, risk factors and consequences among older persons. *Age Ageing.* 2008;37(1):19–24.

160. Balance and Falls Awareness Event Kit: American Physical Therapy Association. Available online at http://iweb.apta. org/Purchase/ProductDetail.aspx?Product_code=PR-294 Accessed 18.07.16.

161. Code of Ethics for the Physical Therapist: American Physical Therapy Association. Available online at https:// www.apta.org/uploadedFiles/APTAorg/About_Us/ Policies/HOD/Ethics/CodeofEthics.pdf Accessed 18.07.16.

162. McCloskey LA. Abused women disclose partner interference with health care: an unrecognized form of battering. *J Gen Intern Med.* 2007;22:1067–1072.

163. Ketter P. Physical therapists need to know how to deal with domestic violence issues. *PT Bulletin.* 1997;12(31):6–7.

164. National Statistics: National Coalition Against Domestic Violence. Available online at http://www.ncadv.org/learn/ statistics Accessed 18.07.16.

165. Domestic violence against men: Know the signs. Mayo Clinic. Available online at http://www.mayoclinic.org/ healthy-lifestyle/adult-health/in-depth/domestic-vio lence-against-men/art-20045149 Accessed 18.07.16.

166. Walters ML, Chen J, Breiding MJ: The national intimate partner and sexual violence survey (NISVS): 2010 findings on victimization by sexual orientation. National Center for Injury Prevention and Control. Centers for Disease Control and Prevention. Available online at https://www. cdc.gov/violenceprevention/pdf/nisvs_sofindings.pdf Accessed 18.07.16.

167. American Physical Therapy Association (APTA): Guidelines for recognizing and providing care for victims of domestic abuse. Available at the APTA Learning Center. Available online at http://learningcenter.apta.org/ student/MyCourse.aspx?id=3c066b92-308c-4cdf-9d5e-291aeaf03507&programid=dcca7f06-4cd9-4530-b9d3-4ef7d2717b5d Accessed 18.07.16.

168. Houry D. Does screening in the emergency department hurt or help victims of intimate partner violence? *Ann Emerg Med.* 2008;51(4):433–442.

169. Brown JB, Lent B, Schmidt G, et al. Application of the woman abuse screening tool (WAST) and WAST-short in the family practice setting. *J Fam Pract.* Oct 2000;49(10):896–903.

170. Hegarty K, Bush R, Sheehan M. The composite abuse scale: further development and assessment of reliability and validity of a multidimensional partner abuse measure in clinical settings. *Violence Vict.* 2005;20:529–547.

171. Cook SL, Conrad L, Bender M, et al. The internal validity of the index of spouse abuse in African American women. *Violence Vict.* 2003;18(6):641–657.

172. Committee opinion no. 498 Adult manifestations of childhood sexual abuse. *Obstet Gynecol.* 2011 Aug;118(2 pt 1):392–395.

173. Leclerc B, Bergeron S, Bibik YM, Khalife S. History of sexual and physical abuse in women with dyspareunia: association with pain, psychosocial adjustment, and sexual functioning. *J Sex Med.* 2010;7(2 pt 2):971–980.

174. Wuest J, Merritt-Gray M, Ford-Gilboe M, Lent B, Varcoe C, Campbell JC. Chronic pain in women survivors of intimate partner violence. *J Pain.* 2008;9(11):1049–1057.

175. Pandya NK, Baldwin K, Wolfgruber H, et al. Child abuse and orthopaedic injury patterns: analysis at a level I pediatric trauma center. *J Pediatr Orthop.* 2009;29(6):618–625.

176. Friedman MJ, Wang S, Jalowiec JE, et al. Thyroid hormone alterations among women with posttraumatic stress disorder due to childhood sexual abuse. *Biol Psychiatry.* 2005;57(10):1186–1192.

177. Paras ML. Sexual abuse and lifetime diagnosis of somatic disorders: a systematic review and meta-analysis. *JAMA.* 2009;302:550–561.

178. Felitti VJ, Anda RF, Nordenberg D, et al. Relationship of childhood abuse and household dysfunction to many of the leading causes of death in adults. The Adverse Childhood Experiences (ACE) Study. *Am J Prev Med.* 1998;14(4):245–258.

179. Hughes K, Bellis MA, Hardcastle KA, et al. The effect of multiple adverse childhood experiences on health: a systematic review and meta-analysis. *Lancet Public Health.* 2017;2(8):e356–e366. https://doi.org/10.1016/ S2468-2667(17)30118-4.

180. Bhandari M. Violence against women health research collaborative: musculoskeletal manifestations of physical abuse after intimate partner violence. *J Trauma.* 2006;61:1473–1479.

181. What is workplace violence?: Occupational Safety and Health Administration. Available online at https://www. osha.gov/OshDoc/data_General_Facts/factsheet-work place-violence.pdf Accessed 18.07.16.

182. Healthcare Wide Hazards: Workplace Violence. Occupational Safety and Health Administration. Available online at https://www.osha.gov/SLTC/etools/hospital/ hazards/workplaceviolence/viol.html Accessed 18.07.16.

183. Schachter Toward sensitive practice: issues for PTs working with survivors of childhood sexual abuse. *Phy Ther.* 1999;79(3):248.

184. Keely BR. Could your patient—or colleague—become violent? *Nursing 2002.* 2002;32(12):32cc1–32cc5.

185. Myers JE, Berliner L, Briere J, et al. *The APSAC handbook on child maltreatment.* ed 3 Thousand Oaks: Sage Publications; 2010.

186. Guidelines for Recognizing and Providing Care for: Victims of Child Abuse. Available at the APTA Learning Center. Available online at http://learningcenter.apta.org/ AdvancedSearch.aspx?KeyWord=child+abuse Accessed 18.07.16.

187. Feldhaus KM. Fighting domestic violence: an intervention plan. *J Musculoskel Med.* 2001;18(4):197–204.

188. Ellis J. Prescription medication borrowing and sharing—risk factors and management. *Aust Fam Phys.* 2009;38(10):816–819.

189. Goldsworthy RC. Prescription medication sharing among adolescents: prevalence, risk, and outcomes. *J Adolesc Health.* 2009;45(6):634–637.

190. Budnitz DS. Medication use leading to emergency department visits for adverse drug events in older adults. *Ann Intern Med.* 2007;148(8):628–629.

191. Hussar D: Genetic makeup and response to drugs. Merck Manual Consumer Edition. Available online at http://www.merckmanuals.com/home/drugs/factors-affecting-response-to-drugs/genetic-makeup-and-response-to-drugs Accessed 18.07.16.

192. Soldin OP, Chung SH, Mattison DR. Sex differences in drug disposition. *J Biomed Biotech 2011 (ePub).* 2011

193. Meredith S, Feldman PH, Frey D, et al. Possible medication errors in home healthcare patients. *J Am Geriatr Soc.* 2001;49(6):719–724.

194. Deadly NSAIDs: Nutrition Digest. American Nutrition Association. Available online at http://americannutritionassociation.org/newsletter/deadly-nsaids Accessed 18.07.16.

195. FDA Drug Safety Communication: FDA strengthens warning that non-aspirin nonsteroidal anti-inflammatory drugs (NSAIDs) can cause heart attacks or strokes. Food and Drug Administration. Available online at http://www.fda.gov/Drugs/DrugSafety/ucm451800.htm Accessed 18.07.16.

196. Preventing Acetaminophen Overdosage: Medscape. Available online at http://www.medscape.com/viewarticle/410911_6 Accessed 19.07.16.

197. Hughes GJ, Patel PN, Saxena N. Effect of acetaminophen on international normalized ratio in patients receiving warfarin therapy. *Pharmacotherapy.* 2011;31(6):591–597.

198. Baggish AL, Weiner RB, Kanayama G, et al. Long term anabolic-androgenic steroid use is associated with left ventricular dysfunction. *Circ Heart Fail.* 2010;3(4):472–476.

199. Benyamin R, Trescot AM, Datta S, et al. Opioid complications and side effects. *Pain Physician.* 2008;11(2 Suppl):S105–S120.

200. Krebs EE, Gravely A, Nugent S, et al. Effect of opioid vs nonopioid medications on pain-related function in patients with chronic back pain or hip or knee osteoarthritis pain: the SPACE randomized clinical trial. *JAMA.* 2018;319(9):872–882. https://doi.org/10.1001/jama.2018.0899.

201. Shah A. Characteristics of initial prescription episodes and likelihood of long-term opioid use — United States, 2006–2015. *MMWR Morb Mortal Wkly Rep.* 2017;66 https://doi.org/10.15585/mmwr.mm6610a1.

202. Benyamin R, Trescot AM, Datta S, et al. Opioid complications and side effects. *Pain Physician.* 2008;11(2 Suppl):S105–S120.

203. Buntin-Mushock C, Phillip L, Moriyama K. Age-dependent opioid escalation in chronic pain patients. *Anesth Analg.* 2005;100(6):1740–1745.

204. Haller C, James L. Out of the medicine closet: time to talk straight about prescription drug abuse. *Clin Pharm Ther.* 2010;88(3):279–282.

205. Boscarino JA. Risk factors for drug dependence among out-patients on opioid therapy in a large US health-care system. *Addiction.* 2010;105(10):1776–1782.

206. Community Anti-Drug Coalitions of America (CADCA): Teen prescription drug abuse: an emerging threat. Available online at http://web.cadca.org/eweb/DynamicPage.aspx?Action=Add&ObjectKeyFrom=1A83491A-9853-4C87-86A4-F7D95601C2E8&WebCode=ProdDetailAdd&DoNotSave=yes&ParentObject=CentralizedOrderEntry&ParentDataObject=Invoice%20Detail&ivd_formkey=69202792-63d7-4ba2-bf4e-a0da41270555&ivd_cst_key=00000000-0000-0000-0000-000000000000&ivd_prc_prd_key=3DB0600B-A410-457D-AF47-7FCCBFAAD5C0 Accessed 19.07.16.

207. Cai R. Emergency department visits involving nonmedical use of selected prescription drugs in the United States. *J Pain Palliat Care Pharmacother.* 2010;24(3):293–297.

208. Hernandez SH. Prescription drug abuse: insight into epidemic. *Clin Pharmacol Ther.* 2010;88(3):307–317.

209. Haller C, James L. Out of the medicine closet: time to talk straight about prescription drug abuse. *Clin Pharm Ther.* 2010;88(3):279–282.

210. Blood Pressure and Women: American Heart Association. Available online at http://www.heart.org/HEARTORG/Conditions/HighBloodPressure/UnderstandYourRiskforHighBloodPressure/High-Blood-Pressure-and-Women_UCM_301867_Article.jsp#.V446APkrKM8 Accessed 19.07.16.

211. Depo-Provera Contraceptive injection (medroxyprogesterone acetate) injectable suspension: US Food and Drug Administration. Available online at http://www.fda.gov/Safety/MedWatch/SafetyInformation/ucm232329.htm Accessed 19.07.16.

212. Information for healthcare professionals: fluoroquinolone antimicrobial drugs [ciprofloxacin (marketed as cipro and generic ciprofloxacin), ciprofloxacin extended-release (marketed as cipro xr and proquin xr), gemifloxacin (marketed as factive), levofloxacin (marketed as levaquin), moxifloxacin (marketed as avelox), norfloxacin (marketed as noroxin), and ofloxacin (marketed as floxin)]. food and drug administration. Available online at http://www.fda.gov/Drugs/DrugSafety/PostmarketDrug SafetyInformationforPatientsandProviders/ucm126085.htm Accessed 19.07.16.

213. Herbal supplements: What to know before you buy. Mayo Clinic. Available online at http://www.mayoclinic.org/healthy-lifestyle/nutrition-and-healthy-eating/in-depth/herbal-supplements/art-20046714 Accessed 19.07.16.

214. Ciccone CD. *Pharmacology in rehabilitation.* ed 5 Philadelphia: FA Davis; 2015.

215. PDR for Herbal Medicines, ed 4. Available online at: http://www.pdrbooks.com/prod/Product-Catalog_92/PDR-for-Herbal-Medicines-4th-Edition_76.aspx?AspxAutoDetectCookieSupport=1. Accessed 19.07.16.

216. Mold JW: Night sweats: a systematic review of the literature. Medscape. Available online at http://www.medscape.com/viewarticle/774526_3 Accessed 19.07.16.

Pain Types and Viscerogenic Pain Patterns

The International Association for the Study of Pain (IASP) defines pain as "an unpleasant sensory and emotional experience associated with, or resembling that associated with, actual or potential tissue damage" (p. 2). This definition is expanded with the addition of six key notes (see Box 3.1) to provide further context. This update in the definition was due to advances in the understanding of pain.

A thorough assessment of pain is critical in optimal physical therapy patient management. Pain is often the primary symptom in patients and clients who access physical therapy services. A thorough examination and evaluation of pain are key features of the physical therapy interview, and serve as a foundation for a multidisciplinary pain management approach. This is crucial in helping solve our current opioid crisis.[1,2] Pain is recognized as the "fifth vital sign,"[3] along with blood pressure, temperature, pulse, and respiration. The physical therapist has the responsibility of investigating the possible sources of the pain complaint, and in understanding the types of pain presented by the patient.

Recognizing pain patterns that are characteristic of systemic disease is a necessary step in the screening process. Understanding how and when diseased organs can refer pain helps the therapist identify suspicious pain patterns.

This chapter includes a detailed overview of pain patterns that can be used as a foundation for the organ systems presented in this text. Information will include a discussion of pain types in general, and viscerogenic pain patterns in particular.

Each section discusses specific pain patterns characteristic of disease entities that can mimic pain that arise from musculoskeletal or neuromuscular conditions. In the clinical decision-making process, the therapist will evaluate information regarding the location, referral pattern, description, frequency, intensity, and duration of systemic pain in combination with knowledge of associated symptoms and aggravating and easing factors. This information is then compared with presenting features of primary musculoskeletal disorders that have similar presentation patterns. Pain patterns of the chest, back, shoulder, scapula, pelvis, hip, groin, and sacroiliac (SI) joint are the most common sites of referred pain from a systemic disease process. These patterns are discussed in greater detail later in this text (see Chapters 15 to 19).

A large component of the screening process is being able to recognize the client demonstrating a significant emotional or psychosocial overlay. Pain patterns from cancer can be very similar to what may be traditionally identified as psychogenic or emotional sources of pain, so it is important to know how to differentiate between these two sources of painful symptoms. To help identify psychogenic sources of pain, discussions of conversion symptoms, symptom magnification, and illness behavior are also included in this chapter.

MECHANISMS OF REFERRED VISCERAL PAIN

The neuroanatomical bases of visceral pain are not well understood, as compared with somatic pain.[4] Current literature provides an understanding of visceral nociceptive mechanisms based on what is known about the somatic (nonvisceral) system.[5] Scientists have not found actual nerve fibers and specific nociceptors in organs, and peripheral visceral neurotransmission is via visceral innervation by afferent fibers projecting to the central nervous system (CNS) via autonomic sympathetic and parasympathetic nerves.[5,6] Afferent supply to internal organs is in close proximity to blood vessels along a path similar to the sympathetic nervous system.[7,8]

Literature continues to identify the sites and mechanisms of visceral nociception. During inflammation, increased nociceptive input from an inflamed organ can sensitize neurons that receive convergent input from an unaffected organ, but the site of visceral cross-sensitivity is unknown.[9]

Viscerosensory fibers ascend the anterolateral system to the thalamus, with fibers projecting to several regions of the brain. These regions encode the site of origin of visceral pain, although they do it poorly because of low receptor density, large overlapping receptive fields, and extensive convergence in the ascending pathway. Thus the cortex cannot very well distinguish where the pain messages originate from in the gut.[10,11]

There are a wide number of gastrointestinal (GI) sensations that are conveyed by the afferent nerves to the CNS ranging from hunger, satiety, fullness, discomfort to pain, urgency, and the need to defecate. The afferent pathway has multiple specialized endings at different levels of the gut that signal these specific sensations to the brain.[12] Studies show there may be multiple mechanisms operating at different

BOX 3.1   ACCOMPANYING NOTES, INTERNATIONAL ASSOCIATION FOR THE STUDY OF PAIN UPDATED DEFINITION OF PAIN

- Pain is always a personal experience that is influenced to varying degrees by biological, psychological, and social factors.
- Pain and nociception are different phenomena. Pain cannot be inferred solely from activity in sensory neurons.
- Through their life experiences, individuals learn the concept of pain.
- A person's report of an experience as pain should be respected.*
- Although pain usually serves an adaptive role, it may have adverse effects on function and social and psychological well-being.
- Verbal description is only one of several behaviors to express pain; inability to communicate does not negate the possibility that a human or a nonhuman animal experiences pain.

Etymology

Middle English, from Anglo-French peine (pain, suffering), from Latin poena (penalty, punishment), in turn from Greek poine (payment, penalty, recompense).

*The Declaration of Montreal, a document developed during the First International Pain Summit on September 3, 2010, states that "Access to pain management is a fundamental human right."

(From Raja SN, Carr DB, Cohen M, et al. The revised International Association for the Study of Pain definition of pain: concepts, challenges, and compromises. Pain 2020;161(9):1976–1982.)

sites to produce the sensation we refer to as "pain." The same symptom can be produced by different mechanisms and a single mechanism may cause different symptoms.[13]

In the case of referred pain patterns of viscera, there are three separate phenomena to consider from a traditional Western medicine approach. These are:

- Embryologic development
- Multisegmental innervation
- Direct pressure and shared pathways

Embryologic Development

Each system has a bit of its own uniqueness in how pain is referred. For example, the viscera in the abdomen comprise a large percentage of all the organs we have to consider. When a person gives a history of abdominal pain, the location of the pain may not be directly over the involved organ (Fig. 3.1).

Functional magnetic resonance imaging (fMRI) and other neuroimaging methods have shown activation of the inferolateral postcentral gyrus by visceral pain so the brain has a role in visceral pain patterns.[14,15] However, it is likely that embryologic development has a primary role in referred pain patterns for the viscera.

Pain is referred to a site where the organ was located in fetal development. Although the organ migrates during fetal development, its nerves persist in referring sensations from the former location. Organs, such as the kidneys, liver, and intestines, begin forming by 3 weeks when the fetus is still less than the size of a raisin. By day 19, the notochord forming the spinal column has closed and by day 21, the heart begins to beat.

Embryologically, the chest is part of the gut; they are formed from the same tissue in utero. This explains symptoms of intrathoracic organ pathology frequently being referred to the abdomen as a viscero-visceral reflex. For example, it is not unusual for disorders of thoracic viscera, such as pneumonia or pleuritis, to refer pain that is perceived in the abdomen instead of the chest.[7,16]

Although the heart muscle starts out embryologically as a cranial structure, the pericardium around the heart is formed from gut tissue. This explains why myocardial infarction or pericarditis can also refer pain to the abdomen.[7,17,18]

For another example of how embryologic development affects the viscera and the soma, consider the ear and the kidney. These two structures have the same shape, come from the same embryologic tissue (otorenal axis of the mesenchyme), and are also formed at the same time (Fig. 3.2). When a child is born with any anomaly of the ear(s), or even a missing ear, the medical staff knows to look for possible similar changes or absence of the kidney on the same side.

A thorough understanding of fetal embryology is not really necessary in order to recognize red flag signs and symptoms of visceral origin, but knowing that it is one of several mechanisms by which the visceral referred pain patterns occur is a helpful start. The more you know about embryologic development of the viscera, the faster you will recognize somatic pain patterns caused by visceral dysfunction. Likewise, the more you know about anatomy, the origins of anatomy, its innervations, and the underlying neurophysiology, the better able you will be to identify the potential structures involved.

Multisegmental Innervation

Multisegmental innervation is the second mechanism used to explain pain patterns of a viscerogenic source (Fig. 3.3). The autonomic nervous system (ANS) is part of the peripheral nervous system and is divided up into sympathetic and parasympathetic divisions (Fig. 3.3 A and B). As shown in this diagram, the viscera have multisegmental innervations.

There is evidence to support referred visceral pain to somatic tissues based on overlapping or same segmental projections of spinal afferent neurons to the spinal dorsal horn. This concept is referred to as ***visceral-organ cross-sensitization***. The mechanism is likely to be sensitization of viscera-somatic convergent neurons.[19,20] Individuals diagnosed with multiple visceral problems obtained relief from pain in all organ systems with overlapping segmental projections when only one visceral area was treated. Therefore, nontreated visceral

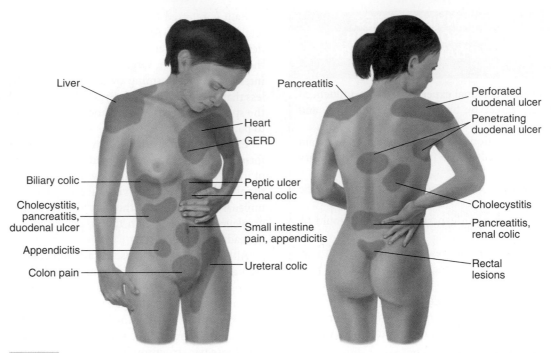

Liver
Heart
GERD
Biliary colic
Cholecystitis, pancreatitis, duodenal ulcer
Appendicitis
Colon pain
Peptic ulcer
Renal colic
Small intestine pain, appendicitis
Ureteral colic

Pancreatitis
Perforated duodenal ulcer
Penetrating duodenal ulcer
Cholecystitis
Pancreatitis, renal colic
Rectal lesions

Fig. 3.1 Common sites of referred pain from the abdominal viscera. When a client gives a history of referred pain from the viscera, the pain's location may not be directly over the impaired organ. Visceral embryologic development is the mechanism of the referred pain pattern. Pain is referred to the site where the organ was located in fetal development. (From Jarvis C. Physical Examination and Health Assessment. 5th ed. Philadelphia: WB Saunders; 2008.)

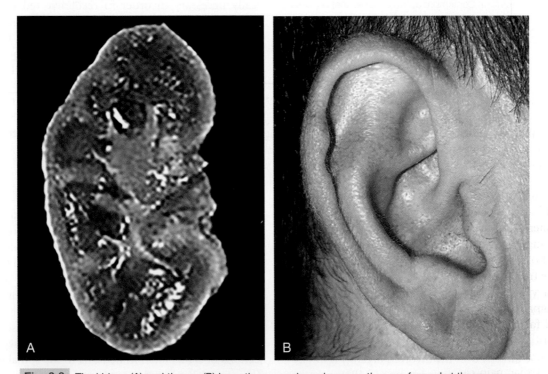

Fig. 3.2 The kidney (A) and the ear (B) have the same shape because they are formed at the same time and from the same embryologic tissue (otorenal axis of the mesenchyme). This is just one example of how fetal development influences form and function. When a child is born with a deformed or missing ear, the medical staff looks for a similarly deformed or missing kidney on the same side. (From (A) Klatt E. The kidneys. Robbins and Cotran Atlas of Pathology. New York: Elsevier; 2021:261-298. (B) From Stetson W and Morgan S. Knee. Arthroscopy: A diagnostic and therapeutic tool for management of ochronotic arthropathy. Arthrosc Tech. 2018;7(11): e1097–e1101.)

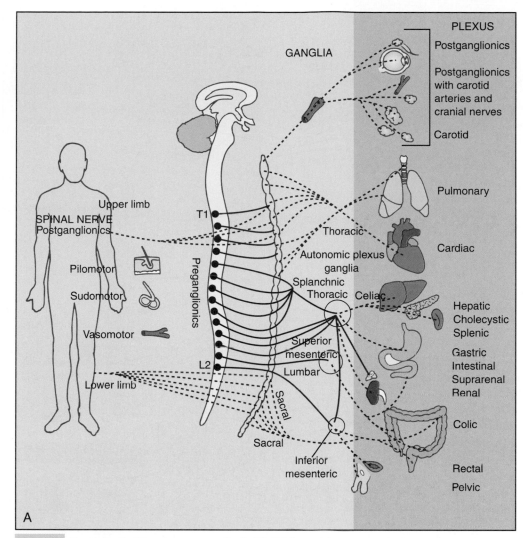

Fig. 3.3 Sympathetic (A) and parasympathetic (B) divisions of the autonomic nervous system. The visceral afferent fibers mediating pain travel with the sympathetic nerves, except for those from the pelvic organs, which follow the parasympathetics of the pelvic nerve. Major visceral organs have multisegmental innervations overlapping innervations of somatic structures. Visceral pain can be referred to the corresponding somatic area because sensory fibers for the viscera and somatic structures enter the spinal cord at the same levels converging on the same neurons. (From Levy MN, Koeppen BM. Berne and Levy Principles of Physiology. 4th ed. St. Louis: Mosby; 2006.)

disease significantly decreased when one viscera of the overlapping segments was addressed. For groups of people with no overlapping segments, spontaneous relief of referred pain was not obtained until and unless all involved visceral systems were treated.[19]

Pain of a visceral origin can be referred to the corresponding somatic areas. The example of cardiac pain is a good model for understanding this concept. Cardiac pain is not felt in the heart, but is referred to areas supplied by the corresponding spinal nerves. Instead of actual physical heart pain, cardiac pain can occur in any structure innervated by C3 to T4 such as the jaw, neck, upper trapezius, shoulder, and arm. Pain of cardiac and diaphragmatic origin is often experienced in the shoulder, in particular, because the C5 spinal segment supplies the heart, respiratory diaphragm, and shoulder.

Direct Pressure and Shared Pathways

A third mechanism by which the viscera refer pain to the soma is the concept of direct pressure and shared pathways (Fig. 3.4). As shown in this illustration, many of the viscera are near the respiratory diaphragm. Any pathologic process that can inflame, infect, or obstruct the organs can bring them in contact with the respiratory diaphragm.

Anything that impinges the **central diaphragm** can refer pain to the **shoulder** and anything that impinges the **peripheral diaphragm** can refer pain to the **ipsilateral costal margins** and/or **lumbar region** (Fig. 3.5).

This mechanism of referred pain through shared pathways occurs as a result of ganglions from each neural system gathering and sharing information through the cord to the plexuses. The visceral organs are innervated through

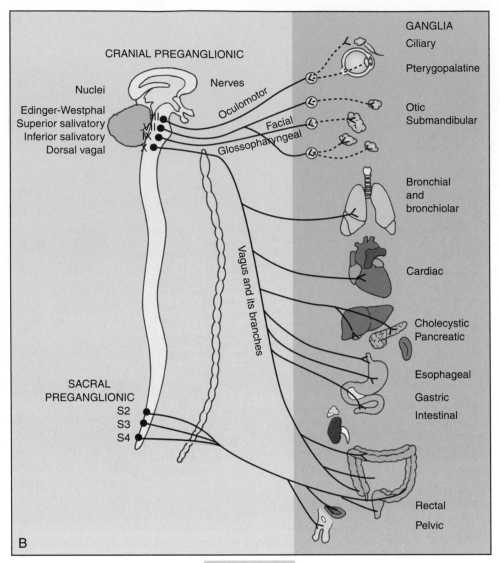

CRANIAL PREGANGLIONIC

Nuclei

Nerves

Edinger-Westphal
Superior salivatory
Inferior salivatory
Dorsal vagal

III
VII
IX
X

Oculomotor

Facial

Glossopharyngeal

GANGLIA

Ciliary

Pterygopalatine

Otic
Submandibular

Bronchial
and
bronchiolar

Cardiac

Cholecystic
Pancreatic

Esophageal

Gastric

Intestinal

Rectal

Pelvic

Vagus and its branches

SACRAL
PREGANGLIONIC

S2
S3
S4

B

Fig. 3.3, Cont'd

the ANS. The ganglions bring in information from around the body. The nerve plexuses decide how to respond to this information and give the body finely tuned, local control over responses.

Plexuses originate in the neck, thorax, diaphragm, and abdomen, terminating in the pelvis. The brachial plexus supplies the upper neck and shoulder, whereas the phrenic nerve innervates the respiratory diaphragm. More distally, the celiac plexus supplies the stomach and intestines. The neurologic supply of the plexuses is from parasympathetic fibers from the vagus and pelvic splanchnic nerves.[7]

The plexuses work independently of each other but not independently of the ganglia. The ganglia collect information derived from both the parasympathetic and the sympathetic fibers. The ganglia deliver this information to the plexuses; it is the plexuses that provide fine, local control in each of the organ systems.[7]

For example, the lower portion of the heart is in contact with the center of the diaphragm. The spleen on the left side of the body is tucked up under the dome of the diaphragm.

The kidneys (on either side) and the pancreas in the center are in easy reach of some portion of the diaphragm.

The body of the pancreas is in the center of the human body. The tail rests on the left side of the body. If an infection, inflammation, or tumor or other obstruction distends the pancreas, it can put pressure on the central part of the diaphragm.

Because the phrenic nerve (C3-C5) innervates the central zone of the diaphragm, as well as part of the pericardium, gallbladder, and pancreas, the client with impairment of these viscera can present with signs and symptoms in any of the somatic areas supplied by C3-C5 (e.g., shoulder).

In other words, the person can experience symptoms in the areas innervated by the same nerve pathways. So a problem affecting the pancreas can look like a heart problem, a gallbladder problem, or a midback/scapular or shoulder problem.

Most often, clients with pancreatic disease present with the primary pain pattern associated with the pancreas (i.e., left epigastric pain or pain just below the xiphoid process).

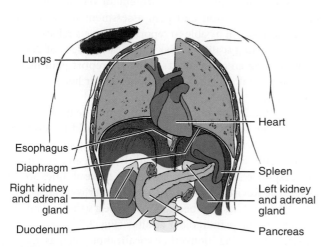

Fig. 3.4   Direct pressure from any inflamed, infected, or obstructed organ in contact with the respiratory diaphragm can refer pain to the ipsilateral shoulder. Note the location of each of the viscera. The spleen is tucked up under the diaphragm on the left side so any impairment of the spleen can cause left shoulder pain. The tail of the pancreas can come in contact with the diaphragm on the left side potentially causing referred pain to the left shoulder. The head of the pancreas can impinge the right side of the diaphragm causing referred pain to the right side. The gallbladder (not shown) is located up under the liver on the right side with corresponding right referred shoulder pain possible. Other organs that can come in contact with the diaphragm in this way include the heart and the kidneys.

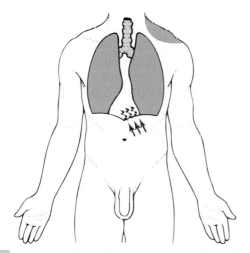

Fig. 3.5   Irritation of the peritoneal (outside) or pleural (inside) surface of the central area of the respiratory diaphragm can refer sharp pain to the upper trapezius muscle, neck, and supraclavicular fossa. The pain pattern is ipsilateral to the area of irritation. Irritation of the peripheral portion of the diaphragm can refer sharp pain to the costal margins and lumbar region (not shown).

The somatic presentation of referred pancreatic pain to the shoulder or back is uncommon, but it is the unexpected, referred pain patterns that we see in a physical or occupational therapy practice.

Another example of this same phenomenon occurs with peritonitis or gallbladder inflammation. These conditions can irritate the phrenic endings in the central part of

the diaphragmatic peritoneum. The client can experience referred shoulder pain as a result of the root origin shared in common by the phrenic and supraclavicular nerves.

Not only is it true that any structure that touches the diaphragm can refer pain to the shoulder, but even structures adjacent to or in contact with the diaphragm in utero can do the same. Keep in mind there has to be some impairment of that structure (e.g., obstruction, distention, inflammation) for this to occur (Case Example 3.1).

CASE EXAMPLE 3.1
Mechanism of Referred Pain

A 72-year-old woman has come to physical therapy for rehabilitation after cutting her hand and having a flexor tendon repair. She uses a walker to ambulate, reports being short of breath "her whole life," and takes the following prescription and over-the-counter (OTC) medications:

* Feldene
* Vioxx*
* Ativan
* Glucosamine
* Ibuprofen "on bad days"
* Furosemide
* And one other big pill once a week on Sunday "for my bones"

During the course of evaluating and treating her hand, she reports constant, aching pain in her right shoulder and a sharp, tingling, burning sensation behind her armpit (also on the right side). She does not have any associated bowel or bladder signs and symptoms, but reports excessive fatigue "since the day I was born."

You suspect the combination of Feldene and ibuprofen along with long-term use of Vioxx may be a problem.

What Is the Most Likely Mechanism of Pain: Embryologic Development, Multisegmental Innervation of the Stomach and Duodenum, or Direct Pressure on the Diaphragm? Even though Vioxx is a cyclooxygenase-2 (COX-2) inhibitor and less likely to cause problems, gastritis and gastrointestinal (GI) bleeding are still possible, especially with chronic long-term use of multiple nonsteroidal antiinflammatory drugs (NSAIDs).

Retroperitoneal bleeding from peptic ulcer can cause referred pain to the back at the level of the lesion (T6–T10) or right shoulder and/or upper trapezius pain. Shoulder pain may be accompanied by sudomotor changes such as burning, gnawing, or cramping pain along the lateral border of the scapula. The scapular pain can occur alone as the only symptom.

Side effects of NSAIDs can also include fatigue, anxiety, depression, paresthesia, fluid retention, tinnitus, nausea, vomiting, dry mouth, and bleeding from the nose, mouth, or under the skin. If peritoneal bleeding is the cause of her symptoms, *the mechanism of pain* is blood in the posterior abdominal cavity irritating the diaphragm through direct pressure.

Be sure to take the client's vital signs and observe for significant changes in blood pressure and pulse. Poor wound healing and edema (sacral, pedal, hands) may be present. Ask if the same doctor prescribed each medication and if her physician (or physicians) knows which medications she is taking. It is possible that her medications have not been checked or coordinated from before her hospitalization to the present time.

*Removed from the market in 2004 by Merck & Co., Inc., due to reports of increased risk of cardiovascular events.

ASSESSMENT OF PAIN AND SYMPTOMS

The interviewing techniques and specific questions for pain assessment are outlined in this section. The information gathered during the interview and examination provides a description of the client that is clear, accurate, and comprehensive. The therapist should keep in mind cultural rules and differences in pain perception, intensity, and responses to pain found among various ethnic groups.[21]

Measuring pain and assessing pain are two separate issues. A measurement assigns a number or value to give dimension to pain intensity.[22] A comprehensive pain assessment includes a detailed health history, physical examination, medication history (including nonprescription drug use and complementary and alternative therapies), assessment of functional status, and consideration of psychosocial-spiritual factors.[23]

The portion of the core interview regarding a client's perception of pain is a critical factor in the evaluation of signs and symptoms. Questions about pain must be understood by the client and should be presented in a nonjudgmental manner. A detailed record of pain may be helpful to standardize pain assessment with each client (Fig. 3.6).

To elicit a complete description of symptoms from the client, the physical therapist may wish to use a term other than *pain*. It is better to use terms such as "symptoms" and then have the patient use descriptors such as burning, tightness, heaviness, discomfort, and aching may be a better approach because patients could personalize and therefore communicate their pain experience better. However, it is important to remember that this could also lead to increased sensitivity of the cortical pain processing areas that may result in increased pain.[24] If the client has completed the McGill Pain Questionnaire (MPQ) (see discussion of **McGill Pain Questionnaire** in this chapter),[25] the physical therapist may choose the most appropriate alternative word selected by the client from the list to refer to the symptoms (Table 3.1).

Pain Assessment in the Older Adult

Physical therapists must be careful to take reports of pain from older persons as serious and very real, and not discount their symptoms as a part of aging, or affected by cognitive disturbances.[26] Joint pain is one of the most prevalent health problems in older adults. The incidence of pain in community dwelling older adults has been reported to be 50%.[27] About one in four adults diagnosed with arthritis report severe joint pain (defined as pain rating of 7 or higher on a scale of 0 being no pain and 10 as worst pain), and nearly half with arthritis report pan of any severity in post or all days within the past 3 months.[28]

As therapists, we are likely to see pain more often as a key feature among older adults as our population continues to age. Older adults may avoid giving an accurate assessment of their pain. [29] For reasons that include concerns of how the pain may be perceived by others, embarrassment and perceptions of exaggerating the symptoms, fear or avoidance, avoidance of medical settings, medications or treatments, and cost, among others.[30]

Sensory and cognitive impairment in older, frail adults makes communication and pain assessment more difficult. The client may still be able to report pain levels reliably using the visual analog scales (VASs) in the early stages of dementia. Improving an older adult's ability to report pain may be as simple as making sure the client has his or her glasses and hearing aid.

The Verbal Descriptor Scale (VDS) could be used to assess pain in older adults, including those with mild-to-moderate cognitive impairment.[31] This scale and other pain scales rely on the client's ability to understand the scale and communicate a response. As dementia progresses, these abilities are lost as well. The Revised Iowa Pain Thermometer is an adaptation of the VDS and has also been shown to be a valid and reliable tool in assessing pain in older adults[32] (Fig. 3.7).

Facial grimacing; nonverbal vocalization such as moans, sighs, or gasps; and verbal comments (e.g., ouch, stop) are the most frequent behaviors among cognitively impaired older adults during painful movement (Box 3.2). Bracing, holding on to furniture, or clutching the painful area are other behavioral indicators of pain. Alternately, the client may resist care by others or stay very still to guard against pain caused by movement.[33]

Pain Assessment in the Young Child

Many infants and children are unable to report pain. Even so the therapist should not underestimate or prematurely conclude that a young client is unable to answer any questions about pain. Even some clients (both children and adults) with substantial cognitive impairment may be able to use pain-rating scales when explained carefully.[34]

The Faces Pain Scale (FACES or FPS) for children (see Fig. 3.6) has been revised from the original version to FPS-R[35] and is used with similar assessment measures.[36]

Most of the pilot work for the FPS was done informally with children from preschool through young school age. Researchers have used the FPS scale with adults, especially the elderly, and have had successful results. Advantages of the cartoon-type FPS scale are that it avoids gender, age, and racial biases.[37] Research shows that use of the word "hurt" rather than "pain" is understood by children as young as 3 years old.[38,39] Use of words such as "owie" or "ouchie" by a child to describe pain is an acceptable substitute.[37] Assessing pain intensity with the FPS scale is fast and easy. The child looks at the faces, the therapist or parent uses the simple words to describe the expression, and the corresponding number is used to record the score.

Fig. 3.8 lists tools that can be used to assess pediatric pain. When using a rating scale is not possible, the therapist may have to rely on the parent's or caregiver's report and/or other measures of pain in children with cognitive or communication impairments and physical disabilities. Look for telltale behavior such as lack of cooperation, withdrawal, acting out, distractibility, or seeking comfort. Altered sleep patterns, vocalizations, and eating patterns provide additional clues.

Pain Assessment Record Form

Client's name: _____   Date: _____

Physician's diagnosis: _____   Physical therapist's diagnosis: _____

Medications: _____   _____
_____   _____
_____   _____

Onset of pain (circle one): Was there an:

Accident   Injury   Trauma (violence)   Specific activity

If yes, describe:

Characteristics of pain/symptoms:

Location (Show me exactly where your pain/symptom is located):

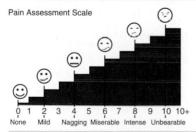

ıııı Numbness
🗲 Severe pain
≋ Moderate pain
↓ Shooting pain

Do you have any pain or symptoms anywhere else?   Yes   No

Description (If yes, what does it feel like):

Circle any other words that describe the client's symptoms:

Knifelike	Dull	Aching	Other (describe):
Boring	Burning	Throbbing	
Heaviness	Discomfort	Sharp	
Stinging	Tingling	Stabbing	

Frequency (circle one):   Constant   Intermittent (comes and goes)

If constant: Do you have this pain right now?   Yes   No

If intermittent: How often is the pain present (circle all that apply):

Hourly   Once/daily   Twice/daily   Unpredictable   Other (please describe): _____

Intensity: *Numeric Rating Scale* and the *Faces Pain Scale*

Instructions: On a scale from 0 to 10 with zero meaning 'No pain' and 10 for 'Unbearable pain,' how would you rate your pain right now?

Pain Assessment Scale

0 1 2 3 4 5 6 7 8 9 10 10+
None Mild Nagging Miserable Intense Unbearable

Alternately: Point to the face that best shows how much pain you are having right now.

Intensity: *Visual Analog Scale*

Instructions: On the line below, put a mark (or point to) the place on the line between 'Pain-free' and 'Worst possible pain' that best describes/shows how much pain you are having right now.

A   **Pain-Free** _____ **Worst Possible Pain**

Fig. 3.6   Pain Assessment Record Form. Use this form to complete the pain history and obtain a description of the pain pattern. The form is printed in the Appendix on for your use. This form may be copied and used without permission. (From Carlsson AM. Assessment of chronic pain. I. Aspects of the reliability and validity of the visual analogue scale. Pain 1983;16(1):87–101.)

Duration:
How long does your pain (name the symptom) last?

Aggravating factors (What makes it worse?)	**Relieving factors** (What makes it better?)

Pattern
Has the pain changed since it first began?   Yes   No
If yes, please explain:

What is your pain/symptom like from morning (am) to evening (pm)?

_____

_____

Circle one: Worse in the morning   Worse midday/afternoon   Worse at night
Circle one: Gradually getting better   Gradually getting worse   Staying the same
Circle all that apply:
Present upon waking up   Keeps me from falling asleep   Wakes me up at night

Therapist: Record any details or description about night pain. See also Appendix on ⓔ for *Screening Questions for Night Pain* when appropriate.

Associated symptoms (What other symptoms have you had with this problem?)

_____

Circle any words the client uses to describe his/her symptoms. If the client says there are no other symptoms ask about the presence of any of the following:

Burning	Difficulty breathing	Shortness of breath	Cough
Skin rash (or other lesions)	Change in bowel/bladder	Difficulty swallowing	Painful swallowing
Dizziness	Heart palpitations	Hoarseness	Nausea/vomiting
Diarrhea	Constipation	Bleeding of any kind	Sweats
Numbness	Problems with vision	Tingling	Weakness
Joint pain	Weight loss/gain	Other:_____	

Final question: Are there any other pain or symptoms of any kind anywhere else in your body that we have not talked about yet?

For the therapist:
Follow-up questions can include:
Are there any positions that make it feel better? Worse?
How does rest affect the pain/symptoms?
How does activity affect the pain/symptoms?
How has this problem affected your daily life at work or at home?
Has this problem affected your ability to care for yourself without assistance (e.g., dress, bathe, cook, drive)?
Has this problem affected your sexual function or activity?
Therapist's evaluation:
Can you reproduce the pain by squeezing or palpating the symptomatic area?
Does resisted motion reproduce the pain/symptoms?
Is the client taking NSAIDs? Experiencing increased symptoms after taking NSAIDs?
If taking NSAIDs, is the client at risk for peptic ulcer? Check all that apply:
☐ Age 65 years   ☐ History of peptic ulcer disease or GI disease
☐ Smoking, alcohol use   ☐ Oral corticosteroid use
☐ Anticoagulation or use of other anticoagulants (even when used for heart patients at a lower dose, e.g., 81 to 325 mg aspirin/day)
☐ Renal complications in clients with hypertension or congestive heart failure (CHF) or who use diuretics or ACE inhibitors
☐ NSAIDs combined with selective serotonin reuptake inhibitors (SSRIs; antidepressants such as Prozac, Zoloft, Celexa, Paxil)
☐ Use of acid suppressants (e.g., H_2-receptor antagonists, antacids)
Other areas to consider:
• Sleep quality   • Bowel/bladder habits   • Depression or anxiety screening score
• Correlation of symptoms with peak effect of medications (dosage, time of day)   • For women: correlation of symptoms with
B • Evaluation of joint pain (see Appendix B-18 on ⓔ: *Screening Questions for Joint Pain*)   menstrual cycle

Fig. 3.6, Cont'd

TABLE 3.1	Recognizing Pain Patterns		
Vascular	Neurogenic	Musculoskeletal	Emotional
Throbbing	Sharp	Aching	Tiring
Pounding	Crushing	Sore	Miserable
Pulsing	Pinching	Heavy	Vicious
Beating	Burning	Hurting	Agonizing
	Hot	Deep	Nauseating
	Searing	Cramping	Frightful
	Itchy	Dull	Piercing
	Stinging		Dreadful
	Pulling		Punishing
	Jumping		Exhausting
	Shooting		Killing
	Electrical		Unbearable
	Gnawing		Annoying
	Pricking		Cruel
			Sickening
			Torturing

(From Melzack R. The McGill pain questionnaire: Major properties and scoring methods. Pain 1975;1:277.)

BOX 3.2 SYMPTOMS OF PAIN IN CLIENTS WITH COGNITIVE IMPAIRMENT

- Verbal comments such as "ouch" or "stop"
- Nonverbal vocalizations (e.g., moans, sighs, gasps)
- Facial grimacing or frowning
- Audible breathing independent of vocalization (labored, short or long periods of hyperventilation)
- Agitation or increased confusion
- Unable to be consoled or distracted
- Bracing or holding on to furniture
- Decreased mobility
- Lying very still, refusing to move
- Clutching the painful area
- Resisting care provided by others, striking out, pushing others away
- Sleep disturbance
- Weight loss
- Depression

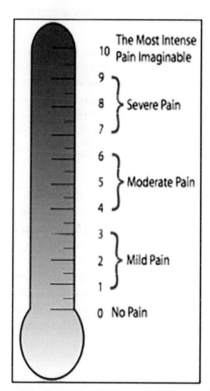

Fig 3.7   Revised Iowa Pain Thermometer. (From Ware L, Herr K, Booker SS, et al. Psychometric evaluation of the revised Iowa Pain Thermometer (IPT-R) in a sample of diverse cognitively intact and impaired older adults: A pilot study. Pain Manage Nurs. 2015;16(4):475–482.)

Vital signs should be documented but not relied upon as the sole determinant of pain (or absence of pain) in infants and young children. The pediatric therapist may want to use several pain measures that correspond to the age of the neonate, infant, or child.

Characteristics of Pain

It is very important to identify how the client's description of pain as a symptom relates to sources and types of pain discussed in this chapter. Many characteristics of pain can be elicited from the client during the Core Interview to help define the source or type of pain in question. These characteristics include:
- Location
- Description of sensation
- Intensity
- Duration
- Frequency and duration
- Pattern

Other additional components are related to factors that aggravate the pain, factors that relieve the pain, and other symptoms that may occur in association with the pain. Specific questions are included in this section for each descriptive component. Keep in mind that an increase in frequency, intensity, or duration of symptoms over time can indicate systemic disease.

Location of Pain

Questions related to the location of pain focus the client's description as precisely as possible. An opening statement might be as follows:

❓ FOLLOW-UP QUESTIONS

- Show me exactly where your symptom/s is/are located.
    Follow-up questions may include:
- Do you have any other symptoms anywhere else?
- If yes, what causes the symptoms to occur in this other area?

Piaget's Developmental Stages	Patients' Understanding of Pain	Nursing Implications
Sensorimotor (birth–24 months)	• Under 6 months: have no understanding of pain • 6–12 months: anticipate a painful event; responsive to parental anxiety	• Provide optimal pain management to reduce psychological and emotional responses to future pain events
Preoperational (2–7 years)	• Understand pain as a physical experience that can magically disappear • Have no concept of cause and effect • Perceive pain as punishment • May hold someone accountable for their pain, striking out physically or verbally	• Help children see the connection between pain treatment and pain relief • Provide reassurance that pain is not a punishment
Concrete operational (7–12 years)	• Can specify location of physical pain • Have increased awareness of their bodies and internal organs • Are developing an understanding of consequences (if they keep ice on an injury, there will be less swelling, for example) • Fear bodily harm and death	• Provide explanations for pain and its treatment • Help calm fears about bodily destruction and death
Formal operational (adolescence–adulthood)	• Begin to problem solve • Valve privacy, control, and trust	• Communicate honestly and in a nonthreatening way that promotes learning and trust

Fig 3.8   Pediatric pain assessment tools. (From Freund D and Bolick BN. Assessing a child's pain. *Am J Nurs.* 2019;119(5):34–41.)

If the client points to a small, localized area and the pain does not spread, the cause is likely to be a superficial lesion and is probably not severe. If the client points to a small, localized area but the pain does spread, this is more likely to be a diffuse, segmental, referred pain that may originate in the viscera or deep somatic structure.

The character and location of pain can change and the client may have several painful areas at once, so repeated pain assessment may be needed.

Description of Pain

To assist the physical therapist in obtaining a clear description of pain sensation, pose the question:

 FOLLOW-UP QUESTIONS

- What does it feel like?
  After giving the client time to reply, offer some additional choices in potential descriptors. You may want to ask: Is your pain/Are your symptoms:

- Knife-like
- Boring
- Throbbing
- Deep aching
- Dull
- Burning
- Prickly
- Sharp

Follow-up questions may include:
- Has the pain changed in quality since it first began?
- Changed in intensity?
- Changed in duration (how long it lasts)?

When a client describes the pain as knife-like, boring, colicky, coming in waves, or a deep aching feeling, this description should be a signal to the physical therapist to consider the possibility of a systemic origin of symptoms. Dull, somatic pain of an aching nature can be differentiated from the aching pain of a muscular lesion by squeezing or pressing the muscle overlying the area of pain. Resisting motion of the limb may also reproduce aching of muscular origin that has no connection to deep somatic aching.

Intensity of Pain

A pain rating scale may be used to assess pain intensity. The therapist may use one or more of these scales, depending on the clinical presentation of each client (see Fig. 3.6). Show the pain scale to the client and ask the client to choose a number and/or a face that best describes his or her current pain level. This scale can quantify symptoms other than pain, such as stiffness, pressure, soreness, discomfort, cramping, aching, numbness, and tingling. Always use the same scale for each follow-up assessment.

The Visual Analog Scale (VAS)[40,41] allows the client to choose a point along a 10-cm (100-mm) horizontal line (see Fig. 3.6). The left end represents "No pain" and the right end represents "Pain as bad as it could possibly be" or "Worst possible pain." This same scale can be presented in a vertical orientation for the client who must remain supine and cannot sit up for the assessment. "No pain" is placed at the bottom, and "Worst possible pain" is put at the top.

The VAS scale is easily combined with the numeric rating scale (NRS) with possible values ranging from 0 (no pain) to 10 (worst imaginable pain). It can be used to assess current pain, worst pain in the preceding 24 hours, least pain in the past 24 hours, or any combination the clinician finds useful.

The Numeric Pain Rating Scale (NPRS; see Fig. 3.6) allows the client to rate the pain intensity on a scale from 0 (no pain) to 10 (the worst pain imaginable). This is probably the most commonly used pain rating scale in both the inpatient and outpatient settings. It is a simple and valid method of measuring pain. Additional information, including psychometric properties of the NPRS can be found at: https://www.sralab.org/rehabilitation-measures/numeric-pain-rating-scale.

Careful assessment of the person's nonverbal behavior (e.g., ease of movement, facial grimacing, guarding movements) may help to clarify the description of the intensity of the pain. Pain of an intense, unrelenting (constant) nature is often associated with systemic disease.

The 36-Item Short-Form Health Survey discussed in Chapter 2 includes an assessment of bodily pain along with a general measure of health-related quality of life. Nurses often use the OPQRST mnemonic to help identify underlying pathology or pain (Box 3.3).

Frequency and Duration of Pain

The frequency of occurrence is related closely to the pattern of the pain, and the client should be asked how often the symptoms occur and whether the pain is constant or intermittent. Duration of pain is a part of this description.

? FOLLOW-UP QUESTIONS

- How long do the symptoms last?
    For example, pain related to systemic disease has been shown to be a *constant* rather than an *intermittent* type of pain experience. Clients who indicate that the pain is constant should be asked:
- Do you have this pain right now?
- Did you notice these symptoms this morning immediately when you woke up?

Further responses may reveal that the pain is perceived as being constant but in fact is not actually present consistently and/or can be reduced with rest or change in position, which are characteristics more common with pain of

BOX 3.3 NURSING ASSESSMENT OF PAIN (OPQRST)

Onset. When did it start and what were you doing?

Provocation and palliation. What causes the pain and what makes it better or worse?

Quality of pain. What type of pain is present (aching, burning, sharp)?

Region and radiation. Where is the pain located? Does it radiate to other parts of the body?

Severity on a scale of 0 to 10. Does the pain interfere with daily activities, mood, function?

Timing. Did the pain come on suddenly or gradually? Is it constant or does it come and go (intermittent)? How often does it occur? How long does it last? Does it come on at the same time of the day or night?

musculoskeletal origin. Symptoms that truly do not change throughout the course of the day warrant further attention.

Pattern of Pain

After listening to the client describe all characteristics of their pain or symptoms, the therapist may recognize a vascular, neurogenic, musculoskeletal, emotional, or visceral pattern (see Table 3.1).

The following sequence of questions may be helpful in further assessing the pattern of pain, especially how the symptoms may change with time.

? FOLLOW-UP QUESTIONS

- Tell me about the pattern of your symptoms.
- *Alternate question:* When does your back/shoulder (name the involved body part) hurt?
- *Alternate question:* Describe your symptoms from first waking up in the morning to going to bed at night. (See special sleep-related questions that follow.)
    Follow-up questions may include:
- Have you ever experienced anything like this before?
- If yes, do these episodes occur more or less often than at first?
- How does your symptom(s) change with time?
- Are your symptoms worse in the morning or evening?

The pattern of pain associated with systemic disease is often a progressive pattern with a cyclical onset (i.e., the client describes symptoms as being alternately worse, better, and worse over a period of months). When there is back pain, this pattern differs from the sudden sequestration of a discogenic lesion that appears with a pattern of increasingly worse symptoms followed by a sudden cessation of all symptoms. Such involvement of the disk occurs without the cyclical return of symptoms weeks or months later, which is more typical of a systemic disorder.

If the client appears to be unsure of the pattern of symptoms or has "avoided paying any attention" to this component of pain description, it may be useful to keep a record at home assisting the client in taking notes of the symptoms for 24 hours.

Medications can alter the pain pattern or characteristics of painful symptoms. Find out how well the client's current medications reduce, control, or relieve pain. Ask how often medications are needed for breakthrough pain.

When using any of the pain rating scales, record the use of any medications that can alter or reduce pain or symptoms such as anti-inflammatories or analgesics. At the same time remember to look for side effects or adverse reactions to any drugs or drug combinations.

Watch for clients taking nonsteroidal anti-inflammatory drugs (NSAIDs) who experience an increase in shoulder, neck, or back pain several hours after taking the medication. Normally, one would expect symptom relief from NSAIDs so any increase in symptoms is a red flag for possible peptic ulcer.

A client will frequently comment that the pain or symptoms have not changed despite 2 or 3 weeks of physical therapy intervention. This information can be discouraging to both client and therapist; however, when the symptoms are reviewed, a decrease in pain, increase in function, reduced need for medications, or other significant improvement in the pattern of symptoms may be seen. However, if no improvement in symptoms or function can be demonstrated, the therapist must again consider a systemic origin of symptoms. Repeating screening questions for medical disease is encouraged throughout the episode of care even if such questions were included in the intake interview.

Because of the progressive nature of systemic involvement, the client may not have noticed any constitutional symptoms at the start of the physical therapy intervention that may now be present. Constitutional symptoms (see Box 1.3) affect the whole body and are characteristic of systemic disease or illness.

Aggravating and Easing Factors

A series of questions addressing aggravating and relieving factors must be included, such as:

 FOLLOW-UP QUESTIONS

- What brings on your pain (symptoms)?
- What kinds of things make your pain (symptoms) worse (e.g., eating, exercise, rest, specific positions, excitement, stress)?
  To assess relieving factors, ask:
- What makes the pain better?
  Follow-up questions include:
- How does rest affect the pain/symptoms?
- Are your symptoms aggravated or relieved by any activities?
- If yes, what?
- How has this problem affected your daily life at work or at home?
- How has this problem affected your ability to care for yourself without assistance (e.g., dress, bathe, cook, drive)?

Systemic pain tends to be relieved minimally, relieved only temporarily, or unrelieved by change in position or by rest. However, musculoskeletal pain is *often* relieved both by a change of position and by rest.

Associated Symptoms

These symptoms may occur alone or in conjunction with the pain of systemic disease. The client may or may not associate these additional symptoms with the chief complaint. The physical therapist may ask:

 FOLLOW-UP QUESTIONS

- What other symptoms have you had that you can associate with this problem?
  If the client denies any additional symptoms, follow-up this question with a series of possibilities, such as:

Burning	Heart palpitations	Numbness/tingling
Difficulty in breathing	Hoarseness	Problems with vision
Difficulty in swallowing	Nausea	Vomiting
Dizziness	Night sweats	Weakness

Whenever the client says "yes" to such associated symptoms, check for the presence of these symptoms bilaterally. Additionally, bilateral weakness, either proximally or distally, should serve as a red flag, possibly indicative of more than a musculoskeletal lesion.

Blurred vision, double vision, scotomas (black spots before the eyes), or temporary blindness may indicate early symptoms of conditions such as multiple sclerosis or may possibly be warning signs of an impending cerebrovascular accident. The presence of any associated symptoms, such as those mentioned here, would require contact with the physician to confirm the physician's knowledge of these symptoms.

In summary, careful, sensitive, and thorough questioning regarding the multifaceted experience of pain can elicit essential information necessary when making a decision regarding treatment or referral. The use of pain assessment tools such as Fig. 3.6 and Table 3.2 may facilitate clear and accurate descriptions of this critical symptom.

SOURCES OF PAIN

Physical therapists frequently see clients whose primary complaint is pain, which often leads to a loss of function. However, focusing on sources of pain does not always help us to identify the causes of tissue irritation.

The most effective physical therapy diagnosis will define the syndrome and address the cause(s) of pain rather than just identifying the source(s) of pain.[42] Usually, a careful assessment of pain behavior is invaluable in determining the nature and extent of the underlying pathology.

The clinical evaluation of pain usually involves identification of the primary disease/etiological factor(s) considered responsible for producing or initiating the pain. The client is placed within a broad pain category usually labeled as nociceptive, inflammatory, or neuropathic. Pain and sensory disturbances associated with central changes (sensitization) may be present with chronic pain.[13,43] It can be difficult in clinical practice to specify which of these, alone or in combination, may be present.[29]

We further classify the pain by identifying its anatomic distribution, quality, and intensity. Such an approach allows for physical therapy intervention for each identified mechanism involved.

From a screening perspective, we look at the possible *sources* of pain and *types* of pain. When listening to the client's description of their pain, consider these possible sources (Table 3.3):
- Cutaneous
- Somatic
- Visceral
- Neuropathic
- Referred

Cutaneous Sources of Pain

Cutaneous pain (related to the skin) includes superficial somatic structures located in the skin and subcutaneous tissue. The pain is well localized as the client can point directly to the area that "hurts." Pain from a cutaneous source can usually be localized with one finger. Skin pain or tenderness can be associated with referred pain from the viscera or from deep somatic structures.

Impairment of any organ can result in sudomotor changes that present as trophic changes, such as itching, dysesthesia, skin temperature changes, or dry skin. The difficulty is that biomechanical dysfunction can also result in these same changes, which is why a careful evaluation of soft tissue structures along with a screening examination for systemic disease is required.

Cutaneous pain perception varies from person to person and is not always a reliable indicator of pathologic etiology. These differences in pain perception may be associated with different pain mechanisms.

Somatic Sources of Pain

Somatic pain can be superficial or deep. Somatic pain is labeled according to its source as deep somatic, somatovisceral, somatoemotional (also referred to as *psychosomatic*), or viscero-somatic.

TABLE 3.2	Comparison of Systemic Versus Musculoskeletal Pain Patterns	
	Systemic Pain	Musculoskeletal Pain
Onset	• Recent, sudden • Does not present as observed for years without progression of symptoms	May be sudden or gradual, depending on the history • Sudden: Usually associated with acute overload stress, traumatic event, repetitive motion; can occur as a side effect of some medications (e.g., statins) • **Gradual:** Secondary to chronic overload of the affected part; may be present off and on for years
Description	• Knife-like quality of stabbing from the inside out, boring, deep aching • Cutting, gnawing • Throbbing • Bone pain • Unilateral or bilateral	• Usually unilateral • May be stiff after prolonged rest, but pain level decreases • Achy, cramping pain • Local tenderness to pressure is present
Intensity	• Related to the degree of noxious stimuli; usually unrelated to presence of anxiety • Mild to severe • Dull to severe	• May be mild to severe • May depend on the person's anxiety level—the level of pain may increase in a client fearful of a "serious" condition
Duration	• Constant, no change, awakens the person at night	• Duration can be modified by rest or change in position • May be constant but is more likely to be intermittent, depending on the activity or the position

Pattern	• Although constant, may come in waves
	• Gradually progressive, cyclical
	• Night pain
	  • Location: chest/shoulder
	  • Accompanied by shortness of breath, wheezing
	  • Eating alters symptoms
	  • Sitting up relieves symptoms (decreases venous return to the heart: possible pulmonary or cardiovascular etiology)
	• Symptoms unrelieved by rest or change in position
	• Migratory arthralgias: Pain/symptoms last for 1 week in one joint, then resolve and appear in another joint
		• Restriction of active/passive/accessory movement(s) observed
		• One or more particular movements "catch" the client and aggravate the pain

Aggravating Factors	• Cannot alter, provoke, alleviate, eliminate, aggravate the symptomsOrgan dependent (examples):
	  • Esophagus—eating or swallowing affects symptoms
	  • Heart—cold, exertion, stress, heavy meal (especially when combined) bring on symptoms
	  • Gastrointestinal (GI)—peristalsis (eating) affects symptoms
		• Altered by movement; pain may become worse with movement or some myalgia decreases with movement

Easing Factors	• Organ dependent (examples):
	  • Gallbladder—leaning forward may reduce symptoms
	  • Kidney—leaning to the affected side may reduce symptoms
	  • Pancreas—sitting upright or leaning forward may reduce symptoms
		• Symptoms reduced or relieved by rest or change in position
		• Muscle pain is relieved by short periods of rest without resulting stiffness, except in the case of fibromyalgia; stiffness may be present in older adults
		• Stretching
		• Heat, cold

TABLE 3.2	Comparison of Systemic Versus Musculoskeletal Pain Patterns—Cont'd	
	Systemic Pain	**Musculoskeletal Pain**
Associated Signs and Symptoms	• Fever, chills • Sweats (at any time day or night) • Unusual vital signs • Warning signs of cancer • GI symptoms: nausea, vomiting, anorexia, unexplained weight loss, diarrhea, constipation • Early satiety (feeling full after eating) • Bilateral symptoms (e.g., paresthesias, weakness, edema, nail bed changes, skin rash) • Painless weakness of muscles: more often proximal but may occur distally • Dyspnea (breathlessness at rest or after mild exertion) • Diaphoresis (excessive perspiration) • Headaches, dizziness, fainting • Visual disturbances • Skin lesions, rashes, or itching that the client may not associate with the musculoskeletal symptoms • Bowel/bladder symptoms • Hematuria (blood in the urine) • Nocturia • Urgency (sudden need to urinate) • Frequency • Melena (blood in feces) • Fecal or urinary incontinence • Bowel smears	• Usually none, although stimulation of trigger points (TrPs) may cause sweating, nausea, blanching

TABLE 3.3	Sources of Pain, Pain Types, and Pain Patterns		
Sources	**Types**	**Characteristics/ Patterns**	

Cutaneous
Deep
   somatic
Visceral
Neuropathic
Referred
	Tension
	Inflammatory
	Ischemic
	Myofascial pain
	   • Muscle tension
	   • Muscle spasm
	   • Trigger points (TrPs)
	   • Muscle deficiency (weakness and stiffness)
	   • Muscle trauma
	Joint pain
	   • Drug-induced
	   • Chemical exposure
	   • Inflammatory bowel disease
	   • Septic arthritis
	   • Reactive arthritis
	Radicular pain
	Arterial, pleural, tracheal
	Gastrointestinal pain
	Pain at rest
	Night pain
	Pain with activity
	Diffuse pain
	Chronic pain
		Client describes:
		   • Location/onset
		   • Description
		   • Frequency
		   • Duration
		   • Intensity
		Therapist recognizes the pattern:
		   • Vascular
		   • Neurogenic
		   • Musculoskeletal/ spondylotic
		   • Visceral
		   • Emotional	

Most of what the therapist treats is part of the somatic system, whether we call that the neuromuscular system or the musculoskeletal system. When psychologic disorders present as somatic dysfunction, we refer to these conditions as psychophysiologic disorders.

Superficial somatic structures involve the skin, superficial fasciae, tendon sheaths, and periosteum. *Deep somatic pain* comes from pathologic conditions of the periosteum and cancellous (spongy) bone, nerves, muscles, tendons, ligaments, and blood vessels. Deep somatic structures also include deep fasciae and joint capsules. Somatic referred pain does not involve stimulation of nerve roots. It is produced by stimulation of nerve endings within the superficial and deep somatic structures just mentioned.

Somatic referred pain is usually reported as dull, aching, or gnawing or described as an expanding pressure that is too diffuse to localize. There are no neurologic signs associated with somatic referred pain because this type of pain is considered nociceptive and is not caused by the compression of spinal nerves or the nerve root.

Deep somatic pain is poorly localized and may be referred to the body surface, becoming cutaneous. It can be associated with an autonomic phenomenon, such as sweating, pallor, or changes in pulse and blood pressure, and is commonly accompanied by a subjective feeling of nausea and faintness.

Pain associated with deep somatic lesions follows patterns that relate to the embryologic development of the musculoskeletal system. This explains why such pain may not be perceived directly over the involved organ (see Fig. 3.1).

Parietal pain (related to the wall of the chest or abdominal cavity) is also considered deep somatic. The visceral pleura (the membrane enveloping the organs) is insensitive to pain, but the parietal pleura is well supplied with pain nerve endings. For this reason, it is possible for a client to have extensive visceral disease (e.g., heart, lungs) without pain until the disease progresses enough to involve the parietal pleura.

The term "psycho-*somatic*" response refers to the mind-*body* connection.

Somatoemotional or *psychosomatic* sources of pain occur when emotional or psychologic distress produces physical symptoms either for a relatively brief period or with recurrent and multiple physical manifestations spanning many months to many years. The person affected by the latter may be referred to as a *somatizer*, and the condition is called a *somatization disorder*.

Alternately, there are *viscero-somatic* sources of pain when visceral structures affect the somatic musculature, such as the reflex spasm and rigidity of the abdominal muscles in response to the inflammation of acute appendicitis or the pectoral trigger point (TrP) associated with an acute myocardial infarction. These visible and palpable changes in the tension of the skin, subcutaneous tissue, and other connective tissues that are segmentally related to visceral pathologic processes are referred to as connective tissue zones or reflex zones.[44]

Somatovisceral pain occurs when a myalgic condition causes functional disturbance of the underlying viscera, such as the TrPs of the abdominal muscles, causing diarrhea, vomiting, or excessive burping (Case Example 3.2).

Visceral Sources of Pain

Visceral sources of pain include the internal organs and the heart muscle. This source of pain includes all body organs located in the trunk or abdomen, such as those of the respiratory, digestive, urogenital, and endocrine systems, as well as the spleen, the heart, and the great vessels.

Visceral pain is not well localized for two reasons: (1) Innervation of the viscera is multisegmental and (2) There are few nerve receptors in these structures (see Fig. 3.3). Visceral pain tends to be poorly localized and diffuse. Visceral pain is well known for its ability to produce referred pain, which is pain perceived in an area other than the site of the stimuli. Referred pain occurs because visceral fibers synapse at the level of the spinal cord close to fibers supplying specific somatic structures. In other words, visceral pain corresponds to dermatomes from which the organ receives its innervations, which may be the same innervations for somatic structures.

For example, the heart is innervated by the C3-T4 spinal nerves. Pain of a cardiac source can affect any part of the soma (body) also innervated by these levels. This is one reason why someone having a heart attack can experience jaw, neck, shoulder, midback, arm, or chest pain and accounts for the many and varied clinical pictures of myocardial infarction (MI) (see Fig. 7.9).

More specifically, the pericardium is adjacent to the diaphragm. Pain of cardiac and diaphragmatic origin is often experienced in the shoulder because the C5-C6 spinal segment (innervation for the shoulder) also supplies the heart and the diaphragm.

CASE EXAMPLE 3.2
Somatic Disorder Mimicking Visceral Disease

A 61-year-old woman reported left shoulder pain for the last 3 weeks. The pain radiates down the arm in the pattern of an ulnar nerve distribution. She had no known injury, trauma, or repetitive motion to account for the new onset of symptoms. She denied any constitutional symptoms (nausea, vomiting, unexplained sweating, or sweats). There was no reported shortness of breath.

Pain was described as "gripping" and occurred most often at night, sometimes waking her up from sleep. Physical activity, motion, and exertion did not bring on, reproduce, or make her symptoms worse.

After Completing the Interview and Screening Examination, What Final Question Should Always Be Asked Every Client?
- Do you have any other pain or symptoms of any kind anywhere else in your body?

Result: In response to this question, the client reported left-sided chest pain that radiated to her nipple and then into her left shoulder and down the arm. Palpation of the chest wall musculature revealed a trigger point (TrP) of the pectoralis major muscle. This TrP was responsible for the chest and breast pain.

Further palpation reproduced a TrP of the left subclavius muscle, which was causing the woman's left arm pain. Releasing the TrPs eliminated all of the woman's symptoms.

Should You Make a Medical Referral for This Client?
Yes, referral should be made to rule out a viscero-somatic reflex causing the TrPs.

The client saw a cardiologist. Her echocardiogram and stress tests were negative. She was diagnosed with pseudocardiac disease secondary to a myofascial pain disorder.

(From Murphy D. Myofascial pain and pseudocardiac disease. *Dynamic chiropractic*, May 10, 1991. http://www.dynamicchiropractic.com/mpacms/dc/article.php?id=44292. Accessed April 30, 2022.)

Other examples of organ innervations and their corresponding sensory overlap are as follows:[7]
- Sensory fibers to the heart and lungs enter the spinal cord from T1-T4 (this may extend to T6).
- Sensory fibers to the gallbladder, bile ducts, and stomach enter the spinal cord at the level of the T7-T8 dorsal roots (i.e., the greater splanchnic nerve).
- The peritoneal covering of the gallbladder and/or the central zone of the diaphragm are innervated by the phrenic nerve originating from the C3-C5 (phrenic nerve) levels of the spinal cord.
- The phrenic nerve (C3-C5) also innervates portions of the pericardium.
- Sensory fibers to the duodenum enter the cord at the T9-T10 levels.
- Sensory fibers to the appendix enter the cord at the T10 level (i.e., the lesser splanchnic nerve).
- Sensory fibers to the renal/ureter system enter the cord at the L1-L2 level (i.e., the splanchnic nerve).

As mentioned earlier, diseases of internal organs can be accompanied by cutaneous hypersensitivity to touch, pressure, and temperature. This viscero-cutaneous reflex occurs during the acute phase of the disease and disappears with its recovery.

Keep in mind that when it comes to visceral pain, the viscera have few nerve endings. The visceral pleura are insensitive to pain. It is not until the organ capsule (deep somatic structure) is stretched (e.g., by a tumor or inflammation) that pain is perceived and possibly localized. This is why changes can occur within the organs without painful symptoms to warn the person. It is not until the organ is inflamed or distended enough from infection or obstruction to impinge nearby structures or the lining of the chest or abdominal cavity that pain is felt.

In the early stage of visceral disease, sympathetic reflexes arising from afferent impulses of the internal viscera may be expressed first as sensory, motor, and/or trophic changes in the skin, subcutaneous tissues, and/or muscles. As mentioned earlier, this can present as itching, dysesthesia, skin temperature changes, dry skin, or sympathetic sudomotor changes.

It appears that there is not one specific group of spinal neurons that respond only to visceral inputs. Because messages from the soma and viscera come into the cord at the same level (and sometimes visceral afferents converge over several segments of the spinal cord), the nervous system has trouble interpreting the input: Is it somatic or visceral? It sends efferent information back out to the plexus for change or reaction, but the input results in an unclear impulse at the cord level.

The body may get skin or somatic responses such as muscle pain or aching periosteum or it may send input to the viscus innervated at the same level to react to the input (e.g., the stomach increases its acid content). This also explains how sympathetic signals from the liver to the spinal cord can result in itching or other sudomotor responses in the area embryologically related to the liver.[7]

This somatization of visceral pain is why we must know the visceral pain patterns and the spinal versus visceral innervations. We examine one (somatic), while screening for the other (viscera).

Because the somatic and visceral afferent messages enter at the same level, it is possible to get somatic-somatic reflex responses (e.g., a bruise on the leg causes knee pain), somato-visceral reflex responses (e.g., a biomechanical dysfunction of the tenth rib can cause gallbladder changes), or viscero-somatic reflex responses (e.g., gallbladder impairment can result in a sore tenth rib; pelvic floor dysfunction can lead to incontinence; heart attack causes arm or jaw pain). These are actually all referred pain patterns originating in the soma or the viscera.

A viscero-viscero reflex (also referred to as *cross-organ sensitization*) occurs when pain or dysfunction in one organ causes symptoms in another organ.[6] For example, the client presents with chest pain and has an extensive cardiac workup with normal findings. The client may be told "it's not in your heart, so don't worry about it."

The problem may really be the gallbladder because the gallbladder originates from the same embryologic tissue as the heart, and gallbladder impairment can cause cardiac changes in addition to shoulder pain from its contact with the diaphragm. This presentation is then confused with cardiac pathology.[7]

On the other hand, the physician may order laboratory tests to investigate gallbladder involvement and find no positive results. The chest pain could be referral from arthritic changes in the cervical spine, as the cervical spine and heart share common sensory pathways from C3 to the spinal cord.

Information from the cardiac plexus and brachial plexus enter the cord at the same level. The nervous system is not able to identify where the input comes from, just what spinal level the message came from. It responds as best it can, based on the information present, sometimes resulting in the wrong symptoms for the problem at hand.

Pain and symptoms of a visceral source are usually accompanied by an ANS response such as a change in vital signs, unexplained perspiration (diaphoresis), and/or skin pallor. Signs and symptoms associated with the involved organ system may also be present. We call these *associated signs and symptoms*. *They are red flags in the screening process.*

Neuropathic Pain

Neuropathic or neurogenic pain results from damage or pathophysiologic changes of the peripheral or CNS.[45] Neuropathic pain can occur as a result of injury or destruction to the peripheral nerves, pathways in the spinal cord, or neurons located in the brain. Neuropathic pain can be acute or chronic depending on the time frame. This type of pain is not elicited by the stimulation of nociceptors or kinesthetic pathways as a result of tissue damage but rather by malfunction of the nervous system itself.[44] Disruptions in the transmission of afferent and efferent impulses in the periphery, spinal cord, and brain can give rise to alterations in sensory modalities (e.g., touch, pressure, temperature), and sometimes motor dysfunction.

Neuropathic pain can be drug-induced, metabolic-based, or brought on by trauma to the sensory neurons or pathways in either the peripheral nervous system or CNS. It can also appear to be idiosyncratic: not all individuals with the same lesion will have pain.[46] Some examples are listed in Table 3.4.

This type of pain is usually described as sharp, shooting, burning, tingling, or producing an electric shock sensation. The pain is steady or evoked by some stimulus that is not normally considered noxious (e.g., light touch, cold). There is no muscle spasm in neurogenic pain.[44] Acute nerve root irritation tends to be severe, described as burning, shooting, and constant. Chronic nerve root pain is more often described as annoying or nagging.

Neuropathic pain is not alleviated by opiates or narcotics, although local anesthesia can provide temporary relief. Medications used to treat neuropathic pain include antidepressants, anticonvulsants, antispasmodics, adrenergics, and anesthetics. Many clients have a combination of neuropathic and somatic pain, making it more difficult to identify the underlying pathology.

TABLE 3.4	Causes of Neuropathic Pain	
Central Neuropathic Pain	**Peripheral Neuropathic Pain**	
Multiple sclerosis	Trigeminal neuralgia (Tic	
Headache (migraine)	douloureux)	
Stroke	Poorly controlled diabetes	
Traumatic brain injury (TBI)	mellitus (metabolic-induced)	
Parkinson's disease	Vincristine (Oncovin) (drug-	
Spinal cord injury	induced, used in cancer	
(incomplete)	treatment)	
	Isoniazid (INH) (drug-induced,	
	used to treat tuberculosis)	
	Amputation (trauma)	
	Crush injury/brachial avulsion	
	(trauma)	
	Herpes zoster (shingles,	
	postherpetic neuralgia)	
	Complex regional pain	
	syndrome (CRPS2,	
	causalgia)	
	Nerve compression syndromes	
	(e.g., carpel tunnel	
	syndrome, thoracic outlet	
	syndrome)	
	Paraneoplastic neuropathy	
	(cancer-induced)	
	Cancer (tumor infiltration/	
	compression of the nerve)	
	Liver or biliary impairment	
	(e.g., liver cancer, cirrhosis,	
	primary biliary cirrhosis)	
	Leprosy	
	Congenital neuropathy (e.g.,	
	porphyria)	
	Guillain-Barré syndrome	

Referred Pain

By definition, referred pain is felt in an area far from the site of the lesion but supplied by the same or adjacent neural segments. Referred pain occurs by way of shared central pathways for afferent neurons and can originate from any somatic or visceral source (primary cutaneous pain is not usually referred to other parts of the body).

Referred pain can occur alone or with accompanying deep somatic or visceral pain. When caused by an underlying visceral or systemic disease, visceral pain usually precedes the development of referred musculoskeletal pain. However, the client may not remember or mention this previous pain pattern so the therapist needs to ask about the presence of any other symptoms.

Referred pain is usually well localized (i.e., the client can point directly to the area that hurts), but it does not have sharply defined borders. It can spread or radiate from its point of origin. Local tenderness is present in the tissue of the referred pain area, but there is no objective sensory deficit. Referred pain is often accompanied by muscle hypertonus over the referred area of pain.

Visceral disorders can refer pain to somatic tissue. On the other hand, as mentioned in the last topic on visceral sources

of pain, some somatic impairments can refer pain to visceral locations or mimic known visceral pain patterns. Finding the original source of referred pain can be quite a challenge (Case Example 3.3).

CASE EXAMPLE 3.3

Type of Pain and Possible Cause

A 44-year-old woman has come to physical therapy with reports of neck, jaw, and chest pain when using her arms overhead. She describes the pain as sharp and "hurting." It is not always consistent. Sometimes she has it, sometimes she does not. Her job as the owner of a window coverings business requires frequent, long periods of time with her arms overhead.

A. Would you classify this as cutaneous, somatic, visceral, neuropathic, or referred pain?

B. What are some possible causes and how can you differentiate neuromusculoskeletal pain from systemic?

A. The client has not mentioned the skin hurting or pointed to a specific area to suggest a cutaneous source of pain. It could be referred pain, but we do not know yet if it is referred from the neuromusculoskeletal system (neck, ribs, shoulder) or from the viscera (given the description, most likely cardiac).

Without further information, we can say it is somatic or referred visceral pain. We can describe it as radiating because it starts in the neck and affects a wide area above and below that. No defined dermatomes have been identified to suggest a neuropathic cause, so this must be evaluated more carefully.

B. This could be a pain pattern associated with *thoracic outlet syndrome* (TOS) because the lower cervical plexus can innervate as far down as the nipple line. This can be differentiated when performing tests and measures for TOS.

Because TOS can affect the neuro- (brachial plexus) or vascular bundle, it is important to measure blood pressure in both arms and compare them for a possible vascular component.

Onset of *anginal pain* occurs in some people with the use of arms overhead. To discern if this may be a cardiac problem, have the client use the lower extremities to exercise without using the arms (e.g., stairs, stationary bike).

Onset of symptoms from a cardiac origin usually has a lag effect. In other words, symptoms do not start until 5 to 10 minutes after the activity has started. It is not immediate as it might be when using impaired muscles. If the symptoms are reproduced 3 to 5 or 10 minutes after the lower extremity activity, consider a cardiac cause. Look for signs and symptoms associated with cardiac impairment. Ask about a personal/family history of heart disease.

At age 44 years, she may be perimenopausal (unless she has had a hysterectomy, which brings on surgical menopause) and still on the young side for cardiac cause of upper quadrant symptoms. Still, it is possible, and would have to be ruled out by a physician if you are unable to find an NMS cause of symptoms.

Chest pain can have a *wide range of causes*, including TrPs, anabolic steroid or cocaine use, breast disease, premenstrual symptoms, assault or trauma, lactation problems, scar tissue from breast augmentation or reduction, and so on. See further discussion, Chapter 18.

Always ask these two questions in your pain interview as a part of the screening process:

❓ FOLLOW-UP QUESTIONS

• Are you having any pain anywhere else in your body?
• Are you having symptoms of any other kind that may or may not be related to your main concern or problem?

Differentiating Sources of Pain[7]

It can be very difficult to differentiate somatic from visceral sources of pain. That is one reason why clients end up in physical therapy even though there is a viscerogenic source of the pain and/or symptomatic presentation.

The superficial and deep somatic structures are innervated unilaterally via the spinal nerves, whereas the viscera are innervated bilaterally through the ANS via visceral afferents. The quality of superficial somatic pain tends to be sharp and more localized. It is mediated by large myelinated fibers, which have a low threshold for stimulation and a fast conduction time. This is designed to protect the structures by signaling a problem right away.

Deep somatic pain is more likely to be a dull or deep aching that responds to rest or a non–weight-bearing position. Deep somatic pain is often poorly localized (transmission via small unmyelinated fibers) and can be referred from some other site.

Pain of a deep somatic nature increases after movement. Sometimes the client can find a comfortable spot, but after moving the extremity or joint, cannot find that comfortable spot again. This is in contrast to visceral pain, which usually is not reproduced with movement, but rather, tends to hurt all the time or with all movements.[7]

Pain from a visceral source can also be dull and aching, but usually does not feel better after rest or recumbency. Keep in mind pathologic processes occurring within somatic structures (e.g., metastasis, primary tumor, infection) may produce localized pain that can be mechanically irritated. This is why movement in general (rather than specific motions) can make it worse. Back pain from metastasis to the spine can become quite severe before any radiologic changes are seen.[7]

Visceral diseases of the abdomen and pelvis are more likely to refer pain to the back, whereas intrathoracic disease refers pain to the shoulder(s). Visceral pain rarely occurs without associated signs and symptoms, although the client may not recognize the correlation. Careful questioning will usually elicit a systemic pattern of symptoms.

Back or shoulder range of motion (ROM) is usually full and painless in the presence of visceral pain, especially in the early stages of disease. When the painful stimulus increases or persists over time, pain-modifying behaviors, such as muscle splinting and guarding, can result in subsequent changes in biomechanical patterns and pain-related disability[47] and may make it more difficult to recognize the systemic origin of musculoskeletal dysfunction.

Mechanisms of Musculoskeletal Pain

It is important to discuss, at this point, the mechanism-based approach to pain management. This approach builds upon the biopsychosocial model, and uses the term "pain mechanisms" to identify and differentiate neurophysiological contributors to the production, maintenance, or enhancement of pain.[48] In the perspective presented by Chimenti, Frey-Law and Sluka, five mechanisms were presented: nociceptive, neuropathic, nociplastic, psychosocial and movement system. The first three mechanisms (nociceptive, neuropathic and nociplastic) were further discussed as mainly originating from the pathobiological processes, and will be discussed below (see Fig. 3.9). Considerations regarding the psychosocial mechanisms are presented later in this chapter.

Nociceptive Pain

Nociceptive pain originates from the peripheral nervous system, and is triggered by injury, inflammation, or mechanical irritant[48] which activates the nociceptors. Pain signals are then related to the spinal cord, through the ascending nociceptive pathways to the cerebral cortex, which results in the perception of pain.[48]

In a study by Smart and colleagues,[49] the dominance of nociceptive pain was predicted by seven criteria, which include:

• The presence of *three* symptoms: (1) pain localized to the area of injury and dysfunction, (2) usually intermittent at rest and sharp with movement or mechanical provocation, and (3) clearly proportionate pain to aggravating easing factors
• The absence of *three* symptoms: (1) pain described as burning, shooting or electric shock-like, (2) pain associated with other dysthesias such as crawling, heaviness, and (3) night pain or disturbed sleep
• The presence of *one* sign: presence of pain-relieving postures or movement pattern.

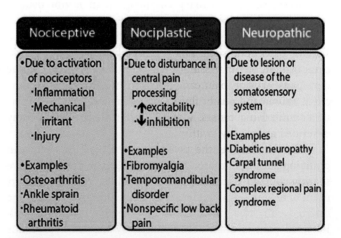

Fig. 3.9 Three pain mechanisms. (From: Chimenti R, Frey-Law L, Sluka K. A mechanism-based approach to physical therapist management of pain. *Phys Ther*. 2018;98(5):302–314.)

Neuropathic Pain

Neuropathic pain (also known as peripheral neuropathic pain) is due to a lesion or disease affecting the somatosensory system,[48] and typically occurs in conditions such as diabetic neuropathy or carpal tunnel syndrome.[48] Additional discussion on neuropathic pain was presented earlier in this chapter. The three criteria that indicate the dominance of neuropathic pain include:[49]

- History of mechanical compromise, nerve injury or pathology
- Presence of constant, unremitting pain
- Pain referred in a dermatomal or cutaneous distribution.

Nociplastic pain (also previously known as central sensitization) is caused by abnormalities in central pain processing, causing either an increase of excitability or decrease in inhibition.[48] The four criteria that indicate the dominance of nociplastic pain include:[49]

- Presence of the following three symptoms:
  - Pain provocation pattern that is disproportional, nonmechanical and unpredictable, that is also disproportionate to the nature or extent of injury or pathology
  - Unpredictable patterns of pain provocation in response to multiple/ nonspecific aggravating or easing factors
  - Strongly associated with maladaptive psychosocial factors including negative emotions, poor self-efficacy, maladaptive beliefs, pain behaviors, altered family, work, social life, medical conflict
- Presence of one sign: diffuse, nonanatomic areas of pain and/or tenderness on palpation.

TYPES OF PAIN

Although there are five sources of most physiologic pain (from a medical screening perspective), many types of pain exist within these categories (see Table 3.3).

When orienting to pain from these main sources, it may be helpful to consider some specific types of pain patterns. Not all pain types can be discussed here, but some of the most commonly encountered are included.

Tension Pain

Organ distention, such as occurs with bowel obstruction, constipation, or the passing of a kidney stone, can cause tension pain. Tension pain can also be caused by blood pooling from trauma and pus or fluid accumulation from infection or other underlying causes. In the bowel, tension pain may be described as "colicky" with waves of pain and tension occurring intermittently as the peristaltic contractile force moves irritating substances through the GI system. Individuals with tension pain will find it difficult to find a comfortable position.

Inflammatory Pain

Inflammation of the viscera or parietal peritoneum (e.g., acute appendicitis) may cause pain that is described as deep or boring. If the visceral peritoneum is involved, then the pain is usually poorly localized. If the parietal peritoneum is the primary area affected, the pain pattern may become more localized (i.e., the affected individual can point to it with one or two fingers). Pain arising from inflammation causes people to seek positions of quiet with little movement.

Ischemic Pain

Ischemia denotes a loss of blood supply. Any area without adequate perfusion will quickly die. Ischemic pain of the viscera is sudden, intense, constant, and progressive in severity or intensity. It is not typically relieved by analgesics, and no position is comfortable. The person usually avoids movement or change in positions.

Myofascial Pain

Myalgia, or muscle pain, can be a symptom of an underlying systemic disorder. Cancer, renal failure, hepatic disease, and endocrine disorders are only a few possible systemic sources of muscle involvement. For example, muscle weakness, atrophy, myalgia, and fatigue that persist despite rest may be early manifestations of thyroid or parathyroid disease, acromegaly, diabetes, Cushing's syndrome, or osteomalacia.

Myalgia can be present in anxiety and depressive disorders. Muscle weakness and myalgia can occur as a side effect of medication. Prolonged use of systemic corticosteroids and immunosuppressive medications has known adverse effects on the musculoskeletal system, including degenerative myopathy with muscle wasting and tendon rupture.

Infective endocarditis caused by acute bacterial infection can present with myalgias and no other manifestation of endocarditis. The early onset of joint pain and myalgia as the first sign of endocarditis is more likely if the person is older and has had a previously diagnosed heart murmur.

Joint pain (arthralgia) can accompany myalgia. Polymyalgia rheumatica (PR), which literally means "pain in many muscles," is a disorder marked by diffuse pain and stiffness that primarily affects muscles of the shoulder and pelvic girdles, in addition to a systemic inflammatory response.[50] With PR, symptoms are vague and difficult to diagnose resulting in delay in medical treatment. The person may wake up one morning with muscle pain and stiffness for no apparent reason or the symptoms may come on gradually over several days or weeks. Adults over 50 years of age are affected; cases peak after 70 years of age.[50]

From a screening point of view, there are many types of muscle-related pain such as tension, spasm, weakness, trauma, inflammation, infection, neurologic impairment, and TrPs (see Table 3.3).[51] The clinical presentation most common with systemic disease is presented here.

Muscle Tension

Muscle tension occurs when prolonged muscular contraction or cocontraction results in local ischemia,[52] increased cellular metabolites, and subsequent pain.

Muscle tension also can occur with physical stress and fatigue. Muscle tension and the subsequent ischemia may occur as a result of faulty ergonomics, prolonged work positions (e.g., as with computer operators), or repetitive motion.

Take for example the person sitting at a keyboard for hours each day. Constant typing with muscle cocontraction does not allow for the normal contract-relax sequence. Muscle ischemia results in greater release of substance P, a pain neurotransmitter (neuropeptide).

Increased substance P levels increase pain sensitivity. Increased pain perception results in more muscle spasm as a splinting or protective guarding mechanism, and thus the pain-spasm cycle is perpetuated. This is an example of a somatic-somatic response.

Muscle tension from a viscero-somatic response can occur when pain from a visceral source results in increased muscle tension and even muscle spasm. For example, the pain from any inflammatory or infectious process affecting the abdomen (e.g., appendicitis, diverticulitis, pelvic inflammatory disease) can cause increased tension in the abdominal muscles.

Given enough time and combined with overuse and repetitive use or infectious or inflammatory disease, muscle tension can turn into muscle spasm. When opposing muscles such as the flexors and extensors contract together for long periods of time (called cocontraction), muscle tension and then muscle spasm can occur.

Muscle Spasm

Muscle spasm is a sudden involuntary contraction of a muscle or group of muscles, usually occurring as a result of overuse or injury of the adjoining neuromusculoskeletal (NMS) or musculotendinous attachments. A client with a painful musculoskeletal problem may also have a varying degree of reflex muscle spasm to protect the joint(s) involved (a somatic-somatic response). A client with painful visceral disease can have muscle spasm of the overlying musculature (a viscero-somatic response).

Spasm pain cannot be attributed to transient increased muscle tension because the intramuscular pressure is insufficiently elevated. Pain with muscle spasm may occur from prolonged contraction under an ischemic situation.

Muscle Trauma

Muscle trauma can occur with acute trauma, burns, crush injuries, or unaccustomed intensity or duration of muscle contraction, especially eccentric contractions. Muscle pain occurs as broken fibers leak potassium into the interstitial fluid. Blood extravasation results from damaged blood vessels, setting off a cascade of chemical reactions within the muscle.[53]

When disintegration of muscle tissue occurs with release of their contents (e.g., oxygen-transporting pigment myoglobin) into the bloodstream, a potentially fatal muscle toxicity called *rhabdomyolysis* can occur. Risk factors and clinical signs and symptoms are listed in Table 3.5. Immediate medical attention is required (Case Example 3.4).

TABLE 3.5	Risk Factors for Rhabdomyolysis	
Risk Factors	Examples	Signs and Symptoms
Trauma	Crush injury Electric shock Severe burns Extended mobility	Profound muscle weakness Pain Swelling Stiffness and cramping Associated signs and symptoms • Reddish-brown urine (myoglobin) • Decreased urine output • Malaise • Fever • Sinus tachycardia • Nausea, vomiting • Agitation, confusion
Extreme Muscular Activity	Strenuous exercise Status epilepticus Severe dystonia	
Toxic Effects	Ethanol Ethylene glycol Isopropanol Methanol Heroin Barbiturates Methadone Cocaine Tetanus Ecstasy (street drug) Carbon monoxide Snake venom Amphetamines	
Metabolic Abnormalities	Hypothyroidism Hyperthyroidism Diabetic ketoacidosis	
Medication-Induced	Inadvertent intravenous (IV) infiltration (e.g., amphotericin B, azathioprine, cyclosporine) Cholesterol-lowering statins (e.g., Zocor, Lipitor, Crestor)	

(Data from Fort CW. How to combat three deadly trauma complications. Nursing 2003;33(5):58–64.)

Muscle Weakness and Stiffness

Muscle weakness and stiffness are common problems as we age and even among younger adults who are deconditioned. Connective tissue changes may occur as small amounts of fibrinogen (produced in the liver and normally converted to

CASE EXAMPLE 3.4
Military Rhabdomyolysis

A 20-year-old soldier reported to the military physical therapy clinic with bilateral shoulder pain and weakness. He was unable to perform his regular duties because of these symptoms. He attributed this to doing many push-ups during physical training 2 days ago.

When asked if there were any other symptoms of any kind to report, the client said that he noticed his urine was a dark color yesterday (the day after the push-up exercises).

The soldier had shoulder active range of motion (ROM) to 90 degrees accompanied by an abnormal scapulohumeral rhythm with excessive scapular elevation on both sides. Passive shoulder ROM was full but painful. Elbow active and passive ROM were also restricted to 90 degrees of flexion secondary to pain in the triceps muscles.

The client was unable to handle manual muscle testing with pain on palpation to the pectoral, triceps, and infraspinatus muscles, bilaterally. The rotator cuff tendon appeared to be intact.

What Are the Red Flags in This Case?
- Bilateral symptoms (pain and weakness)
- Age (for cancer, too young [under 25 years of age] or too old [over 50 years of age] is a red-flag sign)
- Change in urine color

Result: The soldier had actually done hundreds of different types of push-ups, including regular, wide-arm, and diamond push-ups. Although the soldier was not in any apparent distress, laboratory studies were ordered. Serum Creatine Kinase level was measured as 9600 U/L (normal range: 55–170 U/L).

The results were consistent with acute exertional rhabdomyolysis (AER) and the soldier was hospitalized. Early recognition of a potentially serious problem may have prevented serious complications possible with this condition.

Physical therapy intervention for muscle soreness without adequate hydration could have led to acute renal failure. He returned to physical therapy for a recovery program following hospitalization.

(Data from Baxter RE, Moore JH. Diagnosis and treatment of acute exertional rhabdomyolysis. *J Orthop Sports Phys Ther* 2003;33(3): 104–108.)

fibrin to serve as a clotting factor) leak from the vasculature into the intracellular spaces, adhering to cellular structures.

The resulting microfibrinous adhesions among the cells of muscle and fascia cause increased muscular stiffness. Activity and movement normally break these adhesions; however, with the aging process, production of fewer and less efficient macrophages[54] combined with immobility for any reason result in an increase of these adhesions.

Other possible causes of aggravated stiffness include increased collagen fibers from reduced collagen turnover, increased cross-links of aged collagen fibers, changes in the mechanical properties of connective tissues, and structural and functional changes in the collagen protein. Tendons and ligaments also have less water content, resulting in increased stiffness.[55] When muscular stiffness occurs as a result of aging,

increased physical activity and movement can reduce associated muscular pain.

Proximal muscle weakness accompanied by change in one or more deep tendon reflexes is a red flag sign of cancer or neurologic impairment. In the presence of a past medical history of cancer, further screening is advised with possible medical referral required, depending on the outcome of the examination/evaluation.

Trigger Points

TrPs, sometimes referred to as myofascial TrPs (MTrPs), are hyperirritable spots within a taut band of skeletal muscle or in the fascia. Taut bands are rope-like indurations palpated in the muscle fiber.[56] These areas are very tender to palpation and are referred to as local tenderness. There is often a history of immobility (e.g., cast immobilization after fracture or injury), prolonged or vigorous activity such as bending or lifting, or forceful abdominal breathing such as occurs with marathon running.

TrPs are reproduced with palpation or resisted motions. When pressing on the TrP, you may elicit a "jump sign." The jump sign may be a local twitch response of muscle fibers to TrP stimulation The *jump sign* is a general pain response as the client physically withdraws from the pressure on the point and may even cry out or wince in pain. The *local twitch response* is the visible contraction of tense muscle fibers in response to stimulation.[57]

When TrPs are compressed, local tenderness with possible referred pain results. In other words, pain that arises from the TrP is felt at a distance, often remote from its source.

The referred pain pattern is characteristic and specific for every muscle. Knowing the TrP locations and their referred pain patterns is helpful. By knowing the pain patterns, the therapist can go to the site of origin and confirm (or rule out) the presence of the TrP. The distribution of referred TrP pain rarely coincides entirely with the distribution of a peripheral nerve or dermatomal segment.[58]

TrPs as defined by Travell[59] can also produce visceral symptoms without actual organ impairment or disease. This is an example of a somatovisceral response. For example, the client may have an abdominal muscle TrP, but the history is one of upset stomach or chest (cardiac) pain. It is possible to have both tender points and TrPs when the underlying cause is visceral disease.

Pain and dysfunction of myofascial tissues is the subject of several texts to which the reader is referred for more information.[58,60,61]

Joint Pain

Noninflammatory joint pain (no redness, no warmth, no swelling) of unknown etiology can be caused by a wide range of pathologic conditions. Systemic causes of joint pain can be found in Box 3.4. Fibromyalgia,[62] leukemia,[63] sexually transmitted infections (STI),[64] Crohn's disease[65], postmenopausal status or low estrogen levels, and infectious arthritis are all possible causes of joint pain.

BOX 3.4 SYSTEMIC CAUSES OF JOINT PAIN

Infectious and noninfectious systemic causes of joint pain can include, but are not limited to:

- Allergic reactions (e.g., medications such as antibiotics)
- Side effect of other medications such as statins, prolonged use of corticosteroids, aromatase inhibitors
- Delayed reaction to chemicals or environmental factors
- Sexually transmitted infections (STIs) (e.g., human immunodeficiency virus [HIV], syphilis, chlamydia, gonorrhea)
- Infectious arthritis
- Infective endocarditis
- Recent dental surgery
- Lyme disease
- Rheumatoid arthritis
- Other autoimmune disorders (e.g., systemic lupus erythematosus, mixed connective tissue disease, scleroderma, polymyositis)
- Leukemia
- Tuberculosis
- Acute rheumatic fever
- Chronic liver disease (hepatic osteodystrophy affecting wrists and ankles; hepatitis causing arthralgias)
- Inflammatory bowel disease (e.g., Crohn's disease or regional enteritis)
- Anxiety or depression (major depressive disorder)
- Fibromyalgia
- Artificial sweeteners

Joint pain in the presence of fatigue may be a red flag for anxiety, depression, or cancer.[66,67] The client history and screening interview may help the therapist find the true cause of joint pain. Look for risk factors for any of the listed conditions and review the client's recent activities.

When comparing joint pain associated with systemic versus musculoskeletal causes, one of the major differences is in the area of associated signs and symptoms (Table 3.6). Joint pain of a systemic or visceral origin usually has additional signs or symptoms present. The client may not realize there is a connection, or the condition may not have progressed enough for associated signs and symptoms to develop.

The therapist also evaluates joint pain over a 24-hour period. Joint pain from a systemic cause is more likely to be constant and present with all movements. Rest may help at first but over time even this relieving factor will not alter the symptoms. This is in comparison with the client who has osteoarthritis (OA) and often feels better after rest (though stiffness may remain). Morning joint pain associated with OA is less than joint pain at the end of the day after using the joint(s) all day. On the other hand, muscle pain may be worse in the morning and gradually improves as the client stretches and moves about during the day.

The therapist can use the specific screening questions for joint pain to assess any joint pain of unknown cause or with an unusual presentation or history. Joint pain and symptoms that do not fit the expected pattern for injury, overuse, or aging can be screened using a few important questions (Box 3.5).

Drug-Induced

Joint pain as an allergic response, sometimes referred to as "serum sickness," can occur up to 6 weeks after taking a prescription drug (especially an antibiotic). Joint pain is also a potential side effect of statins (e.g., Lipitor, Zocor, Crestor) that are prescribed to lower cholesterol levels.

Musculoskeletal symptoms (e.g., morning stiffness, bone pain, arthralgia, arthritis) are a well-known side effect of chemotherapy in the treatment of breast cancer. Low estrogen concentrations and postmenopausal status are linked with these symptoms. Risk factors for developing joint symptoms may include previous hormone replacement therapy, hormone-receptor positivity, previous chemotherapy, and obesity. Noninflammatory joint pain is also typical of a delayed allergic reaction. The client may report fever, skin rash, and fatigue that dissipate when the drug is stopped.

Chemical Exposure

Likewise, delayed reactions can occur as a result of occupational or environmental chemical exposure. A work and/or military history may be required for anyone presenting with joint or muscle pain or symptoms of unknown cause. These clients can be mislabeled with a diagnosis of autoimmune disease or fibromyalgia. The therapist may recognize and report clues to help the client obtain a more accurate diagnosis.

Inflammatory Bowel Disease

Arthralgias has been reported up to 55% of patients with inflammatory bowel disease (IBD). A person with a known diagnosis of IBD[68] may not know that new onset of joint symptoms can be a part of this condition. The client interview should have brought out the personal history of either ulcerative colitis of Crohn's disease. See the discussion of IBD in Chapter 9.

Arthritis

Joint pain (either inflammatory or noninflammatory) can be associated with a wide range of systemic causes, including bacterial or viral infection, trauma, and sexually transmitted diseases (see Box 3.4). There is usually a positive history or other associated signs and symptoms to help the therapist identify the need for medical referral.

Infectious Arthritis. Joint pain can be a *local* response to an infection. This is called infectious, septic, or bacterial arthritis. Invading microorganisms cause inflammation of the synovial membrane with release of cytokines (e.g., tumor necrosis factor [TNF], interleukin-1 [IL-1]) and proteases.

TABLE 3.6	Joint Pain: Systemic or Musculoskeletal?	
	Systemic	Musculoskeletal
Clinical Presentation	Awakens at night Deep aching, throbbing Reduced by pressure* Constant or waves/spasm Cyclical, progressive symptoms	Decreases with rest Sharp Reduced by change in position Reduced or eliminated when stressful action is stopped Restriction of A/PROM Restriction of accessory motions One or more movements "catch," reproducing or aggravating pain/symptoms
Past Medical History	Recent history of infection: Hepatitis, bacterial infection from staphylococcus or streptococcus (e.g., cellulitis), mononucleosis, measles, URI, UTI, gonorrhea, osteomyelitis, cellulitis History of bone fracture, joint replacement, or arthroscopy History of human bite Sore throat, headache with fever in the last 3 weeks or family/household member with recently diagnosed strep throat Skin rash (infection, medications) Recent medications (last 6 weeks); any drug but especially statins (cholesterol lowering), antibiotics, aromatase inhibitors, chemotherapy Hormone associated (postmenopausal status, low estrogen levels) History of injection drug use/abuse History of allergic reactions History of GI symptoms Recent history of enteric or venereal infection or new sexual contact (e.g., Reiter's) Presence of extensor surface nodules	Repetitive motion Arthritis Static postures (prolonged) Trauma (including domestic violence)
Associated Signs and Symptoms	Jaundice Migratory arthralgias Skin rash/lesions Nodules (extensor surfaces) Fatigue Weight loss Low-grade fever Suspicious or aberrant lymph nodes Presence of GI symptoms Cyclical, progressive symptoms Proximal muscle weakness	Usually none Check for TrPs TrPs may be accompanied by some minimal ANS phenomenon (e.g., nausea, sweating)

*This is actually a cutaneous or somatic response because the pressure provides a counterirritant; it does not really affect the viscera directly.
A/PROM, Active/passive range of motion; *TrPs*, trigger points; *URI*, upper respiratory infection; *UTI*, urinary tract infection.

Bacteria can find its way to the joint via the bloodstream (most common) by:

- Direct inoculation (e.g., surgery, arthroscopy, intraarticular corticosteroid injection, central line placement, total joint replacement)
- Penetrating wound (e.g., fracture)
- Direct extension (e.g., osteomyelitis, cellulitis, abscess)

Staphylococcus aureus, streptococci, and gonococci are the most common infectious causes. A connection between infection and arthritis has been established in Lyme disease. Arthritis can be the first sign of infective endocarditis.[69,77] Viral infections such as Parvovirus, hepatitis B and C, human immunodeficiency virus (HIV), arthropod-borne viruses and Flaviviruses, Herpes zoster and Coronaviruses such as SARS-CoV can be accompanied by arthralgias and arthritis.[70] Joint symptoms appear during the prodromal state of hepatitis (before the clinical onset of jaundice).

Sexually transmitted (infectious) diseases (STIs/STDs) are often accompanied by joint pain and symptoms called *gonococcal arthritis*. Joint pain accompanied by skin lesions at the joint or elsewhere may be a sign of sexually transmitted infections.

In the case of STIs/STDs with joint involvement, skin lesions over or near a joint have a typical appearance with a central black eschar or scab-like appearance surrounded by an area of erythema (Fig. 3.10). Alternately, the skin lesion may have a hemorrhagic base with a pustule in the center. Fever and arthritic-like symptoms are usually present (Fig. 3.11).

Anyone with HIV may develop unusual rheumatologic disorders. Diffuse body aches and pain without joint arthritis

---

BOX 3.5   SCREENING QUESTIONS FOR JOINT PAIN

- Please describe the pattern of pain/symptoms from when you wake up in the morning to when you go to sleep at night.
- Do you have any symptoms of any kind anywhere else in your body? (You may have to explain that these symptoms do not have to relate to the joint pain; if the client has no other symptoms, offer a short list including constitutional symptoms, heart palpitations, unusual fatigue, nail or skin changes, sores or lesions anywhere but especially in the mouth or on the genitals, and so forth.)
- Have you ever had:
  - Cancer of any kind
  - Leukemia
  - Crohn's disease (regional enteritis)
  - Sexually transmitted infection (you may have to prompt with specific diseases such as chlamydia, genital herpes, genital warts, gonorrhea or "the clap," syphilis, Reiter's syndrome, human immunodeficiency virus [HIV])
  - Fibromyalgia
  - Joint replacement or arthroscopic surgery of any kind
- Have you recently (last 6 weeks) had any:
  - Fractures
  - Bites (human, animal)
  - Antibiotics or other medications
  - Infections (you may have to prompt with specific infections such as strep throat, mononucleosis, urinary tract, upper respiratory [cold or flu], gastrointestinal, hepatitis)
  - Skin rashes or other skin changes
  - Do you drink diet soda/pop or use aspartame, Equal, or NutraSweet? (If the client uses these products in any amount, suggest eliminating them on a trial basis

for 30 days; artificial sweetener–induced symptoms may disappear in some people; neurotoxic effects from use of newer products [e.g., Stevia, Splenda] have not been fully investigated.)

To the therapist: You may have to conduct an environmental or work history (occupation, military, exposure to chemicals) to identify a delayed reaction.

Quick Survey
- What kind of work do you do?
- Do you think your health problems are related to your work?
- Are your symptoms better or worse when you are at home or at work?
- Follow-up if worse at work: Do others at work have similar problems?
- Have you been exposed to dusts, fumes, chemicals, radiation, or loud noise?
- Follow-up: It may be necessary to ask additional questions based on past history, symptoms, and risk factors present.
- Do you live near a hazardous waste site or any industrial facilities that give off chemical odors or fumes?
- Do you live in a home built more than 40 years ago? Have you done renovations or remodeling?
- Do you use pesticides in your home, garden, or for your pets?
- What is your source of drinking water?
- Chronology of jobs (type of industry, type of job, years worked)
- How new is the building you are working in?
- Exposure survey (protective equipment used, exposure to dust, radiation, chemicals, biologic hazards, physical hazards)

---

are common among clients with HIV. (See further discussion on HIV in Chapter 13.)

Infectious (septic) arthritis should be suspected in an individual with persistent joint pain and inflammation occurring in the course of an illness of unclear origin or in the course of a well-documented infection such as pneumococcal pneumonia, staphylococcal sepsis, or urosepsis.

Major risk factors include age (older than 80 years), diabetes mellitus, intravenous drug use, indwelling catheters, immunocompromised condition, rheumatoid arthritis, or osteoarthritis.[71] Other predisposing factors are listed in Box 3.6. Look for a history of preexisting joint damage from bone trauma (e.g., fracture) or degenerative joint disease.

Watch for joint symptoms in the presence of skin rash, low-grade fever, and lymphadenopathy. The rash may appear and disappear before the joint symptoms. Joints may be mildly to

severely involved. Fingers, knees, shoulders, and ankles are affected most often (bilaterally). Inflammation is nonerosive, suggestive of rheumatoid arthritis.

Often one joint is involved[72] (knee or hip), but sometimes two or more are also symptomatic, depending on the underlying pathologic mechanism. Symptoms can range from mild to severe. Joint destruction can be rapid so immediate medical referral is required.

With infectious arthritis, the client may be unable to bear weight on the joint. Usually, there is an acute arthritic presentation and the client has a fever (often low grade in older adults or in anyone who is immunosuppressed).

Medical referral is important for the client with joint pain with no known cause and a recent history of infection of any kind. Ask about recent (last 6 weeks) skin lesions or rashes of any kind anywhere on the body, urinary tract infection, or respiratory infection.

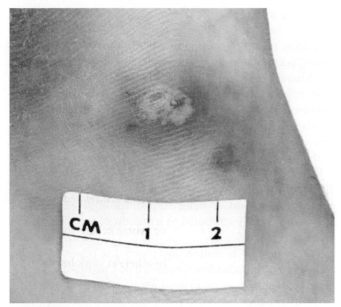

Fig. 3.10 Cutaneous gonococcal lesion secondary to disseminated *Neisseria gonorrhoeae* bacterial infection. Though a sexually transmitted disease, if gonorrhea is allowed to go untreated, the *N. gonorrhoeae* bacteria responsible for the infection can become disseminated throughout the body and form lesions in extragenital locations. This type of lesion can present as (gonococcal) arthritis in any joint; the ankle joint is the target here. (From Goldman L, Schafer AI, et al. Goldman's Cecil Medicine. 24th ed. Philadelphia: Saunders; 2012.)

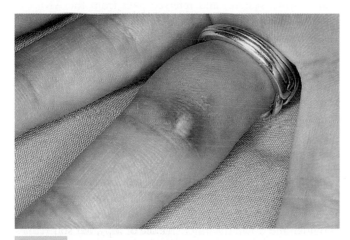

Fig. 3.11 Disseminated gonorrhea. Pustule on a hemorrhagic base. The typical client presents with fever, arthritis, and scattered lesions as shown. Cultures from the lesions are often negative. The therapist should always use standard precautions. Medical referral is required. (From Callen JP, Paller AS, Greer KE, et al. Color Atlas of Dermatology. 2nd ed. Philadelphia: WB Saunders; 2000, Fig. 6.5, p. 148.)

Take the client's temperature and ask about recent episodes of fever, sweats, or other constitutional symptoms. Palpate for residual lymphadenopathy. Early diagnosis and intervention are essential to limit joint destruction and preserve function. Diagnosis can be difficult. The physician must differentiate infectious/septic arthritis from reactive arthritis (Case Example 3.5).

BOX 3.6   RISK FACTORS FOR INFECTIOUS ARTHRITIS

- History of:
  - Previous surgery, especially arthroscopy for joint repair or replacement
  - Human bite, tick bite (Lyme disease), fracture, central line placement
  - Direct, penetrating trauma
  - Infection of any kind (e.g., osteomyelitis, cellulitis, diverticulitis, abscess [located anywhere], hepatitis A or B, *Staphylococcus aureus, Streptococcus pneumoniae, gonococci*, or urinary tract or respiratory tract infection)
  - Rheumatoid arthritis, systemic lupus erythematosus, scleroderma, or mixed connective tissue disease
  - Diabetes mellitus
  - Sarcoidosis (inflammatory pulmonary condition can affect knees, proximal interphalangeal [PIP] joints, wrists, elbows)
- Sexually active, young adult
- Injection drug user
- Chronic joint damage (e.g., rheumatoid arthritis, gout)
- Previous infection of joint prosthesis
- Recent immunization
- Increasing age
- Indwelling catheter (especially in the client with a prosthetic joint)
- Malnutrition, skin breakdown
- Immunosuppression or immunocompromise (e.g., renal failure, steroid treatment, organ transplantation, chemotherapy)

CLINICAL SIGNS AND SYMPTOMS
Infectious Arthritis

- Fever (low grade or high), chills, malaise
- Recurrent sore throat
- Lymphadenopathy
- Persistent joint pain
- Single painful swollen joint (knee, hip, ankle, elbow, shoulder)*
- Multiple joint involvement (often migratory)
- Pain on weight bearing
- Back pain (infective endocarditis)
- Skin lesions (characteristic of the specific underlying infection)
- Conjunctivitis, uveitis
- Other musculoskeletal symptoms depending on the specific underlying infection
  - Myalgias
  - Tenosynovitis (especially wrist and ankle extensor tendon sheaths)
- Elevated C-reactive protein and sedimentation rate

*The particular joint or joints involved and associated signs and symptoms will vary from client to client and are dependent upon the underlying infectious cause. For example, joint involvement with Lyme disease presents differently from Reiter's syndrome or hepatitis B.

CASE EXAMPLE 3.5

Septic Arthritis

A 62-year-old man presented in the physical therapy practice with left wrist pain. There was no redness, warmth, or swelling. Active motion was mildly limited by pain. Passive motion could not be tested because of pain.

All other clinical tests were negative. Neuro screen was negative. Past medical history includes hypertension and non–insulin-dependent diabetes mellitus controlled by diet and exercise.

The client denied any history of fever, skin rashes, or other lesions. He reported a recent trip to Haiti (his native country) 3 weeks ago.

How Do You Screen This Client for Systemic-Induced Joint Pain?

- Review Box 3.6 (Risk Factors for Infectious Arthritis). Besides diabetes, what other risk factors are present? Ask the client about any that apply. Compile a list to review during the Review of Systems.
- Ask the client: Are there any other symptoms of any kind anywhere else in your body?
- Use the client's answer while reviewing clinical signs and symptoms of infectious arthritis for any signs and symptoms of infectious arthritis.
- Review Box 3.5 (Screening Questions for Joint Pain). Are there any further questions from this list appropriate for the screening process?
- Assess the joints above and below (e.g., elbow, shoulder, neck). Assess for trigger points.

Using the information obtained from these steps, look at past medical history, clinical presentation, and associated signs and symptoms. What are the red flags? Review the *Clues to Screening for Viscerogenic Sources of Pain* and *Guidelines for Physician Referral Required* in this chapter.

Based on your findings, decide whether to treat and reevaluate or make a medical referral now.

Result: In this case the therapist did not find enough red flags or suspicious findings to warrant immediate referral. Treatment intervention was initiated. The client missed three appointments because of the "flu." When he returned, his wrist pain was completely gone, but he was reporting left knee pain. There was mild effusion and warmth on both sides of the knee joint. The client stated that he still had some occasional diarrhea from his bout with the flu.

The therapist recognized some additional red flags, including ongoing gastrointestinal (GI) symptoms attributed by the client to the flu and new onset of inflammatory joint pain. The therapist decided to take the client's vital signs and found he was febrile (100° F).

Given his recent travel history, migratory noninflammatory and inflammatory arthralgias, and ongoing constitutional symptoms, the client was referred to his medical doctor. Laboratory tests resulted in a physician's diagnosis of joint sepsis with hematogenous seeding to the wrist and knee; possible osteomyelitis. Probable cause: Exposure to pathogens in contaminated water or soil during his stay in Haiti.

Radicular Pain

Radicular pain results from direct irritation of axons of a spinal nerve or neurons in the dorsal root ganglion and is experienced in the musculoskeletal system in a dermatome, sclerotome, or myotome.

Radicular, radiating, and referred pain are not the same, although a client can have radicular pain that radiates. Radiating means the pain spreads or fans out from the originating point of pain.

Whereas radicular pain is caused by nerve root compression, referred pain results from activation of nociceptive free nerve endings (nociceptors) of the nervous system in somatic or visceral tissue. The physiologic basis for referred pain is convergence of afferent neurons onto common neurons within the CNS.

The term *sciatica* is outdated and reflects our previous (limited) understanding of referred pain. Regional pain anywhere near, around, or along the pathway of the sciatic nerve was automatically attributed to irritation of the sciatic nerve and labeled "sciatica."

Radiculopathy is another symptom that is separate from radicular pain. Radiculopathy describes a neurologic state in which conduction along a spinal nerve or its roots is blocked. Instead of pain, numbness is the primary symptom (when sensory fibers are blocked) or weakness (when there is a motor block). The numbness will be in a dermatomal pattern, whereas the weakness will present in a myotomal distribution. Radiculopathy is determined by these objective neurologic signs and symptoms rather than by pain. It is possible to have radiculopathy and radicular symptoms at the same time. Radiculopathy can occur alone (no pain) and radicular pain can occur without radiculopathy.[73]

Differentiating between radicular (pain from the peripheral nervous system) and referred pain from the ANS can be difficult. Both can start at one point and radiate outward. Both can cause pain distal to the site of pathology.

As mentioned previously, the CNS may not be able to distinguish which part of the body is responsible for the input into these common neurons so, for example, ischemia of the heart results in shoulder pain, one of several somatic areas innervated by the same neural segments as the heart.

Referred pain occurs most often far away from the site of pathologic origin of symptoms, whereas radicular pain does not skip myotomes, dermatomes, or sclerotomes associated with the affected peripheral nerves.

For example, cardiac pain may be described as beginning retrosternally (behind the sternum) and radiating to the left shoulder and down the inner side of the left arm. This radiating referred pain is generated via the pathways of the ANS but follows the somatic pattern of ulnar nerve distribution. It is not radicular pain from direct irritation of a spinal nerve of the peripheral nervous system but rather referred pain from shared pathways in the spinal cord.

Ischemic cardiac pain does not cause arm pain, hand pain, or pain in somatic areas other than those innervated at the C3 to T4 spinal levels of the ANS. Similarly, gallbladder pain may be felt to originate in the right upper abdomen and to radiate to the angle of the scapula. These are the somatic areas innervated by the same level of the ANS as the involved viscera mentioned.

Physical disease can localize pain in dermatomal or myotomal patterns. More often the therapist sees a client who describes pain that does not match a dermatomal or myotomal pattern. This is neither referred visceral pain from ANS involvement nor irritation of a spinal nerve. For example, the client who describes whole leg pain or whole leg numbness may be experiencing *inappropriate illness behavior*.

Inappropriate illness behavior is recognized clinically as illness behavior that is out of proportion to the underlying physical disease and is related more so to the associated psychologic disturbances than to the actual physical disease.[74,75] This behavioral component to pain is discussed in the section on Screening for Systemic Versus Psychogenic Symptoms.

Arterial, Pleural, and Tracheal Pain

Pain arising from arteries, as with arteritis (inflammation of an artery), migraine, and vascular headaches increases with systolic impulse so that any process associated with increased systolic pressure, such as exercise, fever, alcohol consumption, or bending over may intensify the already throbbing pain.

Pain from the pleura and the trachea correlates with respiratory movements. Look for associated signs and symptoms of the cardiac or pulmonary systems. Listen for a description of pain that is "throbbing" (vascular) or sharp and increased with respiratory movements such as breathing, laughing, or coughing.

Palpation and resisted movements will not reproduce the symptoms, which may get worse with recumbency, especially at night or while sleeping.

Gastrointestinal Pain

Pain arising from the GI tract tends to increase with peristaltic activity, particularly if there is any obstruction to forward progress of the food bolus. The pain increases with ingestion and may lessen with fasting or after emptying the involved segment (vomiting or bowel movement).

On the other hand, pain may occur secondary to the effect of gastric acid in the esophagus, stomach, or duodenum. This pain is relieved by the presence of food or by other neutralizing material in the stomach, and the pain is intensified when the stomach is empty and secreting acid. In these cases it is important to ask the client about the effect of eating on musculoskeletal pain. Does the pain increase, decrease, or stay the same immediately after eating and 1 to 3 hours later?

When hollow viscera, such as the liver, kidneys, spleen, and pancreas are distended, body positions or movements that increase intraabdominal pressure may intensify the pain, whereas positions that reduce pressure or support the structure may ease the pain.

For example, the client with an acutely distended gallbladder may slightly flex the trunk. With pain arising from a tense, swollen kidney (or distended renal pelvis), the client flexes the trunk and tilts toward the involved side; with pancreatic pain, the client may sit up and lean forward or lie down with the knees drawn up to the chest.

Pain at Rest

Pain at rest may arise from ischemia in a wide variety of tissue (e.g., vascular disease or tumor growth). The acute onset of severe unilateral extremity involvement accompanied by the "five Ps"—pain, pallor, pulselessness, paresthesia, and paralysis—signifies acute arterial occlusion (peripheral vascular disease [PVD]).[76] Pain in this situation is usually described by the client as burning or shooting and may be accompanied by paresthesia.

Pain related to ischemia of the skin and subcutaneous tissues is characterized by the client as burning and boring. All these occlusive causes of pain are usually worse at night and are relieved to some degree by dangling the affected leg over the side of the bed and by frequent massaging of the extremity.

Pain at rest secondary to neoplasm occurs usually at night. Although neoplasms are highly vascularized (a process called *angiogenesis*), the host organ's vascular supply and nutrients may be compromised simultaneously, causing ischemia of the local tissue. The pain awakens the client from sleep and prevents the person from going back to sleep, despite all efforts to do so. See the next section on Night Pain.

The client may describe pain noted on weight bearing or bone pain that may be mild and intermittent in the initial stages, becoming progressively more severe and more constant. A series of questions to identify the underlying cause of night pain is presented later in this chapter.

Night Pain

Whenever you take a pain history, an evaluation of night pain is important (Box 3.7). Pain at night is a classic red flag symptom of cancer, but it does not mean that all pain at night is caused by cancer or that all people with cancer will have night pain.[77] For example, the person who lies down at night and has not even fallen asleep who reports increased pain may just be experiencing the first moment in the day without distractions. Suddenly, his or her focus is on nothing but the pain, so the client may report the pain is much worse at night.

Bone pain at night is the most highly suspicious symptom, especially in the presence of a previous history of cancer. Neoplasms are highly vascularized at the expense of the host. This produces local ischemia and pain.

Pain with Activity

Pain with activity is common with pathology involving the NMS system. Pain with activity from a systemic or disease process is most often caused by vascular compromise. In this context, activity pain of the upper quadrant is known as *angina* when the heart muscle is compromised and *intermittent vascular claudication* in the case of peripheral vascular compromise (lower quadrant).

Pain from an ischemic muscle (including heart muscle) builds up with the use of the muscle and subsides with rest. Thus, there is a direct relationship between the degree of circulatory insufficiency and muscle work. In other words, the

BOX 3.7   SCREENING QUESTIONS FOR NIGHT PAIN

When screening someone with night pain for the possibility of a systemic or cancerous condition, some possible questions are:

- Tell me about the pattern of your symptoms at night. (Open-ended question.)
- Can you lie on that side? For how long?
- (Alternate question): Does it wake you up when you roll onto that side?
- How are you feeling in general when you wake up?
- Follow-up question: Do you have any other symptoms when the pain wakes you up? Give the client time to answer before prompting with choices such as coughing, wheezing, shortness of breath, nausea, need to go to the bathroom, night sweats.

Always ask the client reporting night pain of any kind (not just bone pain) the following screening questions:

- What makes it better/worse?
- What happens to your pain when you sit up? (Upright posture reduces venous return to the heart; decreased pain when sitting up may indicate a cardiopulmonary cause.)
- How does taking aspirin affect your pain/symptoms? (Disproportionate pain relief can occur using aspirin in the presence of bone cancer.)
- How does eating or drinking affect your pain/symptoms (for shoulder, neck, back, hip, pelvic pain/symptoms; gastrointestinal [GI] system)?
- Does taking an antacid such as Tums change your pain/symptoms? (Some women with pain of a cardiac nature experience pain relief much like men do with nitroglycerin; remember, this would be a woman who is postmenopausal, possibly with a personal and/or family history of heart disease—check vital signs!)

---

interval between the beginning of muscle contraction and the onset of pain depends on how long it takes for hypoxic products of muscle metabolism to accumulate and exceed the threshold of receptor response. Therefore in vascular-induced pain there is usually a delay or lag time between the beginning of activity and the onset of symptoms.

The client complains that a certain distance walked, a certain level of increased physical activity, or a fixed amount of usage of the extremity brings on the pain. When a vascular pathologic condition causes ischemic muscular pain, the location of the pain depends on the location of the vascular pathologic source. This is discussed in greater detail later in this text (see the section on Arterial Disease in Chapter 7).

The timing of symptom onset offers the therapist valuable screening clues when determining when symptoms are caused by musculoskeletal impairment or by vascular compromise.

Look for immediate pain or symptoms (especially when these can be reproduced with palpation, resistance to movement,

and/or a change in position) versus symptoms 5 to 10 minutes after activity begins. Further investigate for the presence of other signs and symptoms associated with cardiac impairment, appropriate risk factors, and positive personal and/or family history.

Diffuse Pain

Diffuse pain that characterizes some diseases of the nervous system and viscera may be difficult to distinguish from the equally diffuse pain so often caused by lesions of the moving parts. The distinction between visceral pain and pain caused by lesions of the vertebral column may be difficult to make and will require a medical diagnosis.

Chronic Pain

It has been reported that chronic pain affects 20% of people globally.[78] In older adults, persistent pain secondary to musculoskeletal disorders is a leading cause of disability.[79]

The IASP defines chronic pain as "pain that lasts or recurs form more than three months.[78]" The association also made the distinction between chronic primary pain, which is "represents chronic pain as a disease in itself," and chronic secondary pain, where "pain is a symptom of an underlying condition.[78]". Diener and colleagues recommends a few "in-depth" questions to ask a patient with persistent pain.[80] (Fig. 3.12)

Persistent or chronic pain can be characterized according to the following: duration, part of body, intensity, functional impact, and mechanism.[81]

Chronic pain syndrome is characterized by a constellation of life changes that produce altered behavior in the individual and persist even after the cause of the pain has been eradicated. This syndrome is a complex multidimensional phenomenon that requires a focus toward maximizing functional abilities rather than treatment of pain.

With chronic pain, the approach is to assess how the pain has affected the person. In patients with chronic pain, it is incorrect to correlate ratings of pain intensity with the severity of tissue damage because pain intensity is linked more with emotional and psychosocial factors than nociception.[82] Physical therapy intervention can be directed toward decreasing the client's emotional response to pain or developing skills to cope with stress and other changes that impair quality of life. In pain neuroscience education (PNE) the approach is to focus on the neurobiological and psychological perspectives to explain pain and manage pain.[81] This could result in a decrease in fear-avoidance behaviors, and an increase in willingness to move.[83] Interventions and approaches such as cognitive behavioral therapy (CBT), motivational interviewing[84] and graded exercise exposure[85] could be combined with PNE to break down pain memories related to movement, and decrease sensitivity of the nervous system.[83] There is increasing evidence on the effectiveness of PNE in managing musculoskeletal pain.[86,87]

Proposed "in-depth" questions

- What do you think is going on with your [*fill in area they are seeking help for*]?
- What do you think should be done for your [*fill in area they are seeking help for*]?
- Why do you think you still hurt?
- What would it take for you to get better?
- Where do you see yourself in 3 years in regard to [*fill in area they are seeking help for*]?
- What have you found to be most helpful for your [*fill in area they are seeking help for*]?
- You have obviously seen many people seeking help. What are your thoughts on this?
- What gives you hope?
- What is your expectation of PT?
- If I could flip a switch and remove all your pain, what things that you have given up on would you do again?
- How has your pain impacted your family and friends?
- Are you angry at anyone about your [*fill in area they are seeking help for*]? Tell me about it.
- Has anyone made you feel like you're "just making it up" or "it's in your head?" Tell me about it.

Fig. 3.12   Proposed in-depth questions ot ask a person with persistent pain. From: Pain mechanisms; From Diener I, Kargela M, Louw A. Listening is therapy: Patient intervlewing from a pain science perspective. *Physiother Theory Pract.* 2016;32(5):356-367.

In acute pain, the pain is proportional and appropriate to the problem and is treated as a symptom. In chronic pain syndrome, uncontrolled and prolonged pain alters both the peripheral nervous system and CNS through processes of neural plasticity and central sensitization and thus the pain becomes a disease itself.[88,89]

Each person may have a unique response to pain called a neuromatrix or neurosignature. The *neuromatrix* is initially determined through genetics and early sensory development. Later, life experiences related to pain and coping shape the neural patterns. Each person develops individual perceptual and behavioral responses to pain that are unique to that person.[90,91]

The person's description of chronic pain is often not well defined and is poorly localized; objective findings are not identified. The person's verbal description of the pain may contain words associated with emotional overlay (see Table 3.1). It may be helpful to ask the client or caregiver to maintain a pain log. This should include entries for pain intensity and its relationship to activity or intervention. Clients can be reevaluated regularly for improvement, deterioration, or complications using the same outcome measures used during the initial evaluation. Always keep in mind that painful symptoms out of proportion to the injury, or that are not consistent with the objective findings, may be a red flag indicating systemic disease. Pain can be triggered by bodily malfunction or severe illness.

Risk Factors

Research evidence has implicated biologic, psychologic, and social variables as key risk factors in chronic pain. These factors do not operate in isolation, but instead often interact with each other.[92] Cognitive processes, such as thoughts, beliefs, and expectations are important in understanding chronic pain, adaptation to chronic pain, response to intervention, and disability.[93]

Catastrophic and/or inflammatory reactivity, which is linked to a tendency to express negative thoughts and emotions, exaggerate the effect of painful experiences, and view of the situation as hopeless (and the person in the situation as helpless) are additional risk factors for the development of chronic pain.[94,95]

The following factors were reported to contribute or influence the development of chronic postoperative pain: anxiety, depression, fear of surgery and postoperative pain, catastrophizing behavior, lack of support and general stress levels.[96]

In a study by Vowles and colleagues, rates of misuse of opioids averaged between 21%-29% in patients with chronic pain.[97] In the 20-year period between 1999-2019, it was estimated that about half a million individuals died from an overdose involving prescription and illicit opioids.[98]

Risk factors for the misuse of opioid analgesics include personal/family history of substance abuse, history of criminal activity and/or legal problems (including driving under the influence [DUI]), heavy tobacco use, history of severe depression or anxiety, and history of rehabilitation for alcohol or other drugs.[99,100] Special screening tools are available, including the 5-item Opioid Risk Tool, Screener and Opioid Assessment for Patients in Pain (SOAPP tool), or the Current Opioid Misuse Measure (COMM). These tools have been validated and provide predictive measures of drug-related behaviors (see articles, discussions, and questionnaires at www.painedu.org).[101]

The therapist should be aware that chronic pain can be associated with physical and/or sexual abuse in both men and women. The abuse may be part of the childhood history and/or a continuing part of the adult experience.

Fear-Avoidance Behavior

Fear-avoidance behavior can also be a part of disability from chronic pain. [3] The concept is based on studies that show a person's fear of pain (not physical impairments) is the most important factor in how he or she responds to musculoskeletal pain. Anxiety, fear of pain, and pain catastrophizing can lead to avoiding physical or social activities. Screening for fear-avoidance behavior to determine whether an individual will resume normal activities (low psychologic distress) or will avoid normal activities because of the anticipation of increased pain and/or reinjury (high psychologic distress) can be done using the Fear-Avoidance Beliefs Questionnaire (FABQ, Table 3.7).[102,103] The therapist should not rely on his or her own perception of the patient's/client's fear-avoidance behaviors. In addition to the FABQ, the Tampa Scale of Kinesophobia (TSK)[104] and Pain Catastrophizing Scale (PSC)[105] are available to identify psychologic beliefs linked with pain.[106]

The FABQ is a 16-item patient-reported questionnaire that assesses how the patient's fear-avoidance behaviors related to their physical activity and work may contribute to and affect their low back pain. The first 5 questions pertain to physical activity and the remaining 11 questions pertain to work. Higher scores are indicative of fear-avoidance behavior. A cut-off score for the work scale indicative of having a decreased chance of returning to work has been proposed. The work subscale of the FABQ is the strongest predictor of work status. There is a greater likelihood of return-to-work for scores less than 30, and less likelihood of return-to-work or increased risk of prolonged work restrictions for scores greater than 34.[107]

Elevated fear-avoidance beliefs are not indicative of a red flag for serious medical pathology. They are indicative of someone who has a poor prognosis for rehabilitation (e.g., poor clinical outcomes, elevated pain symptoms, development of depressive symptoms, greater physical impairments,

---

TABLE 3.7	Fear-Avoidance Beliefs Questionnaire (FABQ)

Here are some of the things other patients have told us about their pain. For each statement, please circle any number from 0 to 6 to say how much physical activities, such as bending, walking, or driving, affect or would affect your back pain.

	Completely Disagree			Unsure		Completely Agree	
1. My pain was caused by physical activity	0	1	2	3	4	5	6
2. Physical activity makes my pain worse	0	1	2	3	4	5	6
3. Physical activity might harm my back	0	1	2	3	4	5	6
4. I should not do physical activities that (might) make my pain worse	0	1	2	3	4	5	6
5. I cannot do physical activities that (might) make my pain worse	0	1	2	3	4	5	6

The following statements are about how your normal work affects or would affect your back pain.

	Completely Disagree			Unsure		Completely Agree	
6. My pain was caused by my work or by an accident at work	0	1	2	3	4	5	6
7. My work aggravated my pain	0	1	2	3	4	5	6
8. I have a claim for compensation for my pain	0	1	2	3	4	5	6
9. My work is too heavy for me	0	1	2	3	4	5	6
10. My work makes or would make my pain worse	0	1	2	3	4	5	6
11. My work might harm my back	0	1	2	3	4	5	6
12. I should not do my normal work with my present pain	0	1	2	3	4	5	6
13. I cannot do my normal work with my present pain	0	1	2	3	4	5	6
14. I cannot do my normal work until my pain is treated	0	1	2	3	4	5	6
15. I do not think I will be back to my normal work	0	1	2	3	4	5	6
16. I do not think that I will ever be able to go back to that work	0	1	2	3	4	5	6

The FABQ is used to quantify the level of fear of pain and beliefs clients with low back pain have about the need to avoid movements or activities that might cause pain. The FABQ has 16 items, each scored from 0 to 6, with higher numbers indicating increased levels of fear-avoidance beliefs. There are two subscales: a seven-item work subscale (sum of items 6, 7, 9, 10, 11, 12, and 15; score range = 0–42) and a four-item physical activity subscale (sum of items 2, 3, 4, and 5; score range = 0–24). The FABQ work subscale is associated with current and future disability and work loss in patients with acute and chronic low back pain.

(From Waddell G, Somerville D, Henderson I, et al. Fear-avoidance beliefs questionnaire (FABQ) and the role of fear-avoidance beliefs in chronic low back pain and disability. Pain 1993;52:157-158.)

continued disability).[108] They are more accurately labeled a "yellow flag" indicating psychosocial involvement and provide insight into the prognosis. Such a yellow flag signals the need to modify intervention and consider the need for referral to a psychologist or behavioral counselor.

When the client shows signs of fear-avoidance beliefs, then the therapist's management approach should include education that addresses the client's fear and avoidance behavior and should consider a graded approach to therapeutic exercise.[109]

The therapist can teach clients about the difference between pain and tissue injury. Chronic ongoing pain does not mean continued tissue injury is taking place. This common misconception can result in movement avoidance behaviors.

Differentiating Chronic Pain from Systemic Disease

Sometimes a chronic or persistent pain can be differentiated from a systemic disease by the nature and description of the pain. Chronic pain is usually dull and persistent, and characterized by multiple complaints, excessive preoccupation with pain, and, frequently, misuse of pharmacological interventions. With chronic pain, there is usually a history of some precipitating injury or event.

Systemic disease is more acute with a recent onset. It is often described as sharp, colicky, knife-like, and/or deep. Look for concomitant constitutional symptoms, any red flags in the personal or family history, and/or any known risk factors. Ask about the presence of associated signs and symptoms characteristic of a particular organ or body system (e.g., GI, GU, respiratory, gynecologic).

Because pain has an affective component, chronic pain could cause anxiety, depression, and anger. The amount of pain behavior and the intensity of pain perceived can change with alterations in environmental reinforcers (e.g., increasing as the time to return to work draws near, decreasing when no one is watching). For more information and assessment tools, see the discussions related to anxiety and depression in this chapter.

Secondary gain may be a factor in perpetuating the problem. This may be primarily financial, but social and family benefits, such as increased attention or avoidance of unpleasant activities or work situations, may be factors (see later discussion of behavior responses to injury/illness).

COMPARISON OF SYSTEMIC VERSUS MUSCULOSKELETAL PAIN PATTERNS

Table 3.2 provides a comparison of the clinical signs and symptoms of systemic pain versus musculoskeletal pain using the typical categories described earlier. The therapist must be very familiar with the information contained within this table. Even with these guidelines to follow, the therapist's job is a challenging one.

In the musculoskeletal setting, physical therapists are very aware that pain can be referred above and below a joint. So, for example, when examining a problem involving the shoulder, the therapist always considers the neck and elbow as potential NMS sources of shoulder pain and dysfunction.

Table 3.8 reflects what is known about referred pain patterns for the musculoskeletal system. Sites for referred pain from a visceral pain mechanism are listed. Lower cervical and upper thoracic impairment can refer pain to the interscapular and posterior shoulder areas.

Likewise, shoulder impairment can refer pain to the neck and upper back, although any condition affecting the upper lumbar spine can refer pain and symptoms to the SI joint and hip. When examining the hip region, the therapist always considers the possibility of an underlying SI or knee joint impairment.

If the client presents with the typical or primary referred pain pattern, he or she will likely end up in a physician's office. A secondary or referred pain pattern can be very deceiving. The therapist may not be able to identify the underlying pathology (in fact, it is not required), but it is imperative to recognize when the clinical presentation does not fit the expected pattern for a NMS impairment.

A few additional comments about systemic versus musculoskeletal pain patterns are important. First, it is unlikely that the client with back, hip, SI, or shoulder pain that has

TABLE 3.8	Common Patterns of Pain Referral	
Pain Mechanism	Lesion Site	Referral Site
Somatic	C7, T1-5 vertebrae	Interscapular area, posterior
	Shoulder	Neck, upper back
	L1, L2 vertebrae	Sacroiliac (SI) joint and hip
	Hip joint	SI and knee
	Pharynx	Ipsilateral ear
	Temporomandibular joint (TMJ)	Head, neck, heart
Visceral	Diaphragmatic irritation	Shoulder, lumbar spine
	Heart	Shoulder, neck, upper back, TMJ
	Urothelial tract	Back, inguinal region, anterior thigh, and genitalia
	Pancreas, liver, spleen, gallbladder	Shoulder, midthoracic or low back
	Peritoneal or abdominal cavity	Hip pain from abscess of psoas or obturator muscle
Neuropathic	Nerve or plexus	Anywhere in distribution of a peripheral nerve
	Nerve root	Anywhere in corresponding dermatome
	Central nervous system	Anywhere in region of body innervated by damaged structure

been present for the last 5 to 10 years is demonstrating a viscerogenic cause of symptoms. In such a case, systemic origins are suspected only if there is a sudden or recent change in the clinical presentation and/or the client develops constitutional symptoms or signs and symptoms commonly associated with an organ system.

Secondly, note the word descriptors used with pain of a systemic nature: knife-like, boring, deep, throbbing. Pay attention any time someone uses these particular words to describe the symptoms.

Third, observe the client's reaction to the information you provide. Often, someone with an NMS problem may gain pain relief just from the examination provided and evaluation offered. The reason? A reduction in the anxiety level. Many people have a need for high control. Pain throws us in a state of fear and anxiety and a perceived loss of control. Knowing what the problem is and having a plan of action can reduce the amplification of symptoms for someone with soft tissue involvement when there is an underlying psychologic component such as anxiety. Signs and symptoms of anxiety are presented later in this chapter. Someone with cancer pain, viscerogenic origin of symptoms, or systemic illness of some kind will not obtain relief from or reduction of pain with reassurance.

Fourth, aggravating and relieving factors associated with NMS impairment often have to do with change in position or a change (increased or decreased) in activity levels. There is usually some way the therapist can alter, provoke, alleviate, eliminate, or aggravate symptoms of an NMS origin. Pain with activity is immediate when there is involvement of the NMS system. There may be a delayed increase in symptoms after the initiation of activity with a systemic (vascular) cause.

Aggravating and relieving factors associated with systemic pain are organ dependent and based on visceral function. For example, chest pain, neck pain, or upper back pain from a problem with the esophagus will likely get worse when the client is swallowing or eating.

Back, shoulder, pelvic, or sacral pain that is made better or worse by eating, passing gas, or having a bowel movement is a red flag. Painful symptoms that start 3 to 5 minutes after initiating an activity and go away when the client stops the activity suggest pain of a vascular nature. This is especially true when the client uses the word "throbbing," which is a descriptor of a vascular origin.

Clients presenting with vascular-induced musculoskeletal complaints are not likely to come to the therapist with a report of cardiac-related chest pain. Rather, the therapist must be alert for the man over the age of 50 years or for the postmenopausal woman with a significant family history of heart disease who is borderline hypertensive. New onset or reproduction of back, neck, temporomandibular joint (TMJ), shoulder, or arm pain brought on by exertion with arms raised overhead or by starting a new exercise program is a red flag.

Leaning forward or assuming a hands and knees position sometimes lessens gallbladder pain. This position moves the distended or inflamed gallbladder out away from its position under the liver. Leaning or side bending toward the painful side sometimes ameliorates kidney pain. Again, for some people, this may move the kidney enough to take the pressure off during early onset of an infectious or inflammatory process.

Finally, notice the long list of potential signs and symptoms associated with systemic conditions (see Table 3.2). At the same time, note the *lack* of associated signs and symptoms listed on the musculoskeletal side of the table. Except for the possibility of some ANS responses with the stimulation of TrPs, there are no comparable constitutional or systemic signs and symptoms associated with the NMS system.

CHARACTERISTICS OF VISCEROGENIC PAIN

There are some characteristics of viscerogenic pain that can occur regardless of which organ system is involved. Any of these by itself is cause for suspicion, and careful listening and observation is warranted. They often occur together in clusters of two or three. Watch for any of the following components of the pain pattern.

Gradual, Progressive, and Cyclical Pain Patterns

Gradual, progressive, and cyclical pain patterns are characteristic of viscerogenic disease. The one time this pain pattern occurs in a musculoskeletal situation is with the client who has low back pain of a discogenic origin. The client is given the appropriate intervention and begins to do his/her exercise program. The symptoms improve, and the client completes a full weekend of gardening, or other excessive activity. The activity aggravates the condition and the symptoms return worse than before. The client returns to the clinic, is given firm reminders by the therapist regarding guidelines for physical activity, and is sent out once again with the appropriate exercise program. The "cooperate—get better—then overdo" cycle may recur until the client completes the rehabilitation process and obtains relief from symptoms and return of function. This pattern can mimic the gradual, progressive, and cyclical pain pattern normally associated with underlying organic pathology. The difference between an NMS pattern of pain and symptoms and a visceral pattern is the NMS problem gradually improves over time, whereas the systemic condition gets worse.

Of course, beware of the client with discogenic back and leg pain who suddenly returns to the clinic completely symptom free. There is always the risk of disc herniation and sequestration when the nucleus detaches and becomes a loose body that may enter the spinal canal. In the case of a "miraculous cure" from disc herniation, be sure to ask about the onset of any new symptoms, especially changes in bowel and bladder function.

Constant Pain

Pain that is constant and intense should raise a red flag. There is a logical and important first question to ask anyone who says the pain is "constant."

❓ FOLLOW-UP QUESTIONS

- Do you have that pain right now?

It is surprising how often the client will answer "No" to this question. Although it is true that pain of an NMS origin can be constant, it is also true that there is usually some way to modulate it up or down. The client often has one or two positions that make it better (or worse).

Constant, intense pain in a client with a previous personal history of cancer and/or in the presence of other associated signs and symptoms raises a red flag.

It is not necessary to have the client complete an entire week's pain log to assess constant pain. A 24- to 48-hour time period is sufficient. Use the recording scale on the right, indicating pain intensity and medications taken (prescription and over-the-counter [OTC]).

Under item number three, include sexual activity. The particulars are not necessary, just some indication that the client was sexually active. The client defines "sexually active" for him- or herself, whether this is just touching and holding or complete coitus. This is another useful indicator of pain levels and functional activity.

Remember to offer clients a clear explanation for any questions asked concerning sexual activity, sexual function, or sexual history. There is no way to know when someone will be offended or claim sexual harassment. It is in your own interest to behave in the most professional manner possible.

There should be no hint of sexual innuendo or humor injected into any of your conversations with clients at any time. The line of sexual impropriety lies where the complainant draws it and includes appearances of misbehavior. This perception differs broadly from client to client.[7]

Finally, the number of hours slept is helpful information. Someone who reports sleepless nights may not actually be awake, but rather, may be experiencing a sleep disturbance. Cancer pain wakes the client up from a sound sleep. An actual record of being awake and up for hours at night or awakened repeatedly is significant (Case Example 3.6). See the discussion on Night Pain earlier in this chapter.

Physical Therapy Intervention "Fails"

If a client does not get better with physical therapy intervention, do not immediately doubt yourself. The lack of progression in treatment could very well be a red-flag symptom. If the client reports improvement in the early intervention phase but later takes a turn for the worse, it may be a red flag. Take the time to step back, reevaluate the client and your intervention, and screen if you have not already done so (or screen again if you have).

Pain Does Not Fit the Expected Pattern

In a primary care practice or under direct access, the therapist may see a client who reports back, hip, or SI pain of systemic

---

CASE EXAMPLE 3.6

Constant Night Pain

A 33-year-old man with left shoulder pain reports "constant pain at night." After asking all the appropriate screening questions related to night pain and constant pain you see the following pattern:

Shoulder pain that is made worse by lying down whether it is at night or during the day. There are no increased pulmonary or breathing problems at night when lying down. Pain is described as a "deep aching." The client cannot find a comfortable position and moves from bed to couch to chair to bed all night long.

He injured his arm 6 months ago in a basketball game when he fell and landed on that shoulder. Symptoms have been gradually getting worse and nothing he does makes them go away. He reports a small amount of relief if he puts a rolled towel under his armpit.

He is not taking any medication; has no significant personal or family history for cancer, kidney, heart, or stomach disease; and has no other symptoms of any kind.

Do You Need to Screen any Further for Systemic Origin of Symptoms?

Probably not, even though there are what look like red flags:

- Constant pain
- Deep aching
- Symptoms beyond the expected time for physiologic healing
- No position is comfortable

Once you complete the objective tests and measures, you will have a better idea if further questions are needed. Although his pain is "constant" and occurs at night, it looks like it may be positional.

An injury 6 months ago with continued symptoms falls into the category of "symptoms persist beyond the expected time for physiologic healing." His description of not being able to find a position of comfort is a possible example of "no position is comfortable."

Given the mechanism of injury and position of mild improvement (towel roll under the arm), it may be more likely that a soft tissue tear is present and physiologic healing has not been possible.

Referral to a physician (or returning the client to the referring physician) may not be necessary just yet. Some clients do not want surgery and opt for a rehabilitation approach. Make sure you have all the information from the primary care physician if there is one involved. Your rehabilitation protocol will depend on a specific diagnosis (e.g., torn rotator cuff, labral tear, impingement syndrome).

If the client does not respond to physical therapy intervention, reevaluation (possibly including a screening component) is warranted with physician referral considered at that time.

---

or visceral origin early on in its development. In these cases, during early screening, the client often presents with full and pain-free ROM. Only after pain has been present long enough to cause splinting and guarding does the client exhibit biomechanical changes (Box 3.8).

> ### BOX 3.8 RANGE OF MOTION CHANGES WITH SYSTEMIC DISEASE
>
> - **Early screening:** Full and pain-free range of motion (ROM)
> - **Late screening:** Biomechanical response to pain results in changes associated with splinting and guarding

SCREENING FOR EMOTIONAL AND PSYCHOLOGIC OVERLAY

Pain, emotion, and pain behavior are all integral parts of the pain experience. There is no disease, illness, or state of pain without an accompanying psychologic component.[7] This does not mean the client's pain is not real or does not exist on a physical level. In fact, clients with behavioral changes may also have significant underlying injury.[110] Physical pain and emotional changes are two sides of the same coin.[111]

Pain is not just a physical sensation that passes up to consciousness and then produces secondary emotional effects. Rather, the neurophysiology of pain and emotions are closely linked throughout the higher levels of the CNS. Sensory and emotional changes occur simultaneously and influence each other.[112]

The sensory discriminative component of pain is primarily physiologic in nature and occurs as a result of nociceptive stimulation in the presence of organic pathology. The motivational-affective dimension of pain is psychologic in nature, subject to the underlying principles of emotional behavior.[113]

The therapist's practice often includes clients with personality disorders, malingering, or other psychophysiologic disorders. Psychophysiologic disorders (also known as *psychosomatic* disorders) include any condition in which the physical symptoms may be caused or made worse by psychologic factors.

Recognizing somatic signs of any psychophysiologic disorder is a part of the screening process. Behavioral, psychologic, or medical treatment may be indicated. Psychophysiologic disorders are generally characterized by subjective complaints that exceed objective findings, symptom development in the presence of psychosocial stresses, and physical symptoms involving one or more organ systems. It is the last variable that can confuse the therapist when trying to screen for medical disease.

It is impossible to discuss the broad range of psychophysiologic disorders that comprise a large portion of the physical therapy caseload in a screening text of this kind. The therapist is strongly encouraged to become familiar with the *Diagnostic and Statistical Manual of Mental Disorders (DSM-V-)*[114] to understand the psychologic factors affecting the successful outcome of rehabilitation.

However, recognizing clusters of signs and symptoms characteristic of the psychologic component of illness is very important in the screening process. Likewise, the therapist will want to become familiar and competent with identifying nonorganic signs indicative of psychologic factors.[115-118]

Three key psychologic components that have important significance in the pain response of many people include anxiety, depression and panic disorder.

Anxiety, Depression, and Panic Disorder

Psychologic factors, such as emotional stress and conflicts leading to anxiety, depression, and panic disorder play an important role in the client's experience of physical symptoms. In the past, physical symptoms caused or exacerbated by psychologic variables were labeled psychosomatic. Today the interconnections between the mind, the immune system, the hormonal system, the nervous system, and the physical body have led us to view psychosomatic disorders as psychophysiologic disorders (Case Example 3.7).

There is considerable overlap, shared symptoms, and interaction between these emotions. They are all part of the normal human response to pain and stress[112] and occur often in clients with serious or chronic health conditions. Intervention is not always needed. However, strong emotions experienced over a long period of time can become harmful if excessive.

Depression and anxiety often present with somatic symptoms that may resolve with effective treatment. Diagnosis of these conditions is made by a medical doctor or trained mental health professional. The therapist can describe the symptoms and relay that information to the appropriate agency or individual when making a referral.

Anxiety

Anyone who feels excessive anxiety may have a generalized anxiety disorder with excessive and unrealistic worry about day-to-day issues that can last months and even longer. Anxiety magnifies physical symptoms, just like the amplifier ("amp") on a sound system. It does not change the sound; it just increases the power to make it louder. The tendency to amplify a broad range of bodily sensations may be an important factor in experiencing, reporting, and functioning with an acute and relatively mild medical illness.[119]

Keep in mind the known effect of anxiety on the *intensity* of pain of a musculoskeletal versus systemic origin. Defining the problem, offering reassurance, and outlining a plan of action with expected outcomes can reduce painful symptoms amplified by anxiety. It does not ameliorate pain of a systemic nature.[120]

Musculoskeletal complaints, such as sore muscles, back pain, headache, or fatigue can result from anxiety-caused tension or heightened sensitivity to pain. Anxiety increases muscle tension, thereby reducing blood flow and oxygen to the tissues, resulting in a buildup of cellular metabolites.

Somatic symptoms are diagnostic for several anxiety disorders, including panic disorder, agoraphobia (fear of open places, especially fear of being alone or of being in public places) and other phobias (irrational fears), obsessive-compulsive disorder (OCD), posttraumatic stress disorder (PTSD), and generalized anxiety disorders.

Anxious persons have a reduced ability to tolerate painful stimulation, noticing it more or interpreting it as more

Post-Total Knee Replacement

A 71-year-old woman has been referred for home health following a left total knee replacement (TKR). Her surgery was 6 weeks ago and she has had severe pain, swelling, and loss of motion. She has had numerous previous surgeries, including right shoulder arthroplasty, removal of the right eye (macular degeneration), rotator cuff repair on the left, hysterectomy, two cesarean sections, and several inner ear surgeries. In all, she proudly tells you she has had 21 operations in 21 years.

Her family tells you she is taking Percocet prescribed by the orthopedic surgeon and Darvon left over from a previous surgery. They estimate she takes at least 10 to 12 pills every day. They are concerned because she complains of constant pain and sleeps 18 hours a day.

They want you to "do something."

What Is the Appropriate Response in This Situation?
As part of the evaluation process, you will be gathering more information about your client's functional level, functional status, mental status, and assessing her pain more thoroughly. Take some time to listen to the client's pain description and concerns. Find out what her goals are and what would help her to reach those goals.

Consider using the McGill Pain Questionnaire to assess for emotional overlay. With a long history of medical care, she may be dependent on the attention she gets for each operation. Addiction to pain-relieving drugs can occur, but it is more likely that she has become dependent on them because of a cycle of pain-spasm-inactivity-pain-spasm and so on.

Physical therapy intervention may help reduce some of this and change around her pain pattern.

Depression may be a key factor in this case. Review the possible signs and symptoms of depression with the client. It may not be necessary to tell the client ahead of time that these signs and symptoms are typical of depression. Read the list and ask her to let you know if she is experiencing any of them. See how many she reports at this time. Afterwards, ask her if she may be depressed and see how she responds to the question.

Medical referral for review of her medications and possible psychologic evaluation may be in her best interest. You may want to contact the doctor with your concerns and/or suggest the family report their concerns as well.

Keep in mind exercise is a key intervention strategy for depression. As the therapist, you may be able to "do something" by including a general conditioning program in addition to her specific knee exercises.

significant than do nonanxious persons. This leads to further complaining about pain and to more disability and pain behavior such as limping, grimacing, or medication seeking.

To complicate matters more, persons with an organic illness sometimes develop anxiety known as *adjustment disorder with anxious mood*. Additionally, the advent of a known organic condition, such as a pulmonary embolus or chronic obstructive pulmonary disease (COPD), can cause an agoraphobia-like syndrome in older persons, especially if the client views the condition as unpredictable, variable, and disabling.

Emotional problems amplify physical symptoms such as ulcerative colitis, peptic ulcers, or allergies. Although allergies may be inherited, anxiety amplifies or exaggerates the symptoms. Symptoms may appear as physical, behavioral, cognitive, or psychologic (Table 3.9).

The Beck Anxiety Inventory (BAI) quickly assesses the presence and severity of client anxiety in adolescents and adults ages 17 and older. It was designed to reduce the overlap between depression and anxiety scales by measuring anxiety symptoms shared minimally with those of depression.

The BAI consists of 21 items, each scored on a 4-point scale between 0 and 3, for a total score ranging from 0 to 63. Higher scores indicate higher levels of anxiety. The BAI is reported to have good reliability and validity for clients with various psychiatric diagnoses.[121-124]

Both physiologic and cognitive components of anxiety are addressed in the 21 items describing subjective, somatic, or panic-related symptoms. The BAI differentiates between anxious and nonanxious groups in a variety of clinical settings and is appropriate for all adult mental health populations.

Depression

Once defined as a deep and unrelenting sadness lasting 2 weeks or more, depression is no longer viewed in such simplistic terms. As an understanding of this condition has evolved, scientists have come to speak of the *depressive illnesses*. This term gives a better idea of the breadth of the disorder, encompassing several conditions, including depression, dysthymia, bipolar disorder, and seasonal affective disorder (SAD).

Although these conditions can differ from individual to individual, each includes some of the symptoms listed. Often the classic signs of depression are not as easy to recognize in people older than 65 years of age, and many people attribute such symptoms simply to "getting older" and ignore them.

Anyone can be affected by depression at any time. There are, in fact, many underlying physical and medical causes of depression (Box 3.9), including medications used for Parkinson's disease, arthritis, cancer, hypertension, and heart disease (Box 3.10). The therapist should be familiar with these.

For example, anxiety and depressive disorders occur at a higher rate in clients with COPD, obesity, diabetes, asthma, arthritis, cancer, and cardiovascular disease.[125,126] Other risk factors for depression include lifestyle choices such as tobacco use, physical inactivity and sedentary lifestyle, and binge drinking.[127] There is also a link between depression and heart disease.[128] It was also reported that up to 85% of patients with chronic pain are also affected by severe depression.[129]

New insights on depression have led scientists to see clinical depression as a biologic disease possibly originating in the brain with multiple visceral involvements (Table 3.10). One error in medical treatment has been to recognize and treat the client's esophagitis, palpitations, irritable bowel, heart disease, asthma, or chronic low back

TABLE 3.9	Symptoms of Anxiety and Panic		
Physical	**Behavioral**	**Cognitive**	**Psychologic**
Increased sighing respirations	Hyperalertness	Fear of losing mind	Phobias
Increased blood pressure	Irritability	Fear of losing control	Obsessive-compulsive behavior
Tachycardia	Uncertainty		
Muscle tension	Apprehension		
Dizziness	Difficulty with memory or concentration		
Lump in throat	Sleep disturbance		
Shortness of breath			
Clammy hands			
Dry mouth			
Diarrhea			
Nausea			
Muscle tension			
Profuse sweating			
Restlessness, pacing, irritability, difficulty concentrating			
Chest pain*			
Headache			
Low back pain			
Myalgia (muscle pain, tension, or tenderness)			
Arthralgia (joint pain)			
Abdominal (stomach) distress			
Irritable bowel syndrome (IBS)			

*Chest pain associated with anxiety accounts for more than half of all emergency department admissions for chest pain. The pain is substernal, a dull ache that does not radiate, and is not aggravated by respiratory movements but is associated with hyperventilation and claustrophobia. See Chapter 18 for further discussion of chest pain triggered by anxiety.

BOX 3.9 PHYSICAL CONDITIONS COMMONLY ASSOCIATED WITH DEPRESSION

Cardiovascular
Atherosclerosis
Hypertension
Myocardial infarction
Angioplasty or bypass surgery

Central Nervous System
Parkinson's disease
Huntington's disease
Cerebral arteriosclerosis
Stroke
Alzheimer's disease
Temporal lobe epilepsy
Postconcussion injury
Multiple sclerosis
Miscellaneous focal lesions

Endocrine, Metabolic
Hyperthyroidism
Hypothyroidism
Addison's disease
Cushing's disease
Hypoglycemia
Hyperglycemia
Hyperparathyroidism
Hyponatremia
Diabetes mellitus
Pregnancy (postpartum)

Viral
Acquired immunodeficiency syndrome (AIDS)
Hepatitis
Pneumonia
Influenza

Nutritional
Folic acid deficiency
Vitamin B_6 deficiency
Vitamin B_{12} deficiency

Immune
Fibromyalgia
Chronic fatigue syndrome
Systemic lupus erythematosus
Sjögren's syndrome
Rheumatoid arthritis
Immunosuppression (e.g., corticosteroid treatment)

Cancer
Pancreatic
Bronchogenic
Renal
Ovarian

Miscellaneous
Pancreatitis
Sarcoidosis
Syphilis
Porphyria
Corticosteroid treatment

(From Goodman CC. Biopsychosocial-spiritual concepts related to health care. In Goodman CC, Fuller K, eds. Pathology: Implications for the Physical Therapist. 4th ed. Philadelphia: WB Saunders; 2015.)

BOX 3.10 DRUGS COMMONLY ASSOCIATED WITH DEPRESSION

For additional information on drugs that can cause depression, see http://www.webmd.com/depression/guide/medicines-cause-depression#2

- Antianxiety medications (e.g., Valium, Xanax)
- Illegal drugs (e.g., cocaine, crack)
- Antihypertensive drugs (e.g., beta-blockers, antiadrenergics)
- Cardiovascular medications (e.g., digitoxin, digoxin)
- Antineoplastic agents (e.g., vinblastine)
- Opiate analgesics (e.g., morphine, Demerol, Darvon)
- Anticonvulsants (e.g., Dilantin, phenobarbital)
- Corticosteroids (e.g., prednisone, cortisone, dexamethasone)
- Nonsteroidal antiinflammatory drugs (NSAIDs) (e.g., indomethacin)
- Alcohol
- Hormone replacement therapy and oral contraceptives

TABLE 3.10 Systemic Effects of Depression

System	Sign or Symptom
General (multiple system crossover)	Persistent fatigue
	Insomnia, sleep disturbance
	See clinical signs and symptoms of depression in the text
Cardiovascular	Chest pain
	• Associated with myocardial infarction
	• Can be atypical chest pain that is not associated with coronary artery disease
Gastrointestinal	Irritable bowel syndrome (IBS)
	Esophageal dysmotility
	Nonulcer dyspepsia
	Functional abdominal pain (heartburn)
Neurologic (often symmetric and nonanatomic)	Paresthesia
	Dizziness
	Difficulty concentrating and making decisions; problems with memory
Musculoskeletal	Weakness
	Fibromyalgia (or other unexplained rheumatic pain)
	Myofascial pain syndrome
	Chronic back pain
Immune	Multiple allergies
	Chemical hypersensitivity
	Autoimmune disorders
	Recurrent or resistant infections
Dysregulation	Autonomic instability
	• Temperature intolerance
	• Blood pressure changes
	Hormonal dysregulation (e.g., amenorrhea)
Other	Migraine and tension headaches
	Shortness of breath associated with asthma or not clearly explained
	Anxiety or panic disorder

(Data from Smith NL. The Effects of Depression and Anxiety on Medical Illness. Sandy, UT: Stress Medicine Clinic, School of Medicine, University of Utah; 2002.)

pain without seeing the real underlying impairment of the CNS (CNS dysregulation: depression) leading to these dysfunctions.[130-132]

A medical diagnosis is necessary because several known physical causes of depression are reversible if treated (e.g., thyroid disorders, vitamin B_{12} deficiency, medications [especially sedatives], some hypertensives, and H_2-blockers for stomach problems). About half of the clients with panic disorder will have an episode of clinical depression during their lifetime.

Depression is not a normal part of the aging process, but it is a normal response to pain or disability and may influence the client's ability to cope. Whereas anxiety is more apparent in acute pain episodes, depression occurs more often in clients with chronic pain.

The therapist may want to screen for psychosocial factors, such as depression, that influence physical rehabilitation outcomes, especially when a client demonstrates acute pain that persists for more than 6 to 8 weeks. Screening is also important because depression is an indicator of poor prognosis.[133] In the primary care setting, the physical therapist has a key role in identifying comorbidities that may have an effect on physical therapy intervention. Depression has been clearly identified as a factor that delays recovery or results in poorer prognosis for clients with low back pain.[134] The longer depression is undetected, the greater the likelihood of prolonged physical therapy intervention and increased disability.[133,140]

The Patient Health Questionnaire (PHQ)-2 is a 2-item questionnaire that can be used as a "first screen approach" for depression (see Fig. 3.13). A person who scores a 3 or above in the PHQ-2 should be further evaluated with the longer 9-item Patient Health Questionnaire-9, another diagnostic instrument or an interview to determine a diagnosis of depressive disorder.[135-137] Additional tests such as the Beck Depression Inventory (BDI) second edition (BDI-II),[138-140] the Zung Depression Scale,[141] or the Geriatric Depression Scale (short form) can be administered by a physical therapist to obtain baseline information that may be useful in determining the need for a medical referral. These tests do not require interpretation that is out of the scope of physical therapist's practice.

Symptoms of Depression. About one third of the clinically depressed clients treated do not feel sad or blue. Instead, they report somatic symptoms such as fatigue, joint pain, headaches, or chronic back pain (or any chronic, recurrent pain present in multiple places). Many of the common GI disorders (e.g., esophageal motility disorder, nonulcer dyspepsia, irritable bowel syndrome [IBS]) are associated with depressive or anxiety disorders[142-144].[132,133,145]

Another red flag for depression is any condition associated with smooth muscle spasm such as asthma, irritable or overactive bladder,[146] Raynaud's disease, and hypertension.[147] Neurologic[148] symptoms with no apparent cause such as paresthesias, dizziness, and weakness may actually be symptoms of depression. This is particularly true if the neurologic symptoms are symmetric or not anatomic.[130]

Instructions: Print out the short form below and ask patients to complete it while sitting in the waiting or exam room.

Use: The purpose of the PHQ-2 is not to establish a final diagnosis or to monitor depression severity, but rather to screen for depression as a "first-step" approach.

Scoring: A PHQ-2 score ranges for 0 to 6; patients with scores of 3 or more should be further evaluated with the PHQ-9 other diagnostic instrument(s), or a direct interview to determine whether they meet criteria for a depressive disorder.

Patient Name: _____ Date of Visit: _____

Over the past 2 weeks, how often have you been bothered by any of the following problems?	Not at all	Several days	More than half of the days	Nearly every day
1. Little interest or pleasure in doing things	0	1	2	3
2. Feeling down, depressed, or hopeless	0	1	2	3

Fig. 3.13 Patient Health Questionnaire (PHQ)-2. (From Kroenke K, Spitzer RL, Williams JR. The patient health questionnaire-2: Validity of a 2-item depression screener. *Med Care.* 2003; 41:1284–1292.)

CLINICAL SIGNS AND SYMPTOMS

Depression (See Also Table 3.10)

- Persistent sadness, low mood, or feelings of emptiness
- Frequent or unexplained crying spells
- A sense of hopelessness
- Feelings of guilt or worthlessness
- Problems in sleeping
- Loss of interest or pleasure in ordinary activities or loss of libido
- Fatigue or decreased energy
- Appetite loss (or overeating)
- Difficulty in concentrating, remembering, and making decisions
- Irritability
- Persistent joint pain
- Headache
- Chronic back pain
- Bilateral neurologic symptoms of unknown cause (e.g., numbness, dizziness, weakness)
- Thoughts of death or suicide
- Pacing and fidgeting
- Chest pain and palpitations

Panic Disorder

Persons with a diagnosis of panic disorder have at least two episodes of panic attacks, characterized by sudden, unprovoked feelings of terror or impending doom with associated physical symptoms such as racing or pounding heartbeat, breathlessness, nausea, sweating, and dizziness. During an attack, people may fear that they are gravely ill, going to die, or going crazy.[149] Panic disorder is characterized by periods of sudden, unprovoked, intense anxiety with associated physical symptoms lasting a few minutes up to a few hours. Dizziness, paresthesias, headaches, and palpitations are common.

The fear of another attack can itself become debilitating so that these individuals avoid situations and places that they believe will trigger the episodes, thus affecting their work, their relationships, and their ability to take care of everyday tasks.

Initial panic attacks may occur when people are under considerable stress, for example, an overload of work or from a loss of a family member or close friend. The attacks may follow surgery, a serious accident, illness, or childbirth. Use of alcohol or drugs to mitigate these symptoms could make the panic disorder worse.[149]

The symptoms of a panic attack can mimic those of other medical conditions, such as respiratory or heart problems. Anxiety or panic is a leading cause of chest pain mimicking a heart attack. Residual sore muscles are a consistent finding after the panic attack and can also occur in individuals with social phobias. People suffering from these attacks may be afraid or embarrassed to report their symptoms to the physician.

The alert therapist may recognize the need for a medical referral. A combination of antidepressants known as selective serotonin reuptake inhibitors (SSRIs) combined with CBT has been proven effective in controlling symptoms.

CLINICAL SIGNS AND SYMPTOMS

Panic Disorder

- Racing or pounding heartbeat
- Chest pains and/or palpitations
- Dizziness, light-headedness, nausea
- Headaches
- Difficulty in breathing
- Bilateral numbness or tingling in nose, cheeks, lips, fingers, toes
- Sweats or chills
- Hand wringing
- Dream-like sensations or perceptual distortions
- Sense of terror
- Extreme fear of losing control
- Fear of dying

Psychoneuroimmunology

When it comes to pain assessment, sources of pain, the mechanisms of pain, and the links between the mind and body, it is impossible to leave out a discussion on *psychoneuroimmunology* (PNI). PNI is the study of the interactions among behavior, neural, endocrine, enteric (digestive), and immune system function. It explains the influence of the nervous system on the immune and inflammatory responses and how the immune system communicates with the neuroendocrine systems. The immune system can activate sensory nerves and the CNS by releasing proinflammatory cytokines, creating an exaggerated pain response.[150,151]

Neuropeptides are chemical messengers that move through the bloodstream to every cell in the body. These information molecules take messages throughout the body to every cell and organ system. For example, the digestive (enteric) system and the neurologic system communicate with the immune system via these neuropeptides. These three systems can exchange information and influence one another's actions.

More than 30 different classes of neuropeptides have been identified. Every one of these messengers is found in the enteric nervous system of the gut. The constant presence of these neurotransmitters and neuromodulators in the bowel suggests that emotional expression of active coping generates a balance in the neuropeptide-receptor network and physiologic healing beginning in the GI system.

The identification of biologic carriers of emotions has also led to an understanding of a concept well known to physical therapists but previously unnamed: cellular memories.[152–154,156,157,186] Many health care professionals have seen the emotional and psychological response of a hands-on approach. These new discoveries help substantiate the idea that cells containing memories are shuttled through the body and brain via chemical messengers. The biologic basis of emotions and memories helps explain how soft tissues respond to emotions; indeed, the soft tissue structures may even contain emotions by way of neuropeptides.

Perhaps this can explain why two people can experience a car accident and whiplash (flexion-extension) or other injury differently. One recovers without any problems, whereas the other develops chronic pain that is resistant to any intervention. The focus of research on behavioral approaches combined with our hands-on intervention may bring a better understanding of what works and why.

Other researchers investigating neuropathic pain see a link between memory and pain. Studies looking at the physical similarities between how a memory is formed and how pain becomes persistent and chronic support such a link.[155,156]

Researchers suggest that when somatic pain persists beyond the expected time of healing the pain no longer originates in the tissue that was damaged. Pain begins in the CNS instead. The experience changes the nervous system. The memory of pain recurs again and again in the CNS.[155]

Other researchers have reported the discovery of a protein that allows nerve cells to communicate and thereby enhance perceptions of chronic pain. The results reinforce the notion that the basic process that leads to memory formation may be the same as the process that causes chronic pain.[157]

Along these same lines, other researchers have shown a communication network between the immune system and the brain. Pain phenomena are actually modulated by immune function. Proinflammatory cytokines (e.g., TNF, IL-1, IL-6) released by activated immune cells signal the brain by both blood-borne and neural routes, leading to alterations in neural activity.[158]

The cytokines in the brain interfere with cognitive function and memory; the cytokines within the spinal cord exaggerate fatigue and pain. By signaling the CNS, these proinflammatory cytokines create exaggerated pain, as well as an entire constellation of physiologic, hormonal, and behavioral changes referred to as the *sickness response*.[159,160]

In essence, immune processes work well when directed against pathogens or cancer cells. When directed against peripheral nerves, dorsal nerve ganglia, or the dorsal roots in the spinal cord, the immune system attacks the nerves, resulting in extreme pain.

Such exaggerated pain states occur with infection, inflammation, or trauma of the skin, peripheral nerves, and CNS. The neuroimmune link may help explain the exaggerated pain state associated with conditions such as chronic fatigue syndrome and fibromyalgia.

With this new understanding that all peripheral nerves and neurons are affected by immune and glial activation, intervention to modify pain will likely change in the near future.[150,161]

SCREENING FOR SYSTEMIC VERSUS PSYCHOGENIC SYMPTOMS

Screening for emotional or psychologic overlay has a place in our examination and evaluation process. Recognizing that this emotion-induced somatic pain response has a scientific basis may help us find better ways to alter or eliminate it.

The key to screening for a systemic versus psychogenic basis of symptoms is to identify the client with a significant emotional or psychologic component influencing the pain experience. Whether to refer the client for further psychologic evaluation and treatment or just modify the physical therapy plan of care is left up to the therapist's clinical judgment.

In all cases of pain, watch for the client who reports any of the following red-flag symptoms:

- Symptoms are out of proportion to the injury
- Symptoms persist beyond the expected time for physiologic healing
- No position is comfortable

These symptoms reflect both the possibility of an emotional or psychologic overlay, as well as the possibility of a more serious underlying systemic disorder (including cancer). In this next section, we will look at ways to screen for emotional content, keeping in mind what has already been said about anxiety, depression, and panic disorder.

Screening Tools for Emotional Overlay

Screening tools for emotional overlay can be used quickly and easily to help screen for emotional overlay in painful symptoms (Box 3.11). The client may or may not be aware that he or she is in fact exaggerating pain responses, catastrophizing the pain experience, or otherwise experiencing pain associated with emotional or psychologic overlay.

This discussion does not endorse physical therapists' practicing as psychologists, which is outside the scope of our expertise and experience. It merely recognizes that in treating the whole client not only the physical but also the psychologic, emotional, and spiritual needs of that person will be represented in his or her magnitude of symptoms, length of recovery time, response to pain, and responsibility for recovery.

Pain Catastrophizing Scale

Pain catastrophizing refers to a negative view of the pain experience or expecting the worst to happen. Catastrophizing boosts anxiety and worry. These emotions stimulate neural systems that produce increased sensitivity to pain so that pain is exaggerated or blown out of proportion. It can occur in a person who already has pain or in individuals who have not even had any pain yet—that person is just anticipating it might happen.

Pain catastrophizing is increasingly being recognized as an important factor in the experience of pain. There is evidence to suggest that pain catastrophizing is related to various levels of pain, physical disability, and psychological disability in individuals with chronic musculoskeletal pain.[162, 163] Without intervention, these pain-related fears can lead to chronic pain and disability over time.[164]

Identifying pain catastrophizing can help in the screening process to make appropriate referral for behavioral therapy and coordinate rehabilitative efforts. The Pain Catastrophizing Scale (PCS)[165] can be used to assist in the screening process. It is significantly predictive of perceived disability and more strongly predictive of function than pain intensity.[164] The PCS is a 13-item self-report scale with items in three different categories (rumination, magnification, and helplessness) that are rated on a scale of 0 to 4. The test has been validated and translated in several languages. The total PCS has reported excellent internal reliability and test-retest reliability.[166] There are also additional reported psychometric values, including normative data and cut-off scores for this test.[167]

McGill Pain Questionnaire

The McGill Pain Questionnaire (MPQ) from McGill University in Canada is a well-known and commonly used tool in assessing chronic pain (Fig. 3.14). The MPQ is designed to measure the subjective pain experience in a quantitative form. It is considered a good baseline for assessing pain and has both high reliability and validity in younger adults.

The MPQ consists primarily of two major classes of word descriptors, sensory and affective (emotional), and can be used to specify the subjective pain experience. It also contains an intensity scale and other items to determine the properties of pain experience.

A variation of the MPQ, the Short Form McGill Pain Questionnaire-2 (SF-MPQ-2),[168] is valid for use in cases of acute low back pain,[169] and in young and older adults with advanced cancer. The original form of the MPQ with all its affective word descriptors to help clients describe their pain gives results that help the therapist identify the source of the pain: vascular (visceral), neurogenic (somatic), musculoskeletal (somatic), or emotional (psychosomatic) (see Table 3.1).

When administering this portion of the questionnaire, the therapist reads the list of words in each box. The client is to choose the *one* word that best describes his or her pain. If no word in the box matches, the box is left blank. The words in each box are listed in order of ascending (rank order) intensity.

For example, in the first box, the words begin with "flickering" and "quivering" and gradually progress to "beating" and "pounding." Beating and pounding are considered much more intense than flickering and quivering. Word descriptors included in group 1 reflect characteristics of pain of a vascular disorder. Knowing this information can be very helpful as the therapist continues the examination and evaluation of the client.

Groups 2 through 8 are words used to describe pain of a neurogenic origin. Group 9 reflects the musculoskeletal system and groups 10 through 20 are all the words a client might use to describe pain in emotional terms (e.g., torturing, killing, vicious, agonizing).

After completing the questionnaire with the client, add up the total number of checks. According to the key, choosing up to eight words to describe the pain is within normal limits. Selecting more than 10 is a red flag for emotional or psychologic overlay, especially when the word selections come from groups 10 through 20.

Illness Behavior Syndrome and Symptom Magnification

Pain in the absence of an identified source of disease or pathologic condition may elicit a behavioral response from the client that is now labeled *illness behavior syndrome*. Illness behavior is what people say and do to show they are ill or perceive themselves as sick or in pain. It does not mean there is nothing wrong with the person. Illness behavior expresses and communicates the severity of pain and physical impairment.[112]

This syndrome has been identified most often in people with chronic pain. Its expression depends on what and how the client thinks about his or her symptoms/illness. Components of this syndrome include:

- Dramatization of complaints, leading to overtreatment and overmedication

---

> ### BOX 3.11   SCREENING TOOLS FOR EMOTIONAL OVERLAY
>
> - McGill Pain Questionnaire (MPQ)
> - Symptom magnification and illness behavior
> - Waddell's nonorganic signs

CLIENT'S NAME_____
DATE_____

DIRECTIONS: There are many words that describe pain. Some of these words are grouped below.
Check (✓) one word in each category that best describes your pain. Any category
that does not describe your pain should remain blank.

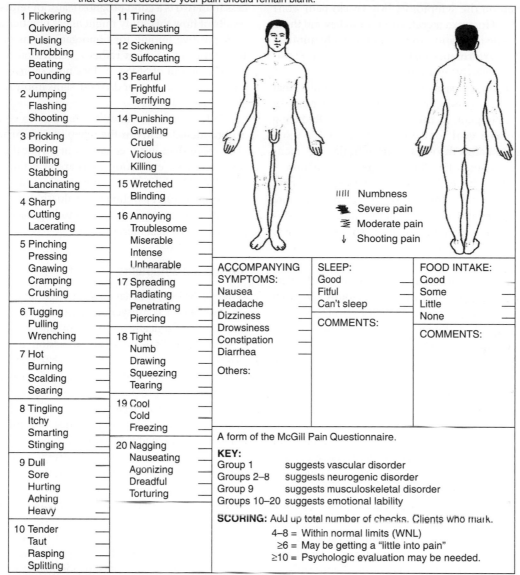

1 Flickering Quivering Pulsing Throbbing Beating Pounding	11 Tiring Exhausting
2 Jumping Flashing Shooting	12 Sickening Suffocating
	13 Fearful Frightful Terrifying
3 Pricking Boring Drilling Stabbing Lancinating	14 Punishing Grueling Cruel Vicious Killing
4 Sharp Cutting Lacerating	15 Wretched Blinding
5 Pinching Pressing Gnawing Cramping Crushing	16 Annoying Troublesome Miserable Intense Unbearable
6 Tugging Pulling Wrenching	17 Spreading Radiating Penetrating Piercing
7 Hot Burning Scalding Searing	18 Tight Numb Drawing Squeezing Tearing
8 Tingling Itchy Smarting Stinging	19 Cool Cold Freezing
9 Dull Sore Hurting Aching Heavy	20 Nagging Nauseating Agonizing Dreadful Torturing
10 Tender Taut Rasping Splitting	

ⅡⅢ Numbness
Severe pain
Moderate pain
↓ Shooting pain

ACCOMPANYING SYMPTOMS:
Nausea
Headache
Dizziness
Drowsiness
Constipation
Diarrhea

Others:

SLEEP:
Good
Fitful
Can't sleep

COMMENTS:

FOOD INTAKE:
Good
Some
Little
None

COMMENTS:

A form of the McGill Pain Questionnaire.

KEY:
Group 1   suggests vascular disorder
Groups 2–8   suggests neurogenic disorder
Group 9   suggests musculoskeletal disorder
Groups 10–20 suggests emotional lability

SCORING: Add up total number of checks. Clients who mark.

4–8 = Within normal limits (WNL)
≥6 = May be getting a "little into pain"
≥10 = Psychologic evaluation may be needed.

Fig. 3.14 McGill-Melzack pain questionnaire. The key and scoring information can be used to screen for emotional overlay or to identify a specific somatic or visceral source of pain. Instructions are provided in the text. (From Melzack R. The McGill pain questionnaire: major properties and scoring methods. Pain 1975;1:277–299.)

- Progressive dysfunction, leading to decreased physical activity and often compounding preexisting musculoskeletal or circulatory dysfunction
- Drug misuse
- Progressive dependency on others, including health care professionals, leading to overuse of the health care system
- Income disability, in which the person's illness behavior is perpetuated by financial gain[170]

Symptom magnification syndrome (SMS) is another term used to describe the phenomenon of illness behavior; conscious symptom magnification is referred to as *malingering*, whereas unconscious symptom magnification is labeled *illness behavior.* Conscious malingering may be described as exaggeration or faking symptoms for external gain. Some experts differentiate symptom amplification from malingering or factitious disorder (i.e., fakery or self-induced symptoms that enable the sick role).[171,172]

By definition, SMS is a self-destructive, socially reinforced behavioral response pattern consisting of reports or displays of symptoms that function to control the life of the sufferer.[173–175]

The amplified symptoms, rather than the physiologic phenomenon of the injury, determine the outcome/function.

The affected person acts as if the future cannot be controlled because of the presence of symptoms. All present limitations are blamed on the symptoms: "My (back) pain won't let me ...." The client may exaggerate limitations beyond those that seem reasonable in relation to the injury, apply minimal effort on maximal performance tasks, and overreact to physical loading during objective examination.

It is important for physical therapists to recognize that we often contribute to SMS by focusing on the relief of symptoms, especially pain, as the goal of therapy. Reducing pain is an acceptable goal for some clients, but for those who experience pain after the injuries have healed, the focus should be restoration, or at least improvement, of function.

In these situations, instead of asking whether the client's symptoms are "better, the same, or worse," it may be more appropriate to inquire about functional outcomes, for example, what can the client accomplish at home that he or she was unable to attempt at the beginning of treatment, last week, or even yesterday.

Conscious or unconscious? Can a physical therapist determine when a client is consciously or unconsciously symptom magnifying? Is it within the scope of the physical therapist's practice to use the label "malingerer" without a psychologist's or psychiatrist's diagnosis of such first?

The American Psychiatric Association and the American Medical Association agree confirmation of malingering is extremely difficult and depends on direct observation. It is safest to assume a person is not malingering unless direct evidence is available.[176,177]

Keep in mind the goal is to screen for a psychologic or emotional component to the client's clinical presentation. The key to achieving this goal is to use objective test measures whenever possible. In this way, the therapist obtains the guidance needed for referral versus modification of the physical therapy intervention.

Compiling a list of nonorganic or behavioral signs and identifying how the client is reacting to pain may be all that is needed. Signs of illness behavior may point the therapist in the direction of more careful "management" of the psychosocial and behavioral aspects of the client's illness.[110]

Waddell's Nonorganic Signs

Waddell et al.[178] identified five nonorganic signs and seven nonanatomic or behavioral descriptions of symptoms (Table 3.11) to help differentiate between physical and behavioral causes of back pain. Each of the nonorganic signs is determined by using one or two of the tests listed. These tests are used to assess a client's pain behavior and detect abnormal illness behavior.

A score of three or more positive signs places the client in the category of *nonmovement dysfunction*. This person is said to have a clinical pattern of nonmechanical, pain-focused behavior. This type of score is predictive of poor outcome and associated with delayed return-to-work or not working.

One or two positive signs is a low Waddell's score and does not classify the client with a nonmovement dysfunction. The value of these nonorganic signs as predictors for return-to-work for clients with low back pain has been investigated.[179] Less than two is a good prognosticator of return-to-work. The results of how this study might affect practice are available.[180]

A positive finding for nonorganic signs does not suggest an absence of pain but rather a behavioral response to pain (see discussion of SMS). It does not confirm malingering or illness behavior, neither do these signs imply the nonexistence of physical pathology.

Waddell and associates[111,178] have given us a tool that can help to identify early in the rehabilitation process those who need more than just mechanical or physical treatment intervention. Other evaluation tools are available (e.g., Oswestry Back Pain Disability Questionnaire, Roland-Morris Disability Questionnaire). A psychologic evaluation and possibly behavioral therapy or psychologic counseling may be needed as an adjunct to physical therapy.[181,182]

Conversion Symptoms

Whereas SMS is a behavioral, learned, inappropriate *behavior*, conversion is a psychodynamic phenomenon and quite rare in the chronically disabled population.

Conversion is a physical expression of an unconscious psychologic conflict such as an event (e.g., loss of a loved one) or a problem in the person's work or personal life. The conversion may provide a solution to the conflict or a way to express "forbidden" feelings. It may be a means of enacting the sick role to avoid responsibilities, or it may be a reflection of behaviors learned in childhood.[25]

Diagnosis of a conversion syndrome is difficult and often requires the diagnostic and evaluative input of the physical therapist. Presentation always includes a motor and/or sensory component that cannot be explained by a known medical or NMS condition.

The clinical presentation is often mistaken for an organic disorder such as multiple sclerosis, systemic lupus erythematosus, myasthenia gravis, or idiopathic dystonias. At presentation, when a client has an unusual limp or bizarre gait pattern that cannot be explained by functional anatomy, family members may be interviewed to assess changes in the client's gait and whether this alteration in movement pattern is present consistently.

The physical therapist can look for a change in the wear pattern of the client's shoes to decide if this alteration in gait has been long-standing. During manual muscle testing, true weakness results in smooth "giving way" of a muscle group; in hysterical weakness the muscle "breaks" in a series of jerks.

Often the results of muscle testing are not consistent with functional abilities observed. For example, the person cannot raise the arm overhead during testing but has no difficulty dressing, or the lower extremity appears flaccid during recumbency but the person can walk on their heels and toes when standing.

TABLE 3.11	Waddell's Nonorganic Signs and Behavioral Symptoms	
Test	**Signs**	**Nonanatomic or Behavioral Description of Symptoms**
Tenderness	*Superficial*—the client's skin is tender to light pinch over a wide area of lumbar skin; unable to localize to one structure. *Nonanatomic*—deep tenderness felt over a wide area, not localized to one structure; crosses multiple somatic boundaries.	1. Pain at the tip of the tailbone 2. Whole leg pain from the groin down to below the knee in a stocking pattern (not dermatomal or sclerotomal, intermittent) 3. Whole leg numbness or whole leg "going dead" (intermittent) 4. Whole leg giving way or collapsing (intermittent, client maintains upright position) 5. Constant pain for years on end without relief 6. Unable to tolerate any treatment, reaction or side effects to every intervention 7. Emergency admission to hospital for back pain without precipitating traumatic event
Simulation tests	*Axial loading*—light vertical loading over client's skull in the standing position reproduces lumbar (not cervical) spine pain. *Acetabular rotation*—lumbosacral pain from upper trunk rotation, back pain reported when the pelvis and shoulders are passively rotated in the same plane as the client stands, considered a positive test if pain is reported within the first 30 degrees.	
Distraction tests	*Straight-leg-raise* (SLR) discrepancy—marked improvement of SLR when client is distracted compared with formal testing; different response to SLR in supine (worse) compared with sitting (better) when both tests should have the same result in the presence of organic pathology. *Double leg raise*—when both legs are raised after straight leg raising, the organic response would be a greater degree of double leg raising; clients with a nonorganic component demonstrate less double leg raise compared with the single leg raise.	
Regional disturbances	*Weakness*—cogwheeling or giving way of many muscle groups that cannot be explained on a neurologic basis. *Sensory disturbance*—diminished sensation fitting a "stocking" rather than a dermatomal pattern.	
Overreaction	Disproportionate verbalization, facial expression, muscle tension, and tremor, collapsing, or sweating. Client may exhibit any of the following behaviors during the physical examination: guarding, bracing, rubbing, sighing, clenching teeth, or grimacing.	

(From Karas R, McIntosh G, Hall H, et al. The relationship between nonorganic signs and centralization of symptoms in the prediction of return to work for patients with low back pain. *Phys Ther.* 1997;77(4):354-360.)

The physical therapist should carefully evaluate and document all sensory and motor changes. Conversion symptoms are less likely to follow any dermatome, myotome, or sclerotome patterns.

CLINICAL SIGNS AND SYMPTOMS

Conversion
- Sudden, acute onset
- Lack of concern about the symptoms
- Unexplainable motor or sensory function impairment

Motor
- Impaired coordination or balance and/or bizarre gait pattern
- Paralysis or localized weakness
- Loss of voice, difficulty swallowing, or sensation of a lump in the throat
- Urinary retention

Sensory
- Altered touch or pain sensation (paresthesia or dysesthesia)
- Visual changes (double vision, blindness, black spots in visual field)
- Hearing loss (mild-to-profound deafness)
- Hallucinations
- Seizures or convulsions
- Absence of significant laboratory findings
- Electrodiagnostic testing within normal limits
- Deep tendon reflexes within normal limits

Screening Questions for Psychogenic Source of Symptoms

Besides observing for signs and symptoms of psychophysiologic disorders, the therapist can ask a few screening questions (Box 3.12). The client may be aware of the symptoms but does not know that these problems can be caused by depression, anxiety, or panic disorder.

Medical treatment for physiopsychologic disorders can and should be augmented with exercise. Physical activity and exercise has a known benefit in the management of mild-to-moderate psychologic disorders, especially depression and anxiety. Aerobic exercise or strength training have both been shown to be effective in moderating the symptoms of these conditions.[81, 182–185]

Patience is a vital tool for therapists when working with clients who are having difficulty adjusting to the stress of illness and disability or the client who has a psychologic disorder. The therapist must develop personal coping mechanisms when working with clients who have chronic illnesses or psychologic disturbances.

Recognizing clients whose symptoms are the direct result of organic dysfunction helps us in coping with clients who are hostile, ungrateful, noncompliant, negative, or adversarial. Whenever possible, involve a psychiatrist, psychologist, or counselor as a part of the management team. This approach will benefit the client and the health care staff.

PHYSICIAN REFERRAL

Guidelines for Immediate Physician Referral

- Immediate medical attention is required for anyone with risk factors for and clinical signs and symptoms of rhabdomyolysis (see Table 3.5).
- Clients reporting a disproportionate relief of bone pain with a simple aspirin may have bone cancer. This red flag requires immediate medical referral in the presence of a personal history of cancer of any kind.
- Joint pain with no known cause and a recent history of infection of any kind. Ask about recent (last 6 weeks) skin lesions or rashes of any kind anywhere on the body, urinary tract infection, or respiratory infection. Take the client's temperature and ask about recent episodes of fever, sweats, or other constitutional symptoms. Palpate for residual lymphadenopathy. Early diagnosis and treatment are essential to limit joint destruction and preserve function.[71]

Guidelines for Physician Referral Required

- Proximal muscle weakness accompanied by change in one or more deep tendon reflexes in the presence of a previous history of cancer.
- The physician should be notified of anyone with joint pain of unknown cause who presents with recent or current skin rash or recent history of infection (hepatitis, mononucleosis, urinary tract infection, upper respiratory infection, STI, streptococcus).
- A team approach to fibromyalgia requires medical evaluation and management as part of the intervention strategy. Therapists should refer clients suspected with fibromyalgia for further medical follow-up.
- Diffuse pain that characterizes some diseases of the nervous system and viscera may be difficult to distinguish from the equally diffuse pain so often caused by lesions of the moving parts. The distinction between visceral pain and pain caused by lesions of the vertebral column may be difficult to make and may require a medical diagnosis.
- The therapist may screen for signs and symptoms of anxiety, depression, and panic disorder. These conditions are often present with somatic symptoms that may resolve with effective intervention. The therapist can describe the symptoms and relay that information to the appropriate agency or individual when making a referral. Diagnosis is made by a medical doctor or trained mental health professional.
- Clients with new onset of back, neck, TMJ, shoulder, or arm pain brought on by a new exercise program or by exertion with the arms raised overhead should be screened for signs and symptoms of cardiovascular impairment. This is especially important if the symptoms are described as "throbbing" and start after a brief time of exercise (3 to 5 up to 10 minutes) and diminish or go away quickly with rest. Look for significant risk factors for cardiovascular involvement. Check vital signs. Refer for medical evaluation if indicated.
- Persistent pain on weight bearing or bone pain at night, especially in the older adult with risk factors such as osteoporosis, postural hypotension leading to falls, or previous history of cancer.

Clues to Screening for Viscerogenic Sources of Pain

We know systemic illness and pathologic conditions affecting the viscera can mimic NMS dysfunction. The therapist who knows pain patterns and types of viscerogenic pain can sort through the client's description of pain and recognize when something does not fit the expected pattern for NMS problems.

We must keep in mind that pain from a disease process or viscerogenic source is often a late symptom rather than a reliable danger signal. For this reason the therapist must remain alert to other signs and symptoms that may be present but unaccounted for.

In this chapter, possible pain types associated with viscerogenic conditions have been presented along with three mechanisms by which viscera refer pain to the body (soma). Characteristics of systemic pain compared with musculoskeletal pain are presented, including a closer look at joint pain.

Pain with the following features raises a red flag to alert the therapist of the need to take a closer look:
- Pain of unknown cause.
- Pain that persists beyond the expected time for physiologic healing.
- Pain that is out of proportion to the injury.
- Pain that is unrelieved by rest or change in position.
- Pain pattern does not fit the expected clinical presentation for a neuromuscular or musculoskeletal impairment.
- Pain that cannot be altered, aggravated, provoked, reduced, eliminated, or alleviated.
- There are some positions of comfort for various organs (e.g., leaning forward for the gallbladder or side bending for the kidney), but with progression of disease the client will obtain less and less relief of symptoms over time.

> ### BOX 3.12 SCREENING QUESTIONS FOR PSYCHOGENIC SOURCE OF SYMPTOMS
>
> - Do you have trouble sleeping at night?
> - Do you have trouble focusing during the day?
> - Do you worry about finances, work, or life in general?
> - Do you feel a sense of dread or worry without cause?
> - Do you ever feel happy?
> - Do you have a fear of being in groups of people? Fear of flying? Public speaking?
> - Do you have a racing heart, unexplained dizziness, or unexpected tingling in your face or fingers?
> - Do you wake up in the morning with your jaw clenched or feeling sore muscles and joints?
> - Are you irritable or jumpy most of the time?

(Data from Davidson J, Dreher H. The Anxiety Book: Developing Strength in the Face of Fear. New York: Penguin Putnam; 2003.)

- Pain, symptoms, or dysfunction are not improved or altered by physical therapy intervention.
- Pain that is poorly localized.
- Pain accompanied by signs and symptoms associated with a specific viscera (e.g., GI, GU, gynecologic [GYN], cardiac, pulmonary, endocrine).
- Pain that is constant and intense no matter the position tried and persists despite rest, eating, or abstaining from food; a previous history of cancer in this client is an even greater red flag necessitating further evaluation.
- Pain (especially intense bone pain) that is disproportionately relieved by aspirin.
- Listen to the client's choice of words to describe their pain. Systemic or viscerogenic pain can be described as deep, sharp, boring, knife-like, stabbing, throbbing, colicky, or intermittent (comes and goes in waves).
- Pain accompanied by full and normal ROM.
- Pain that is made worse 3 to 5 minutes after initiating an activity and relieved by rest (possible symptom of vascular impairment) versus pain that goes away with activity (symptom of musculoskeletal involvement); listen for the word descriptor "throbbing" to describe pain of a vascular nature.
- Pain is a relatively new phenomenon and not a pattern that has been present over several years' time.
- Constitutional symptoms in the presence of pain.
- Pain that is not consistent with emotional or psychologic overlay.
- When in doubt, conduct a screening examination for emotional overlay. Observe the client for signs and symptoms of anxiety, depression, and/or panic disorder. In the absence of systemic illness or disease and/or in the presence of suspicious psychologic symptoms, psychologic evaluation may be needed.
- Pain in the absence of any positive Waddell's signs (i.e., Waddell's test is negative or insignificant).

- Manual therapy to correct an upslip is not successful and the problem has returned by the end of the session or by the next day; consider a somatovisceral problem or visceral ligamentous problem.
- Back, neck, TMJ, shoulder, or arm pain brought on by exertion with the arms raised overhead may be suggestive of a cardiac problem. This is especially true in the postmenopausal woman or in a man over the age of 50 years with a significant family history of heart disease and/or in the presence of hypertension.
- Back, shoulder, pelvic, or sacral pain that is made better or worse by eating, passing gas, or having a bowel movement.
- Night pain (especially bone pain) that awakens the client from a sound sleep several hours after falling asleep; this is even more serious if the client is unable to get back to sleep after changing position, taking pain relievers, or eating or drinking something.
- Joint pain preceded or accompanied by skin lesions (e.g., rash or nodules), following antibiotics or statins, or recent infection of any kind (e.g., GI, pulmonary, GU); check for signs and symptoms associated with any of these systems based on recent client history.
- Clients can have more than one problem or pathology present at one time; it is possible for a client to have both a visceral AND a mechanical problem.[7]
- A careful general history and physical examination is still the most important screening tool; never assume this was done by the referring physician or other staff from the referring agency.[7]
- Visceral problems are unlikely to cause muscle weakness, reflex changes, or objective sensory deficits (exceptions include endocrine disease and paraneoplastic syndromes associated with cancer). If pain is referred from the viscera to the soma, challenging the somatic structure by stretching, contracting, or palpating will not reproduce the symptoms. For example, if a muscle is not sore when squeezed or contracted, the muscle is not the source of the pain.[7]

Key Points To Remember

1. Pain of a visceral origin can be referred to the corresponding somatic areas. The mechanisms of referred visceral pain patterns are not fully known. Information in this chapter is based on proposed models from what is known about the somatic sensory system.

2. Recognizing pain patterns that are characteristic of systemic disease is a necessary step in the screening process. Understanding how and when diseased organs can refer pain to the NMS system helps the therapist identify suspicious pain patterns.

3. At least three mechanisms contribute to referred pain patterns of the viscera (embryologic development, multisegmental innervation, and direct pressure and shared pathways). Being familiar with each one may help the therapist quickly identify pain patterns of a visceral source.

4. The therapist should keep in mind cultural variations in pain perception, intensity, and responses to pain found among various ethnic groups.

5. Pain patterns of the chest, back, shoulder, scapula, pelvis, hip, groin, and SI joint are the most common sites of referred pain from a systemic disease process.

6. Visceral diseases of the abdomen and pelvis are more likely to refer pain to the back, whereas intrathoracic disease refers pain to the shoulder(s). Visceral pain rarely occurs without associated signs and symptoms, although the client may not recognize the correlation. Careful questioning will usually elicit a systemic pattern of symptoms.

7. A comprehensive pain assessment includes a detailed health history, physical examination, medication history (including nonprescription drug use and complementary and alternative therapies), assessment of

functional status, and consideration of psychosocial-spiritual factors. Assessment tools vary from the very young to the very old.

8. Careful, sensitive, and thorough questioning regarding the multifaceted experience of pain can elicit essential information necessary when making a decision regarding treatment or referral. The use of pain assessment tools, such as those in Fig. 3.6 and Table 3.2, may facilitate clear and accurate descriptions of this critical symptom.

9. The client describes the characteristics of pain (location, frequency, intensity, duration, description). It is up to the therapist to recognize sources and types of pain and to know the pain patterns of a viscerogenic origin.

10. Choose alternative words to "pain" when discussing the client's symptoms in order to get a complete understanding of the clinical presentation.

11. Specific screening questions for joint pain are used to assess any joint pain of unknown cause, joint pain with an unusual presentation or history, or joint pain which does not fit the expected pattern for injury, overuse, or aging (see Box 3.5).

12. It is important to know how to differentiate psychogenic and psychosomatic origins of painful symptoms from systemic origins, including signs and symptoms of cancer.

13. Pain described as constant or present at night, awakening the client from sleep must be evaluated thoroughly. When assessing constant and/or night pain, the therapist must know how to differentiate the characteristics of acute versus chronic pain associated with a neuromusculoskeletal problem from a viscerogenic or systemic presentation.

CLIENT HISTORY AND INTERVIEW

SPECIAL QUESTIONS TO ASK

Pain Assessment

Location of Pain
Show me exactly where your pain is located.

Follow-up questions may include:
- Do you have any other pain or symptoms anywhere else?
- *If yes*, what causes the pain or symptoms to occur in this other area?

Description of Pain
What does it feel like?

After giving the client time to reply, offer some additional choices in potential descriptors. You may want to ask: Is your pain/Are your symptoms:

Knife-like	Dull
Boring	Burning
Throbbing	Prickly
Deep aching	Sharp

Follow-up questions may include:
- Has the pain changed in quality since it first began?
- Changed in intensity?
- Changed in duration (how long it lasts)?

Continued

CLIENT HISTORY AND INTERVIEW—*cont'd*

Frequency and Duration of Pain

How long do the symptoms last?

Clients who indicate that the pain is constant should be asked:

- Do you have this pain right now?
- Did you notice these symptoms this morning immediately when you woke up?

Pattern of Pain

Tell me about the pattern of your pain/symptoms.

- *Alternate question:* When does your back/shoulder (name the involved body part) hurt?
- *Alternate question:* Describe your pain/symptoms from first waking up in the morning to going to bed at night. (See special sleep-related questions that follow.) Follow-up questions may include:
- Have you ever experienced anything like this before?

If yes, do these episodes occur more or less often than at first?

- How does your pain/symptom(s) change with time?
- Are your symptoms worse in the morning or evening?

Aggravating and Easing Factors

- What brings your pain (symptoms) on?
- What kinds of things make your pain (symptoms) worse (e.g., eating, exercise, rest, specific positions, excitement, stress)?

To assess easing factors, ask:

- What makes the pain better?

Follow-up questions include:

- How does rest affect the pain/symptoms?
- Are your symptoms aggravated or relieved by any activities? If yes, what?
- How has this problem affected your daily life at work or at home?
- How has this problem affected your ability to care for yourself without assistance (e.g., dress, bathe, cook, drive)?

Associated Symptoms

- What other symptoms have you had that you can associate with this problem?

If the client denies any additional symptoms, follow up this question with a series of possibilities such as:

Burning	Heart palpitations	Numbness/tingling
Difficulty in breathing	Hoarseness	Problems with vision
Difficulty in swallowing	Nausea	Vomiting
Dizziness	Night sweats	Weakness

- Are you having any pain anywhere else in your body?

Alternately: Are you having symptoms of any other kind that may or may not be related to your main problem?

Anxiety/Depression

- Have you been under a lot of stress lately?
- Are you having some trouble coping with life in general and/or life's tensions?
- Do you feel exhausted or overwhelmed mentally or physically?
- Does your mind go blank or do you have trouble concentrating?
- Do you have trouble sleeping at night (e.g., difficulty getting to sleep, staying asleep, restless sleep, feel exhausted upon awakening)? Focusing during the day?
- Do you worry about finances, work, or life in general?
- Do you get any enjoyment in life?
- Do you feel keyed up or restless? Irritable and jumpy? On edge most of the time?
- Do you have a general sense of dread or unknown fears?
- Do you have any of these symptoms: a racing heart, dizziness, tingling, muscle or joint pains?

Joint Pain (See Box 3.5)
Night Pain (See Box 3.7)
Psychogenic Source of Symptoms (See Box 3.12)

CASE STUDY

REFERRAL

A 44-year-old male was referred for physical therapy with a report of right-sided thoracic pain.*

Past Medical History: The client reported a 20-pack year smoking history (one pack per day for 20 years) and denied the use of alcohol or drugs. There was no other significant past medical history reported. He had a sedentary job. The client's symptoms began following chiropractic intervention to relieve left-sided lower extremity radiating pain. Within 6 to 8 hours

after the chiropractor manipulated the client's thoracic spine, he reported sharp shooting pain on the right side of the upper thoracic spine at T4. The pain radiated laterally under the right axilla into the anterior chest. He also reported tension and tightness along the same thoracic level and moderate discomfort during inspiration. There was no history of thoracic pain before the upper thoracic manipulation by the chiropractor.

The client saw his primary care physician who referred him to physical therapy for treatment. No imaging studies were done before physical therapy referral. The client rated the

CASE STUDY—*cont'd*

pain as a constant 10/10 on the NRS during sitting activities at work. He also reported pain waking him at night.

The client was unable to complete a full day at work without onset of thoracic discomfort; pain was aggravated by prolonged sitting.

Evaluation

The client was described as slender in build with forward head and shoulders and kyphotic posture as observed in the upright and sitting positions. There were no significant signs of inflammation or superficial tissue changes observed or palpated in the thoracic spine region. There was palpable tenderness at approximately the T4 costotransverse joint and along the corresponding rib.

A full NMS evaluation was conducted to determine the biomechanical and soft tissue dysfunction that produced the client's signs and symptoms. Active and passive motion and intersegmental mobility were tested. Findings were consistent with a physical therapy diagnosis of hypomobile costotransverse joint at level T4.

This was further evidenced by pain at the posterior costovertebral joint with radiating pain laterally into the chest wall. Pain was increased on inspiration. Patient had a smoker's cough, but reported no other associated signs or symptoms of any kind. See the Pain Assessment Record Form on the companion website.

Result

The client obtained gradual relief from painful symptoms after eight treatment sessions of stretches and costotransverse joint

mobilization (grade 4, nonthrust progressive oscillations at the end of the available range). Pain was reduced from 10/10 to 3/10 and instances of night pain had decreased. The client could sit at work with only mild discomfort, which he could correct with stretching.

The client's thoracic pain returned on the tenth and eleventh treatment sessions. He attributed this to increased stressors at work and long work hours. Night pain and pain with respiratory movements (inhalation) increased again.

Red flags in this case included:
- Age over 40 years
- History of smoking (20-pack-years)
- Symptoms persisting beyond the expected time for physiologic healing
- Pain out of proportion to the injury
- Recurring symptoms (failure to respond to physical therapy intervention)
- Pain is constant and intense; night pain

The client was returned to his primary care physician for further diagnostic studies and later diagnosed with metastatic lung cancer.

Summary

Working with clients several times a week allows the therapist to monitor their symptoms and the effectiveness of intervention. This case study shows the importance of reassessment and awareness of red flags that would lead a practitioner to suspect that the symptoms may be pathologic.

Leanne Lenker, DPT. This case was part of an internship experience at St. Luke's Outpatient Clinic, Allentown, PA, under the supervision of Jeff Bays, MSPT (Clinical Instructor). Dr. Lenker is a graduate of the University of St. Augustine for Health Sciences program in St. Augustine, Florida. Used with permission, 2005.

PRACTICE QUESTIONS

1. What is the best follow-up question for someone who reports constant pain?
   a. Can you use one finger to point to the pain location?
   b. Do you have that pain right now?
   c. Does the pain wake you up at night after you have fallen asleep?
   d. Is there anything that makes the pain better or worse?

2. A 52-year-old woman with shoulder pain tells you that she has pain at night that awakens her. After asking a series of follow-up questions, you are able to determine that she had trouble falling asleep because her pain increases when she goes to bed. Once she falls asleep, she wakes up as soon as she rolls onto that side. What is the most likely explanation for this pain behavior?
   a. Minimal distractions heighten a person's awareness of musculoskeletal discomfort.
   b. This is a systemic pattern that is associated with a neoplasm.

   c. It is impossible to tell.
   d. This represents a chronic clinical presentation of a musculoskeletal problem.

3. Referred pain patterns associated with impairment of the spleen can produce musculoskeletal symptoms in the:
   a. Left shoulder
   b. Right shoulder
   c. Midback or upper back, scapular, and right shoulder areas
   d. Thorax, scapulae, right shoulder, or left shoulder

4. Associated signs and symptoms are a major red flag for pain of a systemic or visceral origin compared with musculoskeletal pain.
   a. True
   b. False

5. Words used to describe neurogenic pain often include:
   a. Throbbing, pounding, beating
   b. Crushing, shooting, pricking

Continued

PRACTICE QUESTIONS—cont'd

c. Aching, heavy, sore

d. Agonizing, piercing, unbearable

6. Pain (especially intense bone pain) that is disproportionately relieved by aspirin can be a symptom of:
    a. Neoplasm
    b. Assault or trauma
    c. Drug dependence
    d. Fracture

7. Joint pain can be a reactive, delayed, or an allergic response to:
    a. Medications
    b. Chemicals
    c. Infections
    d. Artificial sweeteners
    e. All of the above

8. Pain of a viscerogenic nature is not relieved by a change in position.
    a. True
    b. False

9. Referred pain from the viscera can occur alone but is usually preceded by visceral pain when an organ is involved.
    a. True
    b. False

10. A 48-year-old man presented with low back pain of unknown cause. He works as a carpenter and says he is very active, has work-related mishaps (accidents and falls), and engages in repetitive motions of all kinds using his arms, back, and legs. The pain is intense when he has it, but it seems to come and go. He is not sure if eating makes the pain better or worse. He has lost his appetite because of the pain. After conducting an examination including a screening examination, the clinical presentation does not match the expected pattern for a musculoskeletal or neuromuscular problem. You refer him to a physician for medical testing. You find out later he had pancreatitis. What is the most likely explanation for this pain pattern?
    a. Toxic waste products from the pancreas are released into the intestines causing irritation of the retroperitoneal space.
    b. Rupture of the pancreas causes internal bleeding and referred pain called Kehr's sign.
    c. The pancreas and low back structures are formed from the same embryologic tissue in the mesoderm.
    d. Obstruction, irritation, or inflammation of the body of the pancreas distends the pancreas, thus applying pressure on the central respiratory diaphragm.

REFERENCES

1. American Physical Therapy Association. Safe Pain Management Advocacy. Available at: https://www.apta.org/advocacy/issues/opioid-epidemic-safe-pain-management. Accessed June 16, 2021.
2. Scher C, Meador L, Van Cleave JH, et al. Moving beyond pain as the fifth vital sign and patient satisfaction scores to improve pain care in the 21st century. *Pain Manag Nurs.* 2018;19(2):125–129. https://doi.org/10.1016/j.pmn.2017.10.010.
3. Flaherty JH. Who's taking your fifth vital sign? *J Gerontol A Biol Sci Med Sci.* 2001;56:M397–M399.
4. Sengupta JN. Visceral pain: the neurophysiological mechanism. *Handb Exp Pharmacol.* 2009(194):31–74. https://doi.org/10.1007/978-3-540-79090-7_2.
5. Sikandar S, Dickenson AH. Visceral pain: the ins and outs, the ups and downs. *Curr Opin Support Palliat Care.* 2012;6(1):17–26. https://doi.org/10.1097/SPC.0b013e32834f6ec9.
6. Brumovsky PR, Gebhart GF. Visceral organ cross-sensitization—an integrated perspective. *Auton Neurosci.* 2010;153(1-2):106–115.
7. Rex L. *Evaluation and treatment of somatovisceral dysfunction of the gastrointestinal system.* Edmonds, WA: URSA Foundation; 2004.
8. Christianson JA. Development, plasticity, and modulation of visceral afferents. *Brain Res Rev.* 2009;60(1):171–178.
9. Chaban W. Peripheral sensitization of sensory neurons. *Ethn Dis.* 2010;20(1 Suppl 1):S1–S6.
10. Squire LR, ed. *Fundamental neuroscience.* ed 3 Burlington, MA: Academic Press; 2008.
11. Saladin KS. *Personal communication, Distinguished Professor of Biology.* Milledgeville, GA: Georgia College and State University; 2004.
12. de Winter BY, Deiteren A, De Man JG. Novel nervous system mechanisms in visceral pain. *Neurogastroenterol Motil.* 2016;28:309–315.
13. Woolf CJ, Decosterd I. Implications of recent advances in the understanding of pain pathophysiology for the assessment of pain in patients. *Pain Suppl.* 1999;6:S141–S147.
14. Strigio I, Duncan GH, Boivin M, et al. Differentiation of visceral and cutaneous pain in the human brain. *J Neurophysiol.* 2003;89:3294–3303.
15. Aziz Q. Functional neuroimaging of visceral sensation. *J Clin Neurophysiol.* 2000;17(6):604–612.
16. Tsalkidis A, Gardikis S, Cassimos D, et al. Acute abdomen in children due to extra-abdominal causes. *Pediatr Int.* 2008;50:315–318.
17. Koochak HE, Tabibian E, Dehgolan SR. Abdominal pain as extrapulmonary presentation of pneumonia in an adult: a case report. *Acta Medica Iranica.* 2017;55(2). https://acta.tums.ac.ir/index.php/acta/article/view/6234.
18. Ojha N, Dhamoon AS. *Myocardial infarction. [Updated 2020 Nov 21].* In: *StatPearls [Internet].* Treasure Island (FL): StatPearls Publishing; 2021 Jan-. Available from: https://www.ncbi.nlm.nih.gov/books/NBK537076/.
19. Giamberardino M. Viscero-visceral hyperalgesia: characterization in different clinical models. *Pain.* 2010;151(2):307–322.
20. Vergnolle N. Visceral afferents: What role in post-inflammatory pain? *Auton Neurosci.* 2010;153(1–2):79–83. https://doi.org/10.1016/j.autneu.2009.07.015. ISSN 1566-0702. https://www.sciencedirect.com/science/article/pii/S1566070209004202.
21. Leavitt RL. Developing cultural competence in a multicultural world. Part II. *PT Magazine.* 2003;11(1):56–70.
22. O'Rourke D. The measurement of pain in infants, children, and adolescents: from policy to practice. *Phys Ther.* 2004;84(6):560–570.
23. Wentz JD. Assessing pain at the end of life. *Nursing.* 2003;33(8):22.
24. Wilson D, Williams M, Butler D. Language and the pain experience. *Physiother Res Int.* Mar 2009;14(1):56–65.
25. Melzack R. The McGill pain questionnaire: major properties and scoring methods. *Pain.* 1975;1:277.

26. Ali A, Arif AW, Bhan C, et al. Managing chronic pain in the elderly: an overview of the recent therapeutic advancements. *Cureus.* 2018;10(9):e3293. https://doi.org/10.7759/cureus.3293. Published 2018 Sep 13.

27. Buowari DY. Pain management in older persons, Submitted: July 9th 2020 Reviewed: September 8th 2020 Published: April 14th 2021 Update in Geriatrics. DOI: 10.5772/intechopen.93940.

28. Centers for Disease Control and Prevention. Joint Pain and Arthritis. Available online at: https://www.cdc.gov/arthritis/pain/index.htm. Accessed July 15, 2021.

29. Argoff CE, Ferrell B. Pharmacologic therapy for persistent pain in older adults: the updated American Geriatrics Society guidelines and their clinical implications. *Pain Medicine News.* 2010;8(5):1–8.

30. Boring BL, Walsh KT, Nanavaty N, et al. How and why patient concerns influence pain reporting: a qualitative analysis of personal accounts and perceptions of others' use of numerical pain scales. *Front Psychol.* 2021;12:663890. https://www.frontiersin.org/article/10.3389/fpsyg.2021.663890. DOI =10.3389/fpsyg.2021.663890 ISSN=1664-1078.

31. Herr KA, Spratt K, Mobily PR, et al. Pain intensity assessment in older adults: use of experimental pain to compare psychometric properties and usability of selected pain scales with younger adults. *Clin J Pain.* 2004;20(4):207–219.

32. Ware LJ, Herr KA, Booker SS, et al. Psychometric evaluation of the revised iowa pain thermometer (IPT-R) in a sample of diverse cognitively intact and impaired older adults: a pilot study. *Pain Manag Nurs.* 2015;16(4):475–482. https://doi.org/10.1016/j.pmn.2014.09.004. ISSN 1524-9042. https://www.sciencedirect.com/science/article/pii/S1524904214001519.

33. Feldt K. The checklist of nonverbal pain indicators (CNPI). *Pain Manag Nurs.* 2000;1(1):13–21.

34. Ferrell BA. Pain in cognitively impaired nursing home patients. *J Pain Symptom Manage.* 1995;10(8):591–598.

35. Hicks CL, von Baeyer CL, Spafford PA, et al. The faces pain scale-revised: toward a common metric in pediatric pain measurement. *Pain.* 2001;93:173–183.

36. Bieri D. The faces pain scale for the self-assessment of the severity of pain experienced by children: development, initial validation, and preliminary investigation for the ratio scale properties. *Pain.* 1990;41(2):139–150.

37. Wong on Web: *FACES Pain Rating Scale,* Elsevier Health Science Information, 2004.

38. Baker-Lefkowicz A., Keller V., Wong D.L., et al.: *Young children's pain rating using the FACES Pain Rating Scale with original vs abbreviated word instructions,* 1996. unpublished.

39. von Baeyer CL, Hicks CL. Support for a common metric for pediatric pain intensity scales. *Pain Res Manage.* 2000;4(2):157–160.

40. Huskinson EC. Measurement of pain. *Lancet.* 1974;2:1127–1131.

41. Carlsson AM. Assessment of chronic pain: aspects of the reliability and validity of the visual analog scale. *Pain.* 1983;16:87–101.

42. Sahrmann S.: Diagnosis and diagnosticians: the future in physical therapy, Dallas, February 13–16, 1997, Combined Sections Meeting. Available online at www.apta.org.

43. Courtney CA. Interpreting joint pain: quantitative sensory testing in musculoskeletal management. *J Orthop Sports Phys Ther.* 2010;40(12):818–825.

44. Wells PE, Frampton V, Bowsher D. *Pain management in physical therapy.* ed 2 Oxford: Butterworth-Heinemann; 1994.

45. McMahon S, Koltzenburg M, eds. *Wall and Melzack's textbook of pain.* ed 5 New York: Churchill Livingstone; 2005.

46. Tasker RR. Spinal cord injury and central pain. In: Aronoff GM, ed. *Evaluation and treatment of chronic pain.* ed 3 Philadelphia: Lippincott, Williams & Wilkins; 1999:131–146.

47. Prkachin KM. Pain behavior and the development of pain-related disability: the importance of guarding. *Clin J Pain.* 2007;23(3):270–277.

48. Chimenti RL, Frey-Law LA, Sluka KA. A mechanism-based approach to physical therapist management of pain. *Phys Ther.* 2018;98(5):302–314.

49. Smart KM, Blake C, Staines A, Doody C. The discriminative validity of "nociceptive," "peripheral neuropathic," and "central sensitization" as mechanisms-based classifications of musculoskeletal pain. *Clin J Pain.* 2011;27(8):655–663.

50. Milchert M, Brzosko M. Diagnosis of polymyalgia rheumatica usually means a favourable outcome for your patient. *Indian J Med Res.* 2017;145(5):593–600. https://doi.org/10.4103/ijmr.IJMR_298_17.

51. Kraus H. Muscle deficiency. In: Rachlin ES, ed. *Myofascial pain and fibromyalgia.* ed 2 St. Louis: Mosby; 2002.

52. Queme LF, Ross JL, Jankowski MP. Peripheral mechanisms of ischemic myalgia. *Front Cell Neurosci.* 2017;11:419 https://doi.org/10.3389/fncel.2017.00419. Published 2017 Dec 22.

53. Cailliet R, ed. *Low back pain syndrome.* ed 5 Philadelphia: FA Davis; 1995.

54. Linehan E, Fitzgerald DC. Ageing and the immune system: focus on macrophages. *Eur J Microbiol Immunol (Bp).* 2015;5(1):14–24. https://doi.org/10.1556/EUJMI-D-14-00035.

55. Lozano PF, Scholze M, Babian C, et al. Water-content related alterations in macro and micro scale tendon biomechanics. *Sci Rep.* 2019;9(1):7887. https://doi.org/10.1038/s41598-019-44306-z. Published 2019 May 27.

56. Kisilewicz A, Janusiak M, Szafraniec R, et al. Changes in muscle stiffness of the trapezius muscle after application of ischemic compression into myofascial trigger points in professional basketball players. *J Hum Kinet.* 2018;64:35–45. https://doi.org/10.2478/hukin-2018-0043. Published 2018 Oct 15.

57. Donnelly JM, Fernández-de-las-Peñas C, Finnegan M, Freeman JL, eds. *Travell, Simons & Simons' Myofascial Pain and Dysfunction: The Trigger Point Manual.* 3rd ed. Philadelphia: Wolters Kluwer; 2019.

58. Simons D, Travell J, In: *Myofascial pain and dysfunction: the trigger point manual,* 2nd ed., vol. 1 and 2 Baltimore: Williams and Wilkins; 1999.

59. Simons D, Travell J. In: *Myofascial pain and dysfunction: the trigger point manual,* 2nd ed., vol. 1 and 2 Baltimore: Williams and Wilkins; 1999.

60. Kostopoulos D, Rizopoulos K. *The manual of trigger point and myofascial therapy.* Thorofare, NJ: Slack; 2001.

61. Rachlin ES, Rachlin IS, eds. *Myofascial pain and fibromyalgia: trigger point management.* 2nd ed. St. Louis: Mosby; 2002.

62. Ayouni I, Chebbi R, Hela Z, et al. Comorbidity between fibromyalgia and temporomandibular disorders: a systematic review. *Oral Surg Oral Med Oral Pathol Oral Radiol.* 2019;128(1):33–42. https://doi.org/10.1016/j.oooo.2019.02.023. ISSN 2212-4403. https://www.sciencedirect.com/science/article/pii/S2212440319301567.

63. Raj BKA, Singh KA, Shah H. Orthopedic manifestation as the presenting symptom of acute lymphoblastic leukemia. *J Orthop.* 2020;22:326–330. https://doi.org/10.1016/j.jor.2020.05.022. ISSN 0972-978X. https://www.sciencedirect.com/science/article/pii/S0972978X20302075.

64. Carlin E, Flew S. Sexually acquired reactive arthritis. *Clin Med (Lond).* 2016;16(2):193–196. https://doi.org/10.7861/clinmedicine.16-2-193.

65. Annese V. A Review of extraintestinal manifestations and complications of inflammatory bowel disease. *Saudi J Med Med Sci.* 2019;7(2):66–73. https://doi.org/10.4103/sjmms.sjmms_81_18.

66. Kawai K, Kawai AT, Wollan P, et al. Adverse impacts of chronic pain on health-related quality of life, work productivity, depression and anxiety in a community-based study. *Fam Pract.* December 2017;34(6):656–661. https://doi.org/10.1093/fampra/cmx034.

67. Bone and joint pain- Part 1. Leukaemia Care. Available online at: https://www.leukaemiacare.org.uk/support-and-information/latest-from-leukaemia-care/blog/bone-and-joint-pain-part-1/. Accessed July 16, 2021.

68. Feagan BG, Sandborn WJ, Colombel JF, et al. Incidence of arthritis/arthralgia in inflammatory bowel disease with long-term vedolizumab treatment: post hoc analyses of the GEMINI trials. *J Crohns Colitis*. 2019;13(1):50–57. https://doi.org/10.1093/ecco-jcc/jjy125.

69. Soor P, Sharma N, Rao C. Multifocal septic arthritis secondary to infective endocarditis: a rare case report. *J Orthop Case Rep*. 2017;7(1):65–68. https://doi.org/10.13107/jocr.2250-0685.692.

70. Widyadharma IPE, Dewi PR, Wijayanti IAS, et al. Pain related viral infections: a literature review. *Egypt J Neurol Psychiatr Neurosurg*. 2020;56(1):105. https://doi.org/10.1186/s41983-020-00238-4.

71. Issa NC, Thompson RL. Diagnosing and managing septic arthritis: a practical approach. *J Musculoskel Med*. 2003;20(2):70–75.

72. Infectious Arthritis. Arthritis Foundation. Available online at: https://www.arthritis.org/diseases/infectious-arthritis. Accessed July 16, 2021.

73. Bogduk N. On the definitions and physiology of back pain, referred pain, and radicular pain. *Pain*. 2009;147(1-3):17–19.

74. Waddell G, Bircher M, Finlayson D, et al. Symptoms and signs: physical disease or illness behaviour? *BMJ*. 1984;289:739–741.

75. Prior KN, Bond MJ. Patterns of 'Abnormal' illness behavior among healthy individuals. *Am J Health Behav*. 2017;41(2):139–146.

76. Stephens E. What are the peripheral signs of peripheral vascular disease (PVD)? Medscape. Available online at: https://www.medscape.com/answers/761556-89700/what-are-the-peripheral-signs-of-peripheral-vascular-disease-pvd. Accessed July 16, 2021.

77. Saling J. Medically Reviewed by Tyler Wheeler, MD on January 26, 2020. Nighttime back pain. WebMD. Available online at: https://www.webmd.com/back-pain/guide/nightime-back-pain. Accessed July 16, 2021.

78. Chronic Pain has arrived in the ICD-11. International Association for the Study of Pain. Available online at: https://www.iasp-pain.org/PublicationsNews/NewsDetail.aspx?ItemNumber=8340. Accessed July 18, 2021.

79. Hootman JM, Helmick CG, Brady TJ. A public health approach to addressing arthritis in older adults: the most common cause of disability. *Am J Public Health*. 2012;102(3):426–433.

80. Diener I, Kargela M, Louw A. Listening is therapy: patient interviewing from a pain science perspective. *Physiother Theory Pract*. 2016 Jul;32(5):356–367. https://doi.org/10.1080/09593985.2016.1194648. Epub 2016 Jun 28. PMID: 27351690.

81. Johnson H. Psychosocial Elements of Physical Therapy. SLACK, 2019.

82. Ballantyne JC, Sullivan MD. Intensity of chronic pain--The wrong metric? *N Engl J Med*. Nov 26 2015;373(22):2098–2099.

83. Pain neuroscience education. Physiopedia. Available online at: https://www.physio-pedia.com/Pain_Neuroscience_Education_(PNE). Accessed July 19, 2021.

84. Nijs J, Wijma AJ, Willaert W, et al. Integrating motivational interviewing in pain neuroscience education for people with chronic pain: a practical guide for clinicians. *Phys Ther*. 2020;100(5):846–859.

85. Pack MPT, OCS R, Gilliland PhD R, Mecham DPT A. The treatment of central sensitization in an adolescent using pain neuroscience education and graded exposure to activity: a case report. *Physiother Theory Pract*. 2020 Oct;36(10):1164–1174. https://doi.org/10.1080/09593985.2018.1551454. Epub 2018 Dec 12. PMID: 30540222.

86. Louw A, Diener I, Butler DS, et al. The effect of neuroscience education on pain, disability, anxiety, and stress in chronic musculoskeletal pain. *Arch Phys Med Rehabil*. Dec 2011;92(12):2041–2056.

87. Louw A, Zimney K, Puentedura EJ, et al. The efficacy of pain neuroscience education on musculoskeletal pain: a systematic review of the literature. *Physiother Theory Pract*. Jul 2016;32(5):332–355.

88. Turk DC, Melzack R, eds. *Handbook of pain assessment*. ed 3 New York: Guilford; 2010.

89. Simmonds MJ. Pain, mind, and movement—an expanded, updated, and integrated conceptualization. *Clin J Pain*. 2008;24(4):279–280.

90. Melzack R. From the gate to the neuromatrix. *Pain*. 1999;6(Suppl 6):S121–S126.

91. Melzack R. Evolution of the neuromatrix theory of pain. The Prithvi Raj lecture: presented at the third World Congress of World Institute of Pain, Barcelona 2004. *Pain Pract*. 2005;5(2):85–94.

92. Smith BH. Epidemiology of chronic pain, from the laboratory to the bus stop: time to add understanding of biological mechanisms to the study of risk factors in population-based research? *Pain*. 2007;127:5–10.

93. Turk DC. Understanding pain sufferers: the role of cognitive processes. *Spine J*. 2004;4(1):1–7.

94. Berna C. Induction of depressed mood disrupts emotion regulation neurocircuitry and enhances pain unpleasantness. *Biol Psychiatry*. 2010;67(11):1038–1090.

95. Celestin J. Pretreatment psychosocial variables as predictors of outcomes following lumbar surgery and spinal cord stimulation: a systematic review and literature synthesis. *Pain Med*. 2009;10(4):639–653.

96. Richebé P, Capdevila X, Rivat C. Persistent postsurgical pain: pathophysiology and preventative pharmacologic considerations. *Anesthesiology*. 2018;129:590–607. https://doi.org/10.1097/ALN.0000000000002238.

97. Vowles KE, McEntee ML, Julnes PS, et al. Rates of opioid misuse, abuse, and addiction in chronic pain: a systematic review and data synthesis. *Pain*. April 2015;156(4):569–576. https://doi.org/10.1097/01.j.pain.0000460357.01998.f1.

98. Wide-ranging online data for epidemiologic research (WONDER). Atlanta, GA: CDC, National Center for Health Statistics; 2020. Available online at: http://wonder.cdc.gov. Accessed July 19, 2021.

99. Stempniak M. The opioid epidemic. *Hosp Health Netw*. 2016;90(3):22–24.

100. Manchikanti L, Kaye AM, Kaye AD. Current state of opioid therapy and abuse. *Curr Pain Headache Rep*. 2016;20(5):34.

101. Improving Pain Treatment Through Education. Pain EDU. Available online at: https://www.painedu.org/. Accessed July 19, 2021.

102. Waddell G, Somerville D, Henderson I, et al. A fear avoidance beliefs questionnaire (FABQ) and the role of fear avoidance beliefs in chronic low back pain and disability. *Pain*. 1993;52:157–168.

103. George SZ. A psychometric investigation of fear-avoidance model measures in patients with chronic low back pain. *J Orthop Sports Phys Ther*. 2010;40(4):197–205.

104. Swinkels-Meewisse EJ. Psychometric properties of the Tampa scale for kinesiophobia and the fear-avoidance beliefs questionnaire in acute low back pain. *Man Ther*. 2003;8:29–36.

105. Keefe FJ. An objective approach to quantifying pain behavior and gait patterns in low back pain patients. *Pain*. 1985;21:153–161.

106. Calley D. Identifying patient fear-avoidance beliefs by physical therapists managing patients with low back pain. *J Orthop Sports Phys Ther*. 2010;40(12):774–783.

107. Fritz JM, George SZ. Identifying psychosocial variables in patients with acute work-related low back pain: the importance of fear-avoidance beliefs. *Phys Ther*. 2002;82(10):973–983.

108. Leeuw M. The fear-avoidance model of musculoskeletal pain: current state of scientific evidence. *J Behav Med*. 2000;30:77–94.

109. George SZ, Bialosky JE, Fritz JM. Physical therapist management of a patient with acute low back pain and elevated fear-avoidance beliefs. *Phys Ther.* 2004;84(6):538–549.

110. Connelly C. Managing low back pain and psychosocial overlie. *J Musculoskel Med.* 2004;21(8):409–419.

111. Main CJ, Waddell G. Behavioral responses to examination: a reappraisal of the interpretation of "nonorganic signs". *Spine.* 1998;23(21):2367–2371.

112. Waddell G, ed. *The back pain revolution.* ed 2 Philadelphia: Churchill Livingstone; 2004.

113. Lethem J, Slade PD, Troup JDG, et al. Outline of a fear-avoidance model of exaggerated pain perception. *I. Behav Res Ther.* 1983;21(4):401–408.

114. American Psychiatric Association *Diagnostic and Statistical Manual of Mental Disorders (DSM-5).* Arlington, VA: APA; 2013.

115. Scalzitti DA. Screening for psychological factors in patients with low back problems: Waddell's nonorganic signs. *Phys Ther.* 1997;77(3):306–312.

116. Teasell RW, Shapiro AP. Strategic-behavioral intervention in the treatment of chronic nonorganic motor disorders. *Am J Phys Med Rehab.* 1994;73(1):44–50.

117. Waddell G. Symptoms and signs: physical disease or illness behavior? *BMJ.* 1984;289:739–741.

118. Brunner E, Dankaerts W, Meichtry A, et al. Physical therapists' ability to identify psychological factors and their self-reported competence to manage chronic low back pain. *Physical Therapy.* June 2018;98(6):471–479. https://doi.org/10.1093/ptj/pzy012.

119. Barsky AJ, Goodson JD, Lane RS, et al. The amplification of somatic symptoms. *Psychosom Med.* 1988;50(5):510–519.

120. Turk DC. Understanding pain sufferers: the role of cognitive processes. *Spine J.* 2004;4:1–7.

121. Beck AT, Epstein N, Brown G, et al. An inventory for measuring clinical anxiety: psychometric properties. *J Consult Clin Psych.* 1988;56:893–897.

122. Steer RA, Beck AT. Beck Anxiety Inventory. In: Zalaquett CP, Wood RJ, eds. *Evaluating Stress: A Book of Resources.* Lanham, Maryland: Scarecrow Press; 1997.

123. Osman A, Hoffman J, Barrios FX, et al. Factor structure, reliability and validity of the Beck anxiety inventory in adolescent psychiatric inpatients. *J Clin Psychol.* 2002;58(4):443–456.

124. Kwan A, Marzouk S, Ghanean H, et al. Assessment of the psychometric properties of patient-reported outcomes of depression and anxiety in systemic lupus erythematosus. *Semin Arthritis Rheum.* 2019;49(2):260–266. https://doi.org/10.1016/j.semarthrit.2019.03.004. ISSN 0049-0172. https://www.sciencedirect.com/science/article/pii/S004901721830773X.

125. Brenes GA. Anxiety and chronic obstructive pulmonary disease: prevalence, impact, and treatment. *Psychosom Med.* 2003;65(6):963–970.

126. Gonzalez O. Current depression among adults in the United States. *MMWR.* 2010;59(38):1229–1235.

127. Strine TW. Depression and anxiety in the United States: findings from the 2006 behavioral risk factor surveillance system. *Psychiatr Serv.* 2008;59:1383–1390.

128. Carney RM, Freedland KE. Depression and coronary heart disease. *Nat Rev Cardiol.* 2017;14:145–155. https://doi.org/10.1038/nrcardio.2016.181.

129. Sheng J, Liu S, Wang Y, et al. The link between depression and chronic pain: neural mechanisms in the brain. *Neural Plast.* 2017:9724371 https://doi.org/10.1155/2017/9724371. 2017.

130. Smith NL. *The effects of depression and anxiety on medical illness.* Sandy, Utah: University of Utah, Stress Medicine Clinic; 2002.

131. Lespérance F, Jaffe AS. Beyond the blues: understanding the link between coronary artery disease and depression. Retrieved June 15, 2006, from http://www.medscape.com/viewarticle/423461_2. Theheart.org.

132. Lydiard RB. Irritable bowel syndrome, anxiety, and depression: what are the links? *J Clin Psychiatry.* 2001;62(Suppl 8):38–45.

133. Haggman S, Maher CG, Refshauge KM. Screening for symptoms of depression by physical therapists managing low back pain. *Phys Ther.* 2004;84(12):1157–1166.

134. Wong JJ, Tricco AC, Côté P, et al. The association between depressive symptoms or depression and health outcomes in adults with low back pain with or without radiculopathy: protocol of a systematic review. *Syst Rev.* 2019;8:267. https://doi.org/10.1186/s13643-019-1192-4.

135. Maurer DM, Raymond TJ, Davis BN. Depression: screening and diagnosis. *Am Fam Physician.* 2018 Oct 15;98(8):508–515.

136. Staples LG, Dear BF, Gandy M, et al. Psychometric properties and clinical utility of brief measures of depression, anxiety, and general distress: the PHQ-2, GAD-2, and K-6. *Gen Hosp Psychiatry.* 2019;56:13–18. https://doi.org/10.1016/j.genhosppsych.2018.11.003. ISSN 0163-8343. https://www.sciencedirect.com/science/article/pii/S0163834318303712.

137. Kroenke K, Spitzer RL, Williams JB. The PHQ-9 validity of a brief depression severity measure. *J Gen Intern Med.* December 2001;16:606–613. https://doi.org/10.1046/j.1525-1497.2001.016009606.x. Beck AT, Ward CH, Mendelson M, et al. An inventory for measuring depression, *Arch Gen Psychiatry* 4:561–571, 1961.

138. Beck AT, Ward CH, Mendelson M, et al. An inventory for measuring depression. *Arch Gen Psychiatry.* 1961;4:561–571.

139. Williams AC, Richardson PH. What does the BDI measure in chronic pain? *Pain.* 1993;55:259–266.

140. Yesavage JA. The geriatric depression scale. *J Psychiatr Res.* 1983;17(1):37–49.

141. Zung WWK. A self-rating depression scale. *Arch Gen Psychiatry.* 1965;12:63–70.

142. Zamani M, Alizadeh-Tabari S, Zamani V. Systematic review with meta-analysis: the prevalence of anxiety and depression in patients with irritable bowel syndrome. *Aliment Pharmacol Ther.* 2019;50:132–143. https://doi.org/10.1111/apt.15325.

143. Banerjee A, Sarkhel S, Sarkar R, et al. Anxiety and depression in irritable bowel syndrome. *Indian J Psychol Med.* 2017;39:741–745.

144. Simrén M, Törnblom H, Palsson OS, et al. Visceral hypersensitivity is associated with GI symptom severity in functional GI disorders: consistent findings from five different patient cohorts. *Gut.* 2018;67:255–262.

145. Garakani A, Win T, Virk S, et al. Comorbidity of irritable bowel syndrome in psychiatric patients: a review. *Am J Ther.* 2003;10(1):61–67.

146. Melotti IGR, Juliato CRT, Tanaka M, et al. Severe depression and anxiety in women with overactive bladder. *Neurourol Urodyn.* 2018;37:223–228. https://doi.org/10.1002/nau.23277.

147. Choi HG, Kim JH, Park JY, et al. Association between asthma and depression: a national cohort study, *J Allergy Clin Immunol Pract.* 2019;7(4):1239–1245.e1. ISSN 2213-2198, https://doi.org/10.1016/j.jaip.2018.10.046. (https://www.sciencedirect.com/science/article/pii/S2213219818307189).

148. Fábián B, Fábián AK, Bugán A, et al. Comparison of mental and physical health between patients with primary and secondary Raynaud's phenomenon Category: Article. *J Psychosom Res.* 2019;116:6–9. https://doi.org/10.1016/j.jpsychores.2018.11.001. ISSN 0022-3999. https://www.sciencedirect.com/science/article/pii/S0022399918306895.

149. Panic Disorder By Christine Richmond. Medically Reviewed by Neha Pathak, MD on September 21, 2020 WebMD. Available online at: https://www.webmd.com/anxiety-panic/guide/mental-health-panic-disorder. Accessed July 20, 2021.

150. Wieseler-Frank J, Maier SF, Watkins LR. Glial activation and pathological pain. *Neurochem Int.* 2004;45(2-3):389–395.

151. Toljan K, Vrooman B. Psychoneuroimmunological approach to gastrointestinal related pain. *Scand J Pain.* 2017 Oct;17:431–443.

https://doi.org/10.1016/j.sjpain.2017.10.010. Epub 2017 Nov 6. PMID: 29122501.

152. Van Meeteren NLU, et al. Psychoneuroendocrinology and its relevance for physical therapy [Abstract]. *Phys Ther.* 2001;81(5):A66.

153. Jiang Y, Akhavan Aghdam Z, Li Y, et al. A protein kinase A–regulated network encodes short- and long-lived cellular memories. *Sci Signal.* 19 May 2020;13(632):eaay3585. https://doi.org/10.1126/scisignal.aay3585.

154. Liester MB. Personality changes following heart transplantation: the role of cellular memory. *Med Hypotheses.* 2020;135:109468 https://doi.org/10.1016/j.mehy.2019.109468. ISSN 0306-9877. https://www.sciencedirect.com/science/article/pii/S0306987719307145.

155. Yang J. UniSci International Science News, posted July 30, 2001, [http://unisci.com/] Rochester, NY, 2001, source: University of Rochester Medical Center.

156. Price TJ, Inyang KE. Commonalities between pain and memory mechanisms and their meaning for understanding chronic pain. *Prog Mol Biol Transl Sci.* 2015;131:409–434. https://doi.org/10.1016/bs.pmbts.2014.11.010.

157. Wu CM, Lin MW, Cheng JT, et al. Regulated, electroporation-mediated delivery of pro-opiomelanocortin gene suppresses chronic constriction injury-induced neuropathic pain in rats. *Gene Ther.* 2004;11(11):933–940.

158. Maier SF, Watkins LR. Immune-to-central nervous system communication and its role in modulating pain and cognition: implications for cancer and cancer treatment. *Brain Behav Immun.* 2003;17(Suppl 1):S125–S131.

159. Watkins LR, Maier SF. The pain of being sick: implications of immune-to-brain communication for understanding pain. *Annu Rev Psychol.* 2000;51:29–57.

160. Watkins LR, Maier SF. Beyond neurons: evidence that immune and glial cells contribute to pathological pain states. *Physiol Rev.* 2002;82(4):981–1011.

161. Holguin A, O'Connor KA, Biedenkapp J, et al. HIV-1 gp120 stimulates proinflammatory cytokine-mediated pain facilitation via activation of nitric oxide synthase-I (nNOS). *Pain.* 2004;110(3):517–530.

162. Osman A. Factor structure, reliability, and validity of the pain catastrophizing scale. *J Behavioural Med.* 1997;20(6):589–605.

163. Osman A. The pain catastrophizing scale: further psychometric evaluation with adult samples. *J Behav Med.* 2000;23(4):351–365.

164. Swinkels-Meewisse IEJ. Acute low back pain: pain-related fear and pain catastrophizing influence physical performance and perceived disability. *Pain.* 2006;120(1-2):36–43.

165. Sullivan M. The pain catastrophizing scale: development and validation. *Psych Assess.* 1995;7:524–532.

166. Wheeler CHB, Williams ACC, Morley SJ. Meta-analysis of the psychometric properties of the pain catastrophizing scale and associations with participant characteristics. *Pain.* 2019 Sep;160(9):1946–1953. https://doi.org/10.1097/j.pain.0000000000001494. PMID: 30694929.

167. Pain Catastrophizing Scale. Shirley Ryan Ability Lab. Available online at: https://www.sralab.org/rehabilitation-measures/pain-catastrophizing-scale. Accessed June 18, 2021.

168. Gauthier LR, Young A, Dworkin RH, et al. Validation of the short-form McGill pain questionnaire-2 in younger and older people with cancer pain. *J Pain.* 2014;15(7):756–770.

169. Dworkin RH, Turk DC, Trudeau JJ, et al. Validation of the short-form McGill pain questionnaire-2 (SF-MPQ-2) in acute low back pain. *J Pain.* 2015;16(4):357–366.

170. Gersh M, Echternach JL. Management of the individual with pain: part 1–physiology and evaluation. *PT Magazine.* 1996;4(11):54–63.

171. Dohrenwend A, Skillings JL. Diagnosis-specific management of somatoform disorders: moving beyond "vague complaints of pain". *J Pain.* 2009;10(11):1128–1137.

172. Greher MR, Wodushek TR. Performance validity testing in neuropsychology: scientific basis and clinical application—a brief review. *J Psychiatr Pract.* March 2017;23(2):134–140. https://doi.org/10.1097/PRA.0000000000000218.

173. Matheson LN. *Work capacity evaluation: systematic approach to industrial rehabilitation.* Anaheim, CA: Employment and Rehabilitation Institute of California; 1986.

174. Matheson LN. *Symptom magnification casebook.* Anaheim, CA: Employment and Rehabilitation Institute of California; 1987.

175. Matheson LN. Symptom magnification syndrome structured interview: rationale and procedure. *J Occup Rehab.* 1991;1(1):43–56.

176. American Psychiatric Association (APA) *Diagnostic and statistical manual of mental disorders (DSM-IV-TR).* Washington, DC: APA; 2000.

177. Cocchiarella L, Anderson G. *Guides to the evaluation of permanent impairment.* ed 5 Chicago: AMA; 2001.

178. Waddell G, McCulloch JA, Kummer E, et al. Nonorganic physical signs in low back pain. *Spine.* 1980;5(2):117–125.

179. Karas R, McIntosh G, Hall H, et al. The relationship between nonorganic signs and centralization of symptoms in the prediction of return to work for patients with low back pain. *Phys Ther.* 1997;77(4):354–360.

180. Rothstein JM, Erhard RE, Nicholson GG, et al. Conference. *Phys Ther.* 1997;77(4):361–369.

181. Rothstein JM. Unnecessary adversaries (editorial). *Phys Ther.* 1997;77(4):352.

182. Goodwin RD. Association between physical activity and mental disorders among adults in the United States. *Prev Med.* 2003;36:698–703.

183. Lawlor DA, Hopker SW. The effectiveness of exercise as an intervention in the management of depression: systematic review and meta-regression analysis of randomized controlled trials. *BMJ.* 2001;322:1–8.

184. Dunn AL, Trivedi MH, Kampert JB, et al. The DOSE study: a clinical trial to examine efficacy and dose response of exercise as treatment for depression. *Control Clin Trials.* 2002;23:584–603.

185. Dowd SM, Vickers KS, Krahn D. Exercise for depression: physical activity boosts the power of medications and psychotherapy. *Psychiatry Online.* June 2004;3(6).

186. van der Kolk BA. The body keeps the score: memory and the evolving psychobiology of posttraumatic stress. *Harv Rev Psychiatry.* 1994;1(5):253–265.

4

Physical Assessment as a Screening Tool

Brian A. Young, Michael Ross, and Richard Severin

Information gleaned from the patient interview will inform the physical therapist's clinical reasoning decisions regarding which body regions and systems to screen during the physical examination. This screening process is part of the continual determination of patient appropriateness for physical therapist care. It occurs from history, to physical assessment, to response to care throughout a course of treatment. Ongoing screening is essential regardless of the setting of physical therapist practice. In addition, it must occur regardless of the mechanism of patient access to physical therapy, whether direct access or referred.

During an initial screening assessment, the therapist may not need to perform a complete head-to-toe physical assessment. If the initial observations, patient history, screening questions, and screening tests are negative, move on to the next step.

In most situations, it is advised to utilize a regional-interdependence model, which includes assessment of the musculoskeletal, somatovisceral, neurophysiological, and biopsychosocial systems.[1]

When screening for systemic origins of clinical signs and symptoms, the physical therapist first scans the area(s) that directly relate to the patient's history and clinical presentation. For example, a shoulder problem can be caused by a problem in the stomach, heart, liver/biliary, lungs, spleen, kidneys, and ovaries (ectopic pregnancy). Only the physical assessment tests related to these areas would be assessed. These often can be narrowed down by the patient's history, gender, age, presence of risk factors, and associated signs and symptoms linked to a specific system.

More specifically, consider the postmenopausal woman with a primary family history of heart disease who presents with shoulder pain that occurs 3 to 4 minutes after starting an activity and is accompanied by unexplained perspiration. This individual should be assessed for cardiac involvement. Or think about the 45-year-old mother of five children who presents with scapular pain that is worse after she eats. A cardiac assessment may not be as important as a scan for signs and symptoms associated with the gallbladder or biliary system.

Documentation of physical findings is important. From a legal standpoint, if you did not document it, you did not assess it. Look for changes from the expected norm, as well as changes in the patient's baseline measurements. Use simple and clear documentation that can be understood and used by others. Record both normal and abnormal findings for each patient. Keep in mind that the patient's cultural and educational background, beliefs, values, and previous experiences can influence his or her response to questions.

In addition to providing care for illness or injuries, physical therapists may see patients for health and wellness visits. The American Physical Therapy Association provides recommended screening forms for both adult and pediatric patients presenting for health and wellness visits, which are recommended to occur on an annual basis.[2] Performing screening assessments for these patients is equally important, as identification of factors which may influence health and wellness may be found, and offer opportunity for physical therapist to provide education or refer the patient to an appropriate health care provider.

GENERAL SURVEY

Physical assessment begins the moment you meet the patient as you observe body size and type, facial expressions, evaluate self-care, and note anything unusual in appearance or presentation. Keep in mind (as discussed in Chapter 2) that cultural factors may dictate how the patient presents himself (e.g., avoiding eye contact when answering questions, hiding or exaggerating signs of pain).

A few pieces of equipment in a small kit within easy reach can make the screening examination faster and easier (Box 4.1). Using the same pattern in screening each time maintains consistency and will help the therapist avoid missing important screening clues.

As the therapist makes a general survey of each patient, it is also possible to evaluate posture, movement patterns and gait, balance, and coordination. For more involved patients the first impression may be based on level of consciousness, respiratory and vascular function, or nutritional status.

In an acute care or trauma setting the therapist may be using vital signs and the ABCDE (airway, breathing, circulation, disability, exposure) method of quick assessment.[3] A common strategy for history taking in the trauma unit is the mnemonic SAMPLE: Signs and symptoms, Allergies, Medications, Past illnesses, Last meal, and Events of injury.[4]

In any setting, knowing the patient's personal health history will also help guide and direct which components of the physical examination to include. We are not just screening

BOX 4.1 CONTENTS OF A SCREENING EXAMINATION KIT

- Stethoscope
- Sphygmomanometer
- Thermometer
- Pulse oximeter
- Reflex hammer
- Penlight
- Safety pin or sharp object (tongue depressor broken in half gives sharp and dull sides)
- Cotton-tipped swab or cotton ball
- Two test tubes
- Familiar objects (e.g., paper clip, coin, marble)
- Tuning fork (128 Hz)
- Watch with a second counter
- Personal protective equipment to prevent transmission of pathogens (e.g., gloves, gown, mask, googles)
- Ruler or plastic tape measure to measure wound dimensions, skin lesions, leg length
- Goniometer/inclinometer
- Gait belt

for medical disease masquerading as neuromusculoskeletal problems. Many physical illnesses, diseases, and medical conditions directly affect the neuromusculoskeletal system and must be considered. For example, inspection of the integument, limb inspection, and screening of the peripheral vascular system is important for someone at risk for lymphedema.

Therapists in all settings, especially primary care therapists, can use a screening physical assessment to provide education toward primary prevention, as well as intervention and management of current dysfunctions and disabilities.

Mental Status

Level of consciousness, orientation, and ability to communicate are all a part of the assessment of a patient's mental status. Orientation refers to the patient's ability to correctly answer questions about person, place, and time. A healthy individual with normal mental status will be alert, speak coherently, and be aware of the date, day, and time of day.

The therapist must be aware of any factor that can affect a patient's current mental status. Shock, head injury, infection, stroke, hospitalization, surgery (use of anesthesia), medications, age, and the use of substances and/or alcohol (see discussion, Chapter 2) can cause impaired consciousness.

Other factors affecting mental status may include malnutrition, exposure to chemicals, and hypothermia or hyperthermia. Depression and anxiety (see discussion, Chapter 3) also can affect a patient's functioning, mood, memory, ability to concentrate, judgment, and thought processes. Educational and socioeconomic background along with communication skills (e.g., English as a second language, aphasia) can affect mental status and function.

In a hospital, transition unit, or extended care facility, mental status is often evaluated and documented by the social worker or nursing service. It is always a good idea to review the patient's chart or electronic record regarding this information before beginning a physical therapy evaluation. However, independent assessment by the therapist is essential, as it may identify improvements or deteriorations in mental status.

Risk Factors for Delirium

It is not uncommon for older adults to experience a change in mental status or go through a stage of confusion about 24 hours after hospitalization for a serious illness or trauma, including surgery under a general anesthetic. Physicians may refer to this as iatrogenic delirium, anesthesia-induced dementia, or postoperative delirium. It is usually temporary but can last several hours to several weeks.

The cause of deterioration in mental ability is unknown. In some cases, delirium/dementia appears to be triggered by the shock to the body from anesthesia and surgery.[5] It may be a passing phase with complete recovery by the patient, although this can take weeks to months. The likelihood of delirium associated with hospitalization is much higher with hip fractures and hip and knee joint replacements,[6,7] possibly attributed to older age, slower metabolism, and polypharmacy (more than four prescribed drugs at admission).[8]

The therapist should pay attention to risk factors (Box 4.2) and watch out for any of the signs or symptoms of delirium. Physical examination should include vital signs with oxygen concentration measured, neurologic screening (Chapter 5), and surveillance for signs of infection. A medical diagnosis is needed to make the distinction between postoperative delirium, baseline dementia, depression, and withdrawal from drugs and alcohol.[6]

CLINICAL SIGNS AND SYMPTOMS

Iatrogenic Delirium

Cognitive Impairment
- Unable to concentrate during conversation
- Easily distracted or inattentive
- Switches topics often
- Unable to complete simple math or spell simple words backward

Impaired Orientation
- Unable to remember familiar concepts (e.g., say the days of the week, unable to tell time)
- Does not know who or where they are
- Unable to recognize family or close friends without help

Impaired Speech
- Speech is difficult to understand
- Unable to speak in full sentences; sentences do not make sense

Psychologic Impairment
- Anxious and afraid; requires frequent reassurance
- Suspicious of others, paranoid
- Irritable, jumpy, or in constant motion
- Experiencing delusions and hallucinations (e.g., sees objects or people who are not there; smells scents that are not present)

BOX 4.2   RISK FACTORS FOR IATROGENIC OR POSTOPERATIVE DELIRIUM

- Stress, trauma, pain, infection
- Hospitalization (for hip fracture, serious illness, or trauma including surgery) or change in residence
- Older age (65 years old or older)
- Anesthesia
- Hip or knee joint replacement
- Poor cognitive function, underlying dementia, previous cognitive impairment
- Vision or hearing deficits
- Decreased physical function
- History of alcohol abuse
- Medications (e.g., benzodiazepine, narcotics, NSAIDs, anticholinergics prescribed for sleep, psychoactive drugs/antidepressants/antipsychotics, dopamine agents, analgesics, sedative agents for pain and anxiety after surgery)*
- Dehydration
- Urinary retention, fecal impaction, diarrhea
- Sleep deprivation
- Postoperative low hemoglobin, abnormal fluid and/or electrolytes, low oxygen saturation
- Malnutrition, vitamin B_{12}/folate deficiency, low albumin, NSAIDs

*Higher risk medications commonly associated with delirium; lower risk medications associated with delirium include some cardiovascular agents (e.g., antiarrhythmics, beta-blockers, clonidine, digoxin), antimicrobials (e.g., fluoroquinolones, penicillins, sulfonamides, acyclovir), anticonvulsants, and medications for gastroesophageal reflux or nausea.

NSAIDs: nonsteroidal anti-inflammatory drugs.

Data from Alfonso DT. Nonsurgical complications after total hip and total knee arthroplasty. *Am J Orthop* 2006;35(11):503–510; Short M, Winstead PS. Delirium dilemma: pharmacology update. *Orthopedics* 2007;30(4):273–277.

TABLE 4.1	Karnofsky Performance Scale
Score (%)	Description
100	Normal, no complaints; no evidence of disease
90	Able to carry on normal activities; minor signs or symptoms of disease
80	Normal activity with effort; some signs or symptoms of disease
70	Cares for self; unable to carry on normal activity or to do active work
60	Requires occasional assistance but able to care for most of own personal needs
50	Requires considerable assistance and frequent medical care
40	Disabled; requires special care and assistance
30	Severely disabled; hospitalization indicated though death not imminent
20	Very ill; hospitalization required; active supportive treatment necessary
10	Failing rapidly; moribund
0	Dead

Several instruments may be used to assess level of consciousness, performance, and disability. In acute situations, asking the patient a few questions from the Mini-Mental State Examination can provide a brief but valuable assessment.[9] For example, asking the date, day of the week, what city the patient is in, what season it is, or even the current or former president of the United States can provide valuable information regarding the patient's current cognitive state. There are also online calculators that can assist with full administration of the Mini-Mental State Examination.[10]

The Confusion Assessment Method (CAM) is a bedside rating scale physical therapists can use to assess hospitalized or institutionalized individuals for delirium. This tool has been adapted for use with patients who are ventilated and in an intensive care unit (CAM-ICU).[11] There are two parts to the assessment instrument: part one screens for overall cognitive impairment. Part two includes four features that have the greatest ability to distinguish delirium or reversible confusion from other types of cognitive impairment. As a screening tool, the CAM has been validated for use by physicians and nurses in palliative care and intensive care settings (sensitivity of 94% to 100% and specificity of 90% to 95%). Values for positive predictive accuracy were 91% to 94%, and values for negative predictive accuracy were 100% and 90% for the two populations assessed (general medicine, outpatient geriatric center).[12] The CAM-ICU has also been shown to be a valid instrument for the diagnosis of delirium in a variety of medical settings.[13] The Glasgow Outcome Scale (GOS) describes patients on a five-point scale from good recovery (1) to death (5). Vegetative state, severe disability, and moderate disability are included in the continuum. Although it is a commonly used outcome measure, GOS has been reported to have limited sensitivity to detect small but clinically meaningful changes. The GOS-Extended was developed to improve the test's ability to detect those small changes.[14] The Karnofsky Performance Scale in Table 4.1 is used widely to quantify functional status in a wide variety of individuals, but especially among those with cancer. It can be used to compare effectiveness of intervention and to assess individual prognosis. The lower the Karnofsky score, the worse the prognosis for survival.[15]

A practical performance scale originally used for patients with cancer, but can also be applied in other settings, is the Eastern Cooperative Oncology Group Performance Status Scale (Table 4.2).[16] Researchers and health care professionals use these scales and criteria to assess how an individual's disease is progressing, to assess how the disease affects the daily living abilities of the patient, and to determine appropriate treatment and prognosis.

Confusion is not a normal change with aging and must be reported and documented. Confusion is often associated with various systemic conditions (Table 4.3). Increased confusion

TABLE 4.2	Eastern Cooperative Oncology Group Performance Status Scale
Grade	Level of Activity
0	Fully active, able to carry on all predisease performance without restriction (Karnofsky 90%–100%)
1	Restricted in physically strenuous activity but ambulatory and able to carry out work of a light or sedentary nature (e.g., light house work, office work) (Karnofsky 70%–80%)
2	Ambulatory and capable of all self-care but unable to carry out any work activities. Up and about more than 50% of waking hours (Karnofsky 50%–60%)
3	Capable of only limited self-care, confined to bed or chair more than 50% of waking hours (Karnofsky 30%–40%)
4	Completely disabled. Cannot carry on any self-care. Totally confined to bed or chair (Karnofsky 10%–20%)
5	Dead (Karnofsky 0%)

The Karnofsky Performance Scale allows individuals to be classified according to functional impairment. The lower the score, the worse the prognosis for survival for most serious illnesses.
From Oken MM, Creech RH, Tormey DC, et al. Toxicity and response criteria of the Eastern Cooperative Oncology Group. *Am J Clin Oncol* 1982;5:649–655. https://ecog-acrin.org/resources/ecog-performance-status.

CLINICAL SIGNS AND SYMPTOMS

Undernutrition or Malnutrition

- Muscle wasting, loss of fat
- Alopecia (hair loss)
- Dermatitis; dry, flaking skin
- Chapped lips, lesions at corners of mouth
- Brittle nails
- Abdominal distention
- Decreased physical activity/energy level; fatigue, lethargy
- Depression
- Lack of appetite
- Peripheral edema
- Bruising

TABLE 4.3	Systemic Conditions Associated with Confused States
System	Impairment/Condition
Endocrine	Hypothyroidism, hyperthyroidism
	Perimenopause, menopause
Metabolic	Severe anemia
	Fluid and/or electrolyte imbalances; dehydration
	Wilson's disease (copper disorder)
	Porphyria (inherited disorder)
Immune/ Infectious	AIDS
	Cerebral amebiasis, toxoplasmosis, or malaria
	Fungal or tubercular meningitis
	Lyme disease
	Neurosyphilis
Cardiovascular	CHF
Cerebrovascular	Cerebral insufficiency (TIA, CVA)
	Postanoxic encephalopathy
Pulmonary	COPD
	Hypercapnia (increased CO_2)
	Hypoxemia (decreased arterial O_2)
Renal	Renal failure, uremia
	Urinary tract infection
Neurologic	Encephalopathy (hepatic, hypertensive)
	Head trauma
	Cancer
	CVA; stroke
Other	Chronic drug and/or alcohol use
	Medication (e.g., anticonvulsants, antidepressants, antiemetics, antihistamines, antipsychotics, benzodiazepines, narcotics, sedative-hypnotics, Zantac, Tagamet)
	Postoperative
	Severe anemia
	Cancer metastasized to the brain
	Sarcoidosis
	Sleep apnea
	Vasculitis (e.g., SLE)
	Vitamin deficiencies (B_{12}, folate, niacin, thiamine)
	Whipple's disease (severe intestinal disorder)

AIDS, Acquired immunodeficiency syndrome; *CHF*, congestive heart failure; *COPD*, chronic obstructive pulmonary disease; *CVA*, cerebrovascular accident; *SLE*, systemic lupus erythematosus; *TIA*, transient ischemic attack.
Modified from Dains JE, Baumann LC, Scheibel P. *Advanced Health Assessment and Clinical Diagnosis in Primary Care.* 2nd ed. St. Louis: Mosby; 2003:425.

in a patient with any form of dementia can be a symptom of infection (e.g., pneumonia, urinary tract infection), electrolyte imbalance, or delirium. Any observed change in level of consciousness, orientation, judgment, communication or speech pattern, or memory should be documented regardless of which scale is used. The therapist may be the first to notice increased lethargy, slowed motor responses, or disorientation or confusion. Likewise, a sudden change in muscle tone (usually increased tone) in the patient with a neurologic disorder (adult or child) can signal an infectious process. Assessment of these signs and symptoms may help the therapist assess the severity of the condition and determine the need for further medical evaluation.

Nutritional Status

Nutrition is an important part of growth and development and recovery from infection, illness, wounds, and surgery. Patients can exhibit signs of malnutrition or overnutrition (obesity).

Be aware in the health history of any risk factors for nutritional deficiencies (Box 4.3). Remember that some medications can cause appetite changes and that psychosocial factors such as depression, eating disorders, drug or alcohol addictions, and economic variables can affect nutritional status.

BOX 4.3   RISK FACTORS FOR NUTRITIONAL DEFICIENCY

- Economic status
- Living alone
- Older age (metabolic rate slows in older adults; altered sense of taste and smell affects appetite)
- Depression, anxiety
- Eating disorder
- Lactose intolerance (common in Mexican Americans, African Americans, Asians, Native Americans)
- Alcohol/drug addiction
- Chronic diarrhea
- Nausea
- Gastrointestinal impairment (e.g., bowel resection, gastric bypass, pancreatitis, Crohn's disease, pernicious anemia)
- Chronic endocrine or metabolic disorder (e.g., diabetes mellitus, celiac sprue)
- Liver disease
- Dialysis
- Medications (e.g., captopril, chemotherapy, steroids, insulin, lithium) including over-the-counter drugs (e.g., laxatives)
- Chronic disability affecting activities of daily living (e.g., problems with balance, mobility, food preparation)
- Burns
- Difficulty chewing or swallowing (dental problems, stroke or other neurologic impairment)

While undernutrition and malnutrition are serious clinical concerns, individuals who are overweight or obese are at an increased risk for several conditions including type II diabetes mellitus, dyslipidemia, stroke, some cancers, cardiovascular disease (CVD) and hypertension.[17] Therefore, it may be necessary to determine the patient's ideal body weight by calculating the body mass index (BMI), which is a simple and noninvasive screening tool for the general population.[18] The formula for calculating BMI is your weight (in kilograms) divided by the square of your height (in meters) (kg/m^2). Websites are also available to help anyone make this calculation.[18-20] While a normal BMI is between 18.5 and 24.9, overweight is classified as a BMI between 25 and 29.9 and obesity is classified as a BMI of 30 or greater.[18] Since BMI only serves as a surrogate measure of body fat, caution should be used in interpreting an elevated BMI in individuals who have increased muscle mass and low body fat. There is a separate website for children and teens sponsored by the Centers for Disease Control and Prevention. Whenever nutritional deficiencies or concerns are suspected, notify the physician and/or request a referral to a registered dietitian.

Body and Breath Odors

Odors may provide some significant clues to overall health status. For example, a fruity (sweet) breath odor may be a symptom of diabetic ketoacidosis. Bad breath (halitosis) can be a symptom of dental decay, lung abscess, throat or sinus infection, or gastrointestinal (GI) disturbances from food intolerances, *Helicobacter pylori* bacteria, or bowel obstruction. Keep in mind that ethnic foods and alcohol can affect breath and body odor.

Patients who are incontinent (bowel or bladder) may smell of urine, ammonia, or feces. It is important to ask the patient about any unusual odors. It may be best to offer an introductory explanation with some follow-up questions:

FOLLOW-UP QUESTIONS

Mrs. Smith, as a part of the physical therapy examination, we always look at our patient's overall health and general physical condition. Do you have any other health concerns besides your shoulder/back (Therapist: name the involved body part)?

Are you being treated by anyone for any other problems? (Wait for a response but add prompts as needed: chiropractor? acupuncturist? naturopath?)

If you suspect urinary incontinence: Are you having any trouble with leaking urine or making it to the bathroom on time? (Ask appropriate follow-up questions about cause, frequency, severity, triggers, and so on; see Appendix B-5 in the accompanying enhanced eBook version included with print purchase of this textbook.)

If you suspect fecal incontinence: Do you have trouble getting to the toilet on time for a bowel movement?

Do you have trouble wiping yourself clean after a bowel movement? (Ask appropriate follow-up questions about cause, frequency, severity, triggers, and so on.)

If you detect a breath odor: I notice an unusual smell on your breath. Do you know what might be causing this? (Ask appropriate follow-up questions depending on the type of smell you perceive; you may have to conduct an alcohol screening survey [see Chapter 2 or Appendices B-1 and B-2 on in the accompanying enhanced eBook version included with print purchase of this textbook].)

Vital Signs

The need for therapists to assess vital signs, particularly pulse rate and blood pressure (BP), is important,[21] especially without the benefit of laboratory values. Vital signs, observations, and reported associated signs and symptoms are among the best screening tools available to the therapist.

Vital sign assessment is an important tool because high BP is a serious concern in the United States. Many people are unaware they have high BP and are asymptomatic.[22] A study by Severin et al. demonstrated that over 75% of outpatient orthopedic physical therapists report that at least 25% of their current case load included patients either with diagnosed CVD or at moderate or greater risk for CVD and over 50% reported that at least half of their current caseload included such patients.[22] The same study also demonstrated that 69% of outpatient orthopedic physical therapists encounter a new patient either diagnosed with CVD or at moderate risk or greater for CVD at least twice per week and that 30% encounter such patients daily.[22]

BOX 4.4 VITAL SIGNS

The Primary Vital Signs

- Pulse Rate/Heart Rate (beats per minute [bpm])
- Blood pressure (BP)
- Core body temperature (oral or ear)
- Respiratory rate

Additional Vital Signs

- Pulse oximetry (oxygen [O$_2$] saturation)
- Skin temperature
- Pain (now called the fifth vital sign; see Chapter 3 for assessment)
- Walking speed (often considered the sixth vital sign)[78]

TABLE 4.4	Classification of Blood Pressure		
	Systolic Blood Pressure		Diastolic Blood Pressure
FOR ADULTS*			
Normal	Less than 120	And	Less than 80
Elevated	120–129	And	Less than 80
Stage 1 hypertension	130–139	Or	80–89
Stage 2 hypertension	≥140	Or	≥90
Hypertensive crisis	> 180	And/or	>120
FOR CHILDREN AGED 1–<13 YEARS OF AGE†			
Normal	<90th percentile; 50th percentile is the midpoint of the normal range		
Elevated	≥90th percentile to <95th percentile or 120/80 mm Hg to <95th percentile (whichever is lower)		
Stage 1 hypertension	≥95th percentile to <95th percentile + 12 mm Hg, or 130/80 to 139/89 mm Hg (whichever is lower)		
Stage 2 hypertension	≥95th percentile + 12 mm Hg, or ≥140/90 mm Hg (whichever is lower)		
FOR CHILDREN AGED ≥13 YEARS OF AGE†			
Normal	<120/<80 mm Hg		
Elevated	120/<80 to 129/<80 mm Hg)		
Stage 1 Hypertension	130/80 to 139/89 mm Hg		
Stage 2 Hypertension	≥140/90 mm Hg		

*From Whelton PK, Carey RM, Aronow WS, et al. ACC/AHA/AAPA/ABC/ACPM/AGS/APhA/ASH/ASPC/NMA/PCNA guideline for the prevention, detection, evaluation, and management of high blood pressure in adults. *J Am Coll Cardiol* 2018;71(19):e127-e248.
†From Flynn JT, Kaelber DC, Baker-Smith CM, et al. Clinical practice guideline for screening and management of high blood pressure in children and adolescents. *Pediatrics* 2017;140(3):e20171904.

Physical therapists practicing in all settings must know when and how to assess vital signs. The *Guide to Physical Therapist Practice*[23] recommends that heart rate/pulse rate and BP measurements be included in the examination of new patients, and at each follow-up visit.[21,24]

Taking a patient's vital signs remains the single easiest, most efficient way to screen for many systemic illnesses. All vital signs are important (Box 4.4), as they serve as early screening tools for systemic illness or disease, and offer valuable information about the cardiovascular and pulmonary systems.

Assessment of baseline vital signs should be a part of the initial data collected so that correlations and comparisons with future values are available when necessary. The therapist compares measurements taken against normal values and compares future measurements to the baseline units to identify significant changes (normalizing values or moving toward abnormal findings) for each patient.

Normal ranges of values for the vital signs are provided for the therapist's convenience (Table 4.4). BP values warranting further medical examination in children as well (Table 4.5). However, these ranges can be exceeded by a patient and still represent normal for that person. Keep in mind that many factors can affect vital signs, especially pulse rate and BP (Table 4.6). Substances such as alcohol, caffeine, nicotine, and cocaine/cocaine derivatives, and pain and stress/anxiety can cause fluctuations in BP. Adults who monitor their own BP may report wide fluctuations without making the association between these and other factors listed. Additionally, there are several potential sources of error for BP measurement technique which may cause values to appear abnormal (Table). It is the unusual vital sign in combination with other signs and symptoms, medications, and medical status that gives clinical meaning to the pulse rate, BP, and temperature.

Pulse Rate

The pulse rate reveals important information about the patient's heart rate and heart rhythm. A resting pulse rate (normal range: 60 to 100 beats per minute [bpm]) taken at the carotid artery or radial artery pulse point should be available for comparison with the pulse rate taken during treatment or after exercise (Fig. 4.1).[21] A pulse rate above 100 bpm at rest indicates an elevated heart rate (tachycardia); below 60 bpm indicates a slowed heart rate (bradycardia).

Pulse oximeter devices can be used for pulse rate measurement but do have some limitations. The pulse rate provided by a pulse oximeter device often reflects a mean average pulse rate, thus may not reveal dysrhythmias (e.g., a regular irregular pulse rate associated with atrial fibrillation) that could be detected with manual measurement of pulse rate.

Keep in mind that taking the pulse rate measures the peripheral arterial wave propagation generated by the heart's contraction—it is not the same as measuring the true heart rate (and should not be recorded as heart rate when measured by palpation). A true measure of heart rate requires auscultation or recording of the electrical impulses of the heart (such an electrocardiograph). The distinction between pulse rate and heart rate becomes a matter of concern in documentation liability and even greater importance for individuals with dysrhythmias. In such cases, the output of blood by some beats

TABLE 4.5	Blood Pressure Values Warranting Further Medical Evaluation in Children			
		Boys	Girls	
	Age	SBP	DBP	Systolic DBP
1	98	52	98	54
2	100	55	101	58
3	101	58	102	60
4	102	60	103	62
5	103	63	104	64
6	105	66	105	67
7	106	68	106	68
8	107	69	107	69
9	107	70	108	71
10	108	72	109	72
11	110	74	111	74
12	113	75	114	75
≥13	120	80	120	80

[†]From Flynn JT, Kaelber DC, Baker-Smith CM, et al. Clinical practice guideline for screening and management of high blood pressure in children and adolescents. *Pediatrics* 2017;140(3):e20171904.

may be insufficient to produce a detectable pulse wave that would still be discernible on an electrocardiogram.[25]

The resting pulse rate may be higher than normal with fever, anemia, infections, some medications, hyperthyroidism, anxiety, or pain. It is worth nothing that patients even with severe pain may not demonstrate changes in heart rate, and a lack of change in heart rate should not be used to refute a patient's report of pain.[26–28] A low pulse rate (below 60 bpm) is not uncommon among trained athletes. The normal response of pulse rate to physical activity is an increase of approximately 10 bpm per each 1 metabolic equivalent (MET) increase in intensity. The normal recovery of pulse rate to physical activity is a reduction of greater than 12 bpm following 1 minute of seated rest, with the pulse returning to baseline after about 3 minutes. Medications, such as beta-blockers and calcium channel blockers, can also attenuate the normal rise in pulse rate that usually occurs during exercise. In such cases the therapist should also monitor rates of perceived exertion in addition to pulse rate. Other pulse abnormalities are listed in Box 4.5.

When taking the resting pulse or pulse during exercise, some clinicians measure the pulse for 15 seconds and multiply by four to get the rate per minute. However, using shorter periods of measurement can result in an underestimation or overestimation of the pulse rate and may mask dysrhythmias[24] For screening purposes, it is always best to palpate the pulse for a full minute or at minimum 30 seconds. Longer pulse counts give greater accuracy and provide more time for detection of some dysrhythmias (Box 4.6).[24]

TABLE 4.6	Factors Affecting Pulse and Blood Pressure
Pulse	Blood Pressure*
Age	Age
Anemia	Alcohol
Autonomic dysfunction (diabetes, spinal cord injury)	Anxiety
	Blood viscosity
Caffeine	Caffeine
Cardiac muscle dysfunction	Cocaine and cocaine derivatives
Conditioned/deconditioned state	Dehydration
	Diet
Dehydration (decreased blood volume increases heart rate)	Distended urinary bladder
	Force of heart contraction
	Living at higher altitudes
Fear	Medications
Fever, heat	• ACE inhibitors (lowers pressure)
Hyperthyroidism	
Infection	• Adrenergic inhibitors (lowers pressure)
Medications	
• Antidysrhythmic (slows rate)	• Beta-blockers (lowers pressure)
• Atropine (increases rate)	• Diuretics (lowers pressure)
• Beta-blocker (slows rate)	• Narcotic analgesics (lowers pressure)
• Digitalis (slows rate)	
Pain	Nicotine
Sleep disorders or sleep deprivation	Pain
	Sleep disorders or sleep deprivation
Stress (emotional or psychologic)	Stress (emotional or psychologic)
	Time of recent meal (increases SBP)

*Conditions, such as chronic kidney disease, renovascular disorders, primary aldosteronism, and coarctation of the aorta, are identifiable causes of elevated blood pressure. Chronic overtraining in athletes, use of steroids and/or nonsteroidal anti-inflammatory drugs (NSAIDs), and large increases in muscle mass can also contribute to hypertension. Treatment for hypertension, dehydration, heart failure, heart attack, arrhythmias, anaphylaxis, shock (from severe infection, stroke, anaphylaxis, major trauma), and advanced diabetes can cause low blood pressure.
ACE, Angiotensin-converting enzyme; *SBP*, systolic blood pressure.
Modified from Goodman CC, Fuller K. Pathology: Implications for the Physical Therapist. 4th ed. Philadelphia: WB Saunders; 2015.

Pulse Amplitude

Pulse amplitude (weak or bounding quality of the pulse) gives an indication of the circulating blood volume and the strength of left ventricle ejection. Normally, the pulse amplitude increases slightly with inspiration, and decreases with expiration. This slight change is not considered significant. Pulse amplitude can be graded as:

0	Absent, not palpable
1 +	Pulse diminished, barely palpable
2 +	Easily palpable, normal
3 +	Full pulse, increased strength
4 +	Bounding, too strong to obliterate

Pulse amplitude that fades with inspiration instead of strengthening and strengthens with expiration instead of fading

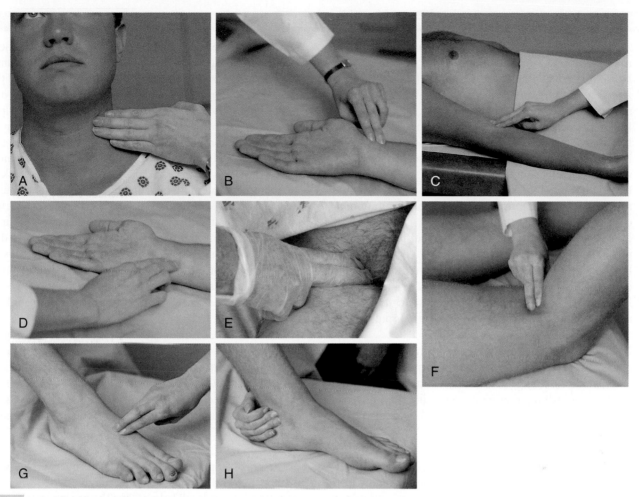

Fig. 4.1 Pulse points. The easiest and most commonly palpated pulses are the (A) carotid pulse and (B) radial pulse. Other pulse points include the brachial pulse (C), ulnar pulse (D), femoral pulse (E), popliteal pulse (knee slightly flexed) (F), dorsalis pedis (G), and posterior tibial (H). The anterior tibial pulse becomes the dorsalis pedis and is palpable where the artery lies close to the skin on the dorsum of the foot. Peripheral pulses are more difficult to palpate in older adults and anyone with peripheral vascular disease. (From Potter PA. Fundamentals of Nursing. 7th ed. St. Louis: Mosby; 2009.)

BOX 4.5 PULSE ABNORMALITIES

- Weak pulse beats alternating with strong beats
- Weak, thready pulse
- Bounding pulse (a cycle of strong throbbing pulsations followed by a sudden collapse or decrease in the force of the pulse felt over one of the arteries)
- Two quick beats followed by a pause (no pulse)
- Irregular rhythm (interval between beats is not equal)
- Pulse amplitude decreases with inspiration/increases with expiration
- Pulse rate too fast (greater than 100 bpm; tachycardia)
- Pulse rate too slow (less than 60 bpm; bradycardia)

is *paradoxic* and should be reported to the physician. Paradoxic pulse occurs most commonly in patients with chronic obstructive pulmonary disease (COPD) but is also observed in patients with constrictive pericarditis.[29]

Constriction or compression around the heart from pericardial effusion, tension pneumothorax, pericarditis with fluid, or pericardial tamponade may be associated with paradoxical pulse. When the person breathes in, the increased mechanical pressure of inspiration added to the physiologic compression from the underlying disease prevents the heart from contracting fully and results in a reduced pulse. When the person breathes out, the pressure from chest expansion is reduced and the pulse increases.

Respiratory/Ventilatory Rate

The normal respiratory rate is between 12 to 20 breaths per minute, and the rise and fall of the chest equals one cycle.[30] When assessing rate it is important to observe excursion (shallow or normal or deep), effort (gasping, straining or relaxed), and pattern. Normally the chest wall and abdomen should move in the same direction during inspiration and expiration. Note any excessive use of accessory muscles (e.g., scalenes and sternocleidomastoid) and whether the patient's breathing is silent or noisy. Watch for puffed cheeks, pursed lips, nasal flaring, or asymmetric chest expansion. Changes in the rate, depth, effort, or pattern of a patient's respirations can be early signs of neurologic, pulmonary, or cardiovascular impairment. For example, asymmetrical expansion between right and left sides of the chest wall could indicate the presence of a pneumothorax.

BOX 4.6   TIPS ON PALPATING PULSE AMPLITUDE

- Assess each pulse for strength and equality for one full minute.
- Normal pulse is 2 + and equal bilaterally (see scale in text).
- Apply gentle pressure; pulses are easily obliterated in some people.
- Popliteal pulse requires deeper palpation.
- Normal veins are flat; pulsations are not visible.
- Flat veins in supine that become distended in sitting may indicate heart disease.
- Pulses should be the same from side to side and should not change significantly with inspiration, expiration, or change in position.
- Pulses tend to diminish with age; distal pulses are not palpable in many older adults.
- If pulses are diminished or absent, listen for a bruit to detect arterial narrowing.
- Pedal pulses can be congenitally absent; the patient may or may not know if absent pulse at this pulse site is normal or a change in pulse pressure.
- In the case of diminished or absent pulses observe the patient for other changes (e.g., skin temperature, texture, color, hair loss, change in toenails); ask about pain in calf or leg with walking that goes away with rest (intermittent claudication, peripheral vascular disease [PVD]).
- Carotid pulse: Assess in the seated position; have patient turn the head slightly toward the side being palpated. Gently and carefully palpate along the medial edge of the sternocleidomastoid muscle (see Fig. 4.1). Palpate one carotid artery at a time; apply light pressure; deep palpation can stimulate carotid sinus with a sudden drop in heart rate and blood pressure causing syncope. Do not poke or mash around to find the pulse; palpation must not provide a massage to the artery because of the risk of liberating a thrombus or plaque, especially in older adults.
- Femoral pulse: Femoral artery is palpable below the inguinal ligament midway between the anterior superior iliac spine and the symphysis pubis. It can be difficult to assess in the obese patient; place fingertips of both hands on either side of the pulse site; femoral pulse should be as strong (if not stronger) than radial pulse.
- Posterior tibial pulse: Foot must be relaxed with ankle in slight plantar flexion (see Fig. 4.1).
- For Pulse Rate measure the number of pulsations felt at either the carotid or radial artery for 1 minute. Measurements can be taken for less than 1 minute and then multiplied by a factor (e.g., 15 seconds × 4, 30 seconds × 2, 6 seconds × 10). It is recommended to measure for no less than 30 seconds when calculating heart rate.

It is often recommended to assess the patient's breathing without drawing attention to what is being done. This is because patients often adjust their breathing rate and pattern if they are aware that they are being examined. One method to examine breathing without the patient made aware is to measure it right after counting the pulse rate. Inform the patient that you are measuring their pulse rate for 1 minute, however only measure the pulse rate for 30 seconds and use the remaining 30 seconds to measure respiratory rate while still holding onto their wrist. In this case, the amount of breathing cycles measured for 30 seconds will be multiplied by two. However, measuring respiratory rate for 30 seconds is only recommended for regular and unlabored breathing. When breathing is labored or irregular, measure for a full minute.

Pulse Oximetry

Arterial blood oxygen saturation of hemoglobin (SaO_2), which is measured via arterial blood gas analysis, can be estimated and monitored using pulse oximetry (SpO_2).[31] This is a noninvasive, photoelectric device with a sensor that can be attached to a well-perfused finger, the bridge of the nose, toe, forehead, or earlobe.[31] Digital readings are less accurate with patients who are anemic, undergoing chemotherapy, or who use fingernail polish or nail acrylics. In such cases, attach the sensor to one of the other accessible body parts.

The sensor probe emits red and infrared light, which is transmitted to the capillaries. When in contact with the skin, the probe measures transmitted light passing through the vascular bed and detects the relative amount of color absorbed by the arterial blood. The SaO_2 level is calculated from this information.

The normal SpO_2 range at rest and during exercise is 95% to 100%. Referral for medical evaluation is advised when resting saturation levels fall below 90%. The exception to the normal range listed here is for patients with a history of tobacco use and/or lung disease such as COPD. Some individuals with COPD may also retain carbon dioxide and can become apneic if the oxygen levels are too high. For this reason, SpO_2 levels for this population may have lower acceptable range of normal.

The drive to breathe in a healthy person results from an increase in the arterial carbon dioxide level ($PaCO_2$). In the normal adult, increased CO_2 levels stimulate chemoreceptors in the brainstem to increase the respiratory rate. With some chronic lung disorders these central chemoreceptors may become desensitized to $PaCO_2$ changes resulting in a dependence on the peripheral chemoreceptors to detect a fall in arterial oxygen levels (PaO_2) to stimulate the respiratory drive.

Too much oxygen delivered as a treatment can depress the respiratory drive in those individuals with COPD who have a dampening of the CO_2 drive. Monitoring the respiratory rate, level of oxygen administered by nasal canula, and SpO_2 levels is very important in this patient population.

Any condition that restricts blood flow (including cold hands) can result in inaccurate SpO_2 readings. Relaxation and physiologic quieting techniques can be used to help restore more normal temperatures in the distal extremities. Since perfusion can impact the accuracy and measurement properties of pulse oximeters, it is recommended to avoid measuring on extremities where a BP cuff is applied.[32]

Oxygen saturation on hemoglobin levels can also be affected by positioning because positioning can affect a person's ability to breathe. Upright sitting position has been reported to provide the highest oxygen saturation value compared with positioning in supine, prone, or sidelying.[33] Upright sitting in individuals with low muscle tone or kyphosis can cause forward flexion of the thoracic spine compromising oxygen intake. Using SpO_2 levels may be a good way to document outcomes of positioning programs for patients with impaired ventilation.

Other factors affecting pulse oximeter readings can include nail polish and nail coverings, irregular heart rhythms, intravascular dyes, electrical interference, and significant venous pulsation.[31] In addition to SpO_2 levels, it is important to assess other signs and symptoms, including vitals, skin and nail bed color and tissue perfusion, mental status, breath sounds, and respiratory pattern for all patients using pulse oximetry.

Blood Pressure

Blood pressure (BP) is the measurement of pressure in an artery at the peak of systole (contraction of the left ventricle) and during diastole (when the heart is at rest after closure of the aortic valve). The units of measurement are in millimeters of mercury (mm Hg) and are recorded as: systolic (contraction phase)/diastolic (relaxation phase).

BP may be influenced by many factors and can vary among individuals (see Table 4.6). Normal systolic BP (SBP) ranges from 100 to 120 mm Hg, and diastolic BP (DBP) ranges from 60 to 80 mm Hg. Highly trained athletes may have lower values. Target ranges for BP are listed in Table 44 and Box 4.7. The baseline BP values can be recorded on the Family/Personal History form (see Fig. 2.2).

Measuring Blood Pressure. There are several options available to measure BP in the clinic. The two most used methods are aneroid devices, which are used for manual auscultatory measurement, and oscillometric devices used for automatic measurement. Both devices measure resting BP accurately.[34-36] However, they utilize slightly different methods.

Manual auscultatory BP measurement utilizes the identification of sounds resulting from the return of arterial blood flow following a period of temporary occlusion produced by an inflatable cuff, which are known as Korotkoff sounds. As the cuff deflates below peak pressure, blood returns into the artery in a turbulent fashion, causing vibration along the arterial wall. This vibration creates a tapping sound that can be heard with auscultation of the artery. Once the cuff pressure falls below the diastolic pressure, laminar blood flow is restored in the artery and the arterial wall no longer vibrates. The lack of vibration causes the tapping sound to disappear, and silence is appreciated on auscultation of the artery. The pressure at the emergence of sound after deflation is used as the SBP, and pressure at the subsequent disappearance of sound is used as the DBP.

Automatic oscillometric devices operate by detecting the vibrations in the arterial wall during cuff inflation and deflation which can be transduced into electrical signals. These devices typically inflate the cuff to a pressure approximately 20 mm Hg above the patient's SBP. As the cuff deflates, the vibrations during deflation are transferred from the arterial wall through the air inside the cuff into a transducer in the device. The

---

BOX 4.7 GUIDELINES FOR BLOOD PRESSURE IN PHYSICAL THERAPY PRACTICE

Consider the following as yellow (caution) flags that require closer monitoring and possible medical referral:

- SBP greater than 120 mm Hg and/or DBP greater than 80 mm Hg, especially in the presence of significant risk factors (age, medications, personal or family history)
- Decrease in DBP below 70 mm Hg in adults aged 75 years or older (risk factor for Alzheimer's)
- Persistent rise or fall in BP over time (at least three consecutive readings over two weeks), especially in a patient taking NSAIDs (check for edema) or any woman taking birth control pills (should be closely monitored by physician)
- Steady fall in BP over several years in adult over 75 years of age (risk factor for Alzheimer's)
- Lower standing SBP (less than 140 mm Hg) in adults over the age of 65 years with a history of falls (increased risk for falls)
- A difference in pulse pressure greater than 40 mm Hg
- More than 10 mm Hg difference (SBP or DBP) from side to side (upper extremities)
- Approaching or more than 40 mm Hg difference (SBP or DBP) from side to side (lower extremities)
- BP in lower extremities is lower than in the upper extremities
- DBP increases more than 10 mm Hg during activity or exercise
- SBP does not rise as workload increases; SBP falls as workload increases
- SBP exceeds 200 mm Hg during exercise or physical activity; DBP exceeds 100 mm Hg during exercise or physical activity; these values represent the upper limits and may be too high for the patient's age, general health, and overall condition
- BP changes in the presence of other warning signs such as first-time onset or unstable angina, dizziness, nausea, pallor, extreme diaphoresis
- Sudden fall in BP (more than 10 to 15 mm Hg SBP) or more than 10 mm Hg DBP with concomitant rise (10% to 20% increase) in pulse (orthostatic hypotension); watch for postural hypotension in hypertensive patients, especially anyone taking diuretics (decreased fluid volume/dehydration)
- Use a manual sphygmomanometer to measure BP during exercise; most automatic units are not designed for this purpose

BP, Blood pressure; *DBP*, diastolic blood pressure; *NSAIDs*, nonsteroidal anti-inflammatory drugs; *SBP*, systolic blood pressure.

---

point of maximal oscillation (vibration) is identified by the device, which corresponds to the mean arterial pressure. Measurements of SBP and DBP are then estimated based on the maximal point of oscillation determined by the device.

Both devices possess unique advantages and disadvantages for BP measurement. The use of automatic oscillometric devices has demonstrated a reduction in the white-coat response (an increase in BP measured in clinic compared to normal BP taken at home) compared with manual measurement[36,37] because it can be done without the clinician present in the room. Automatic oscillometric devices are less susceptible to auscultatory gap (a period of diminished or absent Korotkoff sounds, which can cause SBP to be underestimated) compared to manual measurement.[38] However, due to vibration produced by human movement automatic oscillometric devices cannot accurately measure BP during exercise,[39] while the manual auscultatory method using an aneroid device can be used.

BP Measurement Technique. The standard measurement technique for BP includes having the patient rest in a seated position with their back supported for 5 minutes prior to measurement.[34,40] The patient's feet should be flat on the floor and uncrossed. Considerations for seating options available in each practice setting may vary; however, sitting on the edge of a plinth or treatment table with the feet dangling would be a less than ideal choice since it can cause variations of up to 8 mm Hg.

The arm chosen for measurement should be positioned at the level of the right atrium with the elbow fully extended. The level right atrium can be external located at the midpoint of the sternum or approximately at the midpoint of shoulder flexion. If the measurement site on the arm is placed below the level of the right atrium, the readings will be too high. If the measurement site on the arm is above the level of the right atrium, the readings will be too low.[41] These differences can be attributed to the effects of hydrostatic pressure and may contribute to 2 mm Hg for every inch above or below the heart level.[42] The patient's arm should also be supported to minimize muscle activity during measurement.[41]

The nondominant arm is often recommended for BP measurement, however it is not required and either arm can be used unless it is contraindicated.[41] For the student or clinician learning to take BP, it may be easier to hear the Korotkoff sounds in adults using the left arm because of the closer proximity to the left ventricle. During initial patient encounters, measurement of BP in both arms is often recommended with the higher recording used as the BP for that patient.[29,34] Values should be similar between arms (less than 10 mm Hg difference in SBP between arms).[43] The side and position (supine or sitting or standing) should be documented and BP should be taken in the same arm and in the same position each time it is remeasured. Record BP measurements exactly; do not round numbers up or down as this can result in inaccuracies.[44] Repeated BP measurements should be taken at least 1 minute apart.

Do not apply the BP cuff above an intravenous (IV) line where fluids are infusing or an arteriovenous (AV) shunt, on the same side where breast or axillary surgery has been performed, or when the arm or hand have been traumatized or diseased. Until there is research to support a change, it is recommended that patients who have undergone axillary lymph node dissection (ALND) avoid having BP measurements taken on the affected side. Some oncology staff advise taking BP in the arm with the least amount of nodal dissection. Technique in measuring BP is a key factor in all patients, especially those with ALND (Box 4.8)

Cuff size is important and requires the bladder width-to-length to be at least 1:2. It is generally recommended the cuff should have a bladder length that is 80% and a width that is at least 40% of the arm circumference.[41] BP measurements are overestimated with a cuff that is too small; if a cuff is too small, go to the next size up. Keep in mind that if the cuff is too large, falsely lower BPs may be recorded.[45] It is advised to invest in the purchase of a well-made, reliable stethoscope. Older mod els with tubing long enough to put the earpieces in your ears and still place the bell in a laboratory coat pocket should be replaced. Tubing is normally 65 to 70 cm (26–28 inches), with thicker tubing being better insulated than thinner tubing.[46]

Additional items that may alter the BP measurement and should be controlled for include speaking, sneezing, coughing, and isometric contraction of the surrounding musculature during measurement. Similar to pulse rate, the presence of pain may cause increases in BP but may also have a limited to no effect on BP.[26–28] Furthermore, pain, room temperature, full urinary bladder, overinflated BP cuff bladder, and the speed of cuff deflation (faster than 2–3 mm/s) can impact the reading obtained. Keeping the cuff maximally inflated or deflating the cuff too slowly can also impact BP measurement.

It is more accurate to evaluate consecutive BP readings over time rather than using an isolated measurement for reporting BP abnormalities. BP also should be correlated with any related diet or medication. Before reporting abnormal BP readings, measure both sides for comparison, remeasure both sides, and have another health professional check the readings. Correlate BP measurements with other vital signs, and screen for associated signs and symptoms such as pallor, fatigue, perspiration, and/or palpitations. A persistent rise or fall in BP requires medical attention and possible intervention.

If taking a BP measurement using the leg is the only available alternative, the patient can be seated with the cuff placed on the thigh and the popliteal artery used for auscultation. Systolic BP measured using the leg is reported to be 10% to 20% higher than values taken using the brachial artery.[47]

Pulse Pressure. The difference between the systolic and diastolic pressure readings (SBP–DBP) is called *pulse pressure* normally around 40 mm Hg. Pulse pressure is an index of vascular aging (i.e., loss of arterial compliance and indication of how stiff the arteries are). A widened resting pulse pressure often results from stiffening of the aorta secondary to atherosclerosis. *Resting* pulse pressure consistently greater than 60 to 80 mm Hg is a yellow (caution) flag and is a risk factor for new onset of atrial fibrillation.[48]

Widening of the pulse pressure is linked to a significantly higher risk of stroke and heart failure (HF) after the sixth decade. Some BP medications increase resting pulse pressure width by lowering diastolic pressure more than systolic, whereas others (e.g., angiotensin-converting enzyme [ACE] inhibitors) can lower pulse pressure.[49]

Narrowing of the resting pulse pressure (usually by a drop in SBP as the DBP rises) can suggest HF or a significant blood loss such as occurs during hypovolemic shock. A high pulse pressure accompanied by bradycardia is a sign of increased intracranial pressure and requires immediate medical evaluation.

BOX 4.8 ASSESSING BLOOD PRESSURE

- The patient should avoid tobacco for 30 minutes and caffeine for 60 minutes before BP reading.
- Let the patient sit quietly for 5 minutes; this can help offset the physical exertion of moving to the examination room or the emotional stress of being with a health care professional (white-coat hypertension).
- The patient should be seated comfortably in a chair with the back and arm supported, legs uncrossed, feet on the floor, and not talking.
- Assess for factors that can affect BP (see Table 4.6).
- Position the arm extended in a forward direction (sitting) at the heart's level or parallel to the body (supine); avoid using an arm with a fistula, IV or arterial line, or with a previous history of lymph node biopsy or breast or axillary surgery.
- Wrap the cuff around the patient's upper arm (place over bare skin) so that the lower end of the cuff is 1 inch (2–3 cm) above the antecubital fossa (inside of the elbow); cuff size is critical to accurate measurement.
- The length of the bladder cuff should encircle at least 80% of the upper arm. The width of the cuff should be about 40% of the upper arm circumference. If a cuff is too short or too narrow, the BP reading will be erroneously high; if the cuff is too long or too wide, the BP reading will be erroneously low. BP measurement errors are usually worse in cuffs that are too small compared with those that are too big.
- If you are measuring BP at the ankle, an arm cuff is usually appropriate, but BPs taken at the thigh require a thigh cuff unless the person is very thin.
- Slide your finger under the cuff to make sure it is not too tight.
- Close the valve on the rubber bulb.
- Place the stethoscope (diaphragm or bell side) lightly over the brachial artery which is located slightly lateral to the medial epicondyle at the elbow.

- Inflating the cuff to 180–200 mm Hg should be sufficient for most patients. However, to accurately determine the inflation pression BP use the radial ablation technique.
- Radial Ablation Technique
  1. First palpate the radial artery of the arm you are measuring BP.
  2. Inflate the cuff until you no longer feel a radial artery pulse and then inflate 10–20 mm Hg more g.
  3. Slowly begin to deflate until you feel the radial artery pulse return and record the pressure where it returns.
  4. Add 30 mm Hg to that pressure and use it for your inflation pressure when measuring BP.
- Slowly release the valve on the bulb (deflate at a rate of 2 to 3 mm Hg/second) as you listen for the first Korotkoff sound (two consecutive beats signals the systolic reading) and the last Korotkoff sound (diastolic reading).
- If you are new to BP assessment or if the BP is elevated, check the BP twice. Wait 1–2 minutes and retest. Record date, time of day, patient position, extremity measured (arm or leg, left or right), and results for each reading. Record any factors that might affect BP readings (e.g., recent tobacco use, caffeine intake).
- As soon as the blood begins to flow through the artery again, Korotkoff sounds are heard. The first sounds are tapping sounds that gradually increase in intensity. The initial tapping sound that is heard for at least two consecutive beats is recorded as the SBP.
- The first phase of sound may be followed by a momentary disappearance of sounds that can last from 30 to 40 mm Hg as the needle descends. Following this temporary absence of sound, there are murmuring or swishing sounds (second Korotkoff sound). As deflation of the cuff continues, the sounds become sharper and louder. These sounds represent phase 3. During phase 4, the sounds become muffled rather abruptly and then are followed by silence, which represents phase 5. Phase 5 (the fifth Korotkoff sound or K5), the point at which sounds disappear, is often used as the DBP.

BP, Blood pressure; *DBP*, diastolic blood pressure; *SBP*, systolic blood pressure.
From Pickering TG, Hall JE, Appel LJ, et al. Recommendations for blood pressure measurement in humans and experimental animals. Part 1: blood pressure measurement in humans: a statement for professionals from the subcommittee of professional and public education of the American Heart Association Council on high blood pressure research. *Hypertension.* 2005;45:142–161; Muntner P, Shimbo D, Carey RM, et al. Measurement of blood pressure in humans: a scientific statement from the American Heart Association. *Hypertension.* 2019;73:e35–e66.

In a normal, healthy adult, the pulse pressure generally increases in direct proportion to the intensity of exercise as the SBP increases and DBP stays about the same.[24,50] In a healthy adult, pulse pressure will return to normal within 3 to 10 minutes following moderate exercise.

The key is to watch for pulse pressures that are not accommodating during exercise. Expect to see the systolic rise slightly and the diastolic to stay the same. If the diastolic drops and the systolic rises, or if the pulse width exceeds 100 mm Hg, further assessment and evaluation is needed. Depending on all other parameters (e.g., general health of the patient, past medical history, medications, concomitant associated signs and symptoms), the therapist may monitor pulse pressures over a few sessions and look for a pattern (or lack of pattern) to report if/when generating a medical consult.[51]

Variations in Blood Pressure. There can be some normal variation in SBP from side to side (right extremity compared with left extremity). This is usually no more than 5 to 10 mm Hg DBP or SBP (arms) and 10 to 40 mm Hg SBP (legs). A difference of 10 mm Hg or more in either systolic or diastolic measurements from one extremity to the other may be an indication of vascular problems (look for associated symptoms; in the upper extremity test for thoracic outlet syndrome [TOH]).

Normally the SBP in the legs is 10% to 20% higher than the brachial artery pressure in the arms. BP readings that are lower in the legs compared with the arms are considered abnormal and should prompt a medical referral for assessment of peripheral vascular disease (PVD).[47]

With a change in position (supine to sitting), the normal fluctuation of BP and heart rate increases slightly (about 5 mm Hg for systolic and diastolic pressures and 5 to 10 bpm in heart rate).[52] An orthostatic response to position change would be considered abnormal if the SBP decreases ≥20 mm Hg or the DBP decreases ≥10 mm Hg as the individual moves to a more upright position (sitting to standing). These measures are recommended at a 1- and/or 3-minute time frame after the position change occurs.[53]

Women of reproductive age taking birth control pills may be at an increased risk for hypertension, heart attack, or stroke.[54] The risk of a cardiovascular event is lower with today's low-dose oral contraceptives.[55] However, smoking, hypertension, obesity, undiagnosed cardiac anomalies, and diabetes are factors that increase a woman's risk for cardiovascular events. Any woman using oral contraceptives who presents with consistently elevated BP values must be advised to see her physician for close monitoring and follow-up.

Blood Pressure Changes With Exercise. Systolic pressure increases with exertion in a linear progression. If systolic pressure does not rise as workload increases, or if this pressure falls, it may be an indication that the functional reserve capacity of the heart has been exceeded. Emerging evidence indicates that the measurement of BP during and after exercise may provide a more robust assessment of a patient's hemodynamic stability.[56] As previously mentioned, the SBP increases with an increasing level of activity and exercise in a linear fashion.

The normal SBP response to incremental exercise is a progressive rise, typically 10 mm+2 mm Hg for each MET where 1 MET = 3.5 mL O_2/kg/min with a plateau at peak exercise.[24,50] For example, in a healthy adult an increase in SBP of approximately 20 mm Hg would be expected with light intensity activity (slow walking) and up to a 40 to 50 with moderate to high intensity exercise.[57] Increases in SBP during physical activity and exercise may be attenuated in individuals taking BP medications, and those with cardiac valve disease. Additionally, individuals with hypertension may demonstrate an exaggerated BP response to exercise.[56,57] Normally, diastolic BP should not change much with physical activity and may actually decrease slightly.[24,50]

In an exercise-testing situation, the American College of Sports Medicine (ACSM) recommends stopping the test if the SBP exceeds 250 mm Hg or if DBP exceeds 115 mm Hg.[24] In a clinical setting without the benefit of cardiac monitoring, exercise or activity should be reduced or stopped if the systolic pressure exceeds 200 mm Hg or if diastolic increases greater than 10 mm Hg from baseline. Exercise testing would be contraindicated with a resting SBP exceeds 200 mm Hg systolic or a DBP exceeding 110 mm Hg.[58,59] DBP increases during upper extremity exercise or isometric exercise involving any muscle group.

Activity or exercise should be monitored closely, decreased, or halted if the diastolic pressure exceeds 100 mm Hg.

This is a general (conservative) guideline when exercising a patient without the benefit of cardiac testing (e.g., electrocardiogram [ECG]). This stop-point is based on the ACSM guideline to stop exercise testing at 115 mm Hg DBP.[24,59]

Other warning signs to moderate or stop exercising include the onset of angina, dyspnea, and heart palpitations. Monitor the patient for other signs and symptoms such as fever, dizziness, nausea/vomiting, pallor, extreme diaphoresis, muscular cramping or weakness, and incoordination. Always honor the patient's desire to slow down or stop.

Hypertension. In recent years, an unexpected increase in illness and death caused by hypertension has prompted the National Institutes of Health to issue new guidelines for more effective BP control. The rate of hypertension (HTN)-associated mortality has increased by 23% while the combined mortality rate for all other causes has decreased by 21%.[60,61] (See further discussion of hypertension in Chapter 7).[61] Differences in HTN prevalence have been observed among between socioeconomic and ethnic groups. These concerning figures may due to the asymptomatic nature of HTN even at critical values (>180/120 mm Hg). This asymptomatic nature of HTN has caused awareness, treatment, and effective control to be significant challenges facing the medical system In fact, the Center for Disease Control and Prevention reports that among individuals[61] who are aware of their HTN diagnosis and who receive treatment, only slightly under 50% are effectively controlled.[62] Therefore, it is imperative that physical therapists include routine assessment of BP in the clinic as part of their medical screening.

In adults, hypertension is a systolic pressure above 130 mm Hg or a diastolic pressure above 80 mm Hg.[63] Consistent SBP measurements between 120 and 129 (systolic) with a DBP less than between 80 mm Hg is classified as elevated.[63] The overall goal of treating patients with hypertension is to prevent morbidity and mortality associated with high BP. The specific objective is to achieve and maintain arterial BP below 120/80 mm Hg, if possible[63].

The older adult taking nonsteroidal anti-inflammatory drugs (NSAIDs) is at risk for increased BP because these drugs are potent renal vasoconstrictors. Monitor BP carefully in these patients and look for sacral and lower extremity edema. Document and report these findings to the physician. Always be aware of *masked hypertension* (normal in the clinic but periodically high at home) and *white-coat hypertension*, a clinical condition in which the patient has elevated BP levels when measured in a clinic setting by a health care professional.[21]

The prevalence of masked hypertension ranges between 14% and 30% in adults with normal in-clinic BP readings. Patients with masked hypertension tend to demonstrate an exaggerated BP response to exercise and physical activity.[64] The prevalence of exaggerated BP response to exercise in individuals with masked HTN has been reported to be 41%.[65] Therefore, assessing BP response to exercise may assist with screening for masked hypertension and help facilitate appropriate medical management.[21] White-coat hypertension occurs in 15% to 20% of adults with stage 1 hypertension.[66] Antihypertensive treatment for white-coat hypertension may reduce office BP but may not affect ambulatory BP. The number of adults who develop a sustained high BP is much higher among those who have masked or white-coat hypertension.[66]

At-home BP measurements can help identify adults with masked hypertension, white-coat hypertension, ambulatory hypertension, and individuals who do not experience the usual nocturnal drop in BP (decrease of 15 mm Hg), which is a risk factor for cardiovascular events.[67] Excessive morning BP surge is a predictor of stroke in older adults with known hypertension and is also a red-flag sign.[68] Medical referral is indicated in any of these situations.

Hypertension in Children and Adolescents. Between 2% and 4% of children under the age of 18 years also have hypertension.[69] Guidelines for children and adolescents by age and height have been published by the American Academy of Pediatrics[70] (see Table 4.4).[70] These new guidelines for children and adolescents use terminology and classifications in accordance to the revised guidelines for adults (i.e., replacement of Prehypertension with elevated blood pressure). The guidelines for adolescents between 13 and 18 years are fairly similar to adults (Table 4.4). The guidelines for children under 13 years of age are based on *child height percentiles*. Any child with readings above the 95th percentile for gender, age, and height on three separate occasions is considered to have hypertension. Under the guidelines, children whose readings fall between the 90th and 95th percentile are now considered to have elevated BP (previously pre-HTN).

The long-term health risks for hypertensive children and adolescents can be substantial; therefore, it is important that elevated BP is recognized early and measures are taken to reduce risks and optimize health outcomes.[70] Guidelines for concerning BP measurement values according to age for both boys and girls is provided. Children ages 3 to 18 years seen in any medical setting should have their BP measured at least once during each health care episode. Either manual auscultatory measurement using an aneroid BP cuff and stethoscope or an automatic oscillometric device calibrated for pediatric patients may be used to measure BP in children.[70] Correct measurement requires a cuff that is appropriate to the size of the child's upper arm. If the appropriate cuff size for the child is difficult to determine, the midarm circumference (measured as the midpoint between the acromion of the scapula and olecranon of the elbow, with the shoulder in a neutral position and the elbow flexed to 90°) should be obtained for an accurate determination of the correct cuff size. Clinics managing pediatric cases should have access to a wide range of cuff sizes, including a thigh cuff for use in children and adolescents with severe obesity. If the initial BP is elevated, clinicians should perform two additional BP measurements (either oscillometric or auscultatory) in the same visit and average them. The right arm is preferred with children for comparison with

standard tables unless the child presents with atypical aortic anatomy such as coarctation of the aorta (see Fig. 6.6).

Preparation of the child can affect the BP level as much as technique. The child should be seated with feet and back supported. The right arm should be supported parallel to the floor with the cubital fossa at heart level.[70] Children can be affected by white-coat hypertension as much as adults. Follow the same guidelines for adults as presented in Box 4.8.

See Further Discussion on Hypertension in Chapter 7.

Hypotension. Hypotension is a systolic pressure below 90 mm Hg or a diastolic pressure below 60 mm Hg. A BP level that is borderline low for one person may be normal for another. When the BP is too low, there is inadequate blood flow to the heart, brain, and other vital organs.

The most important factor in hypotension is how the BP changes from the normal condition. Most normal BPs are in the range of 100/60 mm Hg to 120/80 mm Hg, but a significant change, even as little as 20 mm Hg, can cause problems for some people.

Lower standing SBP (less than 140 mm Hg), even within the normotensive range, is an independent predictor of loss of balance and falls in adults over the age of 65 years.[68,71] DBP does not appear to be related to falls. Older adult women with lower standing SBP and a history of falls are at greatest risk. The therapist has an important role in educating patients with these risk factors in preventing falls and related accidents. See discussion in Chapter 2 related to taking a history of falls.

Postural (Orthostatic) Hypotension. A common cause of low BP is postural (orthostatic) hypotension, defined as a sudden drop in BP when changing positions, usually moving from supine to an upright position.

Physiologic responses of the sympathetic nervous system decline with aging, putting them at a greater risk for this condition. Older adults are prone to falls from a combination of postural hypotension and antihypertensive medications. Volume depletion (dehydration) and autonomic dysfunction are the most common causes (see Table 2.5).

Postural (orthostatic) hypotension is more accurately diagnosed as a sustained decrease in SBP of at least 20 mm Hg *or* decrease in diastolic pressure of at least 10 mm Hg within 3 minutes of standing. (Box 4.9 and Case Example 4.1).[72]

The patient should lie supine for at least 5 minutes before BP and pulse check. At least a 1-minute wait is recommended after each subsequent position change before taking the BP and pulse. Standing postural orthostatic hypotension is measured after 2 to 5 minutes of quiet standing. Throughout the procedure assess the patient for signs and symptoms of hypotension, including dizziness, lightheadedness, pallor, diaphoresis, or syncope (or arrhythmias if using a cardiac monitor). Assist the patient to a seated or supine position if any of these symptoms develop and report the results. Do not test the patient in the standing position if signs and symptoms of hypotension occur while sitting. It may be prudent to get the patient from supine to sitting first, then to standing.

BOX 4.9   ORTHOSTATIC HYPOTENSION

For a diagnosis of Orthostatic hypotension, the patient must have:

- Decrease of at least 20 mm Hg of systolic pressure SBP OR
- Decrease of 10 mm Hg (or more) DBP

These changes occur with change in position (within 3 minutes of standing). Another measurement after 1 to 5 minutes of standing may identify orthostatic hypotension missed by earlier readings.

A condition known as initial orthostatic hypotension is defined as a decrease in SBP of >20 mm Hg and/or a decrease in DBP of >20 mm Hg presenting within the first 15 seconds of standing and correcting within 30 to 60 seconds.

Monitor the patient carefully because fainting is a possible risk with low BP, especially when combined with the dehydrating effects of diuretics. Patients receiving chemotherapy who are hypotensive are also at risk for dizziness and loss of balance during the repeated BP measurement in the standing position.

This repetition is useful in the older adult (65 years old or older). Waiting to repeat the BP measurements reveals a patient's inability to regulate BP after a change in position. The presence of low BP after a prolonged time is a red-flag finding. Be sure to check pulse rate.[29]

Postural orthostatic tachycardia syndrome (POTS): Patients with clinical symptoms of orthostatic intolerance who demonstrate a sustained increase in heart rate of ≥30 bpm when moving from a recumbent to a standing position held for more than 30 seconds (or ≥ 40 bpm in individuals 12 to 19 years of age); and the absence of orthostatic hypotension. These patients may also report as well as palpitations, tremulousness, generalized weakness, blurred vision, exercise intolerance, and fatigue to be classified as POTS the symptoms event must occur in the absence of sustained orthostatic hypotension (decrease in systolic blood pressure > 20 mm Hg or diastolic blood pressure > 10 mm Hg within 3 minutes of standing). However, transient initial orthostatic hypotension (lasting < 1 minute) does not preclude or rule out the diagnosis of POTS.

BP, Blood pressure; *DBP*, diastolic blood pressure; *SBP*, systolic blood pressure.

In patients on prolonged bed rest or those taking antihypertensive drug therapy, there may be either no reflexive increase in heart rate or a sluggish vasomotor response. These patients may experience larger drops in BP and often experience light-headedness.

Other patients at risk for postural orthostatic hypotension include those who have just donated blood, anyone with autonomic nervous system disease or dysfunction, and postoperative patients. Other risk factors for orthostatic hypotension in aging adults include hypovolemia associated with dehydration and the overuse of diuretics, anticholinergic medications, antiemetics, and various over-the-counter (OTC) cough/cold preparations.

CASE EXAMPLE 4.1

Vital Signs

A 74-year-old retired homemaker had a total hip replacement (THR) two days ago. She remains as an inpatient with complications related to heart failure (HF). She has a previous medical history of gallbladder removal 20 years ago, total hysterectomy 30 years ago, and surgically induced menopause with subsequent onset of hypertension.

Her medications include intravenous (IV) furosemide (Lasix), digoxin, and potassium replacement.

During the initial physical therapy intervention, the patient complained of muscle cramping and headache but was able to complete the entire exercise protocol. Blood pressure was 100/76 mm Hg. Systolic measurement dropped to 90 mm Hg when the patient moved from supine to standing. Pulse rate was 56 bpm with a pattern of irregular beats. Pulse rate did not change with postural change. Platelet count was 98,000 cells/mm³ when it was measured yesterday.

What is the significance of her vital signs? How would you use vital sign monitoring in a patient like this?

Nurses will be monitoring the patient's signs and symptoms closely. Read the chart to stay up with what everyone else knows about the patient and/or has observed. Read the physician's notes to see what, if any, medical intervention has been ordered based on laboratory values (e.g., platelet levels) or vital signs (e.g., changes in medication).

Do not hesitate to discuss concerns and observations with the nursing staff. This helps them know you are aware of the medical side of care, but also gives you some perspective from the nursing side. What do they see as significant? What requires immediate medical attention?

Be sure to report anything observed but not already recorded in the chart such as muscle cramping, headache, irregular heartbeat with bradycardia, low pulse, and orthostatic hypotension.

Bradycardia is one of the first signs of digitalis toxicity. In some hospitals, a pulse less than 60 bpm in an adult would mean withholding the next dose of digoxin and necessitate physician contact. The protocol may be different from institution to institution.

In this case report and document:

1. Irregular heartbeat with bradycardia (a possible sign of digoxin/digitalis toxicity).
2. Muscle cramping (possible side effect of Lasix) and headache (possible side effect of digoxin).
3. Always chart vital signs; her blood pressure was not too unusual and pulse rate did not change with position change (probably because of medications) so she does not have medically defined orthostatic hypotension.
4. The response of vital signs to exercise must be monitored carefully and charted; monitor vital signs throughout intervention. Record the time it takes for the patient's vital signs to return to normal after exercise or treatment. This can be used as a means of documenting measurable outcomes. The patient may not ambulate any further or faster in the afternoon compared with the morning, but her vital signs may reflect closer to normal values and a faster return to homeostasis as a measurable outcome.

Core Body Temperature

Normal core body temperature is not a specific number but a range of values that depends on factors such as the time of day,

TABLE 4.7	Core Body Temperature	
Location	Men	Women
Oral	Average: 36.7° C (98.1 °F) Range: 35.7 to 37.7° C (96.26 to 99.86° F)	Average: 36.2° C (97.2° F) Range: 33.2 to 38.1° C (91.8 to 100.6° F)
Rectal	Average: 37° C (98.6° F) Range: 36.7 to 37.5° C (98.1 to 99.5° F)	Average: 37.0° C (98.6° F) Range: 36.8 to 37.1° C (98.2 to 98.8° F)
Tympanic membrane	Average: 36.5° C (97.7° F) Range: 35.5 to 37.5° C (95.9 to 99.5° F)	Average: 36.6° C (97.9° F) Range: 35.7 to 37.5° C (96.3 to 99.5° F)

Data from Ng DK, Chan CH, Chan EY, Kwok KL, Chow PY, Lau WF, Ho JC. A brief report on the normal range of forehead temperature as determined by noncon-tact, handheld, infrared thermometer. *Am J Infect Control.* 2005 May;33(4):227-9. doi: 10.1016/j.ajic.2005.01.003. PMID: 15877017; PMCID: PMC7115295.

age, medical status, medication use, activity level, or presence of infection. Core body temperature generally ranges from 36° to 37.5° C (96.8° to 99.5° F), with an average of 37° C (98.6° F)[73] (Table 4.7). Hypothermic core body temperature is defined as less than 35° C (95° F).[74] Hyperthermia/fever is defined as a temperature greater than 38° C (100.4° F).

Older adults (over the age of 65 years) are less likely to have a fever even in the presence of severe infection, so the predictive value of taking the body temperature is less. Because of age-related changes in the thermoregulatory system, they are also more likely to develop hypothermia than young adults. There is a tendency among the aging population to develop an increase in temperature once in response to any change in homeostasis caused by altered thermoregulation. However, some persons with infectious disease remain afebrile, especially the immunocompromised and those with chronic renal disease, and alcoholics. Older adults experience a reduced febrile response due to age-related alterations thermoregulation and a decrease in mean body temperature.[75] A low-grade fever can be an early sign of a life-threatening infection (most commonly pneumonia, urinary tract infection). Unexplained fever in may also be a manifestation of drug abuse.[76]

Postoperative fever is common and may be from an infectious or noninfectious cause. Medical evaluation is needed to make this determination. In the home health setting, wound infection, abscess formation, or peritonitis may appear as a hectic fever pattern 3 to 4 days postoperatively with increases and declines in body temperature but no return to baseline (normal). Such a situation would warrant a telephone consultation with the physician's nurse.

Any patient who has back, shoulder, hip, sacroiliac, or groin pain of unknown cause must have a temperature reading taken. Temperature should also be assessed for any patient who has constitutional symptoms (see Box 1.3), especially gradual increase followed by a sudden drop in body temperature, pain, or symptoms of unknown etiologic basis, and for patients who

have not been medically screened by a physician. Ask about the presence of other signs and symptoms of infection.

When measuring body temperature, the therapist should ask if the person's normal temperature differs from 37° C (98.6° F). A persistent elevation of temperature over time is a red-flag sign; a single measurement may not be sufficient to cause concern. Any measurement outside of normal for that individual should be rechecked.

It is also important to ask whether the patient has taken aspirin (or other NSAIDs) or acetaminophen (Tylenol) to reduce the fever, which might mask an underlying problem. Anyone who is chronically immunosuppressed (such as a recipient of organ transplant, a person being treated with chemotherapy, and any older adult) may have an infection without elevation of temperature.

Temperature can be taken orally, rectally, via armpit (axillary), via ear (tympanic) or at the forehead using an infrared thermometer. Follow the manufacturer information regarding the proper use of the thermometer to obtain the most accurate results. Temperatures can vary from side to side, therefore it is important to record which ear was used and try to use the same ear each time the temperature is recorded. For the patient with hearing aid(s), take the temperature in the ear without an aid. Or, if hearing aids are present in both ears, remove one hearing aid and wait 20 minutes before measuring that side. The presence of excessive earwax will prevent an accurate reading.

Handheld digital forehead infrared thermometers are noninvasive and are quick and easy to use. The forehead plastic temperature strip (fever strip) and the pacifier thermometer for children are not the most reliable methods to take a temperature.

The therapist should use discretionary caution with any patient who has a fever. Exercise with a fever stresses the cardiopulmonary system, which may be further complicated by dehydration. Severe dehydration can occur from vomiting, diarrhea, medications (e.g., diuretics), or heat exhaustion.

CLINICAL SIGNS AND SYMPTOMS
Dehydration

Mild
- Thirst
- Dry mouth, dry lips

Moderate
- Very dry mouth, cracked lips
- Sunken eyes, sunken fontanel (infants)
- Poor skin turgor (see Fig. 4.4)
- Postural hypotension
- Headache

Severe
- All signs of moderate dehydration
- Rapid, weak pulse (more than 100 bpm at rest)
- Rapid breathing
- Confusion, lethargy, irritability
- Cold hands and feet
- Unable to cry or urinate

Patients at greatest risk of dehydration include postoperative patients, aging adults, and athletes. Severe fluid volume deficit can cause vascular collapse and shock. Patients at risk of shock include burn or trauma patients, patients in anaphylactic shock or diabetic ketoacidosis, and individuals experiencing severe blood loss.

CLINICAL SIGNS AND SYMPTOMS
Shock

Stage 1 (Early Stage)
- Restlessness, anxiety, hyperalert
- Listless, lack of interest in play (children)
- Tachycardia
- Increased respiratory rate, shallow breathing, frequent sighs
- Rapid, bounding pulse (not weak)
- Distended neck veins
- Skin warm and flushed
- Thirst, nausea, vomiting

Stage 2
- Confusion, lack of focused eye contact (vacant look)
- Abrupt changes in affect or behavior
- No crying or excessive, unexplained crying in infant
- Cold, clammy skin, profuse sweating, chills
- Weak pulses (not bounding)
- Hypotension (low BP), dizziness, fainting
- Collapsed neck veins
- Weak or absent peripheral pulses
- Muscle tension

Stage 3 (Late Stage)
- Cyanosis (blue lips, gray skin)
- Dull eyes, dilated pupils
- Loss of bowel or bladder control
- Change in level of consciousness

Walking Speed: The Sixth Vital Sign

Walking speed is used by some as a general indicator of function[77] and as such, a reflection of many variables such as health status, motor control, muscle strength, and endurance to name only a few. It is a reliable, valid, and sensitive measure of functional ability with an additional predictive value in assessing future health status, functional decline, potential for hospitalization, and even mortality.[78]

The test involves measuring the time it takes for a patient to walk a specified distance on a level surface. The distances used to measure gait speed are typically short as this is not intended to be used as a measure of endurance. The most used protocol involves measuring gait speed over a course of 5 meters in length with 5 feet on either end for acceleration and deceleration,[79] Another popular protocol involves a 10-meter course with 2 meters on either end for acceleration and deceleration.[79] Complete descriptions of the test and expected results are available.[78] As a screening tool, walking speed may not indicate the presence of systemic pathology, but as specialists in human movement and function, the therapist can use it as a practical and predictive "vital sign" of general health that can be used to monitor change (improvement or decline) in health and function.[78]

TECHNIQUES OF PHYSICAL EXAMINATION

There are four simple techniques used in the medical physical examination: inspection, auscultation, percussion, and palpation. When all are performed together, such as in an abdominal screening examination, they are performed in the order listed. Most percussion and some auscultation techniques require advanced clinical skill and are beyond the scope of a typical screening examination.

The screening examination primarily focuses on the integument, musculoskeletal, neuromuscular, and cardiopulmonary systems, although consideration must made for other systems, such as the GI system. The saying, "What one knows, one sees" underscores the idea that knowledge of physical assessment techniques and experience in performing these are extremely important and come from practice. Assessment techniques are relatively simple; using the finding in a clinical decision-making context is more difficult. The results from inspection, auscultation, percussion (when appropriate), and palpation should always be correlated with the patient's history, risk factors, clinical presentation, and any associated signs and symptoms before making the decision regarding medical referral.

Inspection

Inspection is visual observation. Good lighting and exposure are essential, with clear instruction to the patient for the need of exposure and offer of a chaperone. Always compare one side to the other. Observe for abnormalities in all the following: location, size, position, alignment, color, shape, contour, mobility, and symmetry.

The therapist should try to use a systematic approach to inspection every time to decrease the chance of missing an assessment parameter and to increase accuracy and thoroughness.

Auscultation

Auscultation usually follows inspection, palpation, and percussion (when percussion is performed). The one exception is during examination of the abdomen, which should be assessed in this order: inspection, auscultation, percussion, then palpation, as percussion and palpation can affect the findings of auscultation.

Some sounds of the body can be heard with the unaided ear; others must be heard by auscultation using a stethoscope. Pressing too hard on the skin with the stethoscope can obliterate sounds. The bell side of the stethoscope is used to listen to low-pitched sounds such as heart murmurs and BP (although the diaphragm can also be used for BP). The diaphragm side of the stethoscope is used to listen to high-pitched sounds such as normal heart sounds, bowel sounds, and friction rubs. Avoid placing your thumb on the bell or the diaphragm when holding the stethoscope to avoid hearing your own pulse.

Besides measuring BP, auscultation can be used to listen for breath sounds, heart sounds, bowel sounds, and abnormal sounds in the blood vessels called bruits. Bruits are abnormal blowing or swishing sounds heard during auscultation as blood travels through narrowed or obstructed arteries such as the aorta or the renal, iliac, or femoral arteries. Bruits with both systolic and diastolic components suggest turbulent blood flow due to partial arterial occlusion from a possible aneurysm or vessel constriction. All large arteries in the neck, abdomen, and limbs can be examined for bruits. Physical therapists may assess bowel sounds if performing an abdominal screening examination.

A medical assessment (e.g., physician, nurse, physician assistant) may routinely include auscultation of the temporal and carotid arteries, jugular vein in the head and neck, and vascular sounds in the abdomen (e.g., aorta, iliac, femoral, and renal arteries). The therapist is more likely to assess for bruits when the patient's history (e.g., age over 65 years, history of coronary artery disease), clinical presentation (e.g., neck, back, abdominal, or flank pain), and associated signs and symptoms (e.g., syncopal episodes, signs and symptoms of PVD) warrant additional physical assessment.

Percussion

Percussion (tapping) is used to determine the size, shape, and density of tissue using sound created by vibration. Percussion can also detect the presence of fluid or air in a body cavity, such as the abdominal cavity. Most percussive techniques are beyond the scope of a screening examination and are therefore not discussed in detail.

Percussion can be done directly over the patient's skin using the fingertip of the examiner's index finger. Indirect percussion is performed by placing the middle finger of the examiner's nondominant hand firmly against the patient's skin then striking above or below the interphalangeal joint with the pad of the middle finger of the dominant hand. The palm and other fingers stay off the skin during indirect percussion. Blunt percussion using the ulnar surface of the hand or fist to strike the body surface (directly or indirectly) detects pain from infection or inflammation, such as with Murphy's percussion test (see Fig. 4.53).

The examiner must be careful not to dampen the sound by dull percussing (sharp percussion is needed), holding a finger too loosely on the body surface, or resting the hand on the body surface. Percussive sounds lie on a continuum from tympany to flat, depending on the density of the tissue.

Palpation

Palpation is used to discriminate tenderness, textures, dimensions, shape, contour, consistencies, tissue mobility, and temperature. It is used to define things that are inspected and to reveal things that cannot be inspected. Known tender or painful areas are assessed last while carefully observing the patient's face for nonverbal signs of discomfort. Inspection and palpation are often performed at the same time (other than during the abdominal examination). When performing palpation, be sure to look at the patient for both verbal and nonverbal responses and not just at your hands. Muscle tension interferes with palpation so the patient must be positioned and draped appropriately in a room with adequate lighting and temperature. Patients must be appropriately draped and should be given the opportunity to have a chaperone present, especially for any examination of sensitive areas.

Different parts of the therapist's hands are useful for different aspects of palpation. Assess skin temperature with both hands at the same time. The back of the therapist's hands sense temperature best because of the thin layer of skin. Use the palm or heel of the hand to assess for vibration. The finger pads are best to assess texture, size, shape, position, pulsation, consistency, and turgor. Dimensions or contours are detected using several fingers, the entire hand, or both hands, depending on the area being examined.

Light palpation is used first, assessing for areas of tenderness followed by deep palpation to examine organs, assess for masses, or elicit deep pain. Light palpation (skin is depressed up to ¼ to ½ inch) is also used to assess texture, temperature, moisture, pulsations, vibrations, and superficial lesions. Deep palpation is used for assessing abdominal structures. During deep palpation, enough pressure is used to depress the skin up to 1 inch while assessing patient response and then comfortably releasing the pressure. Heavy or prolonged pressure dulls the examiner's palpatory skill and sensation, and may be uncomfortable for the patient.

INTEGUMENTARY SCREENING EXAMINATION

Therapists should always use standard precautions when assessing skin conditions of any kind, even benign lesions such as psoriasis (Fig. 4.2) or eczema, because any skin disruption increases the risk of infection for both the patient and the therapist. Consideration of all findings in relation to the patient's age, ethnicity, occupation, and general health is essential. Assessment of latex allergy or sensitivity is important, as this will necessitate the use of latex-free equipment during their care.

When screening for systemic disease, the therapist must increase attention to what is observable on the outside via inspection, primarily the skin and nail beds. Changes in the skin and nail beds may be the first sign of inflammatory, infectious, and immunologic disorders. The presence of skin lesions may point to a problem with the integumentary system or may be an integumentary response to a systemic problem. For example, dermatitis can occur 6 to 8 weeks before primary signs and symptoms of pulmonary malignancy develop. Clubbing of the fingers can occur quickly in various acute illnesses and conditions. Skin, hair, and nail bed changes are common with endocrine disorders. Early recognition of the signs and symptoms of herpes zoster virus (Shingles) can result in rapid initiation of medication therapy. Renal disease, rheumatic disorders, and

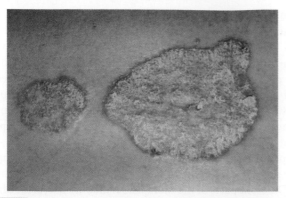

Fig. 4.2   Psoriasis. A common chronic skin disorder characterized by red patches covered by thick, dry silvery scales that are the result of excessive buildup of epithelial cells. Lesions often come and go and can be anywhere on the body but are most common on extensor surfaces, bony prominences, scalp, ears, and genitals. Arthritis of the small joints of the hands often accompanies the skin disease (psoriatic arthritis). (From Lookingbill DP, Marks JG. Principles of Dermatology. 3rd ed. Philadelphia: WB Saunders; 2000.)

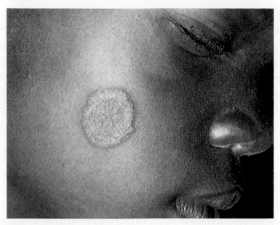

Fig. 4.3   Tinea corporis, or ringworm of the body, presents anywhere on the body of an adult or child but is more commonly seen on the chest, abdomen, back of the arms, face, and dorsum of the feet. The circular lesions with clear centers can form singly or in clusters and represent a fungal infection that is both contagious and treatable. Tinea pedis (not shown), also known as ringworm of the feet or "athlete's foot," occurs most often between the toes, but also along the sides of the feet and the soles (easily spread and treatable). (From Hurwitz S. Clinical Pediatric Dermatology: A Textbook of Skin Disorders of Childhood and Adolescence. 2nd ed. Philadelphia: WB Saunders; 1993.)

autoimmune diseases are all accompanied by skin and nail bed changes in many physical therapy patients.

Pruritus, or itch, is very common among aging adults. The natural attrition of glands that moisturize the skin combined with the effects of sun exposure, medications, excessive bathing, and harsh soaps can result in dry, irritable skin.[80] However, pruritus is the most common manifestation of dermatologic disease, and is also a symptom of underlying systemic disease in 10% to 50% of individuals who seek medical help for the condition.[81] In both situations, skin rash is a common accompanying sign. The most common visceral systems causing pruritus include the renal system in individuals with terminal renal disease undergoing dialysis, and the hepatic systems. Look for associated signs and symptoms of liver or gallbladder impairment such as jaundice, liver flap (asterixis), carpal tunnel syndrome, liver palms (palmar erythema), and spider angiomas (see Fig. 9.3).

The therapist may see scratch marks or even broken skin where the sufferer has scratched violently. Open, red (often bleeding) sores appear most commonly on the face and arms but can be anywhere on the body. These lesions can become inflamed, swollen, and pus-filled in the presence of a *Staphylococcus* infection. Left untreated, pathogens can enter the bloodstream, causing dangerous sepsis or deeper abscess. There is no cure, but medical evaluation is needed; topical treatment and cryotherapy can help, and antibiotic treatment is needed when there is an infection.

New onset of skin lesions, especially in children, should be medically evaluated (Fig. 4.3). Many conditions in adults and children can be treated effectively; some, but not all, can be cured.

Skin Assessment

With the possible exception of a dermatologist, the therapist sees more skin than anyone else in the health care system. Patients are more likely to point out skin lesions or ask the therapist about lumps and bumps. It is important to have a working knowledge of benign versus pathologic skin lesions and know when to refer appropriately.

The hands, arms, feet, and legs can be assessed throughout the physical therapy examination for changes in texture, color, temperature, clubbing, circulation including capillary filling, and edema. Abnormal textural changes include shiny, stiff, coarse, dry, or scaly skin.

Skin mobility and turgor are affected by the fluid status of the patient. Dehydration and aging reduce skin turgor (Fig. 4.4), and edema decreases skin mobility. The physical therapist should have a thorough understanding of signs and symptoms of dehydration, as discussed in the previous section on core body temperature.

The therapist should be aware that many common medications can cause skin to become sensitive to sunlight. Common classes of medications causing skin reactions to sunlight include antibiotics, nonsteroidal anti-inflammatory medications, diuretics, retinoids, hypoglycemics, HMG-CoA reductase inhibitors (statins), neuroleptic drugs, and antifungals.[82] A full understanding of patient medications, the reason for medication use, and possible side effects are important considerations during the screening examination. Mobility-impaired or hospitalized patients should be examined frequently for signs of skin breakdown. Check all pressure points, including the ears, back of the head, scapulae, shoulders, sacrum, area over the greater trochanters, heels, and malleoli. Document staging of any pressure injuries (Table 4.8).

The pressure injury staging system, updated in 2016 by The National Pressure Injury Advisory Panel, is an anatomic description of tissue destruction or wound depth designed for

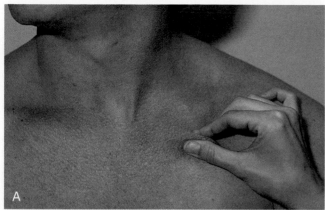

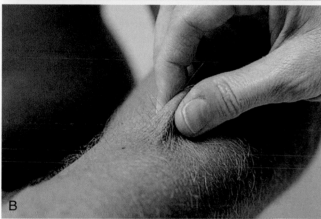

Fig. 4.4   To check skin turgor (elasticity or resiliency), gently pinch the skin between your thumb and forefinger, lifting it up slightly, then release. Skin turgor can be tested on the forehead or sternum, beneath the clavicle (A), and over the extensor surface of the arm (B) or hand. Expect to see the skin lift up easily and return to place quickly. The test is positive for decreased turgor (often caused by dehydration) when the pinched skin remains lifted for 5 seconds or more after its release and returns to normal very slowly. (A From Seidel HM. Mosby's Guide to Physical Examination. 7th ed. St. Louis: Mosby; 2011. B From Potter P, Perry A. Basic Nursing: Essentials for Practice. 6th ed. St. Louis: Mosby; 2007.)

TABLE 4.8	Staging of Pressure Injury

The National Pressure Injury Advisory Panel (NPIAP) now recommends the use of "pressure injury" to replace "pressure ulcer" as localized "damage to the skin and/or underlying tissue usually over a bony prominence or related to a medical or other device. The injury occurs as a result of intense and/or prolonged pressure or pressure in combination with shear" (see citation below).

Stage	Highlights
Stage 1	Skin intact; localized area of nonblanchable erythema
Stage 2	Dermis exposed; partial thickness skin loss
Stage 3	Fat (adipose visible; full-thickness skin loss; visible slough and/or eschar)
Stage 4	Involvement of muscle, bone, tendon, joint capsule, or other supporting structures; full-thickness tissue and skin loss

Complete updated staging system available online at https://npiap.com/page/PressureInjuryStages.

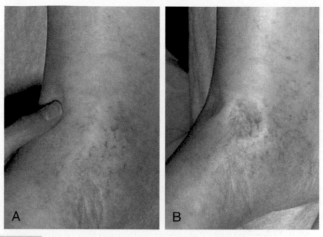

Fig. 4.5   Pitting edema in a patient with cardiac failure. A depression ("pit") remains in the edema for some minutes after firm fingertip pressure is applied. (A) Represents the firm fingertip pressure, (B) represents the depression or pit that remains for an amount of time after the fingertip pressure. (From Forbes CD, Jackson WD. Color Atlas and Text of Clinical Medicine. 3rd ed. London: Mosby; 2003.)

use only with pressure ulcers or wounds created by pressure.[83] Although it is essential to have this information, it is also very important to document other wound characteristics, such as location, size, drainage, and granulation tissue to make the wound assessment complete.

Coordinate with nursing staff to remove prostheses, restraints, and dressings to look beneath them. Anyone with an IV line, catheter, or other insertion site must be examined for signs of infiltration (e.g., pus, erythema), phlebitis, and tape burns.

Observe for signs of edema, which is an accumulation of fluid in the interstitial space. Pitting edema, in which pressing a finger into the skin leaves an indentation, often indicates a chronic condition (e.g., chronic kidney failure, liver failure, congestive heart failure [CHF]) but can occur acutely as well (e.g., face) (Fig. 4.5). The location of edema helps identify the potential cause. Bilateral edema of the legs may be seen in patients with HF or with chronic venous insufficiency.

Abdominal and leg edema can be seen in patients with heart disease, cirrhosis of the liver (or other liver impairment), and protein malnutrition. Edema may also be noted in dependent areas, such as the sacrum, when a person is confined to bed. Localized edema in one extremity may be the result of venous obstruction (thrombosis) or lymphatic blockage of the extremity (lymphedema).

Change in Skin Temperature

Skin temperature can be an indication of vascular supply. A handheld, noninvasive, infrared thermometer can be used to measure skin surface temperature. The most common use of this device is for temperature observation and comparison of both feet in individuals with diabetes for the purpose of identifying increased skin temperatures, intended as an early warning of inflammation, impending infection, and possible foot ulceration. Temperature differences of four or more degrees Fahrenheit between the right and left foot is a predictive risk factor for foot ulcers; self-monitoring has been shown to reduce the risk of ulceration in high-risk individuals.[84]

Other signs and symptoms of vascular changes of an affected extremity may include edema, paresthesia, muscle fatigue and discomfort, or cyanosis with numbness, pain, and loss of hair from a reduced blood supply (Box 4.10).

Change in Skin Color

Capillary filling of the fingers and toes is an indicator of peripheral circulation. Perform a capillary refill test by pressing down on the nail bed and releasing. Observe first for blanching (whitening) followed by return of color within 3 seconds after release of pressure (normal response).

Skin color changes can occur with a variety of illnesses and systemic conditions. Patients may notice a change in their skin color before anyone else does, so be sure and ask about it. Look for pallor; increased or decreased pigmentation; yellow, green, or red skin color; and cyanosis.

Color changes are often observed first in the fingernails, lips, mucous membranes, conjunctiva of the eye, and palms and soles of dark-skinned people.

Skin changes associated with impairment of the hepatic system include jaundice, pallor, and orange or green skin.

In some situations, jaundice may be the first and only manifestation of disease. It is first noticeable in the sclera of the eye as a yellow hue when bilirubin levels reach 2 to 3 mg/dL. Dark-skinned persons may have a normal yellow color to the outer sclera. Jaundice involves the whole sclera up to the iris.

When the bilirubin level reaches 5 to 6 mg/dL, the skin becomes yellow. Other skin and nail bed changes associated with liver disease include palmar erythema (see Fig. 10.6), spider angiomas (see Fig. 9.5), and nails of Terry (see Fig. 10.7; see further discussion in Chapter 10).

A bluish cast to skin color can occur with cyanosis when oxygen levels are reduced in the arterial blood (central cyanosis) or when blood is oxygenated normally but blood flow is decreased and slow (peripheral cyanosis). Cyanosis is first observed in the hands and feet, lips, and nose as a pale blue change in color. The patient may report numbness or tingling in these areas.

Central cyanosis is caused by advanced lung disease, congestive heart disease, and abnormal hemoglobin. Peripheral

---

BOX 4.10   PERIPHERAL VASCULAR ASSESSMENT

Inspection

Compare extremities side to side:
  Size
  Symmetry
  Skin
  Nail beds
  Color
  Hair growth
  Sensation

Palpation
Pulses (see Fig. 4.1)

Upper Quadrant
  Carotid
  Brachial
  Radial
  Ulnar
Lower Quadrant
  Femoral
  Popliteal
  Dorsalis pedis
  Posterior tibial

Characteristics of Pulses
Rate
Rhythm
Strength (amplitude)
  + 4 = bounding
  + 3 = full, increased
  + 2 = normal
  + 1 = diminished, weak
    0 = absent

Check for symmetry (compare right to left)
Compare upper extremity to lower extremity

Arterial Insufficiency of Extremities

Pulses	Decreased or absent
Color	Pale on elevation
	Dusky rubor on dependency
Temperature	Cool/cold
Edema	None
Skin	Shiny, thin pale skin; thick nails; hair loss
	Ulcers on toes
Sensation	Pain: increased with exercise (claudication) or leg elevation; relieved by dependent dangling position
	Paresthesias

Venous Insufficiency of Extremities

Pulses	Normal arterial pulses
Color	Pink to cyanotic
	Brown pigment at ankles
Temperature	Warm
Edema	Present
Skin	Discolored, scaly (eczema or stasis dermatitis)
	Ulcers on ankles, toes, fingers
	Varicose veins
Sensation	Pain: increased with standing or sitting; relieved with elevation or support hose

Special (Quick Screening) Tests
Capillary refill time (fingers and toes)
Arterial-brachial index (ABI)
Rubor on dependency
Allen test

cyanosis occurs with CHF (decreased blood flow), venous obstruction, anxiety, and cold environment.

Rubor (dusky redness) is a common finding in PVD as a result of arterial insufficiency. When the legs are raised above the level of the heart, pallor of the feet and lower legs develops quickly (usually within 1 minute). When the same patient sits up and dangles the feet down, the skin returns to a pink color quickly (usually in about 10 to 15 seconds). A minute later the pallor is replaced by rubor, usually accompanied by pain and diminished pulses. Skin is cool to the touch and trophic changes may be seen (e.g., hair loss over the foot and toes, thick nails, thin skin).

Diffuse hyperpigmentation can occur with Addison's disease, sarcoidosis, pregnancy, leukemia, hemochromatosis, celiac sprue (malabsorption syndrome), scleroderma, and chronic renal failure. This presents as patchy tan to brown spots most often, but may occur as yellow-brown or yellow to tan with scleroderma and renal failure. Any area of the body can be affected, although pigmentation changes in pregnancy tend to affect just the face (melasma or the mask of pregnancy).

Assessing Skin of Color

Patients with darker skin (Black, Asian or Pacific Islander, Hispanic or Latino) may require a different approach to skin assessment than the Caucasian population.[85,86] Observe for any obvious changes in the palms of the hands and soles of the feet; tongue, lips, and gums in the mouth; and in the sclera and conjunctiva of the eyes. An excellent resource for assessing skin of color can be found at https://www.blackandbrownskin.co.uk.

Pallor may present as yellow or ashen-gray as a result of an absence of the normally present underlying red tones in the skin. The palms and the soles show changes more clearly than the skin. Skin rashes may present as a change in skin texture so palpating for changes is important. Edema can be palpated as "tightness" and darker skin may appear lighter. Inflammation may be perceived as a change in skin temperature instead of redness or erythema of the skin.

Jaundice may appear first in the sclera but can be confused for the normal yellow pigmentation of dark-skinned patients. Be aware that the normal oral mucosa (gums, borders of the tongue, and lining of the cheeks) of dark-skinned individuals may appear freckled.

Petechiae are easier to see when present over areas of skin with lighter pigmentation such as the abdomen, gluteal area, and volar aspect of the forearm. Petechiae and ecchymosis (bruising) can be differentiated from erythema by applying pressure over the involved area. Pressure will cause erythema to blanch, whereas the skin will not change in the presence of petechiae or ecchymosis.

Examining a Skin Lesion or Mass

The average lifetime risk of developing melanoma, or skin cancer, is increasing across all races and skin color, with individuals having skin of color at an underestimated risk. In Caucasians, the lifetime risk of developing skin cancer is 1 in 38 for males, and 1 in 58 for females, with projections forecasting increased risk.[87] The risk of developing melanoma is much higher if the patient has any of the risk factors listed in Box 14.3.

When examining the skin, a therapist may identify a skin lesion or mass that is a potential melanoma. In addition to asking about risk factors, the American Cancer Society (ACS) and the Skin Cancer Foundation advocate using the following ABCDEs to assess skin lesions for cancer detection (Fig. 4.6):

A—Asymmetry
B—Border
C—Color
D—Diameter
E—Evolution or Elevation

Early detection and referral by the therapist may result in appropriate diagnosis and treatment.[88,89]

Round, symmetric skin lesions such as common moles, freckles, and birthmarks are considered "normal." If an existing mole or other skin lesion starts to change and a line drawn down the middle shows two different halves, medical evaluation is needed.

Common moles and other "normal" skin changes usually have smooth, even borders or edges. Malignant melanomas, the deadliest form of skin cancer, have uneven, notched borders.

Benign moles, freckles, "liver spots," and other benign skin changes are usually a single color (most often a single shade of brown or tan) (Fig. 4.7). A single lesion with more than one shade of black, brown, or blue may be a sign of malignant melanoma.

Even though some of us have moles we think are embarrassingly large, the average mole is really less than ¼ of an inch (about the size of a pencil eraser). Anything larger than this should be inspected carefully.

For all lesions, masses, or aberrant tissue, observe or palpate for heat, induration, scarring, or discharge. Make note of how long the patient has had the lesion, if it has changed in the last 6 weeks to 6 months, and whether it has been medically evaluated. Always ask appropriate follow-up questions with this assessment:

❓ FOLLOW-UP QUESTIONS

- How long have you had this?
- Has it changed in the last 6 weeks to 6 months?
- Has your doctor seen it?
- Does it itch, hurt, feel sore, or burn?
- Does anyone else in your household have anything like this?
- Have you taken any new medications (prescribed or OTC) in the last 6 weeks?
- Have you traveled somewhere new in the last month?
- Have you been exposed to anything in the last month that could cause this? (Consider exposure to occupational, environmental, and hobby interests.)
- Do you have any other skin changes anywhere else on your body?
- Have you had a fever or sweats in the last 2 weeks?
- Are you having any trouble breathing or swallowing?
- Have you had any other symptoms of any kind anywhere else in your body?

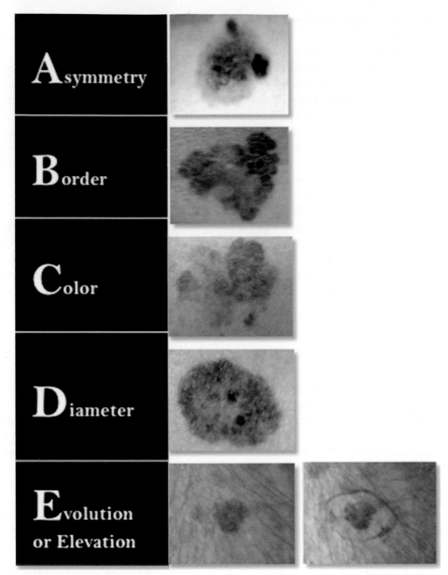

Fig. 4.6   Common characteristics associated with early melanoma are described and shown in this photo. (A) Asymmetry: a line drawn through the middle does not produce matching halves. (B) Borders are uneven, fuzzy, or have notched or scalloped edges. (C) Color changes occur with shades of brown, black, tan, or other colors present at the same time. (D) Diameter is greater than the width of a pencil eraser. (E) Evolution or elevation, in size, shape, color, elevation, or another trait, or any new symptom, such as bleeding, itching, or crusting, requires evaluation. (From Kauffmann RM, Chen SL. Workup and staging of malignant melanoma. Surg Clin N Am 2014;94:963-972. Fig. 1, p. 964. Courtesy of Jae Jung, MD, Department of Dermatology, City of Hope Medical Center, Duarte, CA; and Dr Lynn Cornelius, Washington University, St. Louis, MO.)

How you ask is just as important as *what* you say. Do not frighten people by first telling them you always screen for skin cancer. It may be better to introduce the subject by saying that as health care professionals, therapists are trained to observe many body parts, including the skin, joints, posture, and so on. You notice the patient has an unusual mole (or rash ... or whatever you have observed) and you wonder if this is something that has been there for years. Has it changed in the last 6 weeks to 6 months? Has the patient ever shown it to the doctor?

The Skin Cancer Foundation (www.skincancer.org) has many public education materials available to help the therapist identify suspicious skin lesions. In addition to their website, they have posters, brochures, videos, and other materials available for use in the clinic. It is highly recommended that these types of educational materials be available in waiting rooms as a part of a nationwide primary prevention program.

The Melanoma Education Foundation (www.skincheck. com) provides additional photos of suspicious lesions with more screening guidelines. The therapist must become as familiar as possible with what suspicious skin aberrations may look like in order to refer as early as possible.

Assess Surgical Scars

It is always a good idea to look at surgical scars (Fig. 4.8), especially sites of local cancer removal. Any suspicious scab or tissue granulation, redness, or discoloration must be noted (photographed if possible).

Start by asking the patient if he or she has noticed any changes in the scar. Continue by asking:

❓ FOLLOW-UP QUESTIONS

- Would you have any objections if I looked at (or examined) the scar tissue?

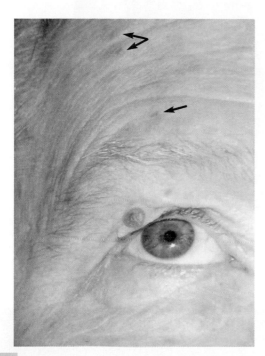

Fig. 4.7 Seborrheic keratosis, a benign well-circumscribed, raised, tan-to-black lesion often presents on the face, neck, chest, or upper back. This lesion represents a buildup of keratin, which is the primary component of the epidermis. There is a family tendency to develop these lesions. The more serious lesions are the red patches located on this patient's forehead (arrows), precancerous lesions called actinic keratosis, are the result of chronic sun exposure. These lesions have a "sandpaper" feel when palpated. Medical treatment is needed for this premalignant lesion. (Courtesy Catherine C. Goodman, 2005. Used with permission.)

If the patient declines or refuses, be sure to follow-up with counsel to perform self-inspection and report any changes to the physician.

In Fig. 4.9, the small scab and granular tissue forming above the scar represent red flags of suspicious local recurrence. Even if the patient suggests this is from "picking" at the scar, a medical evaluation is well advised.

The therapist has a responsibility to report these findings to the appropriate health care professional and make every effort to ensure patient compliance with follow-up.

Common Skin Lesions

Vitiligo

A lack of pigmentation from melanocyte destruction (vitiligo) (Fig. 4.10) can be hereditary and have no significance or it can be caused by conditions such as hyperthyroidism, stomach cancer, pernicious anemia, diabetes mellitus, or an autoimmune disease.

Lesions can occur anywhere on the body but tend to develop in sun-exposed areas, body folds, and around body

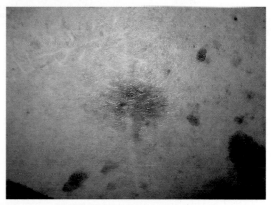

Fig. 4.9 Basal cell carcinoma in a scar. Always ask to see and examine scars from previous surgeries, especially if there is a history of cancer of any kind, including skin cancer. In this photo, basal cell carcinoma can be seen within the scar. (From Wood LD, Ammirati CT. An overview of Mohs micrographic surgery for the treatment of basal cell carcinoma. *Dermatol Clin* 2011;29(2):153–160.)

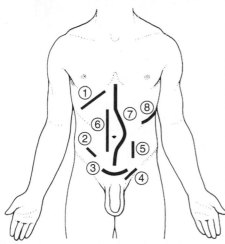

1. Cholecystectomy; a subcostal incision, when made on the right, provides exposure of the gallbladder and common bile duct; used on the left for splenectomy
2. Appendectomy, sometimes called McBurney's or Gridiron incision
3. Transverse suprapubic incision for hysterectomy and other pelvic surgeries
4. Inguinal hernia repair (herniorrhaphy or hernioplasty)
5. Anterior rectal resection (left paramedian incision)
6. Incision through the right flank (right paramedian); called laparotomy or celiotomy; sometimes used to biopsy the liver
7. Midline laparotomy
8. Nephrectomy (removal of the kidney) or other renal surgery

Fig. 4.8 Abdominal surgical scars. Not shown: puncture sites for laparoscopy, usually close to the umbilicus and one or two other sites.

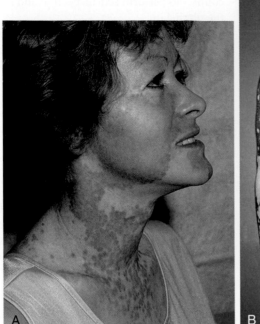
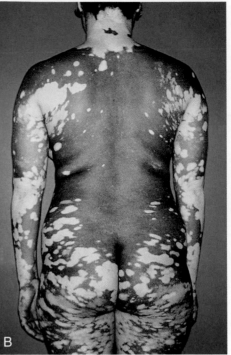

Fig. 4.10 Vitiligo is a term derived from the Greek word for "calf" used to describe patches of light skin caused by loss of epidermal melanocytes. (A) and (B) Note the patchy loss of pigment on the face, trunk, and axilla. This condition can affect any part of the face, hands, or body and can be very disfiguring, especially in dark-skinned individuals. This skin change may be a sign of hyperthyroidism. (From Swartz MH. *Textbook of Physical Diagnosis*. 5th ed. Philadelphia: WB Saunders; 2006.)

openings. Intraarticular steroid injections can cause temporary loss of pigmentation at the injection site. Anyone with any kind of skin type and skin color can be affected by vitiligo.

Café-au-lait

Café-au-lait (coffee with milk) spots describe the light-brown macules (flat lesion, different in color) on the skin as shown in Fig. 4.11. This benign skin condition may be associated with Albright's syndrome or a hereditary disorder called neurofibromatosis. The diagnosis is considered when a child presents with five or more of these skin lesions or if any single patch is greater than 1.5 cm in diameter.

Skin Rash

There are many possible causes of skin rash, including viruses (e.g., chicken pox, measles, Fifth disease, shingles), systemic conditions (e.g., meningitis, lupus, hives), parasites (e.g., lice, scabies), and reactions to chemicals.

A common cause of skin rash seen in a physical therapy practice is a medication, especially antibiotics (Fig. 4.12). The reaction may occur immediately or there may be a delayed reaction of hours up to 6 to 8 weeks after the drug is stopped.

Skin rash can also occur before visceral malignancy of many kinds. Watch for skin rash or hives in someone who has never had hives before, especially if there has been no contact with medications, new foods, new detergents, new perfumes or travel.

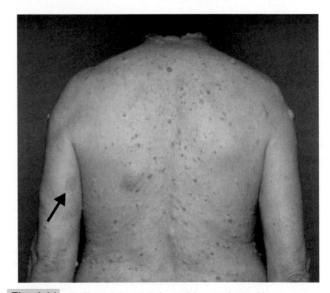

Fig. 4.11 Café-au-lait patch (arrow) in a patient with neurofibromatosis. Occasional (less than five) tan macules are not significant and can occur normally. Patches 1.5 cm in diameter or larger raise the suspicion of underlying pathology even if there is only one present. (From Reynolds RM, Browning GGP, Nawroz I, et al. Von Recklinghausen's neurofibromatosis: neurofibromatosis type 1. *Lancet* 2003;361:1552. Fig. 1.)

Hemorrhagic Rash

Hemorrhagic rash requires medical evaluation. A hemorrhagic rash occurs when small capillaries under the skin start to bleed forming tiny blood spots under the skin (petechiae). The petechiae increase over time as bleeding continues.

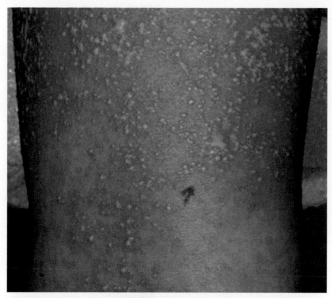

Fig. 4.12   This patient developed a skin rash (reactive erythema) with central pustules caused by a drug reaction to antibiotics for pharyngitis. Hypersensitivity reactions to drugs are most common with antibiotics (especially penicillin), sulfonamides ("sulfa drugs," anti-infectives), and phenobarbital. (From Cohen BA. Chapter 7: Reactive erythema. In: *Pediatric Dermatology*. 4th ed. Philadelphia: Saunders; 2013:169–210.)

This type of rash does not fade under pressure with continued bleeding. Press a clear see-through drinking glass against the skin. Rashes from allergies or viral infections are more likely to fade and the skin will become white or pale. During later stages of hemorrhagic bleeding the rash does not fade or become pale with the pressure test; this test is not as reliable during early onset of hemorrhage. Left untreated, hemorrhagic spots may become bruises and then large red-purple areas of blood. Pressure on a bruise will not cause it to blanch.

Dermatitis

Dermatitis (sometimes referred to as eczema) is characterized by skin that is red, brown, or gray; sore; itchy; and sometimes swollen. The skin can develop blisters and weeping sores. Skin changes, especially in the presence of open lesions, puts the patient at an increased risk of infection. In chronic dermatitis, the skin can become thick and leathery.

There are different types of dermatitis diagnosed on the basis of medical history, etiology (if known), and presenting signs and symptoms. Contributing factors include stress, allergies, genetics, infection, and environmental irritants. For example, contact dermatitis occurs when the skin reacts to something it has come into contact with such as soap, perfume, metals in jewelry, and plants (e.g., poison ivy or oak).

Dyshidrotic dermatitis can affect skin that gets wet frequently. It presents as small, itchy bumps on the sides of the fingers or toes and progresses to a rash. Atopic dermatitis often accompanies asthma or hay fever. It appears to affect genetically predisposed patients who are hypersensitive to

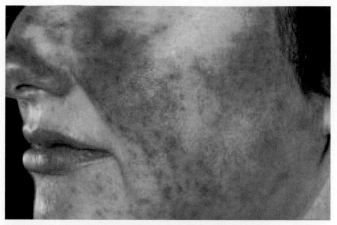

Fig. 4.13   Rosacea, a form of adult acne, may be associated with Helicobacter pylori; medical evaluation and treatment is needed to rule out this possibility. (From Gibson LE. Rosacea, Mayo Clinic Proceedings 2004;79:9. Retrieved from http://www.sciencedirect.com/science/article/pii/S0025619611626049.)

environmental allergens. This type of dermatitis can affect any part of the body, but often involves the skin inside the elbow and on the back of the knees.

Rosacea

Rosacea is a chronic facial skin disorder seen most often in adults between the ages of 30 and 60 years. It can cause a facial rash easily mistaken for the butterfly rash associated with lupus erythematosus. Features include erythema, flushing, telangiectasia, papules, and pustules affecting the cheeks and nose of the face. An enlarged nose is often present, and the condition progressively gets worse (Fig. 4.13).

In some cases, rosacea can be controlled with dermatologic or other medical treatment. Recent studies suggest that rosacea may be linked to GI disease caused by the *H. pylori* bacteria [90-92] Such cases may respond favorably to antibiotics. Medical referral is needed for an accurate diagnosis.

Thrombocytopenia

Decrease in platelet levels can result in thrombocytopenia, a bleeding disorder characterized by petechiae (tiny purple or red spots), multiple bruises, and hemorrhage into the tissues (Fig. 4.14). Joint bleeds, nose and gum bleeds, excessive menstruation, and melena (dark, tarry, sticky stools from oxidized blood in the GI tract) can occur with thrombocytopenia.

There are many causes of thrombocytopenia. In a physical therapy practice, the most common causes seen are bone marrow failure from radiation treatment, leukemia, or metastatic cancer; cytotoxic agents used in chemotherapy; and drug-induced platelet reduction, especially among adults with rheumatoid arthritis treated with gold or inflammatory conditions treated with aspirin or other NSAIDs.

Postoperative thrombocytopenia can be heparin-induced for patients receiving IV heparin. Watch for limb ischemia, cyanosis of fingers or toes, signs and symptoms of a stroke,

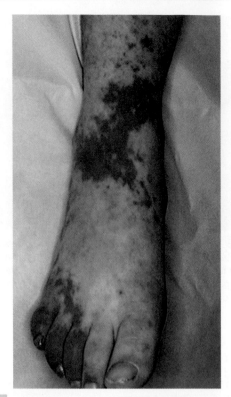

Fig. 4.14 Purpura. Petechiae and ecchymoses are seen in this flat macular hemorrhage from thrombocytopenia (platelet level less than 100,000/mm³). This condition also occurs in older adults as blood leaks from capillaries in response to minor trauma. It can occur in fair-skinned people with skin damage from a lifetime of exposure to ultraviolet (UV) radiation. Exposure to UVB and UVA rays can cause permanent damage to the structural collagen that supports the walls of the skin's blood vessels. Combined with thinning of the skin that occurs with aging, radiation-impaired blood vessels are more likely to rupture with minor trauma. (From Hurwitz S. *Clinical Pediatric Dermatology: A Textbook of Skin Disorders of Childhood and Adolescence*. 2nd ed. Philadelphia: WB Saunders; 1993.)

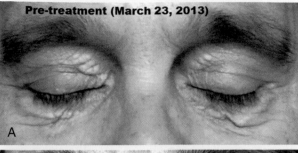

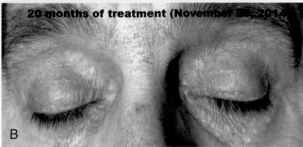

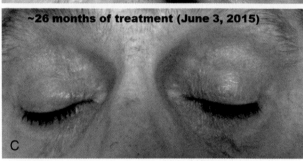

Fig. 4.15 (A)–(C) Xanthelasma. Soft, raised yellow plaques, also known as xanthomas, commonly occur with aging and may be a sign of high cholesterol levels. Shown here on the eyelid, these benign lesions also occur on the extensor surfaces of tendons, especially in the hands, elbows, and knees. They often appear in association with disorders of lipid metabolism. Resolution of the condition is shown after pharmacologic intervention. (From Civeira F, Perez-Calahorra S, Mateo-Gallego R. Rapid resolution of xanthelasmas after treatment with alirocumab. *J Clin Lipidol* 2016;10(5):1933–2874.)

heart attack, or pulmonary embolus. (See further discussion on Thrombocytopenia in Chapter 6.)

Xanthomas

Xanthomas are benign fatty fibrous yellow plaques, nodules, or tumors that develop in the subcutaneous layer of the skin (Fig. 4.15), often around the tendons. The lesion is characterized by the intracellular accumulation of cholesterol and cholesterol esters.

These are seen most often associated with disorders of lipid metabolism, primary biliary cirrhosis, and uncontrolled diabetes (Fig. 4.16). They may have no pathologic significance but can occur in association with malignancy such as leukemia, lymphoma, or myeloma. Xanthomas require a medical referral if they have not been evaluated by a physician. When associated with diabetes, these nodules will resolve with adequate glucose control.

The therapist has an important role in education and prescriptive exercise for the patient with xanthomas from poorly controlled diabetes. Gaining control of glucose levels using the three keys of intervention (diet, exercise, and insulin or

oral hypoglycemic medication) is essential and requires a team management approach.

Rheumatologic Diseases

Skin lesions are often the first sign of an underlying rheumatic disease (Box 4.11). In fact, the skin has been called a "map" to rheumatic diseases. The butterfly rash over the nose and cheeks associated with lupus erythematosus can be seen in the acute (systemic) phase, whereas discoid lesions are more common with the chronic integumentary form of lupus erythematosus (Fig. 4.17).[93]

Individuals with dermatomyositis often have a heliotrope rash and/or Gottron papules. Scleroderma is accompanied by many skin changes; pitting of the nails is common with psoriatic arthritis. Skin and nail bed changes are common with some sexually transmitted diseases (STDs) that also have a rheumatologic component (see Fig. 4.22).[94]

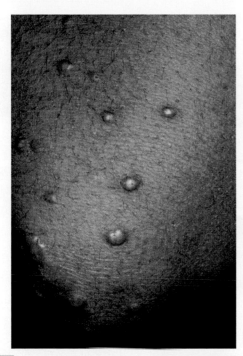

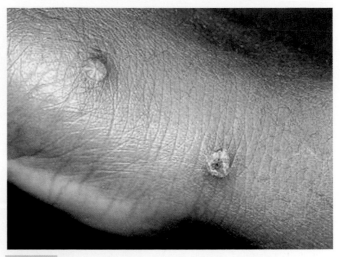

Fig. 4.17 Skin lesions on the lateral aspect of the hand associated with discoid lupus erythematosus. These disk-shaped lesions look like warts or squamous cell carcinoma. A medical examination is needed to make the definitive differential diagnosis. (From Powers DB. Systemic lupus erythematosus and discoid lupus erythematosus. Oral Maxillofac *Surg Clin North Am* 2008;20(4):651–662.)

Fig. 4.16 A slightly different presentation of xanthomas, this time associated with poorly controlled diabetes mellitus. Although the lesion is considered "benign," the presence of these skin lesions in anyone with diabetes signals the need for immediate medical attention. The therapist also plays a key role in patient education and the development of an appropriate exercise program to bring blood glucose levels under adequate control. (From Callen JP, Jorizzo J, Greer KE, et al. *Dermatological Signs of Internal Disease.* 1st ed. Philadelphia: WB Saunders; 1988.)

BOX 4.11 RHEUMATIC DISEASES ACCOMPANIED BY SKIN LESIONS

- Acute rheumatic fever
- Discoid lupus erythematosus
- Dermatomyositis
- Gonococcal arthritis
- Lyme disease
- Psoriatic arthritis
- Reactive arthritis
- Rubella
- Scleroderma
- Systemic lupus erythematosus (SLE)
- Vasculitis

Steroid Skin and Steroid Rosacea

Steroid skin is the name given when bruising or ecchymosis occurs as a result of chronic use of topical or systemic corticosteroids (Fig. 4.18). In the case of topical steroid creams, this is a red flag that the pain is not under control and medical attention for an underlying (probably inflammatory) condition is needed.

The use of topical corticosteroids for more than 2 weeks to treat chronic skin conditions affecting the face can cause a condition characterized by rosacea-like eruptions known as *steroid rosacea*. Attempts to stop using the medication may result in severe redness and burning called *steroid addiction syndrome* (Fig. 4.19).

Whenever signs and symptoms of chronic corticosteroids are seen, a medical evaluation may be needed to review medical management of the problem. In the case of steroid skin from chronic systemic corticosteroid use, ask if the physician has seen (or knows about) the signs and symptoms and how long it has been since medications have been reviewed. The multiple side effects of chronic corticosteroid use are discussed in association with Cushing's syndrome (see Chapter 12).

Erythema Chronicum Migrans

One or more erythema migrans rashes may occur with Lyme disease. There is no one prominent rash. The rash varies in size and shape and may have purple, red, or bruised-looking rings. The rash may appear as a solid red expanding rash, as a blotch, or central red spot surrounded by clear skin that is ringed by an expanding red rash. It may be smooth or bumpy to the touch, and it may itch or ooze. The Centers for Disease Control and Prevention provides a photo gallery of possible rashes associated with Lyme disease.[95]

This rash, which develops in most people with Lyme disease, appears most often 1 to 2 weeks after the disease is transmitted (via tick bite) and may persist for 3 to 5 weeks. It usually is not painful or itchy but may be warm to the touch. The bull's-eye rash may be more difficult to see on darker-skinned people. A dark, bruise-like appearance is more common in those cases. Other symptoms are listed in Chapter 3.

Effects of Radiation

Radiation for the treatment of some cancers has some specific effects on the skin. Pigment producing cells can be affected

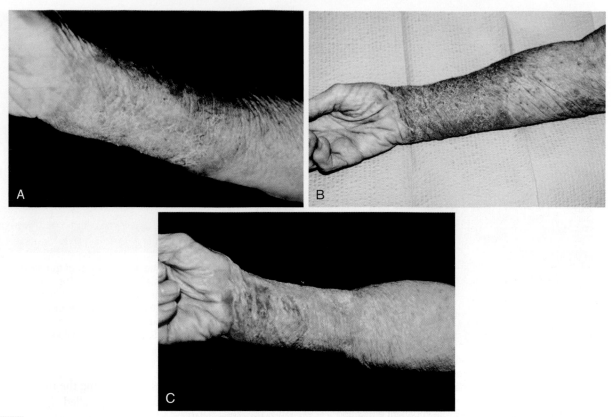

Fig. 4.18   (A)–(C) Ecchymosis as a result of steroid application. Also note the cutaneous atrophy produced by topical steroids. This skin condition is referred to as "steroid skin" when associated with chronic oral or topical steroid use. (**A**) Ecchymosis following six weeks of corticosteroid use; (**B**) five months after cessation of use. Note erythema, exfoliation, and edema. (C) Forearm atrophy nine months after use. Medical referral may be needed for better pain control. (From Rapaport MJ, Lebwohl M. Corticosteroid addiction and withdrawal in the atopic: the red burning skin syndrome. *Clin Dermatol* 2003;21(3):201–214.)

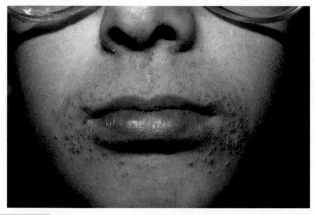

Fig. 4.19   Steroid addiction appearing to be acne. This condition was caused by long-term application of a moderate-potency steroid and Mycostatin combined. (From Weston WL. *Weston Color Textbook of Pediatric Dermatology*. 4th ed. St. Louis: Mosby; 2007.)

by either low-dose radiation causing hyperpigmentation or by high dose radiation resulting in depigmentation (vitiligo). Pigmentation changes can be localized or generalized.

Radiation recall reaction can occur months later as a post-irradiation effect. The physiologic response is much like over-exposure to the sun, with erythema of the skin occurring in the same pattern as the radiation exposure but without evidence of disease progression at that site. It is usually precipitated by some external stimuli or event such as exposure to the sun, infection, or stress.

Radiation recall is also more likely to occur when an individual receives certain chemotherapies (e.g., cyclophosphamide, paclitaxel, doxorubicin, gemcitabine) after radiation.[96] The chemotherapy causes the previously radiated area to become inflamed and irritated.

Radiation dermatitis and *x-ray keratosis*, separate from radiation recall, are terms used to describe acute (expected) skin irritation caused by radiation at the time of radiation.

Skin changes can also occur as a long-term effect of radiation exposure. Radiation levels administered to oncology patients even 10 years ago were much higher than today's current treatment regimes. Always look at previous radiation sites for evidence of long-term effects.

Sexually Transmitted Diseases/Infections

STDs are a variety of clinical syndromes caused by pathogens that can be acquired and transmitted through sexual activity.[97] Over 2.4 million cases of STDs were reported by the U.S. Centers for Disease Control and Prevention in 2018.[98] STDs, also known as sexually transmitted infections (STIs), are often accompanied by skin and/or nail bed lesions and joint pain. Being able to recognize STIs is helpful in the clinic. Someone presenting with joint pain of "unknown cause" and demonstrating signs of an STI (see Fig. 3.10) may help bring the correct diagnosis to light sooner than later.

STIs have been positively identified as a risk factor for cancer. Not all STIs are linked with cancer, but several types of human papillomavirus (HPV) have been attributed to cause the majority of cervical cancers (Fig. 4.20).[99] In 2018, there were 115,045 cases of syphilis reported, a 13.3% increase from 2017.[98] It is highly contagious and spread from person to person by direct contact with a syphilis sore on the body of an infected person. Sores occur at the site of infection, mainly on the external genitals, vagina, anus, or rectum. Sores can also occur on the lips and in the mouth.

Transmission occurs during vaginal, anal, or oral sex. An infected pregnant woman can also pass the disease to her unborn child. Syphilis cannot be spread by contact with toilet seats, doorknobs, swimming pools, hot tubs, bathtubs, shared clothing, or eating utensils.

In the first stage of syphilis, a syphilis chancre may appear (Fig. 4.21) at the site of inoculation (usually the genitals, anus, or mouth). The chancre occurs 4 weeks after initial infection and is often not noticed in women when present in the genitalia. The chancre is often accompanied by lymphadenopathy.

Without treatment, the spread of the bacteria through the blood causes the second stage (secondary syphilis). Therapists may see lesions associated with secondary syphilis (Fig. 4.22). Neurologic (untreated) infection may present as cranial nerve

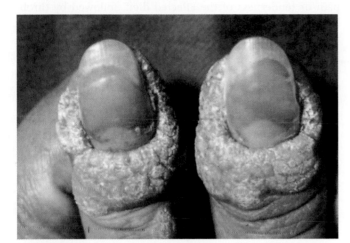

Fig. 4.20   Common warts of the hands caused by human papillomavirus (HPV) via nonsexual transmission. The virus can be transmitted through sexual contact and is a precursor to cancer of the cervix. Genital warts do not typically occur by autoinoculation from the hands. In other words, warts on the fingers caused by HPV are probably NOT transmitted from finger to genitals. They occur with contact of someone else's genital warts. Warts on the fingers caused by sexually transmitted HPV do not transmit the sexually transmitted infection (STI) to the therapist if the therapist shakes hands with the patient or touches the warts. However, standard precautions are always recommended whenever skin lesions of any kind are present. For a summary of standard precautions, see Goodman et al., 2014. (From Cubie HA. Diseases associated with human papillomavirus infection. *Virology* 2013;445:21–34.)

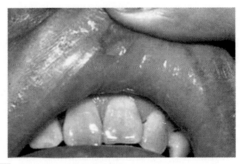

Fig. 4.21   The first stage (primary syphilis) is marked by a very infectious sore called a chancre. The chancre is usually small, firm, round with well-demarcated edges, and painless. It appears at the spot where the bacteria entered the body. Chancres last one to five weeks and heal on their own. (From Cohen SE, Klausner JD, Engelman J, et al. Syphilis in the modern era an update for physicians. *Infect Dis Clin N Am* 2013;27:705–722.)

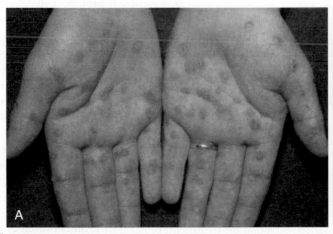
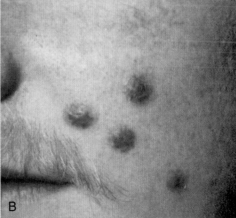

Fig. 4.22   Maculopapular rash associated with secondary syphilis appears as a pink, dusky, brownish-red or coppery, indurated, oval or round lesion with a raised border. These are referred to as "copper penny" spots. The lesions do not bleed and are usually painless. They usually appear scattered on the palms (A) or the bottom of the feet (not shown) but may also present on the face (B). The second stage begins two weeks to six months after the initial chancre disappears. The patient may report joint pain with general flu-like symptoms (e.g., headache, sore throat, swollen glands, muscle aches, fatigue). Patchy hair loss may be described or observed. (From Mir MA. *Atlas of Clinical Diagnosis*. London: WB Saunders; 1995:198.)

dysfunction, meningitis, stroke, auditory or ophthalmic abnormalities.[100]

The patient may report or present with a characteristic rash that can appear all over the body, most often on the palms and soles. The appearance of these skin lesions occurs after the primary chancre disappears.

Syphilis can be tested for with a blood test and treated successfully with antibiotics. Left untreated, tertiary (late stage) syphilis can cause paralysis, blindness, personality changes or dementia, and damage to internal organs and joints. The therapist can facilitate early detection and treatment through immediate medical referral. See further discussion on Infectious Causes of Pelvic Pain in Chapter 15, including special questions to ask concerning sexual activity and STIs. (See also Appendix B-33)

Herpes Virus. Several herpes viruses are accompanied by characteristic skin lesions. Herpes simplex virus (HSV)-1 and -2 are the most common.[101] Most people have been exposed at an early age and already have immunity. In fact, four out of five Americans harbor HSV-1. Because of universal distribution of these viruses, most individuals have developed immunity by the ages of 1 to 2 years.

The HSV-1 and -2 viruses are virtually identical, sharing approximately 50% of their DNA. Both types infect the body's mucosal surfaces, usually the mouth or genitals, and then establish latency in the nervous system.[102] Both can cause skin and nail bed changes.

Cold sores caused by HSV-1 (also known as recurrent herpes labialis; "fever blister") are found on the lip or the skin near the mouth. HSV-1 usually establishes latency in the trigeminal ganglion, a collection of nerve cells near the ear. HSV-1 generally only infects areas above the waistline and occurs when oral secretions or mucous membranes infected with HSV come in contact with a break in the skin (e.g., torn cuticle, skin abrasion).

HSV-1 can be transmitted to the genital area during oral sex. In fact, HSV-1 can be transmitted oral-to-oral, oral-to-genital, anal-to-genital, and oral-to-anal. HSV-1 is predominately orally transmitted, whereas a second herpes virus (genital herpes; HSV-2) is more often transmitted sexually.

HSV-2, also known as "genital herpes" can cause cold sores but usually does not; rather, it is more likely to infect body tissues below the waistline as it resides in the sacral ganglion at the base of the spine.

HSV-1 and HSV-2 infections are typically not a major health threat in most people but slowing the spread of genital herpes is important. The virus is more of a social problem than a medical one. The exception is that genital lesions from herpes can make it easier for a person to become infected with other viruses, including HIV, which increases the risk of developing acquired immunodeficiency syndrome (AIDS).

Nonmedical treatment with OTC products is now available for cold sores. Outbreaks of genital herpes can be effectively treated with medications, but these do not "cure" the virus. HSV-1 is also the cause of herpes whitlow, an infection of the finger and "wrestler's herpes," a herpes infection on the chest or face.

Herpetic Whitlow. Herpetic whitlow, an intense painful infection of the terminal phalanx of the fingers, is caused by HSV-1 (60%) and HSV-2 (40%).[103] The thumb and index fingers are most commonly involved. There may be a history of fever or malaise several days before symptoms occur in the fingers.

Common initial symptoms of infection include tingling pain or tenderness of the affected digit, followed by throbbing pain, swelling, and redness. Fluid-filled vesicles form and eventually crust over, ending the contagious period. The patient with red streaks down the arm and lymphadenopathy may have a secondary infection. Take the patient's vital signs (especially body temperature) and report all findings to the physician. As in other herpes infections, viral inoculation of the host occurs through exposure to infected body fluids via a break in the skin such as a paper cut or a torn cuticle. Autoinoculation can occur in anyone with other herpes infections such as genital herpes. It is an occupational risk among health care workers exposed to infected oropharyngeal secretions of patients, easily prevented by using standard precautions.[104]

Herpes Zoster. Varicella-zoster virus (VZV), or herpes zoster or "shingles," is another herpes virus with skin lesions characteristic of the condition. VZV is caused by the same virus that causes chicken pox. After an attack of chicken pox, the virus lies dormant in the nerve tissue, usually the dorsal root ganglion. If the virus is reactivated, the virus can reappear in the form of shingles.

Shingles is an outbreak of a rash or blisters (vesicles with an erythematous base) on the skin that may be associated with severe pain (Fig. 4.23). Pain is associated with the involved nerve root and associated dermatome and generally presents on one side of the body or face in a pattern characteristic of the involved site (Fig. 4.24). Early signs of shingles include burning or shooting pain and tingling or itching. The rash or blisters are present anywhere from 1 to 14 days.

Complications of shingles involving cranial nerves include hearing and vision loss. Postherpetic neuralgia (PHN), a condition in which the pain from shingles persists for months, sometimes years, after the shingles rash has healed, can also occur. PHN can be very debilitating. Early intervention within the first 72 hours of onset with antiretroviral medication may diminish or eliminate PHN. Early identification and intervention are very important to outcomes.

Adults with shingles are infectious to anyone who has not had chicken pox. Anyone who has had chicken pox can develop shingles when immunocompromised. Other risk factors for VZV include age (young or old) and an immunocompromised status from HIV infection, chemotherapy or radiation treatment, organ transplant, aging, and stress. It is highly recommended that health care professionals with no immunity to VZV receive the varicella vaccine. Therapists who have never had chicken pox (and especially women of childbearing age who have not had chicken pox) should be tested for immune status.

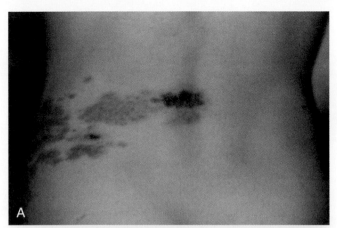
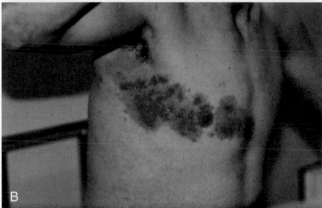

Fig. 4.23   Herpes zoster (shingles). (A) Lesions appear unilaterally along the path of a spinal nerve. (B) Eruptions involving the T4 dermatome. (A From Callen J, Greer K, Hood H, et al. *Color Atlas of Dermatology*. Philadelphia: WB Saunders; 1993; B From Marx J, Hockberger R, Walls R. *Rosen's Emergency Medicine: Concepts and Clinical Practice*. 6th ed. St. Louis: Mosby; 2006.)

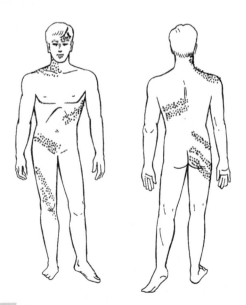

Fig. 4.24   Symptoms of shingles appear on only one side of the body, usually on the torso or face. Most often, the lesions are visible externally. In unusual cases, patients report the same symptoms internally along the dermatome but without a corresponding external skin lesion. (From Malasanos L, Barkauskas V, Stoltenberg-Allen K. *Health Assessment*. 4th ed. St. Louis: Mosby; 1990.)

Cutaneous Manifestations of Abuse

Signs of child abuse, domestic violence in adults, or elder abuse may be seen as skin lesions. Cigarette burns leave a punched-out ulceration with dry, purple crusting. Splash marks or scald lines from thermal (hot water) burns occur most often on the buttocks and distal extremities.[105] Bruising from squeezing and shaking involving the midportion of the upper arms is a suspicious sign. Signs of elder abuse can include atypical bruising, wrist/ankle lesions from inappropriate restraints, malnutrition, dehydration, or pressure sores.[106]

Accidental bruising in young children is common; the therapist should watch for nonaccidental bruising found in atypical areas, such as the buttocks, hands, and trunk, or in a child who is not yet biped (up on two feet) and cruising (walking along furniture or holding an object while taking steps). To make an accurate assessment, it is important to differentiate between inflicted cutaneous injuries and mimickers of physical abuse.

For example, infants with bruising may be demonstrating early signs of bleeding disorders.[107] Mongolian spots can also be mistaken for bruising from child abuse (see next section). The therapist is advised to take photographs of any suspicious lesions in children under the age of 18 years. Document the date and provide a detailed description.

The law requires that professionals report suspected abuse and neglect to the appropriate authorities. It is not up to the health care professional to determine if abuse has occurred; this is left up to investigating officials. See other guidelines regarding child abuse and domestic violence in Chapter 2. Understanding the reporting guidelines helps direct practitioners in their decision-making.[107]

Mongolian Spots.   Discoloration of the skin in newborn infants, called a Mongolian spot (Fig. 4.25), can be mistaken for a sign of child abuse. The Mongolian spot is a congenital, developmental condition exclusively involving the skin and is very common in children of Asian, African, Indian, Native American, Eskimo, Polynesian, or Hispanic origins.

These benign pigmentation changes appear as flat dark blue or black areas and come in a variety of sizes, shapes, and colors. The skin changes result from the entrapment of melanocytes (skin cells containing melanin, the normal pigment of the skin) during their migration from the neural crest into the epidermis.

Cancer-Related Skin Lesions

When screening for primary skin cancer, keep in mind there are other cancer-related skin lesions to watch out for. For example, skin rash can present as an early sign of a paraneoplastic syndrome before other manifestations of cancer or cancer recurrence (Fig. 4.26). See further discussion of paraneoplastic syndromes in Chapter 13.

Pinch purpura, a purplish, brown, or red discoloration of the skin, can be mistaken by the therapist for a birthmark or port wine stain (Fig. 4.27). Using the question "How long have you had this?" can help differentiate between something

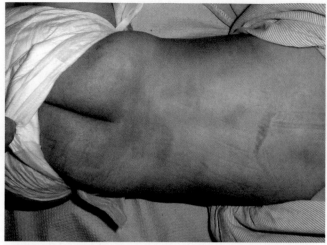

Fig. 4.25 Mongolian spots (congenital dermal melanocytosis). Mongolian spots are common among people of Asian, East Indian, Native American, Inuit, African, and Latino or Hispanic heritage. They are also present in about one in ten fair-skinned infants. Bluish gray to deep brown to black skin markings, they often appear on the base of the spine, on the buttocks and back, and even sometimes on the shoulders, ankles, or wrists. Mongolian spots may cover a large area of the back. When the melanocytes are close to the surface, they look deep brown. The deeper they are in the skin, the more bluish they look, often mistaken for signs of child abuse. These spots "fade" with age as the child grows and usually disappear by the age of five years. (Courtesy Dr. Dubin Pavel, 2004.)

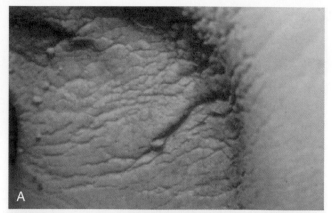

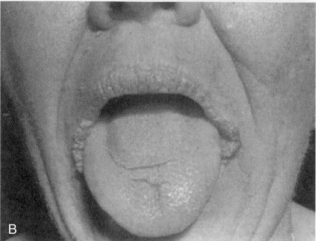

Fig. 4.26 Pigmented, velvety plaques in the axilla (A), mouth (B), neck, or other skin folds indicate acanthosis nigricans, which is seen as a sign of insulin resistance, but could also be associated with malignancy, especially adenocarcinomas. (From Rugo H. Paraneoplastic syndromes and other non-neoplastic effects of cancer. In Goldman L, Schafer A, eds. *Goldman's Cecil Medicine: Approach to Medicine, the Patient, and the Medical Profession*. 24th ed., Philadelphia: Saunders; 2012: Vol. 1; 1192–1200.)

the person has had his or her entire life from a suspicious skin lesion or recent change in the integument.

When purpura causes a raised and palpable skin lesion, it is called *palpable purpura*. The palpable hemorrhage is caused by red blood cells extravasated (escaped) from damaged vessels into the dermis. This type of purpura can be associated with cutaneous vasculitis, pulmonary-renal syndrome, or a drug reaction. The lower extremities are affected most often.

Many older adults assume this is a "normal" sign of aging (and in fact, purpura does occur more often in aging adults; see Fig. 4.14); they do not see a physician when it first appears. Early detection and referral is always the key to a better prognosis. In asking the three important questions, the therapist plays an instrumental part in the cancer screening process.

A patient with a past medical history of cancer now presenting with a suspicious skin lesion (Fig. 4.28) that has not been evaluated by the physician must be advised to have this evaluated as soon as possible. We must be aware of how to present this recommendation to the patient. There is a need to avoid frightening the patient when conveying the importance of early diagnosis of any unusual skin lesions.

Kaposi's Sarcoma

Kaposi's sarcoma is a form of skin cancer common in older Jewish men of Mediterranean descent that presents with a wide range of appearance. It is not contagious to touch and does not usually cause death or disfigurement.

More recently, Kaposi's sarcoma has presented as an opportunistic disease in adults with HIV/AIDS. With the more

successful treatment of AIDS with antiretroviral agents, opportunistic diseases, such as Kaposi's sarcoma, are on the decline.

Even though this skin lesion will not transmit skin cancer or HIV, the therapist is always advised to use standard precautions with anyone who has skin lesions of any type.

Lymphomas

Round patches of reddish-brown skin with hair loss over the area are lymphomas, a type of neoplasm of lymphoid tissue (Fig. 4.29). The most common forms of lymphoma are Hodgkin's disease and non-Hodgkin's lymphoma.

Typically, the appearance of a painless, enlarged lymph node or skin lesion of this type is followed by weakness, fever, and weight loss. A history of chronic immunosuppression (e.g., antirejection drugs for an organ transplant, chronic use of immunosuppressant drugs for an inflammatory or autoimmune disease, cancer treatment) in the presence of this clinical presentation is a major red flag.

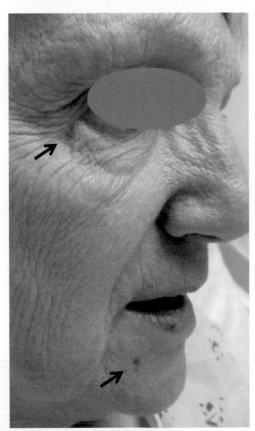

Fig. 4.27 Pinch purpura in an individual with amyloidosis of the skin. Black arrows show the purpuric macules. (From Bhutani M, Shahid Z, Schnebelen A, et al. Cutaneous manifestations of multiple myeloma and other plasma cell proliferative disorders. *Semin Oncol* 2016;43(3):395–400.)

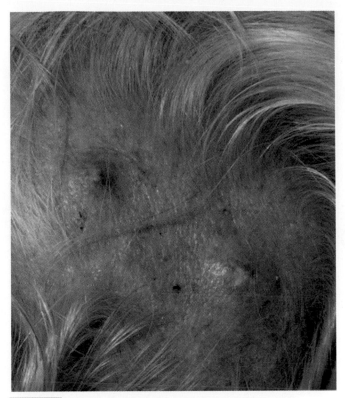

Fig. 4.28 Metastases from follicular thyroid carcinoma presenting as nodules in the scalp. Observing any skin lesions, regardless of what part of the body the therapist is examining, must be followed by the three assessment questions listed in the text. (From Fernández-Antón Martínez MC, Parra-Blanco V, Avilés Izquierdo JA. Cutaneous metastases of internal tumors. *Actas Dermosifiliogr* 2013;104(10):841–853.)

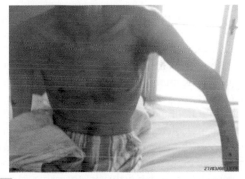

Fig. 4.29 Lymphomas seen on the chest of an adult male arise in individuals who are chronically immunosuppressed for any reason. (From Czepiel J, Kluba-Wojewoda U, Biesiada G, et al. The case of a diffuse large B-cell lymphoma (DLBCL) in a course of HIV. *HIV AIDS Rev* 2010;9(1):25.)

NAIL BED ASSESSMENT

As with assessment of the skin, nail beds (fingers and toes) should be evaluated for color, shape, thickness, texture, and the presence of lesions (Box 4.12). Systemic changes affect both fingernails and toenails, but typically the faster-growing fingernails will more prominently display the signs.[108]

The normal nail consists of three parts: the nail bed, the nail plate, and the cuticle (Fig. 4.30). The nail bed is highly vascularized and gives the nail its pink color. The hard nail is formed at the proximal end (the matrix). About one-fourth of the nail is covered by skin known as the proximal nail fold. The cuticle seals and protects the space between the proximal fold and the nail plate. Many individual variations in color, texture, and grooming of the nails are influenced by factors unrelated to disease, such as occupation, chronic use of nail polish or acrylics, or exposure to chemical dyes and detergents. Longitudinal lines of darker color (pigment) may be seen in the normal nails of patients with darker skin.

In assessing the older adult, minor variations associated with the aging process may be observed (e.g., gradual thickening of the nail plate, appearance of longitudinal ridges, yellowish-gray discoloration).

In the normal individual, pressing or blanching the nail bed of a finger or toe produces a whitening effect; when pressure is released, a return of color should occur within 3 seconds. If the capillary refill time exceeds 3 seconds, the lack of circulation may be as a result of arterial insufficiency from atherosclerosis or spasm.

Nail Bed Changes

Some of the more common nail bed changes seen in a physical therapy practice are included in this chapter. With any

BOX 4.12   HAND AND NAIL BED ASSESSMENT

Observe the Hands for

- Palmar erythema (see Fig. 10.6)
- Tremor (e.g., liver flap or asterixis; see Fig. 10.8)
- Pallor of palmar creases (anemia, gastrointestinal [GI] malabsorption)
- Palmar xanthomas (lipid deposits on palms of hands; hyperlipidemia, diabetes)
- Turgor (lift skin on back of hands; hydration status; see Fig. 4.4)
- Edema

Observe the Fingers and Toenails for

- Color (capillary refill time, nails of Terry: see Fig. 10.7)
- Shape and curvature
- Clubbing:
  - Crohn's or Cardiac/cyanosis
  - Lung (cancer, hypoxia, cystic fibrosis)
  - Ulcerative colitis
  - Biliary cirrhosis
  - Present at birth (harmless)
  - Neoplasm
  - GI involvement
- Nicotine stains
- Splinter hemorrhages (see Fig. 4.34)
- Leukonychia (whitening of nail plate with bands, lines, or white spots; inherited or acquired from malnutrition from eating disorders, alcoholism, or cancer treatment; myocardial infarction [MI], renal failure, poison, anxiety)
- Koilonychia ("spoon nails"; see Fig. 4.32); congenital or hereditary, iron deficiency anemia, thyroid problem, syphilis, rheumatic fever)
- Beau's lines (see Fig. 4.33); decreased production of the nail by the matrix caused by acute illness or systemic insult such as chemotherapy for cancer; recent MI, chronic alcohol abuse, or eating disorders. This can also occur in isolated nail beds from local trauma
- Adhesion to the nail bed. Look for onycholysis (loosening of nail plate from distal edge inward; Graves' disease, psoriasis, reactive arthritis, obsessive-compulsive behavior: "nail pickers")
- Pitting (psoriasis, eczema, alopecia areata)
- Thinning/thickening

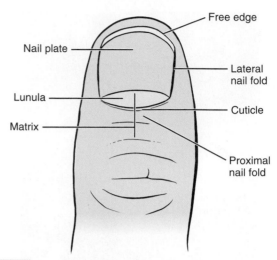

Fig. 4.30 Normal nail structure. The nail matrix forms the nail plate and begins about 5 mm to 8 mm beneath the proximal nail fold and extends distally to the edge of the lunula, where the nail bed begins. The lunula (half-moon) is the exposed part of the nail matrix, distal to the proximal nail fold; it is not always visible.

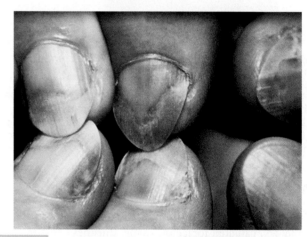

Fig. 4.31 Onycholysis. Loosening of the nail plate, usually from the tip of the nail, progressing inward and from the edge of the nail moving inward. Possible causes include Graves' disease, psoriasis, reactive arthritis, and obsessive-compulsive behaviors (nail pickers). (From Arndt KA, Wintroub BU, Robinson JK, et al. *Primary Care Dermatology*. Philadelphia: WB Saunders; 1997.)

nail or skin condition, ask if the nails have always been like this or if any changes have occurred in the last 6 weeks to 6 months. Referral may not be needed if the physician is aware of the new onset of nail bed changes. Ask about the presence of other signs and symptoms consistent with any of the conditions listed here that can cause any of these nail bed changes.

Again, as with visual inspection of the skin, this section of the text is only a cursory look at the most common nail bed changes. Many more are not included here. A well-rounded library should include at least one text with color plates and photos of various nail bed changes.[109,110] This is not to help the therapist diagnose a medical problem but rather to provide background information, which can be used in the referral decision-making process.

Onycholysis

Onycholysis, a painless loosening of the nail plate occurs from the distal edge inward (Fig. 4.31). Fingers and toes may both be affected as a consequence of dermatologic conditions such as dermatitis, fungal disease, lichen planus, and psoriasis. Systemic diseases associated with onycholysis include myeloma, neoplasia, Graves' disease, anemia, and reactive arthritis.[111]

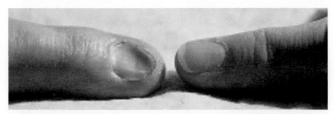

Fig. 4.32 Koilonychia (spoon nails). In this side-by-side view, the affected nail bed is on the left and the normal nail on the right. With a spoon nail, the rounded indentation would hold a drop or several drops of water, hence the name. (From Swartz MH. *Textbook of Physical Diagnosis*. 5th ed. Philadelphia: WB Saunders; 2006.)

Medications, such as tetracycline, fluoroquinolones, anticancer drugs, NSAIDs, psoralens, retinoids, zidovudine, and quinine, can cause photo-onycholysis (toes must be exposed to the sun for the condition to occur).[111]

Local causes from chemical, physical, cosmetic, or traumatic sources can bring on this condition. In the case of trauma, a limited number of nails are affected. For example, in patients with onycholysis as a result of nervous or obsessive-compulsive behaviors, only one or two nails are targeted. The individual picks around the edges until the nail is raised and separated from the nail bed. When there is an underlying systemic disorder, it is more common to see all the nail plates affected.

Koilonychia

Koilonychia or "spoon nails" may be a congenital or hereditary trait and as such is considered "normal" for that individual. These are thin, depressed nails with lateral edges tilted upward, forming a concave profile (Fig. 4.32).

Koilonychia can occur as a result of hypochromic anemia, iron deficiency (with or without anemia), poorly controlled diabetes of more than 15 years duration, chemical irritants, local injury, developmental abnormality, or psoriasis. It can also be an outward sign of thyroid problems, syphilis, and rheumatic fever.

Beau's Lines

Beau's lines are transverse grooves or ridges across the nail plate as a result of a decreased or interrupted production of the nail by the matrix (Fig. 4.33). The cause is usually an acute illness or systemic insult such as cancer chemotherapy. Other common conditions associated with Beau's lines are poor peripheral circulation, eating disorders, cirrhosis associated with chronic alcohol use, and recent myocardial infarction (MI).

Because the nails grow at an approximate rate of 3 mm/month, the date of the initial onset of illness or disease can be estimated by the location of the line. The dent appears first at the cuticle and moves forward as the nail grows. Measure the distance (in millimeters) from the dent to the cuticle and add three to account for the distance from the cuticle to the matrix. This corresponds to the number of weeks ago the person first had the problem.

Beau's lines are temporary until the impaired nail formation is corrected (if and when the individual returns to

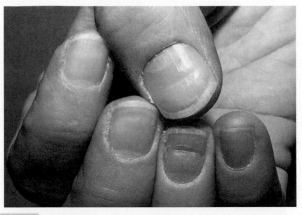

Fig. 4.33 Beau's lines or grooves across the nail plate. A depression across the nail extends down to the nail bed. This occurs with shock, illness, malnutrition, or trauma severe enough to impair nail formation such as acute illness, prolonged fever, or chemotherapy. A dent appears first at the cuticle and moves forward as the nail grows. All nails can be involved, but with local trauma, only the involved nail will be affected. This photo shows a patient postinsult after full recovery. At the time of the illness, nail loss is obvious, often with a change in nail bed color such as occurs with chemotherapy. (From Callen JP, Greer KE, Hood AF, et al. *Color Atlas of Dermatology*. Philadelphia: WB Saunders; 1994.)

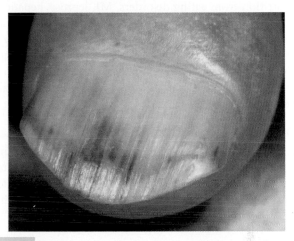

Fig. 4.34 Splinter hemorrhages. These red-brown streaks, embolic lesions, occur with subacute bacterial endocarditis, sepsis, rheumatoid arthritis, vitamin C deficiency, or hematologic neoplasm. They can occur from local trauma in which case only the injured nail beds will have the telltale streak. Splinter hemorrhages also may be a nonspecific sign. (From Hordinsky MK, Sawaya ME, Scher RK. *Atlas of Hair and Nails*. Philadelphia: Churchill Livingstone; 2000.)

normal health). These lines can also occur as a result of local trauma to the hand or fingers.

In the case of an injury, the dent may be permanent. Hand therapists see this condition most often. If it is not the result of a recent injury, the patient may be able to remember sustaining an injury years ago.

Splinter Hemorrhages

Splinter hemorrhages may be the sign of a silent MI or the patient may have a known history of MI. These red-brown linear streaks (Fig. 4.34) can also signal other systemic conditions such as bacterial endocarditis, vasculitis, or renal failure.

In a hospital setting, they are not uncommon in the cardiac care unit or other ICU. In such a case, the therapist may just take note of the nail bed changes and correlate it with the pathologic insult probably already a part of the medical record.

When present in only one or two nail beds, local trauma may be linked to the nail bed changes. Asking the patient about recent trauma or injury to the hand or fingers may bring this to light.

Whenever splinter hemorrhages are observed in the nails, visually inspect both hands and also the toenails. If the patient cannot recall any recent illness, look for a possible cardiac history or cardiac risk factors. In the case of cardiac risk factors with no known cardiac history, proper medical follow-up and diagnosis is essential in the event the patient has had a silent MI.

Leukonychia

Leukonychia, or white nail syndrome, is characterized by dots or lines of white that progress to the free edge of the nail as the nail grows (Fig. 4.35). White nails can be congenital, but more often, they are acquired in association with hypocalcemia, severe hypochromic anemia, Hodgkin's disease, renal failure, malnutrition from eating disorders, MI, leprosy, hepatic cirrhosis, and arsenic poisoning.

Acquired leukonychia is caused by a disturbance to the nail matrix. Repeated trauma, such as keyboard punching, is a more recently described acquired cause of this condition.[112] When the entire nail plate is white, the condition is called *leukonychia totalis* (Case Example 4.2).

Paronychia

Paronychia (not shown) is an infection of the fold of skin at the margin of a nail. There is an obvious red, swollen site of inflammation that is tender or painful. This may be acute as with a bacterial infection or chronic in association with an occupationally induced fungal infection referred to as "wet

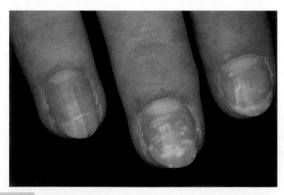

Fig. 4.35 Leukonychia, acquired or inherited white discoloration in the nail. There is a wide range of possibilities in the clinical presentation of leukonychia. Spots, vertical lines, horizontal lines, and even full nail bed changes can occur on individual nail beds of the fingers and/or toes. One or more nails may be affected. (From Jarvis C. *Physical Examination and Health Assessment*. 5th ed. Philadelphia: WB Saunders; 2008.)

CASE EXAMPLE 4.2
Leukonychia

A 24-year-old male (Caucasian) was seen in physical therapy for a work-related back injury. He was asked the final interview questions:

- Are there any other symptoms of any kind anywhere else in your body?
- Is there anything else about your condition that we have not discussed yet?

The patient showed the therapist his nails and asked what could be the cause of the white discoloration in all the nail beds.

He reported the nails seem to grow out from time to time. There was tenderness along the sides of the nails and at the distal edge of the nails. It was obvious the nails were bitten and there were several nails that were red and swollen. The patient admitted to picking at his nails when he was nervous. He was observed tapping his nails on the table repeatedly during the examination. No changes of any kind were observed in the feet.

Past medical history was negative for any significant health problems. He was not taking any medications, over-the-counter drugs, or using recreational drugs. He did not smoke and denied the use of alcohol. His job as a supervisor in a machine shop did not require the mechanical use of his hands. He was not exposed to any unusual chemicals or solvents at work.

Result: When asked, "How long have you had this?" the patient reported for 2 years. When asked, "Have your nails changed in the last 6 weeks to 6 months?" the answer was, "Yes, the condition seems to come and go." When asked, "Has your doctor seen these changes?" the patient did not think so.

The therapist did not know what was causing the nail bed changes and suggested the patient ask his physician about the condition at his next appointment. The physician also observed the patient repeatedly tapping his nails and performed a screening examination for anxiety.

The nail bed condition was diagnosed as leukonychia from repeated microtrauma to the nail matrix. The patient was referred to psychiatry to manage the observed anxiety symptoms. The nails returned to normal in about 3 months (90 to 100 days) after the patient stopped tapping, restoring normal growth to the nail matrix.

From Maino K, Stashower ME: Traumatic transverse leukonychia. Medscape. http://www.medscape.com/viewarticle/467074. Accessed August 7, 2016.

---

work" from having the hands submerged in water for long periods of time.

The patient may also give a history of finger exposure to chemical irritants, acrylic nails or nail glue, or sculpted nails. Paronychia of one or more fingers is not uncommon in people who pick, bite, or suck their nails. Health care professionals with these nervous habits working in a clinical setting (especially hospitals) are at an increased risk for paronychia from infection with bacteria such as *Streptococcus* or *Staphylococcus*. Green coloration of the nail may indicate *Pseudomonas* infection.

Paronychia infections may spread to the pulp space of the finger, developing a painful felon (an infection with localized abscess). Untreated infection can spread to the deep spaces of the hand and beyond.

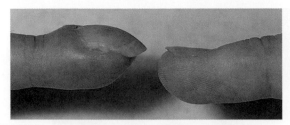

Fig. 4.36 Rapid development of digital clubbing (fingers as shown on the left or toes [not shown]) over the course of a 10-day to two-week period requires immediate medical evaluation. Clubbing can be assessed using the Schamroth method shown in Fig. 4.37. (From Swartz MH. *Textbook of Physical Diagnosis*. 6th ed. Philadelphia: WB Saunders; 2009.)

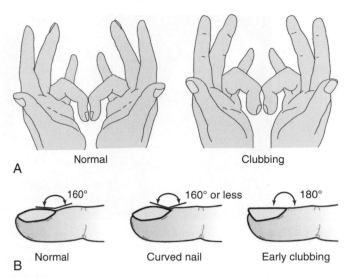

A   Normal   Clubbing

B   Normal   Curved nail   Early clubbing

160°   160° or less   180°

Fig. 4.37 Schamroth method. (A) Assessment of clubbing by the Schamroth method. The patient places the fingernails of opposite fingers together and holds them up to a light. If the examiner can see a diamond shape between the nails, there is no clubbing. Clubbing is identified by the absence of the diamond shape. It occurs first in the thumb and index finger. (B) The index finger is viewed at its profile, and the angle of the nail base is noted (it should be about 160°). The nail base is firm to palpation. Curved nails are a variation of normal with a convex profile. They may look like clubbed nails, but the angle between the nail base and the nail is normal (i.e., 160° or less). Clubbing of nails occurs with congenital chronic cyanotic heart disease, emphysema, cystic fibrosis, and chronic bronchitis. In early clubbing the angle straightens out to 180°, and the nail base feels spongy to palpation. (A From Ignatavicius DD, Bayne MV. Assessment of the cardiovascular system. In Ignatavicius DD, Bayne MV, eds. *Medical-Surgical Nursing*. Philadelphia: WB Saunders; 1993. B From Jarvis C. *Physical Examination and Health Assessment*. Philadelphia: WB Saunders; 2004.)

It is especially important to recognize any nail bed irregularity because it may be a clue to malignancy. Likewise, anyone who has diabetes mellitus, who is immunocompromised, or has a history of steroid and retroviral use is at an increased risk for paronychia formation. Early identification and medical referral are imperative to avoid more serious consequences.

Clubbing

Clubbing of the fingers (Fig. 4.36) and toes usually results from chronic oxygen deprivation in these tissue beds. It is most often observed in patients with advanced COPD, congenital heart defects, and cor pulmonale but can occur within 10 days in someone with an acute systemic condition such as a pulmonary abscess, malignancy, or polycythemia. Clubbing may be the first sign of a paraneoplastic syndrome associated with cancer. Clubbing can be assessed using the Schamroth method (Fig. 4.37).

Any positive findings in the nail beds should be viewed in light of the entire clinical presentation. For example, a positive Schamroth test without observable clinical changes in skin color, capillary refill time, or shape of the fingertips may not signify systemic disease but rather a normal anatomic variation of nail curvature.

Nail Patella Syndrome

Nail patella syndrome (NPS), also called Fong's disease, hereditary onycho-osteodysplasia (HOOD), or Turner-Kieser syndrome, is a genetic disorder characterized by an absence or underdevelopment of nail bed changes as shown here (Fig. 4.38, *A*). Lack of skin creases is also a telltale sign (Fig. 4.39).

Nail abnormalities vary and range from a sliver on each corner of the nail bed to a full nail that is very thick with splits. Some people have brittle, underdeveloped, cracked, or ridged nails, whereas others are absent entirely. They are often concave, causing them to split and flip up, catching on clothing and bedding. Often, the lunula (the light crescent "half-moons" of the nail near the cuticle) are pointed or triangular-shaped (Fig. 4.38, *B*).

The therapist may be the first to see this condition because skeletal and joint problems are a common feature with this condition. The elbows, hips, and knees are affected most often. Absence or hypoplasia (underdevelopment) of the patella and deformities of the knee joint itself often give them a square

shape. Knee instability with patellar dislocation is not uncommon as a result of malformations of the bones, muscles, and ligaments; there is often much instability in the knee joint.

The patient may also develop scoliosis, glaucoma, and kidney disease. Medical referral to establish a diagnosis is important, as patients with NPS need annual screening for renal disease, biannual screening for glaucoma in adulthood, and magnetic resonance imaging (MRI) for orthopedic abnormalities before physical therapy is considered.[113,114]

When a patient presents with skin or nail bed changes of any kind, taking a personal medical history and reviewing recent (last 6 weeks) and current medications can provide the therapist with important clues in deciding whether to make an immediate medical referral. Table 4.9 provides a summary of the most common skin changes encountered in a physical therapy practice and possible causes for each one.

LYMPH NODE ASSESSMENT

Part of the screening process for the therapist may involve visual inspection of the skin overlying lymph nodes and palpation of the lymph nodes. Look for any obvious areas of

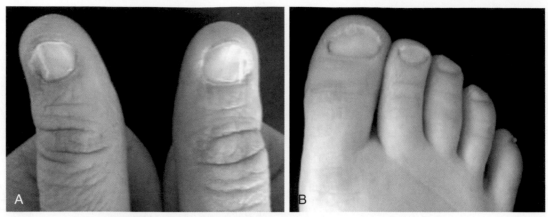

Fig. 4.38   Nail patella syndrome (NPS). Nail bed changes associated with NPS are presented here. Effects vary greatly between individuals but usually involve absence of part or all of the nail bed. For A, the finger and B, the toenails become paper thin in individuals with this condition. (From Lippacher S, Mueller Rossber E, Reichel H, et al. Correction of malformative patellar instability in patients with nail-patella syndrome: a case report and review of the literature. *Orthop Traumatol Surg Res* 2013;99:749–754. Copyright 2013 by Elsevier Masson SAS. All rights reserved.)

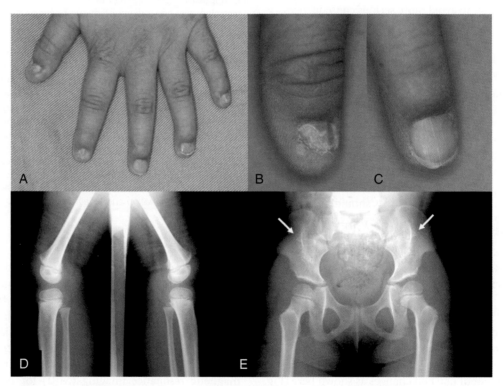

Fig. 4.39   Nail-patella syndrome (NPS). (A) Note the lack of creases in the distal interphalangeal (DIP) joints of the fingers. (B) and (C) Nail changes are the most constant feature of NPS and may be absent, underdeveloped (hypoplastic), or abnormal in size or shape (dysplastic). Alternately, there may be longitudinal ridges, pitting, or discoloration. (D) and (E) are radiographs of the same individual. (D) Note the absence of calcification center in the patella. (E) White arrows indicate iliac horns, which is typical of NPS. The condition may be present at birth and usually presents symmetrically and bilaterally. (From Oshimo T, Fukai K, Higashi N, et al. A novel LMX1B nonsense mutation in a family with nail-patella syndrome. J Dermatol Sci 2008;52(1):57-60.)

swelling or redness (erythema) along with any changes in skin color or pigmentation. Ask the patient about the presence or recent history of sores or lesions anywhere on the body.

Keep in mind the therapist cannot know what the underlying pathology may be when lymph nodes are palpable and questionable. Performing a baseline assessment and reporting the findings is the important outcome of the assessment.[115]

Whenever examining a lump or lesion, document and report findings on location, size, consistency, mobility or fixation, and signs of pain and tenderness (see also Box 4.15). With respect to size, normal lymph nodes should generally be less than 1 cm in diameter. However, the "normal" criteria may vary depending on the lymph node's location and the patient's age. For example, children less than 10 years of age have

TABLE 4.9	Common Causes of Skin and Nail Bed Changes
Skin/Nail Bed Changes	Possible Cause

SKIN CHANGES

Skin/Nail Bed Changes	Possible Cause
Dermatitis	Pulmonary malignancy, allergic reaction
Loss of turgor or elasticity	Dehydration
Rash (see Fig. 4.12)	Viruses (chicken pox, measles, Fifth disease)
	Systemic conditions: meningitis, lupus, hives, rosacea)
	Sexually transmitted diseases
	Lyme disease
	Parasites (e.g., lice, scabies)
	Reaction to chemicals, medications, food
	Malignancy, neoplastic syndromes
Hemorrhage (petechiae, ecchymosis, purpura) (see Fig. 4.14)	NSAIDs
	Anticoagulants (heparin, Coumadin/warfarin, aspirin)
	Hemophilia
	Thrombocytopenia (low platelet level) and anything that can cause thrombocytopenia
	Neoplasm; paraneoplastic syndrome
	Domestic violence
	Aging
Skin color	Jaundice (yellow, green, orange): hepatitis
	Chronic renal failure (yellow-brown)
	Cyanosis (pale, blue): anxiety, hypothermia, lung disease, congestive heart disease, venous obstruction
	Rubor (dusky red): arterial insufficiency
	Sunburn (red): radiation recall or radiation dermatitis
	Tan, black, blue: skin cancer
Hyperpigmentation (see Fig. 4.11)	Addison's disease, ACTH-producing tumors
	Sarcoidosis
	Pregnancy
	Leukemia
	Hemochromatosis
	Celiac sprue (malabsorption)
	Scleroderma
	Chronic renal failure
	Hereditary (nonpathognomonic)
	Low-dose radiation
Café-au-lait (hyperpigmentation; see Fig. 4.11)	Neurofibromatosis (more than five lesions)
	Albright's syndrome
	Urticaria pigmentosa (less than five lesions)
Hypopigmentation (vitiligo; see Fig. 4.10)	Albinism
	Sun exposure
	Steroid injection
	Hyperthyroidism
	Stomach cancer
	Pernicious anemia
	Diabetes mellitus
	Autoimmune disease
	High dose radiation
Xanthomas (see Fig. 4.16)	Disorders of lipid metabolism
	Primary biliary cirrhosis
	Diabetes mellitus (uncontrolled)
Mongolian spots (see Fig. 4.25)	Blue-black discoloration: normal in certain groups

NAIL BED CHANGES

Skin/Nail Bed Changes	Possible Cause
Onycholysis (see Fig. 4.31)	Graves' disease, psoriasis, reactive arthritis, persistent or chronic nail picking
Beau's lines (see Fig. 4.33)	Acute systemic illness
	Chemotherapy
	PVD
	Eating disorder
	Cirrhosis (chronic alcohol use)
	Recent heart attack
	Local trauma

Continued

TABLE 4.9	Common Causes of Skin and Nail Bed Changes—cont'd	
Skin/Nail Bed Changes	**Possible Cause**
Koilonychia (see Fig. 4.32)	Congenital or hereditary
	Hypochromic anemia
	Iron deficiency
	Diabetes mellitus (chronic, uncontrolled)
	Psoriasis
	Syphilis
	Rheumatic fever
	Thyroid dysfunction
Splinter hemorrhages (see Fig. 4.34)	Heart attack
	Bacterial endocarditis
	Vasculitis
	Renal failure
	Any systemic insult
Leukonychia (see Fig. 4.35)	Acquired or congenital
	Acquired: hypocalcemia, hypochromic anemia, Hodgkin's disease, renal failure, malnutrition, heart attack, hepatic cirrhosis, arsenic poisoning
Paronychia	Fungal infection
	Bacterial infection
Digital clubbing (see Fig. 4.36)	Acute: pulmonary abscess, malignancy, polycythemia, paraneoplastic syndrome
	Chronic: COPD, cystic fibrosis, congenital heart defects, cor pulmonale
Absent or underdeveloped nail bed (s) (see)	NPS
	Congenital
Pitting	Psoriasis

ACTH, Adrenocorticotropic hormone; *COPD*, chronic obstructive pulmonary disease; *NPS*, nail patella syndrome; *NSAIDs*, nonsteroidal anti-inflammatory drugs; *PVD*, peripheral vascular disease.

more active immune systems, and lymph nodes up to 2 cm can be considered "normal". However, an epitrochlear node of greater than 0.5 cm is considered "abnormal" in an adult, and warrants physician evaluation.[116] A normal lymph node should also be soft and squishy when palpated; a node that is firm to hard would raise concern. A normal node should be also be mobile and nontender when palpated. One may think that an inflamed lymph node would cause pinpoint pain; however, inflamed lymph nodes are more likely to cause a dull, nonlocalized ache in the region, that is more diffuse in nature. Review Special Questions to Ask: Lymph Nodes at the end of this chapter for appropriate follow-up questions. As a general rule, generalized lymphadenopathy (i.e., two or more noncontiguous locations), especially when combined with the presence of constitutional symptoms, such as fatigue, fever or weight loss, would require a much more extensive investigation than localized adenopathy.[116]

There are several sites where lymph nodes are potentially observable and palpable (Fig. 4.40). Palpation must be done lightly. Excessive pressure can press a node into a muscle or between two muscles. Normal lymph nodes usually are not visible or easily palpable, especially in the supraclavicular, popliteal, and iliac regions.[115] While not all visible or palpable lymph nodes are a sign of cancer, a nontender mass that is firm and nonmobile is often the initial sign of head and neck cancers.[117] Infections, viruses, bacteria, allergies, thyroid conditions, and food intolerances can also cause changes in the lymph nodes, thus abnormal nodes represent an important physical examination finding that warrants a medical evaluation.

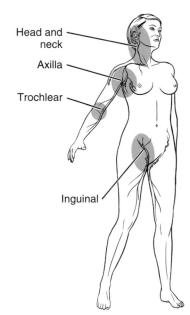

Fig. 4.40 Locations of most easily palpable lymph nodes. Epitrochlear nodes are located on the medial side of the arm above the elbow in the depression above and posterior to the medial condyle of the humerus. Horizontal and vertical chains of inguinal nodes may be palpated in the same areas as the femoral pulse. Popliteal lymph nodes (not shown) are deep but may be palpated in some patients with the knee slightly flexed.

People with seasonal allergies or allergic rhinitis often have enlarged, tender, and easily palpable lymph nodes in the sub-mandibular and supraclavicular areas. This is a sign that the immune system is working hard to stop as many perceived pathogens as possible.

Children often have easily palpable and tender lymph nodes because their developing immune system is continuously filtering out pathogens. Anyone with food intolerances or celiac sprue can have the same lymph node response in the inguinal area.

The therapist is most likely to palpate enlarged lymph nodes in the neck, supraclavicular, and axillary areas during an upper quadrant examination (Fig. 4.41). Virchow's node is located the at the junction of the thoracic duct and the left subclavian vein, where most of the body's lymph drains into the systemic circulation.[118]. Virchow's node, a palpable enlargement of one of the supraclavicular lymph nodes, may be palpated in the supraclavicular area in the presence of primary carcinoma of thoracic or abdominal organs. It is hypothesized that if the thoracic duct is blocked by metastasis, lymph is subsequently regurgitated into the surrounding supraclavicular lymph nodes, which leads to enlargement. Virchow's node is more often found on the left side.

Posterior cervical lymph node enlargement can occur during the icteric stage of hepatitis (see Table 9.3). Swelling of the regional lymph nodes often accompanies the first stage of syphilis that is usually painless. These glands feel rubbery, are freely movable, and are not tender on palpation. This may be followed by a general lymphadenopathy palpable in the posterior cervical or epitrochlear nodes (located in the inner condyle of the humerus).

The axillary lymph nodes are divided into three zones based on regional orientation[120] (Fig. 4.42). Only zones I and II are palpable. Zone I nodes are superficial and palpable with the patient sitting (preferred) or supine with the patient's arm supported by the examiner's hand and forearm. Gently palpate the entire axilla for any lymph nodes.

Zone II lymph nodes are palpated with the patient in sitting position. Zone II lymph nodes are below the clavicle in the area of the pectoralis muscle. The examiner must reach deep into the axilla to palpate for these lymph nodes. As axillary palpation is an extremely sensitive region, the therapist

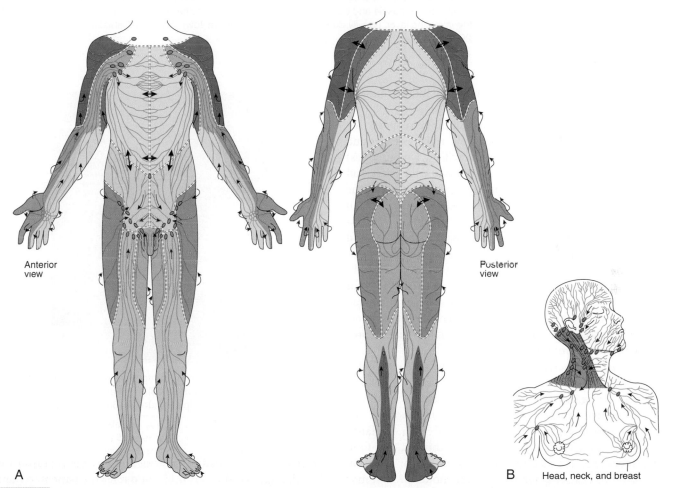

Anterior view

Posterior view

B   Head, neck, and breast

Fig. 4.41 Regional lymphatic system. (A) Superficial and deep collecting channels and their lymph node chains. Lymph territories are indicated by different shadings. Territories are separated by watersheds (marked by== =). Normal drainage is away from the watershed. (B) Lymph nodes of the head, neck, and chest and the direction of their drainage. The head and neck areas are divided into the anterior and posterior triangles divided by the sternocleidomastoid muscle. There are an estimated 75 lymph nodes on each side of the neck. The deep cervical chain is located in the anterior triangle, largely obstructed by the overlying sternocleidomastoid muscle. (From Casley-Smith JR. Modern Treatment for Lymphoedema. 5th ed. Adelaide, Australia: Lymphoedema Association of Australia; 1997. Modified from Földi M, Kubik S. Lehrbuch der lymphologie fur mediziner und physiotherapeuter mit anhang: praktische linweise fur die physiotherape. Stuttgart, Germany: Gustav Fischer Verlag; 1989.)

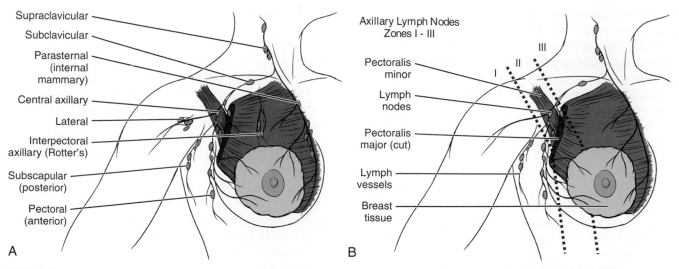

Fig. 4.42 (A) The breast has an extensive network of venous and lymphatic drainage. Most of the lymphatic drainage empties into axillary nodes. The main lymph node chains and lymphatic drainage are labeled as shown here. (B) Axillary lymph nodes are divided into three zones based on anatomic sites. Level I axillary lymph nodes are defined as those nodes lying lateral to the lateral border of the pectoralis minor muscle. Level II nodes are under the pectoralis minor muscle, between its lateral and medial borders. Level III nodes lie medial to the clavipectoral fascia, which invests the pectoralis minor muscle and covers the axillary nodes. Only zones I and II are palpable. Level III nodes are accessed only through penetration of the investing layer, usually during axillary surgery. (From Townsend CM. Sabiston Textbook of Surgery. 18th ed. Philadelphia: Saunders; 2008.)

must ensure appropriate patient instruction and permission, as well as offering of a chaperone.

To examine the right axilla, the examiner supports the patient's right arm with his or her own right forearm and hand (reverse for palpation of the left axillary lymph nodes) (Fig. 4.43). This will help ensure relaxation of the chest wall musculature. Lift the patient's upper arm up from under the elbow while reaching the fingertips of the left hand up as high as possible into the axilla.

The examiner's fingertips will be against the chest wall and the examiner should be able to feel the rib cage (and any palpable lymph nodes). As the patient's arm is lowered slowly, allow the fingertips to move down over the rib cage. Feel for the central nodes by compressing them against the chest wall and muscles of the axilla. The examiner may want to repeat this motion a second or third time until becoming more proficient with this examination technique.

Whenever the therapist encounters enlarged or palpable lymph nodes, ask the patient if they have noticed a lump in the area being evaluated and if a physician has examined it. If the patient is unaware of the lump, ask about a past medical history of cancer (Case Example 4.3), implants, mononucleosis, chronic fatigue, allergic rhinitis, and food intolerances. Ask about a recent illness or cut or infection in the hand or arm. Any tender, movable nodes present may be associated with these conditions, pharyngeal or dental infections, and other infectious diseases, and a referral is warranted. If the patient is aware of the lump and it has been examined by a physician, ask if the lump has changed (e.g., size, consistency, mobility, and signs of pain and tenderness) since they have seen their physician. If it has changed since seeing their physician last, it is important to inquire about

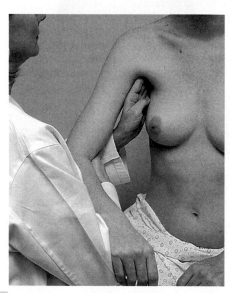

Fig. 4.43 Palpation of zone II lymph nodes in the sitting position. See description in text. (From Seidel HM, Ball JW, Dains JE. Mosby's Physical Examination Handbook. 3rd ed. St. Louis: Mosby; 2003.)

their recent past medical history and any other reason for the change (see also Box 4.15), and refer the patient to their physician.

Lymph nodes that are hard, immobile, and nontender raise the suspicion of cancer, especially in the presence of a previous history of cancer. Previous editions of this textbook mentioned that any change in lymph nodes present for more than 1 month in more than one location was a red flag. This has changed with the increased understanding of cancer

CASE EXAMPLE 4.3
Lymphadenopathy

A 73-year-old woman was referred to a physical therapy clinic by her oncologist with a diagnosis of cervical radiculopathy. She had a history of uterine cancer 20 years ago and a history of breast cancer 10 years ago.

Treatment included a hysterectomy, left radical mastectomy, radiation therapy, and chemotherapy. She has been cancer free for almost 10 years. Her family physician, oncologist, and neurologist actually all evaluated her before she was referred to the physical therapist.

Examination by a physical therapist revealed obvious lymphadenopathy of the left cervical and axillary lymph nodes. When asked if the referring physician (or other physicians) saw the "swelling," she told the therapist that she had not disrobed during her medical evaluation and consultation.

The question for us as physical therapists in a situation like this one is how to proceed.

Several steps must be taken. First, the therapist must document all findings. If possible, photographs of the chest, neck, and axilla should be obtained. The therapist should also screen for constitutional symptoms (Box 4.15).

Second, the therapist must ascertain whether the physician is already aware of the problem and has requested physical therapy as a palliative measure. Requesting the physician's notes from the examination is essential.

Contact with the physician will be important soon after obtaining the records, either to confirm the request as palliative therapy or to report your findings and confirm the need for medical reevaluation.

If it turns out that the physician is, indeed, unaware of these physical findings, it is best to make a problem list identified as "outside the scope of a physical therapist" when returning the patient to the physician. Be careful to avoid making any statements that could be misconstrued as a medical diagnosis.

It is highly advised that the therapist offer to make the appointment for the patient and do so immediately. We recommend writing a brief letter with the pertinent findings and ending with one of two one-liners:

What do you think?

Please advise.

Documentation of findings and recommendations must be complete even if the patient declines. Every effort must be made to get the patient to a physician. This may require follow-up phone calls and some persistence on the part of the therapist. Follow-up with the patient (either in-clinic or via telephone) after they has seen the physician is also indicated to gain an understanding of the patient's disposition.

metastases via the lymphatic system and the potential for cancer recurrence. The most up-to-date recommendation is for physician evaluation of all suspicious lymph nodes.[115,116,121]

❓ FOLLOW-UP QUESTIONS

Lymph Nodes

Assess lymph nodes for size, consistency, mobility and pain/tenderness and report baseline findings.

- [General screening question:] Have you examined yourself for any lumps or nodules and found any thickening or a lump? *If yes*, has your physician examined/treated this?
- Do you have (now or recently) any sores, rashes, or lesions anywhere on your body?
- If any suspicious or aberrant lymph nodes are observed during palpation, ask the following question.
- Have you (ever) had:
- Cancer of any kind?
  If no, have you ever been treated with radiation or chemotherapy for any reason?
- Breast implants
- Recent illness, such as a cold or the flu
- Mastectomy or prostatectomy
- Mononucleosis
- Chronic fatigue syndrome
- Allergic rhinitis
- Food intolerances, food allergies, or celiac sprue
- Recent dental work
- Infection of any kind
- Recent cut, insect bite, or infection in the hand or arm
- A sexually transmitted disease of any kind
- Sores or lesions of any kind anywhere on the body (including genitals)
- Breast: See Chapter 17 and Appendix B-7
- Headache: See Appendix B-17

MUSCULOSKELETAL SCREENING EXAMINATION

Muscle pain, weakness, poor coordination, and joint pain can be caused by many systemic disorders such as hypokalemia, hypothyroidism, dehydration, alcohol or drug use, vascular disorders, GI disorders, cancer, infections, autoimmune disorders, liver impairment, malnutrition, vitamin deficiencies, and psychologic factors.

In a screening examination of the musculoskeletal system, the patient is observed for any obvious deformities, abnormalities, disabilities, and asymmetries. Inspection and palpation of the skin, muscles, soft tissues, and joints often takes place simultaneously.

Assess each patient from the front, back, and each side. Some general examination principles include:[122]

- Let the patient know what to expect; offer simple but clear instructions and feedback.
- When comparing sides, test the "normal" side first.
- Examine the joint above and below the "involved" joint.
- Perform active, passive, and accessory or physiologic movements in that order unless circumstances direct otherwise.
- Resisted isometric movements (break test), which should follow accessory or physiologic motion testing, should be held for a minimum of 5 seconds to see if weakness becomes evident.
- Resisted isometric motion is done in a physiologic neutral position (open pack position); appropriate stabilization should be used to ensure the joint does not move during isometric assessment.

- Painful joint motion or painful empty end feel of a joint should not be forced.
- Inspect and palpate the skin and surrounding tissue for erythema, swelling, masses, tenderness, temperature changes, and crepitus.
- The forward bend and full squat positions, walking on toes and heels, standing one leg, and hopping on one leg are useful general screening tests.
- Perform specific special tests last, based on patient history and results of the screening interview and clinical findings so far.

The *Guide*[23] suggests key tests and measures to include in a comprehensive screening and specific testing process of the musculoskeletal system, including:

- Patient history (demographics, social and employment history, family and personal history, results of other clinical tests)
- Aerobic capacity and endurance
- Anthropometric characteristics
- Arousal, attention, and cognition
- Environmental, home, and work barriers
- Ergonomics and body mechanics
- Gait, locomotion, and balance
- Motor function (motor control and motor learning)
- Muscle performance (strength, power, and endurance)
- Posture
- Range of motion (ROM)
- Self-care and home management
- Work, community, and leisure integration or reintegration

These steps lead to a diagnostic classification or when appropriate, to a referral to another practitioner.[23] Assessing joint or muscle pain is discussed in greater depth in Chapter 3 (see also Appendix B-18 in the accompanying enhanced eBook version included with print purchase of this textbook).

REGIONAL SCREENING EXAMINATION

Head and Neck

Screening of the head and neck areas takes place when patient history and report of symptoms or clinical presentation warrant this type of examination. The head and neck assessment provides information about oral health and the general health of multiple systems including integumentary, neurologic, respiratory, endocrine, hepatic, and GI.

The head, hair and scalp, and face are observed for size, shape, symmetry, cleanliness, and presence of infection. Position of the head over the spine and in relation to midline and range-of-motion testing of the cervical spine and temporomandibular joints can be a part of the screening and posture assessment.

Because the head and neck have a large blood supply, infection from the mouth can quickly spread throughout the body increasing the risk of osteomyelitis, pneumonia, and septicemia in critically ill patients. Evidence of gum disease (e.g., bright red, enlarged, spongy, or bleeding) should be medically evaluated. Ulcerations on the tongue, lips, or gums also require further medical/dental evaluation.

The eyes can be examined for changes in shape, motor function, and color (conjunctiva and sclera). Conducting an assessment of cranial nerves II, III, and IV will also help screen for visual problems. The therapist should be aware that there are changes in the way older adults perceive color. This kind of change can affect function and safety; for example, some older adults are unable to tell when floor tiles end, and the bathtub begins in a bathroom. Stumbling and loss of balance can occur at boundary changes.

Assessment of cranial nerves (see Table 4.10), regional lymph nodes (see discussion, this chapter), carotid artery pulses (see Fig. 4.1), and jugular vein patency (Fig. 4.44) are a part of the head and neck examination. Therapists in a primary care setting may also examine the position of the trachea and thyroid for obvious deviations or palpable lesions.

Headaches are common and often the result of specific foods, stress, muscle tension, hormonal fluctuations, nerve compression, or cervical spine or temporomandibular joint dysfunction. Most headaches are acute and self-limited. Headaches can be a symptom of a serious medical condition and should be assessed carefully (see Appendix B-17 in the accompanying enhanced eBook version included with print purchase of this textbook; see also the discussion of viscerogenic causes of head and neck pain in Chapter 15).

Upper and Lower Extremities

The extremities are examined through a systematic assessment of various aspects of the musculoskeletal, neurologic, vascular, and integumentary systems. Inspection and palpation are two techniques used most often during the examination. A checklist can be very helpful (Box 4.13).

Peripheral Vascular Disease

PVD, both the arterial and venous condition, is a common problem observed in the extremities of older adults, especially those with a history of heart disease. Knowing the risk factors for any condition, but especially problems like PVD, helps the therapist know when to screen. These conditions, including risk factors, are discussed in greater depth in Chapter 7.

The first signs of vascular occlusive disease are often skin changes (see Box 4.10). The therapist must watch out for common risk factors, including bed rest or prolonged immobility, use of IV catheters, obesity, MI, HF, pregnancy, postoperative patients, and any problems with coagulation.

Screening assessment of peripheral arterial disease (PAD) can be done using the ankle-brachial index (ABI) (Fig. 4.45). Patients who would benefit from screening include: patients with risk factors for PAD such as smoking, diabetes, advancing age (over 50 years of age), hypertension, hyperlipidemia, and symptoms of claudication.[123]

Baseline ABI should be taken on both sides for anyone who has (or may have) PAD. Patients with diabetes who have normal ABI levels should be retested periodically.[124] The ABI is the ratio of the SBP in the ankle divided by the SBP in the arm:SBP (ankle)/ SBP (arm)

TABLE 4.10	Cranial Nerve Function and Assessment		
Cranial Nerve (CN)	Type	Function	Assessment
I Olfactory	Sensory	Sense of smell	Able to identify common odors (e.g., coffee, vanilla, orange, or peppermint) with eyes closed
			Close one nostril and test one nostril at a time
II Optic	Sensory	Visual acuity	Visual acuity; test each eye separately with Snellen eye chart
			If literate, able to read printed material
III Oculomotor	Motor	Extraocular eye movement	Assess CNs III, IV, and VI together
		Pupil constriction and dilation	Look for equal pupil size and shape; equal response to light and accommodation; inspect eyelids for drooping (ptosis)
			Ask about blurry or double vision
			Follow finger with eyes without moving head (six points in an H pattern; gaze test)
			Convergence (move finger toward patient's nose)
IV Trochlear	Motor	Upward and downward movement of eyeball	See CN III; assess directions of gaze (eye can move out when intact/ eye remains focused up and out when impaired); visual tracking
			Ask about double vision
V Trigeminal	Mixed	Sensory nerve to skin of face	Corneal reflex: patient looks up and away, examiner lightly touches opposite cornea with wisp of cotton (look for blink in both eyes or a report by patient of blinking sensation)
			Facial sensation: apply sterile, sharp item to forehead, cheek, jaw; repeat with dull object; patient reports "sharp" or "dull"; if abnormal, test for temperature, vibration, and light touch
		Motor nerve to muscles of jaw (mastication)	Ask patient to clench teeth together as you palpate muscles over temples (temporal muscle) and jaw (masseter) on each side
			Look for symmetric tone (normal) or muscle atrophy, deviation of jaw to one side, or fasciculations (abnormal)
VI Abducens	Motor	Lateral movement of eyeballs	See CN III; assess directions of gaze (able to move eyes out laterally when intact/medially deviated when impaired)
VII Facial	Mixed	Facial expression	Look for symmetry with facial expressions (e.g., frown, smile, raise and lower eyebrows, puff cheeks out, close eyes tightly)
VIII Acoustic (auditory, vestibulocochlear)	Sensory	Hearing	Assess ability to hear spoken word and whisper
			Examiner stands behind patient with hands on either side of patient's head/ears; rub candy wrapper or fingers together to make noise on one side, ask patient to identify which side noise is coming from
			Examiner stands 18 inches behind patient and whispers three numbers
			Assess for dizziness and imbalance
			Weber test and Rinne test to distinguish between sensorineural and conductive hearing loss
IX Glossopharyngeal	Mixed	Taste	Patient identifies sour or sweet taste on back of tongue
		Gag, swallow	Gag reflex (sensory IX and motor X) and ability to swallow
X Vagus	Mixed	Pharyngeal sensation, voice, swallow	Patient says, "Ah." Observe for normal palate and pharynx movement
			Listen for hoarseness or nasal quality in voice
			Observe for difficulty swallowing
XI Spinal Accessory	Motor	Movement of head and shoulders	Patient is able to shrug shoulders and turn head against resistance
			Observe shoulders from behind for trapezius atrophy and/or asymmetry (abnormal finding)
			Assess for neck weakness
XII Hypoglossal	Motor	Position and movement of tongue	Patient can stick out tongue to midline and move it from side to side
			Patient can move tongue toward nose and chin
			Clear articulation in speech pattern

Assess ankle SBP using both the dorsalis pedis pulse and the posterior tibial pulse. Divide the higher SBP from each leg by the higher brachial systolic pressure (i.e., if the SBP is higher in the right arm use that figure for the calculation in both legs).

Normal ABI values lie in the range of 0.91 to 1.3. A general guideline is provided in Table 4.11. Recall what was said earlier in this chapter about normal BPs in the legs versus the arms: SBP in the legs is normally 10% to 20% higher than the brachial artery pressure in the arms, resulting in an ABI greater than 1.0. PAD obstruction is indicated when the ABI values fall to less than 1.0.

Buerger's test is another test used to observe the adequacy of arterial circulation. Place the patient in the supine position and observe the color of the soles of the feet. Normal feet should be pink or flesh colored in Caucasians, and tan or brown in patients with dark skin tones. The feet of patients

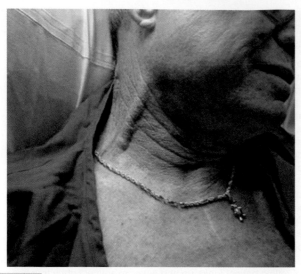

Fig. 4.44 Jugular venous distention is a sign of increased venous return (volume overload) or heart failure, especially congestive heart failure, and requires immediate medical attention if not previously reported. Inspect the jugular veins with the patient sitting up at a 90° angle and again with the head at a 30- to 45° angle. The cervical spine should be in a neutral position. Correlate the findings of this examination with vital signs, breath, heart sounds, peripheral edema, and auscultation of the carotid arteries for bruits. (From Goldman L. Cecil Medicine. 23rd ed. Philadelphia: WB Saunders; 2008.)

BOX 4.13 EXTREMITY EXAMINATION CHECKLIST

- Inspect skin for color, scratch marks, inflammation, track marks, bruises, heat, or other obvious changes
- Observe for hair loss or hair growth
- Observe for asymmetry, contour changes, edema, obvious atrophy, fractures or deformities; measure circumference if indicated
- Assess palpable lesions
- Palpate for temperature, moisture, and tenderness
- Palpate pulses
- Palpate lymph nodes
- Check nail bed refill (normal: capillary refill time under 2–3 seconds for fingers and 3–4 seconds for toes)
- Observe for clubbing, signs of cyanosis, other nail bed changes
- Observe for PVD (see Box 4.10); listen for femoral bruits if indicated; test for thrombophlebitis
- Assess joint ROM and muscle tone
- Perform gross MMT (gross strength test); grip and pinch strength
- Sensory testing: light touch, vibration, proprioception, temperature, pinprick
- Assess coordination (UEs: dysmetria, diadochokinesia; LEs: gait, heel-to-shin test)
- Test deep tendon reflexes

LEs, Lower extremities; *MMT*, manual muscle testing; *PVD*, peripheral vascular disease; *ROM*, range of motion; *UEs*, upper extremities.

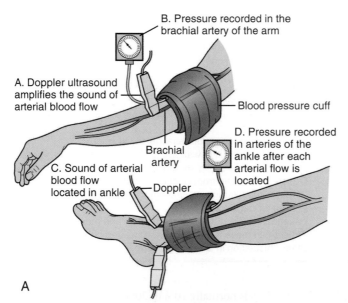

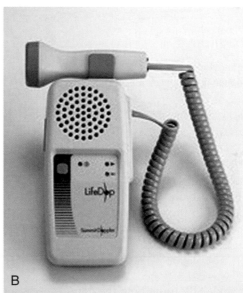

Fig. 4.45 (A) Peripheral vascular testing is usually performed in a vascular laboratory, but an approximation of the integrity of the peripheral arterial circulation can be found by calculating the ankle/brachial index (ABI) by using a Doppler device to compare systolic blood pressure (BP) in the foot and arm. (B) The ABI is measured using a simple, noninvasive tool. Example of a handheld Doppler device with speaker is shown. Devices with an attached stethoscope are also used to measure the ABI. The index correlates well with blood vessel disease severity and symptoms. In the normal individual, the systolic BP in the legs is slightly greater than or equal to the brachial (arm) systolic BP (ABI = 1.0 or above). Where there is arterial obstruction and narrowing, systolic BP is reduced below the area of obstruction. When the ankle systolic blood pressure falls below the brachial systolic BP, the ABI is less than 1.0 (a sign of peripheral vascular obstruction). (From Roberts JR. Clinical Procedures in Emergency Medicine. 5th ed. Philadelphia: WB Saunders; 2010.)

TABLE 4.11	Ankle Brachial Index Reading*
INDICATORS OF PERIPHERAL ARTERIAL DISEASE	
1.0–1.3	Normal (blood pressure at the ankle and arm are the same; no significant narrowing or obstruction of blood flow)
0.8–0.9	Mild peripheral arterial occlusive disease
0.5–<0.8	Moderate peripheral arterial occlusive disease
<0.5	Severe peripheral arterial occlusive disease; critical limb ischemia
<0.2	Ischemic or gangrenous extremity

*Different sources offer slightly different ABI values for normal to severe PAD. Some sources use values between 0.90 and 0.97 as the lower end of normal. Values greater than 1.3 are not considered reliable because calcified vessels show falsely elevated pressures. The therapist should follow guidelines provided by the physician or facility.

Data from Sacks D, et al. Position statement on the use of the ankle brachial index in the evaluation of patients with peripheral vascular disease. A consensus statement developed by the Standards Division of the Society of Interventional Radiology. J Vasc Interv Radiol 2002;13:353.

with impaired circulation are often chalky white (Caucasians) or gray or white in patients with darker skin.

Elevate the legs between 30 to 45 degrees (above the heart level) for 30 to 60 seconds. For patients with compromised arterial blood supply, any color present will quickly disappear in this position; in other words, the elevated foot develops increased pallor. No change (or little change) is observed in the normal individual. Bring the individual to a sitting position with the legs dangling. Normally, the legs in this position may turn slightly pink however in a patient with arterial insufficiency or PAD they will become dark red (dependent rubor).

Venous Thromboembolism

Another condition affecting the extremities is venous thromboembolism (VTE), a common complication seen in patients with cancer or following surgery (especially orthopedic surgery, such as total hip and total knee replacements), major trauma, or prolonged immobilization. Other risk factors are discussed in Chapter 7.

VTE includes deep vein thrombosis (DVT) and pulmonary embolism (PE). A DVT occurs when a blood clot forms in a deep vein, usually in the lower leg, thigh, or pelvis, but may also occur in the upper extremity. A PE occurs when a thrombus dislodges and travels through the bloodstream to the lungs.[125] It is imperative to screen for both conditions in patients at risk for VTE, especially patients following surgery. The revised Wells Clinical Decision Rule (CDR) (Table 4.12) for assessment of DVTs is recommended for the outpatient setting.[126] The Wells CDR incorporates the characteristics of a DVT to include signs, symptoms, and risk factors for DVT. T The revised Wells CDR is a conservative assessment tool that determines whether a DVT is "likely" or "not likely." There are also similar assessment tools for PE.[127,128] It is vital for therapists to stay up to date on the evidence for the use of VTE assessment tools for

TABLE 4.12	Revised Wells Clinical Decision Rule for Deep Vein Thrombosis	
Clinical Presentation		**Score**
Previously diagnosed deep vein thrombosis (DVT)		1
Active cancer (within 6 months of diagnosis or receiving palliative care)		1
Paralysis, paresis, or recent immobilization of lower extremity		1
Bedridden for more than 3 days or major surgery within the previous 12 weeks		1
Localized tenderness in the center of the posterior calf, the popliteal space, or along the femoral vein in the anterior thigh/groin		1
Entire lower extremity swelling		1
Unilateral calf swelling (more than 3 cm larger than uninvolved side)		1
Unilateral pitting edema		1
Collateral superficial veins (nonvaricose)		1
An alternative diagnosis is as likely (or more likely) than DVT (e.g., cellulitis, postoperative swelling, calf strain)		−2
Total points		
Key		
> or equal to 2		DVT likely
<2		DVT unlikely

Medical consultation is advised in the presence of low probability; medical referral is required with moderate or high score.

From Le Gal G, Carrier M, Rodger M. Clinical decision rules in venous thromboembolism. Best Pract Res Clin Haematol 2012;25:303-317.

both the setting and the patient population that the therapist most commonly treats.

The Chest and Back (Thorax)

A screening examination of the thorax requires the same basic techniques of inspection, palpation, and auscultation. Once again, keep in mind this is a screening examination. Being familiar with normal findings of the chest and thorax will help the therapist identify abnormal results requiring further evaluation or referral. Only basic screening tools are included. Specialized training may be required for some acute or primary care settings.

Chest and Back: Inspection[129]

Clinical inspection of the chest and back encompasses both the cardiac and pulmonary systems, but some of the most obvious changes are observed in relation to the respiratory system (Box 4.14). Inspect the patient while he or she is sitting upright without support if possible. Observe the patient's thorax from the front, back, side, and over the shoulder (looking down over the anterior chest). Note any skin changes; signs of skin breakdown; and signs of cyanosis or pallor, scars, wounds, bruises, lesions, nodules, or superficial venous patterns.

Note the shape and symmetry of the thorax from the front and back. Note any obvious anatomic changes or deformities (e.g., pectus excavatum, pectus carinatum, barrel chest).

Record the presence of any substantial deviations of posture from or deformities (e.g., kyphosis, scoliosis, rib hump) that can compromise chest wall excursion. Estimate the anterior-posterior diameter compared with the transverse diameter.

A normal ratio of 1:2 may be replaced by an equal diameter (1:1 ratio) typical of the barrel chest that develops as a result of hyperinflation. Look at the angle of the costal margins at the xiphoid process; for example, anything less than a 90-degree alignment may be indicative of a barrel chest. Observe (and palpate) for equal intercostal spaces and compare sides (right to left). Observe the patient for muscular development and nutritional status by noting the presence of underlying adipose tissue and the visibility of the ribs.

Assess respiratory rate, depth, and rhythm or pattern of breathing while the patient is breathing normally. A description of altered breathing patterns can be found in Chapter 8. Watch for symmetry of chest wall movement, costal versus abdominal breathing, the amount of accessory muscles use,

and bulging or retraction of the intercostal spaces. Remember, the normal ratio of inspiration to expiration is 1:2.

Chest and Back: Palpation

Palpation of the thorax is usually combined with inspection to save time. Lymph node assessment may be a part of the chest examination in males and females (see discussion later in this section).

Palpation can reveal skin changes and alert the therapist to conditions that relate to the patient's respiratory status. Look for crepitus, a crackly, crinkly sensation in the subcutaneous tissue. Feel for vibrations during inspiration as described next.

Palpate the entire thorax (anterior and posterior) for tactile fremitus by placing the palms of both hands over the patient's upper anterior chest at the second intercostal space (Fig. 4.46). The normal response is a feeling of vibrations of equal intensity during vocalizations on either side of the midline, front to back.

Stronger vibrations are felt whenever air is present; the absence of air, such as occurs with atelectasis, is marked by an absence of vibrations. Fluid outside the lung pressing on the lung increases the force of vibration.

Fremitus can be increased or decreased—increased over areas of compression because the dense tissue improves

---

BOX 4.14   CLINICAL INSPECTION OF THE RESPIRATORY SYSTEM

- Respiratory rate, depth, and effort of breathing
  - Tachypnea
  - Dyspnea
  - Gasping respirations
- Breathing pattern or sounds (see also Box 7.1)
  - Cheyne-Stokes respiration
  - Hyperventilation or hypoventilation
  - Kussmaul's respiration
  - Paradoxic breathing
  - Prolonged expiration
  - Pursed-lip breathing
  - Wheezing
  - Rhonchi (low-pitched wheezes)
  - Crackles (formerly called rales)
- Cyanosis
- Pallor or redness of skin during activity
- Clubbing (toes, fingers)
- Nicotine stains on fingers and hands
- Retraction of intercostal, supraclavicular, or suprasternal spaces
- Use of accessory muscles
- Nasal flaring
- Tracheal tug
- Chest wall shape and deformity
  - Barrel chest
  - Pectus excavatum
  - Pectus carinatum
  - Kyphosis
  - Scoliosis
- Cough
- Sputum: clear or white (normal); frothy; red-tinged, green, or yellow (pathologic)

Adapted from Goodman CC, Fuller K. Pathology: Implications for the Physical Therapist. 4th ed. Philadelphia: WB Saunders; 2015.

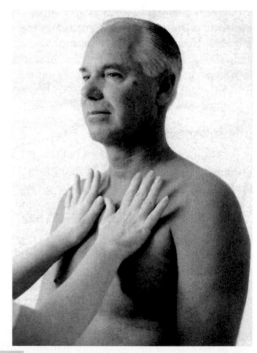

Fig. 4.46 Palpating for tactile fremitus. Place the palmar surfaces of both hands on the patient's chest at the second intercostal space. Ask the patient to say "99" repeatedly as you gradually move your hands over the chest, systematically comparing the lung fields. Start at the center and move out toward the arms. Drop the hands down one level and move back toward the center. Continue until the complete lung fields have been assessed. Repeat the examination on the patient's back. The normal response is a feeling of vibrations of equal intensity during vocalizations on either side of the midline, front to back. (From Expert 10-Minute Physical Examinations. St. Louis: Mosby; 1997.)

transmission of the vibrational wave while being decreased over areas of effusion (decreased density, decreased vibration).

Increased tactile fremitus often accompanies inflammation, infection, congestion, or consolidation of a lung or part of a lung. Diminished tactile fremitus may indicate the presence of pleural effusion or pneumothorax.[129] Record the location, and note whether the tactile fremitus is increased or decreased. It is important to note that it may be challenging to determine if differences are due to an increase in one or a decrease in the other. Therefore, it is important to auscultate the lungs if a difference in tactile fremitus is observed. Confirm all findings with auscultation; a medical evaluation with chest radiographs provides the differential diagnosis.

Assess the symmetry of chest wall excursion with the patient in the sitting position (preferred), or if unable to, assume or maintain an upright position, then in the supine position. The upright position makes it easier to assess all areas of chest wall excursion: upper, middle, and lower. Stand in front of your patient and place your thumbs along the patient's costal margins wrapping your fingers around the rib cage. Observe if the thumbs move apart symmetrically during chest expansion (normal breathing and deep breathing). Measure symmetry at more than one level and front to back. Chest wall excursion demonstrates a wide range variability across the population. The normal range of chest wall excursion measured at the xiphoid process using measuring tape range between 4 and 7 cm. [130,131]

The presence of costovertebral tenderness should be followed up with Murphy's percussion test (see Fig. 4.54). Bone tenderness over the lumbar spinous processes is a red-flag symptom for osseous disorders, such as fracture, infection, or neoplasm, and requires a more complete evaluation.

Chest and Back: Percussion

Chest and back percussion is an important part of the initial examination. The clinician can use percussion of the chest and back to identify the left ventricular border of the heart and the depth of diaphragmatic excursion in the upper abdomen during breathing. Percussion can also help identify disorders that impair lung ventilation such as stomach distention, hemothorax, lung consolidation, and pneumothorax.[129]

Dullness over the lungs during percussion may indicate a mass or consolidation (e.g., pneumonia). Hyperresonance over the lungs may indicate hyperinflated or emphysemic lungs. Decreased diaphragmatic excursion on one side occurs with pleural effusion, diaphragmatic (phrenic nerve) paralysis, tension pneumothorax, stomach distention (left side), hepatomegaly (right side), or atelectasis. Patients with COPD often have decreased excursion bilaterally as a result of a hyperinflated chest depressing the diaphragm.

Chest and Back: Lung Auscultation

During the examination, the therapist should listen for normal breath sounds and air movement through the lungs during inspiration and expiration with the patient breathing through their mouth. Taking a deep breath or coughing clears some sounds. At times the examiner instructs the patient to take a deep breath or cough and listens again for any changes in sound. With practice and training, the therapist can identify the most common abnormal sounds heard in patients with pulmonary involvement: crackles, wheezing, and pleural friction rub.

Crackles (formerly called rales) are the sound of air moving through an airway filled with fluid. It is heard most often during inspiration and sounds like strands of hair being rubbed together under a stethoscope. Crackles/rales are normal sounds in the morning as the alveolar spaces open up. Have the patient take a deep breath to complete this process first before listening.

Abnormal crackles can be heard during exhalation in patients with pneumonia or CHF and during inhalation with the re-expansion of atelectatic areas. Crackles are described as fine (soft and high-pitched), medium (louder and low-pitched), or coarse (moist and more explosive).

Wheezing is the sound of air passing through a narrowed airway blocked by mucous secretions or narrowed due to inflammation. Wheezes usually occur during expiration (wheezing during inspiration is a sign of a more serious problem). It is frequently described as a high-pitched, musical whistling sound but there are different tones to wheezing that can be identified in making the medical differential diagnosis.

There is some debate surrounding the difference between *rhonchi* and wheezing. Some experts consider the low-pitched, rattling sound of rhonchi (similar to snoring) as a form of wheezing. Whether called wheezing or rhonchi, this sound is most often associated with asthma or emphysema. Take careful note when the wheezing goes away in any patient who presents with wheezing. Disappearance of wheezing occurs when the person is not breathing.

Rhonchi are low-pitched wheezes which can be heard during inspiration or expiration, and may be cleared by coughing. It can be difficult to distinguish between high-pitched and low-pitched wheezes (rhonchi) and thus many providers refer to them interchangeably.[132]

Pleural friction rub makes a high-pitched scratchy sound which resembles the sound heard when a hand is cupped over the ear and scratched along the outside of the hand. It is caused by inflamed pleural surfaces and can be heard during inspiration and/or expiration. The pleural linings should move over each other smoothly and easily. In the presence of inflammation (pleuritis, pleurisy, pneumonia, tumors), the inflamed tissue (parietal pleura) is rubbing against other inflamed, irritated tissue (visceral pleura) causing friction.

Assess for *egophony* by asking the patient to say and repeat the "ee" sound during auscultation of the lung fields. The "aa" sound heard as the patient says the "ee" sound indicates pleural effusion or lung consolidation. *Bronchophony*, a clear and audible "99" sound suggests the sound is traveling through fluid or a mass; the sound should be muffled in the healthy adult. Finally, assess for consolidation using *whispered pectoriloquy*. Ask the patient to whisper "1-2-3" as you listen to the chest and back. The examiner should hear a muffled noise (normal) instead of a clear and audible "1-2-3" (consolidation).

Describe sounds heard, the location of the sounds on the thorax, and when the sounds are heard during the respiratory cycle (inspiration versus expiration). Have the patient gently cough (bronchial secretions causing a "gurgle" will often clear with a cough) and listen again. Compare results with the first examination (and with the baseline if available). The decision to treat, treat and consult/refer, or consult/refer a patient for further evaluation is based on history, clinical findings, patient distress, vital signs, and any associated signs and symptoms observed or reported.

Giving the physician details of your physical examination findings is important in order to give a clear idea of the reason for the consult and urgency (if there is one). Sometimes, abnormal findings are "normal" for people with chronic pulmonary problems. For example, always evaluate apparent abnormal breath (and heart) sounds in order to recognize change that is significant for the individual. The physician is more likely to respond immediately when told that the therapist identified crackles in the right lower lung and the patient is producing yellow sputum than if the report is "patient has altered sounds during auscultation."

Chest and Back: Heart Auscultation

The same general principles for auscultation of lung sounds apply to auscultation of heart sounds. The therapist's primary responsibility during the screening is to know what "normal" heart sounds are like and report any changes (absence of normal sounds or presence of additional sounds).

The normal cardiac cycle correlates with the direction of blood flow and consists of two phases: systole (ventricles contract and eject blood) and diastole (ventricles relax and atria contract to move blood into the ventricles and fill the coronary arteries).

Normal heart sounds (S1 and S2) occur in relation to the cardiac cycle. Just before S1, the mitral and tricuspid (AV) valves are open, and blood from the atria fills the relaxed ventricles (see Fig. 7.1). The ventricles contract and raise pressure, beginning the period called systole.

Pressure in the ventricles increases rapidly, forcing the mitral and tricuspid valves to close causing the first heart sound (S1). The S1 sound produced by the closing of the AV valves is *lubb*; it can be heard at the same time the radial or carotid pulse is felt.

As the pressure inside the ventricles increases, the aortic and pulmonic valves open and blood is pumped out of the heart into the lungs and aorta. The ventricle ejects most of its blood and pressure begins to fall causing the aortic and pulmonic valves to snap shut. The closing of these valves produces the *ub* (S2) sound. This marks the beginning of the diastole phase.

S3 (third heart sound), S4 (fourth heart sound), heart murmurs, and pericardial friction rub are the most common extra sounds heard. S3, also known as a ventricular gallop,[133] is a faint, low-pitched *lubb-dup-ah* sound heard directly after S2. It occurs at the beginning of diastole and may be heard in healthy children and young adults as a result of a large volume of blood pumping through a small heart. This

sound is also considered normal in the last trimester of pregnancy. It is not normal when it occurs as a result of anemia, decreased myocardial contractility, or volume overload associated with CHF.

S4, also known as an atrial gallop,[134] occurs in late diastole (just before S1) if there is a vibration of the valves, papillary muscles, or ventricular walls from resistance to filling (stiffness). It is usually considered an abnormal sound (*ta-lup-dubb*) but may be heard in athletes with well-developed heart muscles.

Heart murmurs are swishing sounds made as blood flows across a stiff or incompetent (leaky) valve or through an abnormal opening in the heart wall. Most murmurs are associated with valve disease (stenosis, insufficiency), but they can occur with a wide variety of other cardiac conditions. They may be normal in children and during the third trimester of pregnancy.

A pericardial friction rub associated with pericarditis is a scratchy, scraping sound that is heard louder during exhalation and forward bending. The sound occurs when inflamed layers of the heart viscera (see Fig. 7.5) rub against each other causing friction.

Auscultate the heart over each of the six anatomic landmarks (Fig. 4.47), first with the diaphragm (firm pressure) and then with the bell (light pressure) of the stethoscope. Use a Z-path to include all landmarks while covering the entire surface area of the heart.

Practice at each site until you can hear the rate and rhythm, S1 and S2, extra heart sounds, including murmurs. The high-pitched sounds of S1 and S2 are heard best with the

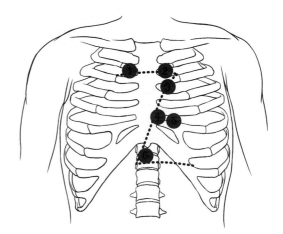

1. Aortic area (right 2nd intercostal space, ICS)
2. Pulmonic area (P1) (left 2nd ICS)
3. Erb's point (P2) (left 3rd ICS); S2 best auscultated here, murmurs are best heard at this point using the stethoscope bell
4. Tricuspid (left 5th ICS at sternum)
5. Mitral or apical point of maximal impulse (PMI), (left 5th ICS medial to the midclavicular line)
6. Epigastric area (just below the tip of the sternum)

Fig. 4.47 Auscultation of cardiac areas using cardiac anatomic landmarks. Inspect and palpate the anterior chest with the patient sitting up. Ask the individual to breathe quietly while you auscultate all six anatomic landmarks shown.

stethoscope diaphragm. Murmurs are not heard with a bell (listen for murmurs with the diaphragm); low-pitched sounds of S3 and S4 are heard with the bell.

As with lung sounds, describe heart sounds heard, rate and rhythm of the sounds, the location of the sounds on the thorax, and when the sounds are heard during the cardiac cycle. The decision to refer a patient for further evaluation is based on history, age, risk factors, presence of pregnancy, clinical findings, patient distress, vital signs, and any associated signs and symptoms observed or reported.

Screening for Early Detection of Breast Cancer. The goal of screening is early detection of breast cancer. Breast cancers that are detected because they are causing symptoms tend to be relatively larger and are more likely to have spread beyond the breast. In contrast, breast cancers found during such examinations are more likely to be small and still confined to the breast.

The size of a breast neoplasm and how far it has spread are the most important factors in predicting the prognosis for anyone with this disease. According to the ACS early detection tests for breast cancer saves many thousands of lives each year; many more lives could be saved if health care providers took advantage of these tests.[135] Following the ACS's guidelines for the early detection of breast cancer improves the chance that breast cancer can be diagnosed at an early stage and treated successfully. Any screening for breast cancer by the PT beyond asking a patient whether they have performed self-screening, received annual mammograms, and/or visited a physician for an examination is beyond the scope of the physical therapist.

Abdomen

Anyone presenting with primary pain patterns from pathology of the abdominal organs will likely see a physician rather than a physical therapist. For this reason, abdominal and visceral assessment is not generally a part of the physical therapy evaluation. When the therapist suspects referred pain from the viscera to the musculoskeletal system, this type of assessment can be helpful in the screening examination.

Abdomen: Inspection

From a screening or assessment point of view, the abdomen is divided into four quadrants centered on the umbilicus (as shown in Figs. 4.48 and 4.49). During the inspection, any abdominal scars (and associated history) should be identified (see Fig. 4.8).

Note the color of the skin and the presence and location of any scars, striae from pregnancy or weight gain/loss, petechiae, or spider angiomas (see Fig. 10.3). A bluish discoloration around the umbilicus (Cullen's sign) or along the lower abdomen and flanks (Grey Turner's sign) (Fig. 1)[136] may be a sign of abdominal pathology and retroperitoneal bleed (e.g., pancreatitis, ruptured ectopic pregnancy, posterior perforated ulcer, splenic rupture in infectious mononucleosis).[136] The color may be a shade of blue-red, blue-purple, or green-brown, depending on the stage of hemoglobin breakdown.[137] Cullen's sign or Grey Turner's sign may appear on an athlete (such as in football after taking a hard hit) or in trauma (such

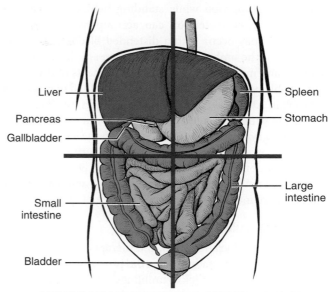

ANTERIOR VIEW OF ABDOMINAL CAVITY

Fig. 4.48 Four abdominal (anterior) quadrants formed by two imaginary perpendicular lines running through the umbilicus. As a general rule, viscera in the right upper quadrant (RUQ) can refer pain to the right shoulder; viscera in the left upper quadrant (LUQ) can refer pain to the left shoulder; viscera in the lower quadrants are less specific and can refer pain to the pelvis, pelvic floor, groin, low back, hip, and sacroiliac/sacral areas (see also Figs. 3.4 and 3.5).

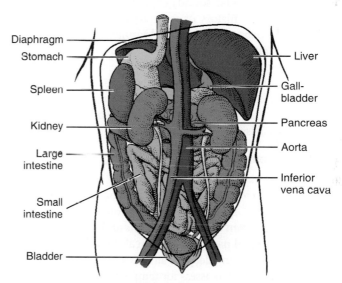

POSTERIOR VIEW OF ABDOMINAL CAVITY

Fig. 4.49 Posterior view of the abdomen. The abdominal aorta passes from the diaphragm through the abdominal cavity, just to the left of the midline. It branches into the left and right common iliac arteries at the level of the umbilicus. Retroperitoneal bleeding from any of the posterior elements (e.g., stomach, spleen, aorta, kidneys) can cause back, hip, and/or shoulder pain.

as a motor vehicle accident). The therapist needs to expediently refer the patient to a physician if one or both of these signs are present.

From a seated position next to the patient, note the contour of the abdomen and look for any asymmetry. Repeat the same visual inspection while standing behind the patient's head. Generalized distention can accompany gas, whereas local bulges may occur with a distended bladder or hernia. Make note if the umbilicus is displaced in any direction or if there are any masses, pulsations, or movements of the abdomen. Visible peristaltic waves are not normal and may signal a GI problem. Document the presence of ascites (see Fig. 10.9).

Patients with an organic cause for abdominal pain usually are not hungry. Ask the patient to point to the location of the pain. Pain corresponding to the epigastric, periumbilical, and lower midabdominal regions is shown in Fig. 9.2. If the finger points to the navel, but the patient seems well and is not in any distress, there may be a psychogenic source of symptoms.[138]

Abdomen: Auscultation

During the initial examination, the therapist may auscultate the four abdominal quadrants for the presence of abdominal sounds. Expect to hear clicks, rumblings, and gurgling sounds every few seconds throughout the abdomen. Auscultation should occur before palpation and/or percussion to avoid altering bowel sounds.

The absence of sounds or very few sounds in any or all of the quadrants is a red flag and is most common in the older adult with multiple risk factors such as recent abdominal, back, or pelvic surgery and the use of opioids or other medications.

As previously mentioned, the therapist may auscultate the abdomen for vascular sounds (e.g., bruits) when the history (e.g., age over 65, history of coronary artery disease), clinical presentation (e.g., neck, back, abdominal, or flank pain), and associated signs and symptoms (e.g., syncopal episodes, signs and symptoms of PVD) warrant this type of assessment.

Listen for pulsations/bruits over the aorta, renal arteries, iliac arteries, and femoral arteries first and remember to do so before palpation because palpation may stir up the bowel contents and increase peristalsis, making auscultation more difficult.

Abdomen: Percussion and Palpation

Remember to auscultate first before percussion and palpation in order to avoid altering the frequency of bowel sounds. Percussion over normal, healthy abdominal organs is an advanced skill, even among physicians and nurses, and is not usually an integral part of the physical therapy examination.

Palpation (light and deep) of all four abdominal quadrants is a separate skill used to assess for temperature changes, tenderness, and large masses. Keep in mind that even a skilled clinician will not be able to palpate abdominal organs in an obese person.

Most viscera in the normal adult are not palpable unless enlarged. Anatomical structures can be mistaken for an abdominal mass. Palpation is contraindicated in anyone with a suspected abdominal aortic aneurysm, appendicitis, or a known kidney disease, or who has had an abdominal organ transplantation.

When palpation is carried out, always explain to your patient what test you are going to perform and why. Make sure the person being examined has an empty bladder. Examine any painful areas last. Use proper draping and warm your hands. Have the patient place their arms at their side and

bend the knees with the feet flat on the examination table to put the abdominal muscles in a relaxed position. During palpation, if the person is ticklish or tense, place his or her hand on top of your palpating hand. Ask him or her to breathe in and out slowly and regularly. The tickle response disappears in the presence of a truly acute abdomen.[139] To help distinguish between voluntary abdominal muscle guarding and involuntary abdominal rigidity, have the patient exhale or breathe through the mouth. Voluntary guarding usually decreases using these techniques.

Start with a light touch, moving the fingers in a circular motion, slowly and gently. If the abdominal muscles are contracted, observe the patient as he or she breathes in and out. The contraction is voluntary if the muscles are more strongly contracted during inspiration and less strong during expiration. Muscles firmly contracted throughout the respiratory cycle (inspiration and expiration) are more likely to be involuntary, possibly indicating an underlying abdominal problem. To check for rebound tenderness, the "pinch-an-inch" test is preferred over the Rebound Tenderness test (Blumberg's sign) (see Figs. 8.11 and 8.12).

A variation of Blumberg's sign (for peritonitis) is the Rovsing sign (suggesting appendicitis).[140] Rovsing sign is elicited by pushing on the abdomen in the left lower quadrant (away from the appendix as in most people the appendix is in the right lower quadrant). Although this maneuver stretches the entire peritoneal lining, it only causes pain in any location where the peritoneum is irritating the muscle. In the case of appendicitis, the pain is felt in the right lower quadrant despite pressure being placed elsewhere.

If left lower quadrant pressure by the examiner leads only to left-sided pain or pain on both the left and right sides, then there may be some other pathologic etiology (e.g., bladder, uterus, ascending [right] colon, fallopian tubes, ovaries, or other structures).

Liver. Liver percussion to determine its size and identify its edges is a skill beyond the scope of a physical therapist for the initial examination. Therapists involved in visceral manipulation will be most likely to develop this advanced skill.

To palpate the liver (Fig. 4.50), have the patient take a deep breath as you feel deeply beneath the costal margin. During inspiration, the liver will move down with the diaphragm so that the lower edge may be felt below the right costal margin.

A normal adult liver is not usually palpable and palpation is not painful. Cirrhosis, metastatic cancer, infiltrative leukemia, right-sided CHF, and third-stage (tertiary) syphilis can cause an enlarged liver. The liver in patients with COPD is more readily palpable as the diaphragm moves down and pushes the liver below the ribs. The liver is often palpable 2 to 3 cm below the costal margin in infants and young children.

If you come in contact with the bottom edge tucked up under the rib cage, the normal liver will feel firm, smooth, even, and rubbery. A palpable hard or lumpy edge warrants further investigation. Some clinicians prefer to stand next to the patient near his head, facing his feet. As the patient breathes in, curl the fingers over the costal margin and up under the ribs to feel the liver (Fig. 4.51).

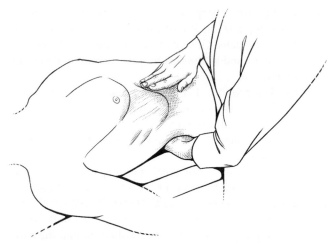

Fig. 4.50   Palpating the liver. Place your left hand under the patient's right posterior thorax (as shown) parallel to and at the level of the last two ribs. Place your right hand on the patient's right upper quadrant (RUQ) over the midclavicular line. The fingers should be pointing toward the patient's head and positioned below the lower edge of liver dullness (previously mapped out by percussion). Ask the patient to take a deep breath while pressing inward and upward with the fingers of the right hand. Attempt to feel the inferior edge of the liver with your right hand as it descends below the last rib anteriorly.

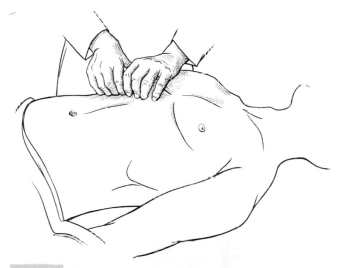

Fig. 4.51   An alternate way to palpate the liver. Hook the fingers of one or both hands (depending on hand size) up and under the right costal border. As the patient breathes in, the liver descends and the therapist may come in contact with the lower border of the liver. If this procedure elicits exquisite tenderness, it may be a positive Murphy's sign for acute cholecystitis (not the same as Murphy's percussion test [costovertebral tenderness] of the kidney depicted in Fig. 4.53).

Spleen.   As with other organs, the spleen is difficult to percuss, even more so than the liver, and is not part of the physical therapist's examination.

Palpation of the spleen is not possible unless it is distended and bulging below the left costal margin (Fig. 4.52). The spleen enlarges with mononucleosis and trauma. Do not continue to palpate an enlarged spleen because it can rupture easily. Report to the physician immediately how far it extends below the left costal margin and request medical evaluation.

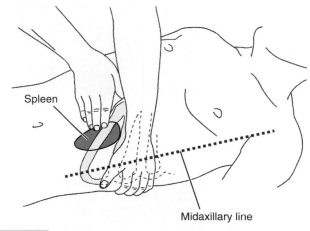

Fig. 4.52   Palpation of the spleen. The spleen is not usually palpable unless it is distended and bulging below the left costal margin. Left shoulder pain can occur with referred pain from the spleen. Stand on the person's right side and reach across the patient with the left hand, placing it beneath the patient over the left costovertebral angle. Lift the spleen anteriorly toward the abdominal wall. Place the right hand on the abdomen below left costal margin. Using findings from percussion, gently press fingertips inward toward the spleen while asking the patient to take a deep breath. Feel for spleen as it moves downward toward the fingers. (From Leasia MS, Monahan FD. A Practical Guide to Health Assessment. 2nd ed. Philadelphia: WB Saunders; 2002.)

Gallbladder and Pancreas.   Likewise, the gallbladder is tucked up under the liver (see Figs. 9.1 and 9.2) is not palpable unless grossly distended. To palpate the gallbladder, ask the person to take a deep breath as you palpate deep below the liver margin. Only an abnormally enlarged gallbladder can be palpated this way.

The pancreas is also inaccessible; as it lies behind and beneath the stomach with its head along the curve of the duodenum and its tip almost touching the spleen (see Fig. 10.1). A round, fixed swelling above the umbilicus that does not move with inspiration may be a sign of acute pancreatitis or cancer in a thin person.

Kidneys.   The kidneys are located deep in the retroperitoneal space in both upper quadrants of the abdomen. Each kidney extends from approximately T12 to L3. The right kidney is usually slightly lower than the left.

Percussion of the kidney is accomplished using Murphy's percussion test (Fig. 4.53). To palpate the kidney, stand on the right side of the supine patient. Place your left hand beneath the patient's right flank. Flex the left metacarpophalangeal joints (MCPs) in the renal angle while pressing downward with the right hand against the right outer edge of the abdomen. This method compresses the kidney between your hands. The left kidney is usually not palpable because of its position beneath the bowel.

Kidney transplants are often located in the abdomen. The therapist should not percuss or palpate the kidneys of anyone with chronic renal disease or organ transplantation.

Bladder.   The bladder lies below the symphysis pubis and is not palpable unless it becomes distended and rises above the pubic bone. Primary pain patterns for the bladder are

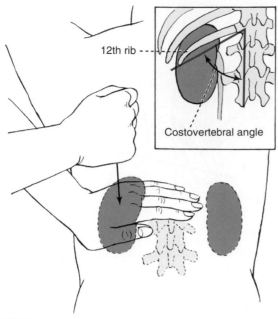

Fig. 4.53 Murphy's percussion, also known as the test for costovertebral tenderness. Murphy's percussion is used to rule out involvement of the kidney and assess for pseudorenal pain (see discussion, Chapter 10). Indirect fist percussion causes the kidney to vibrate. To assess the kidney, position the patient prone or sitting and place one hand over the rib at the costovertebral angle on the back. Give the hand a percussive thump with the ulnar edge of your other fist. The person normally feels a thud but no pain. Reproduction of back and/or flank pain with this test is a red-flag sign for renal involvement (e.g., kidney infection or inflammation). (From Black JM, Matassarin-Jacobs E, eds. Luckmann and Sorensen's Medical-Surgical Nursing. 4th ed. Philadelphia: WB Saunders; 1993.)

shown in Fig. 10.9. Sharp pain over the bladder or just above the symphysis pubis can also be caused by abdominal gas. The presence of associated GI signs and symptoms and lack of urinary tract signs and symptoms may be helpful in identifying this pain pattern.

Aortic Bifurcation. It may be necessary to assess for an abdominal aneurysm, especially in the older patient with back pain and/or who reports a pulsing or pounding sensation in the abdomen during increased activity or while in the supine position.

The ease with which the aortic pulsations can be felt varies greatly with the thickness of the abdominal wall and the anteroposterior diameter of the abdomen. To palpate the aortic pulse, the therapist should press firmly deep in the upper abdomen (slightly to the left of the midline) to find the aortic pulsations (Fig. 4.54A).

The therapist can assess the width of the aorta by using both hands (one on each side of the aorta), pressing deeply, and palpating the aortic pulse. The examiner's fingers along the outer margins of the aorta should remain the same distance apart until the aortic bifurcation. Where the aorta bifurcates (usually near the umbilicus), the width of the pulse should expand (Fig. 4.54B). The normal aortic pulse width is between 2.5 and 4.0 cm (some sources say the width must be no more than 3.0 cm; others list 4.0 cm). Average pulse width is 2.5 cm or about 1.2 inches wide.[141] See Chapter 7 for a more in-depth discussion of aortic pulse width norms.

Throbbing pain that increases with exertion and is accompanied by a sensation of a heartbeat when lying down and of a palpable pulsating abdominal mass requires immediate

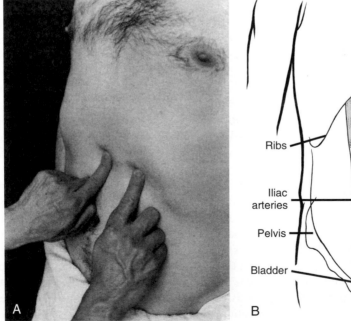

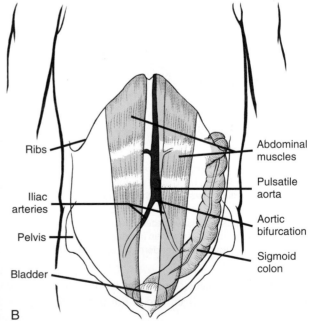

Ribs

Iliac arteries

Pelvis

Bladder

Abdominal muscles

Pulsatile aorta

Aortic bifurcation

Sigmoid colon

Fig. 4.54 (A) Place one hand or one finger on either side of the aorta as shown here. Press firmly deep in the upper abdomen just to the left of the midline. You may feel aortic pulsations. These pulsations are easier to appreciate in a thin person and more difficult to feel in someone with a thick abdominal wall or large anteroposterior diameter of the abdomen. Obesity and abdominal ascites or distention makes this more difficult. Use the stethoscope (bell) to listen for bruits. Bruits are abnormal blowing or swishing sounds heard during auscultation of the arteries. Bruits with both systolic and diastolic components suggest the turbulent blood flow of partial arterial occlusion. If the renal artery is also occluded, the patient will be hypertensive. (B) Visualize the location of the aorta slightly to the left of midline and its bifurcation just below the umbilicus. See text (this chapter and Chapter 6) for discussion of normal and average pulse widths. The pulse width expands at the aortic bifurcation (again, usually just below the umbilicus). An aneurysm can occur anywhere along the aorta; 95% of all abdominal aortic aneurysms occur just below the renal arteries. (A From Boissonnault WG, ed. Examination in Physical Therapy Practice. 2nd ed. New York: Churchill Livingstone; 1995.)

medical attention. Remember, the presence of an abdominal bruit accompanied by risk factors for an aortic aneurysm (see Chapter 7) may be a contraindication to abdominal palpation.

SYSTEMS REVIEW ... OR ... REVIEW OF SYSTEMS?

The *Guide*[2,23] uses the terminology "Review of Systems" (ROS) to perform a series of questions in the patient history to identify signs and symptoms which may be more sinister in nature or beyond the scope of physical therapist treatment. Although the likelihood of serious pathology is low,[142,143] the symptoms may yield a pattern indicating potential system involvement. The identified cluster(s) of associated signs and symptoms are reviewed to search for a potential pattern that may identify the underlying system involved (Box 4.15).

Therapists perform the ROS by categorizing all the complaints and reported or observed associated signs and symptoms. This type of review helps bring to the therapist's attention any signs or symptoms the patient has not recognized, has forgotten, or thought unimportant. After compiling a list of the patient's signs and symptoms, compare those to the list in Box 4.15. Are there any identifying clusters to direct the decision-making process? See Case Example 4.4.

For example, cutaneous (skin) manifestations and joint pain may occur secondary to systemic diseases, such as Crohn's disease (regional enteritis) or psoriatic arthritis, or as a delayed reaction to medications. Likewise, hair and nail changes, temperature intolerance, and unexplained excessive fatigue are cluster signs and symptoms associated with the endocrine system.

Changes in urinary frequency, flow of urine, or color of urine point to urologic involvement. Other groupings of signs and symptoms associated with each system are listed in Box 4.15. If, for example, the patient's signs and symptoms fall primarily within the genitourinary group, then turn to Chapter 11 for additional, pertinent screening questions listed at the end of the chapter. The patient's answers to questions will guide the therapist in the selection of physical examination tests and measures to further the screening process, and aid in making a final decision regarding physician referral (see the Case Study at the end of the chapter).

The *Guide* uses the terminology "Systems Review" to describe a brief or limited hands-on examination of the anatomic and physiologic status of the cardiovascular/pulmonary, integumentary, musculoskeletal, and neuromuscular systems.[2] The patient's ability to communicate and process information is identified as well as any learning barriers, such as hearing or vision impairment, illiteracy, or English as a second language.[2,23] At any point during the ROS or the systems review the therapist may determine a referral to another medical professional is necessary. After the systems review, the therapist may find cause to examine just the upper quadrant or just the lower quadrant more closely. A guide to physical assessment during an examination is provided in Table 4.13.

The therapist is not responsible for identifying the specific pathologic disease underlying the clinical signs and symptoms present. However, the alert therapist who recognizes clusters of signs and symptoms of a systemic nature will be more likely to identify a problem outside the scope of physical therapy practice and make the appropriate referral. It is important to note that medical screening is an ongoing process, and identification of the need for referral may not occur at the initial physical therapist examination.[144] Early identification and intervention for many medical conditions can result in improved outcomes, including decreased morbidity and mortality.

BOX 4.15   REVIEW OF SYSTEMS

When conducting a general review of systems, ask the patient about the presence of any other problems anywhere else in the body. Depending on the patient's answer you may want to prompt him or her about any of the following common signs and symptoms* associated with each system:

General Questions
___Fever, chills, sweating (constitutional symptoms)
___Appetite loss, nausea, vomiting (constitutional symptoms)
___Fatigue, malaise, weakness (constitutional symptoms)
___Excessive, unexplained weight gain or loss
___Vital signs: blood pressure, temperature, pulse, respirations, pain, walking speed
___Insomnia
___Irritability
___Hoarseness or change in voice, frequent or prolonged sore throat
___Dizziness, falls

Integumentary (Include Skin, Hair, and Nails)
___Recent rashes, nodules, or other skin changes
___Unusual hair loss or breakage

___Increased hair growth (hirsutism)
___Change in nail beds
___Itching (pruritus)

Musculoskeletal/Neurologic
___Joint pain, redness, warmth, swelling, stiffness, deformity
___Frequent or severe headache
___Change in vision or hearing
___Vertigo
___Paresthesias (numbness, tingling, "pins and needles" sensation)
___Change in muscle tone
___Weakness; atrophy
___Abnormal deep tendon (or other) reflexes
___Problems with coordination or balance; falling
___Involuntary movements; tremors
___Radicular pain
___Seizure or loss of consciousness
___Memory loss
___Paralysis
___Mood swings; hallucinations

Continued

BOX 4.15 REVIEW OF SYSTEMS—cont'd

Rheumatologic
____Presence/location of joint swelling
____Muscle pain, weakness
____Skin rashes
____Reaction to sunlight
____Raynaud's phenomenon
____Change in nail beds

Cardiovascular
____Chest pain or sense of heaviness or discomfort
____Palpitations
____Limb pain during activity (claudication; cramps, limping)
____Discolored or painful feet; swelling of hands and feet
____Pulsating or throbbing pain anywhere, but especially in the back or abdomen
____Peripheral edema; nocturia
____Sudden weight gain; unable to fasten waistband or belt, unable to wear regular shoes
____Persistent cough
____Fatigue, dyspnea, orthopnea, syncope
____High or low blood pressure, unusual pulses
____Differences in blood pressure from side to side with position change (10 mm Hg or more; increase or decrease/diastolic or systolic; associated symptoms: dizziness, headache, nausea, vomiting, diaphoresis, heart palpitations, increased primary pain or symptoms)
____Positive findings during auscultation

Pulmonary
____Cough, hoarseness
____Sputum, hemoptysis
____Shortness of breath (dyspnea, orthopnea); altered breathing (e.g., wheezing, pursed-lip breathing)
____Night sweats; sweats anytime
____Pleural pain
____Cyanosis, clubbing
____Positive findings during auscultation (e.g., friction rub, unexpected breath sounds)

Psychologic
____Sleep disturbance
____Stress levels
____Fatigue, psychomotor agitation
____Change in personal habits, appetite
____Depression, confusion, anxiety
____Irritability, mood changes

Gastrointestinal
____Abdominal pain
____Indigestion; heartburn
____Difficulty in swallowing
____Nausea/vomiting; loss of appetite
____Diarrhea or constipation

____Change in stools; change in bowel habits
____Fecal incontinence
____Rectal bleeding; blood in stool; blood in vomit
____Skin rash followed by joint pain (Crohn's disease)

Hepatic/Biliary
____Change in taste/smell
____Anorexia
____Feeling of abdominal fullness, ascites
____Asterixis (muscle tremors)
____Change in urine color (dark, cola-colored)
____Light-colored stools
____Change in skin color (yellow, green)
____Skin changes (rash, itching, purpura, spider angiomas, palmar erythema)

Hematologic
____Change in skin color or nail beds
____Bleeding: nose, gums, easy bruising, melena
____Hemarthrosis, muscle hemorrhage, hematoma
____Fatigue, dyspnea, weakness
____Rapid pulse, palpitations
____Confusion, irritability
____Headache

Genitourinary
____Reduced stream, decreased output
____Burning or bleeding during urination; change in urine color
____Urinary incontinence, dribbling
____Impotence, pain with intercourse
____Hesitation, urgency
____Nocturia, frequency
____Dysuria (painful or difficult urination)
____Testicular pain or swelling
____Genital lesions
____Penile or vaginal discharge
____Impotence (males) or other sexual difficulty (males or females)
____Infertility (males or females)
____Flank pain

Gynecologic
____Irregular menses, amenorrhea, menopause
____Pain with menses or intercourse
____Vaginal discharge, vaginal itching
____Surgical procedures
____Pregnancy, birth, miscarriage, and abortion histories
____Spotting, bleeding, especially for the postmenopausal woman 12 months after last period (without hormone replacement therapy)

Endocrine
____Change in hair and nails
____Change in appetite, unexplained weight change

Continued

BOX 4.15   REVIEW OF SYSTEMS—cont'd

___Fruity breath odor
___Temperature intolerance, hot flashes, diaphoresis (unexplained perspiration)
___Heart palpitations, tachycardia
___Headaches
___Low urine output, absence of perspiration
___Cramps
___Edema, polyuria, polydipsia, polyphagia
___Unexplained weakness, fatigue, paresthesia
___Carpal/tarsal tunnel syndrome
___Periarthritis, adhesive capsulitis
___Joint or muscle pain (arthralgia, myalgia), trigger points
___Prolonged deep tendon reflexes
___Sleep disturbance

Cancer
___Constant, intense pain, especially bone pain at night
___Unexplained weight loss (10% of body weight in 10–14 days); most patients in pain are inactive and gain weight
___Loss of appetite

___Excessive fatigue
___Unusual lump(s), thickening, change in a lump or mole, sore that does not heal; other unusual skin lesion or rash
___Unusual or prolonged bleeding or discharge anywhere
___Change in bowel or bladder habits
___Chronic cough or hoarseness, change in voice
___Rapid onset of digital clubbing (10–14 days)
___Proximal muscle weakness, especially when accompanied by change in one or more deep tendon reflexes

Immunologic
___Change in skin or nail beds
___Fever or other constitutional symptoms (especially recurrent or cyclical symptoms)
___Lymph node changes (tenderness, enlargement)
___Anaphylactic reaction
___Symptoms of muscle or joint involvement (pain, swelling, stiffness, weakness)
___Sleep disturbance

*Cluster of three to four or more lasting longer than 1 month.

PHYSICIAN REFERRAL

Medical evaluation is warranted when clinical findings during the ROS, systems review process, or any other time during examination or treatment indicate body system involvement or conditions which are beyond the scope of physical therapist practice. These findings may be the cause of the patient's concerns, may be a contributing factor or comorbidity, or unrelated to the patient's reason for presentation to the therapist. The screening process, therefore, is essential for determining when the patient is not appropriate for physical therapy care, and the results can be used to facilitate follow-on medical care. It is within the clinical judgment of the therapist to determine the urgency of the referral process. Some possible conditions may require emergent care, such as suicidal intentions, vascular suspicion such as DVT, a palpable spleen during an abdominal exam, a patient with a suspicion of a fracture, or a patient with a prior history of cancer with constitutional signs or no progress with therapy. Further information regarding clinical conditions and implications for care is discussed in the following chapter for each body system. It is better to err on the side of being too quick to refer for medical evaluation than to delay and risk progression of underlying disease. The therapist should communicate with the physician the need for the referral and associated examination findings.

REFERRAL FOR IMAGING

There may be times when the physical therapist may determine a need for diagnostic imaging. Some states and health systems allow for physical therapists to submit referrals for imaging within their scope of practice. Although beyond the scope of this text, the reader is referred to a recent article discussing the roles and responsibilities of physical therapists and referral for imaging.[145]

Vital Signs

Vital sign assessment is a very important and valuable screening tool. If the therapist does not conduct any other physical screening assessment, vital signs should be assessed for a baseline value and then monitored. The following findings should always be documented and reported to the primary care provider:

- Any of the yellow caution signs presented in Box 4.7.
- Any patients demonstrating elevated BP not previously diagnosed or patients with HTN who are not at their goal BP.
- Pulse amplitude that fades with inspiration and strengthens with expiration.
- Irregular pulse and/or irregular pulse combined with symptoms of dizziness or shortness of breath (SOB); tachycardia or bradycardia.
- Pulse increase over 20 bpm lasting more than 3 minutes after rest or changing position.
- Persistent low-grade (or higher) fever, especially associated with constitutional symptoms, most commonly sweats but also unintended weight loss, malaise, nausea, vomiting.
- Any unexplained fever without other systemic symptoms, especially in the person taking corticosteroids or who is otherwise immunosuppressed.
- Weak and rapid pulse accompanied by fall in BP (pneumothorax).
- Patients who are neurologically unstable as a result of a recent cerebrovascular accident (CVA), head trauma, spinal cord injury, or other central nervous system insult often exhibit new arrhythmias during the period of instability; when the patient's pulse is monitored, any new arrhythmias noted should be reported to the nursing staff or physician.
- Always take BP in any patient with neck pain, upper quadrant symptoms, or TOS.

CASE EXAMPLE 4.4
Steps in the Screening Process

A 47-year-old man with low back pain of unknown cause has come to you for exercises. After gathering information from the patient's history and conducting the interview, you ask him:

- Are there any other symptoms of any kind anywhere else in your body?

The patient tells you he does break out into an unexpected sweat from time to time but does not think he has a temperature when this happens. He has increased back pain when he passes gas or has a bowel movement, but then the pain goes back to the "regular" pain level (reported as 5 on a scale of 0 to 10).

Other reported symptoms include:

- Heartburn and indigestion
- Abdominal bloating after meals
- Chronic bronchitis from smoking (3 packs/day)
- Alternating diarrhea and constipation

Do these symptoms fall into any one category? See Box 4.15.

What is the next step?

It appears that many of the symptoms are gastrointestinal in nature. Because the patient has mentioned unexplained sweating, but no known fevers, take the time to measure all vital signs, especially body temperature.

Turn to the Special Questions to Ask at the end of Chapter 8 and scan the list of questions for any that might be appropriate with this patient.

For example, find out about the use of nonsteroidal anti-inflammatory drugs (prescription and over-the-counter [OTC]; be sure to include aspirin). Follow up with:

- Have you ever been treated for an ulcer or internal bleeding while taking any of these pain relievers?
- Have you experienced any unexpected weight loss in the last few weeks?
- Have you traveled outside the United States in the last year?
- What is the effect of eating or drinking on your abdominal pain? Back pain?
- Have the patient pay attention to his symptoms over the next 24 to 48 hours:
  - Immediately after eating
  - Within 30 minutes of eating
  - One to 2 hours later
- Do you have a sense of urgency so that you have to find a bathroom for a bowel movement or diarrhea right away without waiting?
- Your decision to refer this patient to a physician depends on your findings from the clinical examination and the patient's responses to these questions. This does not appear to be an emergency because the patient is not in acute distress. An elevated temperature or other unusual vital sign(s) might speed along the referral process. Documentation of the screening process is important, and the physician should be notified appropriately (by phone, fax, and/or report).

Precautions/Contraindications to Therapy

The following parameters are listed as precautions/contraindications rather than one or the other because these signs and symptoms may have different significance depending on the patient's overall health, age, and medications taken. What may be a precaution for one patient may be a clear contraindication for another and vice versa.

- Resting heart rate over 100 bpm
- Resting systolic pressure over 180 mm Hg*
- Resting diastolic pressure over 120 mm Hg*
- Marked dyspnea
- Loss of palpable pulse or irregular pulse with symptoms of dizziness, nausea, or SOB

Anemic individuals may demonstrate an increased normal resting pulse rate that should be monitored during exercise. Anyone with unstable BP may require initial standing with a tilt table or monitoring of the BP before, during, and after treatment. Check the nursing record for pulse rate at rest and BP to use as a guide when taking vital signs in the clinic or at the patient's bedside.

Guidelines for Immediate Physician Referral

- HTN urgency: Patients demonstrating hypertensive crisis (resting SBP over 180 mm Hg and/or DBP over 120 mm Hg) without signs of organ failure.
  - HTN emergency: Patients in HTN crisis (resting SBP over 180 mm Hg and/or DBP over 120 mm Hg) with signs of organ failure, stroke, heart attack or dyspnea should receive emergent medical referral (EMS/911)
- Anyone with diabetes mellitus, who is immunocompromised, or who has a history of steroid and retroviral use who presents with red, inflamed, swollen nail beds or any skin lesion involving the feet must be referred for medical evaluation immediately.
- Any suspicious changes in breast tissue (e.g., unexplained nipple discharge, erythema, contour changes, palpable masses) as reported by the patient must be reported to the physician immediately for evaluation. Breast tissue inspections and examinations are not within the scope of Physical Therapist practice.
- Detection of a palpable, fixed, irregular mass requires medical referral or a recommendation to the patient to contact a physician for evaluation. Suspicious lymph node enlargement or changes, whether singular or generalized changes, should also be evaluated by a physician.
- Unusual or suspicious findings during inspection, palpation, or auscultation of the chest or abdomen including positive Murphy's percussion test, Murphy's sign, the presence of rebound tenderness, or palpable distention of the spleen, liver, or gallbladder should be evaluated by a physician.
- Recurrent cancer can appear as a single lump, a pale or red nodule just below the skin surface, a swelling or dimpling of the skin, or a red rash. Report any of these changes to a physician immediately.
- Immediate medical referral is advised for any patient reporting new onset of SOB who is tachypneic, diaphoretic, or cyanotic; any suspicion of anaphylaxis is also an emergency situation.
- Cough with sputum production that is yellow, green, or rust colored should be evaluated by a physician.
- Abrupt change in mental status, confusion or increasing confusion, and new onset of delirium, especially in the elderly, requires immediate medical attention.
- For an outbreak of vesicular rash associated with herpes zoster, medical referral within 72 hours of the initial

*Unexplained or poorly tolerated by patient.

TABLE 4.13	Guide to Physical Assessment in a Screening Examination	
General Survey	**Upper Quadrant Examination**	**Lower Quadrant Examination**
Level of consciousness	Lymph node palpation	Lymph node palpation
Mental and emotional status	Head and neck	Lower limbs
Vision and hearing	Cranial nerves	• Muscle tone and strength
Speech	Upper limbs	• Trigger points
General appearance	• Muscle tone and strength	• Joint ROM
Nutritional status	• Trigger points	• Reflexes
Level of self-care	• Joint range of motion (ROM)	• Coordination
Body size and type (body mass index [BMI])	• Reflexes	• Motor and sensory function
Obvious deformities	• Coordination	• Vascular assessment
Muscle atrophy	• Vascular assessment	Abdomen
Posture	• Motor and sensory function	• Inspection
Body and breath odors	• Vascular assessment	• Auscultation
Posture	• Chest and back (heart and lungs)	• Percussion
Movement patterns and gait	• Inspection	• Palpation
Use of assistive devices or mobility aids	• Palpation	
Balance and coordination	• Auscultation	
Inspect skin, hair, and nails		
Vital signs		

appearance of skin lesions is needed; the patient will likely begin a course of antiretroviral medication to manage symptoms and help prevent postherpetic neuropathy. The Review of Systems revealed several red flags for the cardiovascular and pulmonary systems. The physical therapist prioritized the Review of Systems to the Cardiovascular system with vital signs assessment. The information gathered from the history, Review of Systems and the limited Systems Review sufficiently raised red flag concerns to necessitate a discussion with the patient regarding referral to the local emergency room.

■ Key Points To Remember

1. A head-to-toe complete physical assessment is an advanced clinical skill and a challenge even to the most skilled physician, physician assistant, or nurse practitioner. The therapist conducts a screening assessment using appropriate portions of the physical assessment.

2. The therapist carries out certain portions of the physical assessment with every patient, referred and direct access, by observing general health and nutrition, mental status, mood or affect, skin and body contours, mobility, and function.

3. The therapist conducts a formal screening examination whenever the patient history, age, gender, or the clinical presentation raise yellow (caution) or red (warning) flags.

4. Measuring vital signs is a key component of the screening assessment. Vital signs, observations, and reported associated signs and symptoms are among the best screening tools available to the therapist. These same tools can be used to plan and progress safe and effective exercise programs for patients who have true neuromuscular or musculoskeletal problems and also have other health concerns or comorbidities.

5. Documentation of physical findings is important. From a legal point of view, if it is not documented, it was not assessed. Record important normal and abnormal findings.

6. The therapist must be able to recognize normal and abnormal results when conducting inspection, auscultation, percussion, and palpation of the chest, thorax, and abdomen.

7. Auscultation usually follows inspection and palpation of the chest and thorax. Examination of the abdomen should be performed in this order: inspection, auscultation, percussion (when performed), and then palpation.

8. The therapist should try to follow the same pattern of examination every time to decrease the chance of missing an assessment parameter and to increase accuracy and thoroughness.

9. Skin and nail bed assessment should be a part of every patient assessment.

10. Changes in the skin and nail beds may be the first sign of inflammatory, infectious, and immunologic disorders and can occur with involvement of a variety of organs.

11. Consider all integumentary and nail bed findings in relation to the patient's age, ethnicity, occupation, and general health. When analyzing any signs and symptoms present, assess if this is a problem with the integumentary system versus an integumentary response to a systemic problem.

12. The therapist may encounter enlarged or palpable lymph nodes. Keep in mind the therapist cannot know what the underlying pathology may be when lymph nodes are palpable and questionable. Performing a baseline assessment and reporting the findings is the important outcome of the assessment.

13. Medical referral is advised for any individual suspected of having a DVT; medical consultation is advised for those even with a low probability of a DVT.

CASE STUDY

To illustrate the integration of the history and physical examination into medical screening, consider this case:[146]

A 60-year-old female presented to PT via physician referral for lower extremity weakness. She was 5 days status-post C5-6 and C6-7 fusion due to cervical spinal stenosis and myelopathy. She ambulated into the clinic with assistance of her husband. Medical history was positive for smoking (stopped 30 years prior) and hypertension. Medications were Lisinopril, Phenergen, and Zyrtec. She annotated shortness of breath, nausea, and poor balance on her health intake form. When questioning her regarding the shortness of breath, she noted it was new since her surgery, as well as new onset of right-sided chest pain between the right breast and right axilla which was noted on her self-completed body chart form. She reported developing a productive cough in the hospital, but no hemoptysis. Two days prior to the PT appointment, she developed a 100.1 F low-grade fever. Due to the findings from the patient history, vital signs of BP (140/93) and pulse rate (89) were obtained.

Key items from the Review of Systems:
- New onset shortness of breath and chest pain since surgery 5 days prior
- Productive cough
- Low-grade fever

Key items from the Systems Review:
- Blood Pressure – elevated despite medications (lisinopril)
- Pulse Rate

Case Disposition: As factors of recent surgery, new onset fever, productive cough, elevated BP despite meds, and new onset of shortness of breath and chest pain could relate to hospital acquired infection, deep vein thrombosis, pulmonary embolism, or other cardiovascular or pulmonary condition, the decision to transport her to the in-house emergency room for work-up was discussed with and agreed to by the patient. The patient was diagnosed with a pulmonary embolism by the emergency room physician, and appropriate medical management was initiated.

PRACTICE QUESTIONS

1. When assessing the abdomen, what sequence of physical assessment is best?
   a. Auscultation, inspection, palpation, percussion
   b. Inspection, percussion, auscultation, palpation
   c. Inspection, auscultation, percussion, palpation
   d. Auscultation, inspection, percussion, palpation
2. A line drawn down the middle of a lesion with two different halves suggests a:
   a. Malignant lesion
   b. Benign lesion
   c. Normal presentation
   d. Skin reaction to medication
3. Pulse strength graded as 1 means:
   a. Easily palpable, normal
   b. Present occasionally
   c. Pulse diminished, barely palpable
   d. Within normal limits
4. During auscultation of an adult patient with rheumatoid arthritis, the heart rate gets stronger as she breathes in and decreases as she breathes out. This sign is:
   a. Characteristic of lung disease
   b. Typical in coronary artery disease
   c. A normal finding
   d. Common in anyone with pain
5. Body temperature should be taken as a part of a vital sign assessment:
   a. Only for patients who have not been seen by a physician
   b. For any patient who has musculoskeletal pain of unknown origin
   c. For any patient reporting the presence of constitutional symptoms, especially fever or sweats
   d. b and c
   e. All of the above
6. A 23-year-old female presents with a new onset of skin rash and joint pain followed 2 weeks later by GI symptoms of abdominal pain, nausea, and diarrhea. She has a previous history of Crohn's disease, but this condition has been stable for several years. She does not think her current symptoms are related to her Crohn's disease. What kind of screening assessment is needed in this case?
   a. Vital signs only.
   b. Vital signs and abdominal auscultation.
   c. Vital signs, neurologic screening, and abdominal auscultation.
   d. No further assessment is needed; there are enough red flags to advise this patient to seek medical attention.
7. A 76-year-old man was referred to physical therapy after a total hip replacement (THR). The goal is to increase his functional mobility. Is a health assessment needed even though he was examined just before the surgery 2 weeks ago? The physician conducted a system's review and summarized the medical record by saying the patient was in excellent health and a good candidate for THR.
8. When would you consider listening for femoral bruits?
9. You notice a new patient has an unusual (strong) breath odor. How do you assess this?
10. Why does postural orthostatic hypotension occur upon standing for the first time in a young adult who has been supine in skeletal traction for 3 weeks?

Common Sources of BP Measurement Error	
Source of Error	**BP Readings can appear higher by**
Full bladder	10–15 mmg
Unsupported back	5–10 mm Hg
Unsupported feet	5–10 mm Hg
Crossed legs	2–8 mm Hg
Cuff placed over clothing	10–40 mm Hg
Unsupported arm	10 mm Hg
Patient talking	10–15 mm Hg

From Severin R, Sabbahi A, Albarrati A, Phillips SA, Arena S. Blood pressure screening by outpatient physical therapists: a call to action and clinical recommendations. Phys Ther. 2020;100(6):1008-1019.

REFERENCES

1. Sueki et al. https://www.ncbi.nlm.nih.gov/pmc/articles/PMC3649356/
2. American Physical Therapy Association. Annual checkup by a physical therapist. http://www.apta.org/AnnualCheckup/. Accessed July 3, 2020.
3. Thim T, Krarup NHV, Grove EL, et al. Initial assessment and treatment with the airway, breathing, circulation, disability, exposure (ABCDE) approach. *Int J Gen Med*. 2012;5:117–121.
4. Honenhaus S, Travers D, Mecham N. Pediatric triage: a review of emergency education literature. *J Emerg Nurs*. 2008;34(4):308–313.
5. Sieber FE. Sedation depth during spinal anesthesia and the development of postoperative delirium in elderly patients undergoing hip fracture repair. *Mayo Clin Proc*. 2010;85(1):18–26.
6. Alfonso DT. Nonsurgical complications after total hip and total knee arthroplasty. *Am J Orthop*. 2006;35(11):503–510.
7. Scott JE, Mathias JL, Kneebone AC. Incidence of delirium following total joint replacement in older adults: a meta-analysis. *Gen Hosp Psychiat*. 2015;37(3):223–229.
8. Björkelund KB, Hommel A, Thorngren KG, et al. Reducing delirium in elderly patients with hip fracture: a multi-factorial intervention study. *Acta Anaesthesiol Scand*. 2010;54(6):678–688.
9. Trivedi D. Cochrane review summary: Mini-Mental State Examination (MMSE) for the detection of dementia in clinically unevaluated people aged 65 and over in community and primary care populations. *Prim Health Care Res Dev*. 2017;18(6):527–528.
10. https://compendiumapp.com/post_4xQIen-Ly. Accessed 29 July, 2020.
11. Sieber FE. Postoperative delirium in the elderly surgical patient. *Anesthesiol Clin*. 2009;27(3):451–464.
12. Wei LA, Fearing MA, Sternberg EJ, et al. The confusion assessment method (CAM): a systematic review of current usage. *J Am Geriatr Soc*. 2008;56(5):823–830.
13. Shi Q, Warren L, Saposnik G, Macdermid JC. Confusion assessment method: a systematic review and meta-analysis of diagnostic accuracy. *Neuropsychiatr Dis Treat*. 2013;9:1359–1370.
14. Weir J, Steyerberg EW, Butcher I, et al. Does the extended Glasgow outcome scale add value to the conventional Glasgow outcome scale? *J Neurotrauma*. 2012;29(1):53–58.
15. Karnofsky performance status scale: medscape. http://emedicine.medscape.com/article/2172510-overview. Accessed October 17, 2020.
16. Jang RW, Caraiscos VB, Swami N, et al. Simple prognostic model for patients with advanced cancer based on performance status. *J Oncol Pract*. 2014;10(5):e335–e341.
17. Williams EP, Mesidor M, Winters K, Dubbert PM, Wyatt SB. Overweight and obesity: prevalence, consequences, and causes of a growing public health problem. *Curr Obes Rep*. 2015;4(3):363–370.
18. National Heart, Lung and Blood Institute. Calculate your body mass index. http://www.nhlbi.nih.gov/health/educational/lose_wt/BMI/bmicalc.htm. Accessed October 17, 2020.
19. Centers for Disease Control and Prevention: BMI Percentile Calculator for Child and Teen English Version.
20. https://www.cdc.gov/healthyweight/bmi/calculator.html. Accessed August 1, 2020.
21. Severin R, Sabbahi A, Albarrati A, Phillips SA, Arena S. Blood pressure screening by outpatient physical therapists: a call to action and clinical recommendations. *Phys Ther*. 2020;100(6):1008–1019.
22. Severin R, Wang E, Wielechowski A, Phillips SA. Outpatient physical therapist attitudes toward and behaviors in cardiovascular disease screening: a national survey. *Phys Ther*. 2019;99:833–848.
23. American Physical Therapy Association. Guide to Physical Therapist Practice 3.0. Alexandria, VA: American Physical Therapy Association; 2014. http://guidetoptpractice.apta.org/. Accessed August 1, 2020.
24. American College of Sports Medicine. Riebe D, Ehrman JK, Liguori G, Magal M. ACSM's Guidelines for Exercise Testing and Prescription. 10th ed. Netherlands: Wolters Kluwer; 2014.
25. Shaw DK. What's so vital about vital signs? *Q Rev*. 2009;44(4):1–5.
26. Marco CA, Plewa MC, Buderer N, Hymel G, Cooper J. Self-reported pain scores in the emergency department: lack of association with vital signs. *Acad Emerg Med*. 2006;13(9):974–979.
27. Dayoub EJ, Jena AB. Does pain lead to tachycardia? Revisiting the association between self-reported pain and heart rate in a national sample of urgent emergency department visits. *Mayo Clin Proc*. 2015;90(8):1165–1166.
28. Bossart P, Fosnocht D, Swanson E. Changes in heart rate do not correlate with changes in pain intensity in emergency department patients. *J Emerg Med*. 2007;32(1):19–22.
29. Bates B, Bickley LS, Hoekelman RA. *A Guide to Physical Examination and History Taking*. 10th ed. Philadelphia: J.B. Lippincott; 2008.
30. Sapra A, Malik A, Bhandari P. Vital sign assessment. [Updated 2020 May 23]. StatPearls [Internet]. Treasure Island, FL: StatPearls Publishing; 2020.
31. Chan ED, Chan MM, Chan MM. Pulse oximetry: Understanding its basic principles facilitates appreciation of its limitations. *Respir. Med*. 2013;107(6):789–799.
32. Kawagishi T, Kanaya N, Nakayama M, Kurosawa S, Namiki A. Comparison of the failure times of pulse oximeters during blood pressure cuff-induced hypoperfusion in volunteers. *Anesth. Anal*. 2004;99(3):793–796.
33. Ceylan B, Khoshid L, Gunes U, et al. Evaluation of oxygen saturation values in different body positions in healthy individuals. *J Clin Nurs*. 2016;25(7-8):1095–1100.
34. Muntner P, Shimbo D, Carey RM, et al. Measurement of blood pressure in humans: a scientific statement from the American Heart Association. *Hypertension*. 2019;73:e35–e66.
35. O'Brien E, Asmar R, Beilin L, et al. European Society of Hypertension recommendations for conventional, ambulatory and home blood pressure measurement. *J Hypertens*. 2003;21:821–848.
36. Roerecke M, Kaczorowski J, Myers MG. Comparing automated office blood pressure readings with other methods of blood pressure measurement for identifying patients with possible hypertension: a systematic review and meta-analysis. *JAMA Intern Med*. 2019;179:351–362.
37. Myers MG, McInnis NH, Fodor GJ, Leenen FHH. Comparison between an automated and manual sphygmomanometer in a population survey. *Am J Hypertens*. 2008;21:280–283.
38. Ogedegbe G, Pickering T. Principles and techniques of blood pressure measurement. *Cardiol Clin*. 2010;28:571–586.

39. Shinohara T, Tsuchida N, Seki K, et al. Can blood pressure be measured during exercise with an automated sphygmomanometer based on an oscillometric method? *J Phys Ther Sci.* 2017;29:1006–1009.

40. Frese EM, Fick A, Sadowsky HS. Blood pressure measurement guidelines for physical therapists. *Cardiopulm Phys Ther J.* 2011;22:5–12.

41. Pickering TG, Hall JE, Appel LJ, et al. Recommendations for blood pressure measurement in humans and experimental animals. Part 1: blood pressure measurement in humans: a statement for professionals from the subcommittee of professional and public education of the American Heart Association Council on high blood pressure research. *Hypertension.* 2005;45:142–161.

42. Mourad A, Carney SL, Gillies A, Jones B, Nanra R, Trevillian P. Arm position and blood pressure: a risk factor for hypertension? *J Hum Hypertens.* 2003;17:389–395.

43. Lane D, Beevers M, Barnes N, et al. Inter-arm differences in blood pressure: when are they clinically significant? *J Hypertens.* 2002;20:1089–1095.

44. Nelson MR. Cluster-randomized controlled trial of oscillometric vs. manual sphygmomanometer for blood pressure management in primary care (CRAB). *Am J Hypertens.* 2009;22(6):598–603.

45. Wolford MR, Harkins KG, King DS, et al. P-175: accurate cuff size in blood pressure measurement. *Am J Hypertens.* 2002;15(S3):92A.

46. Beumont CE. Choosing the best stethoscope. *Nursing.* 2005;35(8):27–28.

47. Frese EM, Fick A, Sadowsky HS. Blood pressure measurement guidelines for physical therapists. *Cardiopulm Phys Ther J.* 2011;22(2):5–12.

48. Mitchell GF. Pulse pressure and risk of new onset atrial fibrillation. *JAMA.* 2007;297(7):709–715.

49. Franklin SS. Pulse pressure as a risk factor. *Clin Exp Hypertens.* 2004;26(7-8):645–652.

50. Pescatello LS, Arena R, Riebe D, Thompson PD. *ACSM's Guidelines for Exercise Testing and Prescription.* 9th ed. Philadelphia, PA: Wolters Kluwer/Lippincott Williams & Wilkins Health; 2014.

51. Lim MA, Townsend RR. Arterial compliance in the elderly: its effect on blood pressure measurement and cardiovascular outcomes. *Clin Geriatr Med.* 2009;25(2):191–205.

52. Netea RT, Lenders JWM, Smits P, Thien T. Both body and arm position significantly influence blood pressure measurement. *J Hum Hypertens.* 2003;17:459–462.

53. Centers for Disease Control and Prevention. Stopping elderly accidents deaths and injuries (STEADI): measuring orthostatic blood pressure. 2017. https://www.cdc.gov/steadi/pdf/STEADI-Assessment-MeasuringBP-508.pdf. Accessed January 6, 2020.

54. Liu H, Yao J, Wang W, Zhang D. Association between duration of oral contraceptive use and risk of hypertension: a meta-analysis. *J Clin Hypertens.* 2017;19:1032–1041.

55. Shufelt CL, Bairey Merz CN. Contraceptive hormone use and cardiovascular disease. *J Am Coll Cardiol.* 2009;53(3):221–231.

56. Schultz MG, Otahal P, Picone DS, Sharman JE. Clinical relevance of exaggerated exercise blood pressure. *J Am Coll Cardiol.* 2015;66:1843–1845.

57. Sabbahi A, Arena R, Kaminsky LA, Myers J, Phillips SA. Peak blood pressure responses during maximum cardiopulmonary exercise testing. *Hypertension.* 2018;71:229–236.

58. Fletcher GF, Ades PA, Kligfield P, et al. Exercise standards for testing and training. *Circulation.* 2013;128(8):873–934.

59. Riebe D, Ehrman JK, Ligouri G, Magal M. What's New in the 10th Edition of ACSM's Guidelines for Exercise Testing and Prescription. Denver, CO: American College of Sports Medicine; 2017.

60. Benjamin EJ, Virani SS, Callaway CW, et al. Heart disease and stroke statistics–2018 update: a report from the American Heart Association. *Circulation.* 2018;137:e67–e492.

61. Benjamin EJ, Muntner P, Alonso A, et al. Heart disease and stroke statistics—2019 update: a report from the American Heart Association. *Circulation.* 2019;139(10):00659.

62. Zhang Y, Moran A. Trends in the prevalence, awareness, treatment, and control of hypertension among young adults in the United States, 1999 to 2014. *Hypertension.* 2017;70:736–742.

63. Whelton PK, Carey RM, Aronow WS, et al. ACC/AHA/AAPA/ABC/ACPM/AGS/APhA/ASH/ASPC/NMA/PCNA guideline for the prevention, detection, evaluation, and management of high blood pressure in adults. *J Am Coll Cardiol.* 2018;71(19):e127–e248.

64. Peacock J, Diaz KM, Viera AJ, Schwartz JE, Shimbo D. Unmasking masked hypertension: prevalence, clinical implications, diagnosis, correlates and future directions. *J Hum Hypertens.* 2014;28:521–528.

65. Ayrak M, Bacaksiz A, Vatankulu MA, et al. Exaggerated blood pressure response to exercise: a new portent of masked hypertension. *Clin Exp Hypertens.* 2010;32:560–568.

66. Mancia G. Long-term risk of sustained hypertension in white-coat or masked hypertension. *Hypertension.* 2009;54(2):226–232.

67. Mancia G, Verdecchia P. Hypertension compendium: clinical value of ambulatory blood pressure, evidence and limits. *Circ Res.* 2015;116:1034–1045.

68. Kario K. Morning surge in blood pressure and cardiovascular risk. *Hypertension.* 2010;56:765–773.

69. Bell CS, Samuel JP, Samuels JA. Prevalence of hypertension in children. *Hypertension.* 2019;73(1):148–152.

70. Flynn JT, Kaelber DC, Baker-Smith CM, et al. Clinical practice guideline for screening and management of high blood pressure in children and adolescents. *Pediatrics.* 2017;140(3):e20171904.

71. Kario K, Tobin JN, Wolfson LI, et al. Lower standing systolic blood pressure as a predictor of falls in the elderly: a community-based prospective study. *J Am Coll Cardiol.* 2001;38(1):246–252.

72. Freeman R, Wieling W, Axelrod FB, et al. Consensus statement on the definition of orthostatic hypotension, neurally mediated syncope and the postural tachycardia syndrome. *Clin Auton Res.* 2011;21(2):69–72.

73. Sund-Levander M, Forsberg C, Wahren LK. Normal oral, rectal, tympanic and axillary body temperature in adult men and women: a systematic literature review. *Scand J Caring Sci.* 2002;16(2):122–128.

74. Del Bene VE. Temperature. In: Walker HK, Hall WD, Hurst JW, eds. *Clinical Methods: The History, Physical, and Laboratory Examinations.* 3rd ed. Boston: Butterworths; 1990. Chapter 218.

75. El Chakhtoura NG, Bonomo RA, Jump RLP. Influence of aging and environment on presentation of infection in older adults. *Infect Dis Clin North Am.* 2017;31(4):593–608.

76. Wurcel AG, Merchant EA, Clark RP, Stone DR. Emerging and underrecognized complications of illicit drug use. *Clin Infect Dis.* 2015;61(12):1840–1849.

77. Montero-Odasso M. Gait velocity as a single predictor of adverse events in healthy seniors aged 75 years and older. *J Gerontol A Biol Sci Med Sci.* 2005;60:1304–1309.

78. Fritz S, Lusardi M. Walking speed: the sixth vital sign. *J Geriatric Phys Ther.* 2009;32(2):2–5.

79. Wilson CM, Kostsuca SR, Boura JA. Utilization of a 5-meter walk test in evaluating self-selected gait speed during preoperative screening of patients scheduled for cardiac surgery. *Cardiopulm Phys Ther J.* 2013;24(3):36–43.

80. Cohen KR, Frank J, Salbu RL, et al. Pruritus in the elderly: clinical approaches to the improvement of quality of life. *PT.* 2012;37(4):227–239.

81. Tarikci N, Kocatürk E, Güngör Ş, Topal IO, Can PÜ, Singer R. Pruritus in Systemic Diseases: A Review of Etiological Factors and New Treatment Modalities. ScientificWorldJournal. 2015; 2015:803752. doi:10.1155/2015/803752.

82. https://emedicine.medscape.com/article/1049648-overview accessed 3 Jul 2020.

83. Edsberg LE, Black JM, Goldberg M, McNichol L, Moore L, Sieggreen M. Revised National Pressure Ulcer Advisory Panel Pressure Injury Staging System: Revised Pressure Injury Staging System. J Wound Ostomy Continence Nurs. 2016;43(6):585-597. doi:10.1097/WON.0000000000000281.

84. Armstrong DG. Skin temperature monitoring reduces the risk for diabetic foot ulceration in high-risk patients. *Am J Med*. 2007;120(12):1042–1046.

85. Houghton VJ, Bower VM, Chant DC. Is an increase in skin temperature predictive of neuropathic foot ulceration in people with diabetes? A systematic review and meta-analysis. J Foot Ankle Res. 2013;6(1):31. Published 2013 Aug 7. doi:10.1186/1757-1146-6-31

86. Alexis AF, Callender VD, Baldwin HE, Desai SR, Rendon MI, Taylor SC. Global epidemiology and clinical spectrum of rosacea, highlighting skin of color: Review and clinical practice experience. J Am Acad Dermatol. 2019;80(6):1722-1729. e7. doi:10.1016/j.jaad.2018.08.049

87. Rigel DS. The evolution of melanoma diagnosis: 25 years beyond the ABCDs. *Ca J Clin*. 2010;60(5):301–316.

88. Wills M. Skin cancer screening. Phys Ther. 2002;82(12):1232-1237.

89. Dundas J. The ABCDEs of Melanoma and Their Applicability to the Field of Physical Therapy. Phys Ther. 2020;100(6):894-896. doi:10.1093/ptj/pzaa051.

90. Rebora A. The management of rosacea. *Am J Clin Dermatol*. 2002;3(7):489–496.

91. Tow A, Wu W, Gallo RL, et al. Part I. Introduction, categorization, histology, pathogenesis, and risk factors. *J Am Acad Dermatol*. 2015;72(5):749–758.

92. Candelli M, Carloni E, Nista EC, et al. Helicobacter pylori eradication and acne rosacea resolution: cause—effect or coincidence? *Dig Liver Dis*. 2004;36(2):163.

93. Yazici Y, Erkan D, Scott R, et al. The skin: a map to rheumatic diseases. *J Musculoskel Med*. 2001;18(1):43–53.

94. Singal A, Arora R. Nail as a window of systemic diseases. *Indian Dermatol Online J*. 2015;6(2):67–74.

95. Lyme Disease Rashes and Look-alikes: Centers for Disease Control and Prevention. http://www.cdc.gov/lyme/signs_symptoms/rashes.html. Accessed July 14 2020.

96. Burris HA, Hurtig J. Radiation recall with anticancer agents. *The Oncologist*. 2010;15(11):1227–1237.

97. https://www.cdc.gov/std/treatment/default.htm. Accessed 14 July 2020

98. https://www.cdc.gov/nchhstp/newsroom/images/multimedia/std/stds-us-2018_higRes.jpg

99. Arbyn M, Tommasino M, Depuydt C, Dillner J. Are 20 human papillomavirus types causing cervical cancer?. J Pathol. 2014;234(4):431-435. doi:10.1002/path.4424

100. Workowski KA, Berman S. Sexually transmitted diseases treatment guidelines. *MMWR*. 2010;59(RR-12):1–110.

101. https://www.who.int/news-room/fact-sheets/detail/herpes-simplex-virus. Accessed 14 July 2020.

102. Herpes simplex virus: World Health Organization. http://www.who.int/mediacentre/factsheets/fs400/en/. Accessed November 7, 2020.

103. Gathier PJ. https://www.ncbi.nlm.nih.gov/pmc/articles/PMC4469579/.

104. Bennett JV, Jarvis WR, Brachman PS. Hospital Infections. 5th ed. Philadelphia: Lippincott Williams & Wilkins; 2014:50.

105. Kos L, Shwayder T. Cutaneous manifestations of child abuse. *Pediatr Dermatol*. 2006;23(4):311–320.

106. Rosen T. https://www.ncbi.nlm.nih.gov/pmc/articles/PMC6057151/

107. Mudd SS, Findlay JS. The cutaneous manifestations and common mimickers of physical child abuse. *J Pediatr Health Care*. 2004;18(3):123–129.

108. Stanley WJ. NAILING a key assessment. *Nurs Crit Care*. 2010;5(5):8–9.

109. Schalock PC. Lippincott's Primary Care. Dermatology. Baltimore: Lippincott, Williams & Wilkins; 2010.

110. Bolognia JL. *Bolognia: Dermatology*. 2nd ed. Philadelphia: Saunders; 2008.

111. Zaias N, Escovar SX, Zaiac MN. Finger and toenail onycholysis. J Eur Acad Dermatol Venereol. 2015;29(5):848-853. doi:10.1111/jdv.12862

112. Maino KL, Stashower M. Traumatic transverse leukonychia. Medscape. http://www.medscape.com/viewarticle/467074. Accessed August 6, 2016.

113. Lemley KV. Kidney disease in nail–patella syndrome. Pediatr Nephrol (Berlin, Germany). 2009;24(12):2345–2354.

114. Sweeney E, Hoover-Fong J, McIntosh I. Nail-patella syndrome. http://www.ncbi.nlm.nih.gov/books/NBK1132/. Accessed August 6, 2016.

115. Gaddey HL, Riegel AM. Unexplained lymphadenopathy: evaluation and differential diagnosis. *Am Fam Physician*. 2016;94(11):896–903.

116. Freeman AM, Matto P. Adenopathy. StatPearls. Treasure Island, FL: StatPearls Publishing; 2020.

117. Concus AP, Singer MI. Head and neck cancer. In: Goldman L, Bennett JC, eds. *Cecil Textbook Of Medicine*. 21st ed. Philadelphia: WB Saunders; 2000:2257–2262.

118. Baumgart DC, Fischer A. Virchow's node. *Lancet*. 2007;370:1568.

119. Siosaki MD, Souza AT. Virchow's node. *N Engl J Med*. 2013;2013:6.

120. Harris J, Lippman M, Osborne K, et al. *Diseases of the Breast*. 4th ed. Philadelphia: Lippincott, Williams & Wilkins; 2009.

121. Bosch X, Coloma E, Donate C, et al. Evaluation of unexplained peripheral lymphadenopathy and suspected malignancy using a distinct quick diagnostic delivery model: prospective study of 372 patients. *Medicine (Baltimore)*. 2014;93(16):e95.

122. Hosford D: On-Line University: The Hosford's differential diagnosis tables. https://www.ptcentral.com/diagnose. Accessed August 1, 2020.

123. US Preventive Services Task Force. Screening for peripheral artery disease and cardiovascular disease risk assessment with the ankle-brachial index: US preventive services task force recommendation statement. *JAMA*. 2018;320(2):177–183.

124. American Diabetes Association. Peripheral arterial disease in people with diabetes. *Diabetes Care*. 2003;26(12):3333–3341.

125. Ortel TL, Neumann I, Ageno W, et al. American Society of Hematology 2020 guidelines for management of venous thromboembolism: treatment of deep vein thrombosis and pulmonary embolism. *Blood Advances*. 2020;4(19):4693–4738.

126. Bates SM, Jaeschke R, Stevens SM, et al. Diagnosis of DVT: antithrombotic therapy and prevention of thrombosis, 9th ed: American College of Chest Physicians evidence-based clinical practice guidelines. *Chest*. 2012;141(2 Suppl):e351S–e418S.

127. Wells PS, Anderson DR, Rodger M, et al. Derivation of a simple clinical model to categorize patients probability of pulmonary embolism: increasing the models utility with the SimpliRED D-dimer. *Thromb Haemost*. 2000;83(3):416–420.

128. Wells PS, Ginsberg JS, Anderson DR, et al. Use of a clinical model for safe management of patients with suspected pulmonary embolism. *Ann Intern Med*. 1998;129:997–1005.

129. Tryniszewski C, ed. *Mosby's Expert 10-Minute Physical Examinations*. 2nd ed. St. Louis: Mosby; 2004.

130. Reddy RS, Alahmari KA, Silvian PS, Ahmad IA, Kakarparthi VN, Rengaramanujam K. Reliability of chest wall mobility and its correlation with lung functions in healthy nonsmokers, healthy smokers, and patients with COPD. *Canadian Respir J*. 2019;2019:1–11.

131. Illeez Memetoğlu Ö, Bütün B, Sezer İ. Chest expansion and modified schober measurement values in a healthy, adult population. *Arch Rheumatol*. 2016;31(2):145–150.

132. Melbye H, Garcia-Marcos L, Brand P, et al. Wheezes, crackles and rhonchi: simplifying description of lung sounds increases the agreement on their classification: a study of 12 physicians' classification of lung sounds from video recordings. *BMJ Open Respir. Res.* 2016;3:e000136.

133. Silverman ME. The Third Heart Sound. In: Walker HK, Hall WD, Hurst JW, eds. *Clinical Methods: The History, Physical, and Laboratory Examinations.* 3rd ed. Boston: Butterworths; 1990. Chapter 24.

134. Williams ES. The fourth heart sound. In: Walker HK, Hall WD, Hurst JW, eds. *Clinical Methods: The History, Physical, and Laboratory Examinations.* 3rd ed. Boston: Butterworths; 1990. Chapter 25.

135. American Cancer Society. Breast cancer early detection and diagnosis. http://www.cancer.org/cancer/breastcancer/more-information/breastcancerearlydetection/breast-cancer-early-detection-toc. Accessed August November 7, 2020.

136. Wright WF. Cullen sign and grey turner sign revisited [published correction appears in J Am Osteopath Assoc. 2016 Aug 1;116(8):501]. *J Am Osteopath Assoc.* 2016;116(6):398–401.

137. Valette X, du Cheyron D. Cullen and Grey Turner's sign in acute pancreatitis. *NEJM.* 2015;373:e28.

138. Potter PA, Weilitz PB. Pocket Guide to Health. Assessment. 6th ed. St. Louis: Mosby; 2006.

139. Schnur W. Tickle me not. *Postgrad Med.* 1994;96(6):35.

140. Snyder MJ, Guthrie M, Cagle S. Acute appendicitis: efficient diagnosis and management. *Am Fam Physician.* 2018;98(1):25–33.

141. Gara PT. Aortic aneurysm. *Circulation.* 2003;107c:e43–e45.

142. Deyo RA, Weinstein JN. Low back pain. *N Engl J Med.* 2001;344(5):363–370.

143. Henschke N, Maher CG, Refshauge KM, et al. Prevalence of and screening for serious spinal pathology in patients presenting to primary care settings with acute low back pain. *Arthritis Rheum.* 2009;60(10):3072–3080.

144. Boissonnault WG, Ross MD. Physical therapists referring patients to physicians: a review of case reports and series. J Orthop Sports Phys Ther. 2012;42(5):446–454. doi:10.2519/jospt.2012.3890

145. Keil AP, Hazle C, Maurer A, et al. Referral for Imaging in Physical Therapist Practice: Key Recommendations for Successful Implementation. Phys Ther. 2021;101(3):pzab013. doi:10.1093/ptj/pzab013

146. Young BA, Flynn TW. Pulmonary emboli: the differential diagnosis dilemma. J Orthop Sports Phys Ther. 2005;35(10):637-644. doi:10.2519/jospt.2005.35.10.637

Screening for Neurologic Conditions

One of the most important factors a physical therapist can do when a patient is being evaluated is to collect data from the patient. Through the history and examination, the therapist determines if the patient has red flags that suggest that the patient has involvement of other systems. As the musculoskeletal system is innervated by the nervous system, there is a complex interplay of possibilities derived from the history and examination to elucidate the involvement of the nervous system. In a patient that has a known nervous system disorder, the therapist would expect involvement of the nervous system during screening for this system. An example of this would be identified as 4+ hyperreflexia in a patient being tested for deep tendon reflexes (DTRs) that should be followed up with a quick stretch reflex of the lower extremity into dorsi flexion to illicit clonus. In this example, it would not be surprising or a red flag if the patient was known to have multiple sclerosis.

In contrast to this scenario, a patient without a known nervous system disorder who presents with a clinical presentation that involves the nervous system becomes a red flag that must be explored and verified. The editors of this textbook recommend performing a complete neurologic exam on this patient as opposed to screening for a neurologic condition to verify the abnormal involvement of the nervous system, and the reader is encouraged to read on for our recommendation that is reinforced by evidence.

The collection of data from the patient helps to determine the response of the therapist from the evaluation of the history and examination to determine if a referral should be emergent or not. An immediate referral to a physician is critical if the patient being examined has emergent or evolving neurologic deterioration. Within this context of referral lie two options for the physical therapist depending on clinical practice setting. If the physical therapist does not work in a hospital setting but instead works in a home health or an independent outpatient orthopedic setting, the therapist has two options, emergent or nonemergent response. For example, a 42-year-old female presenting with progressive worsening of vertiginous episodes that the patient notes were initially episodic but now constant requires immediate referral to a physician that is not an emergent response. This contrasts with the next two examples. A 52-year-old male who presents post complete spinal cord injury to the T-6 level that now presents in an acute care hospital with non-responsive autonomic dysreflexia is an immediate referral that is an emergent situation (Table 5.1). The next example is a 66-year-old male who has been seen for 10 visits for low back pain in an orthopedic outpatient facility that today while warming up on the recumbent bicycle presents with the worst headache of his life which continues to worsen in intensity (Table 5.2; Figs. 5.1–5.3). This is an immediate referral that is an emergent situation, and the therapist should take the patient's vitals to provide to EMS when they arrive on the scene.

In the examples above, the practice setting that the physical therapist works in at the time of the patient encounter may

TABLE 5.1	Spinal Cord Syndromes		
Syndrome	Sensory	Motor	Sphincter Involvement
Central cord syndrome	Variable	Upper extremity weakness, distal > proximal	Variable
Brown-Séquard syndrome	Ipsilateral position and vibration sense loss Contralateral pain and temperature sensation loss	Motor loss ipsilateral to cord lesion	Variable
Anterior cord syndrome	Loss of pin and touch sensation, vibration, position sense preserved	Motor loss or weakness below cord level	Variable
Transverse cord syndrome—complete	Loss of sensation below level of cord injury	Loss of voluntary motor function below cord level	Sphincter control lost
Cauda equina syndrome	Saddle anesthesia may be present, or sensory loss may range from patchy to complete transverse pattern	Weakness may be of lower motor neuron type	Sphincter control impaired

From Marx JA et al: Rosen's emergency medicine, ed 8, Philadelphia, 2014, Saunders.

TABLE 5.2	Physical Examination Findings Associated with Vertebral Fractures and Spinal Cord Injuries	
Injury	**Physical Examination Area**	**Associated Findings**
Vertebral fracture	Spine	Tenderness of the neck and/or back. Examine the entire spine because vertebral fractures may occur in multiples.
	Neurologic	See "Spinal cord injury" later.
	Chest	Thoracic spine fractures: Check for chest tenderness, unequal breath sounds, and arrhythmia, which are suggestive of an associated intrathoracic injury or myocardial contusion.
	Abdomen/pelvis	Thoracolumbar and lumbar spine fractures: Check for abdominal or pelvic tenderness. A transverse area of ecchymosis on the lower abdominal wall (seat belt sign) increases the chance of an abdominopelvic injury.
	Extremity	Thoracolumbar and lumbar spine fractures: Check for calcaneal tenderness because 10% of calcaneal fractures are associated with a low thoracic or lumbar fracture. Mechanistically, these areas are fractured as a result of axial loading.
Spinal cord injury	Neurologic, motor (anterior column)	Assess motor function on a scale of 0–5. The motor level is defined as the most caudal segment with at least 3/5 strength. Injuries to the first eight cervical segments result in tetraplegia (previously known as quadriplegia); lesions below the T1 level result in paraplegia.
	Neurologic, sensory (spinothalamic tract)	Assess sensory function via pinprick and light touch on the following scale: 0 = absent; 1 = impaired; 2 = normal. The sensory level is defined as the most caudal segment of the spinal cord with normal sensory function. The highest intact sensory level should be marked on the patient's spine to monitor for progression.
	Neurologic, sensory (dorsal column)	Assess vibratory sensory function on a scale of 0–2 by using a tuning fork over bony prominences. Assess position sense (proprioception) by flexing and extending the great toe.
	Neurology, deep tendon reflex	On a scale of 0–4, assess the deep tendon reflexes in the upper (biceps, triceps) and lower (patellar, Achilles) extremities.
	Anogenital	Assess rectal tone, sacral sensation, signs of urinary or fecal retention or incontinence, and priapism. Also check the anogenital reflexes. An anal wink (S2-S4) is present if the anal sphincter contracts in response to stroking the perianal skin area. The bulbocavernosus reflex (S3-S4) is elicited by squeezing the glans penis or clitoris (or pulling on an inserted Foley catheter), which results in reflexive contraction of the anal sphincter.
	Head-to-toe examination	A spinal cord injury may mask a patient's ability to perceive and localize pain. Imaging of high-risk areas, such as the abdomen, and areas of bruising or swelling may be required to exclude occult injuries.

From Adams JG et al: Emergency medicine, clinical essentials, ed 2, Philadelphia, 2013, Elsevier.

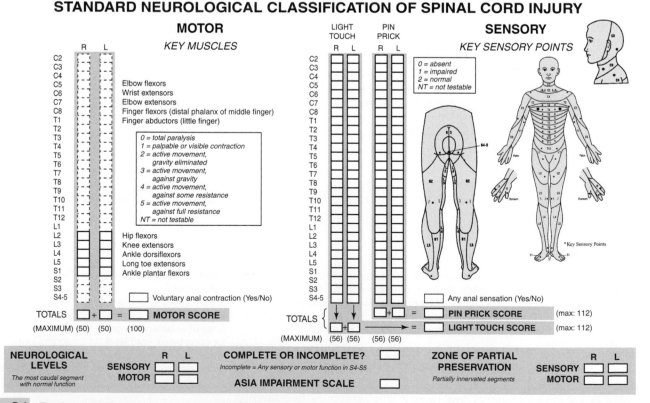

Fig. 5.1 The American Spinal Injury Association (ASIA) neurological classification of spinal cord injury and the ASIA impairment scale are useful tools for precisely mapping motor and sensory deficits to a specific spinal cord level. (From Browner B et al: Skeletal trauma: basic science, management, and reconstruction, ed 6, Philadelphia, 2019, Elsevier.)

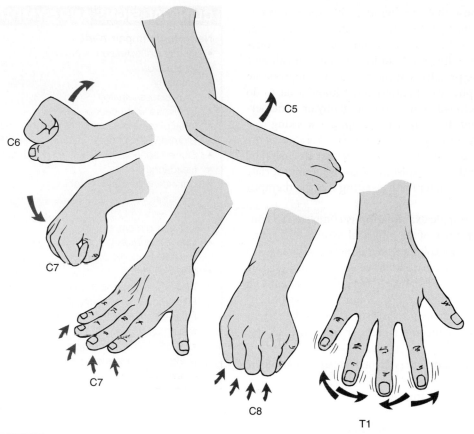

Fig. 5.2 Examination of muscle groups innervated by nerve roots in the upper extremity should include elbow flexion (C5), wrist extension (C6), wrist flexion (C7), finger flexion (C8), and finger abduction (T1). (From Browner B et al: Skeletal trauma: basic science, management, and reconstruction, ed 6, Philadelphia, 2019, Elsevier.)

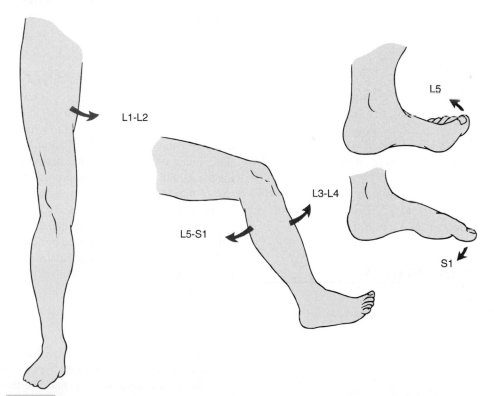

Fig. 5.3 Examination of muscle groups innervated by nerve roots in the lower extremity should include leg adduction (L2), knee extension (L3), ankle dorsiflexion (L4), great toe extension (L5), and great toe flexion (S1). (From Browner B et al: Skeletal trauma: basic science, management, and reconstruction, ed 6, Philadelphia, 2019, Elsevier.)

influence the response that the therapist chooses. For example, a physical therapist working in an acute care setting may not be calling 911 if there is a need for emergent response and instead may be calling out loud for the nurse or calling a code if needed. The practice setting dictates the appropriate response, and the physical therapist must know what to do with a patient if the need arrives to emergently or nonemergently refer a patient. If a physical therapist is working in a home health setting at the patient's home in a rural area, the response may be to activate the emergency response chain by calling 911. The physical therapist must know the appropriate emergent response for each practice setting that the therapist works in.

Much of the neurologic examination is completed in conjunction with other parts of the physical assessment. Acute insult or injury to the neurologic system may cause changes in neurologic status requiring frequent reassessment. Systemic disease can produce nerve damage; careful assessment can help pinpoint the area of pathology. A family history of neurologic disorders or personal history of diabetes, hypertension, high cholesterol, cancer, seizures, or heart disease may be significant.

There are seven major areas to assess in a neurologic examination:

1. Mental and emotional status
2. Cranial nerves
3. Motor function (gross motor and fine motor; coordination, gait, balance)
4. Sensory function (light touch, vibration, pain, pressure, and temperature)
5. Reflexes
6. Neural tension
7. Vision

As always, start with the client's history and note any previous trauma to the head or spine along with reports of headache, confusion (increased confusion), dizziness (see Appendix B-11 in the accompanying enhanced eBook version included with print purchase of this textbook), seizures, difficulty maintaining balance with walking, paresthesias, or other neurologic signs and symptoms. Note the presence of any incoordination, tremors, weakness, or abnormal speech patterns.

As mentioned previously, neurologic symptoms with no apparent cause such as paresthesias, dizziness, and weakness may be symptoms of depression.

❓ FOLLOW-UP QUESTIONS

- Have you ever been in a car accident?
  If yes, did you lose consciousness, have a concussion, or a fractured skull?
- Have you ever been knocked out, unconscious, or had a concussion at any time?
- Have you ever had a seizure?
- Have you ever been paralyzed in your arms or legs?
- Have you ever broken your neck or back?

CLINICAL SIGNS AND SYMPTOMS

Neurologic Impairment

- Confusion/increased confusion
- Depression
- Irritability
- Drowsiness/lethargy
- Dizziness/light-headedness
- Loss of consciousness
- Blurred vision or other change in vision
- Slurred speech or change in speech pattern
- Headache
- Balance/coordination problems
- Paresthesias
- Weakness
- Change in memory
- Change in muscle tone for individual with previously diagnosed neurologic condition
- Seizure activity
- Nerve palsy; transient paralysis. If there are no positive findings upon gross examination of the nervous system (e.g., reflexes, muscle tone assessment, gross manual muscle testing, sensation), further testing may not be required. For example, sensory function is not assessed if motor function is intact and there are no client reports of specific sensory problems or changes.

Keep in mind that fatigue and side effects of medications can affect the results of a neurologic examination. Give instructions clearly and take the time needed to map out any areas of deficit observed during the initial screening examination.

Mental Status

See the previous discussion on General Survey in Chapter 4.

When assessing mental status, it is important to understand the patient's baseline ability to perform fundamental daily tasks. That way you have insight to what the patient knows or does not know. Mental status orientation to person, place, and time should be assessed. Mental status assessment such as asking the patient the name of the president, ability to spell simple words, or adding or subtracting serial threes or sevens should be assessed. The patient can be asked to recall three objects after several minutes after the therapist mentions this to the patient. Attention can be assessed by asking the patient to recall a blocked series of numbers. Mental status assessment through this type of screening provides insight into the patient's memory, attention, and language function.

Cranial Nerves

A neurologic screen may not involve a survey of the cranial nerves unless the therapist finds reason to perform a more focused examination. When the therapist does find a reason to perform a more focused examination, then this must be performed to investigate the full clinical neurologic presentation and especially so when the patient does not have a known neurologic condition. Many of the cranial nerves can be tested during other portions of the physical assessment. When conducting a cranial nerve assessment, follow the information in Table 5.3.

Cranial nerve testing for cranial nerve I or olfactory has become important with COVID-19 as initial presentation involves a loss of smell and taste. Aromatic substances such as vanilla should be used to evaluate the sense of smell.

Cranial nerve testing for cranial nerve II or optic nerve involves visual acuity and pupillary reactivity to light.

Abnormal responses include an afferent pupillary defect or Marcus Gunn pupil (Fig. 5.4). This presentation occurs in an optic nerve abnormality such as after a head injury. A Marcus Gunn presentation is observed during the swinging flashlight test. Light from a penlight is directed towards one eye at a time. In a Marcus Gunn presentation, both pupils dilate inappropriately. A reduced pupillary reaction to light suggests anterior visual pathway lesions such as to the optic nerve, retina, or optic chiasm. Horner syndrome is another optic nerve abnormality that results in a triad clinical presentation of ptosis, miosis, and unilateral facial anhidrosis (Fig. 5.5).

TABLE 5.3	Cranial Nerve Function and Assessment		
Cranial Nerve (CN)	**Type**	**Function**	**Assessment**
I Olfactory	Sensory	Sense of smell	Able to identify common odors (e.g., coffee, vanilla, orange, or peppermint) with eyes closed Close one nostril and test one nostril at a time
II Optic	Sensory	Visual acuity	Visual acuity; test each eye separately with Snellen eye chart If literate, able to read printed material
III Oculomotor	Motor	Extraocular eye movement Pupil constriction and dilation	Assess CNs III, IV, and VI together Look for equal pupil size and shape; equal response to light and accommodation; inspect eyelids for drooping (ptosis) Ask about blurry or double vision Follow finger with eyes without moving head (six points in an H pattern; gaze test) Convergence (move finger toward client's nose)
IV Trochlear	Motor	Upward and downward movement of eyeball	See CN III; assess directions of gaze (eye can move out when intact/eye remains focused up and out when impaired); visual tracking Ask about double vision
V Trigeminal	Mixed	Sensory nerve to skin of face	Corneal reflex: client looks up and away, examiner lightly touches opposite cornea with wisp of cotton (look for blink in both eyes or a report by client of blinking sensation) Facial sensation: apply sterile, sharp item to forehead, cheek, jaw; repeat with dull object; client reports "sharp" or "dull"; if abnormal, test for temperature, vibration, and light touch
		Motor nerve to muscles of jaw (mastication)	Ask client to clench teeth together as you palpate muscles over temples (temporal muscle) and jaw (masseter) on each side Look for symmetric tone (normal) or muscle atrophy, deviation of jaw to one side, or fasciculations (abnormal)
VI Abducens	Motor	Lateral movement of eyeballs	See CN III; assess directions of gaze (able to move eyes out laterally when intact/medially deviated when impaired)
VII Facial	Mixed	Facial expression	Look for symmetry with facial expressions (e.g., frown, smile, raise and lower eyebrows, puff cheeks out, close eyes tightly)
VIII Acoustic (auditory, vestibulocochlear)	Sensory	Hearing	Assess the ability to hear spoken word and whisper Examiner stands behind client with hands on either side of client's head/ears; rub candy wrapper or fingers together to make noise on one side, ask client to identify which side noise is coming from Examiner stands 18 inches behind client and whispers three numbers Assess for dizziness and imbalance
IX Glossopharyngeal	Mixed	Taste Gag, swallow	Client identifies sour or sweet taste on back of the tongue Gag reflex (sensory IX and motor X) and ability to swallow
X Vagus	Mixed	Pharyngeal sensation, voice, swallow	Client says, "Ah." Observe for normal palate and pharynx movement Listen for hoarseness or nasal quality in voice Observe for difficulty swallowing
XI Spinal Accessory	Motor	Movement of head and shoulders	Client is able to shrug shoulders and turn the head against resistance Observe shoulders from behind for trapezius atrophy and/or asymmetry (abnormal finding) Assess for neck weakness
XII Hypoglossal	Motor	Position and movement of tongue	Client can stick out tongue to midline and move it from side to side Client can move tongue toward nose and chin Clear articulation in speech pattern

NORMAL   DEFECT

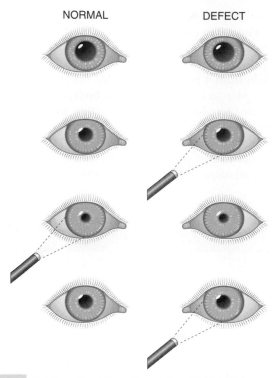

Fig. 5.4   Relative afferent pupillary defect (Marcus Gunn pupil). This patient has an abnormal left optic nerve. In ambient light *(top row)*, the pupils are equal. As the abnormal eye is illuminated *(second row)*, only modest constriction is noted. As the light is swung to the normal eye *(third row)*, the pupils constrict briskly. When the light is swung back to the abnormal eye *(bottom row)*, paradoxical dilation is noted. (From Friedman JN, Kaiser PK, Pineda A: Massachusetts Ear & Eye Infirmary Illustrated manual of ophthalmology, ed 3, Philadelphia, 2009, Saunders.)

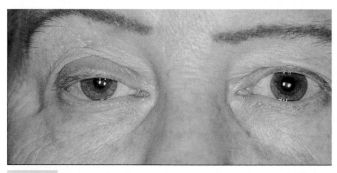

Fig. 5.5   Horner's syndrome with ipsilateral right upper eyelid ptosis and pupillary miosis. (From Yanoff M et al. Ophthalmology, ed 3, Elsevier, 2009.)

Cranial nerve testing for cranial nerve III or oculomotor involves smooth pursuit, convergence, and saccade testing. The oculomotor nerve innervates the superior, inferior, and medial recti, as well as the inferior oblique and levator palpebrae superior muscles. Complete paralysis of this cranial nerve results in ptosis dilation of the pupil, displacement of the eye downward and outward, and impairment of the eye in adduction and elevation (Fig. 5.6). Internuclear ophthalmoplegia (INO), a medial longitudinal fasciculus of the brainstem lesion, results in paralysis of the medial rectus in adducting the eye and nystagmus in the eye that is trying to abduct. INO may occur in patients with multiple sclerosis (Table 5.4).

Cranial nerve testing for cranial nerve IV or trochlear nerve involves assessing adduction with a downward gaze. The trochlear nerve supplies the superior oblique muscle which depresses and intorts the globe of the eye (Fig. 5.7). Abnormality of the trochlear nerve may result in a patient compensating by sidebending their head away from the affected eye to adjust to the resulting double vision or diplopia. Trochlear nerve abnormalities may also result in disconjugate gaze at rest, with one eye vertically displaced 1–2 mm from the other eye, termed strabismus (Table 5.5).

Cranial nerve testing for cranial nerve V or trigeminal nerve involves assessing light touch sensation to the ophthalmic, maxillary, and mandibular areas of the face (Fig. 5.8). As the trigeminal nerve also involves mastication, jaw function is assessed by testing the masseter, pterygoid, and temporalis muscles.

Cranial nerve testing for cranial nerve VI or abducens nerve involves testing smooth pursuit. Abnormalities of this cranial nerve results in the inability for the patient to perform lateral gaze (Table 5.6; Fig. 5.9).

Cranial nerve testing for cranial nerve VII or facial nerve involves testing motor functions of facial expression which includes the buccinator, platysma, stapedius, and stylohyoid muscles and the posterior belly of the digastric muscle (Fig. 5.10). Abnormalities of the facial nerve may occur in Bell's palsy, Guillain-Barré syndrome, Lyme disease, HIV, herpes simplex virus, meningeal inflammation, neoplasm, or trauma. Nasolabial fold or dropping of the corner of the mouth can be seen on observation in these patients (Fig. 5.11).

Cranial nerve testing for cranial nerve VIII or vestibulocochlear nerve involves testing hearing and balance. Abnormalities of this cranial nerve may occur with an acoustic neuroma, vestibular neuritis, or traumatic brain injury. The modified Romberg or sharpened Romberg can be used as a screening test for the vestibular portion of this cranial nerve. Rinne or Weber's test is done to screen for the acoustic portion of this cranial nerve (Fig. 5.12).

Cranial nerve testing for cranial nerve IX or glossopharyngeal nerve involves testing the gag reflex. This nerve supplies motor function to the stylopharyngeus muscle and sensation of the posterior third of the tongue, pharynx, tonsil, internal surface of the tympanic membrane, skin of the external ear, taste fibers from the posterior third of the tongue, parasympathetic innervation to the parotid gland, and general visceral sensory fibers from the carotid bodies. Abnormalities of this cranial nerve may occur in Guillain-Barré syndrome, ischemic events, motor neuron diseases, and tumors.[1]

Cranial nerve testing for cranial nerve X or vagus nerve involves testing palate elevation and the gag reflex. The vagus or wandering nerve supplies 10 terminal branches to include the pharyngeal, carotid body, meningeal, auricular, superior laryngeal, recurrent laryngeal, cardiac, pulmonary,

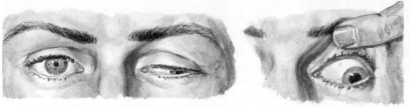

Oculomotor palsy: Ptosis, eye turns laterally and inferiorly, pupil dilated; common finding with cerebral aneurysms, especially carotid-posterior communicating aneurysms

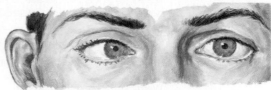

Abducens palsy: Affected eye turns medially. May be first manifestation of intracavernous carotid aneurysm. Pain above eye or on side of face may be secondary to trigeminal (V) nerve involvement.

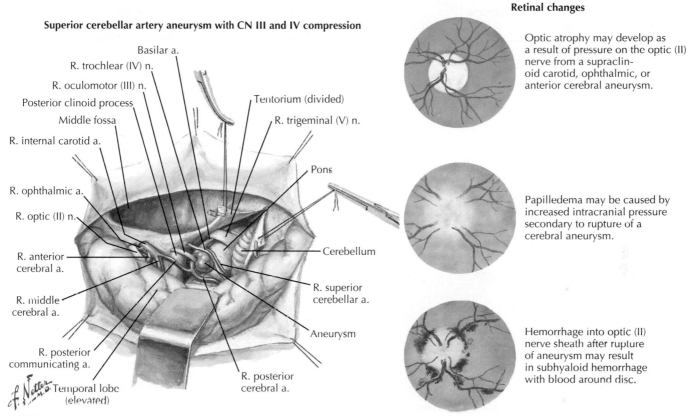

Superior cerebellar artery aneurysm with CN III and IV compression

Basilar a.
R. trochlear (IV) n.
R. oculomotor (III) n.
Posterior clinoid process
Middle fossa
R. internal carotid a.
R. ophthalmic a.
R. optic (II) n.
R. anterior cerebral a.
R. middle cerebral a.
R. posterior communicating a.
Temporal lobe (elevated)

Tentorium (divided)
R. trigeminal (V) n.
Pons
Cerebellum
R. superior cerebellar a.
Aneurysm
R. posterior cerebral a.

Retinal changes

Optic atrophy may develop as a result of pressure on the optic (II) nerve from a supraclinoid carotid, ophthalmic, or anterior cerebral aneurysm.

Papilledema may be caused by increased intracranial pressure secondary to rupture of a cerebral aneurysm.

Hemorrhage into optic (II) nerve sheath after rupture of aneurysm may result in subhyaloid hemorrhage with blood around disc.

Fig. 5.6 Ophthalmologic manifestations of cerebral aneurysms. (From Small JE, Scott BJ, Chaves CJ, Srivivasan J: Netter's Neurology, ed 3, Copyright 2020, Elsevier.)

esophageal, and gastrointestinal. Therefore, abnormalities of the vagus nerve results in a wide spectrum of disorders and can be seen in postoperative thoracotomy surgery.[2]

Cranial nerve testing for cranial nerve XI or spinal accessory nerve involves testing the muscle strength of the trapezius and sternocleidomastoid muscles. Abnormalities to this cranial nerve may occur with motor neuron diseases, myasthenia gravis, myotonic dystrophy, or skull basal fractures.[3]

Cranial nerve testing for cranial nerve XII or hypoglossal nerve involves testing tongue protrusion as this nerve innervates the tongue. Examination of the tongue should include the bulk of the muscle, strength of the muscle, and any abnormal movements such as deviation of the tongue with protrusion. Abnormalities of this cranial nerve may occur most commonly after metastatic cancer such as the base of the skull, subarachnoid space or lesions in the neck, and trauma such as a gunshot wound to the neck.[4]

Motor Function

Motor and cerebellar function can be screened most easily by observation of gait, posture, balance, strength, coordination, muscle tone, and motion. The cerebellum plays a central role in the control of eye movements and gaze stabilization to optimize visual performance and in learning.[5] Most of these tests are performed as a part of the musculoskeletal examination. Vision screening will be covered later in this chapter.

Motor function is a routine physical examination test across all areas of practice for physical therapists. In the patient who presents with muscle weakness, the data gathered from the patient in the history and physical examination are paramount. Muscle weakness has been reported to occur in ~5% of adults in the United States over the age of 60.[6] Contributing systems that may influence muscle weakness include neurologic, rheumatologic, endocrine, genetic,

TABLE 5.4	Lesions of the Oculomotor Nerve	
Anatomic Location	Cause	Associated Symptoms
Nuclear	Infarction, mass, infection, inflammation, compression	Bilateral ptosis and paresis of the contralateral superior rectus; lid function may be spared
	Wernicke-Korsakoff syndrome	Ataxia, abducens palsy, nystagmus, altered mentation
Fascicular	Infarction, mass, infection, inflammation, compression Demyelination	Contralateral hemiparesis or tremor; pupil may be spared
Subarachnoid space	Aneurysm	Headache, stiff neck, pupil-involved
	Vasculopathic	Pupil generally spared
	Meningitis	Headache. cranial nerve involvement, meningismus, fever
	Miller-Fisher syndrome	Areflexia, ataxia, previous viral illness
	Migraine	Headache, family history
	Uncal herniation	Early pupil involvement, altered mentation, ipsilateral hemiparesis
Cavernous sinus	Neoplasm	Cavernous sinus syndrome, pain, sensory changes, ± sympathetic involvement
	Fistula	Exophthalmos, bruit, chemosis
	Thrombosis	Previous infection/trauma, pain, exophthalmos, chemosis
Superior orbital fissure	Neoplasm	Superior division involvement
Neuromuscular junction	Myasthenia gravis	No pupil involvement, frequent fluctuation, ptosis, ophthalmoparesis, orbicularis oculi weakness, dysarthria

From Neuro-Ophthalmology David K Duong MD. MS, Megan M. Leo MD and Elizabeth L. Mitchel MD Emergency Medicine Clinics of North America 2008-02-01. Volume 26, Issue 1, Pages 137-180, Copyright © 2008 Elsevier Inc.

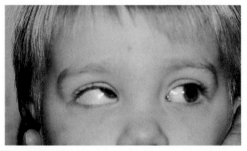

Fig. 5.7 Patient was asked to look to the right side and upwards. Palsy of the trochlear nerve [CN IV] on the left side. (From Zitelli B., McIntire S., Nowalk A.: Zitelli and Davis' Atlas of Pediatric Physical Diagnosis. 6 th ed., Elsevier/Saunders, 2012.)

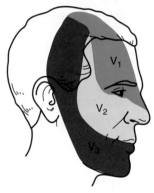

Fig. 5.8 Trigeminal nerve sensory distribution. V1, V2, and V3 sensory distributions in blue, yellow, and red, respectively. (From Massachusetts General Hospital Comprehensive Clinical Psychiatry, 2016, Elsevier.)

TABLE 5.5	Lesions of the Trochlear Nerve	
Anatomic Location	Cause	Associated Symptoms
Nuclear	Infarction	Internuclear ophthalmoplegia, Horner syndrome relative afferent pupillary defect
	Trauma, tumor, infection, inflammation	As above
Fascicular	Infarction	As above
	Trauma, tumor, infection, inflammation	As above
Subarachnoid space	Demyelination	Isolated or with midbrain signs above
	Trauma. hydrocephalus	May be bilateral
	Vasculopathic	Usually isolated
	Mass lesion	Contralateral hemiparesis or ipsilateral ataxia
Cavernous sinus	As with third nerve palsy	Cavernous sinus syndrome
	Herpes zoster ophthalmic	Rash, trigeminal sensory loss V1 or V2 distribution
Orbit	Inflammation, trauma, tumor	Oculomotor. abducens. optic nerve dysfunction proptosis

From Neuro-Ophthalmology David K Duong MD. MS, Megan M. Leo MD and Elizabeth L. Mitchel MD Emergency Medicine Clinics of North America 2008-02-01. Volume 26, Issue 1, Pages 137-180, Copyright © 2008 Elsevier Inc.

TABLE 5.6	Lesions of the Abducens Nerve	

Lesions of the abducens nerve

Anatomic Location	Cause	Associated Symptoms
Nuclear	Infarction	Internuclear ophthalmoplegia, Horner syndrome relative afferent pupillary defect
	Infiltration, trauma, inflammation Wernicke-Korsakoff	Ataxia, nystagmus. altered mentation
Fascicular	Infarction, tumor, inflammation, Multiple sclerosis	Ipsilateral facial nerve paralysis and contralateral hemiplegia
	Anterior inferior cerebellar artery infarction	Ipsilateral facial paralysis, loss of taste, ipsilateral Homer, ipsilateral trigeminal dysfunction, and ipsilateral deafness
Subarachnoid	Mass	Contralateral hemiparesis
	Ischemia	Usually isolated
	Trauma	Papilledema, headache
	Intracranial hypertension or hypotension	Headache
Petrous apex	Mastoiditis, skull fracture, Lateral sinus thrombosis, neoplasms, tumor	Ipsilateral facial paralysis, severe facial pain
Cavernous sinus	As with third nerve palsy	Cavernous sinus syndrome

From Neuro-Ophthalmology David K Duong MD. MS, Megan M. Leo MD and Elizabeth L. Mitchel MD Emergency Medicine Clinics of North America 2008-02-01. Volume 26, Issue 1, Pages 137-180, Copyright © 2008 Elsevier Inc.

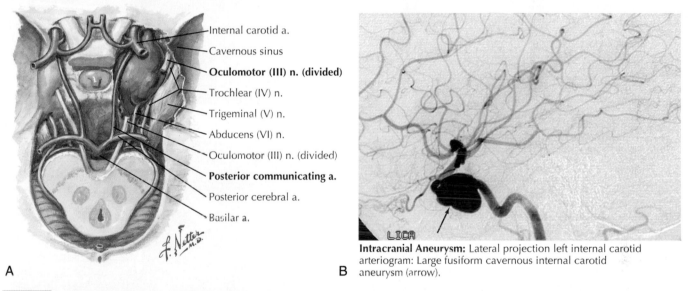

Internal carotid a.
Cavernous sinus
Oculomotor (III) n. (divided)
Trochlear (IV) n.
Trigeminal (V) n.
Abducens (VI) n.
Oculomotor (III) n. (divided)
Posterior communicating a.
Posterior cerebral a.
Basilar a.

A

LICA

Intracranial Aneurysm: Lateral projection left internal carotid arteriogram: Large fusiform cavernous internal carotid aneurysm (arrow).

B

Fig. 5.9 Cranial nerve anatomy (A) and an Arteriogram image (B) showing an Intracranial Aneurysm compressing the oculomotor nerve resulting in a palsy. (From Small JE, Scott BJ, Chaves CJ, Srivivasan J: Netter's Neurology, ed 3, Copyright 2020, Elsevier.)

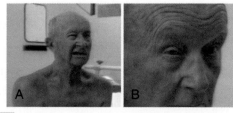

A   **B**

Fig. 5.10 Selective weakness of lower facial muscles after corticobulbar damage. This patient suffered a stroke that resulted in weakness of his left hand (not shown) and the left side of his face. When he tried to bare his teeth (A), weakness of left lower facial muscles was apparent. However, he could not raise his eyebrows symmetrically (B). (From Vanderah TW, Gould DJ: Nolte's Human Brain. 2021. Elsevier. St Louis.)

medication or toxin-related, and infectious etiologies.[6] Physical therapists are well trained on manual muscle testing in entry-level physical therapy programs. It is known that experience plays a factor in application of resistance during manual muscle testing in health care professionals. For example, in medical students and junior residents compared with senior residents and faculty working with patients with known neurologic conditions, inconsistent technique and lower clinical skills have been reported.[7] In the patient with a suspected neurologic condition, manual muscle testing should be repeated more than once on muscles to identify fatigable weakness that may follow conditions that effect the neuromuscular junction.[7] Weakness across multiple muscles during manual muscle testing may indicate involvement of

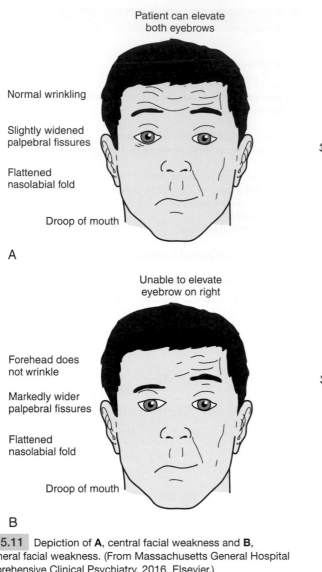

Patient can elevate
both eyebrows

Normal wrinkling

Slightly widened
palpebral fissures

Flattened
nasolabial fold

Droop of mouth

A

Unable to elevate
eyebrow on right

Forehead does
not wrinkle

Markedly wider
palpebral fissures

Flattened
nasolabial fold

Droop of mouth

B

Fig. 5.11 Depiction of **A**, central facial weakness and **B**, peripheral facial weakness. (From Massachusetts General Hospital Comprehensive Clinical Psychiatry, 2016, Elsevier.)

lower motor neurons. Neurologic conditions that present with spasticity during manual muscle testing may indicate upper motor neuron involvement. Manual muscle testing results should be pooled together with the results of the neurologic physical examination to evaluate the potential involvement of the neurologic system. Specific motor tests, such as tandem walking, modified Romberg's test, and diadochokinesia (rapid, alternating movements of the hands or fingers, such as repeatedly alternating forearm pronation to supination, the finger-to-nose/finger-to-finger, thumb-to-finger opposition tests, and pointing/past-pointing test), can be added for a more in-depth screening. Demonstrate all test maneuvers to the patient in order to prevent poor performance from a lack of understanding rather than from neurologic impairment.

Sensory Function

Screening for sensory function can begin with superficial pain (pinprick) and light touch (cotton ball) on the extremities. Show the client the items you will be using and how they

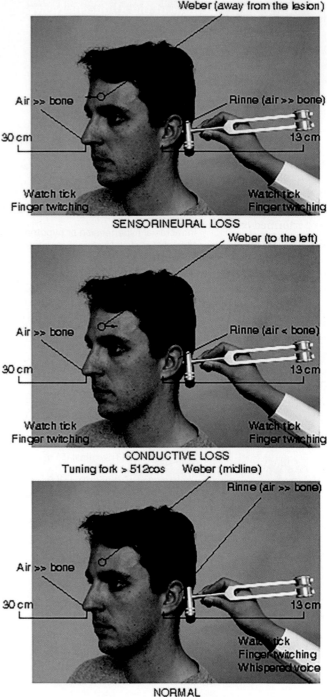

Fig. 5.12 Bedside hearing tests and results with sensorineural or conductive loss in left ear and with normal hearing. (From Magee DJ, Manske RC: Orthopedic Physical Assessment, Elsevier 2021 St Louis.)

will be used. For light touch, dab the skin lightly on the cheek as a demonstration first as you are explaining the test to the client; do not stroke.

Tests are done with the client's eyes closed. Ask the client to tell you where the sensation is felt or to identify "sharp" or "dull." Apply the stimulus randomly and bilaterally over the face, neck, upper arms, hands, thighs, lower legs, and feet. Allow at least 2 seconds between the time the stimulus is applied and the next one is given. This avoids the summation effect.

Follow-up, when appropriate, with temperature using test tubes filled with hot and cold water and vibration using a low-pitch tuning fork over the peripheral joints. Temperature can be omitted if pain sensation is normal. Apply the stem of the vibrating tuning fork to the distal interphalangeal joint of the fingers and interphalangeal joint of the great toe, elbow, and wrist. Ask the client to tell you when vibration is first felt and when it stops. Remember, aging adults often lose vibratory sense in the great toe and ankle both medially and laterally.

Other sensory tests include proprioception (joint position sense), kinesthesia (movement sense), stereognosis (identification of common object placed in the hand), graphesthesia (identifying number or letter when drawn on the palm of the hand), and two-point discrimination. Again, all tests should be performed on both sides after you adequately describe the testing procedure.

The spinal cord extends from the brain stem to the conus medullaris located at L1 or the L2 vertebrae. Inferior to the L2 vertebrae, the spinal cord becomes a series of spinal nerve roots called the cauda equina. If there is compression of any portion of the spinal cord, then symptoms can occur. These symptoms vary depending on the location of the compression (Fig. 5.13). For example, a malignant or a benign tumor could compress the spinal cord or the spinal nerves. In a patient who presents with back pain that worsens at night or with recumbency, a red flag for spinal involvement must be considered. Cauda equina compression often results in saddle anesthesia (Fig. 5.14).

Reflexes

DTRs are tested in a screening examination at the:
- Jaw (cranial nerve V)
- Biceps (C5-C6)
- Brachioradialis (C5-C6)
- Triceps (C7-C8)
- Patella (L3-L4)
- Achilles (S1-S2)

These reflexes are assessed for symmetry and briskness using the following scale:

0	No response, absent
+ 1	Low normal, decreased; slight muscle contraction
+ 2	Normal, visible muscle twitch producing movement of arm/leg
+ 3	More brisk than normal, increased or exaggerated; may not indicate disease
+ 4	Hyperactive; very brisk, clonus; spinal cord disorder suspected

Data from the National Institute of Neurological Disorders and Stroke DTR scale.

A change in one or more DTRs is a yellow (caution) flag. Some individuals have very brisk reflexes normally, whereas others are much more hyporeflexive. Whenever encountering increased (hyper-) or decreased (hypo-) reflexes, the therapist routinely follows several guidelines:

The isolated DTR that does not fit with the client's physiologic pattern must be considered a red flag. As discussed in Chapter 2, one red flag by itself does not require immediate

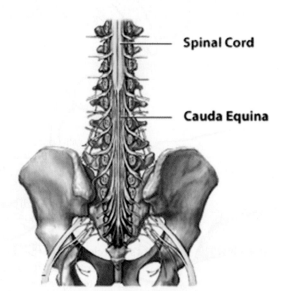

Fig. 5.13 Lower spinal cord anatomy. (From Lower spinal cord. Wikimedia commons. Available at https://commons.wikimedia.org/wiki/File:Onurğa_beyni_at_quyruğu.jpg).

Spinal Cord

Cauda Equina

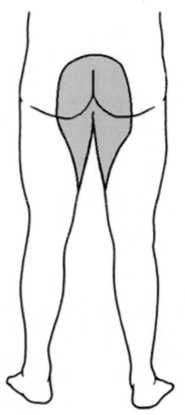

Fig. 5.14 Saddle anesthesia. (From Saddle anesthesia. Wikimedia commons. https://commons.wikimedia.org/wiki/File:Saddle_anesthesia.png.)

? FOLLOW-UP QUESTIONS

- Test reflexes above and below and from side to side in order to gauge overall reflexive response. A "normal" hyperreflexive response will be present in most, if not all, reflexes. The same is true for generalized hyporeflexive responses.
- Offer the client a distraction while testing through conversation or by asking the client to "Count out loud backward by three starting at 89." Alternatively, especially in the case of an absent or hypoactive lower extremity reflex, you could have the client perform the Jendrassik maneuver by having them interlock their fingers, clench their teeth (optional) and then forcefully pull their hands apart while keeping them locked, and then repeat the reflex assessment. Authors have suggested that the effect of the Jendrassik maneuver decreases with age.[8]
- Retest unusual reflexes later in the day or on another day.
- Have another clinician test your client.

medical follow-up. But a hyporesponsive patellar tendon reflex that is reproducible and when added to the patient presentation of back, hip, or thigh pain in the presence of a past history of prostate cancer as one example does become concerning.

A diminished reflex may be interpreted as the sign of a possible "space-occupying lesion"—most often, a disk protruding from the disk space and either pressing on a spinal nerve root or irritating the spinal nerve root (i.e., chemicals released by the herniation in contact with the nerve root can cause nerve root irritation).

Tumors (whether benign or malignant) can also press on the spinal nerve root, mimicking a disk problem. A small lesion can exert enough pressure to irritate the nerve root, resulting in a hyporeflexive DTR. A large tumor can obliterate the reflex arc resulting in diminished or absent reflexes. Either way, changes in DTRs must be considered yellow (caution) or red (warning) flags to be documented, reported, and further investigated.

Superficial (cutaneous) reflexes (e.g., abdominal, cremasteric, plantar) can also be tested using the handle of the reflex hammer. The reliability of superficial or cutaneous reflexes has not been reported in the literature; therefore, they require further investigation in the client to determine the relevance of the reflex response. The abdominal reflex is elicited by applying a stroking motion with a cotton-tipped applicator (or handle of the reflex hammer) toward the umbilicus. A positive sign of neurologic impairment is observed if the umbilicus moves toward the stroke. The test can be repeated in each abdominal quadrant (upper abdominal T7-T9; lower abdominal T11-T12).

The cremasteric reflex is elicited by stroking the thigh downward with a cotton-tipped applicator (or handle of the reflex hammer). A normal response in males is an upward movement of the testicle (scrotum) on the same side. The absence of a cremasteric reflex is an indication of disruption at the T12-L1 level. Testing the cremasteric reflex may help the therapist identify neurologic impairment in any male with

suspicious back, pelvic, groin (including testicular), and/or anterior thigh pain.

The plantar reflex, or Babinski sign, occurs when the sole of the foot is stroked and the toes plantarflex downward (Fig. 5.15). The plantar reflex is normal in children up to 24 months old. The interrater reliability of the Babinski reflex has been reported as a kappa value of 0.72.[9] The Hoffman sign occurs when flicking the nail of the middle digit in a downward direction results in flexion of the index finger and/or the thumb. The Hoffman sign has substantial inter-rater reliability and excellent intra-rater reliability (0.65 and 0.89, respectively).[10] Both the plantar reflex and the Hoffman sign are suggestive of a central nervous system disorder. If they are both present, without a plausible explanation, physician referral and advanced imaging of the brain and spinal cord are indicated.

Neural Tension

Excessive nerve tightness or adhesion can cause adverse neural tension in the peripheral nervous system. When the nerve cannot slide or glide in its protective sheath, neural extensibility and mobility are impaired. The clinical result can be numbness, tingling, and pain. This could be caused by disk

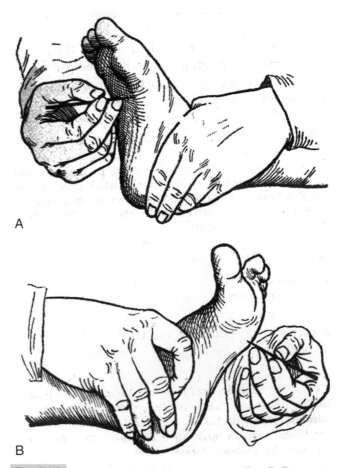

A

B

Fig. 5.15 Babinski's sign. **A,** Normal plantar reflex. **B,** Toe phenomenon. (From Phillipson J, Poirer J. Joseph Babinski: A Biography. New York: Oxford University Press; 2009.)

protrusion, scar tissue, or space-occupying lesions, including cysts, bone spurs, tumors, and cancer metastases.

A positive neural tension test does not tell the therapist what the underlying etiology is—only that the peripheral nerve is involved. History and physical examination are still very important in assessing the clinical presentation.

Someone with full range of motion accompanied by negative articular signs but with impaired neural extensibility and mobility raises a yellow (caution) flag. A second look at the history and a more thorough neurologic examination may be warranted.

Reducing symptoms with neural mobilization does not rule out the possibility of cancer. A red flag is raised with any client who responds well to neural mobilization but experiences recurrence of symptoms. This could be a sign that the tumor has grown larger or cancer metastases have progressed, once again interfering with neural mobility.

Vision

Approximately half of the cortex or real estate of the brain is devoted to vision; therefore, many aspects of vision are vulnerable in clients who have a history of trauma or ischemia.[11] For example, a wide range of visual complaints may follow a client who has incurred head trauma such as photophobia, diplopia, blurred vision, loss of vision, and visual processing problems. The specific neuroanatomical areas of the brain that are involved in vision will not be covered in this chapter or textbook because they are quite complex. The vision system is broken down into specific components that physical therapists can screen to determine the involvement of neuroanatomical locations in the brain to facilitate the referral of the appropriate client or patient for further medical investigation. The vision system components that should be screened by physical therapists include the following:

Saccadic system
Vestibular ocular reflex system
Smooth pursuit system
Convergence system

These vision screening tests can be evaluated in less than 5 minutes in a patient with a history of trauma or a patient with a potential ischemic event.

Saccadic System

In general, the saccadic system directs the eyes to the object of interest in the client and is a ballistic movement of the eyes to the target in the healthy client. Authors have reported abnormalities in saccade generation after multiple forms of brain trauma.[11] Physical therapists can screen the saccadic system by asking the client to rapidly move the eyes back and forth between two targets such as the tip of a pen at arm's distance from the patient and then to a horizontally placed second tip of a pen. The therapist is screening for accuracy of movement, so an abnormal finding would be multiple eye movements such as hypometria or hypermetria to fixate on the target (Fig. 5.16).

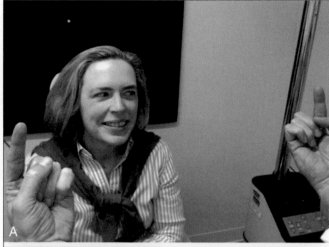
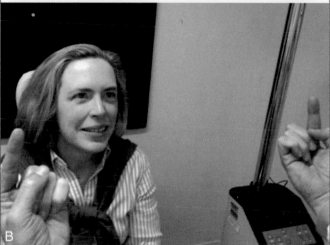

Fig. 5.16 Saccades can be tested by having the patient **A**, look at a target in the periphery and then **B**, look at a target directly in front of their face. Saccades can be assessed for speed and accuracy. (From Ventura RE, Balcer Prof LF, Galletta SL: The neuro-ophthalmology of head trauma, Lancet Neurology, Vol 13, Issue 10, pgs 1006 1016.)

Vestibular Ocular Reflex System

The vestibular ocular reflex (VOR) system allows the client to maintain gaze on a target while moving their head. The VOR involves the interplay of cranial nerves specific to the eyes and the semicircular canals of the vestibular system. Physical therapists can screen the VOR system by asking the patient to fixate on the tip of the therapist's nose at arm's length distance and ask the client to horizontally rotate their head back and forth as if they are saying no (Fig. 5.17). The client who complains of blurred vision or a feeling of dizziness can be followed-up with other tests if the therapist is trained to do so. The head thrust or head impulse test should not be done until the end of the neurological screen in the client with a suspected concussion and should not be done by a therapist who does not have experience with this test. Range of motion of the cervical spine should also be screened prior to performance of the head thrust test. For example, the Canadian Cervical Spine Rules suggest that a patient over the age of 65

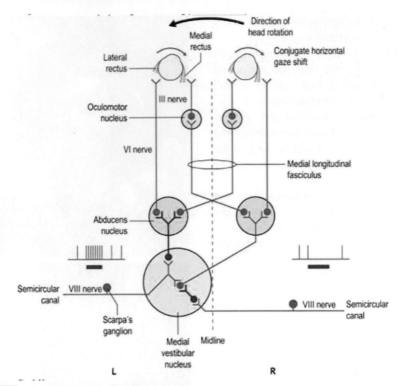

Fig. 5.17 The circuitry of the rotational vestibulo-ocular reflex. Stimulation of the horizontal semicircular canals by leftward head rotation *(red bars)* excites motor neurons to ipsilateral medial rectus and contralateral lateral rectus muscles. Motor neurons to the antagonists are silenced by inhibitory *(red)* neurons. (From Naish J, Syndercombe Court D: Medical Sciences, ed 3, 2019, Elsevier.)

who has had trauma and cannot rotate their neck more than 45 degrees to the right and left and has midline cervical spine tenderness needs to have radiographs prior to any intervention. This patient who is positive for the Canadian Cervical Spine Rules would NOT be appropriate for a head thrust or head impulse test. In the patient who had a positive VOR test for symptoms and did not present with other positive neurologic signs, the head thrust or impulse test can be safely done. The head thrust test is a passive test in which the patient fixates on the therapist's tip of the nose. The therapist slowly oscillates the patient's head back and forth and asks the client to keep focus on the tip of the nose. The therapist passively moves the client's head horizontally in a rapid unpredictable direction to the right or to the left. A left motion of the client's head would be evaluating the left VOR and a right motion would be evaluating the right VOR. A positive response is when the eyes of the client move off of the target of the therapist's nose, thus requiring a corrective saccade back to the therapist's nose. This indicates a vestibular hypofunction. The specificity of the head thrust test has been reported to be 0.85 to 0.90.[12] The sensitivity in a different study was reported as 71% for a vestibular hypofunction and 84% for a bilateral vestibular hypofunction.[13]

Smooth Pursuit System

The smooth pursuit system test involves predictive visual tracking of a target in a horizontal and vertical test. The

TABLE 5.7	Functional Classes of Human Eye Movements
Class of Eye Movement	Main Function
Visual fixation	Holds the image of a stationary object on the fovea
Vestibular	Holds images of the seen world steady on the retina during brief head rotations
Optokinetic	Holds images of the seen world steady on the retina during sustained head rotations
Smooth pursuit	Holds the image of a moving target on the fovea
Nystagmus	The repetition of a compensatory slow-phase and quick-phase resetting movement of the eyes; in quick phases. gaze directed toward the oncoming visual scene
Saccade	Brings images of objects of interest onto the fovea
Vergence	Moves the eyes in opposite directions so that images of a single object are placed simultaneously on both foveae

From Hullar TE et al. Cummings Otolaryngology: Head and Neck Surgery, 166, 2495-2516.e3

smooth pursuit system involves the coordination by the cerebellum based on input from the retina.[14] It also requires higher cortical input to maintain attention on the target[15] as well as anticipation and working memory to fixate on a moving target. Smooth pursuit abnormalities have been reported

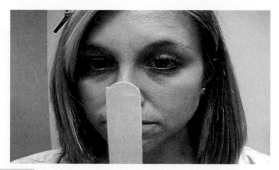

Fig. 5.18 A patient is fixated on the letters as the stick gradually moves toward the nose. (From McGregor ML: Convergence Insufficiency and Vision Therapy. Pediatric Clinics of North America, Volume 61, Issue 3, June 2014, pp 621-630.)

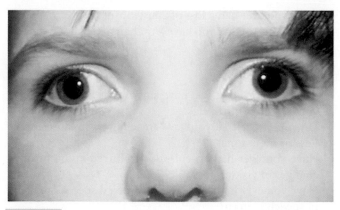

Fig. 5.19 Exotropia, a divergent deviation of the eyes. (From Cheng K P: Zitelli and Davis' Atlas of Pediatric Physical Diagnosis. 7 th ed., Elsevier/Saunders, 2018.)

in patients after a concussion,[11] Parkinson's disease,[16] multiple system atrophy,[16] major depressive disorder,[17] dementia,[18] hypovolemic cerebrospinal fluid,[19] and Alzheimer's disease.[18]

Convergence System

The convergence system test involves tracking a near target toward the patient's eyes and the eyes converge or adduct or move toward the target. To assess near point of convergence, a standardized approach has been suggested[20] (Fig. 5.18). Abnormal convergence has been suggested to be when a patient is unable to see the target clearly at a distance of more than 5 cm from the eye and represents a threshold.[21] Patients with convergence insufficiency commonly complain of blurred vision, diplopia, headaches, dizziness, or nausea.[22]

Interpretation of Neurologic Testing

Performance of these vision tests may be simple, but interpretation is complex as abnormal signs and symptoms implicate specific neuroanatomical areas of the brain as these areas incorporate higher cortical function that is susceptible to trauma and ischemia events such as posterior communicating artery aneurysm. The authors suggest that if the reader is inexperienced or unsure of the results, a referral to another health care provider is warranted. The oculomotor, trochlear, and abducens cranial nerves are screened within these vision tests. Patients should be asked about any symptoms as these visual tests are performed and the therapist should note any abnormal signs such as abnormal tracking during smooth pursuit, nystagmus, or exotropia (Fig. 5.19).

When the seven major areas of the neurologic examination are complete, the physical therapist has gathered enough data to determine the involvement of the neurologic system to include the peripheral and central nervous system. The authors of this textbook recommend a thorough systematic approach to rule in or rule out the involvement of the neurologic system.

CLIENT HISTORY

Special Questions to Ask: Headache

See Appendix C-7 in the accompanying eBook for complete assessment.

HISTORY

Trauma

- Have you ever been in a car accident?
- If yes, did you lose consciousness, have a concussion, or a fractured skull?
- Have you ever been knocked out, unconscious, or had a concussion at any time?
- Have you ever had a seizure?

- Have you ever been paralyzed in your arms or legs?
- Have you ever broken your neck or back?

Mentation

- Do you ever notice times of confusion/increased confusion recently?
- Do you feel that you are depressed?
- Do you ever notice times of being irritable more frequently than in the past?
- Do you ever notice times of being drowsy or lethargic more frequently than in the past?
- Do you ever notice times of being dizzy or light-headed more frequently than in the past?

- Have you ever had a loss of consciousness?
- Do you notice that you have any changes in your memory?

Motor Function

- Do you notice that you have any muscle weakness or that you are dropping things?
- Do you notice that you have any changes in muscle tone? Less or more tone?
- Have you ever had an episode of blurred vision or other changes in vision?
- Have you ever had an episode of slurred speech or change in speech pattern?

- Do you notice that you have frequent headaches?
- Do you notice that you have balance or coordination problems in doing normal activities in your day?

Sensory Function

Do you notice that you have paresthesias, numbness or tingling in your hands, arms, feet , legs, or anywhere else in your body?

Do you have any seizures or does anyone else close to you note any changes in your ability to attend to normal activities?

CASE STUDY

A 44-year-old female registered nurse notes that when she works long hours of a double shift in the intensive care unit of the hospital or when she is very tired, she gets dizzy.

FOLLOW-UP QUESTIONS

Are there any other symptoms of any kind anywhere else in your body? The nurse denies any other symptoms or feelings. When you do get dizzy, do you experience the sensation of spinning? The nurse denies any spinning but complains of a feeling in her eyes and in her head of dizziness.

When you do get dizzy, what are you doing at work? Lifting a patient or carrying equipment? The nurse denies any physical activities that make her dizzy, but she does note that when she gets dizzy, it is only in certain rooms in the intensive care unit that it happens. When asked to explain this, she is unsure why this is the case. I asked her about what she does in these rooms, and she explains typical nursing activities that occur in an intensive care unit. I noted to her that in certain ICU

rooms, the monitors are in different locations in the room. She states that this is probably why she gets dizzy in specific rooms in the intensive care unit.

Do these symptoms fall into any one category? It appears that many of the symptoms may be oculomotor in nature and fall within neurologic for this nurse.

What is the next step in the screening process? As the nurse becomes dizzy when she is very tired, we set up her next appointment for later in the day after she has worked a double shift. The oculomotor examination was performed and revealed an oculomotor palsy. This explains why the nurse becomes dizzy in certain rooms in the intensive care unit as the oculomotor nerve controls the eye movements that correspond to the nurse being able to read the patient's monitors that she cares for and as the oculomotor nerve supplies the motor coordination of specific eye movements, she reports dizziness when the patient's monitor is viewed by the nurse as blurry. The nurse is referred to an ophthalmologist and the physician diagnoses the patient with an oculomotor palsy.

PRACTICE QUESTIONS

1. During a neurologic examination, a patient presents with 3+ reflexes for their bilateral patellar and Achilles reflexes. Which of the following options is the BEST next approach for the therapist?
   a. recheck the reflexes of the upper extremities and lower extremities
   b. consider it normal for this patient and document a 2+ bilateral patellar reflex
   c. perform the Jendrassik maneuver for this patient because there is an abnormal reflex
   d. go right to superficial reflexes such as the abdominal or Beevor's sign
2. During an oculomotor exam, the patient presents with symptoms of double vision and exotropia during convergence testing from 15 centimeters away. The patient does not wear corrective lenses. What is a normal near point of convergence distance?

   a. 10 inches
   b. 10 centimeters
   c. 5 inches
   d. 5 centimeters
3. A patient presents with a + Babinski sign or upgoing toes, clonus during rapid passive dorsiflexion of the right foot, and hyperreflexia of all four extremities deep tendon reflexes. In a patient that it is not known if the patient has a neurologic condition, which of the following is the MOST appropriate action?
   a. document it in the medical record and forget about it
   b. document it in the medical record and refer the patient to a gastroenterologist
   c. document it in the medical record and refer the patient to a neurologist
   d. ask the patient to go to the emergency room immediately

4. In a patient that presents with clonus on a jaw reflex, the cranial nerve involved with this reflex is:
   a. cranial nerve V or trigeminal nerve
   b. cranial nerve VI or abducens nerve
   c. cranial nerve III or oculomotor nerve
   d. cranial nerve II or optic nerve

5. In a patient that presents with an inability to adduct and elevate the right eye, the cranial nerve involved with this patient is:
   a. cranial nerve V or trigeminal nerve
   b. ranial nerve VI or abducens nerve
   c. cranial nerve III or oculomotor nerve
   d. cranial nerve II or optic nerve

REFERENCES

1. Sinnatamby CS. *Last's Anatomy*. 12 ed. St Louis: Elsevier; 2011:455–502.
2. Vanderah TW, Gould DJ. *Nolte's the Human Brain*. 8 ed. St Louis: Elsevier; 2021:286–308.
3. Murray ED, Price BH. *Massachusetts General Hospital Comprehensive Clinical Psychiatry*. 2 ed. Elsevier; 2016:791–804.e4.
4. McGee S. *Evidence-Based Physical Diagnosis*. 5 ed. St Louis: Elsevier; 2022:523–532.
5. Beh SC, Frohman TC, Frohman EM. Cerebellar control of eye movements. *J Neuro-Opthalmol*. 2017;37:87–98.
6. Larson ST, Wilbur J. Muscle weakness in adults: evaluation and differential diagnosis. *Am Fam Physician*. 2020;101(2):95–108.
7. Lewinson RT, Ganesh A, Yeung MMC. The biomechanics of manual muscle testing in the neuromuscular exam. *Can J Neurol Sci*. 2018;45(5):518–521.
8. Burke JR, Schutten MC, Koceja DM, Kamen G. Age-dependent effects of muscle vibration and the Jendrassik maneuver on the patellar tendon reflex response. *Arch Phys Med Rehabil*. 1996;77:600–604.
9. Dafkin C, Green A, Kerr S, Veliotes D, Olivier B, McKinon W. The interrater reliability of subjective assessments of the Babinski reflex. *J Mot Behav*. 2016;48(2):116–121.
10. Annaswamy TM, Sakai T, Goetz LL, Pacheco FM, Ozarkar T. Reliability and repeatability of the Hoffman sign. *PM R*. 2012;4(7):498–503.
11. Ventura RE, Balcer LJ, Galetta SL. The neuro-opthalmology of head trauma. *Lancet Neurol*. 2014;13:1006–1016.
12. Cohen HS, Stitz J, Sangi-Haghpeykar H, et al. Utility of quick oculomotor tests for screening the vestibular system in the subacute and chronic populations. *Acta Otolaryngol*. 2018;138:382–386.
13. Schubert MC, Tusa RJ, Grine LE, Herdman SJ. Optimizing the sensitivity of the head thrust test of identifying vestibular hypofunction. *Phys Ther*. 2004;84(2):151–158.
14. Fukushima K, Yamanobe T, Shinmei Y, Fukushima I, Kurkin S, Peterson BW. Coding of smooth eye movements in three-dimensional space by frontal cortex. *Nature*. 2002;419(6903):157–162.
15. Barnes GR. Cognitive processes involved in smooth pursuit eye movements. *Brain Cogn*. 2008;68:309–326.
16. Zhou H, Wang X, Ma D, et al. The differential diagnostic value of a battery of oculomotor evaluation in Parkinson's Disease and Multiple System Atrophy. *Brain Behav*. 2021;11(7):e02184.
17. Takahashi J, Hirano Y, Miura K, et al. Eye movement abnormalities in major depressive disorder. *Front Psychiatry*. 2021 Aug 10;12:673443.
18. Lage C, López-García S, Bejanin A, et al. Distinctive oculomotor behaviors in Alzheimer's disease and frontotemporal dementia. *Front Aging Neurosci*. 2021 Feb 4;12:603790.
19. Shinmei Y, Takahashi A, Nakamura K, et al. Cerebrospinal fluid hypovolemia syndrome after a traffic accident with abnormal eye movements: a case report. *Am J Ophthalmol Case Rep*. 2020;20:100997.
20. Heick JD, Bay C. Determining near point of convergence: exploring a component of the vestibular/ocular motor screen comparing varied target sizes. *Int J Sports Phys Ther*. 2021;16(1):21–30.
21. Mucha A, Collins MW, Elbin RJ, et al. A brief vestibular/ocular motor screening (VOMS) assessment to evaluate concussions: preliminary findings. *Am J Sports Med*. 2014;42(10):2479–2486.
22. Truong JQ, Ciuffreda KJ. Quantifying pupillary asymmetry through objective binocular pupillometry in the normal and mild traumatic brain injury (mTBI) populations. *Brain Inj*. 2016;30(11):1372–1377.

CHAPTER

6

Screening for Hematologic Disease

The physical therapist must consider several factors when screening for possible hematologic conditions. Symptoms of blood disorders are most common in relation to the use of nonsteroidal antiinflammatory drugs (NSAIDs), neurologic complications associated with pernicious anemia, and complications of chemotherapy or radiation. In addition, bleeding and clotting are the main hematologic considerations in individuals with orthopedic conditions. People who have difficulty with blood clotting (hypocoagulation), or those who clot excessively (hypercoagulation), will require close observation.[1] In addition, patients being seen postsurgically, or those who are immobilized or neurologically compromised, must also be observed carefully for any signs or symptoms of venous thromboembolism.

The hematologic system is composed of the blood, blood vessels, and the organs that produce the blood. Blood contains erythrocytes (red blood cells or RBCs), leukocytes (white blood cells or WBCs), and platelets (thrombocytes) suspended in plasma, a pale yellow or gray-yellow fluid (Fig. 6.1). Blood is the circulating tissue of the body; plasma and its formed elements circulate through the heart, arteries, capillaries, and veins. The *erythrocytes* carry oxygen to and remove carbon dioxide from the tissues. *Leukocytes* act in the inflammatory and immune response. The *plasma* carries antibodies and nutrients to tissues and removes wastes from tissues. *Platelets*, together with *coagulation factors* in plasma, control the clotting of blood.

Primary hematologic diseases are uncommon, but hematologic manifestations secondary to other diseases are common. Cancers of the blood are discussed in Chapter 14.

SIGNS AND SYMPTOMS OF HEMATOLOGIC DISORDERS

From a physical therapy standpoint, the most important indicators of dysfunction in this system include signs and symptoms associated with physical effort (often minimal exertion) such as dyspnea, chest pain, palpitations, severe weakness, and fatigue. In addition, hematologic disorders may cause symptoms affecting the nervous system such as headaches, drowsiness, dizziness, syncope, or polyneuropathy.[2,3]

Hematologic disorders could also affect the integumentary system. The clinician may notice pallor of the face, hands, nail beds, and lips; cyanosis or clubbing of the fingernail beds may also be observed. In addition, wounds or easy bruising or bleeding of the skin, gums, or mucous membranes, often with no reported trauma to the area, may indicate problems in this system. The physical therapist must be aware that the presence of blood in the stool or emesis or severe pain and swelling in joints and muscles can sometimes be a critical indicator of bleeding disorders that can be life-threatening.[4]

In addition, many hematologic-induced signs and symptoms seen in the physical therapy practice occur as a result of medications. For example, chronic or long-term use of steroids and NSAIDs can lead to gastritis and peptic ulcer with gastrointestinal (GI) bleeding and subsequent iron deficiency anemia.[5] Leukopenia, a common problem occurring during chemotherapy, or as a symptom of certain types of cancer, can produce symptoms of infections such as fever, chills, and tissue inflammation; severe mouth, throat, and esophageal pain; and mucous membrane ulcerations.[6]

Thrombocytopenia (decreased platelets) associated with easy bruising and spontaneous bleeding is a result of the pharmacologic treatment of common conditions seen in a physical therapy practice such as rheumatoid arthritis and cancer. More about this condition will be included later in this chapter under thrombocytopenia.

CLASSIFICATION OF BLOOD DISORDERS

Erythrocyte Disorders

Erythrocytes or RBCs consist mainly of hemoglobin and a supporting framework to transport oxygen and carbon dioxide. They comprise 40% of the volume of blood and the total number is determined by gender (women have fewer than men), altitude (less oxygen in the air requires more erythrocytes to carry sufficient amounts of oxygen to the tissues), and physical activity (sedentary people have fewer, athletes have more).

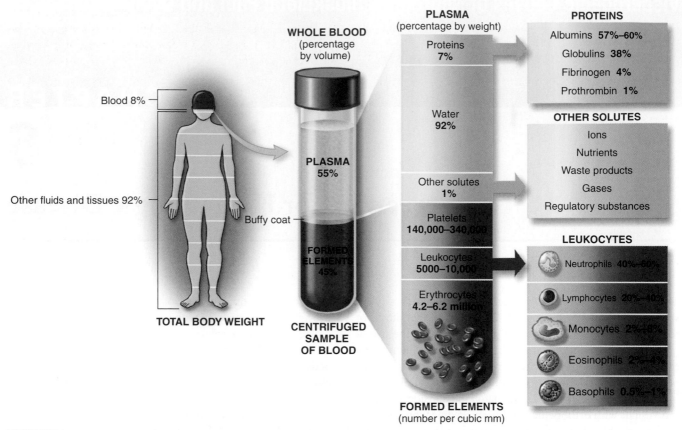

Fig. 6.1 Composition of whole blood and approximate values for each component. (With permission from Huether S, McCance K. Understanding Pathophysiology, 5th ed. Mosby: St. Louis; 2012: p. 479.)

Disorders of erythrocytes are classified as follows. Selected conditions from the list are discussed in this text.

- Anemia (too few erythrocytes)
- Polycythemia (too many erythrocytes)
- Poikilocytosis (abnormally shaped erythrocytes)
- Anisocytosis (abnormal variations in size of erythrocytes)
- Hypochromia (erythrocytes deficient in hemoglobin)

Anemia

Anemia is a reduction in the oxygen-carrying capacity of the blood as a result of an abnormality in the quantity or quality of erythrocytes. Anemia is not a disease but is a symptom of any number of different blood disorders. The most common causes of anemia include excessive blood loss, increased destruction of erythrocytes, and decreased production of erythrocytes.[7]

In the physical therapy practice, anemia-related disorders usually occur in one of four broad categories:

1. Iron deficiency associated with chronic GI blood loss secondary to NSAID use.
2. Chronic diseases (e.g., cancer, kidney disease, liver disease) or inflammatory diseases (e.g., rheumatoid arthritis or systemic lupus erythematosus).
3. Neurologic conditions (pernicious anemia).
4. Infectious diseases, such as tuberculosis or acquired immunodeficiency syndrome (AIDS), and neoplastic disease or cancer (bone marrow failure).

Anemia with neoplasia may be a common complication of chemotherapy, or develop as a consequence of bone marrow metastasis.[8] Anemia can also occur as a symptom of leukemia. Adults with pernicious anemia have significantly higher risks for hip fracture.[9]

Clinical Signs and Symptoms. Decreased capacity of the blood to carry oxygen may result in disturbances in the function of many organs and tissues, and these symptoms may differ from one person to another. Young and healthy individuals could tolerate slowly developing anemia and therefore may be asymptomatic until hemoglobin concentration and hematocrit fall below critical levels. However, rapid onset of anemia will result in an abrupt lack of oxygen transport to the lungs and muscles, and may cause dyspnea, palpitations, weakness and fatigue, and palpitations. Many people can have anemia that is moderate or severe without these symptoms. Although there is no difference in normal blood volume associated with severe anemia, there is a redistribution of blood so that organs most sensitive to oxygen deprivation such as the brain, heart, and muscles receive more blood than organs like the kidneys.

The physical therapist may notice changes in the hands and fingernail beds (Table 6.1 and Fig. 6.2[10]) during the observation portion of the examination (see Boxes 4.13 and 4.15). Observation of the hands should be done at the level of the client's heart to assure optimal circulation. The clinician should also make sure that the hands of the client with anemia are warm, because paleness occurs as a result of vasoconstriction when the hands are cold.

In individuals with darker skin, pallor may be observed by the absence of the underlying red tones that normally give

TABLE 6.1	Changes Associated With Hematologic Disorders
Changes	Causes
SKIN	
Light, lemon-yellow tint	Untreated pernicious anemia
White, waxy appearance	Severe anemia resulting from acute hemorrhage
Gray-green yellow	Chronic blood loss
Gray tint	Leukemia
Pale hands or palmar creases	Anemia
NAIL BED	
Brittle	Long-standing iron deficiency anemia
Concave (rather than convex)	Long-standing iron deficiency anemia
Oral Mucosa/Conjunctiva	
Pale or yellow color	Anemia

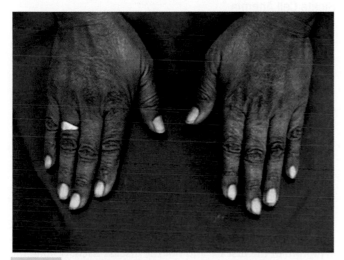

Fig. 6.2 The physical therapist may observe pallor of the hands and fingernail beds in a person with anemia. In individuals with darker skin, pallor may be observed by the absence of the underlying red tones that normally give brown or black skin its luster. (With permission from Rai A, Vaishali V, Naikmasur V, Kumar A, Sattur A. Aplastic anemia presenting as bleeding of gingiva: case report and dental considerations. Saudi J Dent Res 2016; 7(1):69-72.)

brown or black skin its luster. In individuals with brown skin, pallor will be demonstrated with a more yellowish-brown color, whereas in a person with black skin, it will appear ashen or gray.

In individuals with anemia, systolic blood pressure may not be affected, but diastolic pressure may be lower than normal, with an associated increase in the resting pulse rate. Also in individuals with this diagnosis, resting cardiac output is usually normal but increases with exercise more than that of people without anemia. As the anemia becomes more severe, resting cardiac output increases and exercise tolerance progressively decreases until dyspnea, tachycardia, and palpitations occur at rest.

Individuals with anemia demonstrate diminished exercise tolerance. Therefore physical therapists must be cautious during exercise testing and when prescribing, dosing, and progressing exercises in clients with anemia, considering

tolerance and/or perceived exertion levels.[11–13] Consultation, monitoring, and collaboration with the medical team are essential when making clinical decisions regarding exercise interventions in clients with anemia. (Case Example 6.1).

CLINICAL SIGNS AND SYMPTOMS

Anemia

- Skin pallor (palms, nail beds) or yellow-tinged skin (mucosa, conjunctiva)
- Fatigue and listlessness
- Dyspnea on exertion accompanied by heart palpitations and rapid pulse (more severe anemia)
- Chest pain with minimal exertion
- Decreased diastolic blood pressure
- Nervous system manifestations (pernicious anemia):
  - Headache
  - Drowsiness
  - Dizziness, syncope
  - Slow thought processes
  - Apathy, depression
  - Polyneuropathy

CASE EXAMPLE 6.1

Anemia

A 72-year-old woman, status post-open reduction internal fixation (ORIF) due to a hip fracture, was referred to physical therapy before hospital discharge. The physician's preoperative examination and surgical report were unremarkable for physical therapy precautions or contraindications.

She was wearing thigh length support hose, hospital gown, and open-heeled slippers from home. Although the nursing report indicated she was oriented to time and place, the patient seemed confused and required multiple verbal cues to follow the physical therapist's directions.

After ambulating a distance of approximately 50 feet using her wheeled walker and standby assistance from the therapist, the client reported that she could not "catch her breath" and asked to sit down. She placed her hand over her heart and commented that her heart was "fluttering." Blood pressure and pulse measurements were taken and recorded as 145/72 mm Hg (blood pressure) and 90 bpm (pulse rate).

The physical therapist consulted with the interprofessional team regarding this episode and it was decided that it was deemed safe to complete the therapy session. The physical therapist documented the episode in the medical record and left a note for the physician, briefly describing the incident and ending with the question: Are there any medical contraindications to continuing physical therapy?

Result: A significant fall in hemoglobin (Hb) often occurs after hip fracture and surgical intervention secondary to the blood loss caused by the fracture and surgery.

In this case, although the physician did not offer a direct reply to the physical therapist, the physician's notes indicated a suspected diagnosis of anemia. Follow-up blood work was ordered, and the medical diagnosis of anemia was confirmed. The interprofessional team working with the patient monitored signs and symptoms to ensure safe interventions to improve activity tolerance to prepare the patient for discharge.

Polycythemia

Polycythemia (also known as erythrocytosis) is characterized by increases in both the number of RBCs and the concentration of hemoglobin. People with polycythemia have increased whole blood viscosity and increased blood volume.

The increased erythrocyte production results in this thickening of the blood and an increased tendency toward clotting. The viscosity of the blood limits its ability to flow easily, diminishing the supply of blood to the brain and to other vital tissues. Increased platelets in combination with the increased blood viscosity may contribute to the formation of intravascular thrombi.

There are two distinct forms of polycythemia: primary polycythemia (also known as *polycythemia vera*) and secondary polycythemia. *Primary polycythemia* is a relatively uncommon neoplastic disease of the bone marrow of unknown etiology.[14] *Secondary polycythemia* is a physiologic condition resulting from a decreased oxygen supply to the tissues. It is commonly associated with smoking, high altitudes, sleep apnea, chronic arterial hypoxemia, and chronic heart and lung conditions.[8,15,16]

Clinical Signs and Symptoms. The symptoms of this disease are often insidious in onset with vague complaints. The most common first symptoms are shortness of breath and fatigue. The affected individual may be diagnosed only secondary to a sudden complication (e.g., stroke or thrombosis). Increased skin coloration and elevated blood pressure may develop as a result of the increased concentration of erythrocytes and increased blood viscosity.

CLINICAL SIGNS AND SYMPTOMS

Polycythemia

Clinical signs and symptoms of polycythemia (whether primary or secondary) are directly related to the increase in blood viscosity described earlier and may include:

- General malaise and fatigue
- Shortness of breath
- Intolerable pruritus (skin itching; aquagenic pruritus in polycythemia vera)[17]
- Headache
- Dizziness
- Irritability
- Blurred vision
- Fainting
- Decreased mental acuity
- Feeling of fullness in the head
- Disturbances of sensation in the hands and feet
- Weight loss
- Easy bruising
- Cyanosis (blue hue to the skin)
- Clubbing of the fingers
- Splenomegaly (enlargement of spleen)
- Gout
- Hypertension

Gout is sometimes a complication of primary polycythemia[18] and a typical acute attack may be the first symptom of polycythemia. Gout is a metabolic disease marked by increased serum urate levels (hyperuricemia), which cause painfully arthritic joints. Uric acid is an end product of purine metabolism, which is altered by excessive cellular proliferation and breakdown associated with increased RBCs, granulocytes, and platelets. Hyperuricemia is uncommon in secondary polycythemia because the associated cellular proliferation is not as extensive as in primary polycythemia.

Blockage of the capillaries supplying the digits of either the hands or feet may cause peripheral vascular neuropathy with decreased sensation, burning, numbness, or tingling. This small blood vessel occlusion can also contribute to the development of cyanosis and clubbing. If the underlying disorder is not recognized and treated, the person may develop gangrene and have subsequent loss of tissue. The therapist should watch for an increase in blood pressure and elevated hematocrit levels.

Sickle Cell Anemia

Sickle cell disease is a generic term for a group of inherited, autosomal recessive disorders characterized by the presence of an abnormal form of hemoglobin, the oxygen-carrying constituent of erythrocytes. A genetic mutation resulting in a single amino acid substitution in hemoglobin causes the hemoglobin to aggregate into long chains, altering the shape of the cell. This sickled or curved shape causes the cell to lose its ability to deform and squeeze through tiny blood vessels, thereby depriving tissue of an adequate blood supply.[8,19]

The two features of sickle cell disorders, chronic hemolytic anemia and vasoocclusion, occur as a result of obstruction of blood flow to the tissues and early destruction of the abnormal cells. Anemia associated with this condition is merely a symptom of the disease and not the disease itself, despite the term *sickle cell anemia*.

Clinical Signs and Symptoms. A series of "crises," or acute manifestations of symptoms, characterize sickle cell disease. The severity of symptoms varies widely between individuals, with some having only a few symptoms, whereas others are affected severely and have a short lifespan. Recurrent episodes of vasoocclusion and inflammation result in progressive damage to most organs, including the brain, kidneys, lungs, bones, and cardiovascular system. Cerebrovascular accidents (CVAs)[8,20,21] and cognitive impairment[22] are a frequent and severe manifestation.

Stress from viral or bacterial infection, hypoxia, dehydration, emotional disturbance, extreme temperatures, fever, strenuous physical exertion, or fatigue may precipitate a crisis. Pain caused by the blockage of sickled RBCs forming sickle cell clots is the most common symptom. The clots may be in any organ, bone, or joint of the body. Painful episodes of ischemic tissue damage may last 5 or 6 days and manifest in many different ways, depending on the location of the blood clot (Case Example 6.2). Severity of clinical symptoms, and consequently life expectancy, vary significantly in persons with sickle cell anemia.[23]

CASE EXAMPLE 6.2
Sickle Cell Anemia

Adapted with permission from Jennings B. Nursing role in management: hematological problems. In: Lewis S, Collier I, eds. Medical-Surgical Nursing: Assessment and Management of Clinical Problems. Mosby: St Louis; 1992:664–714.

A 20-year-old African-American woman came to physical therapy with severe right knee joint pain. She could recall no traumatic injury but reported hiking 2 days previously in the Rocky Mountains with her brother, whom she was visiting (she was from New York City).

A general screen for systemic illness revealed frequent urination over the past 2 days. She also complained of stomach pain, but she thought this was related to the stress of visiting her family. Past medical history included one other similar episode when she had acute pneumonia at the age of 11 years. She stated that she usually felt fatigued but thought it was because of her active social life and busy professional career. She is a nonsmoker and a social drinker (1 to 3 drinks per week).

On examination, the right knee was enlarged and inflamed, with joint range of motion (ROM) limited by the local swelling. In fact, pain, swelling, and guarded motion in the joint prevented a complete examination. Given that restraint, there were no other physical findings, but not all special tests were completed. The neurologic screen was negative.

This woman was treated for local joint inflammation, but the combination of change in altitude, fatigue, increased urination, and stomach pains alerted the therapist to the possibility of a systemic process despite the client's explanation for the fatigue and stomach upset. Because the client was from out of town and did not have a local physician, the therapist telephoned the hospital emergency department for a telephone consultation. It was suggested that a blood sample be obtained for preliminary screening and the client continue with physical therapy. Laboratory results included the following:

- Hematocrit (Hct) 30% (normal 35%–47%)
- Hemoglobin (Hb) 10 g/dL (normal 12–15 g/dL)
- White blood cells (WBC) 20,000/mm³ (normal 4500–11,000/mm³)

Based on these findings, the client was admitted to the hospital and diagnosed as having sickle cell anemia. It is likely that the change in altitude, the emotional stress of visiting family, and the physical exertion precipitated a "crisis" (now referred to as "episode"). She received continued physical therapy treatment during her hospital stay and was discharged with further follow-up planned in her home city.

Leukocyte Disorders

The blood contains three major groups of leukocytes, including:

1. Lymphoid cells (lymphocytes, plasma cells)
2. Monocytes
3. Granulocytes (neutrophils, eosinophils, basophils)

Lymphocytes produce antibodies and react with antigens, thus initiating an immune response to fight infection. *Monocytes* are the largest circulating blood cells and represent an immature cell until they leave the blood and travel to the tissues where they form macrophages in response to foreign substances such as bacteria. *Granulocytes* contain lysing agents capable of digesting various foreign materials and defend the body against infectious agents by phagocytosing bacteria and other infectious substances.[24]

CLINICAL SIGNS AND SYMPTOMS
Sickle Cell Anemia

- Pain
  - Abdominal
  - Chest
  - Headaches
- Bone and joint episodes from the ischemic tissue, lasting for hours to days and subsiding gradually
  - Low-grade fever
  - Extremity pain
  - Back pain
  - Periosteal pain
  - Joint pain, especially in the shoulder and hip
- Vascular complications
  - Cerebrovascular accidents (affects children and young adults most often)
  - Chronic leg ulcers
  - Avascular necrosis of the femoral head
  - Bone infarcts
- Pulmonary episodes
  - Chest pain
  - Dyspnea
  - Tachypnea
- Neurologic manifestations
  - Seizures
  - Dizziness
  - Drowsiness
  - Stiff neck
  - Paresthesias
  - Cranial nerve palsies
  - Blindness
  - Nystagmus
  - Coma
- Hand-foot syndrome (dactylitis, painful swelling and tenderness of hands and feet)[25]
  - Fever
  - Pain
- Splenic sequestration episode (occurs before adolescence)
  - Liver and spleen enlargement/tenderness due to trapped erythrocytes
  - Subsequent spleen atrophy due to repeated blood vessel obstruction
- Renal complications
  - Enuresis (bed-wetting)
  - Nocturia (excessive urination at night)
  - Hematuria (blood in the urine)
  - Pyelonephritis
  - Renal papillary necrosis
  - End-stage renal failure (older adult population)

Disorders of leukocytes are recognized as the body's reaction to disease processes and noxious agents. The therapist will encounter many clients who demonstrate alterations in the blood leukocyte (WBC) concentration as a result of acute infections or chronic systemic conditions. The leukocyte count may also be elevated (leukocytosis) in women who are pregnant; in clients with bacterial infections, appendicitis, leukemia, uremia, or ulcers; in newborns with hemolytic disease; and normally at birth. The leukocyte count may drop below normal values (*leukopenia*) in clients with viral diseases (e.g., measles), infectious hepatitis, rheumatoid arthritis, cirrhosis of the liver, and lupus erythematosus, and also after treatment with radiation or chemotherapy.

Leukocytosis

Leukocytosis characterizes many infectious diseases and is recognized by a count of more than 10,000 leukocytes/mm[3].[26] It can be associated with an increase in circulating neutrophils (neutrophilia), which are recruited in large numbers early in the course of most bacterial infections.

Leukocytosis is a common finding and is helpful in aiding the body's response to any of the following:
- Bacterial infection
- Inflammation or tissue necrosis (e.g., infarction, myositis, vasculitis)
- Metabolic intoxication (e.g., uremia, eclampsia, acidosis, gout)
- Neoplasm (especially bronchogenic carcinoma, lymphoma melanoma)
- Acute hemorrhage
- Splenectomy
- Acute appendicitis
- Pneumonia
- Intoxication by chemicals
- Acute rheumatic fever

CLINICAL SIGNS AND SYMPTOMS

Leukocytosis

These clinical signs and symptoms are usually associated with symptoms of the conditions listed earlier and may include:
- Fever
- Symptoms of localized or systemic infection
- Symptoms of inflammation or trauma to tissue

Leukopenia

Leukopenia, or reduction of the number of leukocytes in the blood below 5000/mL, can be caused by a variety of factors. Unlike leukocytosis, leukopenia is never beneficial.

Leukopenia can occur in many forms of bone marrow failure such as that following antineoplastic chemotherapy or radiation therapy, in overwhelming infections, in dietary deficiencies, some medications, or in autoimmune diseases.[27,28]

It is important for the physical therapist to be aware of the client's most recent WBC count before and during the course of physical therapy. Infection is a major problem if the client is immunosuppressed. Constitutional symptoms such as fever, chills, or sweats warrant immediate medical referral.

The lowest point the WBC count reaches, is termed *nadir*, and usually occurs 7 to 14 days after chemotherapy or radiation

therapy. During this time, the client is extremely susceptible to opportunistic infections and severe complications. When treating these individuals, the importance of good handwashing and hygiene practices cannot be overemphasized.[29]

CLINICAL SIGNS AND SYMPTOMS

Leukopenia

- Sore throat, cough
- High fever, chills, sweating
- Ulcerations of mucous membranes (mouth, rectum, vagina)
- Frequent or painful urination
- Persistent infections

Leukemia

Leukemia is a disease arising from the bone marrow and involves the uncontrolled growth of immature or dysfunctional WBCs. A complete discussion of this cancer is found in Chapter 14.

Platelet Disorders

Platelets (thrombocytes) function primarily in hemostasis (to stop bleeding) and in the maintenance of capillary integrity (see normal values listed inside book cover). They function in the coagulation (blood clotting) mechanism by forming hemostatic plugs in small ruptured blood vessels or by adhering to any injured lining of larger blood vessels.

A number of substances derived from the platelets that function in blood coagulation have been labeled "platelet factors." Platelets survive approximately 8 to 10 days in circulation and are then removed by the reticuloendothelial cells. *Thrombocytosis* refers to a condition in which the number of platelets is abnormally high, whereas *thrombocytopenia* refers to a condition in which the number of platelets is abnormally low.

Platelets are affected most often by anticoagulant drugs, including aspirin, heparin, warfarin (Coumadin), and other newer antithrombotic drugs such as apixaban (Eliquis), dabigatran (Pradaxa) or rivaroxaban (Xarelto).[30] Platelet levels can also be affected by several other factors. Foods containing lecithin prevent coagulation, whereas those with vitamin K promote it. Furthermore, exercise boosts the production of chemical activators that destroy unwanted clots. Diseases of the liver can affect the supply of vitamin K[31] and finally, platelets are also easily suppressed by radiation and chemotherapy.[32,33]

Thrombocytosis

Thrombocytosis refers to an increase in platelet count that is usually temporary. Primary thrombocytosis, also termed essential thrombocytopenia or ET, results in an increased number of platelets due to abnormal cells in the bone marrow. Secondary thrombocytosis or reactive thrombocytosis results as a compensatory mechanism from surgery, particularly splenectomy; in iron deficiency and polycythemia vera; and as a manifestation of an occult (hidden) neoplasm (e.g., lung cancer).[34]

It is associated with a tendency to clot because blood viscosity is increased by the very high platelet count, resulting in intravascular clumping (or thrombosis) of the sludged platelets. Peripheral blood vessels, particularly in the fingers and toes, are affected.

Thrombocytosis remains asymptomatic until the platelet count exceeds 1 million/mm³. Other symptoms may include splenomegaly and easy bruising.

CLINICAL SIGNS AND SYMPTOMS
Thrombocytosis

- Thrombosis
- Splenomegaly
- Easy bruising

Thrombocytopenia

Thrombocytopenia, a decrease in the number of platelets (less than 150,000/mm³)[26] in circulating blood, can result from decreased or defective platelet production or from accelerated platelet destruction.[35]

There are many causes of thrombocytopenia (Box 6.1). In a physical therapy practice the most common causes seen are from bone marrow failure from radiation treatment, leukemia, or metastatic cancer; cytotoxic agents used in chemotherapy; and drug-induced platelet reduction, especially among adults with rheumatoid arthritis treated with gold or in inflammatory conditions treated with aspirin or other NSAIDs.

Primary bleeding sites include bone marrow or spleen; secondary bleeding occurs from small blood vessels in the skin, mucosa (e.g., nose, uterus, GI tract, urinary tract, respiratory tract), and brain (intracranial hemorrhage).

Clinical Signs and Symptoms. Severe thrombocytopenia results in the appearance of multiple petechiae (small, purple, pinpoint hemorrhages into the skin) (Fig. 6.3),[36] most often observed on the lower legs. GI bleeding and bleeding into the central nervous system (CNS) associated with severe thrombocytopenia may be life-threatening.

The physical therapist must be alert for obvious skin, joint, or mucous membrane symptoms of thrombocytopenia:

BOX 6.1 CAUSES OF THROMBOCYTOPENIA

- Bone marrow failure
- Radiation
- Aplastic anemia
- Leukemia
- Metastatic carcinoma
- Cytotoxic agents (chemotherapy)
  - Medications
  - Nonsteroidal antiinflammatory drugs (NSAIDs), including aspirin
  - Methotrexate
  - Gold
  - Coumadin/warfarin

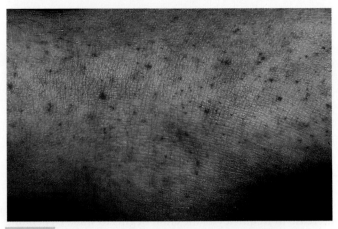

Fig. 6.3 Petechiae are small pinpoint hemorrhages into the skin which may be indicative of capillary bleeding due to thrombocytopenia. (With permission from Smith's Anesthesia for Infants and Children. New York: Elsevier; 2017:1220-1234.)

severe bruising, external hematomas, joint swelling, and the presence of multiple petechiae observed on the skin or gums. These symptoms usually indicate a platelet count well below 100,000/mm³. Strenuous exercise or any exercise that involves straining or bearing down could precipitate a hemorrhage, particularly of the eyes or brain. Blood pressure cuffs must be used with caution and any mechanical compression, visceral manipulation, or soft tissue mobilization is contraindicated without a physician's approval.

People with undiagnosed thrombocytopenia need immediate physician referral. It is important to have an interprofessional collaborative approach in the physical therapy management of patients with this condition, particularly regarding the possible need for transfusion and timing of transfusion prior to mobilization activities.[11]

CLINICAL SIGNS AND SYMPTOMS
Thrombocytopenia

- Bleeding after minor trauma
- Spontaneous bleeding
  - Petechiae (small red dots)
  - Ecchymoses (bruises)
  - Purpura spots (bleeding under the skin)
  - Epistaxis (nosebleed)
- Menorrhagia (excessive menstruation)
- Gingival bleeding
- Melena (black, tarry stools)

Coagulation Disorders

Hemophilia

Hemophilia is a hereditary blood-clotting disorder caused by an abnormality of functional plasma-clotting proteins known as factors VIII and IX.[8] In most cases the person with hemophilia has normal amounts of the deficient factor circulating, but it is in a functionally inadequate state.

Clinical Signs and Symptoms. Bleeding into the joint spaces (hemarthrosis) is one of the most common clinical manifestations of hemophilia. It may result from an identifiable trauma or stress, or may it be spontaneous and most often affects the knee, elbow, ankle, hip, and shoulder (in order of most common appearance).

Recurrent hemarthrosis results in hemophiliac arthropathy (joint disease) with progressive loss of motion, muscle atrophy, and flexion contractures. Bleeding episodes must be treated early with factor replacement and joint immobilization during the period of pain. This type of affected joint is particularly susceptible to being injured again, setting up a cycle of vulnerability to trauma and repeated hemorrhages.[37]

Hemarthroses are not common in the first year of life but increase in frequency as the child begins to walk. Depending on the degree of injury, the severity of the hemarthrosis may vary from mild pain and swelling, which resolves without treatment within 1 to 3 days, to severe pain with an excruciatingly painful, swollen joint that persists for several weeks and resolves slowly with treatment (Fig. 6.4).[38]

The muscle is a common site of bleeding in persons with hemophilia, accounting for 80%–90% of all episodes.[39] Muscle hemorrhages can be more insidious and massive than joint hemorrhages. They may occur anywhere but are common in the large muscles of the lower extremities— flexor muscle groups, predominantly the iliopsoas and gastrocnemius,[39] and flexor surface of the forearm[40]—and they result in deformities such as hip flexion contractures or equinus position of the foot.

When bleeding into the psoas or iliacus muscle puts pressure on the branch of the femoral nerve supplying the skin over the anterior thigh, loss of sensation occurs.[41] Distention of the muscles with blood causes pain that can be felt in the lower abdomen, possibly even mimicking appendicitis if the bleeding is on the right side. In an attempt to relieve the distention and reduce the pain, a position with hip flexion is preferred.

CLINICAL SIGNS AND SYMPTOMS
Acute Hemarthrosis

- Tingling, or prickling sensation
- Stiffening into the position of comfort
- Decreased range of motion
- Pain
- Swelling
- Tenderness
- Heat

CLINICAL SIGNS AND SYMPTOMS
Muscle Hemorrhage

- Gradually intensifying pain
- Protective spasm of the muscle
- Limitation of movement at the surrounding joints
- Muscle assumes the position of comfort (usually shortened)
- Loss of sensation

CLINICAL SIGNS AND SYMPTOMS
CNS Involvement

- Intraspinal hemorrhage (rare)
- Intracranial hemorrhage
  - Irritability, lethargy
  - Seizure
  - Feeding difficulty (children)
  - Unequal pupils
  - Apnea
  - Vomiting
  - Paralysis
  - Tense, bulging fontanelles
  - Death

CLINICAL SIGNS AND SYMPTOMS
GI Involvement

- Abdominal pain and distention
- Melena (blood in stool)
- Hematemesis (vomiting blood)
- Fever
- Low abdominal/groin pain due to bleeding into wall of large intestine or iliopsoas muscle
- Flexion contracture of the hip due to spasm of the iliopsoas muscle secondary to retroperitoneal hemorrhage

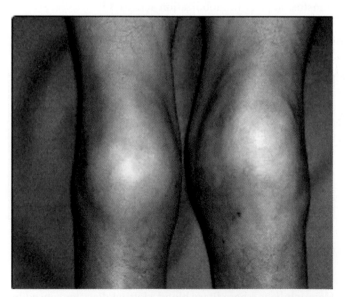

Fig. 6.4 Chronic knee swelling and damage in person with severe hemophilia. (With permission from: Howard MR et al: Haemophilia. In:Howard MR et al, eds:Haematology: An Illustrated Colour Text. 4th ed. Londan, England:Churchill Livingstone; 2013:72-1, Figure 36.1. Copyright Elsevier BV. All rights reserved.

Two tests are used to distinguish an iliopsoas bleed from a hip bleed[42]:

1. When the client flexes the trunk, severe pain is produced in the presence of *iliopsoas bleeding*, whereas only mild pain is found with a hip hemorrhage.
2. When the hip is gently rotated in either direction, severe pain is experienced with a *hip hemorrhage* but is absent or mild with iliopsoas bleeding.

Over time, the following complications may occur:

- Vascular compression causing localized ischemia and necrosis
- Replacement of muscle fibers by nonelastic fibrotic tissue causing shortened muscles and thus producing joint contractures
- Peripheral nerve lesions from compression of a nerve that travels in the same compartment as the hematoma, most commonly affecting the femoral, ulnar, and median nerves
- Pseudotumor formation with bone erosion

A summary of the physical therapy clinical implications for several hematologic-related conditions can be found in Fig. 6.5.

PHYSICIAN REFERRAL

Understanding the components of a client's past medical history that can affect hematopoiesis (production of blood cells) can provide the physical therapist with valuable insight into the client's present symptoms, which are usually already well known to the attending physician.

For example, the effects of certain drugs, exposure to radiation, or recent cytotoxic cancer chemotherapy can affect the bone marrow. The physical therapist is encouraged to contact the physician for discussion and clarification of the client's medical symptoms if several uncertainties are uncovered.

Significant findings include history of excessive menses, folate-poor diet, alcohol abuse, drug ingestion, family history of anemia, and family roots in geographic areas where RBC enzyme or hemoglobin abnormalities are. The presence of any one or more of these factors should alert the physical therapist to the need for medical referral when the client is not already under the care of a physician or when new signs or symptoms develop.

In addition, exercise for clients with anemia must be instituted with extreme caution and should first be approved by the client's physician. Clients with undiagnosed thrombocytopenia need immediate medical referral. The physical therapist must be alert for obvious skin or mucous membrane symptoms of *thrombocytopenia*. The presence of severe bruising, hematomas, and multiple petechiae usually indicates a platelet count well below normal. With clients who have been diagnosed with *hemophilia*, medical referral should be made when any painful episode develops in the muscle(s) or joint(s). Pain usually occurs before any other evidence of bleeding. Any unexplained symptom may be a signal of bleeding.

Guidelines for Immediate Medical Attention

- Signs and symptoms of thrombocytopenia (decreased platelets, e.g., excessive or spontaneous bleeding, petechiae, severe bruising) previously unseen or unreported to the physician

Guidelines for Physician Referral

- Consultation with the interprofessional team may be necessary when establishing or progressing an exercise program for a client with known anemia
- New episodes of muscle or joint pain in a client with hemophilia; pain usually occurs before any other evidence of bleeding. Any unexplained symptom(s) may be a signal of bleeding; coughing up blood in this population group must be reported to the physician.

Clues to Screening for Hematologic Disease

- Previous history (delayed effects) or current administration of chemotherapy or radiation therapy
- Chronic or long-term use of aspirin or other NSAIDs (drug-induced platelet reduction)
- Spontaneous bleeding of any kind (e.g., nosebleed, vaginal/menstrual bleeding, blood in the urine or stool, bleeding gums, easy bruising, hemarthrosis), especially with a previous history of hemophilia
- Recent major surgery or previous transplantation
- Rapid onset of dyspnea, chest pain, weakness, and fatigue with palpitations associated with recent significant change in altitude
- Observed changes in the hands and fingernail beds (see Table 6.1 and Fig. 4.30)

2. Complete Blood Count (CBC)

Complete Blood Count (CBC) Provides results regarding the concentration of red blood cells, white blood cells, and platelets in a blood sample.[1]		Causes	Presentation	Clinical Implications
White Blood Cells Routine test to identify the presence of infection, inflammation, allergens. REFERENCE VALUES[13] 5.0-10.0 10⁹/L	**Trending Upward** *(leukocytosis)*[13] > 11.0 10⁹/L	Infection Leukemia Neoplasm Trauma Surgery Sickle-cell disease Stress/pain Medication-induced Smoking Obesity Congenital Chronic inflammation Connective tissue disease	Fever Malaise Lethargy Dizziness Bleeding Bruising Weight loss (unintentional) Lymphadenopathy Painful inflamed joints	Symptoms-based approach when determining appropriateness for activity, especially in the presence of fever. Consider timing of therapy session due to early-morning low level and late-afternoon high peak.[14]
	Trending Downward *(leukopenia)*[13] < 4.0 10⁹/L	Viral infections Chemotherapy Aplastic anemia Autoimmune disease Hepatitis	Anemia Weakness Fatigue Fever Headache Shortness of breath	Symptoms-based approach when determining appropriateness for activity, especially in the presence of fever.[14]
	Trending Downward *(neutropenia)*[13] < 1.5 10⁹/L 0.5-1.0 10⁹/L = moderate neutropenia < 0.5 10⁹/L= severe neutropenia	Stem cell disorder Bacterial infection Viral infection Radiation	Low-grade fever Skin abscesses Sore mouth Symptoms of pneumonia	Neutropenic precautions (dependent on facility guidelines).[14] Symptoms-based approach when determining appropriateness for activity, especially in the presence of fever.[14]

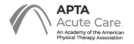

Complete Blood Count (CBC)		Causes	Presentation	Clinical Implications
Platelets REFERENCE VALUES 140-400 k/uL[13]	**Trending Upward** *(thrombocytosis)* > 450 k/uL	Splenectomy Inflammation Neoplasm/cancer Stress Iron deficiency Infection Hemorrhage Hemolysis High altitudes Strenuous exercise Trauma	Weakness Headache Dizziness Chest pain Tingling in hands/feet	Symptoms-based approach when determining appropriateness for activity; monitor symptoms; collaborate with interprofessional team.[13-15] Elevated levels can lead to venous thromboembolism.
	Trending Downward *(thrombocytopenia)* < 150 k/uL	Viral infection Nutrition deficiency Leukemia Radiation Chemotherapy Malignant cancer Liver disease Aplastic anemia Premenstrual and postpartum	Petechiae Ecchymosis Fatigue Jaundice Splenomegaly Risk for bleeding	In presence of severe thrombocytopenia (< 20 k/uL): Symptoms-based approach when determining appropriateness for activity; collaborate with interprofessional team (regarding possible need for/timing of transfusion prior to mobilization)[14] Fall risk awareness (risk of spontaneous hemorrhage).[16,17]
Hemoglobin Assess anemia, blood loss, bone marrow suppression REFERENCE VALUES **Male:** 14-17.4 g/dL[13] **Female:** 12-16 g/dL[13] *Note: Values are slightly decreased in elderly.*[13]	**Trending Upwards** *(polycythemia)*	Congenital heart disease Severe dehydration (or hemoconcentration) Chronic obstructive pulmonary disease (COPD) Congestive heart failure (CHF) Severe burns High altitude	Orthostasis Presyncope Dizziness Arrhythmias CHF onset/exacerbation Seizure Symptoms of transient ischemic attack (TIA) Symptoms of MI Angina	Low critical values (< 5-7 g/dL) can lead to heart failure or death.[13] High critical values (> 20 g/dL) can lead to clogging of capillaries as a result of hemoconcentration.[13] Symptoms-based approach when determining appropriateness for activity, monitor symptoms, collaborate with interprofessional team.[14]

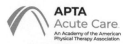

Fig. 6.5 Physical therapy clinical implications for several hematologic-related conditions. (Source: APTA Acute Care and Reprinted with permission, APTA Acute Care)

Complete Blood Count (CBC)		Causes	Presentation	Clinical Implications
Hemoglobin (cont.) Assess anemia, blood loss, bone marrow suppression **REFERENCE VALUES** **Male:** 14-17.4 g/dL[13] **Female:** 12-16 g/dL[13] *Note: Values are slightly decreased in elderly.*[13]	**Trending Downward** *(anemia)*	Hemorrhage Nutritional deficiency Neoplasia Lymphoma Systemic lupus erythematosus Sarcoidosis Renal disease Splenomegaly Sickle cell anemia Stress to bone marrow RBC destruction	Decreased endurance Decreased activity tolerance Pallor Tachycardia	Monitor vitals including SpO_2 to predict tissue perfusion. May present with tachycardia and/or orthostatic hypotension. Medical team might monitor patients with pre-existing cerebrovascular, cardiac, or renal conditions for ineffective tissue perfusion related to decreased hemoglobin.[18] If <8 g/dL: Symptoms-based approach when determining appropriateness for activity; collaborate with interprofessional team (regarding possible need for/timing of transfusion prior to mobilization).[13-15,19] Consultation with the interprofessional team as while as monitoring of signs and symptoms is imperative since hemoglobin levels and blood transfusions is individualized.[18] • hospitalized patients who are hemodynamically stable and asymptomatic may transfuse at 7 g/dL • post surgical cardiac or orthopedic patients and those with underlying cardiovascular disease may transfuse at 8 g/dL. • patients with hematological disorders, oncological disorders and severe thrombocytopenia ,or chronic transfusion-dependent anemia: no transfusion threshold recommendation is available.

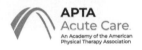

10

Complete Blood Count (CBC)		Causes	Presentation	Clinical Implications
Hematocrit Assess blood loss and fluid balance. **REFERENCE VALUES** **Male:** 42-52%[13] **Female:** 37-47%[13] *Note: Values are slightly decreased in the elderly.*[13]	**Trending Upward** *(polycythemia)*	Burns Eclampsia Severe dehydration Erythrocytosis Tend to be elevated with those living in higher altitude Hypoxia due to chronic pulmonary conditions (COPD, CHF)	Fever Headache Dizziness Weakness Fatigue Easy bruising or bleeding	Low critical value (<15-20%) cardiac failure or death.[13-15] High critical value (>60%) spontaneous blood clotting.[13-15] Symptoms-based approach when determining appropriateness for activity; monitor symptoms; collaborate with interprofessional team[13-15]
	Trending Downward *(anemia)*	Leukemia Bone marrow failure Multiple myeloma Dietary deficiency Pregnancy Hyperthyroidism Cirrhosis Rheumatoid arthritis Hemorrhage High altitude	Pale skin Headache Dizziness Cold hands/feet Chest pain Arrhythmia Shortness of breath	Patient might have impaired endurance; progress slowly with activity. Monitor vitals including SpO_2 to predict tissue perfusion. Might present with tachycardia and/or orthostatic hypotension. Medical team might monitor patients with pre-existing cerebrovascular, cardiac, or renal conditions for ineffective tissue perfusion related to decreased hematocrit.[18] If < 25%: Symptoms-based approach when determining appropriateness for activity; collaborate with interprofessional team (regarding possible need for/timing of transfusion prior to mobilization)[13-15,18]

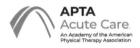

11

Fig. 6.5, cont'd

■ **Key Points to Remember**

1. Anemia may have no symptoms until hemoglobin concentration and hematocrit fall below one half of normal.
2. Weakness, fatigue, and dyspnea are early signs of anemia.
3. Exercise for individuals with anemia must be instituted gradually per tolerance and/or perceived exertion levels with physician approval.
4. Platelet level below 10,000 (thrombocytopenia) can be life-threatening. Platelet transfusions are usually given for platelet counts below this level in adults and children who have chemotherapy-induced thrombocytopenia. Multiple bruises and petechiae may be the only sign.
5. For clients with known thrombocytopenia, exercise programs must avoid the Valsalva (or bearing down) movement, and caution must be used to avoid further injury by bumping against objects.

6. During the observation portion of the examination, screen both hands for skin or nail bed changes that may be indicative of hematologic involvement.
7. For the client with hemophilia, bleeding episodes must be treated early with factor replacement and joint immobilization during the period of pain. Never apply heat to a bleeding or suspected bleeding area.
8. Pain may be the only symptom of a joint or muscle bleed for the client with hemophilia. Any painful or unexplained symptom in this population must be screened medically. Coughing up blood is not a normal finding with hemophilia and should be reported to the physician immediately.
9. The National Hemophilia Foundation (NHF) publishes additional materials for physical therapists. These can be ordered by calling the NHF at (website: https://www.hemophilia.org).

CLIENT HISTORY AND INTERVIEW

Special Questions to Ask

Past Medical History

- Have you recently been told you are anemic?
- Have you recently had any serious blood loss (possibly requiring transfusion)? (**Anemia;** also consider **jaundice/hepatitis post transfusion**)
- Have you ever been told that you have a congenital heart defect (also chronic lung/heart disorders)? (**Polycythemia; also possible with history of heavy tobacco use**)
- Do you have a history of bruising easily, nosebleeds, or excessive blood loss?* (**Polycythemia, hemophilia, thrombocytopenia**)

For example, do you bleed or bruise easily after minor trauma, surgery, or dental procedures?

Has any previous bleeding been severe enough to require a blood transfusion?

- Have you been exposed to occupational or industrial gases, such as chlorine or mustard gas?

Associated Signs and Symptoms

- Do you experience shortness of breath, heart palpitations, or chest pain with slight exertion (e.g., climbing stairs) or even just at rest? (Anemia)
- Alternate or additional questions: Do you ever have trouble catching your breath?
- Are there any activities you have had to stop doing because you do not have enough energy or breath?

(Therapist: Be aware of the clients who stop doing certain activities because they become short of breath.

For example, they no longer go up and down stairs in their homes and choose to avoid this activity...or the client who cannot complete all of his or her shopping at one time. They may not report being short of breath because they have decreased their activity level to accommodate for the change in their pulmonary capacity.)

For persons at elevations above 3500 feet: Have you recently moved from one geographic location to another? (Polycythemia)

Do you ever have episodes of dizziness, blurred vision, headaches, fainting, or a feeling of fullness in your head? (Polycythemia)

Do you have recurrent infections and low-grade fevers, such as colds, influenza-like symptoms, or other upper respiratory infections? (Abnormal leukocytes)

- Do you have black, tarry stools (bleeding into the GI tract) or blood in your urine? (Genitourinary tract)

For women (anemia, thrombocytopenia): Do you frequently have prolonged or excessive bleeding in association with your menstrual flow? (Excessive may be considered to be measured by the use of more than four tampons each day; prolonged menstruation usually refers to more than 5 days—both of these measures are subjective and must be considered along with other factors, such as the presence of other symptoms, personal menstrual history, placement in the life cycle [i.e., in relation to menopause].)

---

*Symptoms beginning in infancy or childhood suggest a congenital hemostatic defect, whereas symptoms beginning later in life indicate an acquired disorder, such as secondary to drug-induced defect of platelet function, a common cause of easy bruising and excessive bleeding. This bruising or bleeding occurs usually in association with trauma, menstruation, dental work, or surgical procedures. Drug-induced bruising or bleeding may also occur with use of aspirin and aspirin-containing compounds; NSAIDs such as ibuprofen and naproxen and penicillins because these drugs inhibit platelet function to some extent.

CASE STUDY

REFERRAL

You are working in a hospital setting and you have received a physician's referral to ambulate and exercise a patient who was involved in a serious automobile accident 10 days ago. The patient had internal injuries that required immediate abdominal surgery and 600 mL of blood transfused within 24 hours postoperatively. His condition is considered to be medically "stable."

CHART REVIEW

What specific medical information should you look for in the medical record before beginning your evaluation?

Name, age, and occupation:

Past medical history:

Previous myocardial infarcts, history of heart disease, diabetes (type)

Surgical report:

Type of surgery, locations of scar, any current contraindications

Were there any other injuries?

If yes, what were these and what is the current status of each?

Body weight:

Pulmonary status:

Is the patient a cigarette or pipe smoker (or other tobacco user)?

Is the patient currently receiving oxygen or respiratory therapy? Is there a recommendation for how many liters (L) of oxygen per minute can be used during exercise?

What was the patient's pulmonary status after the accident and postoperatively?

Laboratory report:

Hematocrit/hemoglobin levels. Anemia?

Current status:

Nursing reports of the patient's complaints of any kind (e.g., symptoms of dyspnea or heart palpitations from rapid loss of blood).

Has the patient been out of bed at all yet?

If yes, when? How far did he or she walk? How much assistance was required? Did he or she have symptoms of orthostatic hypotension?

Does the patient have any GI symptoms?

Is the patient oriented to time, place, and person?

Are there any dietary or fluid restrictions to be observed while the patient is in the physical therapy department? Is he or she on an intravenous line?

Vital signs:

Blood pressure

Presence of fever

Resting pulse rate

Pulse oximetry

Pain assessment

Current medications:

Be aware of the purpose for each medication and potential side effects.

Are there any known discharge plans at this time?

PRACTICE QUESTIONS

1. If rapid onset of anemia occurs after major surgery, which of the following symptom patterns might develop?
   a. Continuous oozing of blood from the surgical site
   b. Exertional dyspnea and fatigue with increased heart rate
   c. Decreased heart rate
   d. No obvious symptoms would be seen
2. Chronic GI blood loss sometimes associated with use of NSAIDs can result in which of the following problems?
   a. Increased incidence of joint inflammation
   b. Iron deficiency
   c. Decreased heart rate and bleeding
   d. Weight loss, fever, and loss of appetite
3. Preoperatively, clients cannot take aspirin or antiinflammatory medications because these:
   a. Decrease leukocytes
   b. Increase leukocytes
   c. Decrease platelets
   d. Increase platelets
   e. None of the above

4. Skin color and nail bed changes may be observed in the client with:
   a. Thrombocytopenia resulting from chemotherapy
   b. Pernicious anemia resulting from Vitamin B_{12} deficiency
   c. Leukocytosis resulting from AIDS
   d. All of the above
5. Bleeding under the skin, nosebleeds, bleeding gums, and black stools require medical evaluation as these may be indications of:
   a. Leukopenia
   b. Thrombocytopenia
   c. Polycythemia
   d. Sickle cell anemia
6. Under what circumstances would you consider asking a client about a recent change in altitude or elevation?
7. In the case of a client with hemarthrosis associated with hemophilia, what physical therapy intervention would be contraindicated?
8. Describe the two tests used to distinguish an iliopsoas bleed from a joint bleed.
9. What is the significance of *nadir*?
10. When exercising a client with known anemia, what two measures can be used as guidelines for frequency, intensity, and duration of the program?

REFERENCES

1. Bushnell BD. Perioperative medical comorbidities in the orthopaedic patient. *J Am Acad Orthop Surg.* 2008;16:216–227.
2. Raza S, Wei J, Abid S, et al. Are blood transfusions useful for non-specific symptoms of anemia in the elderly? *Open Med J.* 2014;1:36–49.
3. Blood disorders. American Society of Hematology. http://www.hematology.org/Patients/Blood-Disorders.aspx. Accessed May 15, 2016.
4. Hillman R. *Hematology in Clinical Practice.* 5th ed. New York: McGraw-Hill; 2011.
5. Sostres C, Gargallo CJ, Lanas A. Nonsteroidal anti-inflammatory drugs and upper and lower gastrointestinal mucosal damage. *Arthritis Res Ther.* 2013;15(Suppl 3):S3.
6. Abeloff M. *Abeloff's Clinical Oncology.* 4th ed. Philadelphia: Churchill Livingstone; 2008.
7. Symptoms and causes-anemia-Mayo Clinic. http://www.mayoclinic.org/diseases-conditions/anemia/symptoms-causes/dxc-20183157. Accessed May 15, 2015.
8. Peterson C. The hematologic system. In: Goodman C, Fuller K, eds. *Pathology: Implications for the Physical Therapists.* 5th ed. New York: Elsevier; 2020.
9. Merriman NA, Putt ME, Metz DC, Yang YX. Hip fracture risk in patients with a diagnosis of pernicious anemia. *Gastroenterology.* 2010;138(4):1330–1337.
10. Rai A, Vaishali V, Naikmasur VG, Kumar A, Sattur A. Aplastic anemia presenting as bleeding of gingiva: case report and dental considerations. *Saudi J Dental Res.* 2016;7(1):69–72.
11. APTA acute care, American Physical Therapy Association. Lab values interpretation resource. Updated 2019. Accessed July 5, 2021.
12. Goodman C, Helgeson K. *Exercise Prescription for Medical Conditions: Handbook for Physical Therapists.* Philadelphia: F. A. Davis; 2011:33.
13. Ebner N, Jankowska EA, Ponikowski P, Lainscak M, Elsner S, Sliziuk V, Steinbeck L, Kube J, Bekfani T, Scherbakov N, Valentova M, Sandek A, Doehner W, Springer J, Anker SD, von Haehling S. The impact of iron deficiency and anaemia on exercise capacity and outcomes in patients with chronic heart failure. Results from the studies investigating co-morbidities aggravating heart failure. *Int J Cardiol.* 2016;205:6–12.
14. Polycythemia vera. Mayo Clinic. http://www.mayoclinic.org/diseases-conditions/polycythemia-vera/basics/definition/con-20031013. Accessed May 20, 2016.
15. Secondary erythrocytosis. Merck Manual Professional Edition. http://www.merckmanuals.com/professional/hematology-and-oncology/myeloproliferative-disorders/secondary-erythrocytosis. Accessed May 21, 2016.
16. Huether S, McCance K. *Understanding Pathophysiology.* 5th ed. St. Louis: Mosby; 2012.
17. Lelonek E, Matusiak Ł, Wróbel T, Szepietowski JC. Aquagenic pruritus in polycythemia vera: clinical characteristics. *Acta Derm Venereol.* 2018;98(5):496–500.
18. US National Library of Medicine. Polycythemia vera. https://medlineplus.gov/genetics/condition/polycythemia-vera/#causes. Accessed June 28, 2021.
19. Bender MA. Sickle cell disease. In: Adam MP, Ardinger HH, Pagon RA, eds. *GeneReviews®.* Seattle, WA: University of Washington; 1993–2021.
20. Talahma M, Sundararajan S. Sickle cell disease and stroke. *Stroke.* 2014;45:e98–e100.
21. Yawn BP, Buchanan GR, Afenyi-Annan AN. Management of sickle cell disease summary of the 2014 evidence-based report by expert panel members. *JAMA.* 2014;312(10):1033–1048.
22. Vichinsky EP, Neumayr LD, Gold JI. Neuropsychological dysfunction and neuroimaging abnormalities in neurologically intact adults with sickle cell anemia. *JAMA.* 2010;303(18):1823–1831.
23. Kato G, Piel F, Reid C, et al. Sickle cell disease. *Nat Rev Dis Primers.* 2018;4:18010.
24. Raynes EA, Pounders V. The immune system. In: Goodman C, Fuller K, eds. *Pathology: Implications for the Physical Therapist.* 5th ed. New York: Elsevier; 2003.
25. Yap Y, Kwok L, Syn N, et al. Predictors of hand-foot syndrome and pyridoxine for prevention of capecitabine–induced hand-foot syndrome: a randomized clinical trial. *JAMA Oncol.* 2017;3(11):1538–1545.
26. Tomkins J, Norris T, Levanhagen K. Laboratory tests and values. In: Goodman C, Fuller K, eds. *Pathology: Implications for the Physical Therapist.* 5th ed. New York: Elsevier; 2003:1681.
27. Mayo Clinic. Low white blood cell count. https://www.mayoclinic.org/symptoms/low-white-blood-cell-count/basics/causes/sym-20050615. Accessed June 29, 2021.
28. Abuirmeileh A. Case report: unexplained chronic leukopenia treated with oral iron supplements. *Int J Clin Pharm.* 2014;36:264–267.
29. Wells C, Lowers S, Koermer B, Ambrosio F. Transplantation. In: Goodman C, Fuller K, eds. *Pathology: Implications for the Physical Therapist.* 5th ed. New York: Elsevier; 2020:1081.
30. Blood thinner basics. WebMD. https://www.webmd.com/dvt/dvt-treatment-tips-for-taking-heparin-and-warfarin-safely. Accessed June 29, 2021.
31. LiverTox: Clinical and Research Information on Drug-Induced Liver Injury. Bethesda, MD: National Institute of Diabetes and Digestive and Kidney Diseases; 2012. Vitamin K. https://www.ncbi.nlm.nih.gov/books/NBK548213/.
32. Stanford children's health. Bone marrow suppression during cancer treatment in children. https://www.stanfordchildrens.org/en/topic/default?id=bone-marrow-suppression-during-cancer-treatment-in-children-90-P02734. Accessed June 29, 2021.
33. Shao L, Wang Y, Chang J, et al. Hematopoietic stem cell senescence and cancer therapy-induced long-term bone marrow injury. *Transl. Cancer Res.* 2013;2(5):397–411.
34. Thrombocytosis. Cleveland Clinic. http://my.clevelandclinic.org/health/diseases_conditions/hic_Thrombocytosis. Accessed May 25, 2016.
35. Cleveland Clinic. Thrombocytopenia. https://my.clevelandclinic.org/health/diseases/14430-thrombocytopenia. Accessed June 29, 2021.
36. Zitelli BJ, Chalifoux TM, et al. *Smith's Anesthesia for Infants and Children.* New York: Elsevier; 2017:1220–1234.
37. Zaiden RA, Nagalla S. *Hemophilia A. Practice Essentials.* Manhattan: Medscape; 2016.
38. From Hemophilia A. Elsevier point of care (see details). Updated March 31, 2021. Copyright Elsevier BV. All rights reserved. https://www.clinicalkey.com/#!/content/clinical_overview/67-s2.0-28c89b23-5bbb-482c-b725-740ac54443cf?scrollTo=%2367-s2.0-28c89b23-5bbb-482c-b725-740ac54443cf-0873f20b-4f8f-46fa-92ff-a18b62d562d1-annotated.
39. Atilla B, Güney-Deniz H. Musculoskeletal treatment in haemophilia. *EFORT Open Rev.* 2019;4(6):230–239.
40. Srivastava A, Brewer AK, Mauser-Bunschoten EP, et al. Guidelines for the management of hemophilia. *Haemophilia.* 2012;19(1):1365–2516.
41. Kawarat V, Javid M, Swaminathan SP, Ross K. A rare case of iliopsoas hematoma in a patient with von Willebrand disease. *Int Surg J.* 2020;7(3):873–875.
42. Hoffman R. Hematology: Basic Principles and Practice. 5th ed. Churchill-Livingstone: Philadelphia; 2008.

Screening for Cardiovascular Disease

The cardiovascular system consists of the heart, capillaries, veins, and lymphatics and functions in coordination with the pulmonary system to circulate oxygenated blood through the arterial system to all cells. This system then collects deoxygenated blood from the venous system and delivers it to the lungs for reoxygenation (Fig. 7.1).

Heart disease remains the leading cause of death in industrialized nations. In the United States alone, 47% of all Americans have at least 1 of the 3 established key risk factors for cardiovascular disease (CVD), which are hypertension, high cholesterol, and smoking.[1] One in three Americans has some form of CVD. The American Heart Association (AHA) reports that about half of all deaths from heart disease are sudden and unexpected.[2]

Known risk factors include advancing age, hypertension, obesity, sedentary lifestyle, excessive alcohol consumption, oral contraceptive use (over age 35, combined with smoking), first-generation family history, tobacco use (including exposure to second-hand smoke), abnormal cholesterol levels, and race (e.g., African Americans, Mexican Americans, Native Americans, and Pacific Islanders are at greater risk).

Fortunately, during the last two decades, cardiovascular research has greatly increased our understanding of the structure and function of the cardiovascular system in health and disease. Despite the formidable statistics regarding the prevalence of CVD, during the last 15 years, a steady decline in mortality from cardiovascular disorders has been witnessed. Effective application of the increased knowledge regarding CVD and its

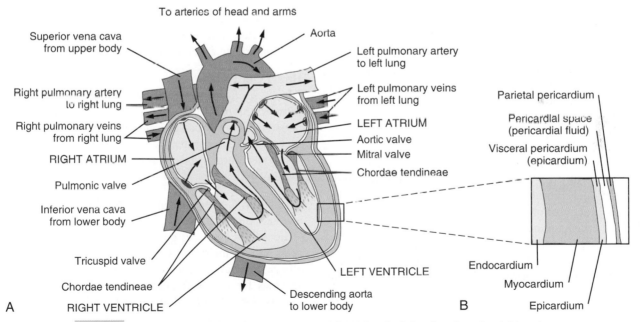

Fig. 7.1 Structure and circulation of the heart. Blood entering the left atrium from the right and left pulmonary veins flows into the left ventricle. The left ventricle pumps blood into the systemic circulation through the aorta. From the systemic circulation, blood returns to the heart through the superior and inferior venae cavae. From there the right ventricle pumps blood into the lungs through the right and left pulmonary arteries. A thick layer of connective tissue called the *septum* separates the left and right chambers of the heart. The top of the heart *(atria)* is also separated from the bottom of the heart *(ventricles)* by connective tissue, which does not conduct electrical activity and serves as an electrical barrier or insulator. (Redrawn from Black JM, Hawks JH: *Luckmann and Sorenson's medical-surgical nursing*, ed 8, Philadelphia, 2009, WB Saunders.)

risk factors will assist health care professionals to educate clients in achieving and maintaining cardiovascular health.

Information about heart disease is changing rapidly. Part of the therapist's intervention includes patient/client education. The therapist can access up-to-date information at many useful websites (Box 7.1). In 2018, a comprehensive study reported that a large proportion of CVD is attributable to dietary risks, high systolic blood pressure, high body mass index, high total cholesterol, high fasting plasma glucose levels, tobacco smoking, and low levels of physical activity.

BOX 7.1 INFORMATIONAL WEBSITES

American Heart Association (AHA)

http://www.americanheart.org

The AHA has also developed a validated tool to assess risk of heart attack, stroke, and diabetes. Available online at http://www.heart.org/HEARTORG/Conditions/More/ToolsForYourHeartHealth/Heart-Health-Risk-Assessments-from-the-American-Heart-Association_UCM_306929_Article.jsp#.WGwNm1MrLcc.

The AHA also has a website just for health care professionals. They offer comprehensive information on cardiovascular and cerebrovascular medicine. You can access clinical summaries of new papers and journal articles from well-known publications. Available online at http://www.my.americanheart.org/portal/professional

American Stroke Association

http://www.strokeassociation.org

The American Stroke Association is a division of the AHA with updated information for consumers on strokes, as well as a special link just for health care professionals.

National Cholesterol Education Program (NCEP)

http://www.nhlbi.nih.gov/about/ncep/

This website offers a risk assessment tool for estimating the 10-year risk of developing coronary vascular disease (heart attack and coronary death) based on recent data from the Framingham Heart Study. Available online at http://hin.nhlbi.nih.gov/atpiii/calculator.asp?usertype=prof

NIHSeniorHealth

http://nihseniorhealth.gov

This website, designed especially for older adults, is a joint effort of the National Institute of Aging (NIA) and the National Library of Medicine (NLM). It contains answers to questions about preventing, detecting, and treating a heart attack. The information is provided in a senior-friendly format. Short, easy-to-read segments of information are featured that can be accessed in large-print type, open-captioned videos, and even an audio version.

Centers for Disease Control and Prevention (CDC)

Division for Heart Disease and Stroke Prevention (DHDSP)
http://www.cdc.gov/dhdsp/

The mission of this group is to provide public health leadership to improve cardiovascular health for all, reduce the burden, and eliminate disparities associated with heart disease and stroke. Its resources include information on heart disease and stroke topics and prevention programs, and publications and statistical information.

American College of Cardiology

http://www.acc.org

The American College of Cardiology offers the latest professional information on heart disease, research, and treatment. A special feature is the availability of clinical statements and guidelines that can be printed or downloaded.

Elsevier Science

http://www.cardiosource.com

This site is offered by collaboration between the American College of Cardiology Foundation and Elsevier Science. It includes a drug database, case studies for self-study, and a library with access to journal abstracts and reference texts.

National Heart, Lung, and Blood Institute (NHLBI)

http://www.nhlbi.nih.gov/index.htm

The NHLBI at the National Institutes of Health (NIH) offers information for health care professionals and consumers. Research results, clinical guidelines, and information for women and heart disease are available.

Heart Center Online

http://www.heartcenteronline.com

Physicians provide patient education on cardiac conditions, medical devices, procedures, and tests. There is also a prevention center with a focus on lifestyle issues and nutrition, video library, and an entire section on transtelephonic monitoring.

American College of Sports Medicine (ACSM)

www.acsm.org

The ACSM provides guidelines for exercise testing and prescription, including screening tests; preexercise evaluations; general principles for exercise prescription; and specifics for mode, frequency, intensity, and duration of exercise for individual diseases and conditions.

Framingham Risk Score

To calculate your Framingham risk score for heart attack in the next 10 years, go to www.health.harvard.edu/heartrisk. A score of 5% to 20% suggests the need for the hs-CRP test (C-reactive protein). Using the results of the CRP test, the Reynolds model will provide a more accurate assessment of risk (www.reynoldsriskscore.org).

In terms of these risks, physical therapists should be at the forefront of changing behavior and providing appropriate exercise prescription for these patients. As movement specialists, we can impact society to improve the human experience![3]

SIGNS AND SYMPTOMS OF CARDIOVASCULAR DISEASE

Cardinal symptoms of cardiac disease usually include chest, neck and/or arm pain or discomfort, palpitations, dyspnea, syncope (fainting), fatigue, cough, diaphoresis, and cyanosis. Edema and leg pain (claudication) are the most common symptoms of the vascular component of a cardiovascular pathologic condition. Symptoms of cardiovascular involvement should also be reviewed by system (Table 7.1).

Chest Pain or Discomfort

Chest pain or discomfort is a common presenting symptom of CVD and must be evaluated carefully. Chest pain may be cardiac or noncardiac in origin and may radiate to the neck, jaw, upper trapezius muscle, upper back, shoulder, or arms (most commonly the left arm).

Radiating pain down the arm commonly follows the pattern of ulnar nerve distribution. Pain of cardiac origin can be experienced in the somatic areas because the heart is supplied by the C3 to T4 spinal segments, referring visceral pain to the corresponding somatic area (see Fig. 3.3). For example,

the heart and the diaphragm, supplied by the C5-C6 spinal segment, can refer pain to the shoulder (see Figs. 3.4 and 3.5).

Cardiac-related chest pain may arise secondary to angina, myocardial infarction (MI), pericarditis, endocarditis, mitral valve prolapse (MVP), or dissecting aortic aneurysm. Location and description (frequency, intensity, and duration) vary according to the underlying pathologic condition (see each condition).

Cardiac chest pain is often accompanied by associated signs and symptoms such as nausea, vomiting, diaphoresis, dyspnea, fatigue, pallor, or syncope. These associated signs and symptoms provide the therapist with red flags to identify musculoskeletal symptoms of a systemic origin.

Cardiac chest pain or discomfort can also occur when coronary circulation is normal, as in the case of clients with anemia, causing lack of oxygenation of the myocardium (heart muscle) during physical exertion.

Noncardiac chest pain can be caused by an extensive list of disorders requiring screening for medical disease. For example, cervical disk disease, rib dysfunction such as a slipped rib, and arthritic changes can mimic atypical chest pain. Chest pain that is attributed to anxiety, trigger points, cocaine use, and other noncardiac causes is discussed in Chapter 18.

Palpitations

Palpitations, the presence of an irregular heartbeat, may also be referred to as arrhythmia or dysrhythmia, which may be caused by a relatively benign condition (e.g., MVP, "athlete's heart," caffeine, anxiety, exercise) or a severe condition (e.g., coronary artery disease [CAD], cardiomyopathy, complete heart block, ventricular aneurysm, atrioventricular valve disease, mitral or aortic stenosis).

The sensation of palpitations has been described as a bump, pound, jump, flop, flutter, or racing sensation of the heart. Associated symptoms may include lightheadedness or syncope. A palpated pulse may feel rapid or irregular, as if the heart "skipped" a beat.

Occasionally, a client will report "fluttering" sensations in the neck. Generally, unless accompanied by other symptoms, these sensations in the neck are caused by anxiety, random muscle fasciculation, or minor muscle strain or overuse.

Palpitations can be considered physiologic (i.e., when less than six occur per minute, this may be considered within normal function of the heart). However, Palpitations lasting for hours or occurring in association with pain, shortness of breath, fainting, or severe light-headedness requires medical evaluation. Palpitations in any person with a history of unexplained sudden death in the family requires medical referral.

Clients describing "palpitations" or similar phenomena may not be experiencing symptoms of heart disease. Palpitations may occur as a result of an overactive thyroid, secondary to caffeine sensitivity, as a side effect of some medications, and with the use of drugs such as cocaine. Encourage the client to report any such symptoms to the physician if this information has not already been brought to the physician's attention.

TABLE 7.1	Cardiovascular Signs and Symptoms by System
System	Symptoms
General	Weakness
	Fatigue
	Weight change
	Poor exercise tolerance
	Peripheral edema
Integumentary	Pressure ulcers
	Loss of body hair
	Cyanosis (lips and nail beds)
Central nervous system	Headache
	Impaired vision
	Dizziness or syncope
Pulmonary	Labored breathing, dyspnea
	Productive cough
Genitourinary	Urinary frequency
	Nocturia
	Concentrated urine
	Decreased urinary output
Musculoskeletal	Chest, shoulder, back, neck, jaw, or arm pain
	Myalgia
	Muscular fatigue
	Muscle atrophy
	Edema
	Claudication
Gastrointestinal	Nausea and vomiting
	Ascites (abdominal distention)

Modified from Goodman CC, Fuller K: *Pathology: implications for the physical therapist*, ed 4, Philadelphia, 2015, WB Saunders.

Dyspnea

Dyspnea, also referred to as breathlessness or shortness of breath, can be cardiovascular in origin, but it may also occur secondary to a pulmonary pathologic condition (see also Chapter 8), fever, certain medications, allergies, poor physical conditioning, or obesity. Early onset of dyspnea may be described as having to breathe too much or as an uncomfortable feeling during breathing after exercise or exertion.

Shortness of breath with mild exertion (dyspnea on exertion), when caused by an impaired left ventricle that is unable to contract completely, results in the lung's inability to empty itself of blood. Pulmonary congestion and shortness of breath then occur. With severe compromise of the cardiovascular or pulmonary systems, dyspnea may occur at rest.

The severity of dyspnea is determined by the extent of disease. Thus the more severe the heart disease is, the easier it is to bring on dyspnea. Extreme dyspnea includes paroxysmal nocturnal dyspnea (PND) and orthopnea (breathlessness that is relieved by sitting upright with pillows used to prop up the trunk and head). Often the degree of severity of orthopnea is measured in how many pillows it takes to breathe comfortably.

PND and sudden, unexplained episodes of shortness of breath frequently accompany heart failure (HF). During the day the effects of gravity in the upright position and the shunting of excessive fluid to the lower extremities permit more effective ventilation and perfusion of the lungs, keeping them relatively fluid free, depending on the degree of HF. PND awakens the sleeping person in the recumbent position because the amount of blood returning to the heart and lungs from the lower extremities increases in this position.

Anyone who cannot climb a single flight of stairs without feeling moderately to severely winded or who awakens at night or experiences shortness of breath when lying down should be evaluated by a physician. Anyone with known cardiac involvement who develops progressively worse dyspnea must also notify the physician of these changes.

Dyspnea relieved by specific breathing patterns (e.g., pursed-lip breathing) or by a specific body position (e.g., leaning forward on the arms to lock the shoulder girdle) is more likely to be pulmonary than cardiac in origin. Because breathlessness can be a terrifying experience for many persons, any activity that provokes the sensation is avoided, thus quickly reducing functional activities.

Cardiac Syncope

Cardiac syncope (fainting) or more mild light-headedness can be caused by reduced oxygen delivery to the brain. Cardiac conditions resulting in syncope include arrhythmias, orthostatic hypotension, poor ventricular function, CAD, and vertebral artery insufficiency.

Light-headedness that results from orthostatic hypotension (sudden drop in blood pressure [BP]) may occur with any quick change in a prolonged position (e.g., going from a supine position to an upright posture or standing up from a sitting position) or physical exertion involving increased abdominal pressure (e.g., straining with a bowel movement, lifting). Any client with aortic stenosis is likely to experience light-headedness as a result of these activities.

Noncardiac conditions, such as anxiety and emotional stress, can cause hyperventilation and subsequent light-headedness (vasovagal syncope). Side effects, such as orthostatic hypotension, may also occur during the period of initiation and regulation of cardiac medications (e.g., vasodilators).

Syncope that occurs without any warning period of light-headedness, dizziness, or nausea may be a sign of heart valve or arrhythmia problems. Because sudden death can thus occur, medical referral is recommended for any unexplained syncope, especially in the presence of heart or circulatory problems or if the client has any risk factors for heart attack or stroke.

Examination of the cervical spine may provoke dizziness. If signs of nystagmus, changes in pupil size, or visual disturbances and symptoms of dizziness or light-headedness occur, the therapist has to determine the cause of the symptoms through a thorough examination (see Chapter 5).

Fatigue

Fatigue provoked by minimal exertion indicates a lack of energy, which may be cardiac in origin (e.g., CAD, aortic valve dysfunction, cardiomyopathy, or myocarditis) or may occur secondary to a neurologic, muscular, metabolic, or pulmonary pathologic condition. Often, fatigue of a cardiac nature is accompanied by associated symptoms such as dyspnea, chest pain, palpitations, or headache.

Fatigue that goes beyond expectations during or after exercise, especially in a client with a known cardiac condition, must be closely monitored. It should be remembered that beta-blockers prescribed for cardiac conditions can also cause unusual fatigue symptoms as a side effect.

For the client experiencing fatigue without a prior diagnosis of heart disease, monitoring vital signs may indicate a failure of the BP to rise with increasing workloads. Such a situation may indicate cardiac output that is inadequate in meeting the demands of exercise. However, poor exercise tolerance is often the result of deconditioning, especially in the older adult population. Further testing (e.g., exercise treadmill test) may help determine whether fatigue is cardiac-induced.

Cough

Cough (see also Chapter 8) is usually associated with pulmonary conditions, but it may occur as a pulmonary complication of a cardiovascular pathologic complex. Left ventricular dysfunction, including mitral valve dysfunction resulting from pulmonary edema or left ventricular CHF, may result in cough when aggravated by exercise, metabolic stress, supine position, or PND. The cough is often hacking and may produce large amounts of frothy, blood-tinged sputum. In the case of HF, a cough develops because a large amount of fluid is trapped in the pulmonary tree, irritating the lung mucosa.

Cyanosis

Cyanosis is a bluish discoloration of the lips and nail beds of the fingers and toes that accompanies inadequate blood oxygen levels (reduced amounts of hemoglobin). Although cyanosis can accompany hematologic or central nervous system disorders, most often, visible cyanosis accompanies cardiac and pulmonary problems.

Edema

Edema in the form of a 3-pound or greater weight gain or a gradual, continuous gain over several days that results in swelling of the ankles, abdomen, and hands combined with shortness of breath, fatigue, and dizziness may be red-flag symptoms of HF.

Other accompanying symptoms may include jugular vein distention (JVD; see Fig. 4.44) and cyanosis (of lips and appendages). Right upper quadrant pain described as a constant aching or sharp pain may occur secondary to an enlarged liver in this condition.

Right-sided HF and subsequent edema can also occur secondary to cardiac surgery, venous valve incompetence or obstruction, cardiac valve stenosis, CAD, or mitral valve dysfunction.

Noncardiac causes of edema may include pulmonary hypertension, kidney dysfunction, cirrhosis, burns, infection, lymphatic obstruction, use of nonsteroidal antiinflammatory drugs (NSAIDs), or allergic reaction.

When edema and other accompanying symptoms persist despite rest, medical referral is required. Edema of a cardiac origin may require electrocardiogram (ECG) monitoring during exercise or activity (the physician may not want the client stressed when extensive ECG changes are present), whereas edema of peripheral origin requires treatment of the underlying etiologic complex.

Claudication

Claudication or leg pain occurs with peripheral vascular disease (PVD; arterial or venous), often simultaneously with CAD. Claudication can be more functionally debilitating than other associated symptoms, such as angina or dyspnea, and may occur in addition to these other symptoms. The presence of pitting edema along with leg pain is usually associated with vascular disease.

Other noncardiac causes of leg pain (e.g., sciatica, pseudoclaudication, anterior compartment syndrome, gout, peripheral neuropathy) must be differentiated from pain associated with PVD. Low back pain associated with pseudoclaudication often indicates spinal stenosis. The discomfort associated with pseudoclaudication is frequently bilateral and improves with rest or flexion of the lumbar spine (see also Chapter 15).

Vascular claudication may occur in the absence of physical findings but is usually accompanied by skin discoloration and trophic changes (e.g., thin, dry, hairless skin) in the presence of vascular disease. Core temperature, peripheral pulses, and skin temperature should be assessed especially in the lower extremities. Cool skin may indicate vascular obstruction; warm to hot skin may indicate inflammation or infection. Abrupt onset of ischemic rest pain or sudden worsening of intermittent claudication may be a result of thromboembolism and must be reported to the physician immediately.

If people with intermittent claudication have normal-appearing skin at rest, exercising the extremity to the point of claudication usually produces marked pallor in the skin over the distal third of the extremity. This postexercise cutaneous ischemia occurs in both upper and lower extremities and is caused by selective shunting of the available blood to the exercised muscle and away from the more distal parts of the extremity.

Vital Signs

Vital signs are vital in our patients! The therapist may see signs of cardiac dysfunction as abnormal responses of heart rate and BP during exercise. The therapist must remain alert to a heart rate that is either too high or too low during exercise, an irregular pulse rate, a systolic BP that does not rise progressively as the work level increases, a systolic BP that falls during exercise, or a change in diastolic pressure greater than 15 to 20 mm Hg.

It should be a standard procedure to take vital signs in our patients because conditions such as hypertension are asymptomatic and without apparent signs. At a minimum, the physical therapist should monitor vital signs in anyone with known heart disease. Some BP-lowering medications can keep a client's heart rate from exceeding 90 bpm. For these individuals the therapist can monitor heart rate, but instead should use perceived rate of exertion (PRE) as a gauge of exercise intensity. See Chapter 4 for more specific information about vital sign assessment.

CARDIAC PATHOPHYSIOLOGY

Three components of cardiac disease are discussed, including diseases affecting the heart muscle, diseases affecting heart valves, and defects of the cardiac nervous system, in Table 7.2.

Conditions Affecting the Heart Muscle

In most cases, a cardiopulmonary pathologic condition can be traced to at least one of three processes:
1. Obstruction or restriction.
2. Inflammation.
3. Dilation or distention.

Any combination of these can cause chest, neck, back, and/or shoulder pain. Frequently, these conditions occur

TABLE 7.2	**Cardiac Diseases**	
Heart Muscle	Heart Valves	Cardiac Nervous System
Coronary artery disease	Rheumatic fever	Arrhythmias
Myocardial infarct	Endocarditis	Tachycardia
Pericarditis	Mitral valve prolapse	Bradycardia
Congestive heart failure	Congenital deformities	
Aneurysms		

sequentially. For example, an underlying *obstruction*, such as pulmonary embolus, leads to *congestion*, and subsequent *dilation* of the vessels blocked by the embolus.

The most common cardiovascular conditions to mimic musculoskeletal dysfunction are angina, MI, pericarditis, and dissecting aortic aneurysm. Other CVDs are not included in this text because they are rare or because they do not mimic musculoskeletal symptoms.

Degenerative heart disease refers to the changes in the heart muscle and blood supply to the heart and the major blood vessels that occur with aging. As the population ages, degenerative heart disease becomes the most prevalent form of cardiovascular disease. Degenerative heart disease is also referred to as atherosclerotic cardiovascular disease, arteriosclerotic cardiovascular disease, coronary heart disease (CHD), and CAD.

Hyperlipidemia

Hyperlipidemia refers to a group of metabolic abnormalities resulting in combinations of elevated serum total cholesterol (hypercholesterolemia), elevated low-density lipoproteins (LDL), elevated triglycerides (hypertriglyceridemia), and decreased high-density lipoproteins (HDL). These abnormalities are the primary risk factors for atherosclerosis and CAD.[4-6]

Statin medications (e.g., Zocor, Lipitor, Crestor, Lescol, Mevacor, Pravachol) are used to reduce LDL cholesterol. Statins are generally well tolerated, but there is a wide body of medical literature that associates the adverse reaction of myalgia and the more serious reaction of rhabdomyolysis with statin medications (see Chapter 10).[6,7] If detected early, statin-related symptoms can be reversible with reduction of dose, selection of another statin, or cessation of statin use.[8-11]

Screening for Side Effects of Statins

Statin-associated muscle symptoms (SAMS) are the most common myotoxic events associated with statins occurring in

---

CASE EXAMPLE 7.1

Importance of Monitoring Vital Signs During Exercise Intervention

Chief Complaint: An 84-year-old woman was referred to outpatient physical therapy due to self-reported decline in balance and multiple falls in the past several weeks. The client would like to improve her balance and walking so she could continue living at home.

Social History: Retired, lives alone in a two-story house.

Past Medical History: Hypertension, arthritis in both hands, visual impairment (right eye), allergies to Novocain and antibiotics, transient ischemic attacks (TIAs), recurrent pneumonia.

Current Medications: Lisinopril, aspirin (nonsteroidal anti-inflammatory), Os-Cal (antacid, calcium supplement)

Clinical Presentation: Client is independent with activities of daily living but slow to complete tasks. She reports that she goes up and down one flight of steep stairs three to four times a day, using a handrail. She also states that she can walk around the house by occasionally holding onto walls and furniture. Baseline testing:

1. Timed-up-and-go test: 17 seconds abnormal, fall risk
2. Functional reach test: 8 inches abnormal, fall risk

Presence of other symptoms includes numbness along both feet that does not change with position. Shortness of breath with activity (short distance walking, ascending and descending six steps); recovers after a short rest. Thoracic kyphosis. Mild strength losses in hips, knees, and ankles. Reports of being "dizzy" and "light-headed," feeling like she is going to "fall out."

Vital signs:

Blood pressure (before activity):	136/79 mm Hg (arm and position not recorded)
Blood pressure (after 10 minutes of activity):	132/69
Pulse (before activity):	82 bpm
Pulse (after activity):	73 bpm

Assessment: This 84-year-old client with risk of falls presented with fairly good bilateral lower extremity strength but had deficits in sensation and vision, increasing her risk for falling. She was quite resistant to using a cane for increased safety. She agreed with the recommendation to continue physical therapy to improve balance and mobility and decrease fall risk.

However during a therapeutic exercise intervention, client experienced an abnormal response to exercise in which the pulse rate and BP decreased. She required several rest breaks during the exercise session because of "fading."

The therapist referred the client to her cardiologist for evaluation to determine medical stability before further intervention.

Result: Nuclear stress testing revealed blockage of two major coronary arteries requiring cardiac catheterization with balloon angioplasty and placement of a stent. The cardiologist confirmed the therapist's suspicion that the client's balance deficits from neuropathy and decreased vision were made worse by shortness of breath and light-headedness from cardiac impairment.

Monitoring vital signs before and during exercise was a simple way to screen for underlying cardiovascular impairment.

Adapted from Goff T: Case report presented in partial fulfillment of DPT 910. *Principles of differential diagnosis*, Institute for Physical Therapy Education, Chester, Pennsylvania, 2005, Widener University. Used with permission.

10% to 25% of patients.[12,13] The incidence of myotoxic events appears to be dose-dependent.

Monitoring for elevated serum liver enzymes and creatine kinase (CK) are significant laboratory indicators of muscle and liver impairment.[12] Symptoms of mild myalgia (muscle ache or weakness without increased CK levels), myositis (muscle symptoms with increased CK levels), or frank rhabdomyolysis (muscle symptoms with marked CK elevation; more than 10 times the normal upper limit) range from 1% to 7%.[6,12]

Muscle soreness after exercise that is caused by statin use may go undetected even by the therapist. Awareness of potential risk factors and monitoring of anyone taking statins and any of these additional risk factors is advised. Muscular symptoms are more common in older individuals (Case Example 7.2).[6,14] Other risk factors include:[15]

- Age over 80 years (women more than men)
- Small body frame or frail
- Kidney or liver disease
- Drinks excessive grapefruit juice daily (more than 1 quart/day)
- Use of other medications (e.g., cyclosporine, some antibiotics, verapamil, human immunodeficiency virus [HIV] protease inhibitors, some antidepressants)[15]
- Alcohol abuse (independently predisposes to myopathy)

Muscle aches and pain, unexplained fever, nausea, vomiting, and dark urine can potentially be signs of myositis and should be referred to a physician immediately. Risk for statin-induced myositis is highest in people with liver disease, acute infection, and hypothyroidism. Severe statin-induced myopathy can lead to rhabdomyolysis (enzyme leakage, muscle cell destruction, and elevated CK levels). Rhabdomyolysis is associated with impaired renal and liver function. Screening for liver impairment (see Chapter 10) of people taking statins is an important part of assessing for rhabdomyolysis (see further discussion of rhabdomyolysis in Chapter 10).[16]

CLINICAL SIGNS AND SYMPTOMS
Statin-Induced Side Effects

- Symptomatic myopathy (muscle soreness, pain, weakness, dyspnea); myositis (elevated CK level); look for weakness in the larger muscle groups bilaterally such as the thigh, back, buttocks, and shoulder musculature[12]
- Unexplained fever
- Nausea, vomiting
- Signs and symptoms of liver impairment:
  - Dark urine
  - Asterixis (liver flap)
  - Bilateral carpal tunnel syndrome
  - Palmar erythema (liver palms)
  - Spider angioma
  - Changes in nail beds, skin color
  - Ascites

CASE EXAMPLE 7.2
Statins and Myalgia

Referral: The client was a 53-year-old woman who complained of right-sided knee pain and stiffness and constant, bilateral thigh pain. She was referred by her orthopedic surgeon for physical therapy with a musculoskeletal diagnosis of osteoarthritis (OA) of both knees.

Medications: Lipitor (antilipemic for high cholesterol), Lopressor (antihypertensive, beta-blocker), Ambien (sedative for insomnia), Naprosyn (antiinflammatory). Dosage of the Lipitor was increased from 20 mg to 40 mg at the last physician visit.

Past Medical History: Hypertension, hypercholesterolemia, insomnia.

Clinical Presentation: Pain pattern—Client reported constant but variable pain in the right knee, ranging from 2/10 at rest and 5/10 during and after weight-bearing activities. Morning stiffness was prominent, and the client described difficulty transitioning from prolonged sitting to standing. The client reported increased pain in the right knee after weight-bearing for approximately 5 minutes.

In addition to the right-sided knee pain, the client also complained of a constant anterior thigh pain. This pain was described as a "flushing" sensation and was unchanged by position or motion. The intensity of the bilateral constant thigh pain was rated 3/10 to 4/10.

Complete physical examination of integument and gait inspection, muscle strength, and joint range of motion (ROM) was conducted, and results were recorded (on file). Findings from the lower quarter screen (LQS) were unremarkable. Lumbar ROM was within normal limits (WNL).

Neurologic screening examination—WNL

Review of Systems (ROS): Unremarkable; no other associated signs or symptoms reported.

What are the red flags in this scenario?
Age
Constant, bilateral myalgic pain unchanged by position or motion
Recent dosage change in medication

Is it safe to treat this client?
Physical therapy intervention can be implemented despite complaints of pain from an unknown origin. In the past 10 weeks before the initial physical therapy examination, this client had been evaluated by a physician four times. The most recent evaluation was by an orthopedic surgeon 1 week before her initial evaluation.

Additionally, the client appeared to be otherwise in good health, and her ROS was unremarkable. The presence of three red flags warrants careful observation of response to intervention, progression of current symptoms, or onset of any new symptoms.

Symptoms related to OA were expected to improve, while symptoms from a nonmusculoskeletal origin were not expected to improve. The plan of care was explained to the client, and it was mutually agreed that if the constant thigh pain did not significantly improve within 4 weeks, the client would be referred back to her physician.

Result: Four weeks after the initial physical therapy visit, symptoms of constant thigh pain had not resolved. The client had a follow-up appointment with her orthopedic surgeon at which time she presented documentation of the physical therapy intervention to date and the therapist's concerns about the thigh pain.

The orthopedic surgeon reiterated his belief that the origin of her symptoms was as a result of OA. The client was instructed to continue physical therapy and to take Naprosyn as prescribed.

The client was discharged after receiving 8 weeks of physical therapy intervention. At this juncture, the therapist believed that the client's right-sided knee symptoms were sufficiently improved and that the client could maintain or improve upon her current status by following her discharge instructions.

Furthermore, the myalgic thigh symptoms had not improved in the last 8 weeks and the therapist did not feel the bilateral thigh myalgia would be improved by further physical therapy intervention.

The client was instructed to contact her primary care physician regarding her myalgic symptoms. Three days later, the client called the physical therapy clinic. She had called her orthopedic surgeon rather than the primary care physician.

According to the client, the orthopedic surgeon dismissed the association between the thigh myalgia and the increased dosage of atorvastatin calcium (Lipitor). The client was again instructed to contact her primary care physician regarding the possibility of an adverse myalgic reaction to atorvastatin calcium (Lipitor). The client was also asked to contact the physical therapy clinic after being evaluated by her primary care physician.

Two weeks later, the client called and indicated her primary care physician evaluated her 2 days following their telephone conversation. The primary care physician discontinued the atorvastatin calcium (Lipitor). The client reported approximately a 50% reduction in the constant bilateral thigh myalgia after discontinuing the atorvastatin calcium (Lipitor).

The client was asked to contact the therapist in 2 or 3 weeks to provide an update of her status. Three weeks passed without hearing from the client. The therapist contacted the client by telephone. The client indicated that approximately 4 weeks following the discontinuation of the atorvastatin calcium (Lipitor) her myalgic thigh complaints were fully resolved.

She stated that she would remain off the atorvastatin calcium (Lipitor) for a total of 12 weeks and then would receive clinical laboratory testing to evaluate serum cholesterol levels. The primary care physician would consider prescribing a different statin to control her hypercholesterolemia based on future cholesterol levels.

Summary: Medication used in many situations may have a significant effect on the health of the client and may alter the clinical presentation or course of the individual's symptoms. It is important to ask if the client is taking any new medication (OTC or by prescription), nutraceutical supplements, and if there have been any recent changes in the dosages of current medications.

There is a wide body of medical literature that associates the adverse reaction of myalgia and the more serious reaction of rhabdomyolysis with statin medications. Therapists must perform good pharmacovigilance.

From Trumbore DJ: Case report presented in partial fulfillment of DPT 910. *Principles of differential diagnosis*, Institute for Physical Therapy Education, Chester, Pennsylvania, 2005, Widener University. Used with permission.

The therapist will need to perform clinical tests and measures to differentiate exercise-related muscle fatigue and soreness from statin-induced symptoms. For example, exercise-induced muscle fatigue and soreness should be limited to the muscles exercised and resolve within 24 to 48 hours. Statin-related weakness may involve muscles not recently exercised, and may progress or fail to show signs of improvement even after several days of rest.[17] Dynamometer testing can be used as a valid and reliable indicator of change in muscle strength.[18,19]

Strength testing, combined with client history, risk factors, and performance on the Stair-Climbing Test and Six-Minute Walk test, may prove to be an adequate means of assessment to detect meaningful declines in functional status; baseline measures are therefore important.[17]

Coronary Artery Disease

The heart muscle must have an adequate blood supply to contract properly. As mentioned, the coronary arteries carry oxygen and blood to the myocardium. When a coronary artery becomes narrowed or blocked, the area of the heart muscle supplied by that artery becomes ischemic and injured, and infarction may result.

The major disorders caused by insufficient blood supply to the myocardium are angina pectoris and MI. CAD includes atherosclerosis (fatty buildup), thrombus (blood clot), and spasm (intermittent constriction).

CAD results from a person's complex genetic makeup and interactions with the environment, including nutrition, activity level, and history of smoking. Susceptibility to CVD may be explained by genetic factors, and it is likely that an "atherosclerosis gene" or "heart attack gene" will be identified.[20] The therapeutic use of drugs that act by modifying gene transcription is a well-established practice in the treatment of CAD and essential hypertension.[21,22]

Atherosclerosis

Atherosclerosis is the disease process often called arteriosclerosis or hardening of the arteries. It is a progressive process that may begin in childhood. It can occur in any artery in the body, but it is most common in medium-sized arteries such as those of the heart, brain, kidneys, and legs. Starting in childhood, the arteries begin to fill with a fatty substance, or lipids such as triglycerides and cholesterol, which then calcify or harden (Fig. 7.2).

This filler, called *plaque*, is made up of fats, calcium, and fibrous scar tissue and lines the usually supple arterial walls, progressively narrowing the arteries. These arteries carry blood rich in oxygen to the myocardium (middle layer of the heart consisting of the heart muscle), but the atherosclerotic process leads to ischemia and necrosis of the heart muscle. Necrotic tissue gradually forms a scar, but before scar formation, the weakened area is susceptible to aneurysm development.

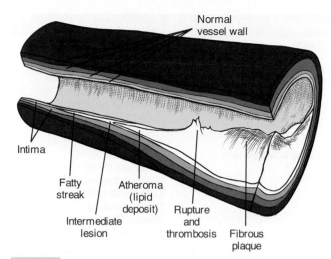

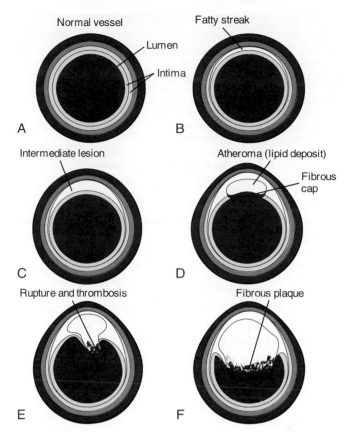

Fig. 7.2 Hardening of the arteries. Atherosclerosis begins with an injury to the endothelial lining of the artery (intimal layer) that makes the vessel permeable to circulating lipoproteins. Penetration of lipoproteins into the smooth muscle cells of the intima produces "fatty streaks." A fibrous plaque large enough to decrease blood flow through the artery develops. Calcification with rupture or hemorrhage of the fibrous plaque is the final advanced stage. Thrombosis (stationary blood clot) may occur, further occluding the lumen of the blood vessel.

Fig. 7.3 Updated model of atherosclerosis. New technology using intravascular ultrasound shows the whole atherosclerotic plaque and has changed the way we view things. The traditional model held that an atherosclerotic plaque in the blood vessel, particularly a coronary blood vessel, kept growing inward and obstructing flow until it closed off and caused a heart attack. This is not entirely correct. It is more accurate to say that in the normal vessel (**A**), penetration of lipoproteins into the smooth muscle cells of the intima produces fatty streaks (**B**) and the start of a coronary lesion forms. **C** and **D**, The coronary lesion grows outward first in a compensatory manner to maintain the open lumen. This is called *positive remodeling*, as the blood vessel tries to maintain an open lumen until it can do so no more. **E**, Only then does the plaque (atheroma) begin to build up, gradually pressing inward into the lumen with obstruction of blood flow and possible rupture and thrombosis, potentially leading to myocardial infarction (MI) or stroke. **F**, Vascular disease today is considered a disease of the wall. Some researchers like to say the disease is in the donut, not the hole of a donut, and that is a new concept.[23]

When fully developed, plaque can cause bleeding, clot formation, and distortion or rupture of a blood vessel (Fig. 7.3). Heart attacks and strokes are the most sudden and often fatal signs of the disease.

Thrombus

When plaque builds up on the artery walls, the blood flow is slowed—a process called hemostasis—and a clot (thrombus) may form on the plaque. When a vessel becomes blocked by a clot, it is called *thrombosis*. Coronary thrombosis refers to the formation of a clot in one of the coronary arteries, usually causing a heart attack.

Spasm

Sudden constriction of a coronary artery is called a *spasm;* blood flow to that part of the heart is cut off or decreased. A brief spasm may cause mild symptoms that never return. A prolonged spasm may cause heart damage such as an infarct. This process can occur in healthy persons who have no cardiac history, as well as in those who have known atherosclerosis. Chemicals like nicotine and cocaine may lead to coronary artery spasm; other possible factors include anxiety and cold air.

Risk Factors

In 1948 the United States government decided to investigate the etiology, incidence, and pathology of CAD by studying the residents of Framingham, Massachusetts. Over the next multiple decades, various aspects of lifestyle, health, and disease were studied. The research revealed important modifiable and nonmodifiable risk factors associated with death caused by CAD. Since that time, an additional category—contributing factors—has been added (Table 7.3). The AHA has also developed a validated health-risk appraisal instrument to assess individual risk of heart attack, stroke, and diabetes (see Box 7.1).

More recent research has identified other possible risk factors for, and predictors of, cardiac events, especially for those persons who have already had a heart attack. These additional risk factors include:

1. Exposure to bacteria such as *Chlamydia pneumoniae, Porphyromonas gingivalis,* and Cytomegalovirus.[24–26]
2. Excess levels of homocysteine, an amino acid by-product of food rich in proteins.
3. High levels of alpha-lipoprotein, a close cousin of LDL that transports fat throughout the body.

TABLE 7.3	Risk Factors for Coronary Artery Disease	
Modifiable Risk Factors	Nonmodifiable Risk Factors	Contributing Factors
Physical inactivity	Advancing age (65 years or older)	Response to stress
Tobacco smoking	Male gender	Personality
Elevated serum Cholesterol	Family history	Peripheral vascular disease
High BP	Race	Hormonal status
Diabetes	Postmenopausal (female)	Alcohol consumption
Obesity		Obesity

AHA Scientific Statements on Prevention of Coronary Heart Disease and Stroke, 2010. Available online at www.heart.org (Risk Factors and Coronary Heart Disease). Accessed September 1, 2010.

TABLE 7.4	Heart Attack Symptoms in Women
Timing	Symptoms
One month before a heart attack	Unusual fatigue (71%)
	Sleep disturbance (48%)
	Dyspnea (42%)
	Indigestion or GERD (39%)
	Anxiety (36%)
	Heart racing (27%)
	Arms weak/heavy (25%)
During a heart attack	Dyspnea (58%)
	Weakness (55%)
	Unusual fatigue (43%)
	Cold sweat (39%)
	Dizziness (39%)
	Nausea (36%)
	Arms weak/heavy (35%)

From McSweeney JC: Women's early warning symptoms of acute myocardial infarction. *Circulation* 108(21):2619–2623, 2003. *GERD*, gastroesophageal reflux disease.

4. High levels of fibrinogen, a protein that binds together platelet cells in blood clots.[27]
5. Large amounts of C-reactive protein (CRP), a specialized protein necessary for repair of tissue injury.[28,29]
6. The presence of troponin T, a regulatory protein that helps heart muscle contract.[30]
7. The presence of diagonal earlobe creases (under continued investigation).[31-35]
8. History of cancer treatment (cardiotoxic chemotherapeutic agents, trunk radiation).[36]

Therapists can assist clients in assessing their 10-year risk for heart attack using a risk assessment tool from the National Cholesterol Education program available online at http://hin.nhlbi.nih.gov/atpiii/calculator.asp?usertype=prof.

Women and Heart Disease

Many women know about the risk of breast cancer, but in truth, they are 10 times more likely to die of CVD. In 2017, 1 in every 5 female deaths was from CVD, and it is the leading cause of death for women in the United States.[1]

Women do not seem to do as well as men after taking medications to dissolve blood clots or after undergoing heart-related medical procedures. Of the women who survive a heart attack, 46% will develop and be disabled by HF within 6 years.[37]

In general, the rate of CAD is rising among women and falling among men. Men develop CAD at a younger age than women, but women make up for it after menopause. The prevalence of CAD among African-American women is 48%, whereas it is 36% for Caucasian women. Therefore whenever screening chest pain, keep in mind the demographics: older men and women, menopausal women, and African-American women are at greatest risk.

Diabetes alone poses a greater risk than any other factor in predicting cardiovascular problems in women. Women with diabetes are seven times more likely to have cardiovascular complications and about half of them will die of CAD.[38]

Studies have shown that women and men differ when it comes to symptoms of CAD, and in the manner in which acute MI can present. Women experience symptoms of CAD, which are more subtle and "atypical" compared with traditional symptoms such as angina and chest pain.

One of the most important primary signs of CAD in women is unexplained, severe episodic fatigue and weakness associated with a decreased ability to carry out normal activities of daily living (ADLs). Because fatigue, weakness, and trouble sleeping are general types of symptoms, they are not as easily associated with cardiovascular events and are many times missed by health care providers when screening for heart disease.[39]

Symptoms of weakness, fatigue and sleeping difficulty, and nausea have been reported as a common occurrence as early as a month before the development of acute MI in women (see Table 7.4). The classic pain associated with CAD is usually substernal chest pain characterized by a crushing, heavy, squeezing sensation commonly occurring during emotion or exertion. CAD pain in women, however, may vary greatly from that in men (see further discussion on MI in this chapter).

Risk reduction in women focuses on lifestyle changes such as: smoking cessation; dietary changes such as increased intake of omega-3 fatty acids, increased fruit, vegetable, whole grain intake, and salt and alcohol limitation; and increased exercise and weight loss. If the woman has diabetes, strict glucose control is extremely important.[40]

Clinical Signs and Symptoms

Atherosclerosis, by itself, does not necessarily produce symptoms. For manifestations to develop, there must be a critical deficit in blood supply to the heart in proportion to the demands of the myocardium for oxygen and nutrients (supply and demand imbalance). When atherosclerosis develops slowly, collateral circulation develops to meet the heart's demands. Often, symptoms of CAD do not appear until the lumen of the coronary artery narrows by 75% (see also Hypertension in this chapter).

Although the arteries are rarely completely blocked, the deposits of plaque are often extensive enough to restrict blood flow to the heart, especially during exercise in clinical practice when there is a need to deliver more oxygen-carrying blood to the heart. Like other muscles, the heart, when deprived of oxygen, may ache, causing chest pain or discomfort referred to as *angina*.

CAD is a progressive disorder, especially if left untreated. If the blood flow is entirely disrupted, usually by a clot that has formed in the obstructed region, some of the tissue that is supplied by the vessel can die, and a heart attack or even sudden cardiac death results.

When tissue loss is extensive enough to disrupt the electrical impulses that stimulate the heart's contractions, HF, chronic arrhythmias, and conduction disturbances may develop.

Angina

Acute pain in the chest, called *angina pectoris*, results from the imbalance between cardiac workload and oxygen supply to myocardial tissue. Angina is a symptom of obstructed or decreased blood supply to the heart muscle primarily from atherosclerosis.

Atherosclerosis is now recognized as an inflammatory condition affecting the coronary arteries and the peripheral vessels. It is often accompanied by hypertension and signs of PVD. Although the primary cause of angina is CAD, angina can occur in individuals with normal coronary arteries and with other conditions affecting the supply/demand balance.

As vessels become lined with atherosclerotic plaque, symptoms of inadequate blood supply develop in the tissues supplied by these vessels. A growing mass of plaque in the vessel collects platelets, fibrin, and cellular debris. Platelet aggregations are known to release prostaglandins capable of causing vessel spasm. This in turn promotes platelet aggregation, and a vicious spasm/pain cycle begins.

The present theory of heart pain suggests that pain occurs as a result of an accumulation of metabolites within an ischemic segment of the myocardium. The transient ischemia of angina or the prolonged, necrotic ischemia of an MI sets off pain impulses secondary to rapid accumulation of these metabolites in the heart muscle.

The imbalance between cardiac workload and oxygen supply can develop as a result of disorders of the coronary vessels, disorders of circulation, increased demands on output of the heart, or damaged myocardium unable to utilize oxygen properly.

Types of Anginal Pain

There are several types of anginal pain, including chronic stable angina (also referred to as walk-through angina), resting angina (angina decubitus), unstable angina, nocturnal angina, atypical angina, new-onset angina, and Prinzmetal's or "variant" angina.

Chronic stable angina occurs at a predictable level of physical or emotional stress and responds promptly to rest or nitroglycerin. No pain occurs at rest, and the location, duration, intensity, and frequency of chest pain are consistent over time.

Resting angina, or *angina decubitus*, is chest pain that occurs at rest in the supine position and frequently at the same time every day. The pain is neither brought on by exercise nor relieved by rest.

Unstable angina, also known as crescendo angina, preinfarction angina, or progressive angina, is an abrupt change in the intensity and frequency of symptoms or decreased threshold of stimulus, such as the onset of chest pain while at rest. The most common trigger of unstable angina is the bursting of a cholesterol-filled plaque in the lining of a coronary artery. A blood clot forms at that site, partially blocking blood flow. The duration of these attacks is longer than the usual 1 to 5 minutes; they may last for up to 20 to 30 minutes and can progress into a full-blown heart attack. Pain or discomfort unrelieved by rest or nitroglycerin signals a higher risk for MI. Such changes in the pattern of angina require immediate medical follow-up by the client's physician.

Nocturnal angina may awaken a person from sleep with the same sensation experienced during exertion. During sleep, this exertion is usually caused by dreams. This type of angina may be associated with underlying CHF.

Atypical angina refers to unusual symptoms (e.g., toothache or earache) related to physical or emotional exertion. These symptoms subside with rest or nitroglycerin. New-onset angina describes angina that has developed for the first time within the last 60 days.

Prinzmetal's (vasospastic or variant) angina produces symptoms similar to those of typical angina but is caused by abnormal or involuntary coronary artery spasm rather than directly by a build-up of plaque from atherosclerosis. These spasms periodically squeeze arteries shut and keep the blood from reaching the heart. About two-thirds of people with Prinzmetal's have severe coronary atherosclerosis in at least one major vessel. The spasm usually occurs close to the blockage.

This form of angina typically occurs at rest, especially in the early hours of the morning, and can be difficult to induce by exercise. It is cyclic and frequently occurs at the same time each day. In postmenopausal women who are not undergoing hormone replacement therapy, the reduction in estrogen may cause coronary arteries to spasm, resulting in vasospastic (Prinzmetal's) angina.

Clinical Signs and Symptoms

The client may indicate the location of the symptoms by placing a clenched fist against the sternum. Angina radiates most commonly to the left shoulder and down the ulnar distribution of the arm to the fingers; but it can also refer pain to the neck, jaw, teeth, upper back, possibly down the right arm, and occasionally to the abdomen (see Fig. 7.8).

Recognizing heart pain in women is more difficult because the symptoms are less reliable and often do not follow the classic pattern described earlier. Many women describe the pain in ways consistent with unstable angina,

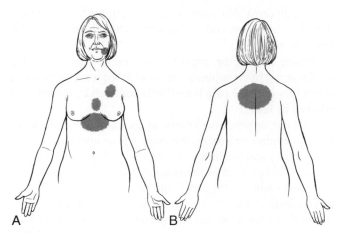

Fig. 7.4 Pain patterns associated with angina in women may differ from patterns in men. Many presenting symptoms are subjective such as extreme fatigue, lethargy, breathlessness, or weakness. Unusual patterns (e.g., TMJ pain) and failure to seek medical diagnosis may delay treatment with less optimal results. More classic pain patterns as shown in Fig. 7.8 are also possible.

suggesting that they first become aware of their chest discomfort or have it diagnosed only after it reaches more advanced stages.

Some experience a sensation similar to inhaling cold air, rather than the more typical shortness of breath. Other women complain only of weakness and lethargy, and some have noted isolated pain in the midthoracic spine or throbbing and aching in the right biceps muscle (Fig. 7.4).

Pain associated with angina and MI occurring along the inner aspect of the arm and corresponding to the ulnar nerve distribution results from common connections between the cardiac and brachial plexuses.

Cardiac pain referred to the jaw occurs through internuncial (neurons connecting other neurons) fibers from cervical spinal cord posterior horns to the spinal nucleus of the trigeminal nerve. Abdominal pain produced by referred cardiac pain is more difficult to explain and may be caused by the overflow of segmental levels to which visceral afferent nerve pathways flow (see Fig. 3.3). This overflow increases the chance that final common pain pathways between the chest and the abdomen may occur.

The *sensation* of angina is described as squeezing, burning, pressing, choking, aching, or bursting. Chest pain can be brought on by a wide variety of noncardiac causes (see discussion of chest pain in Chapter 18).

In particular, angina is often confused with heartburn or indigestion, hiatal hernia, esophageal spasm, or gallbladder disease, but the pain of these other conditions is not described as sharp or knife-like.

The client often says the pain feels like "gas" or "heartburn" or "indigestion." Referred pain from a trigger point in the external oblique abdominal muscle can cause a sensation of heartburn in the anterior chest wall (see Fig. 18.7, D). A physician must make the differentiation between angina and heartburn, hiatal hernia, and gallbladder disease. The therapist can assess for trigger points; relief of symptoms with

the elimination of trigger points is an important diagnostic finding.

CLINICAL SIGNS AND SYMPTOMS
Heartburn

- Frequent "heartburn" attacks
- Frequent use of antacids to relieve symptoms
- Heartburn wakes the client up at night
- Acidic or bitter taste in the mouth
- Burning sensation in the chest
- Discomfort after eating spicy foods
- Abdominal bloating and gas
- Difficulty in swallowing

Severity is usually mild or moderate. Rarely is the pain described as severe. The five-grade angina scale ranks angina as:

Grade 0	No angina
Grade 1	Light, barely noticeable
Grade 2	Moderately bothersome
Grade 3	Severe, very uncomfortable
Grade 4	Most pain ever experienced

As to *location*, 80% to 90% of clients experience the pain as retrosternal or slightly to the left of the sternum. The *duration* of angina as a direct result of myocardial ischemia is typically 1 to 3 minutes, and no longer than 3 to 5 minutes. However, attacks precipitated by a heavy meal or extreme anger may last 15 to 20 minutes. Angina is relieved by rest or nitroglycerin (a coronary artery vasodilator).

People who have had coronary artery stents placed can experience angina if an occlusion occurs above, below, or within the stent. Anyone with a stent who has chest pain should be immediately sent for referral to a physician.

Severity of pain is not a good prognostic indicator; some persons with severe discomfort live for many years, whereas others with mild symptoms may die suddenly. If the pain is not relieved by rest or with up to three nitroglycerin tablets (taken one at a time at 5-minute intervals) in 10 to 15 minutes, the physician should be notified and the client taken to a cardiac care unit.

The client should take his or her nitroglycerin. The therapist should not dispense medication but may assist the client in taking this medication. Nitroglycerin dilates the coronary arteries and improves collateral cardiac circulation, thus providing an increase in oxygen to the heart muscle and a decrease in symptoms of angina.

When screening for chest pain, a lack of objective musculoskeletal findings is always a red flag:

Active range of motion (AROM), such as trunk rotation, side bending, or shoulder motion, does not reproduce symptoms.

Resisted motion (horizontal shoulder abduction/adduction) does not reproduce symptoms.

Heat and stretching do not reduce or eliminate symptoms.

CLINICAL SIGNS AND SYMPTOMS
Angina Pectoris

- Gripping, vise-like feeling of pain or pressure behind the breast bone
- Pain that may radiate to the neck, jaw, back, shoulder, or arms (most often the left arm in men)
- Toothache
- Burning indigestion
- Dyspnea (shortness of breath); exercise intolerance
- Nausea
- Belching

Myocardial Infarction

MI, also known as a heart attack, coronary occlusion, or a "coronary," is the development of ischemia and necrosis of myocardial tissue. It results from a sudden decrease in coronary perfusion or an increase in myocardial oxygen demand without adequate blood supply. If the requirements for blood are not eased (e.g., by decreased activity), the heart attempts to continue meeting the increased demands for oxygen with an inadequate blood supply, which leads to an MI. Myocardial tissue death is usually preceded by a sudden occlusion of one or more of the major coronary arteries.

The myocardium receives its blood supply from the two large coronary arteries and their branches. Occlusion of one or more of these blood vessels (coronary occlusion) is one of the major causes of MI. The occlusion may result from the formation of a clot that develops suddenly when an atheromatous plaque ruptures through the sublayers of a blood vessel, or when the narrow, roughened inner lining of a sclerosed artery leads to complete thrombosis.

Although coronary thrombosis is the most common cause of infarction, many interrelated factors may be responsible, including coronary artery spasm, platelet aggregation and embolism, thrombus secondary to rheumatic heart disease, endocarditis, aortic stenosis, a thrombus on a prosthetic mitral or aortic valve, or a dislodged calcium plaque from a calcified aortic or mitral valve.

Coronary blood flow is affected by the tonus (tone) of the coronary arteries. Arteries "clogged" by plaque formation become rigid like lead pipes, and resultant spasm may be provoked by cold and by exercise, which explains the adverse effect of both factors on clients with angina.

Clinical Signs and Symptoms

There are some well-known pain patterns specific to the heart and cardiac system. Sudden death can be the first sign of heart disease. In fact, according to the AHA, 63% of women who died suddenly of CVD had no previous symptoms. Sudden death is the first symptom for half of all men who have a heart attack.

The onset of an infarct may be characterized by severe fatigue for several days before the infarct. The likelihood of having a heart attack in the morning hours is 40% higher than during the rest of the day[41,42] and is most likely to occur between 6:00 AM and 12:00 PM. The morning is when the body's clotting system is more active, BP surges, heart rate increases, and there may be reduced blood flow to the heart.

Additionally, the level and activity of stress hormones (e.g., catecholamines), which can induce vasoconstriction, increase in the morning. Combined with these factors are the increased mental and physical stresses that typically occur after waking. The shift worker would experience this same phenomenon in the evening or on arising.

Persons who have MIs may not experience any pain and may be unaware that damage is occurring to the heart muscle as a result of prolonged ischemia. The presence of silent infarction (SI) increases with advancing age, especially without a history of CAD.

Cardiac Arrest

Researchers expect the number of Americans living with angina to grow as new treatments improve survival after a heart attack.[43] Failure to recognize prodromal symptoms in men or women may account for many cases of sudden cardiac death.[44]

Cardiac arrest strikes immediately and without warning. Signs of sudden cardiac arrest include[43]:

Sudden loss of responsiveness. No response to gentle shaking.

No normal breathing. The client does not take a normal breath when you check for several seconds.

No signs of circulation. No movement or coughing.

If cardiac arrest occurs, call for emergency help and begin cardiopulmonary resuscitation (CPR) immediately, unless the client has a do not resuscitate (DNR) order on file. Use an automated external defibrillator (AED) if available.

Classic Warning Signs of Myocardial Infarction

Those who do have warning signs of MI may have severe unrelenting chest pain described as "crushing pain" lasting 30 or more minutes that is not alleviated by rest or by nitroglycerin. This chest pain may radiate to the arms, throat, and back, persisting for hours (see Fig. 7.9).

Other symptoms include pallor, profuse perspiration, and possibly nausea and vomiting. The pain of an MI may be misinterpreted as indigestion because of nausea and vomiting. Nausea may be the only prodromal symptom. A medical evaluation may be difficult because many clients have coexisting hiatal hernia, peptic ulcer, or gallbladder disease.

Cardiac pain patterns may differ for men and women. For many men, the most common report is a feeling of pressure or discomfort under the sternum (substernal), in the midchest region, or across the entire upper chest. It can feel like uncomfortable pressure, squeezing, fullness, or pain.

Pain may occur just in the jaw, upper neck, midback, or down the arm without chest pain or discomfort. Pain may also radiate from the chest to the neck, jaw, midback, or down the arm(s). Pain down the arm(s) affects the left arm most often in the pattern of the ulnar nerve distribution. Radiating pain down both arms is also possible.

An MI may occur during exertion, exercise, or exposure to extremes of temperature, or it may occur while the person is at rest. A subtle variation on ischemia during exertion is an important one for the therapist.

The onset of angina and a subsequent MI is known to be precipitated when working with the arms extended over the head. Oxygen requirements of the heart are greater during arm work compared with leg work at the same workload level. If the person becomes weak or short of breath while in this position, ischemia or infarction may be the cause of the pain and associated symptoms; workload should be cut in half to prevent cardiac ischemia.

Because the infarction process may take up to 6 hours to complete, restoration of adequate myocardial perfusion is important if significant necrosis is to be limited. Death generally results from severe arrhythmias, cardiogenic shock, CHF, rupture of the heart, and recurrent MI.

CLINICAL SIGNS AND SYMPTOMS

Myocardial Infarction

- May be silent (smokers, diabetics: reduced sensitivity to pain)
- Sudden cardiac death
- Prolonged or severe substernal chest pain or squeezing pressure
- Pain possibly radiating down one or both arms and/or up to the throat, neck, back, jaw, shoulders, or arms
- Feeling of nausea or indigestion
- Angina lasting for 30 minutes or more
- Angina unrelieved by rest, nitroglycerin, or antacids
- Pain of infarct unrelieved by rest or a change in position
- Nausea
- Sudden dimness or loss of vision or speech
- Pallor
- Diaphoresis (heavy perspiration)
- Shortness of breath
- Weakness, numbness, and feelings of faintness

Warning Signs of Myocardial Infarction in Women

For women, symptoms can be more subtle or "atypical." Chest pain or discomfort is less common in women but still a key feature for some. Women describe heaviness, squeezing, or pain in the left side of the chest, abdomen, midback (thoracic), shoulder, or arm with no midchest symptoms.[45]

They often have prodromal symptoms up to 1 month before having a heart attack (Table 7.4).[44,46]

Fatigue, nausea, and lower abdominal pain may signal a heart attack. Many women pass these off as the flu or food poisoning. Other symptoms for women include a feeling of intense anxiety, isolated right biceps pain, midthoracic pain, or heartburn; sudden shortness of breath, or the inability to talk, move, or breathe; shoulder or arm pain; or ankle swelling or rapid weight gain.

Women may describe palpitations or pain that is sharp and fleeting. Antacids may relieve it rather than rest or nitroglycerin. Women having an acute MI have also described pain in the jaw, neck, shoulder, back, or ear, and a feeling of intense anxiety, nausea, or shortness of breath. Many women do not associate these symptoms with having a heart attack, and they may do nothing to seek help.[45]

CLINICAL SIGNS AND SYMPTOMS

Myocardial Ischemia in Women

- Heart pain in women does not always follow classic patterns
- Many women do experience classic chest discomfort
- Older females: mental status change or confusion may be common
- Dyspnea (at rest or with exertion)
- Weakness and lethargy (unusual fatigue; fatigue that interferes with ability to perform ADLs)
- Indigestion, heartburn, or stomach pain; mistakenly diagnosed or assumed to have gastroesophageal reflux disease (GERD)
- Anxiety or depression
- Sleep disturbance (woman awakens with any of the symptoms listed here)
- Sensation similar to inhaling cold air; unable to talk or breathe
- Isolated, continuous midthoracic or interscapular back pain
- Aching, heaviness, or weakness in one or both arms
- Symptoms may be relieved by antacids (sometimes antacids work better than nitroglycerin)

Pericarditis

Pericarditis is an inflammation of the pericardium, the sac-like covering of the heart. Specifically, it affects the parietal pericardium (fluid-like membrane between the fibrous pericardium and the epicardium) and the visceral (epicardium) pericardium (Fig. 7.5).

This inflammatory process may develop either as a primary condition or secondary to several diseases and conditions (e.g., influenza, HIV infection, tuberculosis, cancer, kidney failure, hypothyroidism, autoimmune disorders). Myocardial injury or trauma such as a heart attack, chest injury, chest radiation, or cardiac surgery can cause pericarditis. Very often the cause is unknown, resulting in a diagnosis of idiopathic pericarditis.

Pericarditis may be acute or chronic (recurring); it is not known why pericarditis may be a single illness in some persons and recurrent in others. Chronic or recurring pericarditis is accompanied by a pericardium that is rigid, thickened, and scarred.

Previous infection may be mild or asymptomatic with postinfectious onset of pain occurring 1 to 3 weeks later. Because this condition can occur in any age group, a history of recent pericarditis in the presence of new onset of chest, neck, or left shoulder pain is important.

Clinical Signs and Symptoms

At first, pericarditis may have no external signs or symptoms. The symptoms of acute pericarditis vary with the cause but usually include chest pain and dyspnea, an increase in the pulse rate, and a temperature rise. Malaise and myalgia may occur.

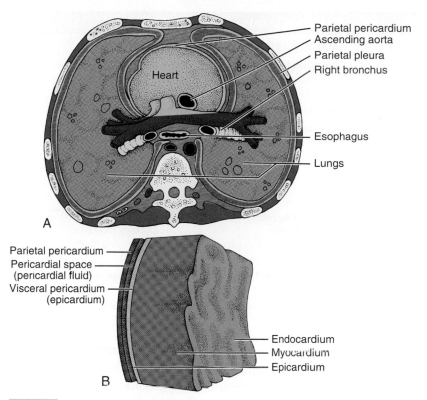

Parietal pericardium
Ascending aorta
Parietal pleura
Right bronchus

Heart

Esophagus

Lungs

A

Parietal pericardium
Pericardial space (pericardial fluid)
Visceral pericardium (epicardium)

Endocardium
Myocardium
Epicardium

B

Fig. 7.5 The heart and associated layers of membranes. **A,** Cross-section through the thorax just above the heart, emphasizing the lining of the cavity that contains the lungs (parietal pleura) and the lining of the cavity that contains the heart (parietal pericardium). **B,** Sagittal view of the layers of the heart.

Over time, the inflammatory process may result in an accumulation of fluid in the pericardial sac, preventing the heart from expanding fully. The inflamed pericardium may cause pain when it rubs against the heart. Chest pain from pericarditis (see Fig. 7.10) closely mimics that of an MI because it is substernal, is associated with cough, and may radiate to the left shoulder or supraclavicular area. It can be differentiated from MI by the pattern of relieving and aggravating factors (Table 7.5).

For example, the pain of an MI is unaffected by position, breathing, or movement, whereas the pain associated with pericarditis may be relieved by kneeling on all fours, leaning forward, or sitting upright. Pericardial chest pain is often worse with breathing, swallowing, belching, or neck or trunk movements, especially sidebending or rotation. The pain tends to be sharp or cutting and may recur in intermittent bursts that are usually precipitated by a change in body position. Pericarditis pain may diminish if the breath is held.

Congestive Heart Failure or Heart Failure

HF, also called *cardiac decompensation* and *cardiac insufficiency*, can be defined as a physiologic state in which the heart is unable to pump enough blood to meet the metabolic needs of the body (determined as oxygen consumption) at rest or during exercise, even though filling pressures are adequate.

The heart fails when, because of intrinsic disease or structural defects, it cannot handle a normal blood volume, or in

CLINICAL SIGNS AND SYMPTOMS
Pericarditis

- Substernal pain that may radiate to the neck, upper back, upper trapezius muscle, left supraclavicular area, down the left arm to the costal margins
- Difficulty in swallowing
- Pain relieved by leaning forward or sitting upright
- Pain relieved or reduced by holding the breath
- Pain aggravated by movement associated with deep breathing (laughing, coughing, deep inspiration)
- Pain aggravated by trunk movements (sidebending or rotation) and by lying down
- History of fever, chills, weakness, or heart disease (a recent MI accompanying the pattern of symptoms may alert the therapist to the need for medical referral to rule out cardiac involvement)
- Cough
- Lower extremity edema (feet, ankles, legs)

the absence of disease cannot tolerate a sudden expansion in blood volume (e.g., exercise). HF is not a disease itself; instead, the term denotes a group of manifestations related to inadequate pump performance from either the cardiac valves or the myocardium.

Whatever the cause, when the heart fails to propel blood forward normally, congestion occurs in the pulmonary circulation as blood accumulates in the lungs. The right ventricle, which is not yet affected by congestive heart disease,

TABLE 7.5	Characteristics of Cardiac Chest Pain		
Angina	**Myocardial Infarction**	**Mitral Valve Prolapse**	**Pericarditis**
Begins 3–5 minutes after exertion or activity ("lagtime"); lasts 1–5 minutes	30 minutes to 1 hour	Minutes to hours	Hours to days
Moderate intensity	Severe (can be painless)	Rarely severe	Varies; mild to severe
Tightness; chest discomfort	Crushing pain; intolerable (can be painless)	May be asymptomatic; "sticking" sensation, not substernal	Asymptomatic; sharp or cutting; can mimic MI
Can occur at rest or during sleep Usually occurs with exertion, emotion, cold, or large meal	Exertion	Often occurs at rest	Worse with breathing, swallowing, belching, neck or trunk movement
Subsides with rest or nitroglycerin; worse when lying down	Unrelieved by rest or nitroglycerin	Unrelieved by rest or nitroglycerin; may be relieved by lying down	Relieved by kneeling on all fours, leaning forward, sitting upright, or breathholding
Pain related to tone of arteries (spasm)	Pain related to ischemia	Mechanism of pain unknown	Pain related to inflammatory process

MI, Myocardial infarction.

continues to pump more blood into the lungs. The immediate result is shortness of breath and, if the process continues, actual flooding of the air space of the lungs with fluid seeping from the distended blood vessels. This last phenomenon is called pulmonary congestion or pulmonary edema.

Because a properly functioning heart depends on both ventricles, failure of one ventricle almost always leads to failure of the other ventricle. This is called *ventricular interdependence.* Right-sided ventricular failure (right-sided HF) causes congestion of the peripheral tissues and viscera. The liver may enlarge, the ankles may swell, and the client develops ascites (fluid accumulates in the abdomen).

Some clients have preexisting mild-to-moderate heart disease with no evidence of CHF. However, when the heart undergoes undue stress or deterioration from risk factors, compensatory mechanisms may be inadequate and the heart fails.

Conditions (risk factors) that precipitate or exacerbate HF include hypertension, CAD, cardiomyopathy, heart valve abnormalities, arrhythmia, fever, infection, anemia, thyroid disorder, pregnancy, Paget's disease, nutritional deficiency (e.g., thiamine deficiency secondary to alcoholism), pulmonary disease, spinal cord injury, and hypervolemia from poor renal function.

Medications are frequently implicated in the development of CHF. Examples include cardiovascular drugs, antibiotics, central nervous system drugs (e.g., sedatives, hypnotics, antidepressants, narcotic analgesics), and antiinflammatory drugs (both nonsteroidal and steroidal).

Chemotherapy used to treat a variety of different types of cancers (including childhood cancers) has also been linked with increased risk of CVD and congestive HF.[36] There may be a significant delay between treatment and the development of left ventricular dysfunction. Signs and symptoms of HF in young adults are unexpected. Consider cancer treatment in children who were treated successfully for cancer years ago a warning flag.

Clinical Signs and Symptoms

The incidence of CHF increases with advancing age. Because of the increasing age of the U.S. population and newer medications and technologies that have increased survival at the expense of increased cardiovascular morbidity, the population affected by CHF is markedly increasing. In view of this increase, many individuals with a wide variety of heart and lung diseases will very likely develop CHF at some time during their lives, manifesting itself as pulmonary congestion or edema.[47] In 2009, 1 in 9 deaths included HF as a contributing cause, and half of the patients who develop HF die within 5 years of diagnosis.[48]

Left Ventricular Failure

Failure of the left ventricle causes either pulmonary congestion or a disturbance in the respiratory control mechanisms. These problems in turn precipitate respiratory distress. The degree of distress varies with the client's position, activity, and level of stress.

However, many persons with severely impaired ventricular performance may have few or no symptoms, particularly if HF has developed gradually. Breathlessness, exhaustion, and lower extremity edema are the most common signs and symptoms of HF.

Dyspnea is subjective and does not always correlate with the extent of HF. To some degree, exertional dyspnea occurs in all clients. The increased fluid in the tissue space causes dyspnea, at first upon effort and then at rest, by stimulation of stretch receptors in the lung and chest wall and by the increased work of breathing with stiff lungs.

PND resembles the frightening sensation of suffocation. The client suddenly awakens with the feeling of severe suffocation. Once the client is in the upright position, relief from the attack may not occur for 30 minutes or longer.

Orthopnea is a more advanced stage of dyspnea. The client often assumes a "three-point position," sitting up with both hands on the knees and leaning forward. Orthopnea develops because the supine position increases the amount of blood returning from the lower extremities to the heart and lungs. This gravitational redistribution of blood increases pulmonary congestion and dyspnea. The client learns to avoid respiratory distress at night by supporting the head and thorax on pillows. Severe HF may have the client resort to sleeping upright in a chair.

Cough is a common symptom of left ventricular failure and is often hacking, producing large amounts of frothy, blood-tinged sputum. The client coughs because a large amount of fluid is trapped in the pulmonary tree, irritating the lung mucosa.

Pulmonary edema may develop when rapidly rising pulmonary capillary pressure causes fluid to move into the alveoli, resulting in extreme breathlessness, anxiety, frothy sputum, nasal flaring, use of accessory breathing muscles, tachypnea, noisy and wet breathing, and diaphoresis.

Cerebral hypoxia may occur as a result of a decrease in cardiac output, causing inadequate brain perfusion. Depressed cerebral function can cause anxiety, irritability, restlessness, confusion, impaired memory, bad dreams, and insomnia.

Fatigue and muscular cramping or weakness is often associated with left ventricular failure (Case Example 7.3). Inadequate cardiac output leads to hypoxic tissue and slowed removal of metabolic waste products, which in turn causes

the client to tire easily. A common report is feeling tired after an activity or type of exertion that was easily accomplished previously. Disturbances in sleep and rest patterns may aggravate fatigue.

The therapist must view this symptom in relation to the bigger picture. Is this someone who is taking diuretics? Is the diuretic a potassium-sparing drug? When does the muscle cramping occur? For example, muscle cramping and fatigue after working out in the garden under a hot sun may be related to fluid loss, dehydration, and exertion, whereas cramping that wakes the person up at night unrelated to exertion (including disturbing dreams) may indicate a different type of electrolyte imbalance.

Nocturia (urination at night) develops as a result of renal changes that can occur in both right- and left-sided HF (but more evident in left-sided failure). During the day the affected individual is upright and blood flow is away from the kidneys with reduced formation of urine. At night, urine formation increases as blood flow to the kidneys improves.

Nocturia may interfere with effective sleep patterns, contributing to the fatigue associated with HF. As cardiac output falls, decreased renal blood flow may result in oliguria (reduced urine output), which is a late sign of HF.

CLINICAL SIGNS AND SYMPTOMS
Left-Sided Heart Failure

- Fatigue and dyspnea after mild physical exertion or exercise
- Persistent spasmodic cough, especially when lying down, when fluid moves from the extremities to the lungs
- Paroxysmal nocturnal dyspnea (occurring suddenly at night)
- Orthopnea (person must be in the upright position to breathe)
- Tachycardia
- Fatigue and muscle weakness
- Edema (especially of the legs and ankles) and weight gain
- Irritability/restlessness
- Decreased renal function or frequent urination at night

CASE EXAMPLE 7.3
Congestive Heart Failure—Muscle Cramping and Headache

A 74-year-old retired homemaker had a total hip replacement (THR) 2 days ago and remains an inpatient with complications related to congestive heart failure (CHF). She has a previous medical history of gallbladder removal 20 years ago, total hysterectomy 30 years ago, and surgically induced menopause with subsequent onset of hypertension. Her medications include intravenous furosemide (Lasix), digoxin, and potassium replacement.

During the initial physical therapy session, the client complained of muscle cramping and headache but was able to complete the entire exercise protocol. Blood pressure was 100/76 mm Hg. Systolic measurement dropped to 90 mm Hg when the client moved from supine to standing. Pulse rate was 56 bpm with a pattern of irregular beats. Pulse rate did not change with postural change. Platelet count was 98,000 cells/mm³.

Result: With CHF, the heart will try to compensate by increasing the heart rate. However, the digoxin is designed to increase cardiac output and lower heart rate. In normal circumstances, postural changes result in an increase in heart rate, but when digoxin is used, this increase cannot occur so the person becomes symptomatic. Most of the clients like this one are also taking beta-blockers, which also prevent the heart rate from increasing when the BP drops.

In a clinical situation such as this one, the response of vital signs to exercise must be monitored carefully and charted. Any unusual symptoms, such as muscle cramping, headaches, and any irregular pulse patterns, must also be reported and documented.

Right Ventricular Failure

Failure of the right ventricle may occur in response to left-sided CHF or as a result of pulmonary embolism (see cor pulmonale in Chapter 8). Right ventricular failure results in peripheral edema and venous congestion of the organs.

For example, as the liver becomes congested with venous blood, it becomes enlarged and abdominal pain occurs. If this occurs rapidly, stretching of the capsule surrounding the liver causes severe discomfort. The client may notice either a constant aching or a sharp pain in the right upper quadrant.

Dependent edema is one of the early signs of right ventricular failure. Edema is usually symmetric and occurs in the dependent parts of the body, where venous pressure is the highest. In ambulatory individuals, edema begins in the feet and ankles and ascends the lower legs. It is most noticeable at the end of a day and often decreases after a night's rest.

Many people experiencing this type of edema assume that it is a normal sign of aging and fail to report it to their physician. In the recumbent person, pitting edema may develop in the presacral area and, as it worsens, progress to the genital area and medial thighs (Case Example 7.4).

Cyanosis of the nail beds appears as venous congestion reduces peripheral blood flow. Clients with CHF often feel anxious, frightened, and depressed. Fears may be expressed as frightening nightmares, insomnia, acute anxiety states, depression, or withdrawal from reality.

CLINICAL SIGNS AND SYMPTOMS
Right-Sided Heart Failure

- Increased fatigue
- Dependent edema (usually beginning in the ankles)
- Pitting edema (after 5 to 10 lbs of edema accumulate)
- Edema in the sacral area or the back of the thighs
- Right upper quadrant pain
- Cyanosis of nail beds

Functional Heart Failure

Heart failure can also be classified as Functional HF and is considered to be due to either systolic or diastolic dysfunction of the left ventricle. It is referred to as HF with reduced ejection fraction (HFrEF) or HF with preserved ejection fraction (HFpEF). Ejection fraction is the percentage of blood in the filled left ventricle that is pumped out during a contraction.

CASE EXAMPLE 7.4
Congestive Heart Failure—Bilateral Pitting Edema

A 65-year-old man came to the clinic with a referral from his family doctor for "hip pain—evaluate and treat." Past medical history included three total hip replacements of the right hip, open heart surgery 6 years ago, and persistent hypertension currently being treated with beta-blockers.

During the interview, it was discovered that the client had experienced many bouts of hip pain, leg weakness, and loss of hip motion. He was not actually examined by his doctor, but had contacted the physician's office by phone, requesting a new physical therapy referral.

During examination, large adhesed scars were noted along the anterior, lateral, and posterior aspects of the right hip, with significant bilateral hip flexion contractures. Pitting edema was noted in the right ankle, with mild swelling also observed around the left ankle. The client was unaware of this swelling. Further questions were negative for shortness of breath, difficulty in sleeping, cough, or other symptoms of cardiopulmonary involvement.

The bilateral edema could have been from compromise of the lymphatic drainage system following the multiple surgeries and adhesive scarring. However, with the positive history for cardiovascular involvement, bilateral edema, and telephone-derived referral, the physician was contacted by phone to notify him of the edema, and the client was directed by the physician to make an appointment.

The client was diagnosed in the early stages of congestive heart failure (CHF). Physical therapy to address the appropriate hip musculoskeletal problems was continued.

Systolic dysfunction in HFrEF refers to a decrease in myocardial contractility characterized by compromised contractility of the ventricles, resulting in reductions in ejection fraction, stroke volume, and cardiac output.[49] Typically, patients with systolic dysfunction present with a compromised left ventricular ejection fraction (LVEF) less than 40%.[50]

Diastolic dysfunction, also known as HFpEF, is characterized by compromised diastolic function of the ventricles.[51] In patients with HFpEF, the ventricles cannot fill adequately during the relaxation (diastolic) phase of the cardiac cycle. This impairs ventricular filling (reduced end diastolic volume [EDV]) thus decreasing the volume of blood ejected with each contraction (stroke volume) and the overall volume of blood ejected per minute (cardiac output).[51] With HFpEF, LVEF is unaltered and remains between 55% and 75%.[51]

Diastolic Heart Failure or HFpEF

Diastolic heart failure describes a condition in which the left ventricle stiffens and hypertrophies. Open space inside the ventricle can become restricted by the thickened ventricle walls. The stiff heart muscle loses some of its flexibility. During diastole (when the muscle fibers relax and stretch), the chambers of the heart expand and fill with blood. Restrictions from a bulky heart muscle caused by overwork or other causes make it more difficult for the muscle to relax between beats and thus unable to fill completely. This is different from systolic heart failure (HFrEF) in which the left ventricle becomes weak and flabby. Both types of heart failure have the same end result: loss of blood supply (and oxygen) to the organs and tissues.

Risk factors for diastolic HF include advancing age, high BP, CAD (atherosclerosis), cardiac muscle damage from a previous heart attack, and valve dysfunction. Other medical conditions, such as diabetes, anemia, and thyroid disease, can also increase the risk of developing diastolic HF.

Physical therapists working with patients with HF are referred to the Clinical Practice Guideline for the management of patients with HF.[52]

CLINICAL SIGNS AND SYMPTOMS
Diastolic Heart Failure

- Fatigue and dyspnea after mild physical exertion or exercise
- Orthopnea (dyspnea when lying down; person must be in the upright position to breathe)
- Edema (especially of the legs and ankles) and weight gain
- Jugular vein distention (see Fig. 4.44)

Aneurysm[53]

An aneurysm is an abnormal dilation (commonly a sac-like formation) in the wall of an artery, vein, or the heart. Aneurysms occur when the vessel or heart wall becomes weakened from trauma, congenital vascular disease, infection, or atherosclerosis. This section could also be discussed under PVDs because aneurysms of arterial blood vessels can result in some form of PVD.

Aneurysms fall under the broader category of *thoracic-aortic disease*, including aortic aneurysm and aortic dissection. Aneurysms can also be designated either venous or arterial and described according to the specific vessel in which they develop. *Thoracic aneurysms* usually involve the ascending, transverse, or descending portion of the aorta from the heart to the top of the diaphragm; *abdominal aneurysms* generally involve the aorta below the diaphragm, between the renal arteries and the iliac branches; *peripheral arterial aneurysms* affect the femoral and popliteal arteries.[53]

Thoracic and Peripheral Arterial Aneurysms

A dissecting aneurysm (most often a thoracic aneurysm) occurs when a tear develops in the inner lining of the aortic wall. The inner and outer layers peel apart, creating an extra channel or "false vessel." Small tears may do no harm but aneurysms divert blood from organs and tissues, and can result in heart attack, stroke, or kidney damage. Thoracic aneurysms occur most frequently in hypertensive men between the ages of 40 and 70 years. Marked elevation of BP may facilitate rapid disruption and final rupture (a break in all three layers of the aortic wall) when a small tear in the intima has occurred. Following a rupture, massive internal hemorrhage occurs as blood flows from the aorta into the chest.

The most common site for peripheral arterial aneurysms is the popliteal space in the lower extremities. Popliteal aneurysms cause ischemic symptoms in the lower limbs and an easily palpable pulse of larger amplitude. An enlarged area behind the knee may be present, seldom with discomfort.

Abdominal Aortic Aneurysms

An aneurysm is an abnormal dilation in a weak or diseased arterial wall causing a sac-like protrusion. Aneurysms can occur anywhere in any blood vessel, but the two most common places are the aorta and cerebral vascular system. The aneurysm may be dissecting, which means a tear has occurred between two layers of the intima and blood is flowing between these two layers rather than through the lumen.

Abdominal aortic aneurysms (AAAs) occur about four times more often than thoracic aneurysms. The natural course of an untreated AAA is expansion and rupture in one of several places, including the peritoneal cavity, the mesentery, behind the peritoneum, into the inferior vena cava, or into the duodenum or rectum.

The most common site for an AAA is just below the kidney (immediately below the takeoff of the renal arteries), with referred pain to the thoracolumbar junction (see Fig. 7.11). Aneurysms can be caused by:

Trauma/weight lifting (aging athletes)
Congenital vascular disease
Infection
Atherosclerosis

Risk Factors

The therapist should look for a history of smoking,[54–56] known congenital heart disease (e.g., bicuspid aortic valve), surgery to replace or repair an aortic valve before age 70 years, recent infection, diagnosis of CAD (atherosclerosis), and some genetic conditions such as Marfan syndrome, Loeys-Dietz syndrome, Turner syndrome, or vascular Ehlers-Danlos syndrome. Many seniors are keeping active and fit by participating in activities at the gym, at home, or elsewhere that involve lifting weights. There is an increased risk of aneurysm in older adults, especially for these active clients. AAAs can be exacerbated by anticoagulant therapy (another risk factor).

The therapist may be prescribing progressive resistive exercises that can have an adverse effect in an older adult with any of these etiologies (Case Example 7.5). Monitoring vital signs is important among exercising older adults. Ideally, physical therapists should take a baseline of vital signs before activity begins to evaluate the stability of the patient. Vital signs should then be reevaluated with activity to determine the patient's response to activity or exercise. Teaching proper breathing and abdominal support without using a Valsalva maneuver is important in any exercise program, but especially for those clients at increased risk for aortic aneurysm.

The U.S. Preventive Services Task Force now recommends one-time ultrasonographic (US) screening for abdominal aortic aneurysm for men ages 65 to 75 years who presently smoke or who have smoked in the past.[58] Guidelines also suggest a US screening for males with significant family history and are over 50 years. The recommendation for females is weak but is present for those over 65 years of age with multiple risk factors, smokers, or those with a significant family history.[59]

CASE EXAMPLE 7.5
Abdominal Aortic Aneurysm—Weight Lifting

A 72-year-old retired farmer has come to the physical therapist for recommendations about weight lifting. He had been following a regular program of weight lifting for almost 30 years, using a set of free weights purchased at a garage sale.

One year ago he experienced an abdominal aortic aneurysm that ruptured and required surgery. Symptoms at the time of diagnosis were back pain at the thoracolumbar junction radiating outward toward the flanks bilaterally. The client is symptom-free and in apparent good health, taking no medications, and receiving no medical treatment at this time.

What are your recommendations for resuming his weight lifting program?

The hemodynamic stresses of weight lifting involve a rapid increase in systemic arterial BP without a decrease in total peripheral vascular resistance. This principle combined with aortic degeneration may have contributed to the aortic dissection.[57]

Weight lifting in anyone with a history of aortic aneurysm is considered a contraindication. The therapist suggested a conditioning program, combining a walking/biking program with resistive exercises using a lightweight elastic band alternating with an aquatic program for cardiac clients. Given this client's history, a medical evaluation before initiating an exercise program is necessary.

Clients who have had orthopedic surgery involving anterior spinal procedures of any kind (e.g., spinal fusion, spinal fusion with cages, artificial disk replacement) are at risk for trauma to the aorta (rather than aortic aneurysm) from damage to blood vessels moved out of the way during surgery. Internal bleeding can result in a distended abdomen, changes in BP, changes in stool (e.g., melena, bloody diarrhea), and possible back and/or shoulder pain.

Clinical Signs and Symptoms

Most AAAs are asymptomatic;[60] discovery occurs during physical or radiographic examination of the abdomen or lower spine for some other reason.[61]

The most common symptom is awareness of a pulsating mass in the abdomen, with or without pain, followed by abdominal pain and back pain. The therapist is most likely to observe rapid onset of severe neck or back pain (Case Example 7.6).

The client may report feeling a heartbeat in the abdomen or stomach when lying down. Back pain may be the only presenting feature. Groin (scrotal), buttock, and/or flank pain may be experienced because of increasing pressure on other structures.

The pain is usually described as sharp, intense, severe, or knife-like in the abdomen, chest, or anywhere in the back (including the sacrum). Pain may radiate to the chest, neck, between the scapulae, or the posterior thighs.

The location of the symptoms is determined by the location of the aneurysm. Most aortic aneurysms (95%) occur just below the renal arteries. Extreme pain described as "tearing" or "ripping" may be felt at the base of the neck along the back, particularly in the interscapular area, while dissection proceeds over the aortic arch and into the descending aorta. Symptoms are not relieved by a change in position.

CASE EXAMPLE 7.6

Abdominal Aortic Aneurysm—Hip Replacement

A therapist was ambulating with a 76-year-old woman post hip arthroplasty in an acute care (hospital) setting. The patient complained of back pain with every step and asked to sit down. The pain went away when she sat down. Once she started walking again, the pain started again.

She asked the therapist to walk her to the bathroom. After helping her onto the toilet, the therapist waited as a standby assist outside the bathroom. When several minutes went by with no call or sound, the therapist knocked on the door. There was no response. The therapist repeated knocking and calling the patient's name.

Upon opening the bathroom door, the therapist found the patient slumped over on the toilet. Emergency help was summoned immediately. She was later diagnosed with an abdominal aortic aneurysm.

What are the red flags in this scenario?

Age

Pain with activity that is relieved with rest

Vital signs should be taken in a case of this type after the first complaint of pain with activity.

The physical therapist can palpate the width of the arterial pulses; these pulses (e.g., aortic, femoral) should be uniform in width from the midline outward on either side (see Fig. 4.54). The normal aortic pulse width is between 2.5 and 4.0 cm (some sources say the width must be no more than 3.0 cm; others list 4.0 cm). Average pulse width is 2.5 cm or about 1.2 inches wide.[62,63]

According to the longitudinal community-based Framingham Heart Study, aortic root diameter increases with age in both men and women but is larger in men at any given age. Each 10-year increase in age is associated with a larger aortic root (by 0.89 mm in men and 0.68 mm in women) after adjustment for body size and BP. A 5-kg/m² increase in body mass index (BMI) was associated with a larger aortic root (by 0.78 mm in men and 0.51 mm in women) after adjustment for age and BP. Each 10-mm Hg increase in pulse pressure is related to age-related increase in stiffness and resultant increase in aortic pressure[64,65] and a smaller aortic root (by 0.19 mm in men and 0.08 mm in women) after adjustment for age and body size.[66] Cadaver studies also show significant reduction in tensile strength and stretch after the age of 30 years.[67]

As the aorta increases in diameter from an expanding aneurysm, the pulse width expands as well. The sensitivity of detection with abdominal palpation increases with the increasing diameter and has been reported as high as 82% with a diameter of 5 cm or more.[68] Sensitivity and specificity for detecting an abdominal aortic aneurysm with palpation have been reported as 28% and 97%, respectively, for a definite pulsatile mass.[69] The risk of rupture approaches 25% for AAAs that are 6.0 cm (2.4 inches).[62]

Palpation is followed by auscultation for bruits (abnormal blowing or swishing sounds heard during auscultation of the arteries). Sensitivity for femoral bruit as a screening tool for detecting an abdominal aortic aneurysm has been reported as 17%, with specificity of 87%. Abdominal bruit has an 11% sensitivity and 95% specificity.[69] Without a careful assessment, smaller diameter aneurysms may escape clinical detection.[70]

The abdominal aorta passes posterior to the diaphragm (aortic hiatus) at the level of the T12 vertebral body and bifurcates at the level of the L4 vertebral body to form the right and left common iliac arteries. Watch for a widening of the pulse width before reaching the umbilicus. The pulse width expands normally at the aortic bifurcation, usually observed just below the umbilicus. Ninety-five percent of all AAAs occur just below the renal arteries.

Systolic BP below 100 mm Hg and a pulse rate over 100 beats per minute may indicate signs of shock. Other symptoms may include ecchymoses in the flank and perianal area; severe and sudden pain in the abdomen, paravertebral area, or flank; and light-headedness and nausea with sudden hypotension.

The therapist may observe cold, pulseless lower extremities and/or BP differences (more than 10 mm Hg) between the arms. Consistent with the model for a screening examination, the therapist must look for screening clues in the history, pain patterns, and associated signs and symptoms. Knowledge of the clinical signs and symptoms of impending rupture or actual rupture of the aortic aneurysm is important.

If a client (usually a postoperative inpatient) has internal bleeding (rather than an aneurysm) from complications of anterior spinal surgery the therapist may note:

- Distended abdomen
- Changes in BP
- Changes in stool
- Possible back and/or shoulder pain

The client's recent history of anterior spinal surgery accompanied by any of these symptoms is enough to notify nursing or medical staff of these observations. Monitoring postoperative vital signs in these clients is essential.

CLINICAL SIGNS AND SYMPTOMS
Aneurysm

Chest pain with any of the following:
- Palpable, pulsating mass (abdomen, popliteal space)
- Abdominal "heartbeat" felt by the client when lying down
- Dull ache in the midabdominal left flank or low back
- Hip, groin, scrotal (men), buttock, and/or leg pain (posterior thigh)
  Weakness or transient paralysis of legs

Ruptured Aneurysm
- Sudden, severe chest pain with a tearing sensation (see Fig. 7.10)
- Pain may extend to the neck, shoulders, between the scapulae, low back, or abdomen; pain radiating to the posterior thighs helps distinguish it from an MI
- Pain is not relieved by a change in position
- Pain may be described as "tearing" or "ripping"
- Pulsating abdominal mass
- Other signs: cold, pulseless lower extremities, BP changes (more than 10 mm Hg difference in diastolic BP between arms; systolic BP less than 100 mm Hg)
- Pulse rate more than 100 bpm
- Ecchymoses in the flank and perianal area
- Light-headedness and nausea

Conditions Affecting the Heart Valves

The second category of heart problems includes those that occur secondary to impairment of the valves caused by disease (e.g., rheumatic fever or coronary thrombosis), congenital deformity, or infection such as endocarditis. Three types of valve deformities may affect aortic, mitral, tricuspid, or pulmonic valves: *stenosis, insufficiency*, or *prolapse*.

Stenosis is a narrowing or constriction that prevents the valve from opening fully, and may be caused by growths, scars, or abnormal deposits on the leaflets. *Insufficiency* (also referred to as *regurgitation*) occurs when the valve does not close properly and causes blood to flow back into the heart chamber. *Prolapse* affects only the mitral valve and occurs when enlarged valve leaflets bulge backward into the left atrium.

These valve conditions increase the workload of the heart and require the heart to pump harder to force blood through a stenosed valve or to maintain adequate flow if blood is seeping back. Further complications for individuals with a malfunctioning valve may occur secondary to a bacterial infection of the valves (endocarditis).

Persons affected by diseases of the heart valves may be asymptomatic, and extensive auscultation with a stethoscope and diagnostic study may be required to differentiate one condition from another. In its early symptomatic stages cardiac valvular disease causes the person to become fatigued easily. As stenosis or insufficiency progresses, the main symptom of HF (breathlessness or dyspnea) appears.

CLINICAL SIGNS AND SYMPTOMS
Cardiac Valvular Disease

- Easy fatigue
- Dyspnea
- Palpitation (subjective sensation of throbbing, skipping, rapid or forcible pulsation of the heart)
- Chest pain
- Pitting edema
- Orthopnea or paroxysmal dyspnea
- Dizziness and syncope (episodes of fainting or loss of consciousness)

Rheumatic Fever

Rheumatic fever is an infection caused by streptococcal bacteria that can be fatal or may lead to rheumatic heart disease, a chronic condition caused by scarring and deformity of the heart valves. It is called rheumatic fever because two of the most common symptoms are fever and joint pain.

The infection generally starts with strep throat in children between the ages of 5 and 15 years, and damages the heart in approximately 50% of cases. Rheumatic fever produces a diffuse, proliferative, and exudative inflammatory process.

The aggressive use of specific antibiotics in the United States had effectively removed rheumatic fever as the primary cause of valvular damage. However, in 1985 a series of epidemics of rheumatic fever occurred in several widely diverse geographic regions of the continental United States. Currently, the prevalence and incidence of cases have not approximated the 1985 record, but they have remained above baseline levels.[71]

Clinical Signs and Symptoms

The most typical clinical profile of a child or young adult with acute rheumatic fever is an initial cold or sore throat, followed 2 or 3 weeks later by a sudden or gradual onset of painful migratory joint symptoms in the knees, shoulders, feet, ankles, elbows, fingers, or neck. Fever of 37.2° C to 39.4° C (99° F to 103° F), palpitations, and fatigue are also present. Malaise, weakness, weight loss, and anorexia may accompany the fever.

The migratory arthralgias may last only 24 hours, or they may persist for several weeks. Joints that are sore, hot, and contain fluid completely resolve, followed by acute synovitis, heat, synovial space tenderness, swelling, and effusion present in a different area the next day. The persistence of swelling, heat, and synovitis in a single joint or joints for more than 2 to 3 weeks is extremely unusual in acute rheumatic fever.

In the acute full-blown sequelae, shortness of breath and increasing nocturnal cough will also occur. A rash on the skin of the limbs or trunk is present in fewer than 2% of clients with acute rheumatic fever. Subcutaneous nodules over the extensor surfaces of the arms, heels, knees, or back of the head may occur.

All layers of the heart (epicardium, endocardium, myocardium, and pericardium) may be involved, and the heart valves are affected by this inflammatory reaction. The most characteristic and potentially dangerous anatomic lesion of rheumatic inflammation is the gross effect on cardiac valves, most commonly the mitral and aortic valves. If untreated, as many as 25% of clients will have mitral valvular disease 25 to 30 years later.

Rheumatic chorea (also called chorea or St. Vitus' dance) may occur 1 to 3 months after the strep infection, and is always noted after polyarthritis. Chorea in a child, teenager, or young adult is almost always a manifestation of acute rheumatic fever. Other uncommon causes of chorea are systemic lupus erythematosus (SLE), thyrotoxicosis, and cerebrovascular accident (CVA), but these are unlikely in a child.

The client develops rapid, purposeless, nonrepetitive movements that may involve all muscles except the eyes. This chorea may last for 1 week, several months or several years without permanent impairment of the central nervous system.

Initial episodes of rheumatic fever last months in children and weeks in adults. Twenty percent of children have recurrences within 5 years. Recurrences are uncommon after 5 years of good health and are rare after 21 years of age.

CLINICAL SIGNS AND SYMPTOMS
Rheumatic Fever

- Migratory arthralgia
- Subcutaneous nodules on extensor surfaces
- Fever and sore throat
- Flat, painless skin rash (short duration)
- Carditis
- Chorea
- Weakness, malaise, weight loss, and anorexia
- Acquired valvular disease

Endocarditis

Bacterial endocarditis, another common heart infection, causes inflammation of the cardiac endothelium (layer of cells lining the cavities of the heart) and damages the tricuspid, aortic, or mitral valve.

This infection may be caused by bacteria entering the bloodstream from a remote part of the body (e.g., skin infection, oral cavity), or it may occur as a result of abnormal

growths on the closure lines of previously damaged or artificial valves. These growths called *vegetations* consist of collagen fibers and may separate from the valve, embolize, and cause infarction in the myocardium, kidney, brain, spleen, abdomen, or extremities.

Risk Factors

In addition to clients with previous valvular damage, injection drug users and postcardiac surgical clients are at high risk for developing endocarditis. Congenital heart disease and degenerative heart disease, such as calcific aortic stenosis, may also cause bacterial endocarditis. The prosthetic cardiac valve (valve replacement) has become more important as a predisposing factor for endocarditis because cardiac surgery is performed on a much larger scale than in the past.

This infection is often the consequence of invasive diagnostic procedures, such as renal shunts and urinary catheters, long-term indwelling catheters, or dental treatment (because of the increased opportunities for normal oral microorganisms to gain entrance to the circulatory system by way of highly vascularized oral structures). Susceptible individuals may take antibiotics as a precaution before undergoing any of these procedures.

Clinical Signs and Symptoms

A significant number of clients (up to 45%) with bacterial endocarditis initially have musculoskeletal symptoms, including arthralgia, arthritis, low back pain, and myalgia. Half of these clients will have only musculoskeletal symptoms without other signs of endocarditis.

The early onset of joint pain and myalgia is more likely if the client is older and has had a previously diagnosed heart murmur. Musculoskeletal problems make up a significant part of the clinical picture of infective endocarditis diagnosed in an injection drug user.

The most common musculoskeletal symptom in clients with bacterial endocarditis is *arthralgia*, generally in the proximal joints. The shoulder is the most commonly affected site, followed (in declining incidence) by the knee, hip, wrist, ankle, metatarsophalangeal, and metacarpophalangeal joints, and acromioclavicular joints.

Most endocarditis clients with arthralgias have only one or two painful joints, although some may have pain in several joints. Painful symptoms begin suddenly in one or two joints, accompanied by warmth, tenderness, and redness. Symmetric arthralgia in the knees or ankles may lead to a diagnosis of rheumatoid arthritis. One helpful clue: as a rule, morning stiffness is not as prevalent in clients with endocarditis as in those with rheumatoid arthritis or polymyalgia rheumatica.

Osteoarticular infections are diagnosed infrequently and most commonly in association with injection drug use. Most commonly affected sites include the vertebrae, the wrist, the sternoclavicular joints, and the sacroiliac joints.[72,73]

Endocarditis may produce destructive changes in the *sacroiliac joint*, probably as a result of seeding the joint by septic emboli. The pain will be localized over the sacroiliac joint, and the physician will use radiographs and bone scans to verify this diagnosis.

Almost one-third of clients with bacterial endocarditis have *low back pain;* in many clients it is the principal musculoskeletal symptom reported. Back pain is accompanied by decreased range of motion (ROM) and spinal tenderness. Pain may affect only one side, and it may be limited to the paraspinal muscles.

Endocarditis-induced low back pain may be very similar to that associated with a herniated lumbar disk; it radiates to the leg and may be accentuated by raising the leg or by sneezing. The key difference is that neurologic deficits are usually absent in clients with bacterial endocarditis.

Widespread diffuse *myalgias* may occur during periods of fever, but these are not appreciably different from the general myalgia seen in clients with other febrile illnesses. More commonly, myalgia will be restricted to the calf or thigh. Bilateral or unilateral leg myalgias occur in approximately 10% to 15% of all clients with bacterial endocarditis.

The cause of back pain and leg myalgia associated with bacterial endocarditis has not been determined. Some suggest that concurrent aseptic meningitis may contribute to both leg and back pain. Others suggest that leg pain is related to emboli that break off from the infected cardiac valves. The latter theory is supported by biopsy evidence of muscle necrosis or vasculitis in clients with bacterial endocarditis.

Rarely, other musculoskeletal symptoms, such as osteomyelitis, nail clubbing, tendinitis, hypertrophic osteoarthropathy, bone infarcts, and ischemic bone necrosis may occur.

CLINICAL SIGNS AND SYMPTOMS
Endocarditis

- Arthralgia
- Arthritis
- Musculoskeletal symptoms
- Low back/sacroiliac pain
- Myalgia
- Petechiae/splinter hemorrhage
- Constitutional symptoms
- Dyspnea, chest pain
- Cold and pain in the extremities

Lupus Carditis

SLE is a multisystem clinical illness associated with the release of a broad spectrum of autoantibodies into the circulation (see Chapter 13). The inflammatory process mediated by the immune response can target the heart and vasculature of the client with SLE.

Except for pericarditis, clinically significant cardiac disease directly associated with SLE is relatively infrequent, but because of the musculoskeletal involvement, it may be of major importance for the therapist. Primary lupus cardiac involvement may include pericarditis, myocarditis, endocarditis, or a combination of the three.

Pericarditis is the most common cardiac lesion associated with SLE, appearing with the characteristic substernal chest pain that varies with posture, becoming worse in recumbency and improving with sitting or bending forward. *Myocarditis* may occur and is strongly associated with skeletal myositis in SLE.

Congenital Valvular Defects

Congenital malformations of the heart occur in approximately 1 of every 100 infants (1%) born in the United States.[74] The most common defects include (Fig. 7.6):

- Ventricular or atrial septal defect (hole between the ventricles or atria)
- Tetralogy of Fallot (combination of four defects)
- Patent ductus arteriosus (shunt caused by an opening between the aorta and the pulmonary artery)
- Congenital stenosis of the pulmonary, aortic, and tricuspid valves

These congenital defects require surgical correction and may be a part of the client's past medical history. They are not conditions that are likely to mimic musculoskeletal lesions and are therefore not covered in detail in this text.

Congenital cardiovascular abnormalities, which are usually asymptomatic and often undiagnosed during life, are the main cause of sudden death in athletes. Aortic stenosis, hypertrophic cardiomyopathy, Marfan syndrome, congenital coronary artery anomalies, and ruptured aorta are the most commonly reported causes of sudden death during the practice of a sports activity.[75,76]

Family history of any of these conditions, premature sudden unexpected syncope, or family member death is an indication for a thorough cardiovascular evaluation of the athlete before participation in sports.[77]

Mitral Valve Prolapse

Echocardiographic studies have advanced our knowledge of MVP in the last two decades. A more precise definition of MVP has resulted in a more accurate estimate of the prevalence rate (2% to 3%).[78-80] This is equally distributed between men and women,[81,82] although men seem to have a higher incidence of complications.

MVP is characterized by mitral leaflet thickness with increased extensibility, decreased stiffness, and decreased strength compared with normal valves. This structural variation has many other names, including floppy valve syndrome, Barlow's syndrome, and click-murmur syndrome.

MVP appears to be caused by connective tissue abnormalities in the valve leaflets or response to abnormalities in left ventricular cavity geometry.[78] Normally, when the lower part of the heart contracts, the mitral valve remains firm and allows no blood to leak back into the upper chambers. In MVP the structural changes in the mitral valve allow one part of the valve, the leaflet, to billow back into the upper chamber during contraction of the ventricle.

One or both of the valve leaflets may bulge into the left atrium during ventricular systole. This protrusion can often

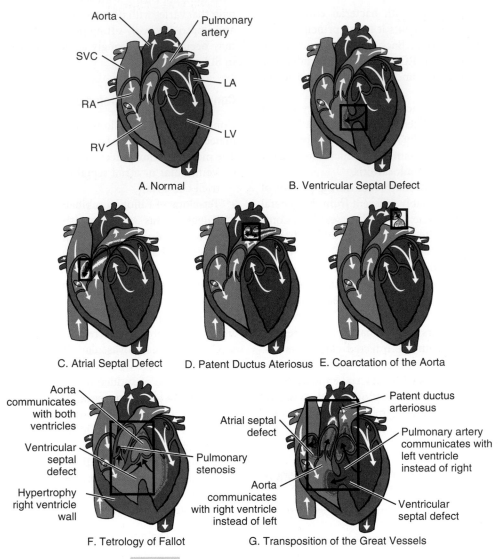

Aorta
Pulmonary artery
SVC
LA
RA
LV
RV

A. Normal

B. Ventricular Septal Defect

C. Atrial Septal Defect

D. Patent Ductus Ateriosus

E. Coarctation of the Aorta

Aorta communicates with both ventricles
Ventricular septal defect
Hypertrophy right ventricle wall
Pulmonary stenosis

F. Tetrology of Fallot

Atrial septal defect
Aorta communicates with right ventricle instead of left

Patent ductus arteriosus
Pulmonary artery communicates with left ventricle instead of right
Ventricular septal defect

G. Transposition of the Great Vessels

Fig. 7.6 Congenital malformations of the heart.

be heard through a stethoscope as a sound known as a "click." Leaking of blood backward through the mitral valve can also be heard and is referred to as a heart murmur.

Risk Factors

MVP is a benign condition in isolation; however, it can be associated with many other conditions, especially the heritable connective tissue disorders such as Ehlers-Danlos syndrome, Marfan syndrome, and osteogenesis imperfecta. Other risk factors include endocarditis, myocarditis, atherosclerosis, SLE, muscular dystrophy, acromegaly, and cardiac sarcoidosis.

Clinical Signs and Symptoms

Two-thirds of the individuals with MVP experience no symptoms. Approximately one-third experience occasional symptoms that are mild to moderately uncomfortable—enough to interfere with the person's ability to enjoy an unrestricted life. Only about 1% suffer severe symptoms and lifestyle restrictions.

Almost all symptoms of MVP syndrome are a result of an imbalance in the autonomic nervous system (ANS), called *dysautonomia*. Frequently, when there is a slight variation in the structure of the heart valve, there is also a slight variation in the function or balance of the ANS.[78] This description in the autonomic innervation of the heart may account for the high incidence of MVP in fibromyalgia, a condition known to be associated with dysregulation or dysautonomia of the ANS.

Symptoms include profound fatigue that cannot be correlated with exercise or stress, cold hands and feet, shortness of breath, chest pain, and heart palpitations. The most common triad of symptoms associated with MVP is fatigue, palpitations, and dyspnea (Fig. 7.7). Frequently occurring

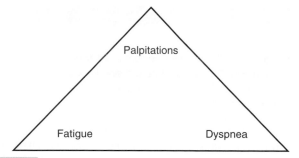

Fig. 7.7 The triad of symptoms associated with mitral valve prolapse.

CLINICAL SIGNS AND SYMPTOMS
Mitral Valve Prolapse

- Profound fatigue; low exercise tolerance
- Chest pain; arm, back, or shoulder discomfort
- Palpitations or irregular heartbeat
- Tachycardia
- Migraine headache
- Anxiety, depression, panic attacks
- Dyspnea

musculoskeletal findings in clients with MVP include joint hypermobility, temporomandibular joint (TMJ) syndrome, and myalgias.

Although the fatigue that accompanies MVP is not related to exertion, deconditioning from prolonged inactivity may develop, further complicating the picture. Chest pain associated with MVP can be severe, but it differs from pain associated with MI (see Table 7.5). When there is an imbalance in the ANS, which controls contraction and relaxation of the chest wall muscles (the muscles of breathing), there may be inadequate relaxation between respirations. Over time these chest wall muscles go into spasm, resulting in chest pain.

The therapist should evaluate the client with chest pain for trigger points. If palpation of the chest reproduces symptoms, especially radiating pain, deactivation of trigger points must be carried out followed by a reevaluation as a part of the screening process for pain of cardiac origin.

MVP is not life-threatening but may be lifestyle threatening for the small number of persons (rare) who have more severe structural problems that may progress to the point at which surgical replacement of the valve is required. Sudden death is a recognized risk for cases of severe mitral regurgitation. To prevent infective endocarditis, the client may be given antibiotics prophylactically before any invasive procedures.

MVP is included in this section because of its increasing prevalence in the physical therapy client population. At presentation, usually, the client with MVP has some other unrelated primary (musculoskeletal) diagnosis. During physical therapy intervention, the symptomatic MVP client may experience symptoms associated with MVP and require assurance or education regarding exercise and MVP.

Most individuals with MVP do not have to restrict their activity level or lifestyle; regular exercise is encouraged. Clients with mitral regurgitation (backward flow of blood into the left atrium) during exercise, but not at rest, have a higher rate of complications, such as HF, syncope, and progressive mitral regurgitation, requiring further medical treatment.[78]

Monitoring vital signs and observing or asking about additional signs and symptoms is important. Caution is advised in the use of weight training for the MVP client. Gradual buildup using light weights and increased repetitions is recommended.

Conditions Affecting the Cardiac Nervous System

The third component of cardiac disease is caused by failure of the heart's nervous system to conduct normal electrical impulses. The heart has an intrinsic conduction system that allows the orderly depolarization of cardiac muscle tissue. Arrhythmias, also called *dysrhythmias*, are disorders of the heart rate and rhythm caused by disturbances in the conduction system.

Arrhythmias may cause the heart to beat too quickly (tachycardia), too slowly (bradycardia), or with extra beats and fibrillations. Arrhythmias can lead to dramatic changes in circulatory dynamics such as hypotension, HF, and shock.

Clients who are neurologically unstable owing to recent CVA, head trauma, spinal cord injury, or a central nervous system insult often exhibit new arrhythmias during the period of instability (Case Example 7.7). These may be as a result of the elevation of intracranial pressure, and once this has been controlled and returned to a normal range, arrhythmias usually disappear.

Arrhythmias may also be triggered by environmental factors, abnormal thyroid function, and some medications. Clients who have preexisting arrhythmias, CAD, or HF, may progress from "transient arrhythmias" to arrhythmias that do not disappear, with the potential for serious complications. Dizziness and loss of consciousness may occur when the arrhythmia results in a serious reduction in cardiac output, owing to loss of brain perfusion (not caused by a transient ischemic attack, as is often suspected).

The therapist should monitor the patient's pulse carefully before, during, and after exercise when working with any client who has had a stroke. Any pulse irregularities not already documented should be reported to the physician immediately and an ECG should be done to determine the nature of the irregularity.

The therapist may be the first health care professional to identify an arrhythmia that appears during exercise. For this reason, the therapist is reminded to obtain a baseline resting set of vital signs to use as a comparison to when the patient performs exercise or activities. In the early recovery period, the therapist should monitor for these arrhythmias by taking the client's pulse. Arrhythmias should be reported to the physician (Case Example 7.8).

CASE EXAMPLE 7.7

Cardiac Arrhythmia Cause of Transient Muscle Weakness

Referral: An 87-year-old man was admitted to a skilled nursing facility for short-term rehabilitation.

Goal: Safely and independently navigate home environment on level surfaces and stairs with discharge to home within 2 to 3 months.

Medical Diagnosis: Mild left hemiparesis secondary to recent cerebrovascular accident (CVA).

Past Medical History: Urosepsis, seizure disorder, deep venous thrombosis (DVT), hypertension (HTN), congestive heart failure (CHF), myocardial infarction (MI), frequent falls, subdural hematoma with evacuation.

Medications: Heparin (anticoagulant, antithrombotic), Lasix (diuretic for hypertension), Os-Cal (antacid, calcium supplement).

Systems Review

Integument: Well-healed scar on head, postsurgical evacuation of subdural hematoma.

Musculoskeletal: Head position in sitting and standing is held in approximately 30 degrees of lateral and forward flexion; full active head and neck range of motion (ROM) present; overall flexed/stooped posture (left more than right); muscle strength in right trunk and right upper extremity: 4–/5; muscle strength in left trunk and left lower extremity: 3–/5.

Neuromuscular: Neurologic screening results consistent with upper motor neuron lesion; Nonambulatory and requires moderate assistance for bed mobility and transfers; able to sit, stand, and walk with assistance of two and the use of a walker; patellar deep tendon reflexes (DTRs): right: within normal limits; left: + 3; positive Babinski response on the left

Cardiovascular/Pulmonary: Blood pressure: 142/80 mm Hg, measured in right upper extremity, sitting; pulse rate: 72 bpm; respiratory rate: 18 breaths per minute; pulse oximeter (oxygen saturation): 97%

First Progress Report: Client made many functional gains during the first 4 weeks of rehab and was planning a trip home for 2 days but experienced multiple falls with several incidences of lacerations to the head requiring stitches.

Client also presented with multiple episodes of transient generalized weakness, increased postural instability, and increased bradykinesia. Episodes of weakness and falling were without warning and unrelated to activity but interfering with progress toward functional independence and discharge plans.

Vital signs: Radial and apical heart rate 72 bpm with periodic and variable drops in heart rate to below 60 bpm with a low measurement of 37 bpm. Episodes of bradycardia lasted from 1 minute to 1 hour. Blood pressure fluctuated from 150/83 mm Hg to 92/40 mm Hg. Respiratory rate remained stable. Pulse oximetry levels varied from 91% to 97% with an occasional drop to 88% during transient episodes of weakness.

There was no complaint of nor apparent shortness of breath, no complaint of dizziness, and no complaint of syncope.

Referral: Client was referred to his primary physician with report of increasingly frequent periods of generalized muscle weakness with poor postural stability (cause unknown). Vital signs were reported.

Physician ruled out dehydration, renal insufficiency, anemia, and active bleeding as possible pathologies. Electrocardiogram (ECG) was obtained. He was eventually hospitalized and diagnosed with episodic bradycardia.

The client returned to the skilled nursing facility and continued to have multiple intermittent episodes of transient weakness and postural instability lasting from several minutes to several hours, affecting his progress toward independent functional mobility.

Second Progress Report: With each episode, vital signs were obtained. A significant drop in radial pulse was noted, along with decreased apical heart rate. This appeared to be the most significant finding. Blood pressure dropped during these incidents; however, it did not drop dangerously low, except during several occurrences (82/40 mm Hg); respiratory rate appeared stable with minimal alteration.

The nursing staff and physician were notified at the time of each occurrence. A 24-hour Holter monitor was ordered. The results were inconclusive because no sustained arrhythmias were noted.

A second cardiac evaluation identified a tachy-brady syndrome. The client received a pacemaker and appropriate medications. The client was discharged to home 6 weeks later, independent in all functional mobility and activities of daily living (ADLs).

Summary: Cardiac arrhythmia may be an underlying concern in patients with diagnosis of CVA. With the increasing population of over 65 years old and the increasing need for rehabilitative services in the aging adult population, understanding the normal aging process versus disease states is imperative. Signs of pathology can be either overlooked or attributed to the age of the client or to the normal aging process.

Cardiac arrhythmia is an elusive state that may or may not produce overt symptoms. This case example suggests that although not documented in the literature yet, cardiac arrhythmia may cause transient weakness.

From Pether bridge A: Case report presented in partial fulfillment of DPT 910. *Principles of differential diagnosis*. Institute for Physical Therapy Education, Chester, Pennsylvania, 2005, Widener University. Used with permission.

Fibrillation

The sinoatrial (SA) node (or cardiac pacemaker) initiates and paces the heartbeat. During an MI, damaged heart muscle cells, deprived of oxygen, can release small electrical impulses that may disrupt the heart's normal conduction pathway. These fibrillation impulses can occur in the atria or the ventricles.

If the heart attack develops suddenly into *ventricular* fibrillation, a potentially lethal arrhythmia, it can result in sudden death. Similarly, a heart damaged by CAD (with or without previous infarcts) can go into ventricular fibrillation. Ventricular fibrillation usually requires resuscitation and emergency electrical countershock (defibrillation) as lifesaving measures.

Atrial fibrillation (AF) is the most common cardiac dysrhythmia and although not immediately lethal, it can increase the risk of HF and stroke. It is characterized by total disorganization of atrial activity without effective atrial contraction. The upper chambers of the heart contract in an unsynchronized pattern, causing the atrium to quiver rather than to

CASE EXAMPLE 7.8

Unstable Cardiac Arrhythmia

Chief Complaint: A 62-year-old woman with a diagnosis of left lower extremity weakness was referred by her cardiologist to physical therapy. She also reported weakness and tingling in both legs from the knees down.

Past Medical History: Recent hospitalization for lung infection. Past history of hypertension, dizziness, and cardiac arrhythmia. Previous surgical history included thoracic outlet release 14 years ago.

Clinical Presentation: The client experienced worsening of symptoms with walking and climbing stairs; rest relieved her symptoms. Manual muscle test revealed weakness in the left hip flexor and external rotator muscles.

Client became diaphoretic with functional strength and exercise tolerance testing (repeated sit to stand and back to sitting). She reported the same response when doing housework.

Review of systems (ROS): Significant for the cardiovascular system. Vital signs were as follows:

Blood pressure:	125/95 mm Hg (left arm, standing) / 150/82 (supine)
	Lower standing BP is a risk factor for falls[00]
Apical pulse:	62 bpm; every third or fourth beat skipped; heart rate speeds up and then slows down after each skipped beat (cardiologist was aware of this pattern of irregularity; client was under medical treatment for cardiac arrhythmia)

What are the red flags in this scenario?

Age

History of cardiac arrhythmia

Diaphoresis is an abnormal response to exercise stress

Irregular heartbeat

Is it safe to proceed with physical therapy intervention because the client was referred by the cardiologist who is treating her for cardiac arrhythmia?

It is not always the case that the referring physician is aware of a client's current cardiovascular status. Referral may not always mean the client is appropriate for participation in an exercise program. Because the therapist noted the irregular heart rate, he was alert to the possibility of other signs of inappropriate exercise response.

The main red flag here is the abnormal response to exercise stress in someone who is already being treated for a cardiac anomaly (arrhythmia). The variable BP and irregular heartbeat suggest an unstable situation.

Result: In this case, it just happened that the client was going from her appointment with the therapist to a visit with her family physician. A note summarizing the therapist's findings, including the vital signs and response to exercise, was sent to the physician.

A copy of the letter was also faxed to the physician's office and to the cardiologist. The therapist followed up with a phone call to the client for an update on her status. The client was given an electrocardiogram (ECG), which was found to be abnormal, and was admitted to the hospital for further testing.

The therapist was very instrumental in referring this client, based on medical screening (i.e., systems review, exercise test) results. Information about the client's cardiovascular status gleaned by the therapist during the assessment was new and important for medical management.

From Vernier DA: The meaning of screening. The application of vital signs should be used in physical therapy practice. *ADVANCE for Physical Therapists & PT Assistants* 15(18):47–49, 2004.

contract and often causing blood to pool, allowing for clots to form. These clots can break loose and travel to the brain, causing a stroke.

Individuals with transient episodes (in and out of AF) or developing a new onset of AF are at greater risk of clot migration than those who have a long-term history, especially if they are already taking blood thinners. Medical consult is more imperative for anyone who has not previously been identified as having AF and/or who is not receiving anticoagulants.

The therapist can easily and quickly screen individuals at risk and teach them to screen themselves by checking the pulse for the telltale signs of an irregular heartbeat. A regular heartbeat is characterized by a series of even and continuous pulsations, whereas an irregular heartbeat often feels like an extra or missed beat. To help determine the steadiness of the heartbeat, the therapist or individual keeps time by tapping the foot. Recently, evidence has been shown to demonstrate the positive impact on decreasing AF burden from modification of risk factors through lifestyle changes [84-86] in patients with AF. Therefore, therapists must educate patients with AF on how modifying risk factors such as obesity, diabetes, alcohol, smoking, physical inactivity, and hypertension positively impacts their AF.

Risk Factors

Persons at risk for fibrillation who require screening include those who have had a previous heart attack or a history that includes high BP, CHF, digitalis toxicity, pericarditis, or rheumatic mitral stenosis.

Other factors that can overstimulate the sinus node include emotional stress, excessive production of thyroid hormone (hyperthyroidism), alcohol and caffeine consumption, and high fevers. In many instances, particularly in younger persons, there is no apparent cause.

Clinical Signs and Symptoms

Symptoms of fibrillation vary, depending on the functional state of the heart and the location of the fibrillation. Fibrillation may exist without symptoms. The affected individual is usually aware of the irregular heart action and reports feeling "palpitations." Careful questioning may be required to pinpoint the exact description of sensations reported by the client.

Some individuals experience the symptoms of inadequate blood flow and low oxygen levels, such as dizziness, chest pain, and fainting. Chronic AF may cause HF, which is often experienced as shortness of breath during exercise and fluid accumulation in the feet and legs.

More than six palpitations occurring in 1 minute or prolonged, repeated palpitations, especially if accompanied by chest pain, dyspnea, fainting, or other associated signs and symptoms, should be reported to the physician.

CLINICAL SIGNS AND SYMPTOMS
Fibrillation

- Subjective report of palpitations
- Sensations of fluttering, skipping, irregular beating or pounding, heaving action
- Dyspnea
- Chest pain
- Anxiety
- Pallor, fatigue
- Dizziness, light-headedness, fainting
- Nervousness
- Cyanosis

Sinus Tachycardia

Sinus tachycardia, defined as an abnormally rapid heart rate to be more than 100 bpm, is the normal physiologic response to such stressors as fever, hypotension, thyrotoxicosis, anemia, anxiety, exertion, hypovolemia, pulmonary emboli, myocardial ischemia, CHF, and shock.

Sinus tachycardia is usually of no physiologic significance; however, in clients with organic myocardial disease, the result may be reduced cardiac output, CHF, or arrhythmias. Because heart rate is a major determinant of oxygen requirements, angina or perhaps an increase in the size of an infarction may accompany persistent tachycardia in clients with CAD.

Clinical Signs and Symptoms

The symptoms of tachycardia vary from one person to another and may range from an increased pulse to a group of symptoms that would restrict normal activity of the client. Anxiety and apprehension may occur, depending on the pain threshold and emotional reaction of the client.

CLINICAL SIGNS AND SYMPTOMS
Sinus Tachycardia

- Palpitation (most common symptom)
- Restlessness
- Chest discomfort or pain
- Agitation
- Anxiety and apprehension

Sinus Bradycardia

In sinus bradycardia, impulses travel down the same pathway as in sinus rhythm, but the sinus node discharges at a rate less than 60 bpm. Bradycardia may be normal in athletes or young adults and is therefore asymptomatic.

In most cases, sinus bradycardia is a benign arrhythmia and may be beneficial by producing a longer period of diastole and increased ventricular filling. In some clients who have acute MI, it reduces oxygen demands and may help minimize the size of the infarction.

Eye surgery, meningitis, intracranial tumors, cervical and mediastinal tumors, and certain disease states (e.g., MI, myxedema, obstructive jaundice, and cardiac fibrosis) may produce sinus bradycardia.

Clinical Signs and Symptoms

Syncope may be preceded by a sudden onset of weakness, sweating, nausea, pallor, vomiting, and distortion or dimming of vision. Signs and symptoms remit promptly when the client is placed in the horizontal position.

Physician referral for sinus bradycardia is needed only when symptoms, such as chest pain, dyspnea, light-headedness, or hypotension occur.

CLINICAL SIGNS AND SYMPTOMS
Sinus Bradycardia

- Reduced pulse rate
- Syncope

CARDIOVASCULAR DISORDERS

Hypertension

BP is the force against the walls of the arteries and arterioles as these vessels carry blood away from the heart. When these muscular walls constrict, reducing the diameter of the vessel, BP rises; when they relax, increasing the vessel diameter, BP falls (see also section on Blood Pressure in Chapter 4).

A high BP reading is usually a sign that the vessels cannot relax fully and remain somewhat constricted, requiring the heart to work harder to pump blood through the vessels. Over time the extra effort can cause the heart muscle to become enlarged and eventually weakened. The force of blood pumped at high pressure can also produce small tears in the lining of the arteries, weakening the arterial vessels. The evidence of this effect is most pronounced in the vessels of the brain, kidneys, and the small vessels of the eye.

Hypertension is a major cardiovascular risk factor, associated with elevated risks of CVDs, especially MI, stroke, PVD, and cardiovascular death. Although diastolic changes were always evaluated closely, research now shows that the risks increase progressively as systolic pressure goes up, especially in adults over the age of 50 years.[87,88]

Hypertension is often considered in conjunction with peripheral vascular disorders for several reasons: both are disorders of the circulatory system, the course of both diseases are affected by similar factors, and hypertension is a major risk factor in atherosclerosis, the largest single cause of PVD.

Hypertension is defined by a pattern of consistently elevated diastolic pressure, systolic pressure, or both measured over a period of time, usually several months. Medical researchers have developed classifications for BP based on risk (see Table 4.5).

See Chapter 4 for more information on this topic.

Blood Pressure Classification

Hypertension can also be classified according to type (systolic or diastolic), cause, and degree of severity. *Primary (or essential) hypertension* is also known as *idiopathic hypertension* and accounts for 90% to 95% of all hypertensive clients.

Secondary hypertension results from an identifiable cause, including a variety of specific diseases or problems such as renal artery stenosis, oral contraceptive use, hyperthyroidism, adrenal tumors, and medication use.

Originally, birth control pills contained higher levels of estrogen, which was associated with hypertension, but today the estrogen and progestin contents of the pill are greatly reduced. The risk of high BP with oral contraceptive use is now considered quite low, but using oral contraceptives does still increase the risk of heart attack, stroke, and blood clots in certain women (e.g., age over 35 years, tobacco use, diabetes).

The risk may be increased for older women who smoke, but the risk for all women returns to normal after they discontinue the pill. The risk of venous thromboembolism associated with newer oral contraceptives remains under investigation.

Drugs that constrict blood vessels can contribute to hypertension. Among the most common are phenylpropanolamine in over-the-counter (OTC) appetite suppressants, including herbal ephedra, pseudoephedrine in cold and allergy remedies, and prescription drugs such as monoamine oxidase (MAO) inhibitors (a class of antidepressant) and corticosteroids when used over a long period.

Intermittent elevation of BP interspersed with normal readings is called *labile hypertension* or *borderline hypertension*. More and more adults over age 50 years and many older adults have a type of high BP called *isolated systolic hypertension* (ISH) characterized by marked elevation of the systolic pressure (140 mm Hg or higher) but normal diastolic pressure (less than 90 mm Hg).[89]

ISH is a risk factor for stroke and death from cardiovascular causes. Elevated systolic pressure also raises the risk of heart attack, CHF, dementia, and end-stage kidney disease.[90] It has been suggested that for every 10 mm Hg rise in systolic pressure there is a 26% increase in mortality.[91]

Two other types of hypertension include *masked hypertension* (normal in the clinic but periodically high at home) and *white-coat hypertension*, a clinical condition in which the client has elevated BP levels when measured in a clinic setting by a health care professional. In such cases, BP measurements are consistently normal outside of a clinical setting.

Masked hypertension may affect up to 10% of adults; white-coat hypertension occurs in 15% to 20% of adults with stage I hypertension.[92] These types of hypertension are more common in older adults. Antihypertensive treatment for white-coat hypertension may reduce office BP but may not affect ambulatory BP. The number of adults who develop

sustained high BP is much higher among those who have masked or white-coat hypertension.[92]

At-home BP measurements can help identify adults with masked hypertension, white-coat hypertension, ambulatory hypertension, and individuals who do not experience the usual nocturnal drop in BP (decrease of 15 mm Hg), which is a risk factor for cardiovascular events.[93] Excessive morning BP surge is a predictor of stroke in older adults with known hypertension and is also a red flag sign.[93] Medical referral is indicated in any of these situations.

Risk Factors

Modifiable risk factors for hypertension are primarily lifestyle factors such as stress, obesity, and poor diet or insufficient intake of nutrients (Table 7.6). Stress has been shown to cause increased peripheral vascular resistance and cardiac output and to stimulate sympathetic nervous system activity. Potassium deficiency can also contribute to hypertension.

The Seventh Report of the Joint National Committee on Prevention, Detection, Evaluation, and Treatment of High Blood Pressure (JNC-7; see Table 4.5) suggested adding a BP category called "prehypertension" to identify adults considered to be at risk for developing hypertension and to alert both individuals and health care providers of the importance of adopting lifestyle changes. Screening for prehypertension provides important opportunities to prevent hypertension and CVD.[94] There have also been suggestions from others such as the Systolic Blood Pressure Intervention Trial (SPRINT) to adopt a lower systolic blood pressure of 120 mm Hg. A finding in the SPRINT was that CVD and death was reduced by 25% and all-cause mortality by 27% in patients who reached the target of <120 mm Hg. This trial did restrict the study to those hypertensive adults, including older adults (>75 years of age), who were at an above-average risk for developing CVD, and diabetic patients and those that already had a CVA.[95-97]

Nonmodifiable risk factors include family history, age, gender, postmenopausal status, and race. The risk of hypertension increases with age as arteries lose elasticity and become less able to relax. There is a poorer prognosis associated with early onset of hypertension.

A sex-specific gene for hypertension may exist[98] because men experience hypertension at higher rates and at an earlier age than women do until after menopause. Hypertension is the most serious health problem for African Americans (both

TABLE 7.6 Risk Factors for Hypertension	
Modifiable	**Nonmodifiable**
Smoking or tobacco	African American ethnicity
Type 2 diabetes	Age (60 years or older)
High cholesterol	Postmenopausal status
Chronic alcohol use/abuse	(including surgically induced
Obesity	menopause)
Sedentary lifestyle	Family history of cardiovascular
Stress	disease (women younger than
Diet, nutritional status;	age 65 years; men younger
potassium deficiency	than age 55 years)

men and women and at earlier ages than for white people) in the United States (see further discussion of hypertension in African Americans in Chapter 4).

Clinical Signs and Symptoms

Clients with hypertension are usually asymptomatic in the early stages, but when symptoms do occur, they include occipital headache (usually present in the early morning), vertigo, flushed face, nocturnal urinary frequency, spontaneous nosebleeds, and blurred vision (see Case Example 7.9).

CLINICAL SIGNS AND SYMPTOMS

Hypertension

- Occipital headache
- Vertigo (dizziness)
- Flushed face
- Spontaneous epistaxis
- Vision changes
- Nocturnal urinary frequency

Transient Ischemic Attack

Hypertension is a major cause of HF, stroke, and kidney failure. Aneurysm formation and CHF are also associated with hypertension. Persistent elevated diastolic pressure damages the intimal layer of the small vessels, which causes an accumulation of fibrin, local edema, and possibly intravascular clotting.

CASE EXAMPLE 7.9

Hypertension

Chief Complaint: A 70-year-old woman came to physical therapy with a diagnosis of left supraspinatus tendon strain.

Past Medical History: Cortisone injection to shoulder; recent normal electrocardiogram (ECG)

Clinical Presentation: The client reported posterior left shoulder pain and lateral arm pain with occasional radiating pain down the arm to her hand. No other symptoms were reported. Vital signs were assessed:

Blood pressure:	170/95 (left arm, sitting)
Pulse:	82 bpm, regular

Should the client be referred for high BP based on this information?

Hypertension is a medical diagnosis. However, one high reading is not sufficient to render this diagnosis. Many other factors can influence BP and should be evaluated (see Table 4.4).

The client was asked if she was ever diagnosed with high BP or hypertension. She denied any personal history of known elevated BP.

The client decided to have her BP checked at the local health department once a week for the next 2 weeks. Each time the readings were above normal. She made a self-referral to her medical doctor. After a medical evaluation, she was placed on appropriate medication.

Data from Vernier DA: The meaning of screening. The application of vital signs should be used in physical therapy practice. *ADVANCE for Physical Therapists & PT Assistants* 15(18):47–49, 2004.

Eventually, these damaging changes diminish blood flow to vital organs, such as the heart, kidneys, and brain, resulting in complications such as HF, renal failure, and cerebrovascular accidents or stroke.

Many persons have brief episodes of transient ischemic attacks (TIAs). The attacks occur when the blood supply to part of the brain has been temporarily disrupted. These ischemic episodes last from 5 to 20 minutes, although they may last for as long as 24 hours. TIAs are considered by some as a progression of cerebrovascular disease and may be referred to as "ministrokes."

TIAs are important warning signals that an obstruction exists in an artery leading to the brain. Without treatment, 10% to 20% of people will go on to have a major stroke within 3 months, many within 48 hours.[99] Immediate medical referral is advised for anyone with signs and symptoms of TIAs, especially anyone with a history of heart disease, hypertension, or tobacco use. Other risk factors for TIAs include age (over 65 years), diabetes, and being overweight. The ABCD[100] score is used and supported by the AHA and American Stroke Association guidelines to triage patients with a TIA for hospitalization. The ABCD score is calculated as follows: age greater than or equal to 60 years (1 point); BP greater than or equal to 140/90 mm Hg upon presentation (1 point); clinical features: unilateral weakness (2 points) or speech/language impairment without weakness (1 point); duration greater than or equal to 60 minutes (2 points) or 10 to 59 minutes (1 point); and diabetes mellitus (1 point). The ABCD[100] score can vary from 0 to 7 and increasing scores predict increased risk of a CVA.

CLINICAL SIGNS AND SYMPTOMS

Transient Ischemic Attack

- Slurred speech, sudden difficulty with speech, or difficulty understanding others
- Sudden confusion, loss of memory, even loss of consciousness
- Temporary blindness or other dramatic visual change
- Dizziness
- Sudden, severe headache
- Paralysis or extreme weakness, usually affecting one side of the body
- Difficulty walking, loss of balance or coordination
- Symptoms are usually brief, lasting only a few minutes but can persist up to 24 hours

Orthostatic Hypotension (See also discussion on Hypotension in Chapter 4)

Orthostatic hypotension is an excessive fall in BP of 15 mm Hg or more in systolic BP or a drop of at least 7 mm Hg or more of diastolic arterial BP on assumption of an erect standing position (Case Example 7.10).[101] This is an update from the previously accepted definition of orthostatic hypotension. The previous definition was a significant reduction in systolic (greater than 20 mmHg) or diastolic (greater than 10 mmHg)

CASE EXAMPLE 7.10
Monitoring Vital Signs

Referral: An 83-year-old woman was referred to physical therapy for mobility training.

Goal: Improve balance to prevent nursing home placement.

Chief Complaints: Forgetfulness, two falls during the past 3 months, and inability to complete independent activities of daily living (ADLs).

Past/Current Medical History: Pernicious anemia, chronic venous insufficiency, non–insulin-dependent diabetes, hypercholesterolemia, osteoporosis, progressive dementia, gastroesophageal reflux (GERD).

Medications/Supplements: Lasix for chronic edema in lower extremities secondary to venous insufficiency, Lipitor for elevated cholesterol, calcium for osteoporosis, Prilosec for GERD.

Systems Review

Integument: Integument intact with good turgor.

Musculoskeletal: Strength 4/5 upper and lower extremities. Range of motion (ROM) within functional limits (WNLs). Thoracic kyphosis present.

Neuromuscular: Intact cranial nerves, independent transfers, impaired gait and balance.

Cardiovascular/Pulmonary: Heart rate: 65 bpm at rest; respiratory rate: 16 breaths per minute; BP: 100/70 mm Hg (measured in sitting, right upper extremity).

Vital Signs: Oral temperature: 100° F with a regular pulse rate; finger pulse oximeter (oxygen saturation)—88% (rest) and 85% (walking with wheeled walker).

Further BP assessment was conducted comparing measures in supine (110/70 mm Hg), sitting (100/70 mm Hg), and standing (90/65 mm Hg) with only slight increase in pulse rate (from 16 to 20 bpm) suggesting postural orthostatic hypotension (for discussion on postural orthostatic hypotension, see Chapter 4). Client became diaphoretic during BP testing.

Decreased breath sounds heard in right lower lobe during auscultation. Client reported productive cough and unusual fatigue.

What are the red flags in this scenario?

Age

Constitutional symptoms (low-grade fever, fatigue, unexplained diaphoresis)

Abnormal vital signs (BP changes with change in position accompanied by increase in pulse rate, low oxygen saturation levels)

Productive cough, decreased breath sounds, right lower lobe

Result: The primary physician was contacted to discuss the therapist's concerns regarding the client's vital signs, constitutional symptoms, and signs and symptoms associated with the pulmonary system. The client was treated for unstable BP and pneumonia.

Physical therapists can take a leadership role in the management of their clients. Every physical therapy examination should include, at a minimum, a baseline measurement of vital signs even without red flags or specific symptoms to suggest it.

From Heins P: Case report presented in partial fulfillment of DPT 910. *Principles of differential diagnosis.* Institute for Physical Therapy Education, Chester, Pennsylvania, 2005, Widener University. Used with permission.

BP within 3 minutes of standing from a sitting or supine position.[102] Orthostatic hypotension is not a disease but a manifestation of abnormalities in normal BP regulation.

This condition may occur as a normal part of aging or secondary to the effects of drugs such as hypertensives, diuretics, and antidepressants; as a result of venous pooling (e.g., pregnancy, prolonged bed rest, or standing); or in association with neurogenic origins. The last category includes diseases affecting the ANS, such as Guillain-Barré syndrome, diabetes mellitus, or multiple sclerosis.

Orthostatic intolerance is the most common cause of light-headedness in clients, especially in those who have been confined to prolonged bed rest or those who have had prolonged anesthesia for surgery. When such a client is getting up out of bed for the first time, BP and heart rate should be monitored with the client in the supine position and repeated after the person is upright. If the legs are dangled off the bed, a significant drop in BP may occur with or without compensatory tachycardia. This drop may provoke light-headedness, and standing may even produce a loss of consciousness.

These postural symptoms are often accentuated in the morning and are aggravated by heat, humidity, heavy meals, and exercise.

CLINICAL SIGNS AND SYMPTOMS
Orthostatic Hypotension

- Change in BP (decrease) and pulse (increase)
- Light-headedness, dizziness
- Pallor, diaphoresis
- Syncope or fainting
- Mental or visual blurring
- Sense of weakness or "rubbery" legs

Peripheral Vascular Disorders

Impaired circulation may be caused by many acute or chronic medical conditions known as PVDs. PVDs can affect the arterial, venous, or lymphatic circulatory system.

Vascular disorders secondary to occlusive arterial disease usually have an underlying atherosclerotic process that causes disturbances in the circulation to the extremities and can result in significant loss of function of either the upper or lower extremities.

Peripheral arterial occlusive diseases also can be caused by embolism, thrombosis, trauma, vasospasm, inflammation, or autoimmunity. The cause of some disorders is unknown.

Arterial (Occlusive) Disease

Arterial diseases include acute and chronic arterial occlusion (Table 7.7). Acute arterial occlusion may be caused by:

1. Thrombus, embolism, or trauma to an artery.
2. Arteriosclerosis obliterans.
3. Thromboangiitis obliterans or Buerger's disease.
4. Raynaud's disease.

Clinical manifestations of chronic arterial occlusion caused by PVD may not appear for 20 to 40 years. The lower

TABLE 7.7	Comparison of Acute and Chronic Arterial Symptoms	
Symptom Analysis	Acute Arterial Symptoms	Chronic Arterial Symptoms
Location	Varies; distal to occlusion; may involve entire leg	Deep muscle pain, usually in calf, may be in lower leg or dorsum of foot
Character	Throbbing	Intermittent claudication; feels like cramp, numbness, and tingling; feeling of cold
Onset and duration	Sudden onset (within 1 hour)	Chronic pain, onset gradual following exertion
Aggravating factors	Activity such as walking or stairs; elevation	Same as acute arterial symptoms
Relieving factors	Rest (usually within 2 minutes); dangling (severe involvement)	Same as acute arterial symptoms
Associated symptoms	6 P's: Pain, pallor, pulselessness, paresthesia, poikilothermia (coldness), paralysis (severe)	Cool, pale skin
At risk	History of vascular surgery, arterial invasive procedure, abdominal aneurysm, trauma (including injured arteries), chronic atrial fibrillation	Older adults; more males than females; inherited predisposition; history of hypertension, smoking, diabetes, hypercholesterolemia, obesity, vascular disease

From American Heart Association (AHA): *Heart and stroke encyclopedia*. Available online at http://www.americanheart.org. Accessed November 11, 2010.

limbs are far more susceptible to arterial occlusive disorders and atherosclerosis than are the upper limbs.

Risk Factors

Diabetes mellitus increases the susceptibility to CHD. People with diabetes have abnormalities that affect several steps in the development of atherosclerosis. Only the combination of factors, such as hypertension, abnormal platelet activation, and metabolic disturbances affecting fat and serum cholesterol account for the increased risk.

Other risk factors include smoking, hypertension, hyperlipidemia (elevated levels of fats in the blood), and older age. Peripheral artery disease most often afflicts men older than the age of 50 years, although women are at significant risk because of their increased smoking habits.

Clinical Signs and Symptoms

The first sign of vascular occlusive disease may be the loss of hair on the toes. The most important symptoms of chronic arterial occlusive disease are intermittent claudication (limping resulting from pain, ache, or cramp in the muscles of the lower extremities caused by ischemia or insufficient blood flow) and ischemic rest pain.

The pain associated with arterial disease is generally felt as a dull, aching tightness deep in the muscle, but it may be described as a boring, stabbing, squeezing, pulling, or even burning sensation. Although the pain is sometimes referred to as a cramp, there is no actual spasm in the painful muscles.

The location of the pain is determined by the site of the major arterial occlusion (see Table 15.7). Aortoiliac occlusive disease induces pain in the gluteal and quadriceps muscles. The most frequent lesion, which is present in about two-thirds of clients, is occlusion of the superficial femoral artery between the groin and the knee, producing pain in the calf that sometimes radiates upward to the popliteal region and lower thigh. Occlusion of the popliteal or more distal arteries causes pain in the foot.

In the typical case of superficial femoral artery occlusion, there is a 2 + or normal femoral pulse at the groin but arterial pulses are absent (0) at the knee and foot, although resting circulation appears to be good in the foot.

After exercise, the client may have numbness in the foot and pain in the calf. The foot may be cold, pale, and chalky white, which is an indication that the circulation has been diverted to the arteriolar bed of the leg muscles. Blood in regions of sluggish flow becomes deoxygenated, inducing a red-purple mottling of the skin.

Painful cramping symptoms occur during walking and disappear quickly with rest. Ischemic rest pain is relieved by placing the limb in a dependent position, using gravity to enhance blood flow. In most clients, the symptoms are constant and reproducible (i.e., the client who cannot walk the length of the house because of leg pain one day but can walk indefinitely the next, does not have intermittent claudication).

Intermittent claudication is influenced by the speed, incline, and surface of the walk. Exercise tolerance decreases over time, so that episodes of claudication occur more frequently with less exertion. The differentiation between vascular claudication and neurogenic claudication is presented in Chapter 17 (see Table 17.5).

CLINICAL SIGNS AND SYMPTOMS
Arterial Disease

- Intermittent claudication
- Burning, ischemic pain at rest
- Rest pain aggravated by elevating the extremity; relieved by hanging the foot over the side of the bed or chair
- Change in color, temperature, skin, nail beds
- Decreased skin temperature
- Dry, scaly, or shiny skin
- Poor nail and hair growth
- Possible ulcerations and gangrene on weight-bearing surfaces (e.g., toes, heel)
- Change in vision (diabetic atherosclerosis)
- Fatigue upon exertion (diabetic atherosclerosis)

Ulceration and gangrene are common complications and may occur early in the course of some arterial diseases (e.g., Buerger's disease). Gangrene usually occurs in one extremity at a time. In advanced cases, the extremities may be abnormally red or cyanotic, particularly when dependent. Edema of the legs is fairly common. Color or temperature changes and changes in the nail beds and skin may also appear.

Raynaud's Phenomenon and Disease

The term *Raynaud's phenomenon* refers to intermittent episodes during which small arteries or arterioles in extremities constrict, causing temporary pallor and cyanosis of the digits and change in skin temperature.

These episodes occur in response to cold temperature or strong emotion (anxiety, excitement). As the episode passes, the color change is replaced by redness. If the disorder is secondary to another disease or underlying cause, the term *secondary Raynaud's phenomenon* is used.

Secondary Raynaud's phenomenon is often associated with connective tissue or collagen vascular diseases, such as scleroderma, polymyositis/dermatomyositis, SLE, or rheumatoid arthritis. Raynaud's may occur as a long-term complication of cancer treatment. Unilateral Raynaud's phenomenon may be a sign of hidden neoplasm.

Raynaud's phenomenon may occur after trauma or use of vibrating equipment such as jackhammers, or it may be related to various neurogenic lesions (e.g., thoracic outlet syndrome) and occlusive arterial diseases.

Raynaud's disease is a primary vasospastic or vasomotor disorder, although it is included in this section under occlusive arterial disease because of arterial involvement. It appears to be caused by:
1. Hypersensitivity of digital arteries to cold.
2. Release of serotonin.
3. Congenital predisposition to vasospasm.

Eighty percent of clients with Raynaud's disease are women between the ages of 20 and 49 years. Primary Raynaud's disease rarely leads to tissue necrosis.

Idiopathic Raynaud's disease is differentiated from secondary Raynaud's phenomenon by a history of symptoms for at least 2 years with no progression of symptoms and no evidence of underlying cause.

Clinical Signs and Symptoms

The typical progression of Raynaud's phenomenon is pallor in the digits, followed by cyanosis accompanied by feelings of cold, numbness, and occasionally pain, and finally, intense redness with tingling or throbbing.

The pallor is caused by vasoconstriction of the arterioles in the extremity, which leads to decreased capillary blood flow. Blood flow becomes sluggish and cyanosis appears; the digits turn blue. The intense redness (rubor) results from the end of vasospasm and a period of hyperemia as oxygenated blood rushes through the capillaries.

CLINICAL SIGNS AND SYMPTOMS
Raynaud's Phenomenon and Disease

- Pallor in the digits
- Cyanotic, blue digits
- Cold, numbness, pain of digits
- Intense redness of digits

Venous Disorders

Venous disorders can be separated into acute and chronic conditions. Acute venous disorders include thromboembolism. Chronic venous disorders can be separated further into varicose vein formation and chronic venous insufficiency.

Acute Venous Disorders

Acute venous disorders are caused by the formation of thrombi (clots), which obstruct venous flow. Blockage may occur in both superficial and deep veins. Superficial thrombophlebitis is often iatrogenic, resulting from the insertion of intravenous catheters or as a complication of intravenous sites.

Pulmonary emboli (see Chapter 8), most of which start as thrombi in the large deep veins of the legs, are an acute and potentially lethal complication of deep venous thrombosis (DVT).

Thrombus formation results from an intravascular collection of platelets, erythrocytes, leukocytes, and fibrin in the blood vessels, often the deep veins of the lower extremities. When thrombus formation occurs in the deep veins, the production of clots can cause significant morbidity and mortality resulting in a floating mass (embolus) that can occlude blood vessels of the lungs and other critical structures.[103]

Risk Factors

DVT, defined as blood clots in the pelvis, leg, or major upper extremity veins, is a common disorder, affecting men more than women and adults more than children.[104] Approximately one-third of clients older than 40 years of age who have had either major surgery or an acute MI develop DVT. Clinical decision rules (CDR's) to determine pretest probability of having a DVT have investigated both inpatient[105] and outpatient[104] settings and depending on the setting there are specific significant clinical risk factors that influence the development of DVT's. For example, the prevalence of cancer was 17% in the hospital setting compared with 4% in outpatients. The Wells CDR for DVT has been validated for outpatients and there are several inpatient CDR's in development.[106] The development of CDR's for the sequelae of a DVT leading to pulmonary embolism have also been published[104,106,107] (see Chapter 8 and Box 8.2).

Thrombus formation is usually attributed to (1) venous stasis, (2) hypercoagulability, or (3) injury to the venous wall. *Venous stasis* is caused by prolonged immobilization or absence of the calf muscle pump (e.g., because of illness, paralysis, or inactivity). Other risk factors include traumatic spinal cord injury, multiple trauma, CHF, obesity, pregnancy,

---

BOX 7.2 RISK FACTORS FOR PULMONARY EMBOLISM (PE) AND DEEP VENOUS THROMBOSIS (DVT)

Previous personal/family history of thromboembolism
Congestive heart failure
Age (over 50 years)
Oral contraceptive use
Immobilization or inactivity (blood stasis)
Obstetric/gynecologic conditions
Obesity
Neoplasm
Pacemaker
Trauma
- Recent surgical procedures
- Indwelling central venous catheter (upper extremity DVT)
- Fracture
- Burns
- Spinal cord injury
- Endothelial injury, stroke

Blood disorders (e.g., hypercoagulable state, clotting abnormalities)
History of infection, diabetes mellitus

---

and major surgery (orthopedic, oncologic, gynecologic, abdominal, cardiac, renal, or splenic)[108] (Case Example 7.11).

Hypercoagulability often accompanies malignant neoplasms, especially visceral and ovarian tumors. Oral contraceptives, selective estrogen receptor modulators (SERMs; e.g., raloxifene) often used for osteoporosis related to menopause, and hematologic (clotting) disorders also may increase the coagulability of the blood. In addition, previous spontaneous thromboembolism and increased levels of homocysteine are risk factors for venous and arterial thrombosis.[110]

The observed relationship of higher venous thrombosis risk with the use of third-generation oral contraceptives is an important consideration.[111,112] Third-generation contraceptives refer to the newest formulation of oral contraceptives with much lower levels of estrogen than those first administered.

The risk of having a blood clot depends on several factors and increases with age. It also depends on what kind of oral contraceptive is being taken. Women using progestogen-only pills are at little or no increased risk of blood clots. The venous clots associated with the newest oral contraceptives typically develop in superficial leg veins and rarely result in pulmonary emboli.

Injury or trauma to the venous wall may occur as a result of intravenous injections, Buerger's disease, fractures and dislocations, sclerosing agents, and opaque mediator radiography.

Clinical Signs and Symptoms

Superficial thrombophlebitis appears as a local, raised, red, slightly indurated (hard), warm, tender cord along the course of the involved vein.

CASE EXAMPLE 7.11
Deep Venous Thrombosis in a Patient with a Spinal Cord Injury

Referral: An 18-year-old male with Down syndrome fell and sustained a fracture at C2 with resultant spinal cord injury and flaccid quadriparesis. After medical treatment and stabilization, he was transferred to a rehabilitation facility.

Medications: Lovenox (anticoagulant, antithrombotic for DVT prevention)

Summary: This client had a long and extensive recovery and rehabilitation because of his diagnosis of Down syndrome, high-level spinal cord injury, chronic pressure ulcers, and cardiovascular complications.

Eight months after the start of rehabilitation he developed unilateral swelling, pain, and warmth in the left lower extremity. Elevating the leg did not relieve symptoms.

Circumference measurements around the left thigh, calf, and foot were 1 inch greater compared to the right leg.

A deep venous thrombosis (DVT) was highly suspected because the leg symptoms were unilateral. If the swelling was simply as a result of his legs being in the dependent position, one would expect swelling in both of his legs. The client was in a high-risk category for developing a DVT.

He was also taken off Lovenox injections just 1 month before developing his symptoms. Weaning a client off percutaneous anticoagulation therapy by 6 months is a generally accepted practice, continuing only with oral anticoagulation therapy such as Coumadin.[109] The client had been on Lovenox for 9 months.

Result: The client was diagnosed and treated for DVT and returned to the rehabilitation hospital. Repeat ultrasound the following month showed interval improvement without resolution of the DVT. Further medical treatment was instituted.

Although the risk of DVT is greater in the acute care phase, the therapist must remain alert to symptoms of DVT in at-risk clients with multiple comorbidities and complications. Use of the revised Wells' Clinical Decision Rule (see Table 4.11) is advised.

Even with medical treatment, it should not be assumed that the condition has resolved until confirmed by medical testing. All precautions must remain in effect until released by the physician.

In contrast, symptoms of DVT are less distinctive; about one half of clients are asymptomatic. The most common symptoms are pain in the region of the thrombus and unilateral swelling distal to the site (Case Example 7.12).

Other symptoms may include redness or warmth of the arm or leg, dilated veins, or low-grade fever, possibly accompanied by chills and malaise. Unfortunately, the first clinical manifestation may be pulmonary embolism. Frequently, clients have thrombi in both legs even though the symptoms are unilateral. For further discussion on DVT of the upper extremity, see Chapter 19.

Homans' sign (discomfort in the upper calf during gentle, forced dorsiflexion of the foot) and Pratt's sign (compression

CASE EXAMPLE 7.12

Deep Venous Thrombosis (DVT)

Referral: A 96-year-old woman was discharged from a hospital to a subacute center for rehabilitation.

Goal: Return to previous level of function if possible.

Chief Complaint: Fall with fracture of left pelvis; diffuse pain around left pelvic area rated 5/10 on the numeric rating scale; pain increases with weight-bearing and movement. Conservative nonsurgical treatment was employed.

Past Medical History: Dementia, colon cancer

Current Medications: Acetaminophen 500 mg prn (for pain), warfarin daily (anticoagulant), Risperidone (for dementia), calcium carbonate/vitamin D (for osteoporosis)

Systems Review

Integument: Skin integrity within normal limits for client's age

Musculoskeletal: Muscle strength 3+/5 in both lower extremities; range of motion within functional limits for all but left hip; left hip flexion limited by pain at end of range; functional transfers, bed mobility, ambulation, and stairs with assistance; antalgic gait with decreased base of support, decreased stride/step length, minimal weight bearing on left leg

Neuromuscular: Standing balance fair, dynamic standing balance fair minus (F −) with a wheeled walker

Cardiovascular/pulmonary: Lower extremity pulses and circulation within normal limits for client's age (baseline). Two weeks later, affected foot and calf were edematous but reportedly pain free. Calf was tender to touch; leg was warm with discoloration of the affected limb.

Further Screening: revised Wells' Clinical Decision Rule for DVT*

Result: Client was referred for medical evaluation of sudden change in the involved lower extremity. Recent pelvic fracture is a major risk factor for deep venous thrombosis, a potentially life-threatening condition. Duplex ultrasonography confirmed provisional medical diagnosis of DVT.

Clinical Presentation	Possible Score	Client's Score
Active cancer (within 6 months of diagnosis or receiving palliative care)	1	0

Clinical Presentation	Possible Score	Client's Score
Paralysis, paresis, or recent immobilization of lower extremity	1	1
Bedridden for more than 3 days or major surgery within the previous 12 weeks	1	0
Localized tenderness in the center of the posterior calf, the popliteal space, or along the femoral vein in the anterior thigh/groin	1	1
Lower extremity swelling	1	0
Unilateral calf swelling (more than 3 cm larger than uninvolved side) measured 10 cm below tibial tuberosity	1	1
Pitting edema confined to symptomatic leg	1	0
Collateral superficial veins (nonvaricose)	1	0
Previously documented DVT	1	0
An alternative diagnosis is as likely (or more likely) than DVT (e.g., cellulitis, postoperative swelling, calf strain)	−2	0
Total Points	3	

Key:

> or equal to 2	DVT likely
< 2	DVT unlikely

Medical referral is required with a "likely" score of above 2.

*Le Gal G, Carrier M, Rodger M. Clinical decision rules in venous thromboembolism. *Best Practice & Research Clinical Hematol* 2012;25:303-317. From Kehinde JA: Case report presented in partial fulfillment of DPT 910. *Principles of differential diagnosis*. Institute for Physical Therapy Education, Chester, Pennsylvania, 2005, Widener University. Used with permission.

of the calf) is still commonly assessed during physical examination. Homans' sign is insensitive and nonspecific. It is present in less than one-third of clients with documented DVT. Also, more than 50% of clients with a positive finding of Homans' sign do not have evidence of venous thrombosis.

Other more specific risk and physical assessment tools are available for valuation of DVT and PVD (see ankle-brachial index [ABI], Wells' CDR for DVT and PE in Chapter 4). A simple model to predict upper extremity DVT has also been proposed and remains under investigation (see Table 19.3).[113]

Symptoms of superficial thrombophlebitis are relieved by bed rest with elevation of the legs and the application of heat for 7 to 15 days. When local signs of inflammation subside, the client is usually allowed to ambulate wearing elastic stockings with appropriate compression specific to the individual patient need.

Sometimes, antiinflammatory medications are required. Anticoagulants, such as heparin and warfarin, are used to prevent clot extension.

CLINICAL SIGNS AND SYMPTOMS

Superficial Venous Thrombosis

- Subcutaneous venous distention
- Palpable cord
- Warmth, redness
- Indurated (hard)

CLINICAL SIGNS AND SYMPTOMS
Deep Venous Thrombosis

- Unilateral tenderness or leg pain
- Unilateral swelling (>3 cm difference in leg circumference)
- Warmth
- Discoloration

Chronic Venous Disorders

Chronic venous insufficiency, also known as postphlebitic syndrome, is identified by chronic swollen limbs; thick, coarse, brownish skin around the ankles; and venous stasis ulceration. Chronic venous insufficiency is the result of dysfunctional valves that reduce venous return, which thus increases venous pressure and causes venous stasis and skin ulcerations.

Chronic venous insufficiency follows the most severe cases of DVT but may take as long as 5 to 10 years to develop. Education and prevention are essential, and clients with a history of DVT must be monitored periodically for life.

Lymphedema

The final type of peripheral vascular disorder, lymphedema, is defined as an excessive accumulation of fluid in the tissue spaces. Lymphedema typically occurs secondary to an obstruction of the lymphatic system from trauma, infection, radiation, or surgery.

Postsurgical lymphedema is usually seen after surgical excision of axillary, inguinal, or iliac nodes, usually performed as a prophylactic or therapeutic measure for a metastatic tumor. Lymphedema secondary to primary or metastatic neoplasms in the lymph nodes is common.

CLINICAL SIGNS AND SYMPTOMS
Lymphedema

- Edema of the dorsum of the foot or hand
- Decreased range of motion, flexibility, and function
- Usually unilateral
- Worse after prolonged dependency
- No discomfort or a dull, heavy sensation; sense of fullness

LABORATORY VALUES

The results of diagnostic tests can provide the therapist with information to assist in client education. The client often reports test results to the therapist and asks for information regarding the significance of those results. The information presented in this text discusses potential reasons for abnormal laboratory values relevant to clients with cardiovascular problems.

A basic understanding of laboratory tests used specifically in the diagnosis and monitoring of cardiovascular problems can provide the therapist with additional information regarding the client's status.

Some of the tests commonly used in the management and diagnosis of cardiovascular problems include lipid screening (cholesterol levels, LDL levels, HDL levels, and triglyceride levels), serum electrolytes, and arterial blood gases.

Other laboratory measurements of importance in the overall evaluation of the client with CVD include red blood cell values (e.g., red blood cell count, hemoglobin, and hematocrit). Those values (see Chapter 6) provide valuable information regarding the oxygen-carrying capability of the blood and the subsequent oxygenation of body tissues such as the heart muscle.

Serum Electrolytes

Measurement of serum electrolyte values is particularly important in diagnosis, management, and monitoring of the client with CVD because electrolyte levels have a direct influence on the function of cardiac muscle (like that of skeletal muscle). Abnormalities in serum electrolytes, even in noncardiac clients, can result in significant cardiac arrhythmias and even cardiac arrest.

Certain medications prescribed for cardiac clients can alter serum electrolytes in such a way that rhythm problems can occur as a result of the medication. The electrolyte levels most important to monitor include potassium, sodium, calcium, and magnesium (see inside back cover).

Potassium

Serum potassium levels can be lowered significantly as a result of diuretic therapy (particularly with loop diuretics such as Lasix [furosemide]), vomiting, diarrhea, sweating, and alkalosis. Low potassium levels cause increased electrical instability of the myocardium, life-threatening ventricular arrhythmias, and increased risk of digitalis toxicity.

Serum potassium levels must be measured frequently by the physician in any client taking a digitalis preparation (e.g., digoxin), because most of these clients are also undergoing diuretic therapy. Low potassium levels in clients taking digitalis can cause digitalis toxicity and precipitate life-threatening arrhythmias.

Increased potassium levels most commonly occur because of renal and endocrine problems, or as a result of potassium replacement overdose. Cardiac effects of increased potassium levels include ventricular arrhythmias and asystole/flat line (complete cessation of electrical activity of the heart).

Sodium

Serum sodium levels indicate the client's state of water/fluid balance, which is particularly important in CHF and other pathologic states related to fluid imbalances. A low serum sodium level can indicate water overload or extensive loss of sodium through diuretic use, vomiting, diarrhea, or diaphoresis.

A high serum sodium level can indicate a water deficit state such as dehydration or water loss (e.g., lack of antidiuretic hormone).

Calcium

Serum calcium levels can be decreased as a result of multiple transfusions of citrated blood, renal failure, alkalosis, laxative or antacid abuse, and parathyroid damage or removal. A decreased calcium level provokes serious and often life-threatening ventricular arrhythmias and cardiac arrest.

Increased calcium levels are less common but can be caused by a variety of situations, including thiazide diuretic use (e.g., Diuril [chlorothiazide]), acidosis, adrenal insufficiency, immobility, and vitamin D excess. Calcium excess causes atrioventricular conduction blocks or tachycardia and ultimately can result in cardiac arrest.

Magnesium

Serum magnesium levels are rarely changed in healthy individuals because magnesium is abundant in foods and water. However, magnesium deficits are often seen in alcoholic clients or clients with critical illnesses that involve shifting of a variety of electrolytes.

Magnesium deficits often accompany potassium and calcium deficits. A decrease in serum magnesium results in myocardial irritability and cardiac arrhythmias, such as atrial or ventricular fibrillation or premature ventricular beats.

SCREENING FOR THE EFFECTS OF CARDIOVASCULAR MEDICATIONS

When a client is physically challenged, as often occurs in physical therapy, signs and symptoms develop from side effects of various classes of cardiovascular medications (Table 7.8).

For example, medications that cause peripheral vasodilation can produce hypotension, dizziness, and syncope when combined with physical therapy interventions that also produce peripheral vasodilation (e.g., hydrotherapy, aquatics, aerobic exercise).

On the other hand, cardiovascular responses to exercise can be limited in clients who are taking beta-blockers because these drugs limit the increase in heart rate that can occur as exercise increases the workload of the heart. The available pharmaceuticals used in the treatment of the conditions listed in Table 7.8 are extensive. Understanding of drug interactions and implications requires a more specific text.

The therapist must especially keep in mind that NSAIDs, often used in the treatment of inflammatory conditions, can negate the antihypertensive effects of angiotensin-converting enzyme (ACE) inhibitors. Anyone being treated with both NSAIDs and ACE inhibitors must be monitored closely during exercise for elevated BP.

Likewise, NSAIDs can decrease the excretion of digitalis glycosides (e.g., digoxin [Lanoxin] and digitoxin [Crystodigin]). Therefore levels of these glycosides can increase, thus producing digitalis toxicity (e.g., fatigue, confusion, gastrointestinal problems, arrhythmias).

Digitalis and diuretics in combination with NSAIDs exacerbate the side effects of NSAIDs. Anyone receiving any of these combinations must be monitored for lower-extremity (especially ankle) and abdominal swelling.

TABLE 7.8	Cardiovascular Medications
Condition	Drug Class
Angina pectoris	Organic nitrates Beta-blockers Calcium channel (Ca^{2+}) blockers
Arrhythmias	Sodium channel blockers Beta-blockers Calcium channel (Ca^{2+}) blockers Agents prolonging depolarization
Congestive heart failure	Cardiac glycosides (digitalis) Diuretics ACE inhibitors Vasodilators
Hypertension	Diuretics Beta-blockers ACE inhibitors Vasodilators Calcium (Ca^{2+}) channel blockers Alpha (α-^{1})-blockers

Courtesy Susan Queen, Ph.D., P.T., University of New Mexico School of Medicine, Physical Therapy Program, Albuquerque, New Mexico. *ACE*, angiotensin-converting enzyme.

Diuretics

Diuretics, usually referred to by clients as "water pills," lower BP by eliminating sodium and water and thus reducing the blood volume. Thiazide diuretics may also be used to prevent osteoporosis by increasing calcium reabsorption by the kidneys. Some diuretics remove potassium from the body, causing potentially life threatening arrhythmias.

The primary adverse effects associated with diuretics are fluid and electrolyte imbalances such as muscle weakness and spasm, dizziness, headache, incoordination, and nausea (Box 7.3).

Beta-Blockers

Beta-blockers relax the blood vessels and the heart muscle by blocking the beta receptors on the SA node and myocardial cells, producing a decline in the force of contraction and a reduction in heart rate. This effect eases the strain on the heart by reducing its workload and reducing oxygen consumption.

The therapist must monitor the client's perceived exertion and watch for excessive slowing of the heart rate (bradycardia) and contractility, resulting in depressed cardiac function. Other potential side effects include depression, worsening of asthma symptoms, sexual dysfunction, and fatigue. The generic names of beta-blockers end in "olol" (e.g., propranolol, metoprolol, atenolol). Trade names include Inderal, Lopressor, and Tenormin.

BOX 7.3   POTENTIAL SIDE EFFECTS OF CARDIOVASCULAR MEDICATIONS

Abdominal pain*
Asthmatic attacks
Bradycardia
Cough
Dehydration
Difficulty swallowing
Dizziness or fainting
Drowsiness
Dyspnea (shortness of breath or difficulty breathing)
Easy bruising
Fatigue
Headache
Insomnia†
Joint pain
Loss of taste
Muscle cramps
Nausea
Nightmares
Orthostatic hypotension
Palpitations
Paralysis
Sexual dysfunction
Skin rash
Stomach irritation
Swelling of feet or abdomen
Symptoms of congestive heart failure
Shortness of breath
Swollen ankles
Coughing up blood
Tachycardia
Unexplained swelling, unusual or uncontrolled bleeding
Vomiting
Weakness
   *Immediate physician referral.
   †Notify physician.

Alpha-1 Blockers

Alpha-1 blockers lower BP by dilating blood vessels. The therapist must be observant for signs of hypotension and reflex tachycardia (i.e., the heart rate increases to compensate for the hypotension). The generic names of alpha-1 blockers end in "zosin" (e.g., prazosin, terazosin, doxazosin; trade names include Minipress, Hytrin, Cardura).

ACE Inhibitors

Angiotensin-converting enzyme (ACE) inhibitors are highly selective drugs that interrupt a chain of molecular messengers that constrict blood vessels. They can improve cardiac function in individuals with heart failure and are used in persons with diabetes or early kidney damage. Rash and a persistent dry cough are common side effects. The generic names of ACE inhibitors end in "pril" (e.g., benazepril, captopril, enalapril, lisinopril). Trade names include Lotensin, Capoten, Vasotec, Prinivil, and Zestril. The newest on the market are ACE II inhibitors, such as Cozaar (losartan potassium) and Hyzaar (losartan potassium-hydrochlorothiazide).

Calcium Channel Blockers

Calcium channel blockers inhibit calcium from entering the blood vessel walls, where calcium works to constrict blood vessels. Side effects may include swelling in the feet and ankles, orthostatic hypotension, headache, and nausea.

There are several groups of calcium channel blockers. Those in the group that primarily interact with calcium channels on the smooth muscle of the peripheral arterioles all end with "pine" (e.g., amlodipine, felodipine, nisoldipine, nifedipine). Trade names include Norvasc, Plendil, Sular, and Adalat or Procardia.

A second group of calcium channel blockers works to dilate coronary arteries to lower BP and suppress some arrhythmias. This group includes verapamil (Verelan, Calan, Isoptin) and diltiazem (Cardizem, Dilacor).

Nitrates

Nitrates, such as nitroglycerin (e.g., nitroglycerin [Nitrostat, Nitro-Bid], isosorbide dinitrate [Iso-Bid, Isordil]), dilate the coronary arteries and are used to prevent or relieve the symptoms of angina. Headache, dizziness, tachycardia, and orthostatic hypotension may occur as a result of the vasodilating properties of these drugs.

There are other classes of drugs to treat various aspects of CVDs separate from those listed in Table 7.8. Hyperlipidemia is often treated with medications to inhibit cholesterol synthesis. Platelet aggregation and clot formation are prevented with anticoagulant drugs, such as heparin, warfarin (Coumadin), and aspirin, whereas thrombolytic drugs, such as streptokinase, urokinase, and tissue-type plasminogen activator (t-PA), are used to break down and dissolve clots already formed in the coronary arteries.

Anyone receiving cardiovascular medications, especially in combination with other medications or OTC drugs, must be monitored during physical therapy for red flag signs and symptoms and any unusual vital signs.

The therapist should be familiar with the signs or symptoms that require immediate physician referral and those that must be reported to the physician. Special Questions to Ask: Medications are available at the end of this chapter.

PHYSICIAN REFERRAL

Referral by the therapist to the physician is recommended when the client has any combination of systemic signs or symptoms discussed throughout this chapter at presentation. These signs and symptoms should always be correlated with the client's history to rule out systemic involvement or to identify musculoskeletal or neurologic disorders that would be appropriate for physical therapy intervention.

Clients often confide in their therapists and describe symptoms of a more serious nature. Cardiac symptoms unknown to the physician may be mentioned to the therapist during the opening interview or in subsequent visits.

The description and location of chest pain associated with pericarditis, MI, angina, breast pain, gastrointestinal disorders, and anxiety are often similar. The physician can distinguish among these conditions through a careful history, and medical examination and testing.

For example, compared with angina, the pain of true musculoskeletal disorders may last for seconds or hours, is not relieved by nitroglycerin, and may be aggravated by local palpation or by exertion of just the upper body.

It is not the therapist's responsibility to differentiate diagnostically among the various causes of chest pain, but rather to recognize the systemic origin of signs and symptoms that may mimic musculoskeletal disorders.

The physical therapy interview presented in Chapter 2 is the primary mechanism used to begin exploring a client's reported symptoms; this is accomplished by carefully questioning the client to determine the location, duration, intensity, frequency, associated symptoms, and relieving or aggravating factors related to pain or symptoms.

Guidelines for Immediate Medical Attention

Sudden worsening of intermittent claudication may be as a result of thromboembolism and must be reported to the physician immediately. Symptoms of TIAs in any individual, especially those with a history of heart disease, hypertension, or tobacco use, warrant immediate medical attention.

In the clinical setting, the onset of an anginal attack requires immediate cessation of exercise. Symptoms associated with angina may be reduced immediately, but should subside within 3 to 5 minutes of cessation of activity.

If the client is currently taking nitroglycerin, self-administration of medication is recommended. Relief from anginal pain should occur within 1 to 2 minutes of nitroglycerin administration; some women may obtain similar results with an antacid. The nitroglycerin may be repeated according to the prescribed directions. If anginal pain is not relieved in 20 minutes or if the client has nausea, vomiting, or profuse sweating, immediate medical intervention may be indicated.

Changes in the pattern of angina, such as increased intensity, decreased threshold of stimulus, or longer duration of pain, require immediate intervention by the physician. Pain associated with an MI is not relieved by rest, change of position, or administration of nitroglycerin or antacids.

A client in treatment under these circumstances should either be returned to the care of the nursing staff or, in the case of an outpatient, should be encouraged to contact their physician by telephone for further instruction before leaving the physical therapy department. The client should be advised not to leave unaccompanied.

Guidelines for Physician Referral

When a client has any combination of systemic signs or symptoms at presentation, refer him or her to a physician.

Women with chest or breast pain who have a positive family history of breast cancer or heart disease should always be referred to a physician for a follow-up examination.

Palpitation in any person with a history of unexplained sudden death in the family requires medical evaluation. More than six episodes of palpitations in 1 minute, or palpitations lasting for hours or occurring in association with pain, shortness of breath, fainting, or severe light-headedness require medical evaluation.

Anyone who cannot climb a single flight of stairs without feeling moderately to severely winded, or who awakens at night or experiences shortness of breath when lying down should be evaluated by a physician.

Fainting (syncope) without any warning period of light-headedness, dizziness, or nausea may be a sign of heart valve or arrhythmia problems. Unexplained syncope in the presence of heart or circulatory problems (or risk factors for heart attack or stroke) should be evaluated by a physician.

Clients who are neurologically unstable as a result of a recent CVA, head trauma, spinal cord injury, or other central nervous system insult often exhibit new arrhythmias during the period of instability. When the client's pulse is monitored, any new arrhythmias noted should be reported to the nursing staff or physician.

Cardiac clients should be sent back to their physician under the following conditions:
- Nitroglycerin tablets do not relieve anginal pain
- Pattern of angina changes is noted
- Client has abnormally severe chest pain with nausea and vomiting
- Anginal pain radiates to the jaw or to the left arm
- Anginal pain is not relieved by rest
- Upper back feels abnormally cool, sweaty, or moist to touch
- Client develops progressively worse dyspnea
- Individual with coronary artery stent experiencing chest pain
- Client demonstrates a difference of more than 40 mm Hg in pulse pressure (systolic BP minus diastolic BP = pulse pressure)
- Client has any doubt about his or her present condition

Clues to Screening for Cardiovascular Signs and Symptoms

Whenever assessing chest, breast, neck, jaw, back, or shoulder pain for cardiac origins, look for the following clues:
- Personal or family history of heart disease including hypertension
- Age (postmenopausal woman; anyone over 65 years)
- Ethnicity (African-American women)

- Other signs and symptoms such as pallor, unexplained profuse perspiration, inability to talk, nausea, vomiting, sense of impending doom, or extreme anxiety
- Watch for the three Ps.
  1. Pleuritic pain (exacerbated by respiratory movement involving the diaphragm, such as sighing, deep breathing, coughing, sneezing, laughing, or the hiccups; this may be cardiac if pericarditis or it may be pulmonary); have the client hold his or her breath and reassess symptoms—any reduction or elimination of symptoms with breathholding or the Valsalva maneuver suggests a pulmonary or cardiac source of symptoms.
  2. Pain on palpation (musculoskeletal origin).
  3. Pain with changes in position (musculoskeletal or pulmonary origin; pain that is worse when lying down and improves when sitting up or leaning forward is often pleuritic in origin).
- If two of the three P's are present, an MI is very unlikely. An MI or anginal pain occurs in approximately 5% to 7% of clients whose pain is reproducible by palpation. If the symptoms are altered by a change in position, this percentage drops to 2%, and if the chest pain is reproducible by respiratory movements, the likelihood of a coronary event is only 1%.[73]
- Chest pain may occur from intercostal muscle or periosteal trauma with protracted or vigorous coughing. Palpation of local chest wall will reproduce tenderness. However, a client can have both a pulmonary/cardiac condition with subsequent musculoskeletal trauma from coughing. Look for associated signs and symptoms (e.g., fever, sweats, blood in sputum).
- Angina is activated by physical exertion, emotional reactions, a large meal, or exposure to cold and has a lag time of 5 to 10 minutes. Angina does not occur immediately after physical activity. Immediate pain with activity is more likely musculoskeletal, thoracic outlet syndrome, or psychologic (e.g., "I do not want to shovel today").
- Chest pain, shoulder pain, neck pain, or TMJ pain occurring in the presence of CAD or previous history of MI, especially if accompanied by associated signs and symptoms, may be cardiac.
- Upper quadrant pain that can be induced or reproduced by lower quadrant activity, such as biking, stair climbing, or walking without using the arms, is usually cardiac in origin.
- Recent history of pericarditis in the presence of a new onset of chest, neck, or left shoulder pain; observe for additional symptoms of dyspnea, increased pulse rate, elevated body temperature, malaise, and myalgia(s).
- If an individual with known risk factors for congestive heart disease, especially a history of angina, becomes weak or short of breath while working with the arms extended over the head, ischemia or infarction is a likely cause of the pain and associated symptoms.
- Insidious onset of joint or muscle pain in the older client who has had a previously diagnosed heart murmur may be caused by bacterial endocarditis. Usually, there is no morning stiffness to differentiate it from rheumatoid arthritis.
- Back pain similar to that associated with a herniated lumbar disk, but without neurologic deficits, especially in the presence of a diagnosed heart murmur, may be caused by bacterial endocarditis.
- Watch for arrhythmias in neurologically unstable clients (e.g., spinal cord, new CVAs, or new traumatic brain injuries); check pulse and ask about/observe for dizziness.
- Anyone with chest pain must be evaluated for trigger points. If palpation of the chest reproduces symptoms, especially symptoms of radiating pain, deactivation of the trigger points must be carried out and followed by a reevaluation as a part of the screening process for pain of a cardiac origin (see Fig. 18.7 and Table 18.4).
- Symptoms of vascular occlusive disease include exertional calf pain that is relieved by rest (intermittent claudication), nocturnal aching of the foot and forefoot (rest pain), and classic skin changes, especially hair loss on the ankle and foot. Ischemic rest pain is relieved by placing the limb in a dependent position.
- Throbbing pain at the base of the neck and/or along the back into the interscapular areas that increases with exertion requires monitoring of vital signs and palpation of peripheral pulses to screen for aneurysm. Check for a palpable abdominal heartbeat that increases in the supine position.
- See also section on clues to differentiating chest pain in Chapter 18.

CARDIAC CHEST PAIN PATTERNS

ANGINA (FIG. 7.8)

Location:	Substernal/retrosternal (beneath the sternum)
	Left chest pain in the absence of substernal chest pain (women)
	Isolated midthoracic back pain (women)
	Aching in one or both upper arm (biceps)
Referral:	Neck, jaw, back, shoulder, or arms (most commonly the left arm)
	May have only a toothache
	Occasionally to the abdomen

CARDIAC CHEST PAIN PATTERNS—cont'd

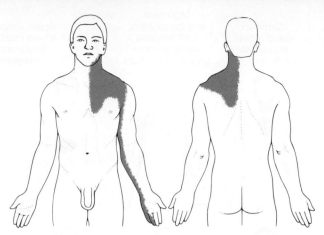

Fig. 7.8 Pain patterns associated with angina. *Left,* Area of substernal discomfort projected to the left shoulder and arm over the distribution of the ulnar nerve. Referred pain may be present only in the left shoulder or in the shoulder and along the arm only to the elbow. *Right,* Occasionally, anginal pain may be referred to the back in the area of the left scapula or the interscapular region. Women can have the same patterns as shown for men in this figure or they may present as shown in Fig. 7.4. There may be no pain but rather a presenting symptom of extreme fatigue, weakness, or breathlessness.

Description:	Vise-like pressure, squeezing, heaviness, burning indigestion
Intensitya:	Mild to moderate Builds up gradually or may be sudden
Duration:	Usually less than 10 minutes Never more than 30 minutes Average: 3–5 minutes
Associated signs and symptoms:	Extreme fatigue, lethargy, weakness (women) Shortness of breath (dyspnea) Nausea Diaphoresis (heavy perspiration) Anxiety or apprehension Belching (eructation) "Heartburn" (unrelieved by antacids) (women) Sensation similar to inhaling cold air (women) Prolonged and repeated palpitations without chest pain (women)
Relieving factors:	Rest or nitroglycerin Antacids (women)
Aggravating factors:	Exercise or physical exertion Cold weather or wind Heavy meals Emotional stress

^aFor each pattern reviewed, intensity is related directly to the degree of noxious stimuli.

MYOCARDIAL INFARCTION (FIG. 7.9)

Location:	Substernal, anterior chest
Referral:	May radiate like angina, frequently down both arms
Description:	Burning, stabbing, vise-like pressure, squeezing, heaviness
Intensity:	Severe
Duration:	Usually at least 30 minutes; may last 1–2 hours Residual soreness 1–3 days

CARDIAC CHEST PAIN PATTERNS—cont'd

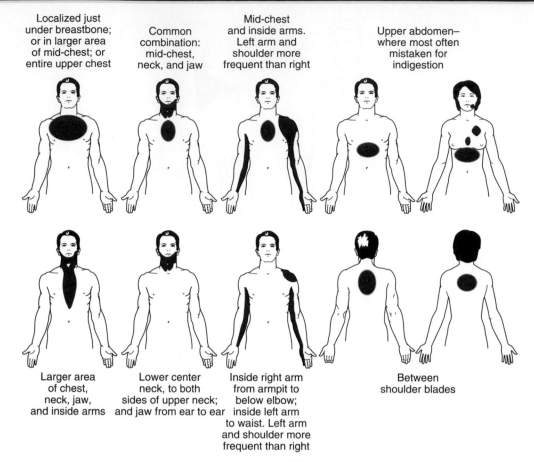

Localized just under breastbone; or in larger area of mid-chest; or entire upper chest

Common combination: mid-chest, neck, and jaw

Mid-chest and inside arms. Left arm and shoulder more frequent than right

Upper abdomen—where most often mistaken for indigestion

Larger area of chest, neck, jaw, and inside arms

Lower center neck, to both sides of upper neck; and jaw from ear to ear

Inside right arm from armpit to below elbow; inside left arm to waist. Left arm and shoulder more frequent than right

Between shoulder blades

Most common warning signs of heart attack

- Uncomfortable pressure, fullness, squeezing or pain in the center of the chest (prolonged)
- Pain that spreads to the throat, neck, back, jaw, shoulders, or arms
- Chest discomfort with light-headedness, dizziness, sweating, pallor, nausea, or shortness of breath
- Prolonged symptoms unrelieved by antacids, nitroglycerin, or rest

Atypical, less common warning signs (especially women)

- Unusual chest pain (quality, location, e.g., burning, heaviness; left chest), stomach or abdominal pain
- Continuous midthoracic or interscapular pain
- Continuous neck or shoulder pain (not shown in Fig. 7.9)
- Pain relieved by antacids; pain unrelieved by rest or nitroglycerin
- Nausea and vomiting; flu-like manifestation without chest pain/discomfort
- Unexplained intense anxiety, weakness, or fatigue
- Breathlessness, dizziness

Fig. 7.9 Early warning signs of a heart attack. Multiple segmental nerve innervations shown in Fig. 3.3 account for varied pain patterns possible. A woman can experience any of the various patterns described but is just as likely to develop atypical symptoms of pain as depicted here. (From Goodman CC, Fuller K: *Pathology: implications for the physical therapist*, ed 3, Philadelphia, 2009, WB Saunders.)

Associated signs and symptoms:	None with a silent MI
	Dizziness, feeling faint
	Nausea, vomiting
	Pallor
	Diaphoresis (heavy perspiration)
	Apprehension, severe anxiety
	Fatigue, sudden weakness
	Dyspnea
	May be followed by painful shoulder-hand syndrome (see text)
Relieving factors:	None; unrelieved by rest or nitroglycerin taken every 5 minutes for 20 minutes
Aggravating factors:	Not necessarily anything; may occur at rest or may follow emotional stress or physical exertion

CARDIAC CHEST PAIN PATTERNS—cont'd

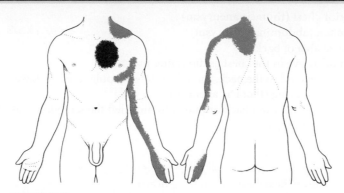

Fig. 7.10 Substernal pain associated with pericarditis *(dark red)* may radiate anteriorly *(light red)* to the costal margins, neck, upper back, upper trapezius muscle, and left supraclavicular area or down the left arm.

PERICARDITIS (FIG. 7.10)

Location:	Substernal or over the sternum, sometimes to the left of midline toward the cardiac apex
Referral:	Neck, upper back, upper trapezius muscle, left supraclavicular area, down the left arm, costal margins
Description:	More localized than pain of MI Sharp, stabbing, knife-like
Intensity:	Moderate-to-severe
Duration:	Continuous; may last hours or days followed by residual soreness
Associated signs and symptoms:	Usually medically determined associated symptoms (e.g., by chest auscultation using a stethoscope); cough
Relieving factors:	Sitting upright or leaning forward
Aggravating factors:	Muscle movement associated with deep breathing (e.g., laughter, inspiration, coughing) Left lateral (side) bending of the upper trunk Trunk rotation (either to the right or to the left) Supine position

DISSECTING AORTIC ANEURYSM (FIG. 7.11)

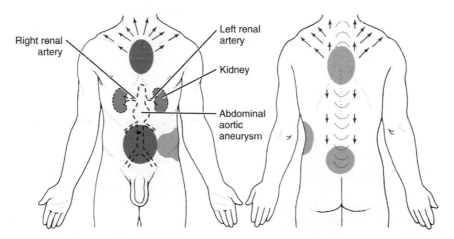

Right renal artery

Left renal artery

Kidney

Abdominal aortic aneurysm

Fig. 7.11 Most aortic aneurysms (more than 95%) are located just below the renal arteries and extend to the umbilicus, causing low back pain. Chest pain *(dark red)* associated with thoracic aneurysms may radiate *(arrows)* to the neck, interscapular area, shoulders, low back, or abdomen. Early warning signs of an impending rupture may include an abdominal heartbeat when lying down (not shown) or a dull ache in the midabdominal left flank or low back *(light red)*.

CARDIAC CHEST PAIN PATTERNS—cont'd

Location:	Anterior chest (thoracic aneurysm)
	Abdomen (abdominal aneurysm)
	Thoracic area of back
Referral:	Pain may move in the chest as dissection progresses
	Pain may extend to the neck, shoulders, interscapular area, or lower back
Description:	Knife-like, tearing (thoracic aneurysm)
	Dull ache in the lower back or midabdominal left flank (abdominal aneurysm)
Intensity:	Severe, excruciating
Duration:	Hours
Associated signs and symptoms:	Pulses absent
	Person senses "heartbeat" when lying down
	Palpable, pulsating abdominal mass
	Lower BP in one arm
	Other medically determined symptoms
Relieving factors:	None
Aggravating factors:	Supine position accentuates symptoms

NONCARDIAC CHEST PAIN PATTERNS

- Musculoskeletal disorders; see Chapters 15 to 19.
- Neurologic disorders; see Chapters 15 to 19.
- Pleuropulmonary disorders; see Chapter 8.
- Gastrointestinal disorders; see Chapter 9.
- Breast diseases; see Chapter 18.
- Anxiety states; see Chapter 3.

■ Key Points to Remember

1. Fatigue beyond expectation during or after exercise is a red-flag symptom.
2. Be on the alert for cardiac risk factors in older adults, especially women, and begin a conditioning program before an exercise program.
3. The client with stable angina typically has a normal BP; it may be low, depending on medications. BP may be elevated when anxiety accompanies chest pain or during acute coronary insufficiency; systolic BP may be low if there is HF.
4. Cervical disk disease and arthritic change can mimic atypical chest pain of angina pectoris, requiring screening through questions and musculoskeletal evaluation.
5. If a client uses nitroglycerin, make sure that he or she has a fresh supply, and check that the physical therapy department has a fresh supply in a readily accessible location.
6. Anyone being treated with both NSAIDs and ACE inhibitors must be monitored closely during exercise for elevated BP.
7. A person taking medications, such as beta-blockers or calcium channel blockers, may not be able to achieve a target heart rate (THR) above 90 bpm. To determine a safe rate of exercise, the heart rate should return to the resting level 2 minutes after stopping exercise.
8. Make sure that a client with cardiac compromise has not smoked a cigarette or eaten a large meal just before exercise.
9. A 3-pound or greater weight gain, or a gradual, continuous gain over several days resulting in swelling of the ankles, abdomen, and hands, combined with shortness of breath, fatigue, and dizziness that persists despite rest, may be red-flag symptoms of CHF.
10. The pericardium (sac around the entire heart) is adjacent to the diaphragm. Pain of cardiac and diaphragmatic origin is often experienced in the shoulder because the heart and the diaphragm are supplied by the C5-C6 spinal segment. The visceral pain is referred to the corresponding somatic area.
11. Watch for muscle pain, cramps, stiffness, spasms, and weakness that cannot be explained by arthritis, recent strenuous exercise, a fever, a recent fall, or other common causes in clients taking statins to lower cholesterol.

CLIENT HISTORY AND INTERVIEW

Special Questions To Ask

Past Medical History

- Has a doctor ever said that you have heart trouble? High BP?
- Have you ever had a heart attack?
  If yes, when? Please describe.
- Do you associate your current symptoms with your heart problems?
- Have you ever had rheumatic fever, twitching of the limbs called St. Vitus' dance, or rheumatic heart disease?
- Have you ever had an abnormal electrocardiogram (ECG)?
- Have you ever had an ECG taken while you were exercising (e.g., climbing up and down steps or walking on a treadmill) that was not normal?
- Do you have a pacemaker, artificial heart, or any other device to assist your heart?
- For the therapist: Remember to review smoking, diet, lifestyle, exercise, and stress history (see family/personal history, Chapter 2).

Angina/Myocardial Infarct

- Do you have angina (pectoris), chest pain, or tightness?
  If yes, please describe the symptoms and tell me when they occur.
  If no, have you ever had chest pain, dizziness, or shortness of breath during or after activity, exercise, or sport?
- Can you point to the area of pain with one finger? (Anginal pain is characteristically demonstrated with the hand or fist on the chest.)
- Is the pain close to the surface or deep inside? (Pleuritic pain is close to the surface; anginal pain can be close to the surface but also always has a "deep inside" sensation.)
  If yes, what makes it better?
  If no, pursue further with the following questions:
- Do you ever have discomfort or tightness in your chest?
- Have you ever had a crushing sensation in your chest with or without pain down your left arm?
- Do you have pain in your jaw either alone or in combination with chest pain?
- If you climb a few flights of stairs fairly rapidly, do you have tightness or a pressing pain in your chest?
- Do you get pressure, pain, or tightness in the chest as if you were walking in the cold wind or facing a cold blast of air?
- Have you ever had pain, pressure, or a squeezing feeling in the chest that occurred during exercise, walking, or any other physical or sexual activity?
- Have you been unusually tired lately (possible new onset of angina in women)?
- Do you get tired faster than others doing the same things?

- Has anyone in your family ever had or died from heart problems?
  If yes, did he or she die suddenly before the age of 50 years?

Associated Symptoms

- Do you ever have bouts of rapid heart action, irregular heartbeats, or palpitations of your heart?
- Have you ever felt a "heartbeat" in your abdomen when you lie down? *If yes*, is this associated with low back pain or left flank pain? (**Abdominal aneurysm**)
- Do you ever notice sweating, nausea, or chest pain when your current symptoms (e.g., back pain, shoulder pain) occur?
- Do you have frequent attacks of heartburn, or do you take antacids to relieve heartburn or acid indigestion? (**Noncardiac cause of chest pain [men], abdominal muscle trigger point, gastrointestinal disorder**)
- Do you get very short of breath during activities that do not make other people short of breath? (**Dyspnea**)
- Do you ever wake up at night gasping for air or have short breaths? (**Paroxysmal nocturnal dyspnea**)
- Do you ever need to sleep on more than one pillow to breathe comfortably? (**Orthopnea**)
- Do you ever get cramps in your legs if you walk for several blocks? (**Intermittent claudication**)
- Do you ever have swollen feet or ankles? *If yes*, are they swollen when you get up in the morning? (**Edema/CHF; NSAIDs**)
- Have you gained unexpected weight during a fairly short period of time (i.e., less than 1 week)? (**Edema, CHF**)
- Do you ever feel dizzy or have fainting spells? (**Valvular insufficiency, bradycardia, pulmonary hypertension, orthostatic hypotension**)
- Have you had any significant changes in your urine (e.g., increased amount, concentrated urine, frequency at night, or decreased amount)? (**CHF, diabetes, hypertension**)
- Do you ever have sudden difficulty with speech, temporary blindness, or other changes in your vision? (**TIAs**)
- Have you ever had sudden weakness or paralysis down one side of your body or just in an arm or a leg? (**TIAs**)

Medications

- Have you ever taken digitalis, nitroglycerin, or any other drug for your heart?
- Have you been on a diet or taken medications to lower your blood cholesterol?
  For the therapist
- Any clients taking anticlotting drugs should be examined for hematoma, nosebleed, or other sites of bleeding. Protect client from trauma.

CLIENT HISTORY AND INTERVIEW—cont'd

- Anyone taking cardiovascular medications (especially ACE inhibitors or digitalis glycosides) in combination with NSAIDs must be monitored closely (see text explanation).
- Any woman older than 35 years of age and taking oral contraceptives who has a history of smoking should be monitored for increases in BP.
- Any woman taking third-generation oral contraceptives should be monitored for venous thrombosis.

  For clients taking nitroglycerin
- Do you ever have headaches, dizziness, or a flushed sensation after taking nitroglycerin? (Most common side effects)
- How quickly does your nitroglycerin reduce or eliminate your chest pain? (Use as a guideline in the clinic when the client has angina during exercise; refer to a physician if angina is consistently unrelieved with nitroglycerin or rest after the usual period of time.)

  For clients with breast pain, see questions in Chapter 17
  For clients with joint pain
- Have you had any recent skin rashes or dot-like hemorrhages under the skin? (**Rheumatic fever, endocarditis**) *If yes*, did this occur after a visit to the dentist? (**Endocarditis**)
- Do you notice any increase in your joint pain or symptoms 1 to 2 hours after you take your medication? (**Allergic response**)
- For new onset of left upper trapezius muscle/left shoulder pain: Have you been treated for any infection in the last 3 weeks?

CASE STUDY

REFERRAL

A 30-year-old woman with five children comes to you for an evaluation after a recommendation from her friend, who received physical therapy from you last year. She has not been to a physician since her last child was delivered by her obstetrician 4 years ago.

Her chief complaint is pain in the left shoulder and left upper trapezius muscle with pain radiating into the chest and referred pain down the medial aspect of the arm to the thumb and first two fingers.

When the medical history is being taken, the client mentions that she was told 5 years ago that she had MVP secondary to rheumatic fever, which she had when she was 12 years old. She is not taking any medication, denies any palpitations, but she complains of fatigue and has dyspnea after playing ball with her son for 10 or 15 minutes.

There is no reported injury or trauma to the neck or shoulder, and the symptoms subside with rest. Physical exertion, such as carrying groceries up the stairs or laundry outside, aggravates the symptoms, but she is uncertain whether just using her upper body has the same effect.

Despite the client's denial of injury or trauma, the neck and shoulder should be screened for any possible musculoskeletal or neurologic origin of symptoms. Your observation of the woman indicates that she is 30 to 40 pounds overweight. She confides that she is under physical and emotional stress by the daily demands made by seven people in her house.

She is not involved in any kind of exercise program outside of her play activities with the children. These two factors (obesity and stress) could account for her chronic fatigue and dyspnea, but that determination must be made by a physician. Even if you can identify a musculoskeletal basis for this woman's symptoms, the past medical history of rheumatic heart disease and absence of medical follow-up would support your recommendation that the client should go to the physician for a medical checkup.

How do you rule out the possibility that this pain is not associated with MVP and is caused instead by true cervical spine or shoulder pain?

It should be pointed out here that the therapist is not equipped with the skills, knowledge, or expertise to determine that the MVP is the cause of the client's symptoms.

However, a thorough subjective and objective evaluation can assist the therapist both in making a determination regarding the client's musculoskeletal condition and in providing clear and thorough feedback for the physician on referral.

SCREENING FOR MITRAL VALVE PROLAPSE

- Pain of MVP must be diagnosed by a physician.
- MVP may be asymptomatic.
- Positive history for rheumatic fever.
- Carefully ask the client about a history of possible neck or shoulder pain, which the person may not mention otherwise.
- Musculoskeletal pain associated with the neck or shoulder is more superficial than cardiac pain.
- Total body exertion causing shoulder pain may be secondary to angina or myocardial ischemia and subsequent infarction, whereas movements of just the upper extremity causing shoulder pain are more indicative of a primary musculoskeletal lesion.
- Ask the client: Does your shoulder pain occur during exercise, such as walking, climbing stairs, mowing the lawn, or during any other physical or sexual activity that does not require the use of your arm or shoulder?
- Presence of associated signs and symptoms such as dyspnea, fatigue, or heart palpitations.

CASE STUDY—cont'd

- Medical imaging reports, if available, may confirm osteophyte formation with decreased intraforaminal spaces, which may contribute to cervical spine pain.
- History of neck injury or overuse.
- History of shoulder injury or overuse.
- Results of objective tests to clear or rule out the cervical spine and shoulder as the cause of symptoms.

- Presence of other neurologic signs to implicate the cervical spine or thoracic outlet type of symptoms (e.g., abnormal deep tendon reflexes, subjective report of numbness and tingling, objective sensory changes, muscle wasting or atrophy).
- Pattern of symptoms; a change in position may relieve symptoms associated with a cervical disorder.

PRACTICE QUESTIONS

1. Pursed-lip breathing in the sitting position while leaning forward on the arms relieves symptoms of dyspnea for the client with:
   a. Orthopnea
   b. Emphysema
   c. HF
   d. a and c
2. Briefly describe the difference between myocardial ischemia, angina pectoris, and MI.
3. What should you do if a client complains of throbbing pain at the base of the neck that radiates into the interscapular areas and increases with exertion?
4. What are the 3Ps? What is the significance of each one?
5. When are palpitations clinically significant?
6. A 48-year-old woman with TMJ syndrome has been referred to you by her dentist. How do you screen for the possibility of medical (specifically cardiac) disease?
7. A 55-year-old male grocery store manager reports that he becomes extremely weak and breathless when he is stocking groceries on overhead shelves. What is the possible significance of this complaint?
8. You are seeing an 83-year-old woman for a home health evaluation after a motor vehicle accident (MVA) that required a long hospitalization followed by transition care in an intermediate care nursing facility and now home health care. She is ambulating short distances with a wheeled walker, but she becomes short of breath quickly and requires lengthy rest periods. At each visit the client is wearing her slippers and housecoat, so you suggest that she start dressing each day as if she intended to go out. She replies that she can no longer fit into her loosest slacks and she cannot tie her shoes. Is there any significance to this client's comments, or is this consistent with her age and obvious deconditioning? Briefly explain your answer.

9. Peripheral vascular disease includes:
   a. Arterial and occlusive diseases
   b. Arterial and venous disorders
   c. Acute and chronic arterial diseases
   d. All of the above
   e. None of the above
10. Which statement is the most accurate?
    a. Arterial disease is characterized by intermittent claudication, pain relieved by elevating the extremity, and history of smoking.
    b. Arterial disease is characterized by loss of hair on the lower extremities and throbbing pain in the calf muscles that goes away by using heat and elevation.
    c. Arterial disease is characterized by painful throbbing of the feet at night that goes away by dangling the feet over the bed.
    d. Arterial disease is characterized by loss of hair on the toes, intermittent claudication, and redness or warmth of the legs that is accompanied by a burning sensation.
11. What are the primary signs and symptoms of HF?
    a. Fatigue, dyspnea, edema, nocturia
    b. Fatigue, dyspnea, varicose veins
    c. Fatigue, dyspnea, tinnitus, nocturia
    d. Fatigue, dyspnea, headache, night sweats
12. When would you advise a client in physical therapy to take his/her nitroglycerin?
    a. 45 minutes before exercise
    b. When symptoms of chest pain do not subside with 10 to 15 minutes of rest
    c. As soon as chest pain begins
    d. None of the above
    e. All of the above

REFERENCES

1. Virani AHA Statistical Update. Heart Disease and stroke statistics—2020 update. *Circulation.* 2020;141:e139–e596. https://doi.org/10.1161/CIR.00000000007571.
2. Heart disease & stroke statistics A report from the American Heart Association Statistics Committee and Stroke Statistics Subcommittee 2009. *Circulation.* 2009;119:e21–e181.
3. Roth GA, Johnson CO, Abate KH, Abd-Allah F, Ahmed M, Alam K, Alam T, Alvis-Guzman N, Ansari H, Arnlov J, et al. Global Burden of Cardiovascular Diseases Collaboration. The burden of cardiovascular diseases among US states, 1990–2016. *JAMACardiol.* 2018;3:375–389. http://doi.org/10.1001/jamacardio.2018.0385.
4. Trumbore DJ. *Statins and myalgia: a case report of pharmacovigilance with implications for physical therapy case report presented in partial fulfillment of DPT 910, Principles of Differential*

Diagnosis. Chester, Pennsylvania: Institute for Physical Therapy Education; 2005. Widener University.

5. Zhao H, Thomas G, Leung Y, et al. Statins in lipid-lowering therapy. *Acta Cardiologica Sinica.* 2003;19:1–11.

6. Rosenson RS. Current overview of statin-induced myopathy. *Am J Med.* 2004;116:408–416.

7. Roten L, Schoenenberger RA, Krahenbuhl S, et al. Rhabdomyolysis in association with simvastatin and amiodarone. *Ann Pharmacother.* 2004;38:978–981.

8. Iwere RB, Hewitt J. Myopathy in older people receiving statin therapy: a systematic review and meta-analysis. *Br J Clin Pharmacol.* 2015;80(3):363–371.

9. Tomlinson S, Mangione K. Potential adverse effects of statins on muscle: update. *Phys Ther.* 2005;85(5):459–465.

10. Pasternak RC, Smith SC, Bairey-Merz CN, et al. ACC/AHA/NHLBI clinical advisory on the use and safety of statins. *Circulation.* 2002;106:1024.

11. Mills EJ, et al. Efficacy and safety of statin treatment for cardiovascular disease: a network meta-analysis of 170,255 patients from 76 randomized trials. *QJM.* 2011;104(2):109–124.

12. Thompson PD, Panza G, Zaleski A, et al. Statin-associated side effects. *J Am Coll Cardiol.* 2016;67(20):2395–2410.

13. Leibowitz M, Karpati T, Cohen-Stavi CJ, et al. Association between achieved low-density lipoprotein levels and major adverse cardiac events in patients with stable ischemic heart disease taking statin treatment. *JAMA Intern Med.* 2016;176(8):1105–1113.

14. Evans M, Rees A. Effects of HMG-CoA reductase inhibitors on skeletal muscle: are all statins the same? *Drug Saf.* 2002;25:649–663.

15. Using Crestor—and all statins—safely: *Harvard Heart Letter.* p. 3. More information available online at www.health.harvard.edu/heartextra, September 2005. Accessed: October 17, 2010.

16. Cholesterol drugs: very safe and highly beneficial, *Johns Hopkins Medical Letter: health After 50* 13(12):3, 2002.

17. DiStasi SL. Effects of statins on skeletal muscle: a perspective for physical therapists. *Phys Ther.* 2010;90(10):1530–1542.

18. Dobkin BH. Underappreciated statin-induced myopathic weakness causes disability. *Neurorehabil Neural Repair.* 2005;19:259–263.

19. Kelln BM. Hand-held dynamometry: reliability of lower extremity muscle testing in healthy, physically active, young adults. *J Sport Rehab.* 2008;17:160–170.

20. Prager GW, Binder BR. Genetic determinants: is there an "atherosclerosis gene"? *Acta Med Austriaca.* 2004;31(1):1–7.

21. Kurtz TW, Gardner DG. Transcription-modulating drugs: a new frontier in the treatment of essential hypertension. *Hypertension.* 1998;32(3):380–386.

22. Benson SC, Pershadsingh HA, Ho CI. Identification of telmisartan as a unique angiotensin II receptor antagonist with selective PPAR gamma-modulating activity. *Hypertension.* 2004;43(5):993–1002.

23. Horn H.R.: The impact of cardiovascular disease. Available online at http://www.medscape.com/viewarticle/466799_2, April 2004. Accessed November 05, 2011.

24. Davidson M. Confirmed previous infection with Chlamydia pneumoniae (TWAR) and its presence in early coronary atherosclerosis. *Circulation.* 1998;98(7):628–633.

25. Muhlestein JB. Bacterial infections and atherosclerosis. *J Invest Med.* 1998;46(8):396–402.

26. Grayston JT, Kronmal RA, Jackson LA, et al. Azithromycin for the secondary prevention of coronary events. *N Engl J Med.* 2005;352(16):1637–1645.

27. Toss H, Gnarpe J, Gnarpe H. Increased fibrinogen levels are associated with persistent Chlamydia pneumoniae infection in unstable coronary artery disease. *Eur Heart J.* 1998;19(4):570–577.

28. Anderson JL, Carlquist JF, Muhlestein JB, et al. Evaluation of C-reactive protein, an inflammatory marker, and infectious serology as risk factors of coronary artery disease and myocardial infarction. *J Am Coll Cardiol.* 1998;32(1):35–41.

29. Toth PP. C-reactive protein as a potential therapeutic target in patients with coronary heart disease. *Curr Atheroscler Rep.* 2005;7(5):333–334.

30. Morrow DA, Rifai N, Antman EM, et al. C-reactive protein is a potent predictor of mortality independently of and in combination with troponin T in acute coronary syndromes: a TIMI 11A substudy-thrombolysis in myocardial infarction. *J Am Coll Cardiol.* 1998;31(7):1460–1465.

31. Elliot WJ, Powel LH. Diagonal earlobe creases and prognosis in patients with suspected coronary artery disease. *Am J Med.* 1996;100(2):205–211.

32. Bahcelioglu M, Isik AF, Demirel D, et al. The diagonal ear lobe crease as sign of some diseases. *Saudi Med.* 2005;26(6):947–951.

33. Shrestha I. Diagonal ear-lobe crease is correlated with atherosclerotic changes in carotid arteries. *Circ J.* 2009;73(10):1945–1949.

34. Friedlander AH, Scully C. Diagonal ear lobe crease and atherosclerosis: a review of the medical literature and oral and maxillofacial implications. *J Oral Maxillofac Surg.* 2010;68(12):3043–3050.

35. Koracevic G. Point of disagreement in evidence-based medicine. *Am J Forensic Med Pathol.* 2009;30(1):89.

36. Yeh ET, Bickford CL. Cardiovascular complications of cancer therapy: incidence, pathogenesis, diagnosis, and management. *J Am Coll Cardiol.* 2009;53(24):2231–2247. 16.

37. Gender matters Heart disease risk in women. *Harvard Women's Health Watch.* 2004;11(9):1–3.

38. Cheek D. What's different about heart disease in women? *Nursing.* 2003;33(8):36–42.

39. LaGrossa J.: Heart attack in women, *Advance Online Editions for Physical Therapists,* February 2, 2004. Available online at www.advanceforpt.com. Accessed October 17, 2010.

40. Barclay L., Vega C.: AHA updates guidelines for cardiovascular disease prevention in women, *CME,* 2004. Available online at www.medscape.com. Accessed October 17, 2010.

41. Cohen MC, Rohtla KM, Mittleman MA, et al. Meta-analysis of the morning excess of acute myocardial infarction and sudden cardiac death. *Am J Cardiol.* 1997;79(11):1512–1516.

42. Willich SN, Linderer T, Wegscheider K, et al. Infarction in the ISAM study: absence with prior b-adrenergic blockade. *Circulation.* 1989;80(4):853–858.

43. American Heart Association (AHA): Heart and stroke encyclopedia. Available online at http://www.americanheart.org. Accessed November 11, 2010.

44. McSweeney JC. Women's early warning symptoms of acute myocardial infarction. *Circulation.* 2003;108(21):2619–2623.

45. Is it a heart attack?: If you're a woman, will you know? *Berkeley Wellness Letter* 17(2):10, 2000.

46. Marrugat J. Mortality differences between men and women following first myocardial infarction. *JAMA.* 1998;280:1405–1409.

47. Cahalin LP. Heart failure. *Phys Ther.* 1996;76(5):517–533.

48. Mozaffarian D. Dietary and Policy Priorities for Cardiovascular Disease, Diabetes, and Obesity: A Comprehensive Review. *Circulation.* 2016;133(2):187–225.

49. Yancy CW, Jessup M, Bozkurt B, et al. ACCF/AHA guideline for the management of heart failure: executive summary. A report of the American College of Cardiology Foundation/American Heart Association Task Force on practice guidelines. *Circulation.* 2013;128(16):1810–1852.

50. Sharma K, Kass DA. Heart failure with preserved ejection fraction: mechanisms, clinical features, and therapies. *Circ Res.* 2014;115(1):79–96.

51. Shoemaker MJ, Dias KJ, Heick JD, Lefevbre KM, Collins SM. Physical therapy for adults following acutely decompensated

chronic heart failure. *Physical Therapy Journal*. 2020;100(1):14–43. Doi 10.1093/ptj/pzz127. PMID 31972027.

52. Hiratzka LF, Bakris GL, Beckman JA, et al. Guidelines for the diagnosis and management of patients with thoracic aortic disease: executive summary. A report of the American College of Cardiology Foundation/American Heart Association Task Force on Practice Guidelines, American Association for Thoracic Surgery, American College of Radiology, American Stroke Association, Society of Cardiovascular Anesthesiologists, Society for Cardiovascular Angiography and Interventions, Society of Interventional Radiology, Society of Thoracic Surgeons, and Society for Vascular Medicine. *Catheter Cardiovasc Interv*. 2010;76(2):E43–E86.

53. Lederle FA. Smokers' relative risk for aortic aneurysm compared with other smoking-related diseases: a systematic review. *J Vasc Surg*. 2003;38:329–334.

54. Dua MM, Dalman RL. Identifying aortic aneurysm risk factors in postmenopausal women. *Womens Health*. 2009;5(1):33–37.

55. Lederle FA. Abdominal aortic aneurysm events in the women's health initiative: cohort study. *BMJ*. 2008;337:1724–1734.

56. de Virgilio C. Ascending aortic dissection in weight lifters with cystic medial degeneration. *Ann Thorac Surg*. 1990;49(4):638–642.

57. Guirguis-Blake JM, Beil TL, Sun X, et al. *Primary care screening for abdominal aortic aneurysm: a systematic evidence review for the US preventive services task force*. Rockville, MD: Agency for Healthcare Research and Quality; 2014:1–145. www.ncbi.nlm.nih.gov/books/NBK184793/.

58. Scaife M, Giannakopoulos T, Al-Khoury GE, et al. Contemporary applications of ultrasound in abdominal aortic aneurysm management. *Front Surg*. 2016;27(3):29.

59. Edwards JZ. Chronic back pain caused by an abdominal aortic aneurysm: case report and review of the literature. *Orthopedics*. 2003;26:191–192.

60. Chervu A. Role of physical examination in detection of abdominal aortic aneurysms. *Surgery*. 1995;117(4):454–457.

61. O'Gara P.T.: Aortic aneurysm, *Circulation* 107(e43), 2003. Available online at http://circ.ahajournals.org/cgi/content/full/107/6/e43. Accessed January 6, 2010.

62. Moore KL. *Clinically oriented anatomy*. ed 6 Philadelphia: Wolters Kluwer/Lippincott Williams & Wilkins; 2010.

63. O'Rourke MF. The cardiovascular continuum extended: aging effects on the aorta and microvasculature, *Vasc Med*. 2010;15(6):461–468.

64. Hickson SS. The relationship of age with regional aortic stiffness and diameter. *J Am Coll Cardiol: Cardiovascular Imaging*. 2010;3(12):1247–1255.

65. Lam CS. Aortic root remodeling over the adult life course: longitudinal data from the Framingham Heart Study. *Circulation*. 2010;122(9):884–890.

66. Guinea GV. Factors influencing the mechanical behavior of healthy human descending thoracic aorta. *Physiol Meas*. 2010;31:1553–1565.

67. Fink HA. The accuracy of physical examination to detect abdominal aortic aneurysm. *Arch Intern Med*. 2000;160:833–836.

68. Lederle FA. Selective screening for abdominal aortic aneurysms with physical examination and ultrasound. *Arch Intern Med*. 1988;148:1753.

69. Mechelli F. Differential diagnosis of a patient referred to physical therapy with low back pain: abdominal aortic aneurysm. *J Orthop Sports Phys Ther*. 2008;38(9):551–557.

70. Hillman ND, Tani LY, Veasy LG, et al. Current status of surgery for rheumatic carditis in children. *Ann Thoracic Surg*. 2004;78(4):1403–1408.

71. Sapico FL, Liquette JA, Sarma RJ. Bone and joint infections in patients with infective endocarditis: review of a 4-year experience. *Clin Infect Dis*. 1996;22:783–787.

72. Vlahakis NE, Temesgen Z, Berbari EF, et al. Osteoarticular infection complicating enterococcal endocarditis. *Mayo Clin Proc*. 2003;78(5):623–628.

73. Petrini JR. Racial differences by gestational age in neonatal deaths attributable to congenital heart defects in the United States. *MMWR*. 2010;59(37):1208–1211.

74. Cava JR, Danduran MJ, Fedderly RT, et al. Exercise recommendations and risk factors for sudden cardiac death. *Pediatr Clin North Am*. 2004;51(5):1401–1420.

75. Berger S, Kugler JD, Thomas JA, et al. Sudden cardiac death in children and adolescents: introduction and overview. *Pediatr Clin North Am*. 2004;51(5):1201–1209.

76. Bader RS, Goldberg L, Sahn DJ. Risk of sudden cardiac death in young athletes: which screening strategies are appropriate? *Pediatr Clin North Am*. 2004;51(5):1421–1441.

77. Hayek E, Gring CN, Griffin BP. Mitral valve prolapse. *Lancet*. 2005;365(9458):507–518.

78. Freed LA, Leby D, Levine RA, et al. Prevalence and clinical outcome of mitral valve prolapse. *N Engl J Med*. 1999;341:1–7.

79. Devereux RB, Jones EC, Roman MJ, et al. Prevalence and correlates of mitral valve prolapse in a population-based sample of American Indians: the Strong Heart Study. *Am J Med*. 2001;111:679–685.

80. Freed LA, Benjamin EJ, Levy D, et al. Mitral valve prolapse in the general population: the benign nature of echocardiographic features in the Framingham Heart Study. *J Am Coll Cardiol*. 2002;40(7):1298–1304.

81. Freed LA, Levy D, Levine RA, et al. Prevalence and clinical outcome of mitral valve prolapse. *N Engl J Med*. 1999;341(1):1–7.

82. Kairo K, Tobin J, Wolfson L, et al. Lower standing systolic blood pressure as a predictor of falls in the elderly: a community-based prospective study. *J Am Coll Cardiol*. 2001;38(1):246–252.

83. Pathak RK, Middeldorp ME, Lau DH, et al. Aggressive risk factor reduction study for atrial fibrillation and implications for the outcome of ablation: The ARREST-AF cohort study. *J Am Coll Cardiol*. 2014;64(21):2222–2231. https://doi.org/10.1016/j.jacc.2014.09.028.

84. Pathak RK, Middeldorp ME, Meredith M, et al. Long-term effect of goal-directed weight management in an atrial fibrillation cohort: A long-term follow-up study (LEGACY). *J Am Coll Cardiol*. 2015 https://doi.org/10.1016/j.jacc.2015.03.002.

85. Pathak RK, Elliott A, Middeldorp ME, et al. Impact of CARDIOrespiratory FITness on arrhythmia recurrence in obese individuals with atrial fibrillation. The CARDIO-FIT study. *J Am Coll Cardiol*. 2015 https://doi.org/10.1016/j.jacc.2015.06.488.

86. Strandberg TE. Isolated systolic blood pressure measurement. *Lancet*. 2008;372(9643):1033–1034.

87. Ntatsaki E. Isolated systolic blood pressure measurement. *Lancet*. 2008;372(9643):1033.

88. Chaudhry SI, Krumholz HM, Foody JM. Systolic hypertension in older persons. *JAMA*. 2004;292(9):1074–1080.

89. Your blood pressure: check that top number, *Johns Hopkins Medical Letter: Health After 50* 16(11):6–7, 2005.

90. Staessen JA, Fagard R, Thijs L, et al. Randomised double-blind comparison of placebo and active treatment for older patients with isolated systolic hypertension. The Systolic Hypertension in Europe (Syst-Eur) Trial Investigators. *Lancet*. 1997;350(9080):757–764.

91. Mancia G. Long-term risk of sustained hypertension in white-coat or masked hypertension. *Hypertension*. 2009;54(2):226–232.

92. Furie KL, et al. Guidelines for the prevention of stroke in patients with stroke and transient ischemic attack. A guideline for healthcare professionals from the American Heart Association/American Stroke Association. *Stroke*. 2010;42(1):227–276.

93. Miller ER, Jehn ML. New high blood pressure guidelines create new at-risk classification: changes in blood pressure classification by JNC 7. *J Cardiovasc Nurs*. 2004;19(6):367–371.

94. Wright Jr. JT, Williamson JD, Whelton PK, et al. A randomized trial of intensive versus standard blood pressure control SPRINT Research Group. *N Engl J Med*. 2015;373:2103–2116.

95. Xie X, Atkins E, Lv J, et al. Effects of intensive blood pressure lowering on cardiovascular and renal outcomes: updated systematic review and meta-analysis. *Lancet*. 2016;387(10017):435–443.

96. Ettehad D, Emdin CA, Kiran A, et al. Blood pressure lowering for prevention of cardiovascular disease and death: a systematic review and meta-analysis. *Lancet*. 2016;387(10022):957–967.

97. O'Donnell CJ, Lindpaintner K, Larson MG, et al. Evidence for association and genetic linkage with hypertension and blood pressure in men but not women in the Framingham heart study. *Circulation*. 1998;97(18):1766–1772.

98. Treating a "mini stroke" to prevent a "major" stroke, *Johns Hopkins Medical Letter: Health After 50* 17(8):6–7, 2005.

99. Johnston SC, Rothwell PM, Nguyen-Huynh MN, et al. Validation and refinement scores to predict early stroke risk after transient ischaemic attack. *Lancet*. 2007;369(9558):283–292.

100. Shaw BH, Garland EM, Black BK, Paranjape SY, et al. Optimal diagnostic thresholds for diagnosis of orthostatic hypotension with a "sit-to'stand test". *J Hypertens*. 2017;35(5):1019–1025.

101. Kim HA, Yi HA, Lee H. Recent advances in orthostatic hypotension presenting orthostatic dizziness or vertigo. *Neurol Sci*. 2015;36:1995–2002.

102. Tepper S, McKeough M. Deep venous thrombosis: risks, diagnosis, treatment interventions, and prevention. *Acute Care Perspectives*. 2000;9(1):1–7.

103. Constans J, Boutinet C, Salmi R, et al. Comparison of four clinical prediction scores for the diagnosis of lower limb deep venous thrombosis in outpatients. *Am J Med*. 2003;115:436–440.

104. Constans J, Nelzy ML, Salmi LR, et al. Clinical prediction of lower limb deep vein thrombosis in symptomatic hospitalized patients. *Thromb Haemost*. 2001;86:985–990.

105. Le Gal G, Carrier M, Rodger M. Clinical decision rules in venous thromboembolism. *Best Pract Res Clin Haemat*. 2012;25:303–317.

106. Powell M. Duplex ultrasound screening for deep vein thrombosis in spinal cord injured patients at rehabilitation admission. *Arch Phys Med Rehab*. 1999;80:1044–1046.

107. Agnelli G, Sonaglia F. Prevention of venous thromboembolism. *Thromb Res*. 2000;97(1):V49–V62.

108. Ageno W. Treatment of venous thromboembolism. *Thromb Res*. 2000;97(1):V63–V72.

109. Bauer K. Hypercoagulable states. *Hematology*. 2005;10(Suppl 1):39.

110. Wu O, Robertson L, Langhorne P, et al. Oral contraceptives, hormone replacement therapy, thrombophilias, and risk of venous thromboembolism: a systematic review. The Thrombosis: Risk and Economic Assessment of Thrombophilia Screening (TREATS) Study. *Thromb Haemost*. 2005;94(1):17–25.

111. Gomes MP, Deitcher SR. Risk of venous thromboembolic disease associated with hormonal contraceptives and hormone replacement therapy: a clinical review. *Arch Intern Med*. 2004;164(18):1965–1976.

112. Constans J. A clinical prediction score for upper extremity deep venous thrombosis. *Thromb Haemost*. 2008;99:202–207.

113. Mozaffarian D, et al. Heart disease and stroke statistics—2016 update: A report from the American Heart Association. *Circulation*. 2015;134(15):E38–360.

114. High blood pressure in adults. *JAMA*. 2014;311(5):507–520.

Screening for Pulmonary Disease

For the client presenting with neck, shoulder, or back pain, it may be necessary to consider the possibility of a pulmonary cause requiring medical referral. The most common pulmonary conditions to mimic those of the musculoskeletal system include pneumonia, pulmonary embolism (PE), pleurisy, pneumothorax, and pulmonary arterial hypertension (PAH).

The information gathered from the client—such as the past medical history, risk factor assessment, clinical presentation, as well as asking about the presence of any associated signs and symptoms—guides the screening process to determine the potential involvement of the pulmonary system. In the case of pleuropulmonary disorders, the client's recent personal medical history may include a previous or recurrent upper respiratory infection or pneumonia.

Each pulmonary condition will have unique risk factors that can predispose clients to a specific respiratory disease or illness. For example, a pneumothorax may be preceded by trauma, overexertion, or recent scuba diving.

A previous history of cancer, especially primary lung cancer or cancers that metastasize to the lungs (e.g., breast, bone), is a red flag and a risk factor for cancer recurrence. Risk factor assessment also helps identify increased risk for other respiratory conditions or illnesses that can present as a primary musculoskeletal problem.

The material in this chapter will assist the therapist in assessing both the client with a known pulmonary condition and the client with musculoskeletal signs and symptoms that may have an underlying systemic basis (Case Example 8.1).

SIGNS AND SYMPTOMS OF PULMONARY DISORDERS

Signs and symptoms of pulmonary disorders can be many and varied; the most common symptoms associated with pulmonary disorders are cough and dyspnea. Other manifestations include chest pain, abnormal sputum, hemoptysis, cyanosis, digital clubbing, altered breathing patterns, and chest pain.

Cough

As a physiologic response, cough occurs frequently in healthy people, but a persistent dry cough may be caused by a tumor, congestion, or hypersensitive airways (allergies). A productive cough with purulent sputum (yellow or green) may indicate infection, whereas a productive cough with nonpurulent sputum (clear or white) is nonspecific and indicates airway irritation. Rust-colored sputum may be a sign of pneumonia and should also be investigated. Hemoptysis (coughing and spitting blood) indicates a pathologic condition—infection, inflammation, abscess, tumor, or infarction.

CASE EXAMPLE 8.1

Bronchopulmonary Pain

A 67-year-old woman with a known diagnosis of rheumatoid arthritis has been treated as needed in a physical therapy clinic for the last 8 years. She has reported occasional chest pain described as "coming on suddenly, like a knife pushing from the inside out—it takes my breath away."

She missed 2 days of treatment because of illness, and when she returned to the clinic, the physical therapist noticed that she had a newly developed cough and that her rheumatoid arthritis was much worse. She says that she missed her appointments because she had the "flu."

Further questioning to elicit the potential development of chest pain during inspiration, presence of ongoing fever and chills, and the change in breathing pattern is recommended.

Positive findings beyond the reasonable duration of influenza (7 to 10 days) or an increase in pulmonary symptoms (shortness of breath [SOB], hacking cough, hemoptysis, wheezing or other changes in breathing pattern) raise a red flag, indicating the need for medical referral.

This clinical case points out that clients currently undergoing physical therapy for a known musculoskeletal problem may be describing signs and symptoms of systemic disease.

Dyspnea

Shortness of breath (SOB), or dyspnea, usually indicates hypoxemia but can be associated with emotional states, particularly fear and anxiety. Dyspnea is usually caused by diffuse and extensive rather than focal pulmonary disease; PE is the exception. Factors contributing to the sensation of dyspnea include increased work of breathing (WOB), respiratory muscle fatigue, increased systemic metabolic demands, and decreased respiratory reserve capacity. Dyspnea when the person is lying down is called *orthopnea* and is caused by redistribution of body water. Fluid shift leads to increased fluid in the lung, which interferes with gas exchange and leads to orthopnea. In supine, the abdominal contents also exert pressure on the diaphragm, increasing the WOB and often limiting vital capacity.

The therapist must be careful when screening for dyspnea or SOB, either with exertion or while at rest. If a client denies compromised breathing, look for functional changes as the client accommodates for difficulty breathing by reducing activity or exertion.

Cyanosis

The presence of cyanosis, a bluish color of the skin and mucous membranes, depends on the oxygen saturation of arterial blood and the total amount of circulating hemoglobin. It may be observed as a bluish discoloration in the oral mucous membranes, lips, and conjunctivae and pale (white) or blue nail beds and nose.

Clubbing (see Chapter 4)

Thickening and widening of the terminal phalanges of the fingers and toes result in a painless club-like appearance recognized by the loss of the angle between the nail and the nail bed (see Figs. 4.36 and 4.37).Conditions that chronically interfere with tissue perfusion and nutrition may cause clubbing, including cystic fibrosis (CF), chronic obstructive pulmonary disease (COPD), lung cancer, bronchiectasis, pulmonary fibrosis, congenital heart disease, and lung abscess. Most of the time, clubbing occurs as a result of pulmonary disease and resultant hypoxia (diminished availability of blood to the body tissues), but clubbing can be a sign of heart disease, peripheral vascular disease, and disorders of the liver and gastrointestinal tract.

Altered Breathing Patterns

Changes in the rate, depth, regularity, and effort of breathing occur in response to any condition affecting the pulmonary system. Breathing patterns can vary, depending on the neuromuscular or neurologic disease or trauma (Box 8.1). Breathing pattern abnormalities seen with head trauma, brain abscess, diaphragmatic paralysis of chest wall muscles and thorax (e.g., generalized myopathy or neuropathy), heat stroke, spinal meningitis, and encephalitis can include apneustic breathing, ataxic breathing, or Cheyne-Stokes respiration (CSR).

Apneustic breathing (gasping inspiration with short expiration) localizes damage to the midpons and is most commonly a result of a basilar artery infarct. *Ataxic*, or *Biot's*,

---

BOX 8.1 BREATHING PATTERNS AND ASSOCIATED CONDITIONS

Hyperventilation

- Anxiety
- Acute head injury
- Hypoxemia
- Fever

Kussmaul's

- Strenuous exercise
- Metabolic acidosis

Cheyne-Stokes

- Congestive heart failure
- Renal failure
- Meningitis
- Drug overdose
- Increased intracranial pressure
- Infants (normal)
- Older people during sleep (normal)

Hypoventilation

- Fibromyalgia syndrome
- Chronic fatigue syndrome
- Sleep disorder
- Muscle fatigue
- Muscle weakness
- Malnutrition
- Neuromuscular disease
  - Guillain-Barré
  - Myasthenia gravis
  - Poliomyelitis
  - Amyotrophic lateral sclerosis (ALS)
- Pickwickian or obesity hypoventilation syndrome
- Severe kyphoscoliosis

Apneustic

- Midpons lesion
- Basilar artery infarct

Biot's Respiration (Ataxia)

- Exercise
- Shock
- Cerebral hypoxia
- Heat stroke
- Spinal meningitis
- Head injury
- Brain abscess
- Encephalitis

From Ikeda B, Goodman CC, Fuller K: The respiratory system. In Goodman CC: *Pathology: implications for the physical therapist*, ed 3, St Louis, 2009, Elsevier.

breathing (irregular pattern of deep and shallow breaths with abrupt pauses) is caused by a disruption of the respiratory rhythm generator in the medulla.

CSR may be evident in healthy older adults and compromised clients. The most common cause of CSR is severe congestive heart failure (CHF), but it can also occur with renal failure, meningitis, drug overdose, and increased intracranial pressure. It may be a normal breathing pattern in infants and older persons during sleep.

Exercise may induce pleural pain, coughing, hemoptysis, SOB, and/or other abnormal changes in breathing patterns. When asked if the client is ever short of breath, the individual may say "no" because he or she has reduced activity levels to avoid dyspnea (see Appendix B-12 in the accompanying enhanced eBook version included with print purchase of this textbook).

Pulmonary Pain Patterns

The most common sites for referred pain from the pulmonary system are the chest, ribs, upper trapezius, shoulder, and thoracic spine. The first symptoms may not appear until the client's respiratory system is stressed by the addition of exercise during physical therapy. On the other hand, the client may present with what appears to be primary musculoskeletal pain in any one of those areas. Auscultation may reveal the first signs of pulmonary distress (see Chapter 4 for screening examination by auscultation).

Pulmonary pain patterns are usually localized in the substernal or chest region over the involved lung fields that may include the anterior chest, side, or back (Fig. 8.1). However, pulmonary pain can radiate to the neck, upper trapezius muscle, costal margins, thoracic region, scapulae, or shoulder. Shoulder pain may radiate along the medial aspect of the arm, mimicking other neuromuscular causes of neck or shoulder pain (see Fig. 8.11).

Pulmonary pain usually increases with inspiratory movements, such as laughing, coughing, sneezing, or deep breathing, and the client notes the presence of associated symptoms, such as dyspnea (exertional or at rest), persistent cough, fever, and chills. Palpation and resisted movements will not reproduce the symptoms, which may get worse with recumbency, especially at night or while sleeping.

The thoracic cavity is lined with pleura, or serous membrane. One surface of the pleura lines the inside of the rib cage (parietal) and the other surface covers the lungs (visceral). The parietal pleura is sensitive to painful stimulation, but the visceral pleura is insensitive to pain. Extensive disease may occur in the lung without the occurrence of pain until the process extends to the parietal pleura. This explains why pathology of the lungs may be painless until obstruction or inflammation is enough to press on the parietal pleura.

Pleural irritation then results in sharp, localized pain that is aggravated by any respiratory movement. Clients usually note that the pain is alleviated by autosplinting, that is, lying on the affected side or applying pressure to that painful side, which diminishes the movement of that side of the

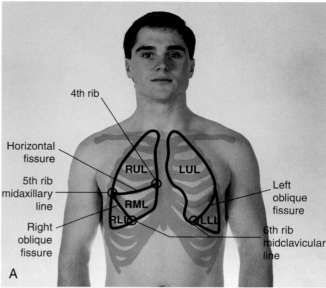

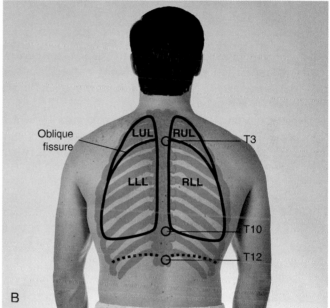

Fig. 8.1 *Pulmonary pain patterns are localized over involved lung fields affecting the anterior chest, side, or back. Radiating pain can also cause neck, shoulder, upper trapezius, rib, and/ or scapular pain.* **A,** Anterior chest. **B,** Posterior chest. The posterior chest is comprised primarily of lower lung lobes. The upper lobes occupy a small area from T1 to T3 or T4. (From Jarvis C: *Physical examination and assessment,* ed 5, Philadelphia, 2007, WB Saunders.)

chest (see further discussion of pleural pain in this chapter).[1]

Tracheobronchial Pain

Within the pulmonary system, the trachea and large bronchi are innervated by the vagus trunks, whereas the finer bronchi and lung parenchyma appear to be free of pain innervation. Tracheobronchial pain is referred to sites in the neck or anterior chest at the same levels as the points of irritation in the air passages (Fig. 8.2). This irritation may be caused by inflammatory lesions, irritating foreign materials, or cancerous tumors.

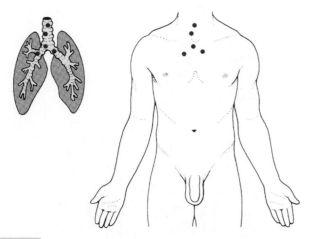

Fig. 8.2 *Tracheobronchial pain is referred to sites in the neck or anterior chest at the same levels as the points of irritation in the air passages.* The points of pain are on the same side as the areas of irritation.

Pleural Pain

When the disease progresses enough to extend to the parietal pleura, pleural irritation occurs and results in sharp, localized pain that is aggravated by any respiratory movement and is diminished by *autosplinting*.

Debate continues concerning the mechanism by which pain occurs in the parietal membrane. It has been long thought that friction between the two pleural surfaces (when the membranes are irritated and covered with fibrinous exudate) causes sharp pain. Other theories suggest that intercostal muscle spasm resulting from pleurisy or stretching of the parietal pleura causes this pain.

Pleural pain is present in pulmonary diseases such as pleurisy, pneumonia, pulmonary infarct (when it extends to the pleural surface, thus causing pleurisy), tumor (when it invades the parietal pleura), and pneumothorax. Tumor, especially bronchogenic carcinoma, may be accompanied by severe, continuous pain when the tumor tissue, extending to the parietal pleura through the lung, constantly irritates the pain nerve endings in the pleura.

Diaphragmatic Pleural Pain

The *diaphragmatic pleura* receives dual pain innervation through the phrenic and intercostal nerves. Damage to the phrenic nerve produces paralysis of the corresponding half of the diaphragm. The phrenic nerves are sensory and motor from both surfaces of the diaphragm.

Stimulation of the peripheral portions of the diaphragmatic pleura results in sharp pain felt along the costal margins, which can be referred to the lumbar region by the lower thoracic somatic nerves. Stimulation of the central portion of the diaphragmatic pleura results in sharp pain referred to the upper trapezius muscle and shoulder on the ipsilateral side of the stimulation (see Figs. 3.4 and 3.5).

Pain of cardiac and diaphragmatic origin is often experienced in the shoulder because the heart and diaphragm are

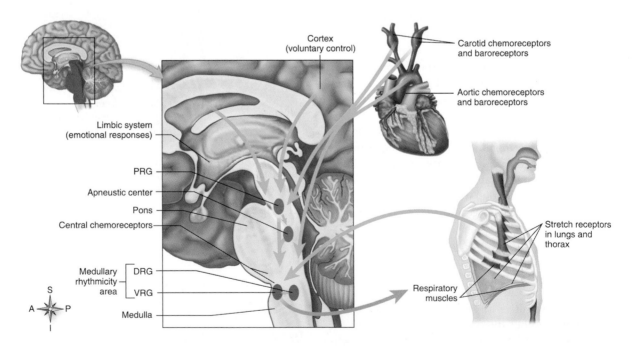

Fig 8.3 *Regulation of Breathing.* The dorsal respiratory group (DRG) and ventral respiratory group (VRG) of the medulla represent the medullary rhythmicity area. The pontine respiratory group (PRG, or pneumotaxic center) and apneustic center of the pons influence the basic respiratory rhythm by means of neural input to the medullary rhythmicity area. The brainstem also receives input from other parts of the body; information from chemoreceptors, baroreceptors, and stretch receptors can alter the basic breathing pattern, as can emotional (limbic) and sensory input. Despite these subconscious reflexes, the cerebral cortex can override the "automatic" control of breathing to some extent to do such activities as sing or blow up a balloon. Green arrows show the flow of information to the respiratory control centers. The purple arrow shows the flow of information from the control centers to the respiratory muscles that drive breathing. From Patton KT, Thibodeau GA, eds. The human body in health & disease. 7th ed. St Louis: Elsevier; 2018

supplied by the C5-C6 spinal segment, and the visceral pain is referred to the corresponding somatic area.

Diaphragmatic pleurisy secondary to pneumonia is common and refers sharp pain along the costal margins or upper trapezius, which is aggravated by any diaphragmatic motion, such as coughing, laughing, or deep breathing.

There may be tenderness to palpation along the costal margins, and sharp pain occurs when the client is asked to take a deep breath. A change in position (sidebending or rotation or the combination of sidebending with rotation of the trunk) does not reproduce the symptoms, which would be the case with a true intercostal lesion or tear.

Forceful, repeated coughing can result in an intercostal lesion in the presence of referred intercostal pain from diaphragmatic pleurisy, which can make differentiation between these two entities impossible without a medical referral and further diagnostic testing.

Pulmonary Physiology

The primary function of the respiratory system is to provide oxygen to and to remove carbon dioxide (CO_2) from cells in the body. The act of breathing, in which the oxygen and CO_2 exchange occurs, involves the two interrelated processes of ventilation and respiration.

Ventilation is the movement of air from outside of the body to the alveoli of the lungs. Respiration is the process of oxygen uptake and CO_2 elimination between the body and the outside environment.

Breathing is an automatic process by which sensors detect changes in the levels of CO_2 and continuously direct data regarding the composition of blood and cerebrospinal fluid concentration to the medulla. The medulla then directs respiratory muscles that adjust ventilation. Breathing patterns can be altered voluntarily when this automatic response is overridden by conscious thought.

The major sensors mentioned here are the central chemoreceptors (located near the medulla) and the peripheral sensors (located in the carotid body and aortic arch) (Fig. 8.3). The central chemoreceptors respond to increases in CO_2 and decreases in pH in cerebrospinal fluid.

As CO_2 increases, the medulla signals a response to increase respiration. The peripheral chemoreceptor system responds to low arterial blood oxygen and is believed to function only in pathologic situations such as when there are chronically elevated CO_2 levels (e.g., COPD).

Acid-Base Regulation

The proper balance of acids and bases in the body is essential to life. This balance is very complex and must be kept within the narrow parameters of a pH of 7.35 to 7.45 in the extracellular fluid. This number (or pH value) represents the hydrogen ion concentration in body fluid.

A reading of less than 7.35 is considered *acidosis*, and a reading greater than 7.45 is called *alkalosis*. Life cannot be sustained if the pH values are less than 7 or greater than 7.8.

Living human cells are extremely sensitive to alterations in body fluid pH (hydrogen ion concentration); thus various mechanisms are in operation to keep the pH at a relatively constant level.

Acid-base regulatory mechanisms include chemical buffer systems, the respiratory system, and the renal system. These systems interact very closely to maintain a normal acid-base ratio of 20 parts of bicarbonate to 1 part of carbonic acid and thus to maintain normal body fluid pH.

The blood test used most often to measure the effectiveness of ventilation and oxygen transport is the arterial blood gas (ABG) test (Table 8.1). The measurement of arterial blood gases is important in the diagnosis and treatment of ventilation, oxygen transport, and acid-base problems.

The ABG test measures the amount of dissolved oxygen and CO_2 in arterial blood and indicates acid-base status by measurement of the arterial blood pH. In simple terms, a low

TABLE 8.1	Arterial Blood Gas Values*
pH	7.35–7.45
PCO_2 (partial pressure of carbon dioxide)	35–45 mm Hg
HCO_3 (bicarbonate ion)	22–31 mEq/L
PO_2 (partial pressure of oxygen)	75–100 mm Hg
Oxygen (O_2) saturation	96%–100%
Panic Values	
pH	≤7.20 or >7.6
PCO_2	<20 or >70 mm Hg
HCO_3	<10 or >40 mEq/L
PO_2	<40 mm Hg
O_2 saturation	≤60%

Normal pH level: The pH is inversely proportional to the hydrogen ion concentration in the blood. As the hydrogen ion concentration increases (acidosis), the pH decreases; as the hydrogen ion concentration decreases (alkalosis), the pH increases.

Normal PCO_2: The PCO_2 is a measure of the partial pressure of carbon dioxide (CO_2) in the blood. As the CO_2 increases, the pH decreases (respiratory acidosis); as the CO_2 level decreases, the pH increases (respiratory alkalosis). PCO_2 measures the effectiveness of the body's ventilation system as CO_2 is removed.

Bicarbonate ion: HCO_3 is a measure of the metabolic portion of the acid-base function. As the bicarbonate value increases, the pH increases (metabolic alkalosis); as the bicarbonate value decreases, the pH decreases (metabolic acidosis).

Partial pressure of oxygen: PO_2 is a measure of the partial pressure of O_2 in the blood and represents the status of alveolar gas exchange.

Oxygen saturation: O_2 saturation is an indication of the percentage of hemoglobin saturated with oxygen. When 95% to 100% of the hemoglobin binds and carries oxygen, the tissues are adequately perfused with oxygen. As the PO_2 decreases, the percentage of hemoglobin saturation also decreases. At O_2 saturation levels of less than 70%, the tissues are unable to carry out vital functions.

*Modified from Chernecky C, Berger B: *Laboratory tests and diagnostic procedures*, ed 5, Philadelphia, 2008, WB Saunders.

pH reflects increased acid buildup and a high pH reflects an increased base buildup.

Acid buildup occurs when there is an ineffective removal of CO_2 from the lungs or when there is excess acid production from the tissues of the body. These problems are corrected by adjusting the ventilation or buffering the acid with bicarbonate.

Pulmonary Pathophysiology

Respiratory Acidosis

Any condition that decreases pulmonary ventilation increases the retention and concentration of CO_2, hydrogen, and carbonic acid; this increases the amount of circulating hydrogen and is called respiratory acidosis.

If ventilation is severely compromised, CO_2 levels become extremely high and respiration is depressed even further, causing hypoxia.

During respiratory acidosis, potassium moves out of cells into the extracellular fluid to exchange with circulating hydrogen. This results in hyperkalemia (abnormally high potassium concentration in the blood) and cardiac changes that can cause cardiac arrest.

Respiratory acidosis can result from pathologic conditions that decrease the efficiency of the respiratory system. These pathologies can include damage to the medulla, which controls respiration, obstruction of airways (e.g., neoplasm, foreign bodies, pulmonary disease such as COPD, pneumonia), loss of lung surface ventilation (e.g., pneumothorax, pulmonary fibrosis), weakness of respiratory muscles (e.g., poliomyelitis, spinal cord injury, Guillain-Barré syndrome), or overdose of respiratory depressant drugs.

As hypoxia becomes more severe, diaphoresis, shallow rapid breathing, restlessness, and cyanosis may appear. Cardiac arrhythmias may also be present as the potassium level in the blood serum rises.

Treatment is directed at restoration of efficient ventilation. If the respiratory depression and acidosis are severe, injection of intravenous sodium bicarbonate and use of a mechanical ventilator may be necessary. Any client with symptoms of inadequate ventilation or CO_2 retention needs immediate medical referral and intervention.

CLINICAL SIGNS AND SYMPTOMS

Respiratory Acidosis

- Decreased ventilation
- Confusion
- Sleepiness and unconsciousness
- Diaphoresis
- Shallow, rapid breathing
- Restlessness
- Cyanosis

Respiratory Alkalosis

An increased respiratory rate and depth decrease the amount of available CO_2 and hydrogen and create a condition of increased pH, or alkalosis. When pulmonary ventilation is increased, CO_2 and hydrogen are eliminated from the body too quickly and are not available to buffer the increasingly alkaline environment.

Respiratory alkalosis is usually caused by *hyperventilation*. Rapid, deep respirations are often caused by neurogenic or psychogenic problems, including anxiety, pain, and cerebral trauma or lesions. Other causes can be related to conditions that greatly increase metabolism (e.g., hyperthyroidism) or overventilation of clients who are using a mechanical ventilator.

If the alkalosis becomes more severe, muscular tetany and convulsions can occur. Cardiac arrhythmias caused by serum potassium loss through the kidneys may also occur. The kidneys keep hydrogen in exchange for potassium.

Treatment of respiratory alkalosis includes reassurance, assistance in slowing breathing and facilitating relaxation, sedation, pain control, CO_2 administration, and use of a rebreathing device such as a rebreathing mask or paper bag. A rebreathing device allows the client to inhale and "rebreathe" the exhaled CO_2.

Respiratory alkalosis related to hyperventilation is a relatively common condition and might be present more often in the physical therapy setting than respiratory acidosis. Pain and anxiety are common causes of hyperventilation and treatment needs to be focused on reduction of both of these interrelated elements. If hyperventilation continues in the absence of pain or anxiety, serious systemic problems may be the cause and immediate physician referral is necessary.

If either respiratory acidosis or alkalosis persists for hours to days in a chronic and not life-threatening manner, the kidneys then begin to assist in the restoration of normal body fluid pH by selective excretion or retention of hydrogen ions or bicarbonate. This process is called *renal compensation*. When the kidneys compensate effectively, blood pH values are within normal limits (7.35 to 7.45) even though the underlying problem may still cause the respiratory imbalance.

CLINICAL SIGNS AND SYMPTOMS

Respiratory Alkalosis

- Hyperventilation
- Light-headedness
- Dizziness
- Numbness and tingling of the face, fingers, and toes
- Syncope (fainting)

Chronic Obstructive Pulmonary Disease

COPD, also called chronic obstructive lung disease (COLD), refers to several disorders that have in common abnormal airway structures resulting in obstruction of air in and out of the lungs. The most important of these disorders are obstructive bronchitis, emphysema, and asthma.

Although bronchitis, emphysema, and asthma may occur in a "pure form," these conditions most commonly coexist. For example, adults with active asthma are as much as 12 times more likely to acquire COPD over time than adults with no active asthma.[2-5]

COPD is a leading cause of morbidity and mortality among cigarette smokers. Other predisposing factors to COPD include air pollution; occupational exposure to aerosol pesticides, irritating dusts or gases, or art materials (e.g., paint, glass, ceramics, sculpture); hereditary factors; infection; allergies; aging; and potentially harmful drugs and chemicals.[6]

COPD rarely occurs in nonsmokers; however, only a minority of cigarette smokers develop symptomatic disease, suggesting that genetic factors or some other underlying predisposition may contribute to the development of COPD.[7]

In all forms of COPD, narrowing of the airways obstructs airflow to and from the lungs (Table 8.2). This narrowing impairs ventilation by trapping air in the bronchioles and alveoli. The obstruction increases the resistance to airflow. The severity of symptoms depends on how much of the lung parenchyma has been damaged or destroyed.

Trapped air hinders normal gas exchange and causes distention of the alveoli. Other mechanisms of COPD vary with each form of the disease. In the healthy adult, the bottom margin of the respiratory diaphragm sits at T9 when the lungs are at rest. Taking a deep breath expands the diaphragm (and lungs) inferiorly to T11. For the client with COPD the lower lung lobes are already at T11 when the lungs are at rest from overexpansion as a result of alveoli distention and hyperinflation.

COPD develops earlier in life than is usually recognized, making it the most underdiagnosed and undertreated pulmonary disease. Smoking cessation is the only intervention shown to slow a decline in lung function. Identifying risk factors and recognizing early signs and symptoms of COPD increases the affected individual's chance of reduced morbidity through early intervention.[6]

Bronchitis.

Acute. Acute bronchitis is an inflammation of the trachea and bronchi (tracheobronchial tree) that is self-limiting and of short duration with few pulmonary signs. This condition may result from chemical irritation (e.g., smoke, fumes, gas) or may occur with viral infections such as influenza, measles, chickenpox, or whooping cough.

These predisposing conditions may become apparent during the subjective examination (i.e., Personal/Family History form or the Physical Therapy Interview). Although bronchitis is usually mild, it can become complicated in older adults and clients with chronic lung or heart disease. Pneumonia is a critical complication to acute bronchitis.

TABLE 8.2	Respiratory Diseases: Summary of Differences	
Disease	Primary Area Affected	Results
Bronchitis	Membrane lining bronchial tubes	Inflammation of lining
Bronchiectasis	Bronchial tubes (bronchi or air passages)	Bronchial dilation with inflammation
Pneumonia	Alveoli (air sacs)	Causative agent invades alveoli with resultant outpouring from lung capillaries into air spaces and continued healing process
Emphysema	Air spaces beyond terminal bronchioles (small airways)	Breakdown of alveolar walls; air spaces enlarged
Asthma	Bronchioles (small airways)	Bronchioles obstructed by muscle spasm, swelling of mucosa, thick secretions
Cystic fibrosis	Bronchioles	Bronchioles become obstructed and obliterated. Later, larger airways become involved. Plugs of mucus cling to airway walls, leading to bronchitis, bronchiectasis, atelectasis, pneumonia, or pulmonary abscess

CLINICAL SIGNS AND SYMPTOMS

Acute Bronchitis

- Mild fever from 1 to 3 days
- Malaise
- Back and muscle pain
- Sore throat
- Cough with sputum production, followed by wheezing
- Possibly laryngitis

Chronic. Chronic bronchitis is a condition associated with prolonged exposure to nonspecific bronchial irritants and is accompanied by mucous hypersecretion and structural changes in the bronchi (large air passages leading into the lungs). This irritation of the tissue usually results from exposure to cigarette smoke or long-term inhalation of dust or air pollution and causes hypertrophy of the goblet cells, the mucous-producing cells in the bronchi.

In bronchitis, partial or complete blockage of the airways from mucous secretions causes insufficient oxygenation in the alveoli (Fig. 8.4). The swollen mucous membrane and thick sputum obstruct the airways, causing wheezing, and the client develops a cough to clear the airways. The clinical definition of a person with chronic bronchitis is anyone who coughs for at least 3 months per year for 2 consecutive years without having had a precipitating disease.

To confirm that the condition is chronic bronchitis, tests are performed to determine whether the airways are obstructed and to exclude other diseases that may cause similar symptoms such as silicosis, tuberculosis, or a tumor

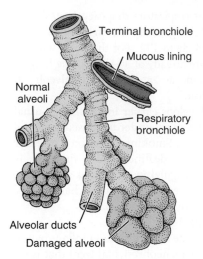

Fig. 8.4 *Chronic bronchitis may lead to the formation of misshapen or large alveolar sacs with reduced space for oxygen and carbon dioxide exchange.* The client may develop cyanosis and pulmonary edema.

in the upper airway. Sputum samples will be analyzed and lung function tests may be performed. A common approach of testing clients with COPD to predict mortality in clients is the BODE.[8] The BODE is a 0–10 scale based on the BMI (*B*), the degree of airflow obstruction (*O*; assessed via FEV_1 [forced expiratory volume of air in 1 second] in a pulmonary function test), dyspnea (*D*; assessed by the dyspnea scale), and exercise capacity (*E*; assessed by the Six-Minute Walk Test distance).

Treatment is aimed at keeping the airways as clear as possible. Smokers are encouraged and helped to stop smoking. A combination of drugs may be prescribed to relieve the symptoms, including bronchodilators to open the obstructed airways and to thin the obstructive mucus so that it can be coughed up more easily.

Chronic bronchitis may develop slowly over years, but it will not go away if untreated. Eventually, the bronchial walls thicken and the number of mucous glands increases. The client is increasingly susceptible to respiratory infections, during which the bronchial tissue becomes inflamed and the mucus becomes even thicker and more profuse.

Chronic bronchitis can be incapacitating and lead to more serious and potentially fatal lung disease. Influenza and pneumococcal vaccines are recommended for these clients.

CLINICAL SIGNS AND SYMPTOMS
Chronic Bronchitis

- Persistent cough with production of sputum (worse in the morning and evening than midday)
- Reduced chest expansion
- Wheezing
- Fever
- Dyspnea (SOB)
- Cyanosis (blue discoloration of skin and mucous membranes)
- Decreased exercise tolerance

Bronchiectasis. Bronchiectasis is a form of obstructive lung disease that is a type of bronchitis. It is a progressive and chronic pulmonary condition that occurs after infections such as childhood pneumonia or CF.

Although bronchiectasis was once a common disease because of measles, pertussis, tuberculosis, and poorly treated bacterial pneumonias, the prevalence of bronchiectasis has diminished greatly since the introduction of antibiotics. It is characterized by abnormal and permanent dilation of the large air passages leading into the lungs (bronchi) and by destruction of bronchial walls.

Bronchiectasis is caused by repeated damage to bronchial walls. The resultant destruction and bronchial dilation reduce bronchial wall movement so that secretions cannot be removed effectively from the lungs, and the client is predisposed to frequent respiratory infections.

This vicious cycle of bacterial infection and inflammation of the bronchial wall leads to loss of ventilation and irreversible lung damage. Advanced bronchiectasis may cause pneumonia, cor pulmonale, or right-sided ventricular failure.

All pulmonary irritants, especially cigarette smoke, should be avoided. Postural drainage, adequate hydration, good nutrition, and bronchodilator therapy in bronchospasm are important components in treatment. Antibiotics are used during disease exacerbations (e.g., increased cough, purulent sputum, hemoptysis, malaise, and weight loss). The use of immunomodulatory therapy to alter the host response directly, and thereby reduce tissue damage, is under investigation.[9,10]

CLINICAL SIGNS AND SYMPTOMS
Bronchiectasis

Clinical signs and symptoms of bronchiectasis vary widely, depending on the extent of the disease and on the presence of complicating infection, but may include:
- Chronic "wet" cough with copious foul-smelling secretions; generally worse in the morning after the individual has been recumbent for a length of time
- Hemoptysis (bloody sputum)
- Occasional wheezing sounds
- Dyspnea
- Sinusitis (inflammation of one or more paranasal sinuses)
- Weight loss
- Anemia
- Malaise
- Recurrent fever and chills
- Fatigue

Emphysema. Emphysema may develop in a person after a long history of chronic bronchitis in which the alveolar walls are destroyed, leading to permanent overdistention of the air space and loss of normal elastic tension in the lung tissue.

Air passages are obstructed as a result of these changes (rather than as a result of mucous production, as in chronic bronchitis). Difficult expiration in emphysema is caused by the destruction of the walls (septa) between the alveoli, by partial airway collapse, and by the loss of elastic recoil.

As the alveoli and septa collapse, pockets of air form between the alveolar spaces (called *blebs*) and within the lung parenchyma (called *bullae*). This process leads to increased ventilatory "dead space," or areas that do not participate in gas or blood exchange. The WOB is increased because there is less functional lung tissue to exchange oxygen and CO_2. Emphysema also destroys the pulmonary capillaries, further decreasing oxygen perfusion and ventilation.

In advanced emphysema, oxygen therapy is usually necessary to treat the progressive hypoxemia that occurs as the disease worsens. Oxygen therapy is carefully titrated and monitored to maintain venous oxygen saturation levels at or slightly above 90%. Too much oxygen can depress the respiratory drive of a person with emphysema.

The drive to breathe in a healthy person results from an increase in the arterial CO_2 level (PCO_2). In the normal adult, increased CO_2 levels stimulate chemoreceptors in the brainstem to increase the respiratory rate. In some chronic lung disorders, these central chemoreceptors may become desensitized to PCO_2 changes, resulting in a dependence on the peripheral chemoreceptors to detect a fall in arterial oxygen levels (PO_2) to stimulate the respiratory drive. Therefore too much oxygen delivered as a treatment can depress the respiratory drive in those individuals with COPD who have a dampening in their CO_2 drive.

Monitoring respiratory rate, level of oxygen administered by nasal cannula, and oxygen saturation levels are very important in this client population. Some pulmonologists agree that supplemental oxygen levels can be increased during activity without compromising the individual because they will "blow it (CO_2) off" anyway. To our knowledge, there is no evidence yet to support this clinical practice.

Types of Emphysema. There are three types of emphysema. *Centrilobular emphysema* (Fig. 8.5), the most common type, destroys the bronchioles, usually in the upper lung regions. Inflammation develops in the bronchioles, but usually the alveolar sac remains intact.

Panlobular emphysema destroys the more distal alveolar walls, most commonly involving the lower lung. This destruction of alveolar walls may occur secondary to infection or irritants (most commonly cigarette smoke). These two forms of emphysema, collectively called centriacinar emphysema, occur most often in smokers.

Paraseptal (or *panacinar*) *emphysema* destroys the alveoli in the lower lobes of the lungs, resulting in isolated blebs along the lung periphery. Paraseptal emphysema is believed to be the likely cause of spontaneous pneumothorax.

Clinical Signs and Symptoms. The irreversible destruction reduces the elasticity of the lung and increases the effort to exhale trapped air, causing marked dyspnea on exertion, later progressing to dyspnea at rest. Cough is uncommon.

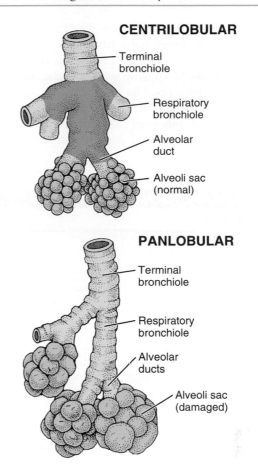

Fig. 8.5 *Emphysema traps air in the lungs so that expelling air becomes increasingly difficult.* Centrilobular emphysema affects the upper airways and produces a destructive change in the bronchioles. Panlobular emphysema affects the lower airways and is more diffusely scattered throughout the alveoli.

The client is often thin, has tachypnea with prolonged expiration, and uses the accessory muscles for respiration. The client often leans forward with the arms braced on the knees to support the shoulders and chest for breathing. The combined effects of trapped air and alveolar distention change the size and shape of the client's chest, causing a barrel chest and increased expiratory effort.

As the disease progresses, there is a loss of surface area available for gas exchange. In the final stages of emphysema, cardiac complications, especially enlargement and dilation of the right ventricle, may develop. The overloaded heart reaches its limit of muscular compensation and begins to fail (cor pulmonale).

The most important factor in the treatment of emphysema is smoking cessation. The main goals for the client with emphysema are to improve oxygenation and decrease CO_2 retention.

Pursed-lip breathing causes resistance to outflow at the lips, which in turn maintains intrabronchial pressure and improves the mixing of gases in the lungs. This type of breathing should be encouraged to help the client get rid of the stale air trapped in the lungs.

Exercise has not been shown to directly improve pulmonary function but is used indirectly to enhance cardiovascular fitness and train skeletal muscles to function more effectively. Routine progressive walking is the most common form of exercise prescribed for these clients.

Lung volume reduction surgery is available for clients and improves not only lung function and exercise performance, but also activities of daily function and quality of life.[11,12]

CLINICAL SIGNS AND SYMPTOMS
Emphysema

- SOB
- Dyspnea on exertion
- Orthopnea (only able to breathe in the upright position) immediately after assuming the supine position
- Chronic cough
- Barrel chest
- Weight loss
- Malaise
- Use of accessory muscles of respiration
- Prolonged expiratory period (with grunting)
- Wheezing
- Pursed-lip breathing
- Increased respiratory rate
- Peripheral cyanosis

INFLAMMATORY/INFECTIOUS DISEASE

Asthma

Asthma is a reversible obstructive lung disease caused by an increased reaction of the airways to various stimuli in certain clients. It is a chronic inflammatory condition with acute exacerbations that can be life-threatening if not properly managed. Our understanding of asthma has changed dramatically over the last decade.[57,58,59]

Asthma was once viewed as a bronchoconstrictive disorder in which the airways narrowed, causing wheezing and breathing difficulties. Treatment with bronchodilators to open airways was the primary focus. Evidence now supports the idea that asthma is primarily an inflammatory disorder in which the constriction of airways is a symptom of the underlying inflammation.

Asthma and other atopic disorders are the result of complex interactions between genetic predisposition and multiple environmental influences. The marked increase in asthma prevalence in the last three decades suggests environmental factors as a key contributor in the process of allergic sensitization.[13]

Approximately twenty-four million Americans are affected by asthma, with 9.49% of adults and 7.5% children.[14-16] Asthma has decreased in children from 2001 to 2016 even though it is the most common chronic lung disease in childhood. Asthma prevalence among adults varies across specific states in the United States, ranging from 7.3% in Texas to 13.2% in New Hampshire. Adult women are affected more than men, but boys are affected more than girls from aged 0 to 4. Asthma prevalence is similar for males and females aged 5 to 24.[17-19]

Immune Sensitization and Inflammation

There are two major components of asthma. When the immune system becomes sensitized to an allergen, usually through heavy exposure in early life, an inflammatory cascade occurs, extending beyond the upper airways into the lungs.

The lungs become hyperreactive, responding to allergens and other irritants exaggeratedly. This hyperresponsiveness causes the muscles of the airways to constrict, making breathing more difficult (Fig. 8.6). The second component is inflammation, which causes the air passages to swell and the cells lining the passages to produce excess mucus, further impairing breathing.

Asthma may be categorized as conventional asthma, occupational asthma, or exercise-induced asthma (EIA), but the underlying pathophysiologic complex remains the same. As the triggers or allergens vary, each person reacts differently.

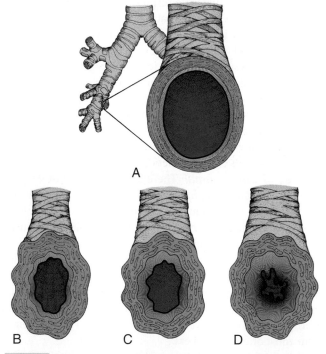

Fig. 8.6 *Airway changes with asthma.* **A,** Normal bronchus: cross-section of a normal bronchus (mucous membrane in color). Healthy bronchioles accommodate a constant flow of air when open and relaxed. **B,** Asthma: airway inflammation begins. The smooth muscle surrounding the bronchus contracts and causes narrowing of the airway, called *bronchospasm*. **C,** The airway tissue swells; this edema of the mucous membrane further narrows the airways. **D,** Mucus is produced, further compromising airflow.

SOB, wheezing, tightness in the chest, and cough are the most commonly reported symptoms, but other symptoms may also occur.

Clinical Signs and Symptoms

Anytime a client experiences SOB, wheezing, and cough and comments, "I am more out of shape than I thought," the therapist should ask about past medical history of asthma and review the list of symptoms with the client. Therapists working with clients with known asthma should encourage them to maintain hydration by drinking fluids to prevent mucous plugs from hardening and to take prescribed medications.

EIA or hyperventilation-induced asthma potentially can be prevented by exercising in a moist, humid environment and by grading exercise according to client tolerance using diaphragmatic breathing. Any type of sustained running or cycling or activity in the cold is more likely to precipitate EIA (Box 8.2).

BOX 8.2 FACTORS THAT MAY TRIGGER ASTHMA

- Respiratory infections, colds
- Cigarette smoke
- Allergic reactions to pollen, mold, animal dander, feather, dust, food, insects
- Indoor and outdoor air pollutants, including ozone
- Physical exertion or vigorous exercise
- Exposure to cold air or sudden temperature change
- Excitement or strong emotion, psychologic or emotional stress

---

Complications. Status asthmaticus is a severe, life-threatening complication of asthma. With severe broncho spasm, the workload of breathing increases five to ten times, which can lead to acute cor pulmonale. When air is trapped, a severe paradoxical pulse develops as venous return is obstructed. This condition is seen as a blood pressure drop of more than 10 mm Hg during inspiration.

A pneumothorax may develop. If status asthmaticus continues, hypoxemia worsens and acidosis begins. If the condition is untreated or not reversed, respiratory or cardiac arrest will occur. An acute asthmatic episode may constitute a medical emergency.

Medical treatment for the underlying inflammation and resulting airway obstruction is with antiinflammatory agents and bronchodilators to prevent, interrupt, or terminate ongoing inflammatory reactions in the airways. Antiinflammatory agents known as leukotriene modifiers work by blocking the activity of chemicals called leukotrienes, which are involved in airway inflammation.[20] Reducing, eliminating, and avoiding allergens or triggers is important in self-care (see Box 8.2).

CLINICAL SIGNS AND SYMPTOMS
Asthma

Listen for:

- Wheezing, however light
- Irregular breathing with prolonged expiration
- Noisy, difficult breathing
- Episodes of dyspnea
- Clearing the throat (tickle at the back of the throat or neck)
- Cough with or without sputum production, especially in the absence of a cold and/or occurring 5 to 10 minutes after exercise

Look for:

- Skin retraction (clavicles, ribs, sternum)
- Hunched-over body posture; inability to stand, sit straight, or relax
- Pursed-lip breathing
- Nostrils flaring
- Unusual pallor or unexplained sweating

Ask about:

- Restlessness during sleep
- Vomiting
- Fatigue unrelated to working or playing

Pneumonia

Pneumonia is an inflammation of the lungs and can be caused by (1) aspiration of food, fluids, or vomitus; (2) inhalation of toxic or caustic chemicals, smoke, dust, or gases; or (3) a bacterial, viral, or mycoplasmal infection. It may be primary or secondary (a complication of another disease); it often follows influenza.

The common feature of all types of pneumonia is an inflammatory pulmonary response to the offending organism or agent. This response may involve one or both lungs at the level of the lobe (lobar pneumonia) or more distally beginning in the terminal bronchioles and alveoli (bronchopneumonia). Bronchopneumonia is seen more frequently than lobar pneumonia and is common in clients postoperatively and in clients with chronic bronchitis, particularly when these two situations coexist.

There are three main types of pneumonia: hospital-acquired pneumonia (HAP; also known as nosocomial pneumonia), ventilator-associated pneumonia (VAP), and community-acquired pneumonia (CAP). By definition, HAP occurs 48 hours or more after hospital admission; when HAP develops in a mechanically ventilated patient after endotracheal intubation, it becomes VAP.

Risk Factors

Infectious agents responsible for pneumonia are typically present in the upper respiratory tract and cause no harm unless resistance is lowered severely by some other factor such as smoking, a severe cold, disease, alcoholism, or generally poor health (e.g., poorly controlled diabetes, chronic renal problems, compromised immune function).

Risk factors for developing HAP are age older than 70 years, serious comorbidities, malnutrition, impaired consciousness, prolonged hospitalization, and COPD.[21] Older or bedridden clients are particularly at risk because of physical inactivity and immobility. Limited mobility causes normal secretions to pool in the airways and facilitates bacterial growth. Other risk factors predisposing a client to pneumonia are listed in Box 8.3.

BOX 8.3   RISK FACTORS FOR PNEUMONIA

- Age: very young, very old
- Have not received a pneumococcal vaccination
- Smoking
- Air pollution
- Upper respiratory infection (URI)
- Altered consciousness: alcoholism, head injury, seizure disorder, drug overdose, general anesthesia
- Endotracheal intubation, nasogastric tube
- Recent chest surgery
- Prolonged immobility
- Immunosuppressive therapy: corticosteroids, cancer chemotherapy
- Nonfunctional immune system: acquired immunodeficiency syndrome (AIDS)
- Severe periodontal disease
- Prolonged exposure to virulent organisms
- Malnutrition, dehydration
- Chronic diseases: diabetes mellitus, heart disease, chronic lung disease, renal disease, cancer
- Prolonged debilitating disease
- Inhalation of noxious substances
- Aspiration of oral/gastric material (food or fluid), foreign materials (e.g., petroleum products)
- Chronically ill, older clients who have poor immune systems, often residing in group-living situations; transfer from one health care facility to another (hospital-acquired or nosocomial pneumonia); hospitalization in the fall or winter

---

Pneumocystis carinii is a protozoan organism that rarely causes pneumonia in healthy individuals. *Pneumocystis carinii* pneumonia (PCP) has been the most common life-threatening opportunistic infection in persons with acquired immunodeficiency syndrome (AIDS). PCP also is the first indicator of conversion from human immunodeficiency virus (HIV) infection to the designation of AIDS.

Clinical Signs and Symptoms

The onset of all types of pneumonia is generally marked by any of the following: fever, chills, sweats, pleuritic chest pain, cough, sputum production, hemoptysis, dyspnea, headache,

or fatigue. PCP causes a dry, hacking cough without sputum production.

The older client can have full-blown pneumonia and may appear with altered mental status (especially confusion) rather than fever or respiratory symptoms because of the changes in temperature regulation as we age. Anytime an older person has shoulder pain and confusion at presentation, consider the possibility of diaphragmatic impingement by an underlying lung pathologic condition (Case Example 8.2).

The clinical manifestations of PCP are slow to develop; they include fever, tachypnea, tachycardia, dyspnea, nonproductive cough, and hypoxemia. A diffuse, bilateral pattern of alveolar infiltration is apparent in a chest radiograph.

Hospitalization may be required for the immunocompromised client. Otherwise, if the client has an intact defense system and good general health, recuperation can take place at home with rest and supportive treatment. In the hospital,

---

CASE EXAMPLE 8.2
Pneumonia

A 42-year-old man came to an outpatient physical therapy clinic with complaints of painful, swollen knees. Symptoms were first observed 10 days ago, and the left knee was reportedly worse than the right. Stiffness was reported in the morning when rising, with pain increasing as the day progressed. As a nonsmoker, the man reported his general health as "good" and noted that he had sprained his left ankle 2 months before the onset of knee pain.

The knee joints were not tender, warm, or red. Observable and palpable "boggy" fluid could be demonstrated in the popliteal spaces bilaterally. There was no sign of effusion when viewed anteriorly, and the test for a wave of fluid was negative.

All special tests for the hip and knee were negative, with full active and passive range of motion present. There was no known history of Baker's cysts (herniation of synovial tissue through a weakening in the posterior capsule wall) reported. There were no palpable myalgias of the lower leg musculature and no trigger points present.

The left ankle demonstrated some residual stiffness with a mild loss of plantar flexion. Joint accessory motions were consistent with a grade 1 lateral ankle sprain. Standing posture was unremarkable for possible contributing alignment problems.

The clinical presentation of this client was puzzling to the evaluating therapist. A brief screening for possible systemic origin of symptoms elicited no red-flag symptoms or history. Ongoing evaluation continued as treatment for both knees and the left ankle was initiated. After 3 weeks, there were no changes in the clinical presentation of the knees. At that time the client developed a noticeable productive cough with greenish/yellow sputum but no other reported symptoms. Vital signs (including temperature) were unremarkable.

Given the unusual clinical presentation, lack of progress with treatment, and development of a productive cough, this client was referred to his family physician for a medical evaluation. A one-page letter outlining the therapist's findings and treatment protocol was sent with the client. A medical diagnosis of pneumonia was established. The physician noted that although the clinical presentation was unusual, knee involvement can occur with pneumonia. The pathophysiologic mechanism for this is unknown.

rigorous handwashing by medical personnel is essential for reducing the transmission of infectious agents.

CLINICAL SIGNS AND SYMPTOMS

Pneumonia

- Sudden and sharp pleuritic chest pain that is aggravated by chest movement
- Shoulder pain
- Hacking, productive cough (rust-colored or green, purulent sputum)
- Dyspnea
- Tachypnea (rapid respirations associated with fever or pneumonia) accompanied by decreased chest excursion on the affected side
- Cyanosis
- Headache
- Fever and chills
- Generalized aches and myalgia that may extend to the thighs and calves
- Knees may be painful and swollen
- Fatigue
- Confusion in older adult or increased confusion in client with dementia or Alzheimer's disease

Tuberculosis

Tuberculosis (TB) is a bacterial infectious disease transmitted by the gram-positive, acid-fast bacillus *Mycobacterium tuberculosis*. Despite improved methods of detection and treatment, TB remains a worldwide health problem with increasing spread of a highly drug-resistant strain of TB present in almost every state of the United States.

Before the development of anti-TB drugs in the late 1940s, TB was the leading cause of death in the United States. Drug therapy, along with improvements in public health and general living standards, resulted in a marked decline in incidence. However, recent influxes of immigrants from developing Third World nations, rising homeless populations, and the emergence of HIV led to an increase in reported cases in the mid-1980s, reversing 40 years of decline.

Risk Factors

Although TB can affect anyone, certain segments of the population have an increased risk of contracting the disease (Box 8.4). The mycobacterium is usually spread by airborne droplet nuclei, which are produced when actively infected persons sneeze, speak, sing, or cough.

Once released into the atmosphere, the organisms are dispersed and can be inhaled by a susceptible host. Brief exposure to a few bacilli rarely causes an infection. More commonly, it is spread with repeated close contact with an infected person.

Drug-resistant strains of TB develop when the full course of treatment, lasting 6 to 9 months, is not completed. Once the infected person feels better and stops taking the prescribed medication, a new drug-resistant strain is passed along. Incomplete treatment among inner-city residents and the homeless presents a major factor in the failure to eradicate TB.

BOX 8.4   RISK FACTORS FOR TUBERCULOSIS

- Health care workers, especially those working in older hospitals (centralized ventilation), homeless shelters, or extended care facilities. Health care workers, including physical therapists, must be alert to the need to use a special mask (particulate respirator) when cough-inducing procedures are being performed on any client who is at risk for, or who has, active tuberculosis (TB).
- Older adults, who constitute nearly half of the newly diagnosed cases of TB in the United States.
- Overcrowded housing, most common among the economically disadvantaged; homeless, especially those in crowded homeless shelters.
- People who are incarcerated.
- U.S.-born non-Hispanic Blacks.[22]
- Immigrants (including adopted children) from Southeast and Central Asia, Ethiopia, Mexico, Latin America, Eastern Europe.
- Clients who are dependent on alcohol or other chemicals with resultant malnutrition, debilitation, and poor health.
- Infants and children under the age of 5 years.
- Clients with reduced immunity or malnutrition (e.g., anyone undergoing cancer therapy or steroid therapy) and those with human immunodeficiency virus (HIV)-positive lung cancer or head and neck cancer.
- Persons with diagnosed rheumatoid arthritis. Data suggests increases in incidence could be as a result of new immunosuppressive treatments.[22]
- Persons with diabetes mellitus and/or end-stage renal disease.
- People with a history of gastrointestinal disease (e.g., chronic malabsorption syndrome, upper gastrointestinal carcinomas, gastrectomy, intestinal bypass).

Drug-resistant strains are also developing globally. Areas of the world with increased rates of drug-resistant disease include countries of the former Soviet Union (e.g., Estonia, Kazakhstan, Latvia, Lithuania, Uzbekistan) and Central Asia.

Families who adopt internationally should be aware of potential TB infection in children from some of the high-risk areas of the world. The bacille Calmette-Guerin (BCG) vaccine has been used in many foreign countries to attempt to prevent the serious dissemination of TB infection in those countries.

The value of the BCG vaccine is controversial because the protection it confers is short term. The Centers for Disease Control and Prevention (CDC) and the American Academy of Pediatrics strongly recommend that history of BCG vaccination in a child from a high-risk part of the world usually be ignored and that all children adopted internationally be skin tested for TB and treated if the disease is latent or active.[23]

TB most often involves the lungs, but extrapulmonary TB (XPTB) can also occur in the kidneys, bone growth plates, lymph nodes, and meninges and can be disseminated throughout the body.

Widespread dissemination throughout the body is termed *miliary tuberculosis* and is more common in people 50 years or older and very young children with unstable or underdeveloped immune systems.

On rare occasions, TB will affect the hip joints and vertebrae, resulting in severe, arthritis-like damage, possibly even avascular necrosis of the hip. TB of the spine, referred to as Pott's disease, is rare but can result in compression fracture of the vertebrae.

Pyogenic vertebral osteomyelitis can be caused by atypical organisms such as TB. As with other pyogenic infection, back pain is the most common symptom, but it is less severe than in other infections. Individuals from high-risk areas of the world, high-risk living conditions, and the immunocompromised and malnourished should be considered suspect for this condition.[24]

Clinical Signs and Symptoms

Clinical signs and symptoms are absent in the early stages of TB. Many cases are found incidentally when routine chest radiographs are made for other reasons. When systemic manifestations of active disease initially appear, the clinical signs and symptoms listed here may appear.

Tuberculin skin testing is done to determine whether the body's immune response has been activated by the presence of the bacillus. A positive reaction develops 3 to 10 weeks after the initial infection. A positive skin test reaction indicates the presence of a TB infection but does not show whether the infection is dormant or is causing a clinical illness.

Chest radiographs and sputum cultures are done as a follow-up to positive skin tests. All cases of active disease are treated, and certain cases of inactive disease are treated prophylactically.

CLINICAL SIGNS AND SYMPTOMS
Tuberculosis

- Fatigue
- Malaise
- Anorexia
- Weight loss
- Low-grade fever (especially in late afternoon)
- Night sweats
- Frequent productive cough
- Dull chest pain, tightness, or discomfort
- Dyspnea

Systemic Sclerosis Lung Disease

Systemic sclerosis (SS), or scleroderma, is a restrictive lung disease of unknown etiologic origin characterized by inflammation and fibrosis of many organs (see Chapter 13). Fibrosis affecting the skin and the visceral organs is the hallmark of SS.

The lungs, highly vascularized and composed of abundant connective tissue, are a frequent target organ, ranking second only to the esophagus in visceral involvement.

The most common pulmonary manifestation of SS is interstitial fibrosis, which is clinically apparent in more than 50% of cases. Autopsy results suggest a prevalence of 75%, indicating the insensitivity of traditional tests such as the pulmonary function test and chest radiographs.

Clinical Signs and Symptoms

As discussed in Chapter 13, skin changes associated with SS generally precede visceral alterations. Dyspnea on exertion and nonproductive cough is the most common clinical findings associated with SS. Rarely, these symptoms precede the occurrence of cutaneous changes of scleroderma.

Clubbing of the nails rarely occurs in SS because of the nearly universal presence of sclerodactyly (hardening and shrinking of the connective tissue of the fingers and toes). Peripheral edema may develop secondary to cor pulmonale, which occurs as the pulmonary fibrosis becomes advanced.

Pulmonary manifestations in SS include:
- *Common:* Interstitial pneumonitis and fibrosis and pulmonary vascular disease
- *Less common:* Pleural disease, aspiration pneumonia, pneumothorax, neoplasm, pneumoconiosis, pulmonary hemorrhage, and drug-induced pneumonitis

Pleural effusions may appear with orthopnea, edema, and paroxysmal nocturnal dyspnea if CHF occurs. Cystic changes in the parenchyma may progress to form pneumatoceles (thin-walled air-containing cysts) that may rupture spontaneously and produce a pneumothorax. Clients with SS have an increased incidence of lung cancer. Hemoptysis is often the first sign of a pulmonary malignancy in individuals with SS.

The course of SS is unpredictable, from a mild, protracted course to rapid respiratory failure and death. Treatment of pulmonary complications, pulmonary hypertension, and interstitial lung disease remains difficult.

CLINICAL SIGNS AND SYMPTOMS
Systemic Sclerosis Lung Disease

- Dyspnea on exertion
- Nonproductive cough
- Peripheral edema (secondary to cor pulmonale)
- Orthopnea
- Paroxysmal nocturnal dyspnea (CHF)
- Hemoptysis

Neoplastic Disease

Lung Cancer (Bronchogenic Carcinoma)

Lung cancer is a malignancy in the epithelium of the respiratory tract. At least a dozen different tumor cell types are included under the classification of lung cancer.

Clinically, lung cancers are grouped into two divisions: small cell lung cancer (15% of all lung cancers) and non–small cell lung cancer. The four major types of lung cancer include small cell carcinoma (oat cell carcinoma), and the subtypes of non–small cell lung cancer (e.g., squamous cell carcinoma [25% to 30%], adenocarcinoma [40%], and large cell carcinoma [10% to 15%]).

Since the mid-1950s, lung cancer has been the most common cause of death from cancer in men. In 1987 lung cancer surpassed breast cancer to become the leading cause of cancer death in women in the United States. It is now the second most commonly diagnosed cancer in both men and women and remains the number one cause of death in both groups.[25]

The incidence of lung cancer and mortality rates in the United States has been declining since the 1990s. This decline is attributed to a continued reduction in the number of those who start to smoke across men and women.[26]

Risk Factors. Smoking is the major risk factor for lung cancer, accounting for 82% of deaths caused by lung cancer.[27] Other risk factors are listed in Box 8.5. Compared with non-smokers, heavy smokers (i.e., those who smoke more than 25 cigarettes a day) have a twentyfold greater risk of developing cancer.[26]

BOX 8.5 RISK FACTORS FOR LUNG CANCER

- Age greater than 50 years
- Smoking or other tobacco use
- Previous tobacco-related cancer
- Passive (environmental) smoke
- Low consumption of fruits and vegetables
- Genetic predisposition
- Exposure to air pollution, toxic chemicals (e.g., asbestos, uranium), fumes, radon gas
- Previous lung disease (e.g., chronic obstructive pulmonary disease [COPD], tuberculosis, pulmonary fibrosis, sarcoidosis)

States with strong antitobacco programs (e.g., Arizona, California) have the fewest current smokers, the most people who have quit smoking in some age groups, and the greatest drop in the death rate from lung cancer.[28] Quitting smoking lowers the risk, but the decrease is gradual and does not approach that of a nonsmoker.

The risk of lung cancer is increased in the smoker who is exposed to other carcinogenic agents such as radon, asbestos, and chemical carcinogens. Internationally, the incidence of lung cancer has decreased in the United States and the United Kingdom but emerging nations including Brazil, Russia, India, China, and South Africa continue to have a high rate of cigarette smoking, a lower incidence of cancer but a higher mortality burden compared with developed countries.[26]

The increase in lung cancer mortality in the last decade in developing countries can be entirely attributed to the trend of tobacco consumption. However, there is a lag time of many years between beginning smoking and the clinical manifestation of cancer. The therapist can have a key role in the prevention of lung cancer through risk-factor assessment and client education (see Chapter 2).

Metastases. Metastatic spread of pulmonary tumors is usually to the long bones, vertebral column (especially the thoracic vertebrae), liver, and adrenal glands. Brain metastasis is also common, occurring in as many as 50% of cases.

Local metastases by direct extension may involve the chest wall, pleura, pulmonary parenchyma, or bronchi. Further local tumor growth may erode the first and second ribs and associated vertebrae, causing bone pain and paravertebral pain associated with the involvement of sympathetic nerve ganglia.

The respiratory system is a common site for complications associated with cancer and cancer therapy. Several factors can lead to pulmonary complications. Immunosuppression caused by the underlying disease or cancer therapy can lead to infectious disease.

Also, the lungs contain an enormous capillary bed through which flows the entire venous circulation, making it a common site of metastasis from other primary cancers and pulmonary emboli. Carcinomas of the kidney, breast, pancreas, colon, and uterus are especially likely to metastasize to the lungs.

Clinical Signs and Symptoms. Clinical signs and symptoms of lung cancer often remain silent until the disease process is at an advanced stage. In many instances, lung cancer may mimic other pulmonary conditions or may initially appear as chest, shoulder, or arm pain (Case Example 8.3).

Chest pain is a vague aching, and depending on the type of cancer, the client may have pleuritic pain on inspiration that limits lung expansion. Anorexia and weight loss occur in many clients with lung cancer and can be a symptom of advanced disease.[29]

Hemoptysis (coughing or spitting up blood) may occur secondary to ulceration of blood vessels. Wheezing occurs when the tumor obstructs the bronchus. Dyspnea, either unexplained or out of proportion, is a red flag indicating the need for medical screening, as is unexplainable weight loss accompanied by dyspnea.

Centrally located tumors cause increased cough, dyspnea, and diffuse chest pain that can be referred to the shoulder, scapulae, and upper back. This pain is the result of peribronchial or perivascular nerve involvement.

Other symptoms may include postobstructive pneumonia with fever, chills, malaise, anorexia, hemoptysis, and fecal breath odor (secondary to infection within a necrotic tumor mass). If these tumors extend to the pericardium, the client may develop a sudden onset of arrhythmia (tachycardia or atrial fibrillation), weakness, anxiety, and dyspnea.

Peripheral tumors are most often asymptomatic until the tumor extends through visceral and parietal pleura to the chest wall. Irritation of the nerves causes localized sharp, pleuritic pain that is aggravated by inspiration.

Metastases to the mediastinum (tissue and organs between the sternum and the vertebrae, including the heart and its large vessels; trachea; esophagus; thymus; lymph nodes) may cause hoarseness or dysphagia secondary to vocal cord paralysis as a result of entrapment or local compression of the laryngeal nerve.

CASE EXAMPLE 8.3

Neurologic Deficits in a Smoker

A 66-year-old man was referred by his primary care physician to physical therapy for weakness in the lower extremities. He also reported dysesthesia (pain with touch) in both legs from the knees down. The symptoms had been present for about 1 month before he saw his doctor. At the time of his physical therapy evaluation, symptoms had been present for almost 2 months (client was delayed getting in to see a therapist because of his scheduling conflicts).

The client was a social worker who had never been married but had two children out of wedlock, had a history of chronic alcohol use, and reported a 60-pack year history of tobacco use (pack-years = number of packs/day × number of years; in this case the client had smoked two packs a day for the last 30 years).

Past medical history was negative for any previous significant injuries, illnesses, or hospitalizations. Both parents were killed in a car accident when the client was a child. Any other family history was unknown for the parents and unremarkable for the siblings.

Clinical examination revealed mild weakness in the distal muscle groups of the lower extremities (left weaker than right). Altered sensation was circumferential and included both lower legs equally. Tests for clonus and Babinski were negative. Deep tendon reflexes were equal bilaterally and within normal limits (WNL). Other neurologic screening tests were negative. There were no constitutional signs or symptoms reported or observed.

A program of strengthening and conditioning was started based on the physician's referral, requesting strength training and clinical findings of muscular weakness. In the first 2 weeks of treatment, the client's weakness increased and he developed bilateral foot drop.

He started reporting episodes of dropping anything he lifted over 2 lbs. A quick screening examination showed bilateral weakness developing in the hands and wrists, as well as the feet and ankles.

What are all the red flags in this case?
- Age (over 50 years)
- Significant smoking history
- Alcohol use
- Bilateral symptoms (hands and feet)
- Progressive neurologic symptoms

Are there any other screening tests that can/should be done?

A screening physical examination should be conducted (see Chapter 4) and any significant findings noted and reported to the physician.

A general survey, vital signs, and chest auscultation would be a good place to start. It is possible that the client presentation (and certainly the new onset of symptoms) is unknown to the physician who saw him almost 1 month ago.

In fact, the therapist observed signs of digital clubbing (hands only), reported oxygen saturation levels (SaO_2) consistently at 90%, and noted bilateral basilar crackles during lung auscultation.

The client was advised to make a follow-up appointment with the physician, and the therapist faxed a letter of request for follow-up based on these new findings. The client also hand carried a copy of the therapist's letter to the medical appointment.

Result: The client was diagnosed with lung cancer with accompanying paraneoplastic syndrome (see discussion of paraneoplastic syndromes, Chapter 14). His condition worsened rapidly and he died 6 weeks later.

The family later came back to the therapist and expressed their appreciation for finding the problem early enough to make end-of-life decisions. Both children and three of the four siblings were able to visit with the gentleman before he died suddenly in his sleep.

Apical (Pancoast's) tumors of the lung apex do not usually cause symptoms if confined to the pulmonary parenchyma. They can extend into surrounding structures and frequently involve the eighth cervical and first thoracic nerves within the brachial plexus.

A constellation of symptoms referred to as Pancoast's syndrome present in the distribution of the C8, T1, and T2 dermatomes, mimicking thoracic outlet syndrome.[30] Tumor invasion of any anatomic structures of the lower trunks of the brachial plexus and/or the C8 and T1 nerve roots can result in significant disability and loss of hand function.[30] Extension of the tumor into the paravertebral sympathetic nerves results in Horner's syndrome, which consists of enophthalmos (backward displacement of the eye), ptosis (drooping eyelid), and miosis (pupil constriction).

The most common initial symptom is sharp (often posterior) shoulder pain produced by invasion of the brachial plexus and/or extension of the tumor into the parietal pleura, endothoracic fascia, first and second ribs, or vertebral bodies. There may be pain in the axilla and subscapular areas on the affected side (Case Example 8.4).

CASE EXAMPLE 8.4

Pancoast's Tumor

A 55-year-old man presented with shoulder pain radiating down the arm present for the last 3 months. His job as a mechanic required many hours with his arms raised overhead, which is what he thought was causing the problem.

He was diagnosed with cervical radiculopathy after cervical radiographs showed moderate osteoarthritic changes at the C6, C7, and C8 levels. Electromyographic (EMG) studies confirmed the diagnosis, and he was sent to physical therapy.

The client gave a history as a nonsmoker but mentioned his parents were chain-smokers and his wife of 35 years also smokes heavily. There was no other significant social or personal history. The client was adopted and did not know his family history.

CASE EXAMPLE 8.4, cont'd

The therapist conducted a physical screening examination and noted a slight drooping of the left eyelid, which the client attributed to fatigue and changes with middle age. Vital signs were within normal limits. Muscle atrophy and weakness were present in the left hand consistent with a C7-C8 neurologic impairment. There were changes in the thumbs and index fingers on both sides with what looked like early signs of digital clubbing. The nail beds were spongy with a definite change in the shape of the distal phalanx.

When asked if there were any other symptoms of any kind anywhere else in the body, the client mentioned a change in the way he perspires. He noticed his left face and armpit do not perspire like the right side. He could not remember when this change began but knew it was not something he had his whole life.

What are the red-flag signs in this case?
- Age
- Exposure to passive tobacco smoke
- Nail bed changes
- Anhydrosis (lack of sweating)
- Questionable change in eyelid

What other screening tests might be appropriate?

A more careful neurologic examination is in order. Any findings to suggest impairment outside the parameters of the C6, C7, and C8 nerve function might raise a yellow flag. Upper limb neurodynamic and neural tension tests are important; trigger point assessment is often helpful. A cranial nerve assessment is also advised because of the possible eye drooping observed.

Although the vital signs were unremarkable, the nail bed changes should prompt lung auscultation and a closer look at skin color, capillary refill time, and peripheral vascular assessment.

Result: No other neurologic findings were observed and the cranial nerve assessment was within normal limits, with the exception of the eyelid drooping. The therapist also noticed the pupil in the left eye seemed smaller than the pupil in the right. Repeated attempts to use a penlight or darkness to change pupil size were unsuccessful.

Based on the objective findings, the therapist started an intervention of neural mobilizations and gave the client a home program of postural exercises and self-neural mobilizations. A plan was outlined to integrate a strengthening program as soon as time would allow.

All findings were documented and sent to the physician. The client was not sent back to the physician, but the physician, upon reading the therapist's notes, called the therapist and asked for further explanation of the therapist's findings. The physician was concerned and asked to have the client make a follow-up appointment.

Further medical testing brought about a diagnosis of Pancoast's tumor in the left upper lung lobe involving the brachial plexus and the first and second ribs. Horner's syndrome was also recognized as the cause of his drooping eye and anhydrosis.

Symptoms from the Horner's syndrome resolved after radiotherapy; pain and weakness also improved after medical therapy. Physical therapy for rehabilitation was initiated after medical treatment, but the client developed progressive regional disease with distant metastases and died within 2 months.

Pain may radiate up to the head and neck, across the chest, and/or down the medial aspect of the arm and hand (ulnar nerve distribution) (Fig. 8.7). There may be subsequent atrophy of the upper extremity muscles with weakness in the muscles of the hand.

Pulmonary symptoms, such as cough, hemoptysis, and dyspnea, are uncommon until late in the disease. Affected individuals are often treated for presumed cervical osteoarthritis or shoulder bursitis resulting in delay of diagnosis. The pain eventually progresses to become severe and constant, resulting in more thorough testing and accurate diagnosis.[31] The onset of pulmonary symptoms in any client with neck, shoulder, and/or arm pain should be a red-flag symptom for the therapist.

Trigger points of the serratus anterior muscle (see Fig. 18.7) also mimic the distribution of pain caused by the eighth cervical nerve root compression. Trigger points can be ruled out by palpation and lack of neurologic deficits and

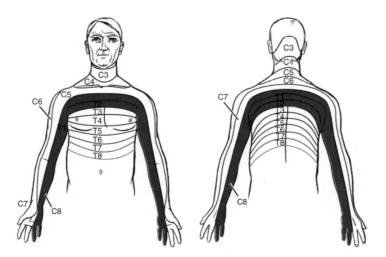

Fig. 8.7 *Pancoast's tumors can present with changes in cutaneous dermatomal innervation.* The shaded areas show the dermatomes affected when the superior (apical) sulcus tumors associated with Pancoast's syndrome invade the brachial plexus. Direct extension to the brachial plexus involving C8 and T1 result in symptoms affecting the C8, T1, and T2 dermatomes.

may be confirmed by elimination with appropriate physical therapy intervention.

Paraneoplastic syndromes (remote effects of a malignancy; see explanation in Chapter 14) occur in 10% to 20% of lung cancer clients and represent a feature of advanced disease. These usually result from the secretion of hormones by the tumor acting on target organs, producing a variety of symptoms. Occasionally, symptoms of paraneoplastic syndrome occur before detection of the primary lung tumor.

As mentioned earlier, brain metastasis is common and can be seen as often as 50% of all cases. About 10% of all individuals with lung cancer have central nervous system (CNS) involvement at the time of diagnosis. CNS symptoms, such as muscle weakness, muscle atrophy, loss of lower extremity sensation, and localized or radicular back pain may be associated with lung cancer and must be investigated by a physician to establish a medical diagnosis.

Other clinical symptoms of brain metastasis resulting from increased intracranial pressure may include headache, nausea, vomiting, malaise, anorexia, weakness, and alterations in mental processes. Localized motor or sensory deficits occur, depending on the location of lesions (see Chapter 14).

Metastasis to the spinal cord produces signs and symptoms of cord compression (see Table 14.5 and Appendix A-2 in the accompanying enhanced eBook version included with print purchase of this textbook), including back pain (localized or radicular), muscle weakness, loss of lower extremity sensation, bowel and bladder incontinence, and diminished or absent lower extremity reflexes (unilateral or bilateral).

CLINICAL SIGNS AND SYMPTOMS
Lung Cancer[60,61]

- Any change in respiratory patterns
- Recurrent pneumonia or bronchitis
- Hemoptysis
- Persistent cough
- Change in cough or development of hemoptysis in a chronic smoker
- Hoarseness or dysphagia
- Sputum streaked with blood
- Dyspnea (SOB)
- Wheezing
- Sharp chest, upper back, shoulder, scapular, rib, or arm pain aggravated by inspiration or accompanied by respiratory signs and symptoms
- Sudden, unexplained weight loss; anorexia; fatigue
- Chest, shoulder, or arm pain; bone aching, joint pain
- Atrophy and weakness of the arm and hand muscles
- Fecal breath odor
- See also Clinical Signs and Symptoms of Paraneoplastic Syndrome, Brain Metastasis, and Metastasis to the Spinal Cord in Chapter 14; Table 14.5; and Appendix A-2 in the accompanying enhanced eBook version included with print purchase of this textbook

GENETIC DISEASE OF THE LUNG

Cystic Fibrosis

CF is an inherited disease of the exocrine ("outward-secreting") glands primarily affecting the digestive and respiratory systems.

This disease is the most common genetic disease in the United States, inherited as a recessive trait: both parents must be carriers, each having a defective copy of the CF gene. Each time two carriers conceive a child, there is a 25% chance that the child will have CF, a 50% chance that the child will be a carrier, and a 25% chance that the child will be a noncarrier. In the United States 5% of the population, or 12 million people, carry a single copy of the CF gene.

Because cysts and scar tissue on the pancreas were observed during autopsy when the disease was first being differentiated from other conditions, it was given the name *cystic fibrosis of the pancreas*. Although this term describes a secondary rather than primary characteristic, it has been retained.[62]

In 1989, scientists isolated the CF gene located on chromosome 7. In healthy people, a protein called CF transmembrane conductance regulator (CFTR) provides a channel by which chloride (a component of salt) can pass in and out of cells.

Persons with CF have a defective copy of the gene that normally enables cells to construct that channel. As a result, salt accumulates in the cells lining the lungs and digestive tissues, making the surrounding mucus abnormally thick and sticky. These secretions, which obstruct ducts in the pancreas, liver, and lungs, and abnormal secretion of sweat and saliva are the two main features of CF.

Usually, CF manifests itself in early childhood, but some individuals have a variant form of the disease in which symptoms can appear during adolescence or adulthood. Symptoms tend to be milder and sweat chloride concentration may be normal.[32]

Obstruction of the bronchioles by mucous plugs and trapped air predisposes the client to infection, which starts a destructive cycle of increased mucous production with increased bronchial obstruction, infection, and inflammation with eventual destruction of lung parenchyma.

Clinical Signs and Symptoms

Pulmonary involvement is the most common and severe manifestation of CF. Obstruction of the airways leads to a state of hyperinflation and bronchiectasis. In time, fibrosis develops, and restrictive lung disease is superimposed on the obstructive disease.

Over time, pulmonary obstruction leads to chronic hypoxia, hypercapnia, and acidosis. Pneumothorax, pulmonary hypertension, and eventually cor pulmonale may develop. These are very poor prognostic indicators in adults. The course of CF varies from one client to another depending on the degree of pulmonary involvement.

Advances in treatment, including aerosolized antibiotics, mucous thinning agents, antiinflammatory agents, chest physical therapy, enzyme supplements, and nutrition programs have extended the average life expectancy for CF sufferers. As of 2018 the life expectancy of people born with CF between 2014 and 2018 is 44 years.[33]

Because the genetic abnormality has been identified, considerable progress has been made in the development of gene therapy and preventive gene transfer for this disease.[34-37] Lung transplantation in older childhood and adolescence is a possible treatment option based on rapidly declining lung function.[38]

CLINICAL SIGNS AND SYMPTOMS
Cystic Fibrosis

In Early or Undiagnosed Stages:
- Persistent coughing and wheezing
- Recurrent pneumonia
- Excessive appetite but poor weight gain
- Salty skin/sweat
- Bulky, foul-smelling stools (undigested fats caused by a lack of amylase and tryptase enzymes)

In Older Child and Young Adult:
- Infertility
- Nasal polyps
- Periostitis
- Glucose intolerance

CLINICAL SIGNS AND SYMPTOMS
Pulmonary Involvement in Cystic Fibrosis

- Tachypnea (very rapid breathing)
- Sustained chronic cough with mucous production and vomiting
- Barrel chest (caused by trapped air)
- Use of accessory muscles for respiration and intercostal retraction
- Cyanosis and digital clubbing
- Exertional dyspnea with decreased exercise tolerance

Further complications include
- Pneumothorax
- Hemoptysis
- Right-sided heart failure secondary to pulmonary hypertension

OCCUPATIONAL LUNG DISEASES

Lung diseases are among the most common occupational health problems. They are caused by the inhalation of various chemicals, dusts, and other particulate matter present in certain work settings. Not everyone exposed to occupational inhalants will develop lung disease. Prolonged exposure combined with smoking increases the risk of developing occupational lung disease and increases the severity of these diseases.[39]

During the interview process, the therapist will ask questions about occupational and smoking history to identify the possibility of an underlying pulmonary pathologic condition (see Chapter 2 and Appendix B-14 in the accompanying enhanced eBook version included with print purchase of this textbook).

The most commonly encountered occupational lung diseases are occupational lung cancer, occupational asthma (also known as work-related asthma), asbestosis, mesothelioma, and byssinosis (brown lung disease). Other less common occupational lung diseases include hypersensitivity pneumonitis, acute respiratory irritation, and pneumoconiosis (black lung disease, silicosis).

The greatest number of occupational agents causing *asthma* are those with known or suspected allergic properties such as plant and animal proteins (e.g., wheat, flour, cotton, flax, and grain mites). Exposure within the workplace can aggravate preexisting asthma.[40]

Asbestosis and *mesothelioma* occur as a result of asbestos exposure. Asbestos is the name of a group of naturally occurring minerals that separate into strong, very fine fibers. The fibers are heat-resistant and extremely durable, which are qualities that made asbestos useful in construction and industry.

Scarring of the lung tissue occurs in asbestosis as a result of exposure to the microscopic fibers of asbestos. Under certain circumstances, fibers can be released and pose a health risk such as lung cancer from inhaling the fibers. Mesothelioma is an otherwise rare cancer of the chest lining caused by asbestos exposure.

Byssinosis (brown lung disease) caused by dust from hemp, flax, and cotton processing, results in chronic obstruction of the small airways impairing lung function. Textile workers are at the greatest risk of disability from byssinosis.

Hypersensitivity pneumonitis, or allergic alveolitis, is most commonly caused by the inhalation of organic antigens of fungal, bacterial, or animal origin. *Acute respiratory irritation* results from the inhalation of chemicals such as ammonia, chlorine, and nitrogen oxides in the form of gases, aerosols, or particulate matter. If such irritants reach the lower airways, alveolar damage and pulmonary edema can result. Although the effects of these acute irritants are usually short-lived, some may cause chronic alveolar damage or airway obstruction.

Pneumoconioses, or "the dust diseases," result from inhalation of minerals, notably silica, coal dust, or asbestos. These diseases are most commonly seen in miners, construction workers, sandblasters, potters, and foundry and quarry workers. Occupational exposure to dust, fumes, or gases (including diesel) increases mortality as a result of COPD, even among workers who have never smoked.[41]

Pneumoconioses usually develop gradually over years, eventually leading to diffuse pulmonary fibrosis, which diminishes lung capacity and produces restrictive lung disease.[41]

Home Remodeling

Home remodeling projects in the United States have increased dramatically in the last decade. Whether it is a do-it-yourself project or the occupants remain in the home during remodeling, problems can occur from dust inhalation and exposure to hazardous materials such as lead, asbestos, and creosote.

Creosote is toxic (inhaled as fumes) and is a skin and eye irritant.

Lead poisoning is a serious problem in home remodeling projects throughout the United States. Special precautions to avoid lead poisoning must be followed if the home was built before 1978.

Lead poisoning can occur from inhaling paint dust (the result of sanding or scraping painted surfaces) and lead can be found in soil (children come into contact during play). Both sources of poisoning are common problems associated with remodeling projects.

Anyone presenting with a constellation of integumentary, musculoskeletal, and/or neurologic symptoms accompanied by pulmonary involvement should be asked about the possibility of recent home remodeling projects and exposure to any of these materials.

Clinical Signs and Symptoms

Early symptoms of occupational-related lung disease depend on the specific exposure but may include noninflammatory joint pain, myalgia, cough, and dyspnea on exertion.

Chest pain, productive cough, and dyspnea at rest develop as the condition progresses. The therapist needs to be alert for the combination of significant arthralgias and myalgias with associated respiratory symptoms, accompanied by a past occupational and smoking history (see Appendix B-14 in the accompanying enhanced eBook version included with print purchase of this textbook).

CLINICAL SIGNS AND SYMPTOMS

Occupational Lung Diseases

- Arthralgia
- Myalgia
- Chest pain
- Cough
- Dyspnea on exertion (progresses to dyspnea at rest)
- See also signs and symptoms of lung cancer in this chapter

PLEUROPULMONARY DISORDERS

Pulmonary Embolism and Deep Venous Thrombosis

PE involves pulmonary vascular obstruction by a displaced thrombus (blood clot), an air bubble, a fat globule, a clump of bacteria, amniotic fluid, vegetations on heart valves that develop with endocarditis, or other particulate matter. Once dislodged, the obstruction travels to the blood vessels supplying the lungs, causing SOB, tachypnea (very rapid breathing), tachycardia, and chest pain.

The most common cause of PE is deep venous thrombosis (DVT) originating in the proximal deep venous system of the lower legs. The embolism causes an area of blockage, which then results in a localized area of ischemia known as a *pulmonary infarct*. The infarct may be caused by small emboli that extend to the lung surface (pleura) and result in acute pleuritic chest pain.

Risk Factors

Three major risk factors linked with DVT are blood stasis (e.g., immobilization because of bed rest, such as with burn clients, obstetric and gynecologic clients, and older or obese populations), endothelial injury (secondary to neoplasm, surgical procedures, trauma, or fractur7s of the legs or pelvis), and hypercoagulable states (see Box 7.2).

Other people at increased risk for DVT and PE include those with CHF, trauma, surgery (especially hip, knee, and prostate surgery), age over 50 years, previous history of thromboembolism, malignant disease, infection, diabetes mellitus, inactivity or obesity, pregnancy, clotting abnormalities, and oral contraceptive use (see Chapter 7).

Prevention

Given the mortality of PE and the difficulties involved in its clinical diagnosis, prevention of DVT and PE is critical. A careful review of the Personal/Family History form (outpatient) or hospital medical chart (inpatient) may alert the therapist to the presence of factors that predispose a client to have a PE. Risk factor assessment is an important part of screening and prevention.

Although frequent changing of position, exercise, and early ambulation are necessary to prevent thrombosis and embolism, sudden and extreme movements should be avoided. Under no circumstance should the lower extremity be massaged to relieve "muscle cramps," especially when the pain is located in the calf and the client has not been up and about.

Restrictive clothing and prolonged sitting or standing should be avoided. Elevating the legs should be accomplished with caution to avoid continuous severe flexion of the hips, which will slow blood flow and increase the risk of new thrombi.

Deep Venous Thrombosis (see also Chapter 7)

Unfortunately, at least half the cases of DVT are asymptomatic,[42] and in up to one-third of all clients with apparent clinical appearance of DVT, there is no DVT demonstrable. If there are signs and symptoms, they may include tenderness, leg pain, swelling (a difference in leg circumference of 1.4 cm in men and 1.2 cm in women is significant), and warmth.

Homans' sign (pain elicited from passive dorsiflexion) is an unreliable test to diagnose DVT. The therapist should be aware that using the Homans' test to assess for DVT is no longer recommended or supported by evidence.[42-45] Only about half of all clients with DVT experience pain and Homans' sign.

A more sensitive and specific tool for predicting DVT is the Wells Clinical Decision Rule for DVT.

Pulmonary Embolism

The signs and symptoms of PE are important to watch for in our clients as PE is the result of DVT. Signs and symptoms of PE are nonspecific and vary greatly, depending on the extent to which the lung is involved, the size of the clot, and the general condition of the client.

Clinical presentation does not differ between younger and older persons. Dyspnea, pleuritic chest pain, and cough are the most common symptoms reported. Pleuritic pain is caused by an inflammatory reaction of the lung parenchyma or by pulmonary infarction or ischemia caused by obstruction of small pulmonary arterial branches.

Typical pleuritic chest pain is sudden in onset and aggravated by breathing. The client may also report hemoptysis, apprehension, tachypnea, and fever (temperature as high as 39.5° C, or 103.5° F). The presence of hemoptysis indicates that the infarction or areas of atelectasis have produced alveolar damage.

The therapist can use the *simplified Wells CDR criteria* for PE to clinically assess for PE when determining the need for referral for possible PE (Table 8.3). The *modified Wells CDR* for assessing clinical probability of exclusion of PE used 1 to 3 points assigned for the variables listed[46] but has now become easier to use as the simplified Wells rule assigning "likely" or "unlikely" to the original variables.[47-49]

The Wells criteria also outline factors that constitute the PE rule-out criteria (PERC). Combining information from the list below with the PE score can help the therapist recognize low versus high priority for medical consultation.[46] The following parameters reduce the likelihood of a PE:

- Age less than 50 years
- Heart rate less than 100 bpm
- Oxyhemoglobin saturation equal to or greater than 95%
- No hemoptysis
- No estrogen use
- No prior DVT or PE

TABLE 8.3	Simplified Wells Criteria for the Clinical Assessment of Pulmonary Embolism	
Criteria		**Score**
Clinical symptoms of DVT (leg swelling, pain with palpation)		1.0
Other diagnosis less likely than pulmonary embolism		1.0
Heart rate greater than 100 bpm		1.0
Immobilization for 3 or more days or surgery in the past 4 weeks		1.0
Previous history of DVT/PE		1.0
Hemoptysis		1.0
Malignancy		1.0
Screening Clinical Probability Assessment		
PE likely; medical consult advised		Total score: 2 or more
PE unlikely; review all other factors then document findings		Total score: 0 or 1

Data from Douma RA: Validity and clinical utility of the simplified Wells rule for assessing clinical probability for the exclusion of pulmonary embolism, *Thromb Haemost* 101(1):197–200, 2009, and Gibson NS: Further validation and simplification of the Wells clinical decision rule in pulmonary embolism, *Thromb Haemost* 99:229–234, 2008.
DVT, Deep venous thrombosis; *PE*, pulmonary embolism.

- No unilateral leg swelling
- No surgery or trauma requiring hospitalization within the past 4 weeks

The PERC approach has a high negative predictive value and sensitivity when combined with a low probability of PE using the *simplified* Wells criteria, but a low positive predictive value and specificity. In other words, low-risk patients who have all of the PERC are highly unlikely to have PE, but the absence of one or more of the PERC does not mean that PE exists.[50]

CLINICAL SIGNS AND SYMPTOMS
Pulmonary Embolism

- Dyspnea
- Pleuritic (sharp, localized) chest pain
- Diffuse chest discomfort
- Persistent cough
- Hemoptysis (bloody sputum)
- Apprehension, anxiety, restlessness
- Tachypnea (increased respiratory rate)
- Tachycardia
- Fever

Cor Pulmonale

When PE is sufficiently massive and obstructs 60% to 75% of the pulmonary circulation, the client may have central chest pain, and acute cor pulmonale occurs. Cor pulmonale is a serious cardiac condition and an emergency arising from sudden dilation of the right ventricle as a result of PE.

As cor pulmonale progresses, edema, and other signs of right-sided heart failure develop. Symptoms are similar to those of CHF from other causes: dyspnea, edema of the lower extremities, distention of the veins of the neck, and liver distention. The hematocrit is increased as the body attempts to compensate for impaired circulation by producing more erythrocytes.

CLINICAL SIGNS AND SYMPTOMS
Cor Pulmonale

- Peripheral edema (bilateral legs)
- Chronic cough
- Central chest pain
- Exertional dyspnea or dyspnea at rest
- Distention of neck veins
- Fatigue
- Wheezing
- Weakness

Pulmonary Arterial Hypertension

PAH is a condition of vasoconstriction of the pulmonary arterial vascular bed. PAH is medically defined as a mean pulmonary artery pressure of 25 mm Hg or more with a pulmonary capillary wedge pressure of 15 mm Hg or less (measured by cardiac catheterization).[51]

It can be either *primary* (rare), occurring three times more often in women in their 30s and 40s compared with men, or *secondary*, occurring as a result of other clinical conditions such as PE, chronic lung disease, sickle-cell disease, Graves' disease, polycythemia, collagen vascular disease, portal hypertension, heart abnormalities, and sleep apnea. Along with thromboemboli, tumors can also obstruct pulmonary circulation. Either type is probably a combination of genetic and environmental factors.[51,52]

Normally, the pulmonary circulation has a low resistance and can accommodate large increases in blood flow during exertion. When pulmonary arterial vasoconstriction occurs and pulmonary arterial pressure rises above normal, the condition becomes self-perpetuating inducing further vasoconstriction in the pulmonary vasculature, structural abnormalities, and eventual right-sided heart failure (cor pulmonale).

Clinical Signs and Symptoms

There may not be any symptoms in the early stages of PAH. The onset of symptoms can be very subtle and difficult to recognize initially, especially in secondary PAH as underlying lung disease is usually present. PAH may present as progressive dyspnea (present upon exertion first and later develop at rest). Dull retrosternal chest pain, fatigue, and dizziness upon exertion are common and often mimic angina pectoris.[51,52]

The right ventricle must pump very hard against a narrowed, resistant pulmonary vascular bed, thus resulting in pump failure. The right ventricle enlarges in its effort to overcome abnormally high PA pressure. Ascites (increased abdominal girth) is a common visible sign. With auscultation, there may be an accentuated pulmonic component of S2 caused by the increased force of pulmonary valve closure in the presence of PAH. There may be a pulmonary regurgitation murmur as well.[51]

Pleurisy

Pleurisy is an inflammation of the pleura (serous membrane enveloping the lungs) and is caused by infection, injury, or tumor. The membranous pleura that encases each lung consists of two close-fitting layers: the visceral layer encasing the lungs and the parietal layer lining the inner chest wall. A lubricating fluid lies between these two layers.

If the fluid content remains unchanged by the disease, the pleurisy is said to be dry. If the fluid increases abnormally, it is a wet pleurisy or pleurisy with effusion (pleural effusion). If the wet pleurisy becomes infected with the formation of pus, the condition is known as purulent pleurisy or empyema.

Pleurisy may occur as a result of many factors, including pneumonia, TB, lung abscess, influenza, systemic lupus erythematosus (SLE), rheumatoid arthritis, and pulmonary infarction. Any one of these conditions is a risk factor for the development of pleurisy, especially in the aging adult population.

Pleurisy, with or without effusion associated with SLE, may be accompanied by acute pleuritic pain and dysfunction of the diaphragm.

Clinical Signs and Symptoms

The chest pain is sudden and may vary from vague discomfort to an intense stabbing or knife-like sensation in the chest. The pain is aggravated by breathing, coughing, laughing, or other similar movements associated with deep inspiration.

The visceral pleura is insensitive; pain results from inflammation of the parietal pleura. Because the latter is innervated by the intercostal nerves, chest pain is usually felt over the site of the pleuritis, but pain may be referred to the lower chest wall, abdomen, neck, upper trapezius muscle, and shoulder because of irritation of the central diaphragmatic pleura (Fig. 8.8).

CLINICAL SIGNS AND SYMPTOMS

Pleurisy

- Chest pain
- Cough
- Dyspnea
- Fever, chills
- Tachypnea (rapid, shallow breathing)

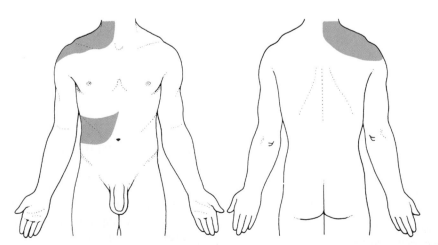

Fig. 8.8 *Chest pain over the site of pleuritis is usually perceived by the client.* Referred pain *(light red)* associated with pleuritis may occur on the same side as the pleuritic lesion affecting the shoulder, upper trapezius muscle, neck, lower chest wall, or abdomen.

Pneumothorax

Pneumothorax, or free air in the pleural cavity between the visceral and parietal pleurae, may occur secondary to pulmonary disease (e.g., when an emphysematous bulla or other weakened areas in the lung ruptures) or as a result of trauma and subsequent perforation of the chest wall. Other risk factors include scuba diving and overexertion.

Pneumothorax is not uncommon after surgery or after an invasive medical procedure involving the chest or thorax. Air may enter the pleural space directly through a hole in the chest wall (open pneumothorax) or diaphragm. Pneumothorax associated with surgical management of patent ductus arteriosus in neonates has been reported.[53]

Air may escape into the pleural space from a puncture or tear in an internal respiratory structure (e.g., bronchus, bronchioles, or alveoli). This form of pneumothorax is called closed or spontaneous pneumothorax.

Pneumothorax associated with scuba diving occurs as a result of arterial gas embolism (AGE). AGE is caused by pulmonary overinflation if the breathing gas cannot be exhaled adequately during the ascent. Inert gas bubbles cause impairment of pulmonary functions as a result of hypoxia.[54]

Extraalveolar air (pulmonary barotrauma) from scuba diving can be overlooked, resulting in serious neurologic sequelae. Scuba diving is contraindicated in anyone with asthma, hypertension, coronary heart disease, diabetes, or a history of pneumothorax.

Spontaneous pneumothorax occasionally affects the exercising individual and occurs without preceding trauma or infection. In a healthy individual, abrupt onset of dyspnea raises the suspicion of spontaneous pneumothorax. Peak incidence for this type of pneumothorax is in adults between 20 and 40 years. Spontaneous pneumothorax in term newborn infants is significantly more likely in males with higher birth weights and with vacuum delivery.[55]

Idiopathic spontaneous pneumothorax (SP) is the result of leakage of air from the lung parenchyma through a ruptured visceral pleura into the pleural cavity. This rupture may be caused by an increased pressure difference between parenchymal airspace and pleural cavity. Another theory is that peripheral airway inflammation leads to obstruction with airtrapping in the lung parenchyma, which precedes spontaneous pneumothorax.[56]

Clinical Signs and Symptoms

Symptoms of pneumothorax, whether occurring spontaneously or as a result of injury or trauma vary depending on the size and location of the pneumothorax and the extent of lung disease. When air enters the pleural cavity, the lung collapses, producing dyspnea and a shift in tissues and organs to the unaffected side.

The client may have severe pain in the upper and lateral thoracic wall, which is aggravated by any movement and by the cough and dyspnea that accompany it. The pain may be referred to the ipsilateral shoulder (corresponding shoulder on the same side as the pneumothorax), across the chest, or over the abdomen (Fig. 8.9). The client may be most comfortable when sitting in an upright position.

Other symptoms may include a fall in blood pressure, a weak and rapid pulse, and cessation of normal respiratory movements on the affected side of the chest (Case Example 8.5).

CLINICAL SIGNS AND SYMPTOMS

Pneumothorax

- Dyspnea
- Change in respiratory movements (affected side)
- Sudden, sharp chest pain
- Increased neck vein distention
- Weak and rapid pulse (>100 bpm)
- Fall in blood pressure
- Dry, hacking cough
- Shoulder pain
- Sitting upright is most comfortable

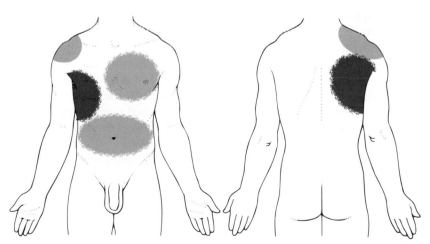

Fig. 8.9 *Possible pain patterns associated with pneumothorax:* upper and lateral thoracic wall with referral to the ipsilateral shoulder, across the chest, or over the abdomen.

CASE EXAMPLE 8.5
Tension Pneumothorax

An 18-year-old male who was injured in a motor vehicle accident (MVA) has come into the hospital physical therapy department with orders to begin ambulation. He had a long leg cast on his left leg and has brought a pair of crutches with him. This is the first time he has been out of bed in the upright position; he has not ambulated in his room yet.

Blood pressure measurement taken while the client was sitting in the wheelchair was 110/78 mm Hg. Pulse was easily palpated and measured at 72 bpm. The therapist gave the necessary instructions and assisted the client to the standing position in the parallel bars. Immediately once standing, this young man began to experience the onset of sharp midthoracic back pain and shortness of breath (SOB). He became pale and shaky, breaking out in a cold sweat.

The therapist assisted him to a seated position and asked the client if he was experiencing pain anywhere else (e.g., chest, shoulder, abdomen) while reassessing blood pressure. His blood pressure had fallen to 90/56 mm Hg, and he was unable to respond verbally to the questions asked. A clinic staff person was asked to telephone for immediate emergency help. While waiting for a medical team, the therapist noted a weak and rapid pulse, distention of the client's neck veins, and diminished respiratory movements.

This young man was diagnosed with tension pneumothorax caused by a displaced fractured rib. Untreated, tension pneumothorax can quickly produce life-threatening shock and bradycardia. Monitoring of the client's vital signs by the therapist resulted in fast action to save this young man's life.

PHYSICIAN REFERRAL

It is more common for a therapist to be treating a client with a previously diagnosed musculoskeletal problem who now has chronic, recurrent pulmonary symptoms than to be the primary evaluator and health care provider of a client with pulmonary symptoms.

In either case, the therapist needs to know what further questions to ask and which of the client's responses represent serious symptoms that require medical follow-up.

Shoulder or back pain can be referred from diseases of the diaphragmatic or parietal pleura or secondary to metastatic lung cancer. When clients have chest pain, they usually fall into one of two categories: those who demonstrate chest pain associated with pulmonary symptoms and those who have true musculoskeletal problems, such as intercostal strains and tears, myofascial trigger points, fractured ribs, or myalgias secondary to overuse.

Clients with chronic, persistent cough, whether productive or dry and hacking, may develop sharp, localized intercostal pain similar to pleuritic pain. Both intercostal and pleuritic pain is aggravated by respiratory movements, such as laughing, coughing, deep breathing, or sneezing. Clients who have intercostal pain secondary to insidious trauma or repetitive movements, such as coughing, can benefit from physical therapy.

For the client with asthma, it is important to maintain contact with the physician if the client develops signs of asthma or any bronchial activity during exercise. The physician must be informed to help alter the dosage of their medications to maintain optimal physical performance.

The therapist will want to screen for medical disease through a series of questions to elicit the presence of associated systemic (pulmonary) signs and symptoms. Aggravating and relieving factors may provide further clues that can assist in making a treatment or referral decision.

In all of these situations, the referral of a client to a physician is based on the family/personal history of pulmonary disease, the presence of pulmonary symptoms of a systemic nature, or the absence of substantive objective findings indicating a musculoskeletal lesion.

Guidelines for Immediate Medical Attention

- Abrupt onset of dyspnea accompanied by weak and rapid pulse and fall in blood pressure (pneumothorax), especially following motor vehicle accident, chest injury, or other traumatic event
- Chest, rib, or shoulder pain with neurologic symptoms following recent recreational or competitive scuba diving
- Clients with symptoms of inadequate ventilation or CO_2 retention (see Respiratory Acidosis)
- Any red-flag signs and symptoms in a client with a previous history of cancer, especially lung cancer

Guidelines for Physician Referral

- Shoulder pain aggravated by respiratory movements; have the client hold his or her breath and reassess symptoms; any reduction or elimination of symptoms with breath-holding or the Valsalva maneuver suggests a pulmonary or cardiac source of symptoms.
- Shoulder pain that is aggravated by supine positioning; pain that is worse when lying down and improves when sitting up or leaning forward is often pleuritic in origin; abdominal contents push up against diaphragm and, in turn, against the parietal pleura.
- Shoulder or chest (thorax) pain that subsides with autosplinting (lying on the painful side).
- For the client with asthma: signs of asthma or bronchial activity during exercise.
- Weak and rapid pulse accompanied by a fall in blood pressure (pneumothorax).
- Presence of associated signs and symptoms such as persistent cough, dyspnea (rest or exertional), or constitutional symptoms (see Box 1.3).

Clues to Screening for Pulmonary Disease

These clues will help the therapist in the decision-making process:

- Age over 40 years.
- History of cigarette smoking for many years.
- Past medical history of breast, prostate, kidney, pancreas, colon, or uterine cancer.
- Recent history of upper respiratory infection, especially when followed by noninflammatory joint pain of unknown cause.
- Musculoskeletal pain exacerbated by respiratory movements (e.g., deep breathing, coughing, laughing).
- Respiratory movements are diminished or absent on one side (pneumothorax).
- Dyspnea (unexplained or out of proportion), especially when accompanied by unexplained weight loss.
- Unable to localize pain by palpation.
- Pain does not change with spinal motions (e.g., no change in symptoms with sidebending, rotation, flexion, or extension).
- Pain does not change with alterations in position (possible exceptions: sitting upright is preferred with pneumothorax; symptoms may be worse at night with recumbency, sitting upright eases or relieves symptoms).
- Symptoms are increased with recumbency (lying supine shifts the contents of the abdominal cavity in an upward direction, thereby placing pressure on the diaphragm and in turn the lungs, referring pain from a lower lung pathologic condition).
- Presence of associated signs and symptoms, especially persistent cough, hemoptysis, dyspnea, and constitutional symptoms, most commonly sore throat, fever, and chills.
- Autosplinting decreases pain.
- Elimination of trigger points resolves symptoms, confirming a musculoskeletal problem (or conversely, trigger point therapy does NOT resolve symptoms, raising a red flag for further examination and evaluation).
- Range of motion does not reproduce symptoms* (e.g., trunk rotation, trunk sidebending, shoulder motions).
- Anytime an older person has shoulder pain and confusion at presentation, consider the possibility of diaphragmatic impingement by an underlying lung pathologic condition, especially pneumonia.

PULMONARY PAIN PATTERNS

PLEUROPULMONARY DISORDERS (FIG. 8.10)

Location:	Substernal or chest over involved lung fields—anterior, side, back
Referral:	Often well localized (client can point to exact site of pain) without referral
	May radiate to neck, upper trapezius muscle, shoulder, costal margins, or upper abdomen
	Thoracic back pain occurs with irritation of the posterior parietal pleura
Description:	Sharp ache, stabbing, angina-like pressure, or crushing pain with pulmonary embolism

ANGINA-LIKE CHEST PAIN WITH SEVERE PULMONARY HYPERTENSION

Intensity:	Moderate
Duration:	Hours to days
Associated signs and symptoms:	Preceded by pneumonia or upper respiratory infection
	Wheezing
	Dyspnea (exertional or at rest)
	Hyperventilation
	Tachypnea (increased respirations)
	Fatigue, weakness
	Tachycardia (increased heart rate)
	Fever, chills
	Edema
	Apprehension or anxiety, restlessness
	Persistent cough or cough with blood (hemoptysis)
	Dry hacking cough (occurs with the onset of pneumothorax)
	Medically determined signs and symptoms (e.g., by chest auscultation and chest radiograph)
Relieving factors:	Sitting
	Some relief when at rest, but most comfortable position varies (pneumonia)
	Pleuritic pain may be relieved by lying on the affected side

* There are two possible exceptions to this guideline. Painful symptoms from an intercostal tear (secondary to forceful coughing caused by diaphragmatic pleurisy) will be reproduced by trunk sidebending to the opposite side and trunk rotation to one or both sides. In such a case there is an underlying pulmonary pathologic condition, and a musculoskeletal component. Pleuritic pain can also be reproduced by trunk movements, but the therapist will be unable to localize the pain during palpation.

Aggravating factors:	Breathing at rest
	Increased inspiratory movement (e.g., laughter, coughing, sneezing)
	Symptoms accentuated with each breath

LUNG CANCER

Location:	Anterior chest
Referral:	Scapulae, upper back, ipsilateral shoulder radiating along the medial aspect of the arm
	First and second ribs and associated vertebrae and paravertebral muscles (apical or Pancoast's tumors)
Description:	Localized, sharp pleuritic pain (peripheral tumors)
	Dull, vague aching in the chest
	Neuritic pain of shoulders/arm (apical or Pancoast's tumors)
	Bone pain caused by metastases to adjacent bone or the vertebrae
Intensity:	Moderate-to-severe
Duration:	Constant
Associated signs and symptoms:	Dyspnea or wheezing
	Hemoptysis (coughing up or spitting up blood)
	Fever, chills, malaise, anorexia, weight loss
	Fecal breath odor
	Tachycardia or atrial fibrillation (palpitations)
	Muscle weakness or atrophy (e.g., Pancoast's tumor may involve the shoulder and arm on affected side)
	Associated CNS symptoms:
	• Headache
	• Nausea
	• Vomiting
	• Malaise
	Signs of cord compression:
	• Localized or radicular back pain
	• Weakness
	• Loss of lower extremity sensation
	• Bowel/bladder incontinence
	Hoarseness, dysphagia (peripheral tumors)
Relieving factors:	None without medical intervention
Aggravating factors:	Inspiration: deep breathing, laughing, coughing

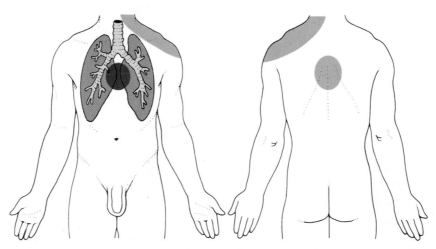

Fig. 8.10 *Primary pain patterns (dark red)* associated with pleuropulmonary disorders, such as pulmonary embolus, cor pulmonale, pleurisy, or spontaneous pneumothorax may vary, but they usually include substernal or chest pain. Pain over the involved lung fields (anterior, lateral, or posterior) may occur (not shown). Pain may radiate *(light red)* to the neck, upper trapezius muscle, ipsilateral shoulder, thoracic back, costal margins, or upper abdomen (the latter two areas are not shown).

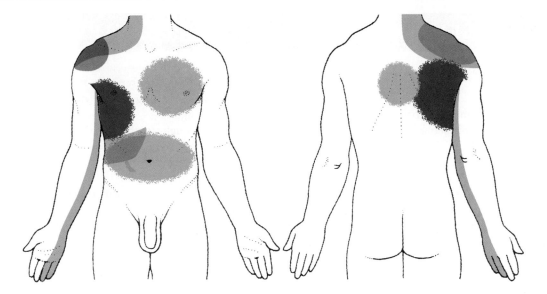

Fig. 8.11 *A composite picture of the pain patterns associated with many different impairments of the pulmonary parenchyma including pleuritis, pneumothorax, pulmonary embolism, cor pulmonale, and pleurisy.* No single individual will present with all of these patterns at the same time. A composite illustration gives an idea of the wide range of referred pain patterns possible with pulmonary diseases or conditions. Remember that viscerogenic pain patterns do not usually present as discrete circles or ovals of pain as depicted here. This figure is an approximation of what the therapist might expect to hear the client describe associated with a pulmonary problem.

■ Key Points to Remember

1. Pulmonary pain patterns are usually localized in the substernal or chest region over involved lung fields, which may include the anterior chest, side, or back (Fig. 8.11; see also Fig. 8.10).

2. Pulmonary pain can radiate to the neck, upper trapezius muscle, costal margins, thoracic back, scapulae, or shoulder.

3. Shoulder pain caused by pulmonary involvement may radiate along the medial aspect of the arm, mimicking other neuromuscular causes of neck or shoulder pain.

4. Pulmonary pain usually increases with inspiratory movements such as laughing, coughing, sneezing, or deep breathing.

5. Shoulder pain that is relieved by lying on the involved side may be "autosplinting," a sign of a pulmonary cause of symptoms.

6. Shoulder pain that is aggravated when lying supine (arm/elbow supported) may be an indication of a pulmonary cause of symptoms.

7. For anyone with pain patterns pictured here as presenting symptoms, especially in the absence of trauma or injury, check the client's personal medical history for previous or recurrent upper respiratory infection or pneumonia.

8. Any client with symptoms of inadequate ventilation, pneumothorax, or CO_2 retention needs immediate medical referral.

9. Clients with COPD who tend to retain CO_2 must be monitored carefully. Because clients with CO_2 retention have a decreased ventilatory drive unless oxygen levels are low, oxygen delivered by nasal cannula cannot get too high or the client will become apneic. There is a standard practice to increase oxygen levels administered by cannula during exercise with some clients who are compromised. Maintaining these levels around 1 L/min to 2 L/min may be required with some clients who have COPD. Consult with respiratory therapy or nursing staff for optimal levels for this particular group of clients.

10. CNS symptoms, such as muscle weakness, muscle atrophy, headache, loss of lower extremity sensation, and localized or radicular back pain may be associated with lung cancer.

11. Any CNS symptom may be the silent presentation of a lung tumor.

12. Posterior leg or calf pain postoperatively may be caused by a thrombus and must be reported to the physician before physical therapy begins or continues.

13. Hemoptysis or exertional/at rest dyspnea, either unexplained or out of proportion to the situation or person, is a red-flag symptom requiring medical referral.

14. Change in cough or change in sputum requires further assessment.

15. Any client with chest pain should be evaluated for trigger points and intercostal tears.

CLIENT HISTORY AND INTERVIEW

SPECIAL QUESTIONS TO ASK

Past Medical History

- Have you ever had trouble with breathing or lung disease such as bronchitis, emphysema, asthma, pneumonia, or blood clots?
  - *If yes:* Describe what this problem was, when it occurred, and how it was treated.
  - If the person answered yes to asthma, either on the Personal/Family History form or to this question, ask:
    - How can you tell when you are having an asthma episode?
    - What triggers an asthma episode for you?
    - Do you use medications during an episode?
    - Do you have trouble with asthma during exercise?
    - Do you time your medications with your exercise to prevent an asthma episode during exercise?
- Have you ever had tuberculosis?
  - *If yes:* When did it occur, and how was it treated? What is your current status?
  - When was your last test for tuberculosis? What was the test result?
- Have you had a chest radiograph film taken in the last 5 years?
  - *If yes:* What were the results?
- Have you ever broken your nose, been told that you have a deviated septum (nasal passageway), nasal polyps, or sleep apnea? **(Hypoxia)**
- Have you ever had lung or heart surgery?
- *If yes:* What and when? **(Decreased vital capacity)**

ASSOCIATED SIGNS AND SYMPTOMS

- Are you having difficulty breathing now?
- Do you ever have SOB or breathlessness or cannot quite catch your breath?
  - *If yes:* When does this happen? When you rest? When you lie flat, walk on level ground, or walk up stairs?
- How far can you walk before you feel breathless?
- What symptoms stop your walking (e.g., SOB, heart pounding, chest tightness, or weak legs)?
- Are these episodes associated with night sweats, cough, chest pain, or bluish color around your lips or fingernails?
- Does your breathlessness seem to be related to food, pollen, dust, animals, season, stress, or strong emotion? **(Asthma)**
- Do you have any breathing aids (e.g., oxygen, continuous positive airway pressure [CPAP], nebulizer, inhaler, humidifier, air cleaner, or other aid)?
- Do you have a cough? (Note whether the client smokes, for how long, and how much.)

- *If yes* to cough, separate this cough from a smoker's cough by asking: When did it start? Is it related to smoking?
- Do you cough anything up? *If yes:* Describe the color, amount, and frequency.
- Are you taking anything to prevent this cough? *If yes,* does it seem to help?
- Are there occasions when you cannot seem to stop coughing?
- Do you ever cough up blood or anything that looks like coffee grounds? (Bright red fresh blood; brown or black older blood)
- Have you strained a muscle or your lower back from coughing?
- Does it hurt to touch your chest or take a deep breath, cough, sneeze, or laugh?
- Have you unexpectedly lost or gained 10 or more pounds recently?

Gained: **Pulmonary edema, CHF, fat deposits under the diaphragm in the obese client reduces ventilation**

Lost: **Emphysema, cancer**

- Do your ankles swell? **(CHF)**
- Have you been unusually tired lately? **(CHF, emphysema)**
- Have you noticed a change in your voice? **(Pathology of left hilum or trachea)**

Environmental and Work History

Quick Survey (For full survey, see Appendix B-14 in the accompanying enhanced eBook version included with print purchase of this textbook):

- What kind of work do you do?
- Do you think your health problems are related to your work?
- Do you wear a mask at work?
- Are your symptoms better or worse when you are at home or at work?

  Follow-up if worse at work: Do others at work have similar problems?

  Follow-up if worse at home: Have you done any remodeling at home in the last 6 months?
- Have you been exposed to dusts, asbestos, fumes, chemicals, radiation, or loud noise?
- Have you ever served in any branch of the military?
  - *If yes,* were you ever exposed to dusts, fumes, chemicals, radiation, or other substances?

Follow-up: It may be necessary to ask additional questions based on past history, symptoms, and risk factors present.

CASE STUDY

REFERRAL

A 65-year-old man has come to you for an evaluation of low back pain, which he attributes to lifting a heavy box 2 weeks ago. During the medical history, you notice that the client has a persistent cough and that he sounds hoarse.

After reviewing the Personal/Family History form, you note that the client smokes two packs of cigarettes each day and that he has smoked at least this amount for at least 50 years. (One pack per day for 1 year is considered "one pack-year.") This person has smoked an estimated 100 pack-years; anyone who has smoked for 20 pack-years or more is considered to be at risk for the development of serious lung disease.

What questions will you ask to decide for yourself whether his back pain is systemic?

PHYSICAL THERAPY INTERVIEW

Introduction to Client

It is important for me to make certain that your back pain is not caused by other health problems, such as prostate problems or respiratory infection, so I will ask a series of questions that may not seem to be related to your back pain, but I want to be very thorough and cover every possibility to obtain the best and most effective treatment for you.

Pain

From your history form, I see that you associate your back pain with lifting a heavy box 2 weeks ago. When did you first notice your back pain (sudden or gradual onset)?

Have you ever hurt your back before or have you ever had pain similar to this episode in the past? **(Systemic disease: recurrent and gradually increases over time)**

Please describe your pain (supply descriptive terms if necessary).

How often do you have this pain?

 Follow-ups (FUPs): How long does it last when you have it?
 What aggravates your pain/symptoms?
 What relieves your pain/symptoms?
 How does rest affect your pain?
 Have you noticed any change in your pain/symptoms since they first started to the present time?

Do you have any numbness in the groin or inside your legs? (Saddle anesthesia: **cauda equina**)

Pulmonary

I notice you have quite a cough and you sound hoarse to me. How long have you had this cough and hoarseness (when did it first begin)?

Do you have any back pain associated with this cough? Any other pain associated with your cough?

If yes: Have the person describe where, when, intensity, aggravating and relieving factors.

How does it feel when you take a deep breath? Does your low back hurt when you laugh or take a deep breath?

When you cough, do you produce phlegm or mucus?

If yes: Have you ever noticed any red streaks or blood in it?

Does your coughing or back pain keep you awake at night?

Have you been examined by a physician for either your cough or your back pain?

Have you had any recent chest or spine x-rays taken?

If yes: When and where? What were the results?

General Systemic

Have you had any night sweats, daytime fevers, or chills?

Do you have difficulty in swallowing (**Esophageal cancer, anxiety, cervical disc protrusion**)? Have you had laryngitis over and over? **(Oral cancer)**

Urologic

Have you ever been told that you have a prostate problem or prostatitis?

If yes: Determine when this occurred, how it was treated, and whether the person had the same symptoms at that time that he is now describing to you.

Have you noticed any change in your bladder habits?

Follow-up questions (FUPS): Have you had any difficulty in starting or continuing to urinate?

Is there any burning or discomfort during urination?

Have you noticed any blood in your urine?

Have you recently had any difficulty with kidney stones or bladder or kidney infections?

Gastrointestinal

Have you noticed any change in your bowel pattern?

Have you had difficulty having a bowel movement?

Do you find that you have soiled yourself without even realizing it? (Cauda equina lesion—this would require immediate referral to a physician)

Does your back pain begin or increase when you are having a bowel movement?

Is your back pain relieved after having a bowel movement?

Have you noticed any association between when you eat and when your pain/symptoms increase or decrease?

Final Question

Is there anything about your current back pain or your general health that we have not discussed that you think is important for me to know?

(Refer to Special Questions to Ask in this chapter for other questions that may be pertinent to this client, depending on the answers to these questions.)

PHYSICIAN REFERRAL

As always, correlation of findings is important in making a decision regarding medical referral. If the client has a positive family history for respiratory problems (especially lung cancer) and if clinical findings indicate pulmonary involvement, the client should be strongly encouraged to see a physician for a medical check-up.

If there are positive systemic findings, such as difficulty in swallowing, persistent hoarseness, SOB at rest, night sweats,

CASE STUDY—cont'd

fever, bloody sputum, recurrent laryngitis, or upper respiratory infection, *either in addition to or in association with* the low back pain, the client should be advised to see a physician, and the physician should receive a copy of your findings.

This guideline covers the client who has a true musculoskeletal problem, but also has other health problems, as well as the client who may have back pain of systemic origin that is unrelated to the lifting injury 2 weeks ago.

PRACTICE QUESTIONS

1. If a client reports that the shoulder/upper trapezius muscle pain increases with deep breathing, how can you assess whether this results from a pulmonary or musculoskeletal cause?

2. Neurologic symptoms such as muscle weakness or muscle atrophy may be the first indication of:
   a. Cystic fibrosis
   b. Bronchiectasis
   c. Neoplasm
   d. Deep vein thrombosis

3. Back pain with radiating numbness and tingling down the leg past the knee does not occur as a result of:
   a. Postoperative thrombus
   b. Bronchogenic carcinoma
   c. Pott's disease
   d. Trigger points

4. Pain associated with pleuropulmonary disorders can radiate to the:
   a. Anterior neck
   b. Upper trapezius muscle
   c. Ipsilateral shoulder
   d. Thoracic spine
   e. a and c
   f. All of the above

5. The presence of a persistent dry cough (no sputum or phlegm produced) has no clinical significance to the therapist. True or false?

6. Dyspnea associated with emphysema is the result of:
   a. Destruction of the alveoli
   b. Reduced elasticity of the lungs
   c. Increased effort to exhale trapped air
   d. a and b
   e. All of the above

7. What is the significance of autosplinting?

8. Which symptom has greater significance: dyspnea at rest or exertional dyspnea?

9. The presence of pain and anxiety in a client can often lead to hyperventilation. When a client hyperventilates, the arterial concentration of carbon dioxide will do which of the following?
   a. Increase
   b. Decrease
   c. Remain unchanged
   d. Vary depending on potassium concentration

10. Common symptoms of respiratory acidosis would be most closely represented by which of the following descriptions?
    a. Presence of numbness and tingling in face, hands, and feet
    b. Presence of dizziness and light-headedness
    c. Hyperventilation with change in level of consciousness
    d. Onset of sleepiness, confusion, and decreased ventilation

REFERENCES

1. Scharf SM. History and physical examination. In: Baum GL, Wolinsky E, eds. *Textbook of pulmonary diseases.* ed 5 Boston: Little, Brown; 1989.
2. Guerra S. Overlap of asthma and chronic obstructive pulmonary disease. *Curr Opin Pulm Med.* 2005;11(1):7–13.
3. Zuskin E. Respiratory function in pesticide workers. *J Occup Environ Med.* 2008;50(11):1299–1305.
4. Zuskin E. Occupational health hazards of artists. *Acta Dermatovenerol Croat.* 2007;15(3):167–177.
5. Schachter EN. Gender and respiratory findings in workers occupationally exposed to organic aerosols: a meta analysis of 12 cross-sectional studies. *Environ Health.* 2009;12(8):1–9.
6. Pauwels RA, Rabe KF. Burden and clinical features of chronic obstructive pulmonary disease (COPD). *Lancet.* 2004;364(9434):613–620.
7. Meyers DA, Larj MJ, Lange L. Genetics of asthma and COPD. Similar results for different phenotypes. *Chest.* 2004;126(2 Suppl):105S–110S.
8. Pirard L, Marchand E. *Int J Chron Obstruct Pulmon Dis.* 2018;10(13):3963–3970. https://doi.org/10.2147/COPD. S182483. eCollection 2018. PMID: 30573956.

9. Amsden GW. Anti-inflammatory effects of macrolides: an under-appreciated benefit in the treatment of community-acquired respiratory tract infections and chronic inflammatory pulmonary conditions? *J Antimicrob Chemother.* 2005;55(1):10–21.
10. Rubin BK, Henke MO. Immunomodulatory activity and effectiveness of macrolides in chronic airway disease. *Chest.* 2004;125(2 Suppl):70S–78S.
11. Goto Y, Kurosawa H, Mori N, et al. Improved activities of daily living, psychological state and health-related quality of life for 12 months following lung volume reduction surgery in patients with severe emphysema. *Respirology.* 2004;9(3):337–344.
12. Trow TK. Lung-volume reduction surgery for severe emphysema: appraisal of its current status. *Curr Opin Pulm Med.* 2004;10(2):128–132.
13. Upham JW, Holt PG. Environment and development of atopy. *Curr Opin Allergy Clin Immunol.* 2005;5(2):167–172.
14. Zhou Y, Liu Y. Recent trends in current asthma prevalence among US adults, 2009-2018. *J Allergy Clin Immunol Pract.* 2020:S2213–2198. 30398-6.
15. NHIS, Centers for Disease Control and Prevention: Most recent national asthma data. Available at: https://www.cdc.gov/asthma/most_recent_national_asthma_data.htm (2020.)

16. Asthma in US children *The Lancet 17.* 2018;391(10121):632 https://doi.org/10.1016/S0140-6736(18)30258-7. PMID: 29617249.

17. CDC National Center for Health Statistics: National Health Interview Survey (NHIS). National Surveillance of Asthma: United States, 2001–2017.

18. Moorman JE, Akinbami LJ, Bailey CM, et al. National Surveillance of Asthma: United States, 2001–2010. National Center for Health Statistics. *Vital Health Stat 3.* 2012(35).

19. NHIS Asthma Data Tables: https://www.cdc.gov/asthma/nhis/default.htm Current Asthma and Asthma Attack Prevalence (2011–2017): United States

20. Schauberger E, Peinhaupt M, Cazares T, et al. Lipid mediators of allergic disease: pathways, treatments, and emerging therapeutic targets. *Curr Allergy Asthma Rep.* 2016;16:48.

21. Abouelela A, Al-Badawy T, Abdel Gawad M. Predictive value of different scoring systems for critically ill patients with hospital acquired pneumonia. *Intensive Care Med Exp.* 2015;3(Suppl 1): A345.

22. Racial disparities in tuberculosis, selected Southeastern States, 1991–2002, *MMWR* 53(25):556–559, 2004.

23. Wisniewski A. Chronic bronchitis and emphysema: clearing the air. *Nursing.* 2003;33(5):44–49.

24. Tay B, Deckey J, Hu S. Spinal infections. *J Am Acad Orthop Surg.* 2002;10(3):188–197.

25. Siegel RL, Miller KD, Jemal A. Cancer statistics. *CA Cancer J Clin.* 2016;66:7–30.

26. Barta JA, Powell CA, Wisnivesky JP. Global Epidemiology of Lung Cancer. *Ann Glob Health 22.* 2019;85(1):8 https://doi.org/10.5334/aogh.2419. PMID: 30741509.

27. American Lung Association: Trends in tobacco use. February 2010. Available online at http://www.lungusa.org/finding-cures/ our-research/trend-reports/Tobacco-Trend-Report.pdf. Posted on October 27, 2010. Accessed January 28, 2011.

28. Jemal A. Lung cancer trends in young adults: an early indicator of progress in tobacco control (United States). *Cancer Causes Control.* 2003;14(6):579–585.

29. Kreamer K. Getting the lowdown on lung cancer. *Nursing.* 2003;33(11):36–42.

30. Davis GA. Pancoast tumors. *Neurosurg Clin N Am.* 2008;19:545–557.

31. Arcasoy S.M., Jett J.R., Schild S.E.: Pancoast's syndrome and superior (pulmonary) sulcus tumors. UpToDate Patient Information. Sponsored by the American Society of General Internal Medicine and the American College of Rheumatology. Available online at: http://patients.uptodate.com/topic.asp?file=lung_ca/12055 (version 13.2), Updated September 2010. Accessed January 28, 2011.

32. Donaldson SH. Update on pathogenesis of cystic fibrosis lung disease. *Curr Opin Pulm Med.* 2003;9(6):486–491.

33. Cystic Fibrosis Foundation Patient Registry *2018 annual data report to the center directors.* Bethesda, MD: Cystic Fibrosis Foundation; 2018.

34. Mitomo K. Toward gene therapy for cystic fibrosis using lentivirus pseudotyped with Sendai virus envelopes. *Mol Ther.* 2010;18(6):1173–1182.

35. Ostedgaard LS, Rokhlina T, Karp PH, et al. A shortened adeno-associated virus expression cassette for CFTR gene transfer to cystic fibrosis airway epithelia. *Proc Natl Acad Sci U S A.* 2005;102(8):2952–2957.

36. Sloane PA. Cystic fibrosis transmembrane conductance regulator protein repair as a therapeutic strategy in cystic fibrosis. *Curr Opin Pulm Med.* 2010;16(6):591–597.

37. De Boeck K, Amaral MD. Progress in therapies for cystic fibrosis. *Lancet Respir Med.* 2016;4(8):662–674.

38. Rosenbluth DB, Wilson K, Ferkol T, et al. Lung function decline in cystic fibrosis patients and timing for lung transplantation referral. *Chest.* 2004;126(2):412–419.

39. American Lung Association: Occupational lung disease fact sheet, January 2004. Available online at: http://www.lungusa.org/. Accessed January 28, 2011.

40. National Institute for Occupational Safety and Health Respiratory diseases. *Worker Health Chartbook.* 2004:142–146.

41. Bergdahl IA, Toren K, Eriksson K, et al. Increased mortality in COPD among construction workers exposed to inorganic dust. *Eur Respir J.* 2004;23(3):402–406.

42. Delis KT. Incidence, natural history, and risk factors of deep vein thrombosis in elective knee arthroscopy. *Thromb Haemost.* 2001;86(3):817–821.

43. O'Donnell T, Abbott W, Athanasoulis C, et al. Diagnosis of deep venous thrombosis in the outpatient by venography. *Surg Gynecol Obstet.* 1980;150:69–74.

44. Molloy W, English J, O'Dwyer R, et al. Clinical findings in the diagnosis of proximal deep venous thrombosis. *Ir Med J.* 1982;75:119–120.

45. Shah NB. 82-year-old man with bilateral leg swelling. *Mayo Clin Proc.* 2010;85(9):859–862.

46. van Belle A, Buller HR, Huisman MV, et al. Effectiveness of managing suspected pulmonary embolism using an algorithm combining clinical probability, D-dimer testing, and computed tomography. *JAMA.* 2006;295:172.

47. Wells PS. Derivation of a simple clinical model to categorize patients probability of pulmonary embolism: increasing the models utility with the simplified D-dimer. *Thromb Haemost.* 2000;83:416–430.

48. Douma RA. Validity and clinical utility of the simplified Wells rule for assessing clinical probability for the exclusion of pulmonary embolism. *Thromb Haemost.* 2009;101(1):197–200.

49. Gibson NS. Further validation and simplification of the Wells clinical decision rule in pulmonary embolism. *Thromb Haemost.* 2008;99(6):1134–1136.

50. Wolf SJ. Assessment of the pulmonary embolism rule-out criteria rule for evaluation of suspected pulmonary embolism in the emergency department. *Am J Emerg Med.* 2008;26:181.

51. Badesch DB. Medical therapy for pulmonary arterial hypertension: updated ACCP evidence-based clinical practice guidelines. *Chest.* 2007;131(6):1917–1928.

52. Pulmonary Hypertension Association: What is pulmonary hypertension? Available online at http://www.phassociation.org. Accessed December 21, 2010.

53. Jog SM, Patole SK. Diaphragmatic paralysis in extremely low birthweight neonates: is waiting for spontaneous recovery justified? *J Paediatr Child Health.* 2002;38(1):101–103.

54. Taylor DM, O'Toole KS, Ryan CM. Experienced, recreational scuba divers in Australia continue to dive despite medical contraindications. *Wilderness Environ Med.* 2002;13(3):187–193.

55. Al Tawil K, Abu-Ekteish FM, Tamimi O, et al. Symptomatic spontaneous pneumothorax in term newborn infants. *Pediatr Pulmonol.* 2004;37(5):443–446.

56. Smit HJ, Golding RP, Schramel FM, et al. Lung density measurements in spontaneous pneumothorax demonstrate air trapping. *Chest.* 2004;125(6):2083–2090.

57. Centers for Disease Control. Asthma. http://www.cdc.gov/asthma/default.htm.

58. National Center for Health Statistics Centers for Disease Control. *Asthma.* 2014 http://www.cdc.gov/nchs/fastats/asthma.htm.

59. National Institute of Allergy and Infectious Disease. Asthma. http://www.niaid.nih.gov/topics/asthma/Pages/default.aspx.

60. Porello P.: Neoplasms, Lung. eMedicine. Available online at www.emedicine.com/emerg/topic335.htm. Accessed January 28, 2011.

61. Jemal A, Ward E, Thun MJ. Contemporary lung cancer trends among U.S. women. *Cancer Epidemiol Biomarkers Prev.* 2005;14(3):582–585.

62. Cystic Fibrosis Foundation Patient Registry *Annual Data Report to the Center Directors.* Bethesda, MD: Cystic Fibrosis Foundation;

The gastrointestinal (GI) system functions to digest and absorb nutrients which are ingested, and excrete the waste products following the process of digestion.[1] The four functions of the digestive system include: (1) motility; (2) secretion; (3) digestion; and (4) absorption.[2] The GI tract is comprised of a series of hollow organs joined by a long twisting tube that begins in the mouth and terminates in the anus (Fig. 9.1).[3] The GI tract has its own independent nervous system called the enteric nervous system (ENS), the only internal organ to have evolved its own nervous system.[1] Over the past decade, there has been significant interest in understanding the ENS. For example, it is now known that the lining of the digestive tract from the esophagus through the large intestine (Fig. 9.2)[4] is composed of approximately 100 million nerve cells that contain neuropeptides and their receptors. This neural network has been called the ENS and provides the connection between digestion, mood, and health.[5,6]

In addition to the classic hormonal and neural negative feedback loops, there are direct actions of gut hormones on the dorsal vagal complex. The person experiencing a "gut reaction" or "gut feeling" may indeed be experiencing the direct effects of gut peptides on brain function.[5] It can therefore be said that humans have a "brain-in-the-gut"[7].

The association between the enteric system, the immune system, and the brain (now a part of the research referred to as psychoneuroimmunology [PNI])[8] has been clearly established and forms an integral part of GI symptoms associated with immune disorders such as fibromyalgia, systemic lupus erythematosus, rheumatoid arthritis, and chronic fatigue syndrome.

About 70% to 80% of all immune cells are located in the gut.[9] There are more T cells in the intestinal epithelium than in all other body tissues combined. The gamma delta T cells form the forefront of the immune defense mechanism. They act as an early warning system for the cells lining the intestines, which are heavily exposed to microorganisms and toxins.[10] In some people the wall of the gut seems to have been breached, either because the network of intestinal cells develops increased permeability (a syndrome referred to as "leaky gut") or perhaps because bacteria and yeast overwhelm it and migrate into the bloodstream.[11,12]

All of these associations and new findings support the need for the physical therapist to carefully assess the possibility of GI symptoms being present but unreported. This is especially important when considering the fact that GI tract problems can sometimes imitate musculoskeletal dysfunction.

Disorders affecting the GI system can refer pain to the sternal region, shoulder and neck, scapular region, midback, lower back, hip, pelvis, and sacrum. This pain can mimic primary musculoskeletal or neuromuscular dysfunction, causing confusion for the physical therapist or for the physician assessing the client's chief complaints.

Although these neuromusculoskeletal symptoms can occur alone and far from the actual site of the disorder, the client usually has other systemic signs and symptoms associated with GI disorders that should give the therapist grounds for suspicion. A careful interview to screen for systemic illness should include a few important questions concerning the client's history, prescribed medications, and the presence of any associated signs or symptoms that would immediately alert the therapist to the need for medical follow-up. The most common intraabdominal diseases that refer pain to the musculoskeletal system are those that involve ulceration or infection of the mucosal lining. Drug-induced GI symptoms can also occur with delayed reactions as much as 6 or 8 weeks after exposure to the medication. The most common occurrences are antibiotic colitis; nausea, vomiting, and anorexia from digitalis toxicity[13]; and nonsteroidal antiinflammatory drug (NSAID)–induced ulcers.[14]

SIGNS AND SYMPTOMS OF GASTROINTESTINAL DISORDERS

Any disruption of the digestive system can create symptoms such as nausea, vomiting, pain, diarrhea, and constipation. The bowel is susceptible to altered patterns of normal motility caused by food, alcohol, caffeine, drugs, physical and emotional stress, and lifestyle (e.g., lack of regular exercise, tobacco use). Effects of chemotherapy in the GI system include nausea and vomiting, anorexia, taste alteration, weight loss, oral mucositis, diarrhea, and constipation.

Symptoms, including pain, can be related to various GI organ disturbances and differ in character, depending on the affected organ. The most clinically meaningful GI symptoms reported in a physical therapy practice include:
- Abdominal pain
- Dysphagia

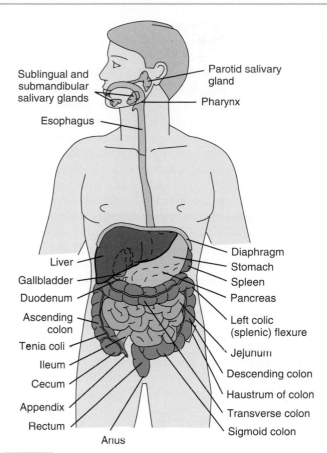

Fig. 9.1 Organs of the digestive system (From Hall JE: *Guyton and Hall textbook of medical physiology*, ed 12, Philadelphia, 2010, WB Saunders.)

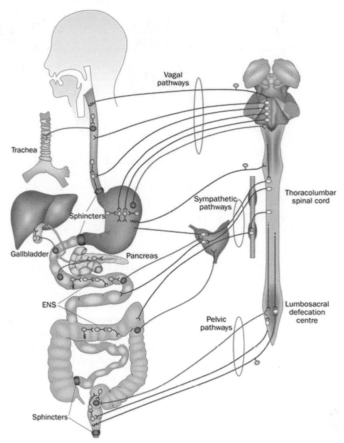

Fig. 9.2 The enteric system and its connections to the central nervous system. (From: Furness, J. The enteric nervous system and neurogastroenterology. *Nat Rev Gastroenterol* Hepatol 9, 286–294 (2012).)

- Odynophagia
- GI bleeding (emesis, melena, red blood)
- Epigastric pain with radiation to the back
- Symptoms affected by food
- Early satiety with weight loss
- Constipation
- Diarrhea
- Fecal incontinence
- Arthralgia
- Referred shoulder pain
- Psoas abscess
- Tenderness over McBurney's point (see Appendicitis section in this chapter)
- Neuropathy

Abdominal Pain

When discussing primary and referred abdominal pain patterns, be aware that each pain pattern has listed with it both the sympathetic nerve distribution to the viscera (i.e., autonomic nervous system innervation of the structure) and the anatomic location of radiating or referred pain from the viscera or GI segment involved in the primary pain patterns. Whenever possible, labels are used to differentiate between sympathetic nerve innervations of the viscera and anatomic locations of the pain. For example, the small intestine (viscera) is innervated by T9 to T11 but refers (somatic) pain to the L3 to L4 (anatomic) lumbar spine.

Primary Gastrointestinal Visceral Pain Patterns

Visceral pain (internal organs) occurs in the midline because the digestive organs arise embryologically in the midline and receive sensory afferents from both sides of the spinal cord. The site of pain generally corresponds to dermatomes from which the visceral organs receive their innervation (see Fig. 3.3). Pain is not well localized because innervation of the viscera is multisegmental over up to eight segments of the spinal cord with fewer nerve endings than other sensitive organs.

The most common primary pain patterns associated with organs of the GI tract are depicted in Fig. 9.3. Reasons for abdominal pain fall into three broad categories: inflammation, organ distention (tension pain), and necrosis (ischemic pain). The underlying cause can be life-threatening, requiring a quick examination and evaluation and fast referral.

Pain in the *epigastric region* occurs anywhere from the midsternum to the xiphoid process from the heart, esophagus, stomach, duodenum, gallbladder, liver, and other mediastinal

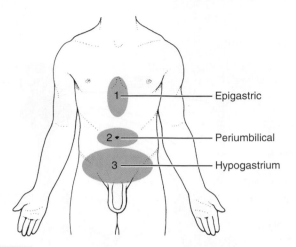

Fig. 9.3 Visceral pain. *1*, The epigastric region from the heart, esophagus, stomach, duodenum, gallbladder, liver, or pancreas and corresponding to T3 to T5 sympathetic nerve distribution; *2*, the periumbilical region from the pancreas, small intestine, appendix, or proximal colon (T9 to T11 sympathetic nerve distribution; the umbilicus is level with the disk located between the L3 and L4 vertebral bodies in the adult who is not overweight); and *3*, the lower midabdominal or hypogastrium region from the large intestine, colon, bladder, or uterus (T10 to L2 sympathetic nerve distribution).

organs corresponding to the T3 to T5 sympathetic nerve distribution. The client may report that pain radiates around the ribs or straight through the chest to the thoracic spine at the T3 to T6 or T7 anatomic levels.

Pain in the *periumbilical region* (T9 to T11 nerve distribution) occurs with impairment of the small intestine (see Fig. 9.17), pancreas, and appendix. Primary pain in the periumbilical region usually sends the client to a physician. However, pain around the umbilicus may be accompanied by low back pain. In the healthy adult who is not obese and does not have a protruding abdomen, the umbilicus is at the same level as the disk located anatomically between the L3 and L4 vertebral bodies.

The physical therapist is more likely to see a client with anterior abdominal and low back pain at the same level but with alternating presentation. In other words, the client experiences first periumbilical pain with or without associated GI signs and symptoms, then the painful episode resolves. Later, the client develops low back pain with or without GI symptoms but does not realize there is a link between these painful episodes. It is at this point that the client would present in a physical therapy practice.

Pain in the *lower abdominal region* (hypogastrium) from the large intestine and/or colon may be mistaken for bladder or uterine pain (and vice versa) by its suprapubic location. Referred pain at the same anatomic level posteriorly corresponds to the sacrum (see Fig. 9.18). The large intestine and colon are innervated by T10 to L2, depending on the location (e.g., ascending, transverse, descending colon).

The abdominal viscera are ordinarily insensitive to many stimuli, such as cutting, tearing, or crushing, that when applied to the skin evokes severe pain. Visceral pain fibers are

sensitive only to stretching or tension in the wall of the gut from neoplasm, distention, or forceful muscular contractions secondary to bowel obstruction or spasm.

Tension pain can occur as a result of bowel obstruction; constipation; and pus, fluid, or blood accumulation from infection or other causes. The rate that tension develops must be rapid enough to produce pain; gradual distention, such as with malignant obstruction, may be painless unless ulceration occurs. Rapid, peristalsis forces of the bowel trying to eliminate irritating substances can cause tension pain described as "colicky" pain. Individuals with tension pain have trouble finding a comfortable position; often shifting positions decreases the offending symptoms.

Visceral organs of the GI tract (particularly hollow organs such as the intestines) respond to stretching and distention as pain, more so than typical tissue injury caused by cutting or crushing. Because of similar innervation, it is often difficult to distinguish pain associated with the heart from pain caused by an esophageal disorder.

One difference between visceral organ pain and pain from the parietal peritoneum is that the parietal peritoneum is innervated by nerves that travel with the somatic nerves, providing a more precise location of pain. This is noted with acute appendicitis, when early, vague pain (from inflammation of the appendix) is replaced by more localized pain at McBurney's point once the inflammation involves the parietal peritoneum.

Inflammatory pain arising from the visceral or parietal peritoneum (e.g., acute appendicitis) is described as steady, deep, and boring. It can be poorly localized as when the visceral peritoneum is involved or more localized with parietal peritoneum involvement. Individuals with inflammatory pain seek a quiet position (often with the knees bent or in a curled up/fetal position) without movement.

Ischemia (deficiency of blood) may produce visceral pain by increasing the concentration of tissue metabolites in the region of the sensory nerve. Pain associated with ischemia is steady pain, whether this ischemia is secondary to vascular disease or from an obstruction causing strangulation of bowel tissue. The pain is sudden in onset and extremely intense. It progresses in severity and is not relieved by analgesics.

Additionally, although the viscera experience pain, the visceral peritoneum (membrane enveloping organs) is not sensitive to cutting. Except in the presence of widespread inflammation or ischemia, it is possible to have extensive disease without pain until the disease progresses enough to involve the parietal peritoneum.

Visceral pain is usually described as deep aching, boring, gnawing, vague burning, or deep grinding as opposed to the sharp, pricking, and knife-like qualities of cutaneous pain. When referred to the somatic regions of the low back, hip, or shoulder, the sensation is vague and poorly localized because visceral afferents provide input over multiple segments of the spinal cord. As mentioned, afferents from different abdominal locations converge on the same dorsal nerve roots, which may be shared with the more precisely developed somatic sensory pathways.

Referred Gastrointestinal Pain Patterns

Sometimes visceral pain from a digestive organ is felt in a location remote from the usual anterior midline presentation. The referred pain site still lies within the dermatomes of the dorsal nerve roots serving the painful viscera. Referred pain is often more intense and localized than typical visceral pain. Afferent nerve impulses transmit pain from the esophagus to the spinal cord by sympathetic nerves from T5 to T10. Integration of the autonomic and somatic systems occurs through the vagus and the phrenic nerves. There can be referred pain from the esophagus to the midback and referred pain from the midback to the esophagus. For example, esophageal dysfunction can present as anterior neck pain or midthoracic spine pain and disk disease of the midthoracic spine can masquerade as esophageal pain.

Client history and the presence or absence of associated signs and symptoms will help guide the therapist. For example, a client with midback pain from esophageal dysfunction will not likely report numbness and tingling in the upper extremities or bowel and bladder changes such as you might see with disk disease. Likewise, disk involvement with referred pain to the esophagus will not cause melena or symptoms associated with meals.

Visceral afferent nerves from the liver, respiratory diaphragm, and pericardium are derived from C3 to C5 sympathetics and reach the central nervous system (CNS) via the phrenic nerve (see Fig. 3.3). The visceral pain associated with these structures is referred to the corresponding somatic area (i.e., the shoulder).

Afferent nerves from the gallbladder, stomach, pancreas, and small intestine travel through the celiac plexus (network of ganglia and nerves supplying the abdominal viscera) and the greater splanchnic nerves and enter the spinal cord from T6 to T9. Referred visceral pain from these visceral structures may be perceived in the midback and scapular regions.

Afferent stimuli from the colon, appendix, and pelvic viscera enter the 10th and 11th thoracic segments through the mesenteric plexus and lesser splanchnic nerves. Finally, the sigmoid colon, rectum, ureters, and testes are innervated by fibers that reach T11 to L1 segments through the lower splanchnic nerve and through the pelvic splanchnic nerves from S2 to S4. Referred pain may be perceived in the pelvis, flank, low back, or sacrum (Case Example 9.1).

Hyperesthesia (excessive sensibility to sensory stimuli) of skin and hyperalgesia (excessive sensibility to painful stimuli) of muscle may develop in the referred pain distribution. As mentioned in Chapter 3, in the early stage of visceral disease, sympathetic reflexes arising from afferent impulses of the internal viscera can be expressed first as sensory, motor, and/or trophic changes in the skin, subcutaneous tissues, and/or muscles. The client may present with itching, dysesthesia, skin temperature changes, perspiration, or dry skin.

The viscera do not perceive pain, but the sensory side is trying to get the message out that something is wrong by creating sympathetic sudomotor changes. When the afferent visceral pain stimuli are intense enough, discharges at synapses within the spinal cord cause this reflex phenomenon,

---

CASE EXAMPLE 9.1
Colon Cancer

A 66-year-old university professor consulted with a physical therapist after twisting his back as he was taking the garbage out three weeks ago. He reported experiencing ongoing, painful, low back symptoms. The evaluation was consistent with a strain of the right paraspinal muscles with overall diminished lumbar spinal motion consistent with this gentleman's age. Given the reported mechanism of injury and the results of the examination consistent with a musculoskeletal problem, a medical screening examination was not included in the interview. A home exercise program was initiated, including stretching and conditioning components.

When the client did not return for his follow-up appointment, telephone contact was made with his family. The client had been hospitalized after collapsing at work. A medical diagnosis of colon cancer was determined. The family reported he had been experiencing digestive difficulties "off and on" and low back pain for the past 3 years, always alternately and never simultaneously. The client died 6 weeks later.

In this case the only red flag suggesting the need for medical screening was the client's age. However, the therapist did not ask about any associated signs and symptoms. We must always remember that even with a known and plausible reason for the injury, the client may wrongfully attribute symptoms to a logical event or occurrence. This man had been experiencing both abdominal symptoms and referred back pain, but because these episodes did not occur at the same time, he did not see a connection between them.

Always finish every interview with the question: "Are you having any other symptoms of any kind anywhere else in your body?"

---

usually transmitted by peripheral nerves of the same spinal segment(s). Thus the sudomotor changes occur as an automatic reflex along the distribution of the somatic nerve.

Remember from the discussion of viscerogenic pain patterns in Chapter 3 that any structure touching the respiratory diaphragm can refer pain to the shoulder, usually to the ipsilateral shoulder, depending on where the direct pressure occurs. Anyone with upper back or shoulder pain and symptoms should be asked a few general screening questions about the presence of GI symptoms.

Referred pain to the musculoskeletal system can occur alone, without accompanying visceral pain, but usually visceral pain (or other symptoms) precedes the development of referred pain. The therapist will find that the client does not connect the two sets of symptoms or fails to report abdominal pain and GI symptoms when experiencing pain in the shoulder or low back, thinking these are two separate problems. For a more complete discussion of the mechanisms behind viscerogenic referred pain patterns, see Chapter 3.

Most of what has been presented in this text has dealt with the sensory side of the clinical presentation. There can also be motor effects of GI dysfunction. For example, contraction, guarding, and splinting of the rectus abdominis and muscles above the umbilicus can occur with dysfunction of the stomach, gallbladder, liver, pylorus, or respiratory diaphragm.

Impairment of the ileum, jejunum, appendix, cecum, colon, and rectum are more likely to result in muscle spasm of the rectus abdominis below the umbilicus.[15]

At the same time, impairment of these GI structures can cause muscle dysfunction in the back (thoracic and lumbar spine) with loss of motion of the involved spinal segments. The clinical picture is one that is easily confused with the primary pathology of the spinal segment.[15] Once again, the history and associated signs and symptoms help the therapist sort through the clinical presentation to reach a differential diagnosis. A thorough screening process is essential in such cases.

Dysphagia

Dysphagia (difficulty swallowing) is the sensation of food catching or sticking in the esophagus. This sensation may occur (initially) just with coarse, dry foods and may eventually progress to include anything swallowed, even thin liquids and saliva. Dysphagia may be caused by achalasia, a process by which the circular and longitudinal muscular fibers of the lower esophageal sphincter fail to relax, producing an esophageal obstruction.[16]

Other possible GI causes of dysphagia include peptic esophagitis (inflammation of the esophagus) with stricture (narrowing), gastroesophageal reflux disease (GERD), and neoplasm (Case Example 9.2). Dysphagia may be a symptom of many other disorders unrelated to GI disease (e.g., stroke, Alzheimer's disease, Parkinson's disease). Certain types of drugs[17], including antidepressants, antisychotics,[18] antihypertensives, and asthma drugs[19] can make swallowing difficult.[20]

The presence of dysphagia requires prompt attention by the physician. Medical intervention is based on a subsequent endoscopic examination.

Odynophagia

Odynophagia, or pain during swallowing, can be caused by esophagitis or esophageal spasm. Esophagitis may occur secondary to GERD, the herpes simplex virus, or fungus caused by prolonged use of strong antibiotics.[21] Pain after eating may occur with esophagitis or may be associated with coronary ischemia[22].

To differentiate esophagitis from coronary ischemia: *upright positioning relieves esophagitis pain*, whereas *cardiac pain* is relieved by nitroglycerin or by supine positioning. Both conditions require medical attention.

Gastrointestinal Bleeding

Occult (hidden) GI bleeding can appear as midthoracic back pain with radiation to the right upper quadrant. Bleeding may not be obvious; serial hemoccult tests and laboratory tests (checking for anemia and iron deficiency) are needed. Ask about the presence of other signs such as blood in the client's vomit or stools (Box 9.1). *Coffee-ground emesis* (vomit) may indicate a perforated peptic or duodenal ulcer. A physician should evaluate any type of bleeding.

Bloody diarrhea may accompany other signs of ulcerative colitis (UC). Diarrhea and UC are discussed in greater depth separately in this chapter. *Bright red blood* usually represents pathology close to the rectum or anus and may be an indication of rectal fissures or hemorrhoids, but can also occur as a result of colorectal cancer.

Melena, or black, tarry stool, occurs as a result of large quantities of blood in the stool. When asked about changes in bowel function, clients may describe black, tarry stools that have an unusual, noxious odor. The odor is caused by the presence of blood, and the black color arises as the digestive acids in the bowel oxidize red blood cells (e.g., bleeding esophageal varices, stomach or duodenal ulceration). Melena is very sticky and does not clean well.

It may be necessary to ask about bowel smears on the undergarments or difficulty getting wiped clean after a bowel movement. The following series may guide the therapist in this area:

❓ FOLLOW-UP QUESTIONS

I would like to ask a few questions that may not seem related to your shoulder (back, hip, pelvic) pain, but they are very important in finding out what is causing your symptoms.

- Have you noticed any blood in your stools or change in the color or consistency of your bowel movements?
- Do you have any trouble wiping yourself clean after a bowel movement?
- Have you noticed any bowel smears on your underwear later after a bowel movement?

After going through the questions, it may be helpful to leave the conversation open. Perhaps leave the client with this thought:

- If you do not know the answer right now or if you just have not noticed, please feel free to let me and your physician know if you notice any changes.

CASE EXAMPLE 9.2

Esophageal Cancer

An 88-year-old woman with a total knee replacement (TKR) was referred for rehabilitation because of loss of motion, joint swelling, and persistent knee pain. She was accompanied to the clinic for each session by one of her three daughters. Over a period of 2 or 3 weeks, each daughter commented on how much weight the mother had lost. When questioned, the client complained of a loss of appetite and difficulty in swallowing, but she had been evaluated and treated only for her knee pain by the orthopedist. She was encouraged to contact her family doctor for evaluation of these red-flag symptoms and was subsequently diagnosed with esophageal cancer.

BOX 9.1 SIGNS OF GASTROINTESTINAL BLEEDING

Coffee-ground emesis (vomit)
Bloody diarrhea
Bright red blood
Melena (dark, tarry stools)
Reddish or mahogany-colored stools

Esophageal varices are dilated blood vessels, most commonly due to alcoholic cirrhosis of the liver. Blood that would normally be pumped back to the heart must bypass the damaged liver. The blood then "backs up" through the esophagus. Ruptured esophageal varices are an emergent, life-threatening condition. Vascular abnormalities of the stomach causing bleeding may include ulcers.

The therapist should ask the client about the presence of any blood in the stool to determine whether it is melenic (from the upper GI tract; ask about a history of NSAID use) or bright red (from the distal colon or rectum). Bleeding from internal or external hemorrhoids (enlarged veins inside or outside the rectum), rectal fissures, or colorectal carcinoma can cause bright red blood in the stools. Rectal bleeding from anal lesions or fissures can occur in individuals who engage in anal sexual intercourse. A brief sexual history may be indicated in some cases.

Reddish or mahogany-colored stools can occur from eating certain foods, such as beets, or significant amounts of red food coloring but can also represent bleeding in the lower GI/colon. Medications that contain bismuth (e.g., Kaopectate, Pepto-Bismol, Bismatrol, Pink Bismuth) can cause darkened or black stools and the client's tongue may also appear black or "hairy."

Clients who have received pelvic radiation for gynecologic, rectal, or prostate cancers have an increased risk for radiation proctitis, which can cause subsequent (delayed) rectal bleeding episodes. Be sure to ask about a past history of cancer and radiation treatment.

Epigastric Pain with Radiation

Epigastric pain perceived as intense or sharp pain behind the breastbone with radiation to the back may occur secondary to long-standing ulcers. For example, the client may be aware of an ulcer but does not relate the back pain to the ulcer. Close questioning related to GI symptoms can provide the therapist with knowledge of underlying systemic disease processes.

Anyone with epigastric pain accompanied by a burning sensation that begins at the xiphoid process and radiates up toward the neck and throat may be experiencing heartburn. Other common symptoms may include a bitter or sour taste in the back of the throat, abdominal bloating, gas, and general abdominal discomfort. Heartburn is often associated with GERD. It can be confused with angina or heart attack when accompanied by chest pain, cough, and shortness of breath (SOB). A physician must evaluate and diagnose the cause of epigastric pain or heartburn.

A screening interview and evaluation is especially helpful when clients have not sought medical treatment for a long-standing problem. For example, long-standing epigastric back pain will cause the individual to assume postures to reduce symptoms. If sustained for a long time, biomechanical changes in the spine can occur, potentially causing musculoskeletal dysfunction. A good medical history can be a valuable tool in revealing the actual cause of the back pain.

Symptoms Affected by Food

Clients may or may not be able to relate pain to meals. Pain associated with gastric ulcers (located more proximally in the GI tract) may begin within 30 to 90 minutes after eating, whereas pain associated with duodenal or pyloric ulcers (located distally beyond the stomach) may occur 2 to 4 hours after meals (i.e., between meals). Alternatively stated, food may relieve the symptoms of a duodenal ulcer but will not likely relieve the pain of a gastric ulcer.

The client with a duodenal ulcer or cancer-related pain may report pain during the night between midnight and 3:00 AM. Ulcer pain may be differentiated from the nocturnal pain associated with cancer by its intensity (7 or higher on a scale of 0 to 10) and duration (constant). More specifically, the gnawing pain of an ulcer may be relieved by eating, but the intense, boring pain associated with cancer is not relieved by any measures.

Ask the client with nighttime shoulder, neck, or back pain to eat something and assess the effect of food on these symptoms. Anyone whose musculoskeletal pain is altered (increased or decreased) or eliminated by food should be screened more thoroughly and referred for further medical evaluation when appropriate. Anyone with a previous history of cancer and nighttime pain must also be evaluated more closely. This is true even if eating has no effect on the client's symptoms.

Early Satiety

Early satiety occurs when the client feels hungry, takes one or two bites of food, and feels full. The sensation of being full is out of proportion with the time of the previous meal and the initial degree of hunger experienced. This can be a symptom of obstruction, stomach cancer, gastroparesis (slowing down of stomach emptying),[23] peptic ulcer disease, and other tumors. Vertebral compression fractures can occur from a variety of disorders including osteoporosis and can result in severe spinal deformity. This deformity, along with severe back pain, can cause early satiety resulting in malnutrition.[24]

Constipation

Constipation is defined clinically as being a condition of prolonged retention of fecal content in the GI tract resulting from decreased motility of the colon or difficulty in expelling stool.

The Rome IV Diagnostic criteria for functional constipation defines this condition using several criteria, and must include two of the following examples of which include the following: straining during defecation, hard, lumpy stools; sensation of incomplete evacuation, sensation of anorectal obstruction; manual maneuvers to facilitate defecation; fewer than three defecations per week; loose stools rarely present without laxatives and insufficient criteria for irritable bowel syndrome.[25] Intractable constipation is called *obstipation* and can result in a fecal impaction that must be removed. Back pain may be the overriding symptom of obstipation, especially in older adults who do not have regular bowel movements or who cannot remember if their last bowel movement was several weeks ago (Case Example 9.3).

CASE EXAMPLE 9.3

Obstipation

A 75-year-old Caucasian male was transported from his home to a hospital emergency department with acute onset of shortness of breath (SOB). He was intubated en route by ambulance personnel, secondary to hypoxemia and acute respiratory distress. Family members state that the patient has severe chronic obstructive pulmonary disorder (COPD) and uses continuous supplemental oxygen at home (usually 3 L per minute). The client had no complaints of chest pain leading up to or during the episode.

While in the hospital, the client was hypotensive. Chest x-ray revealed acute pulmonary edema consistent with congestive heart failure (CHF). He was treated with intravenous Lasix. Following removal of the nasogastric (NG) tube, the client began to complain of severe low back pain and was started on Vicodin. Magnetic resonance imaging (MRI) of the lumbar/sacral spine showed multiple levels of lumbar stenosis and facet sclerosis.

Four days post hospital admission, the client's oxygen saturation was 90% on 4 L per minute of supplemental oxygen. The decision was made to transfer the client to a skilled nursing facility (SNF) with orders for activity as tolerated and physical therapy (evaluate and treat accordingly).

Medical Diagnoses	Past Medical History
Acute respiratory failure	Pulmonary asbestosis
Hypoxemia	Hypotension
Congestive heart failure (CHF)	Benign prostatic
Pulmonary edema	hypertrophy (BPH)
COPD	Non-Q myocardial
Chronic low back pain	infarction (MI)
Degenerative joint disease (DJD)	
Spinal stenosis	

Medications

Bactrim (antiinfective)
Ketoconazole (antifungal)
Plavix (coronary artery disease prophylaxis; platelet aggregation inhibitor)
Aspirin (ASA; coronary artery disease prophylaxis)
Magnesium oxide (supplement)
K-Dur (supplement)
Vasotec (antihypertensive; angiotensin-converting enzyme [ACE] inhibitor)
Lasix (loop diuretic; CHF)
Percocet (opiate analgesic; back pain)
Colace (laxative)

Current Complaints

Client reports increased SOB with minor exertion and severe lumbar/sacral pain that has been constant over the last 3 days and appears to be getting worse.

Pain is described as "a dull ache" and is aggravated by movement. Minor relief is obtained through rest and use of pain medication. The client also reported recent lower abdominal discomfort, which he attributed to something he "ate for breakfast."

When asked about elimination patterns, he states that his bowel movements are not regular, but he "must have had one in the hospital." He "urinates frequently," has trouble starting a flow of urine, and does not void completely as a result of an enlarged prostate.

He reports a long history of progressive back pain without traumatic onset, starting in his 40s. His immediate goal is relief of back pain. His "normal" back pain is described as a 4 to 6 on a 0 to 10 scale. His current level of intensity is described as an 8/10 on pain medication.

Review of Systems

General

Oxygen saturation (pulse oximeter) while on 4 L oxygen per minute: 92%
Blood pressure (BP): 110/65 (seated, left arm)
Respiratory rate (RR): 16/minute
Heart rate (HR): 86 bpm (regular taken for 1 full minute)
Body temperature: 99.4° F

Neurologic

History of radicular pain symptoms in both lower extremities (LEs) above the knee but not present at this time
No observable atrophy of LE musculature
Deep tendon reflexes (DTRs): + 1 in bilateral patellar tendon; 0 for bilateral Achilles
Manual muscle test (MMT): Unable to perform as a result of back pain; decreased functional strength observed
Proprioception: Decreased in feet and ankles, bilaterally

Cardiovascular

Mild pitting edema (pedal: feet and ankles bilaterally) with 15- to 20-second rebound
History of claudication with prolonged standing and ambulation

Pulmonary

Diminished breath sounds, especially at bases (auscultation)
Early exertional dyspnea
2-3 pillow orthopnea
Digital clubbing, bilaterally

Gastrointestinal

Lower abdominal pain/discomfort
Constipation

Genitourinary

Frequent urge to urinate
Difficulty starting flow
Decreased urine output

Musculoskeletal

Flexed postural stance (unable to straighten up because of pain)
Mild age-related range of motion (ROM) limitations noted
Muscle guarding and spasm in paravertebral musculature from T4 to L2
Balance, mobility, ambulation assessed and recorded

Evaluation: Although the client's back pain was made worse by movement, the presence of intense pain and constitutional symptoms (low-grade fever) alerted the therapist to a possible systemic or viscerogenic cause of pain. The fact that the client could not remember his last bowel movement combined with

Continued

CASE EXAMPLE 9.3—Cont'd
Obstipation

abdominal pain was of concern. Change in bladder function was also of concern.

Before initiation of physical therapy services, the client was referred back to the attending physician. A brief summary of the client's neuromusculoskeletal impairments was presented, along with a description of the proposed intervention. A simple statement at the end was highlighted:
- Intense back pain accompanied by low-grade fever
- Abdominal pain and no recall of last bowel movement
- Difficulty initiating and maintaining a flow of urine
- Urinary frequency without a sense of void completion

Doctor XXX: These symptoms are outside the scope of physical therapy practice. Would you please evaluate before we begin rehab? Thank you

Outcome
Physician ordered a urine culture, but attempts to obtain a sample were unsuccessful. The physician was unable to insert a straight

catheter, so the resident was sent to the hospital and a suprapubic catheter was inserted. He returned to the SNF 4 days later with the following diagnoses:
- Bladder outlet obstruction
- Urinary tract infection with *Escherichia coli*
- Prostate cancer, probably metastatic
- Obstipation

When the resident returned to the SNF and was seen by physical therapy, there were no complaints of low back pain (beyond his lifetime baseline) and no lower abdominal discomfort. The neurologic deficits previously identified in both lower extremities were absent.

Summary: This is a good case to point out that medical personnel occasionally miss things that a physical therapist can find when conducting a screening examination and a review of systems. Recognizing red flags sent this client back to the physician sooner rather than later and ended needless painful suffering on his part.

(Courtesy of Joseph R. Clemente, DPT, submitted as part of a tDPT requirement), New York, 2003.)

TABLE 9.1	**Causes of Constipation**			
Neurogenic	Muscular	Mechanical	Rectal Lesions	Drugs/Diet
Cortical, voluntary, or involuntary evacuation	Atony (loss of tone)	Bowel obstruction	Thrombosed hemorrhoids	Anesthetic agents (recent general surgery)
Central nervous system lesions	Severe malnutrition	Neoplasm	Perirectal abscess	Antacids (containing aluminum or calcium)
Multiple sclerosis	Metabolic defects	Volvulus (intestinal twisting)		Anticholinergics
Cord tumors	Hypothyroidism	Diverticulitis		Anticonvulsants
Tabes dorsalis	Hypercalcemia	Extra-alimentary tumors		Antidepressants
Spinal cord lesions or tumors	Potassium depletion	Pregnancy		Antihistamines
Parkinson's	Hyperparathyroidism	Colostomy		Antipsychotics
Irritable bowel syndrome	Inactivity; chronic back pain			Barium sulfate
Dementia				Cancer chemotherapy (e.g., Oncovin)
				Iron compounds
				Diuretics
				Narcotics
				Lack of dietary bulk
				Renal failure (caused by fluid restriction, phosphate binders)
				Myocardial infarction (narcotics for pain control)

Keep in mind the individual who has low back pain with constipation could also be manifesting symptoms of pelvic floor muscle overactivity or spasm. In such cases, pelvic floor assessment should be a part of the screening examination. Consultation with a physical therapist skilled in this area should be considered if the primary care therapist is unable to perform this examination.

Changes in bowel habit may be a response to many other factors such as diet (decreased fluid and bulk intake), smoking, side effects of medication (especially constipation associated with opioids), acute or chronic diseases of the digestive system, extra-abdominal diseases, personality, mood (depression), emotional stress, inactivity, prolonged bed rest, and lack of exercise (Table 9.1). Commonly

implicated medications include narcotics, aluminum- or calcium-containing antacids (e.g., Tums, Rolaids), anticholinergics, tricyclic antidepressants, phenothiazines, calcium channel blockers, and iron salts.

Diets that are high in refined sugars and low in fiber discourage bowel activity. Transit time of the alimentary bolus from the mouth to the anus is influenced mainly by dietary fiber and is decreased with increased fiber intake. Additionally, motility can be decreased by emotional stress that has been correlated with personality. Constipation associated with severe depression can be improved by exercise.

People with low back pain may develop constipation as a result of muscle guarding and splinting that causes reduced bowel motility. Pressure on sacral nerves from stored fecal content may cause an *aching discomfort in the sacrum, buttocks, or thighs* (Case Example 9.4).

Because there are many specific organic causes of constipation, it is a symptom that may require further medical evaluation. It is considered a red-flag symptom when clients with unexplained constipation have sudden and unaccountable changes in bowel habits or blood in the stools.

Diarrhea

Diarrhea is defined as an abnormal increase in stool frequency and liquidity. This may be accompanied by urgency, perianal discomfort, and fecal incontinence. The causes of diarrhea vary widely from one person to another, but food, alcohol, use of laxatives and other drugs, medication side effects, and travel may contribute to the development of diarrhea (Table 9.2).

Acute diarrhea, especially when associated with fever, cramps, and blood or pus in the stool, can accompany invasive enteric infection. Chronic diarrhea associated with weight loss is more likely to indicate neoplastic or inflammatory bowel disease (IBD). Extraintestinal manifestations such as arthritis or skin or eye lesions are often present in IBD. Any of these combinations of symptoms must be reported to the physician.

Drug-induced diarrhea is associated most commonly with antibiotics. Diarrhea may occur as a direct result of antibiotic use and the GI symptom resolves when the drug is discontinued. Symptoms may also develop 6 to 8 weeks after first ingestion of an antibiotic. A more serious antibiotic-induced colitis with severe diarrhea is caused by *Clostridium difficile*[26,27]

This anaerobic bacterium colonizes the colon of 5% of healthy adults and over 20% of hospitalized patients. Clients receiving enteral (tube) feedings are at higher risk for acquisition of *C. difficile* and associated severe diarrhea. *C. difficile* is the major cause of diarrhea in patients hospitalized for more than 3 days. It is spread in an oral-fecal manner and is readily transmitted from patient to patient by hospital personnel. Fastidious handwashing, use of gloves, and extremely careful

---

CASE EXAMPLE 9.4

Constipated Biker with Leg Pain

A 29-year-old male presented in the physical therapy clinic with inner thigh pain of the left leg of unknown cause over the last 3 weeks. The pain occurred most often when he had a bowel movement. He was training for an iron man competition (swimming, biking, running) but did not have any known injury or accident to attribute the symptom to.

When asked if there were any other symptoms anywhere else in his body, the client reported an inability to get an erection and a tendency toward constipation with hard stools. The therapist could find no clinical signs of muscle weakness, atrophy, or dysfunction. Postural alignment was symmetrical and without apparent problems. All provocation tests for hip, spine, sacrum, sacroiliac (SI), and pelvis were negative. The client could complete a full squat without difficulty. Hop test and heel strike were both negative.

The client was screened for signs and symptoms associated with other possible causes of erectile dysfunction such as diabetes, past history of testicular or prostate problems, past history of cancer, and possible sexual abuse. No red-flag history or red-flag signs and symptoms were found. Visual inspection of the lower half of the body revealed no signs of vascular compromise. The client denied any bladder problems or urinary incontinence.

Knowing that the pudendal nerve is responsible for penile erection, the therapist asked to see the client on his bicycle. Pressure on the nerve from a poorly constructed and minimally padded seat was a possible cause. The client was advised to change bike seats, change the seat height and tilt, and reassess symptoms in 2 weeks.

The client was also encouraged to stand up intermittently to relieve perineal pressure.

Result: The client reported complete cessation of all symptoms with the purchase of a bicycle seat with a cut-away middle. Because the obturator nerve passes below the symphysis pubis, it is likely that the bicycle seat compression on the nerve contributed to the inner thigh pain as well.

Bicycle seat neuropathy is not uncommon among long-distance bikers and results from the cyclist supporting their body weight on a narrow seat. Vascular and/or neurologic compromise of the pudendal nerve is the most likely explanation for these symptoms.[106–108]

TABLE 9.2	Causes of Diarrhea			
Malabsorption	**Neuromuscular**	**Mechanical**	**Infectious**	**Nonspecific**
Pancreatitis	Irritable bowel	Incomplete obstruction	Viral	Ulcerative colitis
Pancreatic	syndrome	Neoplasm	Bacterial	Diverticulitis
carcinoma	Diabetic enteropathy	Adhesions	Parasitic	Diet
Crohn's disease	Hyperthyroidism	Stenosis	Protozoal	Laxative abuse
	Caffeine	Fecal impaction	*(Giardia)*	Food allergy
		Muscular incompetency		Antibiotics (*Clostridium difficile*)
		Postsurgical effect (ileal		Creatine use
		bypass)		Cancer chemotherapy (e.g., Fluorouracil)
				Lactose (milk) intolerance
				Psychogenic (nervous tension)

cleaning of the bathroom, bed linens, and associated items are helpful in decreasing transmission.[28]

Athletes using creatine supplements to enhance power and strength in performance may experience minor GI symptoms such as diarrhea, stomach upset, and belching.[29] Therapists working with athletes should keep this in mind when hearing reports of GI distress. Many sports players do not even know how much creatine they are taking or are taking more than the recommended dose.

For the client describing chronic diarrhea, it may be necessary to probe further about the use of laxatives as a possible contributor to this condition. Laxative abuse contributes to the production of diarrhea and begins a vicious cycle as chronic laxative users experience excessive secretion of aldosterone and resultant edema when they attempt to stop using them. This edema and increased weight forces the person to continue to rely on laxatives[30]. The abuse of laxatives is common in individuals with eating disorders (e.g. anorexia, bulimia), and in the elderly, especially those in institutional facilities.[31]

Questions about laxative use can be asked tactfully during the Core Interview when asking about medications, including over-the-counter (OTC) drugs. Encourage the client to discuss bowel management without drugs at the next appointment with the physician.

Fecal Incontinence

Fecal incontinence may be described as an inability to control evacuation of stool and is associated with a sense of urgency, diarrhea, and abdominal cramping. It has been reported that about 1 in 12 adults in the United States have fecal incontinence.[32] Causes include partial obstruction of the rectum (cancer), colitis, and radiation therapy, especially in the case of women treated for cervical or uterine cancer. The radiation may cause trauma to the rectum, resulting in incontinence and diarrhea. Anal distortion secondary to traumatic childbirth, hemorrhoids, and hemorrhoidal surgery may also cause fecal incontinence.

Arthralgia

The relationship between "gut" inflammation and joint inflammation is well known but not fully understood. Many inflammatory GI conditions have an arthritic component affecting the joints. For example, IBD (UC and Crohn's disease [CD]) is often accompanied by rheumatic manifestations. There is a high occurrent of inflammatory bowel disease and subclinical gut inflammation in patients with spondyloarthritis[33].

It is hypothesized that an antigen crosses the gut mucosa and enters the joint, which sets up an immunologic response. Arthralgia with synovitis and immune-mediated joint disease may occur as a result of this immunologic response.[34] Joint arthralgia associated with GI infection is usually asymmetric, migratory, and oligoarticular (affecting only one or two joints). This type of joint involvement is termed *reactive arthritis* when triggered by microbial infection such as *C.*

difficile from the GI (and sometimes genitourinary or respiratory) tract. Other accompanying symptoms may include fever, malaise, skin rash or other skin lesions, nail bed changes (nails separate from the nail beds and become thin and discolored), iritis, or conjunctivitis.

The bowel and joint symptoms may or may not occur at the same time. Usually, this type of arthralgia is preceded by 1 to 3 weeks of diarrhea, urethritis, regional enteritis (CD), or other bacterial infection. The larger joints of the arms and legs are more frequently involved.[35]

A large knee effusion is a common presentation, but some clients have joint pain with minimal or no signs of inflammation. Muscle atrophy occurs when a chronic condition is present; in which case, there will be a history of previous GI and joint involvement. Stiffness, pain, tenderness, and reduced range of motion may be present, but with proper medical intervention, there is no permanent deformity.

Spondylitis with sacroiliitis may present as low back pain and morning stiffness that improves with activity and restriction of chest and spinal movement. Radiographic findings are consistent with those of classic ankylosing spondylitis with bilateral SI joint involvement and bony erosion and sclerosis of the symphysis pubis, ischial tuberosities, and iliac crests. Ultimately, "bamboo spine" will result.

Inflammation involving the sites of bony insertion of tendons and ligaments termed *enthesitis* is a classic sign of reactive arthritis.[36] Tendon sheaths and bursae may also become inflamed. Ligaments along the spine and SI joints and around the ankle and midfoot may also show evidence of inflammation.

Heel pain is a frequent complaint, with swelling and tenderness located either posteriorly at the Achilles tendon insertion site, or inferiorly where the plantar fascia attaches to the calcaneus. Plantar fasciitis is common.[37] For a more complete discussion of joint pain and how to evaluate joint pain, see Chapter 3. A list of screening questions for joint pain is also reproduced in the Appendix

in the accompanying enhanced eBook version included with print purchase of this textbook as a quick reference in clinical practice.

Shoulder Pain

Pain in the left shoulder (Kehr's sign: pain with pressure placed on the upper abdomen[38]; Danforth sign: shoulder pain with inspiration) can occur as a result of free air following laparoscopic surgery or blood in the abdominal cavity, usually from a ruptured spleen or retroperitoneal bleeding causing distention. Retroperitoneum refers to a position external or posterior to the peritoneum, the serous membrane lining the abdominopelvic walls. Retroperitoneal organs refer to viscera that lie against the posterior body wall and are covered by peritoneum on the anterior surface only (e.g., thoracic portion of the esophagus, pancreas, duodenal cap, ascending and descending colon, rectum).

The screening interview may help the client recall any precipitating trauma or injury such as a sharp blow during an athletic event, a fall, or perhaps even a minor automobile accident causing pressure from the steering wheel. The client may not connect these seemingly unrelated events with the present shoulder pain.

Perforated duodenal or gastric ulcers can leak gastric juices to the posterior wall of the stomach and irritate the diaphragm, referring pain to the shoulder; although the stomach is on the left side of the body, the referral pattern is usually to the right shoulder.

A ruptured ectopic pregnancy with retroperitoneal bleeding into the abdominal cavity can also present as lower abdominal and/or shoulder pain. Usually there is a history of sexual activity and missed menses in a woman of reproductive age.

Pancreatic cancer can refer pain to the shoulder and is often missed as the cause. Fluid in the pleural space as a result of pancreatitis can present as shoulder pain. When the head of the pancreas is involved, the client could have right shoulder pain, but more often it manifests as midback or midthoracic pain sometimes lateralized from the spine on either side. When the tail of the pancreas is diseased, pain can be referred to the left shoulder (see Fig. 3.4). Pain may also occur in the right shoulder when blood is present in the abdominal cavity as a result of liver trauma (Case Example 9.5). Accumulation of blood in this area from a slow bleed of the spleen, liver, or stomach can produce bilateral shoulder pain.

Obturator or Psoas Abscess

Abscess of the obturator or psoas muscle is a possible cause of lower abdominal pain, usually the consequence of spread of inflammation or infection from an adjacent structure. Because these muscles lie behind abdominal structures with no protective barrier, any infectious or inflammatory process affecting the abdominal or pelvic cavity can cause an obturator or psoas abscess (Figs. 9.4 and 9.5).

CASE EXAMPLE 9.5
Ruptured Spleen

A 23-year-old soccer player sustained a blow to the side as he was moving down the soccer field. He fell on his left side with the full force of his own body weight and the weight of the other player on top of him. He reported having "the wind knocked out of me" and sat out on the sideline for 20 minutes. He resumed playing and completed the game. The next morning, he awoke with severe left shoulder pain and stopped by the office of a physical therapist located in the same building as his office. The examination was unremarkable for shoulder movement dysfunction, which was inconsistent with the client's complaint of "constant pain." The client was treated symptomatically.

He made a follow-up appointment with the therapist for the next day, but before noon, he collapsed at work and was taken to a hospital emergency department. A diagnosis of ruptured spleen was made during emergency surgery. A ruptured spleen would have sent the typical adult for medical care much sooner, but this client was in excellent physical condition with a high tolerance for pain.

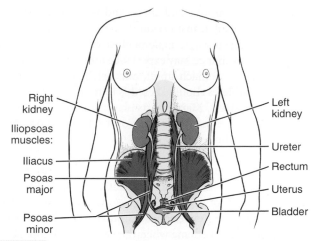

Fig. 9.4 The iliopsoas muscle is not separated from the abdominal or pelvic cavity. As this illustration shows, most of the viscera in the abdominal and pelvic cavities can come in contact with the iliopsoas muscle. Any infectious or inflammatory process present in either of these cavities can seed itself to the psoas muscle by direct extension.

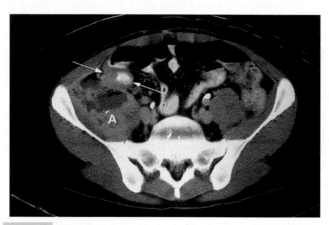

Fig. 9.5 Abscess secondary to Crohn's disease. CT scan shows a right psoas muscle abscess (*A*) containing fluid and gas adjacent to a thick-walled small-bowel loop *(arrows)*. (From Haaga JR, Lanzieri CF, Gilkeson RC, eds: *CT and MR. Imaging of the whole body*, ed 4, St Louis, 2003, Mosby.)

Psoas abscesses most commonly result from direct extension of intraabdominal infections such as diverticulitis, CD,[39] pelvic inflammatory disease (PID), appendicitis, and colorectal carcinoma (see also the discussion on McBurney's point later in this chapter under Appendicitis).[25,40] Kidney infection or abscess can also cause psoas abscess. *Staphylococcus aureus* (staph infection) is the most common cause of psoas abscess secondary to vertebral osteomyelitis.

Peritonitis, as a result of any infectious or inflammatory process, can result in psoas abscess. Besides the diseases and conditions mentioned here, peritonitis can occur as a surgical complication. Look for a history of abdominal surgery of any kind, especially the anterior approach to spinal surgery for disk removal, spinal fusion, and insertion of a cage or artificial disk implant.[41]

Regardless of the etiology, the abscess is usually confined to the psoas fascia but can spread to the hip, upper thigh, or buttock. The iliacus muscle in the iliac fossa joins with the lower portion of the psoas muscle. Osteomyelitis of the ilium or septic arthritis of the SI joint can penetrate the muscle sheath of either muscle, producing an abscess of either the iliacus or psoas portion of the muscle.[42]

In addition, abscesses of the pelvis, retroperitoneal area, and abdomen can spread bacteria or fungi to local vertebral areas, causing spinal infections such as pyogenic vertebral osteomyelitis. Clinical manifestations of a psoas or iliacus abscess include fever; night sweats; lower abdominal, pelvic, or back pain; or pain referred to the hip, medial thigh or groin (femoral triangle area), or knee. The right side is affected most often when associated with appendicitis. Both sides can be involved with generalized peritonitis, but usually that person has a clear systemic presentation and seeks medical evaluation. It is the unusual cases that a therapist will see, making it necessary to know both the typical and atypical pain patterns associated with systemic disease.

Antalgic gait may develop with a psoas abscess secondary to a reflex spasm pulling the leg into internal rotation and causing a functional hip flexion contracture. The affected individual may have pain with hip extension. Often a tender mass can be palpated in the groin. The therapist must assess for dysfunction of the iliopsoas muscle, as a psoas minor syndrome can be mistaken for appendicitis

Four tests can be performed to assess the possibility of systemic origin of painful hip or thigh symptoms (Box 9.2). Gently pick up the client's leg on the involved side and tap the heel. A painful expression and report of right lower quadrant pain may accompany peritoneal inflammation. If the client is willing and able, have him or her hop on one leg. The person with an inflamed peritoneum will clutch that side and be unable to complete the movement. The *iliopsoas muscle test* (Fig. 9.6) is performed when acute abdominal pain is a possible cause of hip or thigh pain. When an abscess forms on the iliopsoas muscle from an inflamed or perforated appendix or inflamed peritoneum, the iliopsoas muscle test causes pain felt in the right lower abdominal quadrant. (Pain and tenderness in the lower left side of the abdomen and pelvis may be caused by bowel perforation associated with diverticulitis, constipation, or obstipation [impaction] of the sigmoid, or appendicitis when the appendix is located on the left side of the midline.)

Alternately, the client lies on the pain-free side, and the therapist gently hyperextends the involved leg to stretch the psoas major muscle. Additionally, palpate the iliopsoas

muscle by placing the client in a supine position with hips and knees flexed and fully supported in a 90-degree position (Fig. 9.7). Palpate one third of the distance between the anterior superior iliac spine (ASIS) and the umbilicus. The client is asked to flex the hip gently to assist in isolating the iliopsoas muscle. Muscular tightness in the iliopsoas may

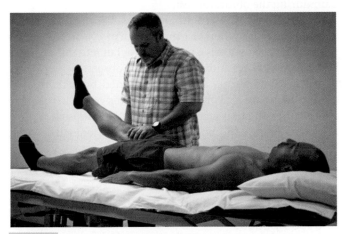

Fig. 9.6 Iliopsoas muscle test. In the supine position, have the client actively perform a straight leg raise; apply resistance to the distal thigh as the client tries to hold the leg up. Alternately, ask the client to turn onto his or her side. Extend the person's uppermost leg at the hip. Increased abdominal, flank, or pelvic pain on either maneuver constitutes a positive sign, suggesting irritation of the psoas muscle by an inflamed appendix or peritoneum. Only a handful of studies have been done to validate the accuracy of this test for appendicitis/peritonitis. One systematic review reported sensitivity value at 0.16 and specificity as 0.95 with a positive likelihood ratio (LR +) of 2.38 (reported range: 1.21-4.67) and negative likelihood range (LR−) of 0.90 (range: 0.83-0.98).[105]

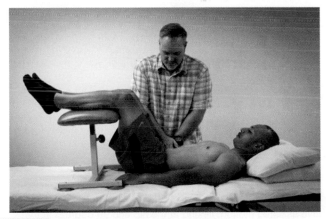

Fig. 9.7 Palpating the iliopsoas muscle. Place the client in a supine position with the hips and knees both flexed and supported at a 90-degree angle. Slowly press fingers into abdomen approximately one third the distance from the anterior superior iliac spine (ASIS) toward the umbilicus. It may be necessary to ask the client to initiate slight hip flexion to help isolate the muscle and avoid palpating the bowel. Reproducing or causing lower quadrant, pelvic, or abdominal pain is considered a positive sign for iliopsoas abscess. Palpation may produce back pain or local muscular pain from shortened or contracted muscle.

BOX 9.2 SCREENING TESTS FOR PSOAS ABSCESS

- Heel tap
- Hop test
- Iliopsoas muscle test
- Palpate iliopsoas muscle

result in radiating pain to the low back region during palpation, whereas inflammation or abscess will bring on painful symptoms in the right (or left depending on the underlying pathology) lower abdominal quadrant.

The *obturator muscle test* (Fig. 9.8) is also performed when the appendix could be the cause of referred pain to the hip. A perforated appendix or inflamed peritoneum can irritate the obturator muscle, producing right lower quadrant abdominal pain during the obturator test.

Although uncommon, psoas abscess still can be confused with a hernia. The therapist may perform evaluative tests to screen for a psoas abscess, but the physician must differentiate between an abscess and a hernia. Psoas abscess is often softer than a femoral hernia and has ill-defined borders, in contrast to the more sharply defined margins of the hernia. The major differentiating feature is the fact that a psoas abscess lies lateral to the femoral artery, whereas the femoral hernia is located medial to the femoral artery.[43]

CLINICAL SIGNS AND SYMPTOMS
Psoas Abscess

- Fever ("hectic" fever pattern: up and down)
- Night sweats
- Abdominal pain
- Loss of appetite or other GI upset
- Back, pelvic, abdominal, hip, and/or knee pain
- Antalgic gait
- Palpable, tender mass

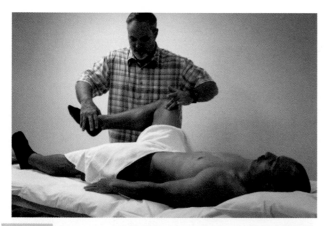

Fig. 9.8 Obturator muscle test. In the supine position, perform active assisted motion, flexing at the hip and 90 degrees at the knee. Hold the ankle and rotate the leg internally to stretch the obturator muscle. A negative or normal response is no pain. A positive test for muscle affected by peritoneal infection or inflammation from a perforated appendix reproduces right lower quadrant abdominal or pelvic pain with irritation of the muscle. Although the obturator test has not been studied independently of the psoas test, this sign is assumed to have a sensitivity and specificity similar to the psoas sign. Further research is needed to verify this as a valid and reliable evidence-based test for appendicitis/peritonitis.

Neuropathy

Vitamin B_{12} deficiency following bariatric surgery may cause symptoms of numbness and weakness of the lower extremities.[44] Additional neurological symptoms following vitamin B_{12} deficiency include symmetric paresthesias and ataxia associated with loss of vibration and position sense.

Other symptoms can include irritability, memory loss, and dementia. Besides neuropathy, presentation may include confusion, nystagmus, seizures, unsteady gait and ataxia, hearing loss, and lower limb hypotonia.[45,46] Symptoms may resolve with medical treatment.

GASTROINTESTINAL DISORDERS
Gastroesophageal Reflux Disease

Gastroesophageal Reflux Disease (GERD) is an array of problems related to the backward movement of stomach acids and other stomach contents, such as pepsin and bile, into the esophagus, a phenomenon called *acid reflux*. Normally, some gastric contents move or reflux from the stomach into the esophagus, but in GERD, the process becomes pathologic, producing symptoms that point to tissue injury in the esophagus and sometimes the respiratory tract.[47] About 10% to 20% of U.S. adults have GERD with males and females being equally affected.[41]

Clinical Signs and Symptoms

Symptoms can include heartburn, chest pain, dysphagia, and a sense of a lump in the throat. Symptoms are sometimes mistaken for a heart attack. Less frequent symptoms can include wheezing, hoarseness, coughing, earache, sore throat, and difficulty swallowing. Sleep disturbance from nighttime coughing and heartburn can lead to fatigue and decreased daytime functioning. Complications of GERD may range from discomfort to severe strictures of the esophagus, esophagitis, aspiration pneumonia, and asthma.

Other serious consequences can be related to weight loss, GI blood loss, and Barrett's esophagus, a precancerous condition. The relationship between GERD and asthma is poorly understood but is thought to be a consequence of aspiration of gastric acid contents into the lung, causing bronchospasm.

Watch for frequent, forceful spitting up or vomiting, accompanied by irritability. Other alarm symptoms include respiratory distress, apnea, dysphagia, or failure to thrive. Watch for change in color, change in muscle tone, or choking and gagging.

Children may experience GERD in the same way adults do with abdominal or epigastric pain. Nighttime coughing, vomiting, and/or nausea are also possible. Neurologically impaired children and adults are at increased risk for reflux with aspiration. Fluid enters the upper airways from the esophagus, causing chronic respiratory problems, including recurrent pneumonia.

GERD should be treated in order to prevent a chronic condition from occurring with more serious consequences. Symptoms may be mild at first, but have a cumulative effect with increasing symptoms after the age of 40. Chronic GERD is a major risk factor for adenocarcinoma, an increasingly common cancer in white males in the United States.

Medical referral is advised for anyone who reports signs and symptoms of GERD. Some clients may need surgical treatment, now available with less invasive endoscopic techniques, but most can be treated with some simple changes in eating patterns, positioning, and medications. Drug treatment includes antacids, H$_2$-receptor blockers, and proton pump inhibitors (PPIs). Antacids, such as Mylanta, Maalox, Tums, and Rolaids, are available OTC and do not reduce the acid, but merely neutralize it. H$_2$-receptor blockers, such as Tagamet (cimetidine), Zantac (ranitidine), and Pepcid (famotidine) reduce the amount of stomach acid produced by the stomach and are available OTC.

PPIs, such as omeprazole (Prilosec), lansoprazole (Prevacid), or esomeprazole (Nexium), are the most potent acid-suppressing agents available. These drugs actually inhibit acid formation rather than just neutralize it. The first PPI is now available OTC; others are expected to become available as well. Caution is needed when using PPIs to self-treat without medical supervision. They can mask symptoms of serious GI disorders such as esophageal or stomach cancer. Diagnosis at an early, treatable stage may be delayed with serious implications.

Therapists must listen for client reports of headache, constipation or diarrhea, abdominal pain, or dizziness in anyone taking these medications. The client should be advised to notify his or her medical doctor with a report of these side effects.

CLINICAL SIGNS AND SYMPTOMS
Gastroesophageal Reflux Disease

Typical Symptoms
- Heartburn
- Regurgitation with bitter taste in mouth
- Belching

Atypical Symptoms
- Chest pain unrelated to activity
- Sensation of a lump in the throat
- Difficulty swallowing (dysphagia)
- Painful swallowing (odynophagia)
- Wheezing, coughing, hoarseness
- Asthma
- Sore throat, laryngitis
- Weight loss
- Anemia

Peptic Ulcer

Peptic ulcer is a loss of tissue lining the lower esophagus, stomach, and duodenum. Gastric and duodenal ulcers are considered together in this section. Acute lesions that do not extend through the mucosa are called erosions. Chronic ulcers involve the muscular coat, destroying musculature, and replacing it with permanent scar tissue at the site of healing.

Originally, all ulcers in the upper GI tract were believed to be caused by the aggressive action of hydrochloric acid and pepsin on the mucosa. They thus became known as "peptic ulcers," which is actually a misnomer.

It is now known that many of the gastric and duodenal ulcers are caused by infection with *Helicobacter pylori*, a corkscrew-shaped bacterium that bores through the layer of mucus that protects the stomach cavity from stomach acid. Chronic use of NSAIDs such as aspirin, ibuprofen, and naproxen may develop ulcers[48] (Table 9.3).[49,50] Additionally,

TABLE 9.3	Nonsteroidal Antiinflammatory Drugs
Generic	Common Brand Names
OVER-THE-COUNTER	
Aspirin	Anacin, Bayer*, Bufferin*, Ecotrin*, Excedrin*, various generic store brands
Diclofenac (topical cream)	Aspercreme, Voltaren
Ibuprofen	Motrin, Advil, various generic store brands
Magnesium salicylate	DeWitt's pain reliever, Doan's, Percogesic
Naproxen	Aleve, various generic store brands
PRESCRIPTION COX-2 SELECTIVE NSAIDS	
Celecoxib	Celebrex
PRESCRIPTION NONSELECTIVE NSAIDS	
Choline magnesium trisalicylate	Tricosal, Trilisate
Diclofenac	Flector, Cataflam, Voltaren, Cambia
Diflunisal	Dolobid
Etodolac	Lodine, Lodine XL
Fenoprofen	Nalfon
Flurbiprofen	Ansaid
Ibuprofen	None
Indomethacin	Indocin, Indocin SR
Ketoprofen	Oruvail, Orudis
Ketorolac	Toradol, Acular
Meclofenamate	Meclomen
Mefenamic acid	Ponstel
Meloxicam	Mobic
Nabumetone	Relafen
Naproxen	Naprosyn, Anaprox, Anaprox DS
Oxaprozin	Daypro
Piroxicam	Feldene
Salsalate	Salsitab, Salflex, Disalcid
Sulindac	Clinoril
Tolmetin	Tolectin, Tolectin DS

COX, Cyclooxygenase; *NSAIDs*, nonsteroidal antiinflammatory drugs.
Several nonselective (standard) NSAIDs are available over-the-counter (OTC) at lower doses (e.g., 200 mg) and by prescription at higher doses (e.g., 500 mg).
Information in this table was reviewed and updated by the University of Montana College of Health Professions and Biomedical Sciences Drug Information Service 2021 (Jordan Willis, PharmD candidate).
*These products have additives to minimize gastrointestinal (GI) side effects but are known as aspirin products.

26% of users of OTC NSAIDS report taking more than the recommended dose of the medication[51].

H. pylori ulcers are primarily located in the lining of the duodenum (upper portion of the small intestine that connects to the stomach) (Fig. 9.9). NSAID-induced ulcers occur primarily in the lining of the stomach, most frequently on the posterior wall, which can account for shoulder (usually right shoulder; depending on the extent of retroperitoneal bleeding) or back pain as an associated symptom.

Ulcers can be dangerous if left untreated, eroding into the stomach arteries and causing life-threatening bleeding or perforating the stomach and spreading infection. *H. pylori*-induced ulcers can recur after treatment. A past medical history of peptic ulcers in anyone with new onset of back or shoulder pain is a red flag requiring further screening and possible medical referral.

Clinical Signs and Symptoms

The cardinal symptom of peptic ulcer is epigastric pain that may be described as "heartburn" or as burning, gnawing, cramping, or aching located over a small area near the midline in the epigastrium near the xiphoid. Gastric ulcers are found along the distribution of the eighth thoracic nerve, which causes pain in the upper epigastrium about one to two inches to the right of a spot halfway between the xiphoid and the umbilicus (see Fig. 9.16). Duodenal pain tends to present more in the right epigastrium, specifically a localized spot one to two inches above and to the right of the umbilicus because of its innervation by the tenth thoracic nerve.

The pain comes in waves that last several minutes (rather than hours) and may radiate below the costal margins into the back or to the right shoulder. The daily pattern of pain is related to the secretion of acid and the presence of food in the stomach to act as a buffer.

Pain associated with duodenal ulcers is prominent when the stomach is empty such as between meals and in the early morning. The pain may last from minutes to hours and may be relieved by antacids. Gastric ulcers are more likely to cause pain associated with the presence of food. Symptoms often appear for 3 or 4 days or weeks and then subside, reappearing weeks or months later.

Other symptoms of uncomplicated peptic ulcer include nausea, vomiting, loss of appetite, sometimes weight loss, and occasionally back pain. In duodenal ulcers, steady pain near the midline of the back (see Fig. 9.16) between T6 and T10 with radiation to the right upper quadrant may indicate perforation of the posterior duodenal wall.

Back pain may be the first and only symptom. Complications of hemorrhage, perforation, and obstruction may lead to additional symptoms that the client does not relate to the back pain. Bleeding may occur when the ulcer erodes through a blood vessel. It may present as vomited bright red blood or coffee-ground vomitus and by dark tarry stools (melena). The bleeding may vary from massive hemorrhage to occult (hidden) bleeding that occurs over a long period of time.

Symptoms associated with *H. pylori* include halitosis (bad breath)[52] and a form of facial acne called *rosacea*.[53] Rosacea is characterized by a rosy appearance of the cheeks, nose, and chin. Facial flushing, red lines, and bumps over the nose may accompany rosacea.

CLINICAL SIGNS AND SYMPTOMS
Peptic Ulcer

- "Heartburn" or epigastric pain aggravated by food (gastric ulcer); relieved by food, milk, antacids, or vomiting (duodenal ulcer)
- Night pain (12 midnight to 3:00 AM)—same relief as for epigastric pain (duodenal ulcer)
- Radiating back pain
- Stomach pain
- Right shoulder pain
- Light-headedness or fainting
- Nausea
- Vomiting
- Anorexia
- Weight loss
- Bloody stools
- Black, tarry stools

Gastrointestinal Complications of Nonsteroidal Antiinflammatory Drugs

NSAIDs (see Table 9.3) use is widespread because of its analgesic, antiinflammatory, antipyretic, and antithrombotic (platelet-inhibitory) actions. More than 70 million prescriptions are written and 30 billion over-the counter doses of NSAIDs are consumed annually in the United States.[54]

The most commonly taken NSAIDs have few toxic effects. Taking large doses of NSAIDs or using them long term

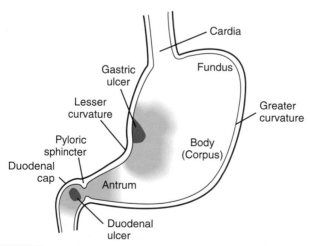

Fig. 9.9 Most common sites for peptic ulcers. Gastric ulcers are found along the distribution on the eighth thoracic nerve with a corresponding pain pattern as described in Fig. 9.15. Pain patterns associated with duodenal ulcers correspond to the tenth thoracic nerve. (Adapted from Ignatavicius DD, Bayne MV: *Medical-surgical nursing*, Philadelphia, 1991, WB Saunders.)

increase the risk of side effects. They can have deleterious effects on the entire GI tract from the esophagus to the colon, with the most obvious clinical effect on the gastroduodenal mucosa, causing subclinical erosions which can progress to ulcerations with life-threatening bleeding and perforation.

People with NSAID-induced GI impairment can be asymptomatic until the condition is advanced. NSAID-induced GI bleeding is a major cause of morbidity and mortality among the aging adult population.[55,56]

For those who are symptomatic, the most common side effects of NSAIDs are stomach upset and pain, possibly leading to ulceration. GI complications of NSAID use include ulcerations, hemorrhage, perforation, stricture formation, and exacerbation of IBD. Each NSAID has its own pharmacodynamic characteristics, and clients' responses to each drug may vary greatly.

Other possible adverse side effects of NSAIDs may include suppression of cartilage repair and synthesis, fluid retention and kidney damage, liver damage, skin reactions (e.g., itching, rashes, acne), and impairment of the nervous system such as headache, depression, confusion or memory loss, mood changes, and ringing in the ears.[54]

Many people diagnosed with painful musculoskeletal conditions, especially arthritis, rely on NSAIDs to relieve pain and improve function. Anyone with a recent history of NSAID use presenting with back or shoulder pain, especially when accompanied by any of the associated signs and symptoms listed for peptic ulcer, must be evaluated by a physician. The therapist should remain alert for the client taking multiple NSAIDs and simultaneously combining prescription and OTC NSAIDs or other drugs.

These drugs are potent renal vasoconstrictors, so look for increased blood pressure and ankle/foot edema. Take vital signs and visually inspect clients at risk for NSAID-induced impairments. Ask about muscle weakness, unusual fatigue, restless legs syndrome, polyuria, nocturia, or pruritus (signs of renal failure). In the aging adult, NSAID use may be associated with confusion and memory loss or increased confusion in the client with dementia or Alzheimer's disease. Teach clients to recognize signs and symptoms of adverse effects from NSAIDs and report any associated signs and symptoms to the physician. Changing the dosage or switching to a different NSAID at the first sign of side effects can help clients avoid serious complications that can occur with prolonged use of an inappropriate dose or poorly tolerated NSAID.

Risk factor assessment is especially important in the primary care setting. Any identified risk factors should serve as red flags in any setting. The most predictive risk factors of serious GI events include age, disability, NSAID use, previous GI hospitalization, prior GI symptoms with NSAIDs, and use of prednisone (Case Example 9.6).

CASE EXAMPLE 9.6

Nonsteroidal Antiinflammatory Drugs

Outpatient Orthopedic Client: A 72-year-old client is status-post (s/p) left total knee replacement (TKR) ×2 weeks. She did not attain 90-degree knee flexion and continues to walk with a stiff leg. Her orthopedic surgeon has sent her to physical therapy for rehab.

Past Medical History: Client reports generalized osteoarthritis. Previous left shoulder replacement 18 months ago. Very slow recovery and still does not have full shoulder range of motion (ROM). Long-standing hearing impairment for 60 years. Lost her left eye to macular degeneration 2 years ago.

Medications: Client reports the following drug use—Aleve for pain; Vioxx daily for arthritis. Also takes Feldene when her shoulder bothers her and daily ibuprofen.

Walks with a Trendelenburg gait and drags left leg using wheeled walker.

Current symptoms include left knee and shoulder pain, intermittent dizziness, sleep disturbance, finger/hand swelling in the afternoon, and early morning nausea.

How do you assess for nonsteroidal antiinflammatory drug (NSAID) complications?

Review risk factors:
>65 years old
Shoulder pain
Ask about tobacco and alcohol use
Nausea … ask about other gastrointestinal (GI) symptoms and previous history of peptic ulcer disease
Take blood pressure
Observe for peripheral edema (sacral and pedal)

How do you carry out a Review of Systems from a screening perspective and a Systems Review?

After gathering all of the subjective and objective data, make a list of all the signs and symptoms. Are there any clusters or groups of signs and symptoms that fall into any particular category? These may or may not be associated with the primary neuromusculoskeletal problem as many clients have one or more other diseases, illnesses, or conditions (referred to as comorbidities) with additional clinical manifestations.

Start with general health. Client reports:

Hearing and vision loss
Intermittent dizziness
Early morning nausea
Finger/hand swelling
Sleep disturbance

There is not much in the report about her general health. Make a note to consider asking a few more questions about her past and current general health. Ask how she would describe her overall health in one or two words.

Review her medications. She reports:

Aleve for pain
Vioxx daily (cyclooxygenase-2 [COX-2] NSAID)
Feldene prn (standard or nonselective NSAID)
Ibuprofen daily (standard or nonselective NSAID)

Given how many forms of NSAIDs she is taking, ask yourself: Did I ask if there were any other symptoms or problems of any kind anywhere else in the body?

CASE EXAMPLE 9.6—Cont'd

Nonsteroidal Antiinflammatory Drugs

The remaining symptoms noted (positive Trendelenburg gait and antalgic gait, left shoulder and knee pain) fall into the musculoskeletal category. No other symptoms are noted.

Knowing what we do about the potential for GI and renal complications in some clients taking NSAIDs, make a mental note to ask about the presence of previously unreported GI or renal signs and symptoms (see discussion of Clinical Signs and Symptoms of NSAID-Induced Disease). If appropriate you can go through this list and ask:

Do you have any nausea? Stomach pain? Indigestion or heartburn?

Have you had any skin changes? You may want to prompt with: itching? Rash anywhere on your body?

Any ringing in the ears? Headaches? Depression or mood changes? Memory loss or confusion?

Have you had any trouble getting up out of a chair or bed? Difficulty with stairs? (muscle weakness) Shortness of breath? Unusual fatigue?

Are you urinating more often during the day? Getting up at night to empty your bladder? Do you have any trouble wiping yourself clean after a bowel movement? Any change in the color or smell of your stools?

Documentation, communication, and medical referral will be based on the results of your evaluation using a review mechanism like the one we just completed.

Diverticular Disease

The terms *diverticulosis* and *diverticulitis* have distinct meanings and should not be used interchangeably. *Diverticulosis* is a benign condition in which the mucosa (lining) of the colon balloons out through weakened areas in the wall. Up to 58% of people over age 60- have these sac-like protrusions.[57] Someone with diverticulosis is typically asymptomatic; the diverticula are diagnosed when screening for colon cancer or other problems.[58]

About 15% to 20% of patients with diverticulosis develop symptomatic diverticular disease.[59] *Diverticulitis* describes the infection and inflammation that accompany a microperforation of one of the diverticula. Perforation and subsequent infection result in left lower abdominal or pelvic pain and tenderness. For the therapist performing the iliopsoas and obturator tests, abdominal pain in the left lower quadrant may be caused by diverticular disease and should be reported to the physician. The diagnosis of diverticulitis is confirmed by accompanying fever, bloody stools, elevated white blood cell count, and imaging studies.

CLINICAL SIGNS AND SYMPTOMS

Diverticulitis

- Generalized abdominal pain often with loss of appetite, nausea, abdominal bloating
- Left lower quadrant pain (present in 70% of patients); [60]possible positive pinch-an-inch test (see Fig. 9.12)
- Right lower abdominal pain (especially of people of Asian descent)[61]
- Decreased or absent bowel sounds; palpable abdominal mass
- Flatulence (passing gas)
- Bloody stools
- Constipation or irregular bowel movements; diarrhea is less common[62]
- Fever Nausea and vomiting

Appendicitis

Appendicitis is an inflammation of the vermiform appendix that occurs most commonly in adolescents and young adults. It is a serious disease usually requiring surgery. When the appendix becomes obstructed, inflamed, and infected, rupture may occur, leading to peritonitis.

Differential diagnoses for appendicitis include, but are not limited to, the following: CD (regional enteritis), abdominal abscesses, gallbladder attacks, and kidney infections on the right side, and for women, ectopic pregnancy, ovarian cyst or torsion, and cystitis.[63]

Clinical Signs and Symptoms

The classic symptoms of appendicitis are pain preceding nausea and vomiting and low-grade fever in adults. Children tend to have higher fevers. Other symptoms may include coated tongue and bad breath.

The pain usually begins in the umbilical region and eventually localizes in the right lower quadrant of the abdomen over the site of the appendix. In retrocecal appendicitis, the pain may be referred to the thigh or right testicle (see Fig. 9.11). Groin and/or testicular pain may be the only symptoms of appendicitis, especially in young, healthy, male athletes. The pain comes in waves, becomes steady, and is aggravated by movement, causing the client to bend over and tense the abdominal muscles or to lie down and draw the legs up to relieve abdominal muscle tension (Case Example 9.7).

Generalized peritonitis, whether caused by appendicitis or some other abdominal or pelvic inflammatory condition, can result in a "board-like" abdomen because of the spasm of the rectus abdominis muscles. Lean muscle mass deteriorates with aging, especially evident in the abdominal muscles of the aging population. The very old person may not present with this classic sign of generalized peritonitis because of the lack of toned abdominal muscles.

For this reason, the nursing home, skilled care facility, or home health therapist must evaluate the aging client who presents with hip or thigh pain for possible systemic origin

CASE EXAMPLE 9.7

Appendicitis

Remember the 32-year-old female university student featured in Fig. 1.6 (see Chapter 1)? She had been referred to physical therapy with the provisional diagnosis: *Possible right oblique abdominis muscle tear/possible right iliopsoas muscle tear*. Her history included the sudden onset of "severe pain" in the right lower quadrant with accompanying nausea and abdominal distention. Aggravating factors included hip flexion, sit-ups, fast walking, and movements such as reaching, turning, and bending. Painful symptoms could be reproduced by resisted hip or trunk flexion, and tenderness/tightness was elicited on palpation of the right iliopsoas muscle compared with the left. A neurologic screen was negative. Screening questions for general health revealed constitutional symptoms, including fatigue, night sweats, nausea, and repeated episodes of severe, progressive pain in the right lower abdominal quadrant.

Although she presented with a musculoskeletal pattern of symptoms at the time of her initial evaluation with the physician, by the time she entered the physical therapy clinic her symptoms had taken on a definite systemic pattern. She was returned for further medical follow-up, and a diagnosis of appendicitis complicated by peritonitis was established. This client recovered fully from all her symptoms following an emergency appendectomy.

(assess for signs of peritonitis and/or appendicitis as appropriate; see also McBurney's point, and specific tests for iliopsoas or obturator abscess).

CLINICAL SIGNS AND SYMPTOMS

Appendicitis

- Periumbilical and/or epigastric pain
- Right lower quadrant or flank pain
- Right thigh, groin, or testicular pain
- Abdominal involuntary muscular guarding and rigidity
- Positive McBurney's point and/or positive pinch-an-inch test
- Rebound tenderness (peritonitis)
- Positive hop test (hopping on one leg or jumping on both feet reproduces painful symptoms)
- Nausea and vomiting
- Anorexia
- Dysuria (painful/difficult urination)
- Low-grade fever
- Coated tongue and bad breath

McBurney's Point

Parietal pain caused by inflammation of the peritoneum in acute appendicitis or peritonitis (from appendicitis or other inflammatory/infectious causes) may be located at McBurney's point (Fig. 9.11). The vermiform appendix receives its sympathetic supply from the 11th thoracic segment. In some people, a branch of the 11th thoracic nerve pierces the rectus abdominis muscle and innervates the skin over McBurney's point. This may explain the hyperalgesia seen at this point of appendicitis.[15]

McBurney's point is located by palpation with the client in a fully supine position. Isolate the ASIS and the umbilicus, then palpate for tenderness halfway between these two surface anatomic points. This method differs from palpation of the iliopsoas muscle because the position used to locate the iliopsoas muscle has the client in a supine position, with hips and knees flexed in a 90-degree position, whereas McBurney's point is palpated with the client in the fully supine position.

The palpation point for the iliopsoas muscle is one third the distance between the ASIS and the umbilicus, whereas McBurney's point is halfway between these two points. Be aware that the location of the vermiform appendix can vary from individual to individual, making the predictive value of this test less accurate (Fig. 9.11). Because the appendix develops at the descent of the colon, its final position can be posterior to the cecum or colon. These positions of the appendix are called *retrocecal* or retrocolic, respectively. In about 50% of cases, the appendix is retrocecal or retrocolic.[64] Atypical locations of the appendix can lead to unusual clinical findings with backache, left lower quadrant pain, groin pain, and urologic symptoms.[65,66]

Both McBurney's point and the iliopsoas muscle are palpated for reproduction of symptoms to rule out appendicitis or iliopsoas abscess associated with appendicitis or peritonitis. Alternately, instead of palpating for McBurney's point (these tests can be very painful when positive), perform a pinch-an-inch test (Fig. 9.12). This test is a new technique for detecting peritonitis/appendicitis that is more comfortable and statistically equivalent to the traditional rebound tenderness technique.[67-69] Like a rebound tenderness test, a positive pinch-an-inch test is a classic sign of peritonitis and represents aggravation by stretching or moving the parietal layer of the peritoneum. A positive pinch-an-inch test, or alternately, rebound tenderness, may occur with any disease or condition affecting the peritoneum (including appendicitis when it has progressed to include peritonitis). If the pinch-an-inch test is negative, then proceed with the rebound tenderness test (Fig. 9.13) and/or palpation of McBurney's point.

Pancreatitis

Pancreatitis is an inflammation of the pancreas that may result in autodigestion of the pancreas by its own enzymes. Pancreatitis can be acute or chronic, but the therapist is most likely to see individuals with referred pain patterns associated with acute pancreatitis. The pancreas is both an exocrine gland and an endocrine gland. Its function in digestion is primarily exocrine. This chapter focuses on digestive disorders associated with the pancreas. See Chapter 12 for pancreatic disorders associated with endocrine function.

The most common cause of acute pancreatitis is gallstones, comprising 40% to 70% of cases[70]. Chronic alcoholism, high triglyceride blood levels[71] or toxicity from some other agent, such as glucocorticoids, thiazide diuretics, or acetaminophen can bring on an acute attack of pancreatitis. Chronic pancreatitis is primarily caused by alcohol use and smoking.[72] The long-standing inflammation of the pancreas results

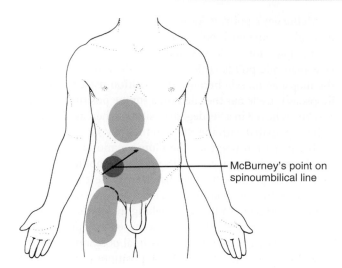

Fig. 9.10 The vermiform appendix and colon can refer pain to the area of sensory distribution for the eleventh thoracic nerve (T11). Primary *(dark red)* and referred *(light red)* pain patterns associated with the vermiform appendix are shown here with McBurney's point halfway between the ASIS and the umbilicus, usually on the right side. Gentle palpation of McBurney's point produces pain or exquisite tenderness. Pinch-an-inch test should also be assessed (see Fig. 9.12).

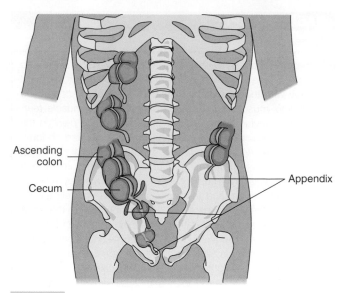

Fig. 9.11 Variations in the location of the vermiform appendix. Negative tests for appendicitis using McBurney's point may occur when the appendix is located somewhere other than at the end of the cecum. In 50% of cases the appendix is retrocecal (behind the cecum) or retrocolic (behind the colon).

in irregular fibrosis irreversible damage to the structure and function of the pancreas.[72,73]

Clinical Signs and Symptoms

The clinical course of most clients with *acute pancreatitis* follows a self-limited pattern. Symptoms can vary from mild, nonspecific abdominal pain to profound shock with coma and possible death. Abdominal pain begins abruptly in the midepigastrium, increases in intensity for several hours, and can last from days to more than a week. The pain has a penetrating quality and radiates to the back. Pain is made worse by walking and lying supine and is relieved by sitting and leaning forward. The client may have a bluish discoloration of the periumbilical area (Cullen sign)[63,74,75] as a physical manifestation of acute pancreatitis. This occurs in cases of severe hemorrhagic pancreatitis. Grey Turner's sign is a reddish-brown discoloration of the flanks, also present in hemorrhagic pancreatitis.[74,75]

Symptoms associated with *chronic pancreatitis* include persistent or recurrent episodes of epigastric and left upper quadrant pain with referral to the upper left lumbar region. Pathology of the head of the pancreas is more likely to cause epigastric and midthoracic pain from T5 to T9. Impairment of the tail of the pancreas can refer pain to the left shoulder.

Nausea, vomiting, weight loss, oily or fatty stools, and clay-colored or pale stools are common symptoms of chronic pancreatitis.[76] Attacks may last only a few hours or as long as 2 weeks; pain may be constant. In clients with alcohol-associated pancreatitis, the pain often begins 12 to 48 hours after an episode of inebriation. Clients with gallstone-associated pancreatitis typically experience pain after a large meal. Nausea and vomiting accompany the pain. Other symptoms include fever, tachycardia, jaundice, and malaise.

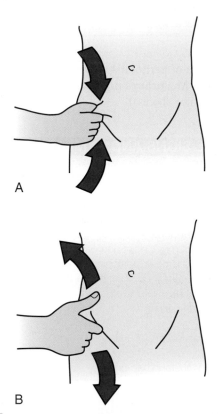

Fig. 9.12 Pinch-an-inch test. **A**, To avoid the discomfort of the classic rebound tenderness (Blumberg's) test, the pinch-an-inch test is recommended to assess for appendicitis or generalized peritonitis. To perform the test, a fold of abdominal skin over McBurney's point is gently grasped and elevated away from the peritoneum. **B**, The skin is then allowed to recoil back against the peritoneum quickly. If the individual has increased pain when the skin fold strikes the peritoneum (upon release of the skin), the test is positive for possible peritonitis. If the person being tested reacts to the pinch in an excessive fashion, he or she may have a very low pain threshold, a factor that should be taken into consideration when assessing the results.[68,69]

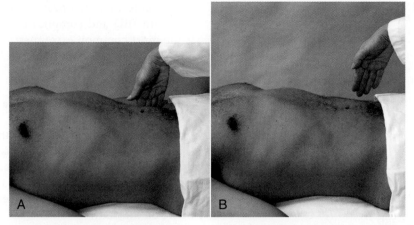

Fig. 9.13 Rebound tenderness or Blumberg's sign. **A**, To assess for appendicitis or generalized peritonitis, press your fingers gently but deeply over the right lower quadrant for 15 to 30 seconds. **B**, The palpating hand is then quickly removed. Pain induced or increased by quick withdrawal results from rapid movement of inflamed peritoneum and is called rebound tenderness. When rebound tenderness is present, the client will have pain or increased pain on the side of the inflammation when the palpatory pressure is released. Ask the client if it hurts as you are palpating or during the release. Because abdominal pain is increased uncomfortably with this test, save it for last when assessing abdominal pain during the physical examination. (From Jarvis C: *Physical examination and health assessment*, ed 5, Philadelphia, 2007, WB Saunders.)

CLINICAL SIGNS AND SYMPTOMS
Acute Pancreatitis

- Epigastric pain radiating to the back
- Nausea, vomiting, diarrhea; anorexia
- Abdominal distention and pain
- Fever and sweating
- Tachycardia
- Malaise
- Weakness
- Bluish discoloration of abdomen or flanks (severe hemorrhagic acute pancreatitis)
- Jaundice

CLINICAL SIGNS AND SYMPTOMS
Chronic Pancreatitis

- Epigastric pain radiating to the back
- Upper left lumbar region pain
- Nausea and vomiting
- Weight loss
- Oily or fatty stools
- Clay-colored or pale stools

Pancreatic Carcinoma

Pancreatic carcinoma is the fourth most common cause of death, accounting for 3% of all cancer deaths[77] and 7% of all cancer-related deaths.[78] According to the American Cancer Society, the average lifetime risk of pancreatic cancer is about 1 in 64, but the person's chances of getting pancreatic cancer can be affected by the following modifiable risk factors: tobacco use, being overweight, diabetes, chronic pancreatitis, and exposure to certain chemicals at the workplace.[77]

Nonmodifiable risk factors include increasing age, gender (men are slightly of higher risk), race (African Americans are slightly of higher risk), and family history, which includes selected inherited genetic syndromes.[79]

Clinical Signs and Symptoms

The clinical features of pancreatic cancer initially are non-specific and vague, contributing to a delay in diagnosis and high mortality. It is difficult to diagnose early the presence of pancreatic cancer. Symptoms do not usually appear until the tumor obstructs nearby bile ducts or grows large enough to cause abdominal pressure or pain, or has spread to other organs. Genetic testing could be performed in people with increased risk of pancreatic cancer. Newer tests like endoscopic ultrasound or MRI could also be performed in people with high risk of developing this cancer.[80]

The most common symptoms of pancreatic cancer are anorexia and weight loss, midepigastric pain sometimes with radiation to the midlower back region, and painless jaundice secondary to obstruction of the bile duct.[78] Jaundice is characterized by fatigue and yellowing of the skin and sclera of the eye. The urine may become dark like the color of a cola soft drink.

As with any pancreatic impairment, involvement of the head of the pancreas is more likely to cause epigastric and midthoracic pain (T5-T9), whereas impairment of the tail of the pancreas (located to the left of midline; see Fig. 3.4) can refer pain to the left shoulder. Epigastric pain is often vague and diffuse. Radiation of pain into the lumbar region is sometimes the only symptom of the disease.[81]

The pain may become worse after the person eats or lies down. Sitting up and leaning forward may provide some relief, and this usually indicates that the lesion has spread beyond the pancreas and is inoperable. Other signs and symptoms include light-colored stools, constipation, nausea, vomiting, loss of appetite, weight loss, and weakness.

CLINICAL SIGNS AND SYMPTOMS
Pancreatic Carcinoma

- Epigastric pain radiating to the back
- Back pain may be the only symptom
- Jaundice
- Anorexia and weight loss
- Light-colored stools
- Constipation
- Nausea and vomiting
- Weakness

Inflammatory Bowel Disease

IBD (*not* the same as irritable bowel syndrome [IBS]) collectively refers to two inflammatory conditions discussed separately:

- Ulcerative colitis
- CD (also referred to as regional enteritis or ileitis)

CD and ulcerative colitis (UC) are disorders of unknown etiology which involves genetic, immunologic and environmental influences on the GI tract.[41] UC affects the large intestine (colon). CD can affect any portion of the intestine from the mouth to the anus.[82] Both diseases not only cause inflammation inside the intestine but can also cause significant problems in other parts of the body.[83] These two diseases share many epidemiologic, clinical, and therapeutic features. Both are chronic, medically incurable conditions.

Extraintestinal manifestations occur frequently in clients with IBD and complicate its management. Arthritis is the most common extraintestinal complication of IBD, affecting about 30% of those with CD or UC,[84] and the client may not know these signs and symptoms are associated with the conditions.. Therefore a client with new onset of joint pain should be asked about a previous history of CD or UC.

Skin lesions may occur as either erythema nodosum (Fig. 9.14A) (red or violet bumps located primarily over the shins)[85] or pyoderma gangrenosum[86] (Fig. 9.14B) (deep ulcers or canker sores) of the shins, ankles, and calves. Ask about a recent history (last 6 weeks) of skin lesions anywhere on the body.

Nutritional deficiencies are the most common complications of IBD because of decreased nutrient intake, decreased absorption, and/or increased losses.[87] Inflammation alone and the decrease in functioning surface area of the small intestine, increases food requirements, causing poor absorption. These micronutrient deficiencies could increase risk for conditions such as bone disease, cognitive decline, anemia and arterial and venous thromboembolism, among others.[88] In addition, nutritional problems associated with the medical treatment of IBD may occur. For example, he use of prednisone decreases vitamin D metabolism, impairs calcium absorption, decreases potassium supplies, and increases the nutritional requirement for protein and calories. Decreased vitamin D metabolism and impaired calcium absorption subsequently result in bone demineralization and osteoporosis.

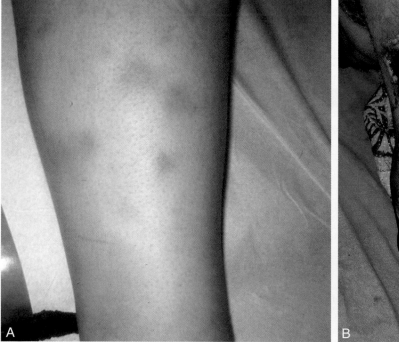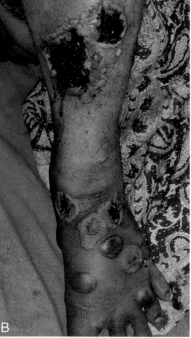

Fig. 9.14 Erythema nodosum and pyoderma gangrenosum in Crohn's disease. **A**, erythema nodosum are red of violet bumps located primarily over the shins; **B**, pyoderma gangrenosum are deep ulcers of the shins, ankles and calves. (From: (A): Strong S. Surgery for Crohn's disease. Colorectal Surgery. Elsevier, 2013. (B): Bhanja DB. Bullous pyoderma gangrenosum in Crohn's disease. Surgery: Official Journal of the Society of Universal Surgeons, Central Surgical Association, and the American Association of Endocrine Surgeons. 2020. 167(5):ell-e12.)

Crohn's Disease

CD is an inflammatory disease that can affect any portion of the intestinal tract but most commonly attacks the distal portion of the small intestine (ileum) and the colon. It can appear at any age but is more likely to develop in persons between 20 to 29 years, those who have a family member (sibling or parent) with IBD, and smokers.[89]

Clinical Signs and Symptoms

CD may have acute manifestations, but the condition is usually slow and nonaggressive. The client may present with mild intermittent symptoms months before the diagnosis is made. Fever may occur, with acute inflammation, abscesses, or rheumatoid manifestations.

Terminal ileum involvement produces pain in the periumbilical region with possible referred pain to the corresponding segment of the low back. Pain of the ileum is intermittent and felt in the lower right quadrant with possible associated iliopsoas abscess causing hip pain (see previous discussion of Psoas Abscess). The client may experience relief of discomfort after passing stool or flatus. For this reason, it is important to ask whether low back pain is relieved after passing stool or gas.

Inflammatory arthritis and arthralgias are present in 40% to 50% of patients with IBD, with 15% to 20% of these patients having CD.[90] The person may present with monoarthritis (i.e., asymmetric pattern affecting one joint at a time), usually involving an ankle or knee, although elbows and wrists can be included.

Polyarthritis (involving more than one joint) or sacroiliitis (arthritis of the lower spine and pelvis) is common and may lead to ankylosing spondylitis in rare cases. Whether monoarthritic or polyarthritic, this condition comes and goes with the disease process and may precede repeat episodes of bowel symptoms by 1 to 2 weeks. With proper medical intervention, there is no permanent joint deformity.

Ulcerative Colitis

By definition, UC is an inflammation and ulceration of the inner lining of the large intestine (colon) and rectum. UC is not the same as IBS or spastic colitis (another term for IBS).

Colorectal cancer is more common among those who have had conditions resulting in inflammation of the colon compared with the general population. The incidence is greatly increased 8 years after being diagnosed with IBD.[91]

Clinical Signs and Symptoms

The predominant symptom of UC is diarrhea with blood or pus and abdominal discomfort.[92] Mainly the left colon is involved; the small intestine is never involved. Clients often experience diarrhea, possibly 20 or more stools per day. Nausea, vomiting, anorexia, weight loss, and decreased serum potassium may occur with severe disease. Fever is present during acute disease. Nocturnal diarrhea is usually present when daytime diarrhea is prominent.

The development of anemia depends on the degree of blood loss, severity of the illness, and dietary iron intake. Ankylosing spondylitis, anemia, and clubbing of the fingers are occasional findings.

Medical testing and diagnosis are required to differentiate between these inflammatory conditions. Most often, the therapist is faced with clients presenting complaints of pain located in the shoulder, back, or groin that may have a GI origin and not be true musculoskeletal dysfunction at all.

CLINICAL SIGNS AND SYMPTOMS

Ulcerative Colitis and Crohn's Disease

- Diarrhea
- Constipation
- Fever
- Abdominal pain
- Rectal bleeding
- Night sweats
- Decreased appetite, nausea, weight loss
- Skin lesions
- Uveitis (inflammation of the eye)
- Arthritis
- Migratory arthralgias
- Hip pain (iliopsoas abscess)

Irritable Bowel Syndrome

IBS affects between 25 to 45 million Americans.[93] It is a functional disorder of motility in the small and large intestines diagnosed according to specific bowel symptom clusters.

IBS is classified as a "functional" disorder because the abnormal muscle contraction identified in people with IBS cannot be attributed to any identifiable structural or biomechanical abnormalities of the bowel.[94] However, latest research has proposed possible organic causes, such as the role of the enteric nervous system and changes in the neuroendocrine system of the gut.[94]

Other descriptive names for this condition are spastic colon, irritable colon, nervous indigestion, functional dyspepsia, pylorospasm, spastic colitis, intestinal neuroses, and laxative or cathartic colitis.

IBS is the most common GI disorder in Western society, affecting 20% of the population[95] The condition affects individuals of all ages but most persons with the diagnosis are aged 50 years and below. The condition affects women more than men (2 in 3 individuals with IBS are women).[93] Reported risk factors include the following: (1) family history of IBS; (2) emotional stress, tension or anxiety (3) food intolerance; (4) history of physical or sexual abuse; and (5) severe digestive tract infection.[96]

Clinical Signs and Symptoms

There is a highly variable complex of intermittent GI symptoms, including nausea and vomiting, anorexia, foul breath, sour stomach, flatulence, cramps, abdominal bloating, and constipation and/or diarrhea. The client may report white mucus in the stools.[96,97] Within the Rome IV classification, there are four bowel patterns that could be seen in IBS: (1) IBS-D (diarrhea predominant; (2) IBS-C (constipation predominant); (3) IBS-M (mixed diarrhea and constipation); and (4) IBS-U (unclassified)[98].

Pain may be steady or intermittent, and there may be a dull deep discomfort with sharp cramps in the morning or after eating. The typical pain pattern consists of lower left quadrant abdominal pain, constipation, and diarrhea. Symptoms seem to come and go with no apparent cause and effect that can be identified by the affected individual. Abdominal pain or discomfort is relieved by defecation. Possible gas pockets in the splenic fissure may masquerade as in the anterior chest area or in the left upper abdominal quadrant[99].

The therapist should also be alert for the client with a known history of IBS now experiencing unexplained weight loss or persistent, severe diarrhea, possibly signaling disorders such as malignancy, IBD, or celiac disease. Symptoms of IBS tend to disappear at night when the client is asleep. Nocturnal diarrhea, awakening the client from a sound sleep, is more often a result of organic disease of the bowel and is less likely to occur in IBS.

CLINICAL SIGNS AND SYMPTOMS
Irritable Bowel Syndrome

- Painful abdominal cramps
- Constipation
- Diarrhea
- Nausea and vomiting
- Anorexia
- Flatulence
- Foul breath

Colorectal Cancer

Colorectal cancer is the third leading cause of deaths related to cancer in the United States.[100] In 2021 it is estimated that there will be 104,270 new cases of colon cancer and 45,230 new cases of rectal cancer.[101] Screening programs and changes in lifestyle-related risk factors have resulted in a decrease in the overall colorectal cancer rates since the mid-1980s.[101] The population of patients diagnosed with colorectal cancer has shifted toward the younger population, with increasing incidence in younger individuals, and decreasing incidence in the older population.[102] Compared with other racial groups in the United States, non-Hispanic blacks have the highest colorectal cancer incidence and mortality, followed by American Indians and Alaska Natives.[102]

The American Cancer Society recommends regular early screening starting at age 45 through a stool-based (fecal occult blood test) test or a visual examination[103] (colonoscopy). More frequent screening or screening before age 45 is recommended for individuals belonging to high-risk groups, particularly those with a personal or strong family history of colorectal cancer or certain types of polyps, previous history

of chronic IBD (e.g., CD, UC), known family history of adenomatous polyps, hereditary nonpolyposis colon cancer, and history of radiation to the abdomen or pelvic region secondary to a prior cancer diagnosis.[103].

Clinical Signs and Symptoms

The presentation of colorectal carcinoma is related to the location of the neoplasm within the colon. Individuals are asymptomatic in the early stages, then develop minor changes in their bowel habits (diarrhea, constipation or narrowing of stool, lasting for more than a few days), and present symptoms such as rectal bleeding; blood in the stool that causes dark brown or black stools; abdominal pain; weight loss, weakness and fatigue.[104] Many cases of colon cancer do not show any symptoms until metastases has occurred, and can manifest as right quadrant pain.[41] Acute pain is often indistinguishable from that of cholecystitis or acute appendicitis. Fatigue and SOB may occur secondary to the iron deficiency anemia that develops with chronic blood loss. Mahogany-colored stools may be present when there is blood mixed with the stool. The reddish-mahogany color associated with bleeding in the lower GI/colon differs from the melena or dark, tarry stools that occur when blood loss in the upper GI tract is oxidized before being excreted. Bleeding with bright red blood is more common with a carcinoma of the left side of the colon. Pencil-thin stool may be described with cancer of the rectum.

When rectal tumors enlarge and invade the perirectal tissue, a sensation of rectal fullness develops and may progress to a dull, aching perineal or sacral pain that can radiate down the legs when peripheral nerves are involved.

CLINICAL SIGNS AND SYMPTOMS
Colorectal Cancer

Early Stages
- Rectal bleeding, hemorrhoids
- Abdominal, pelvic, back, or sacral pain
- Back pain that radiates down the legs
- Changes in bowel patterns

Advanced Stages
- Constipation progressing to obstipation
- Diarrhea with copious amounts of mucus
- Nausea, vomiting
- Abdominal distention
- Weight loss
- Fatigue and dyspnea
- Fever (less common)

PHYSICIAN REFERRAL

A 67-year-old man was referred to home health physical therapy after being discharged from the hospital for a total hip replacement. His recovery has been slowed by chronic diarrhea.

A 25-year-old woman who is diagnosed as having SI pain and joint dysfunction is being seen in outpatient physical therapy. She stated to the therapist that she has read somewhere that exercises will help for constipation and would like to know what exercises she could to for this condition.

A 44-year-old man with a medical diagnosis of bicipital tendinopathy is being seen by a physical therapist. During the interview, the patient reports several episodes of fever and chills, diarrhea, and abdominal pain, which he attributes to "the stress of meeting deadlines on the job."

These are common examples of symptoms of a GI nature that are described by clients and are unrelated to current physical therapy treatment. These people may be seeking the therapist's advice as the only medical person with whom they have contact. Knowing the pain patterns associated with GI involvement and which follow-up questions to ask can assist the therapist in deciding when to suggest that the client return to a physician for a medical examination and treatment.

The client may not associate GI symptoms or already diagnosed GI disease with his or her musculoskeletal pain, which makes it necessary for the therapist to initiate questions to determine the presence of such GI involvement.

Taking the client's temperature and vital signs during the initial evaluation is recommended for any person who has musculoskeletal pain of unknown origin. Fever, low-grade fever over a long period (even if cyclic), or sweats are indicative of systemic disease.

When appendicitis or peritonitis from any cause is suspected because of the client's symptoms, a physician should be notified immediately. The client should lie down and remain as quiet as possible. It is best to give her or him nothing by mouth because of the danger of aggravating the condition, possibly causing rupture of the appendix, or in case surgery is needed. Applications of heat are contraindicated for the same reason.

On the other hand, the therapist may be evaluating a client who presents with shoulder, back, or groin pain and limitations that are not caused by true musculoskeletal lesions but rather the result of GI involvement. The presence of associated GI symptoms in the absence of conclusive musculoskeletal findings will alert the therapist to the possible need for medical referral. Correlate the *history* with *pain patterns* and any *unusual findings* that may indicate systemic disease.

Guidelines for Immediate Medical Attention

- Anytime appendicitis or iliopsoas/obturator abscess is suspected (positive McBurney's test, positive iliopsoas/obturator test, positive pinch-an-inch test, positive test for rebound tenderness).
- Anytime the therapist suspects retroperitoneal bleeding from an injured, damaged, or ruptured spleen or ectopic pregnancy; or there is a history of trauma; missed menses; positive Kehr's sign.

Guidelines for Physician Referral

- Clients who chronically rely on laxatives should be encouraged to discuss bowel management without drugs with their physician.

- Joint involvement accompanied by skin or eye lesions may be reflective of inflammatory bowel disease and should be reported to the physician if the physician is unaware of these extraintestinal manifestations.
- Anyone with a history of NSAID use presenting with back or shoulder pain, especially when accompanied by any of the associated signs and symptoms listed for peptic ulcer, must be evaluated by a physician.
- Back pain associated with meals or relieved by a bowel movement (especially if accompanied by rectal bleeding) or with back pain and abdominal pain at the same level requires medical evaluation.
- Back pain of unknown cause that does not fit a musculoskeletal pattern, especially in a person with a previous history of cancer.

Clues to Screening for Gastrointestinal Disease

These clues will help the therapist in the decision-making process:
- Age over 45 years.
- Previous history of NSAID-induced GI bleeding; NSAID use, especially chronic or multiple prescriptions and OTC NSAIDs taken simultaneously.
- Symptoms increase within 2 hours after taking NSAIDs or other medication.
- Symptoms are affected (increased or decreased) by food anywhere from immediately up to 2 to 4 hours later.
- Presence of abdominal or GI symptoms occurring within 4 to 6 weeks of musculoskeletal symptoms, especially recurring or cyclical symptoms (systemic pattern).
- Back pain and abdominal pain at the same level, simultaneously or alternately, especially when accompanied by constitutional symptoms.
- Shoulder, back, pelvic, or sacral pain:
  - Of unknown origin, especially with a past history of cancer.
  - Affected by food, milk, antacids, or vomiting.
  - Accompanied by constitutional symptoms.
- Back, pelvic, or sacral pain that is relieved or reduced by a bowel movement or accompanied by rectal bleeding.
- Low back pain accompanied by constipation may be a manifestation of pelvic floor overactivity or spasm; this requires a pelvic floor screening examination.
- Shoulder pain within 24 to 48 hours of laparoscopy, ruptured ectopic pregnancy, or traumatic blow or injury to the left side (Kehr's sign; see Chapter 19).
- Positive iliopsoas or obturator sign; positive McBurney's point; right (or left) lower quadrant abdominal or pelvic pain produced when palpating the iliopsoas muscle or tapping the heel of the involved side.
- Joint pain or arthralgias preceded by skin rash, especially in the presence of a history of CD.
- When evaluated during early onset of referred pain, there is usually full and painless range of motion, but as time goes on, muscle splinting and guarding secondary to pain can produce altered movements as well.

GASTROINTESTINAL PAIN PATTERNS

ESOPHAGEAL PAIN (FIG. 9.15)

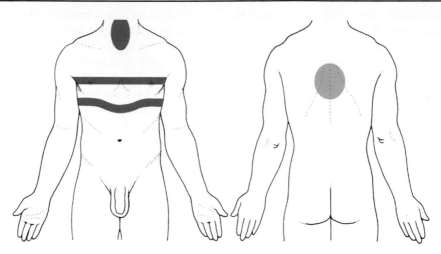

Fig. 9.15 Nerve distribution of the esophagus is through T5 to T6 with primary pain around the xiphoid. Esophageal pain may be projected around the chest at any level corresponding to the esophageal lesion. Only two of the possible bands of pain around the chest are shown here. Similar symptoms can occur anywhere a lesion appears along the length of the esophagus.

Location:	Substernal discomfort at the level of the lesion Lesion of upper esophagus: pain in the (anterior) neck Lesion of lower esophagus: pain originating from the xiphoid process, radiating around the thorax
Referral:	Severe esophageal pain: pain referred to the middle of the back Back pain may be the only symptom or may be the earliest symptom of esophageal cancer
Description:	Sharp, sticking, knife-like, stabbing Strong burning pain (esophagitis)
Intensity:	Varies from mild discomfort to severe pain
Duration:	May be constant; associated with meals
Associated signs and symptoms:	Dysphagia, odynophagia, melena
Possible etiology:	Obstruction of the esophagus (neoplasm) Esophageal stricture secondary to acid reflux (peptic esophagitis) Esophageal stricture of unknown cause Achalasia Esophagitis or esophageal spasm Esophageal varices (usually asymptomatic except bleeding)

STOMACH AND DUODENAL PAIN (FIG. 9.16)

Location:	Pain in the midline of the epigastrium Upper abdomen just below the xiphoid process One to two inches above and to the right of the umbilicus
Referral:	Common referral pattern to the back at the level of the lesion (T6 to T10) Right shoulder/upper trapezius Lateral border of the right scapula
Description:	Aching, burning ("heartburn"), gnawing, cramp-like pain (true visceral pain)
Intensity:	Can be mild or severe
Duration:	Comes in waves

Continued

GASTROINTESTINAL PAIN PATTERNS—*cont'd*

Associated signs and symptoms:

Early satiety
Melena
Symptoms may be associated with meals

Possible etiology:

Peptic ulcers: gastric, pyloric, duodenal (history of NSAIDs)
Stomach carcinoma
Kaposi's sarcoma (most common malignancy associated with acquired immunodeficiency syndrome [AIDS])

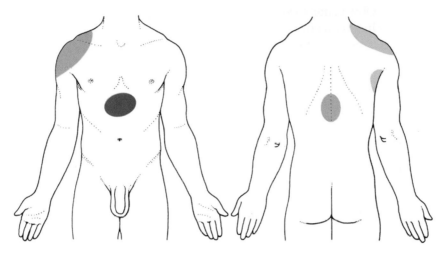

Fig. 9.16   Stomach or duodenal pain *(dark red)* may occur anteriorly in the midline of the epigastrium or upper abdomen just below the xiphoid process. There is a tendency for the stomach and duodenum to refer pain posteriorly. Referred pain *(light red)* to the back occurs at the anatomic level of the abdominal lesion (T6 to T10). Other patterns of referred pain *(light red)* may include the right shoulder and upper trapezius or the lateral border of the right scapula.

SMALL INTESTINE PAIN (FIG. 9.17)

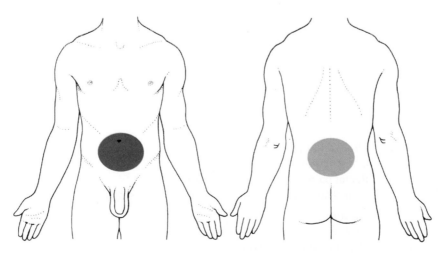

Fig. 9.17   Midabdominal pain *(dark red)* caused by disturbances of the small intestine is centered near the umbilicus (T9 to T11 nerve distribution) and may be referred *(light red)* to the low back area at the same anatomic level. Keep in mind the umbilicus is at the same level as the L3-L4 disk space in the average adult who is not obese or who has a protruding abdomen.

GASTROINTESTINAL PAIN PATTERNS—*cont'd*

Location: Midabdominal pain (about the umbilicus)

Referral: Pain referred to the back if the stimulus is sufficiently intense or if the individual's pain threshold is low

Description: Cramping pain

Intensity: Moderate to severe

Duration: Intermittent (pain comes and goes)

Associated signs and symptoms: Nausea, fever, diarrhea
Pain relief may not occur after passing stool or gas

Possible etiology: Obstruction (neoplasm)
Increased bowel motility
Crohn's disease (regional enteritis)

LARGE INTESTINE AND COLON PAIN (FIG. 9.18)

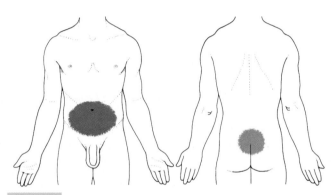

Fig. 9.18 Pain associated with the large intestine and colon *(dark red)* may occur in the lower abdomen across either or both abdominal quadrants. Pain may be referred to the sacrum *(light red)* when the rectum is stimulated. The pattern of nerve supply varies depending on the segment: vermiform appendix, cecum, and ascending colon are supplied by the T10 to T12 sympathetic fibers. Nerve distribution to the transverse colon is T12 to L1 and the descending colon is supplied by L1 to L2.

Location: Lower midabdomen (across either or both quadrants)
Poorly localized

Referral: Pain may be referred to the sacrum when the rectum is stimulated

Description: Cramping

Intensity: Dull

Duration: Steady

Associated signs and symptoms: Bloody diarrhea, urgency
Constipation
Rectal pain; pain during defecation
Pain relief may occur after defecation or passing gas

Possible etiology: Ulcerative colitis
Crohn's disease (regional enteritis)
Carcinoma of the colon
Long-term use of antibiotics
Irritable bowel syndrome

Continued

GASTROINTESTINAL PAIN PATTERNS—*cont'd*

PANCREATIC PAIN (FIG. 9.19)

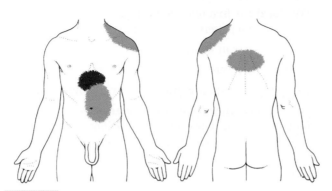

Fig. 9.19   Pancreatic pain *(dark red)* occurs in the midline or left of the epigastrium, just below the xiphoid process, but may be referred *(light red)* to the left shoulder or to the midthoracic spine. Posterior pain may radiate or lateralize from the spine away from the midline. Sensory nerve distribution is from T5 to T9.

Location:	Midline or to the left of the epigastrium, just below the xiphoid process
Referral:	Referred pain in the middle or lower back is typical with pancreatic disease; more rarely, pain may be referred to the upper back, midscapular region.
	Somatic pain felt in the left shoulder may result from activation of pain fibers in the left diaphragm by an adjacent inflammatory process in the tail of the pancreas. Less often, pain is perceived in the right shoulder if/when the head of the pancreas is involved.
Description:	Burning or gnawing abdominal pain
Intensity:	Severe
Duration:	Constant pain, sudden onset
Associated signs and symptoms:	Sudden weight loss
	Jaundice
	Nausea and vomiting
	Constipation
	Flatulence
	Tachycardia
	Light-colored stools (carcinoma)
	Symptoms may be unrelated to digestive activities (carcinoma)
	Weakness
	Symptoms may be related to digestive activities (pancreatitis)
	Fever
	Malaise
Aggravating factors:	Walking and lying supine (pancreatitis)
	Alcohol, large meals
Relieving factors:	Sitting and leaning forward (pancreatitis, pancreatic carcinoma)
Possible etiology:	Pancreatitis
	Pancreatic carcinoma (primarily disease of men, occurs during the sixth and seventh decade)

GASTROINTESTINAL PAIN PATTERNS—*cont'd*

APPENDICEAL PAIN (SEE FIG. 9.10)

Location:	Right lower quadrant pain
Referral:	Well localized; first referred to epigastric or periumbilical area
	Referred pain pattern to the right hip and/or right testicle
Description:	Aching, comes in waves
Intensity:	Moderate to severe
Duration:	Steadily progresses over time (usually 12 hours with acute appendicitis)
Associated signs and symptoms:	Positive McBurney's point for tenderness
	Iliopsoas abscess may occur; positive iliopsoas muscle test or positive obturator test
	Anorexia, nausea, vomiting, low-grade fever
	Coated tongue and bad breath
	Dysuria (painful/difficult urination)

Figs. 9.20 and 9.21 provide a summary of all the GI pain patterns described that can mimic the pain and dysfunction usually associated with musculoskeletal lesions.

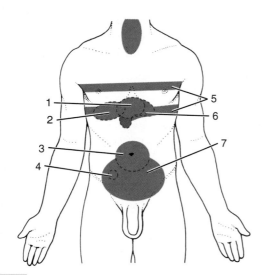

Fig. 9.20 Full-figure **primary** pain pattern. *1*, Stomach/duodenum; *2*, liver/gallbladder/common bile duct; *3*, small intestine; *4*, appendix; *5*, esophagus; *6*, pancreas; and *7*, large intestine/colon.

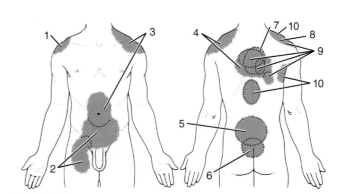

Fig. 9.21 Full-figure **referred** pain patterns. *1*, Liver/gallbladder/common bile duct; *2*, appendix; *3*, pancreas; *4*, pancreas; *5*, small intestine; *6*, colon; *7*, esophagus; *8*, stomach/duodenum; *9*, liver/gallbladder/common bile duct; and *10*, stomach/duodenum.

■ Key Points To Remember

1. GI disorders can refer pain to the sternum, neck, shoulder, scapula, low back, sacrum, groin, and hip.
2. When evaluated during early onset of referred pain, there is usually full and painless range of motion, but as time goes on, muscle splinting and guarding secondary to pain or as a component of motor nerve involvement will produce altered movements as well.
3. The membrane that envelops organs (visceral peritoneum) is insensitive to pain so that, except in the presence of inflammation/ischemia, it is possible to have extensive disease without pain.
4. Clients may not relate known GI disorders to current (or new) musculoskeletal symptoms.
5. Sudden and unaccountable changes in bowel habits, blood in the stool, or vomiting red blood or coffee-ground vomitus are red-flag symptoms requiring medical follow-up.
6. Antibiotics and NSAIDs are the drugs that most commonly induce GI symptoms.
7. Kehr's sign (left shoulder pain) occurs as a result of free air or blood in the abdominal cavity causing distention (e.g., trauma, ruptured spleen, laparoscopy, ectopic pregnancy).
8. Epigastric pain radiating to the upper back, or upper back pain alone, can be the primary symptom of peptic ulcer, pancreatitis, or pancreatic carcinoma.
9. Appendicitis and diseases of the intestines, such as Crohn's disease and ulcerative colitis can cause abscess of the iliopsoas muscle, resulting in hip, thigh, or groin pain.
10. Arthritis and migratory arthralgias occur in 25% of Crohn's disease cases.

CLIENT HISTORY AND INTERVIEW

SPECIAL QUESTIONS TO ASK

After completing the initial intake interview, if there is cause to suspect GI involvement, include any of the following additional questions that seem pertinent. It may be helpful to let the client know you will be asking some questions about overall health issues that may seem unrelated to their current symptoms but that are nevertheless important.

When asking questions about medications, look for long-term use of antibiotics, corticosteroids, or other hepatotoxic drugs. See Table 9.1 for a list of medications that can cause constipation.

PAST MEDICAL HISTORY

- For the client with left shoulder pain: Have you sustained any injuries in the last week during a sports activity, fall, or automobile accident? Were you pushed down or pushed against something hard (assault)? (**Ruptured spleen: positive Kehr's sign**)
- Have you experienced any abdominal or intestinal problems, nausea, vomiting, episodes of night sweats, or fever?
  - *If yes*, have you seen a physician about these problems or reported them to your physician?
  - For further follow-up questions related to this area, see Associated Signs and Symptoms.
- Have you ever had an upset stomach or heartburn while taking (NSAID) pain relievers like ibuprofen, naproxen (name the specific drug)?
- Have you ever been treated for an ulcer or internal bleeding while taking (NSAID) pain relievers?

- *If so*, when?
- Do you still have any pain from your ulcer? Please describe.
- Have you ever had a colonoscopy, proctoscopy, or endoscopy?
  - *If yes*, why and how long ago?
- Have you ever been diagnosed with cancer of any kind?
  - *If yes*, what, when, and has there been any follow-up?
- Have you ever had radiation treatment? (**Rectal bleeding is a sign of radiation proctitis**)
- Have you ever had abdominal or spinal (anterior retroperitoneal approach) surgery?
  - *If yes*, when and what type was it?
- Do you have hemorrhoids?
  - *If yes*, have you had surgery for your hemorrhoids? (**Most common cause of bright red blood coating stools**)

ASSOCIATED SIGNS AND SYMPTOMS: EFFECTS OF EATING/DRINKING

- Do you have any problems chewing or swallowing food? Do you have any pain when swallowing food or liquids? (**Dysphagia, odynophagia**)
- Have you been vomiting? (**Esophageal varices, ulcers**)
  - *If so*, how often?
  - Is your vomitus ever dark brown or black or look like it has coffee grounds in it? (**Blood**)
- Have you ever vomited, coughed up, or spit up blood?

- Have you experienced any loss of appetite or sudden weight loss in the last few weeks? (i.e., 10 to 15 pounds in 2 weeks without trying)
- Does eating relieve your symptoms? (**Duodenal or pyloric ulcer**)
  - *If yes*, how soon after eating?
- Does eating aggravate your symptoms? (**Gastric ulcer, gallbladder inflammation**)
- Does your pain occur 1 to 3 hours after eating or between meals? (**Duodenal or pyloric ulcers, gallstones, pancreatitis**)
- Have you ever had gallstones?
- Have you noticed any change in your symptoms after drinking alcohol? (**Alcohol-associated pancreatitis**)
- Have you ever awakened at night with pain? (**Duodenal ulcer, cancer**)
  - Approximately what time does this occur? (**12 midnight to 3:00 AM: ulcer**)
  - Can you relieve the pain in any way and get back to sleep. *If yes*, how? (**Ulcer: eating and antacids relieve/ Cancer: nothing relieves**)
- Do you have a feeling of fullness after only one or two bites of food? (**Early satiety: esophagus, stomach and duodenum, or gallbladder**)

ASSOCIATED SIGNS AND SYMPTOMS: CHANGE IN BOWEL HABITS

- Have you had any changes in your bowel movements (Normal frequency varies from three times a day to once every 3 or more days)? (**Constipation/bowel obstruction**)
  - *If yes* to constipation, do you use laxatives or stool softeners? How often?

- Do you have diarrhea? (**Ulcerative colitis, Crohn's disease, long-term use of antibiotics, colonic obstruction, amebic colitis, angiodysplasia, creatine supplementation**)
  - Do you have more than two loose stools a day? *If so*, do you take medication for this problem? What kind of medication do you use?
  - Have you traveled outside of the United States within the last 6 months to 1 year? (**Amebic colitis associated with bloody diarrhea**)
- Do you have a sense of urgency so that you have to find a bathroom immediately without waiting?
- Do you ever have any blood in your stool, reddish-mahogany-colored stools, or dark, tarry stools that are hard to wipe clean? (**Bleeding ulcer, esophageal varices, colon or rectal cancer, hemorrhoids or rectal fissures; rectal lesions with bleeding can be caused by homosexual activity [men] or anal intercourse [women]**)
  - *If yes*, how often?
  - For the therapist: *If yes*, assess NSAID use and risk factors for NSAID-induced gastropathy.
  - Is the blood mixed in with the stool or does it coat the surface? (**Distal colon or rectum versus melena**)
- Do you ever have white mucus around or in your stools? (**Irritable bowel syndrome**)
- Do you ever have gray-colored stools? (**Lack of bile or caused by biliary obstruction such as hepatitis, gallstones, cirrhosis, pancreatic carcinoma, hepatotoxic drugs**)
- Are your stools ever pencil thin? (**Indicates bowel obstruction such as tumor or rectocele [prolapsed rectum] in women after childbirth**)
- Is your pain relieved after passing stool or gas? (**Yes: large intestine and colon; No: small intestine**)

CASE STUDY

Crohn's Disease

REFERRAL

A 21-year-old woman comes to physical therapy with complaints of pain on hip flexion when she lifts her right foot off the brake in the car. There are no other aggravating factors, and she is unaware of any way to relieve the pain when she is driving her car. Before the onset of symptoms, she jogged 5 to 6 miles/day but could not recall any injury or trauma that might contribute to this pain. The Family/ Personal History form indicates no personal illness but shows a complex, positive family history for heart disease, diabetes, ulcerative colitis, stomach ulcers, stomach cancer, and alcoholism.

PHYSICAL THERAPY INTERVIEW

It is suggested that the therapist use the physical therapy interview to assess the client's complaints today and follow-up with appropriate additional questions such as those noted here.

Introduction to Client

From your family history form, I noticed that a number of your family members have reportedly been diagnosed with various diseases.

- Do you have any other medical or health-related problems?

Continued

CASE STUDY—*cont'd*

Crohn's Disease

- Have you sustained any injuries to the lower back, side, or abdomen in the last week—for example, during a sports activity, fall, or automobile accident? Were you pushed, kicked, or shoved against something?

Although the symptoms that you have described appear to be a musculoskeletal problem, I would like to check out the possibility of a urologic, abdominal, or gynecologic source for your complaints. I will ask you some additional questions that may seem to be unrelated to the problem with your hip, but which will help me put together the whole picture of your history, symptoms, and actual physical results from my examination today.

General Systemic

What other symptoms have you had with this problem? (After allowing the client to answer, you may prompt her by asking: For example, have you had any…)

- Numbness
- Fatigue
- Legs giving out from under you
- Burning, tingling sensation
- Weakness

Gastrointestinal

- Nausea
- Diarrhea
- Loss of appetite
- Feeling of fullness after only one or two bites of a meal
- Unexpected weight gain or loss (10 to 15 pounds without trying)
- Vomiting
- Constipation
- Blood in your stool

(If yes to any of these, follow-up with *Special Questions to Ask* in the Client History and Interview box.)

Have you noticed any association between when you eat and your symptoms? (After allowing the client to respond, you may want to prompt her by asking whether eating relieves or aggravates the pain.)

Is your pain relieved or aggravated during or after you have a bowel movement?

Gynecologic

Since your hip/groin/thigh symptoms started, have you been examined by a gynecologist to rule out any gynecologic causes of this problem?

If no

- Have you ever been told that you have ovarian cysts, uterine fibroids, retroverted uterus, endometriosis, an ectopic pregnancy, or any other gynecologic problem?

- Are you pregnant or have you recently terminated a pregnancy either by miscarriage or abortion?
- Are you using an intrauterine contraceptive device (IUD)?
- Are you having any unusual vaginal discharge?

(If yes to any of these questions, see the follow-up questions for women in Appendix B-37 in the accompanying enhanced eBook version included with print purchase of this textbook

Urologic

- Have you had any problems with your kidneys or bladder?
- If yes, please describe.
- Have you noticed any changes in your ability to urinate since your pain or symptoms started? (If no, it may be necessary to provide examples of what changes you are referring to; for example, difficulty in starting or continuing the flow of urine, numbness or tingling in the groin or pelvis, painful urination, urinary incontinence, blood in the urine.)
- Have you had burning with urination during the last 1 to 3 weeks?

Physical Examination

Your physical examination reveals tenderness or palpation over the right anterior upper thigh muscles to the groin, with reproduction of the pain on resisted trunk flexion only. This woman attends daily ballet classes, stretches daily, and seems to be very active physically. All tests for flexibility were negative for tightness, including the Thomas' test for tight hip flexors.

Other special tests for a hip and a neurologic screen had negative results. The client's temperature was normal when it was taken during the intake screen of vital signs today, but during the physical therapy interview, when specifically asked about fevers and night sweats, she indicated several recurrent episodes of night sweats during the last 3 months.

RESULTS

Although the client's complaints are primarily musculoskeletal, the absence of trauma, positive family history for systemic disease, limited musculoskeletal findings, and the client's remark concerning the presence of night sweats will alert the physical therapist to the need for a medical referral to rule out the possibility of a systemic origin of symptoms.

The client's condition gradually worsened during a 3-week period and reexamination by the physician led to an eventual diagnosis of Crohn's diseas e (regional gastroenteritis). The client was treated with medications that reduce abdominal inflammation and subjective reports of pain on active hip flexion were eliminated. Performing the special tests for iliopsoas abscess may have provided valuable information and earlier medical referral if assessed during the initial evaluation.

PRACTICE QUESTIONS

1. Bleeding in the gastrointestinal (GI) tract can be manifested as:
   a. Dysphagia
   b. Melena
   c. Psoas abscess
   d. Tenderness over McBurney's point
2. What is the significance of Kehr's sign?
   a. Gas, air, or blood in the abdominal cavity
   b. Infection of the peritoneum (peritonitis, appendicitis)
   c. Esophageal cancer
   d. Thoracic disk herniation masquerading as chest or anterior neck pain
3. What areas of the body can GI disorders refer pain to?
   a. Sternum, shoulder, scapula
   b. Anterior neck, midback, low back
   c. Hip, pelvis, sacrum
   d. All of the above
4. A 56-year-old client was referred to physical therapy for pelvic floor rehab. His primary symptoms are obstructed defecation and puborectalis muscle spasm. He wakes nightly with left flank pain. The pattern is low thoracic, laterally, but superior to iliac crest. Sometimes he has buttock pain on the same side. He does not have any daytime pain but is up for several hours at night. Advil and light activity do not help much. The pain is relieved or decreased with passing gas. He has very tight hamstrings and rectus femoris. Change in symptoms with gas or defecation is possible with:
   a. Thoracic disk disease
   b. Obturator nerve compression
   c. Small intestine disease
   d. Large intestine and colon dysfunction
5. Name two of the most common medications taken by clients seen in a physical therapy practice likely to induce GI bleeding.
   a. Corticosteroids
   b. Antibiotics and antiinflammatories
   c. Statins
   d. None of the above
6. Which of the following are clues to the possible involvement of the GI system?
   a. Abdominal pain alternating with TMJ pain within a 2-week period
   b. Abdominal pain at the same level as back pain, occurring either simultaneously or alternately
   c. Shoulder pain alleviated by a bowel movement
   d. All of the above
7. A 65-year-old client is taking OxyContin for a "sore shoulder." She also reports aching pain of the sacrum that radiates. The sacral pain can be caused by:
   a. Psoas abscess caused by vertebral osteomyelitis
   b. GI bleeding causing hemorrhoids and rectal fissures
   c. Crohn's disease manifested as sacroiliitis
   d. Pressure on sacral nerves from stored fecal content in the constipated client taking narcotics
8. Body temperature should be taken as part of vital sign assessment:
   a. For every client evaluated
   b. For any client who has musculoskeletal pain of unknown origin
   c. For any client reporting the presence of constitutional symptoms, especially fever or night sweats
   d. b and c
9. What is the significance of the psoas sign?
10. What is the significant of the Kehr sign?

REFERENCES

1. Spencer NJ, Hu H. Enteric nervous system: sensory transduction, neural circuits and gastrointestinal motility. *Nat Rev Gastroenterol Hepatol.* 2020;17(6):338–351. https://doi.org/10.1038/s41575-020-0271-2.
2. Cunha J. What Are the Four Main Functions of the Digestive System? Emedicine health.com. Reviewed 2/01/2021. Available at: https://www.emedicinehealth.com/four_main_functions_of_the_digestive_system/article_em.htm. Accessed July 5, 2021.
3. National Institute of Diabetes and Digestive and Kidney Diseases: Your Digestive System and How it Works. Available at: https://www.niddk.nih.gov/health-information/digestive-diseases/digestive-system-how-it-works. Accessed July 5, 2021.
4. Furness J. The enteric nervous system and neurogastroenterology. *Nat Rev Gastroenterol Hepatol.* 2012;9:286–294. https://doi.org/10.1038/nrgastro.2012.32.
5. The Brain-Gut Connection: Health Aging. Johns Hopkins Medicine. Available online at: http://www.hopkinsmedicine.org/health/healthy_aging/healthy_body/the-brain-gut-connection. Accessed July 5, 2021.
6. Goldstein AM, Hofstra RMW, Burns AJ. Building a brain in the gut: development of the enteric nervous system. *Clin Genet.* 2013;83(4):307–316.
7. Wood J. Enteric Nervous System: Brains-in-the-Gut. In: Said HM, ed. *Physiology of the Gastrointestinal Tract.* Elsevier; 2018:6e.
8. Moraes LJ, Miranda MB, Loures LF, et al. A systematic review of psychoneuroimmunology-based interventions. *Psychol Health Med.* 2018;23(6):635–652. https://doi.org/10.1080/13548506.2017.1417607. | Received 20 Feb 2017, Accepted 24 Nov 2017, Published online: 20 Dec 2017.
9. Vighi G, Marcucci F, Sensi L, et al. Allergy and the gastrointestinal system. *Clin Exp Immunol.* 2008;153(Suppl 1):3–6. https://doi.org/10.1111/j.1365-2249.2008.03713.x.
10. Sourav P, Lal S, Lal G. Role of gamma-delta (γδ) T cells in autoimmunity. *J Leukoc Biol.* 2015;97(2):259–271.
11. Fasano A. Leaky gut and autoimmune diseases. *Clin Rev Allergy Immunol.* 2012;42(1):71–78.
12. Fasano A. All disease begins in the (leaky) gut: role of zonulin-mediated gut permeability in the pathogenesis of some chronic inflammatory diseases. *F1000Res* 9:F1000 Faculty Rev-69, 2020. https://doi.org/10.12688/f1000research.20510.1. Published 2020 Jan 31.
13. Yang EH, Shah S, Criley JM. Digitalis toxicity: a fading but crucial complication to recognize. *Am J Med.* 2012;125(4):337–343.
14. Shin SJ, Noh CK, Lim SG, et al. Non-steroidal anti-inflammatory drug-induced enteropathy. *Intest Res.* 2017;15(4):446–455. https://doi.org/10.5217/ir.2017.15.4.446.
15. Rex L. *Evaluation and Treatment of Somatovisceral Dysfunction of the Gastrointestinal System.* Edmonds, WA: URSA Foundation; 2004.
16. Vaezi MF, Pandolfino JE, Vela MF. Diagnosis and management of achalasia. *American College of Gastroenterology.* Available

online at: http://gi.org/guideline/diagnosis-and-management-of-achalasia. Accessed on July 5, 2021.

17. Dysphagia: Mayo Clinic. Available online at: http://www.mayoclinic.org/diseases-conditions/dysphagia/basics/causes/con-20033444. Accessed July 5, 2021.

18. Cicala G, Barbieri MA, Spina E, et al. A comprehensive review of swallowing difficulties and dysphagia associated with antipsychotics in adults. *Expert Rev Clin Pharmacol.* 2019;12(3):219–234. https://doi.org/10.1080/17512433.2019.1577134. | Received 18 Jul 2018, Accepted 29 Jan 2019, Accepted author version posted online: 31 Jan 2019, Published online: 08 Feb 2019.

19. Stegemann S, Gosch M, Bretkreutz J. Swallowing dysfunction and dysphagia is an unrecognized challenge for oral drug therapy. *Int J Pharm.* 2012;430(1–2):197–206.

20. Schwemmle C, Jungheim M, Miller S, et al. [Medication-induced dysphagia: a review]. *HNO.* 2015;63(7):504–510. https://doi.org/10.1007/s00106-015-0015-8.

21. Davis K, Prater A, Fluker SA, et al. A difficult case to swallow: herpes esophagitis after epidural steroid injection. *Am J Ther.* 2014;2(1):e9–e14.

22. Hwang C, Desai B, Desai A. Dysphagia and Odynophagia. In: Desai B, Desai A, eds. *Primary Care for Emergency Physicians.* Springer, Cham; 2017. http://doi.org/10.1007/978-3-319-44360-7_8.

23. WebMD: Early Satiety: Why Do I Feel So Full After a Few Bites? Medically Reviewed by Michael W. Smith, MD on May 05, 2021. Available at: https://www.webmd.com/digestive-disorders/early-satiety. Accessed July 7, 2021.

24. Krishnakumar R, Lenke L. "Sternum-into-abdomen" deformity with abdominal compression following osteoporotic vertebral compression fractures managed by 2-level vertebral column resection and reconstruction. *Spine.* 2015;40(18):E1035–E1039.

25. Rome IV. Diagnostic Criteria for Functional Gastrointestinal Disorders. Available online at: https://theromefoundation.org/rome-iv/rome-iv-criteria/. Accessed July 6, 2021.

26. Aberra FN. Medscape. *Which antibiotics increase the risk of developing Clostridium difficile (C diff) colitis?* In: Anand BS. ed. Updated: Jul 25, 2019 Available at: https://www.medscape.com/answers/186458-154808/which-antibiotics-increase-the-risk-of-developing-clostridium-difficile-c-diff-colitis. Accessed July 6, 2021.

27. Surawicz CM, Brandt LJ, Binion DG, et al. Guidelines for diagnosis, treatment, and prevention of clostridium difficile infections. *Am J Gastroenterol.* 2013;108:478–498.

28. 2007 Guideline for Isolation Precautions: Preventing Transmission of Infectious Agents in Healthcare Settings. Centers for Disease Control and Prevention. Available online at: http://www.cdc.gov/hicpac/2007IP/2007isolationPrecautions.html. Accessed July 5, 2021.

29. Ostojic SM, Ahmetovic Z. Gastrointestinal distress after creatine supplementation in athletes: are side effects dose dependent? *Res Sports Med.* 2008;16(1):15–22.

30. Ragunathan A, Singh P, Gosal K, et al. Laxative abuse cessation leading to severe edema. *Cureus.* June 23, 2021;13(6):e15847. https://doi.org/10.7759/cureus.15847.

31. Roerig JL, Steffen KJ, Mitchell JE, et al. Laxative abuse. epidemiology, diagnosis and management. *Drugs.* 2010;70(12):1487–1503.

32. Fecal Incontinence: National Institute of Diabetes and Digestive and Kidney Diseases. Available online at: https://www.niddk.nih.gov/health-information/digestive-diseases/bowel-control-problems-fecal-incontinence. Accessed July 6, 2021.

33. Gracey E, Vereecke L, McGovern D, et al. Revisiting the gut–joint axis: links between gut inflammation and spondyloarthritis. *Nat Rev Rheumatol.* 2020;16:415–433. https://doi.org/10.1038/s41584-020-0454-9.

34. Baeten D, De Keyser F, Van Damme N, et al. Influence of the gut and cytokine patterns in spondyloarthropathy. *Clin Exp Rheumatol.* 2002(6 Suppl 28):S38–S42. 2002.

35. Crohn's and Colitis Foundation of America: Fact Sheet. Arthritis and Joint Pain. Available online at: http://www.ccfa.org/assets/pdfs/arthritiscomplications.pdf. Accessed July 3, 2016.

36. Selmi C, Gershwin ME. Diagnosis and classification of reactive arthritis. *Autoimmun Rev.* 2014;13(4–5):546–549.

37. Psoriatic Arthritis: Patient. Available online at: http://patient.info/doctor/psoriatic-arthritis-pro. Accessed July 5, 2021.

38. Söyüncü S, Bektaş F, Cete Y. Traditional Kehr's sign: left shoulder pain related to splenic abscess. *Turkish J Trauma Emerg Surg.* 2012;18(1):87–88.

39. Doukas SG, Bhandari K, Dixon K. Psoas abscess presented as right hip pain in a young adult with Crohn's disease. *Cureus.* 2021;13(2):e13162. https://doi.org/10.7759/cureus.13162. Published 2021 Feb 5.

40. Sields D, Robinson P, Crowley TP. Danforth sign inspiration. *Int J Surg.* 2012;10(9):466–469.

41. Peterson C, Shelly E. The gastrointestinal system. In: Goodman CC, Fuller KS, eds. *Pathology: Implications for the Physical Therapist.* Elsevier; 2020:5e.

42. Mandell GL. *Mandell, Douglas, and Bennett's Principles and Practice of Infectious Diseases.* ed 7 Philadelphia: Churchill Livingstone; 2009.

43. Femoral Hernia: Patient. Available online at: http://patient.info/doctor/femoral-hernias. Accessed July 5, 2021.

44. Lupoli R, Lembo E, Saldalamacchia G, et al. Bariatric surgery and long-term nutritional issues. *World J Diabetes.* 2017;8(11):464–474. https://doi.org/10.4239/wjd.v8.i11.464.

45. Manzoni AP, Weber M. Skin changes after bariatric surgery. *An Bras Dermatol.* 2015;90(2):157–168.

46. Teitleman M, Katzka DA. A Case of Polyneuropathy After Gastric Bypass Surgery. *Medscape.* July 5, 2021 Available online at: http://www.medscape.com/viewarticle/499484_2. Accessed.

47. Griffiths TL, Nassar M, Soubani AO. Pulmonary manifestations of gastroesophageal reflux disease. *Expert Rev Respir Med.* 2020;14(8):767–775. https://doi.org/10.1080/17476348.2020.1758068.

48. Drini M. Peptic ulcer disease and non-steroidal anti-inflammatory drugs. *Aust Prescr.* 2017;40(3):91–93. https://doi.org/10.18773/austprescr.2017.037.

49. Lanza FL, Chan FK, Quigley EM, et al. Guidelines for prevention of NSAID-related ulcer complications. *Am J Gastroenterol.* 2009;104:728–738.

50. Peptic Ulcer. US National Library of Medicine. *Medline Plus.* July 5, 2021 Available online at: https://www.nlm.nih.gov/medlineplus/pepticulcer.html. Accessed.

51. Goldstein JL, Cryer B. Gastrointestinal injury associated with NSAID use: a case study and review of risk factors and preventative strategies. *Drug Health Patient Saf.* 2015;7:31–41. https://doi.org/10.2147/DHPS.S71976. Published 2015 Jan 22.

52. HajiFattahi F, Hesari M, Zojaji H, et al. Relationship of halitosis with gastric helicobacter pylori infection. *J Dent (Tehran).* 2015;12(3):200–205.

53. Yang X. Relationship between Helicobacter pylori and Rosacea: review and discussion. *BMC Infect Dis.* 2018;18(1):318 https://doi.org/10.1186/s12879-018-3232-4. Published 2018 Jul 11.

54. Wiegand T. Nonsteroidal Anti-inflammatory Drug (NSAID) Toxicity. *Medscape.* July 5, 2021 Updated May 30, 2020nm. Available online at: http://emedicine.medscape.com/article/816117-overview. Accessed.

55. Cryer B, Mahaffey KW. Gastrointestinal ulcers, role of aspirin, and clinical outcomes: pathobiology, diagnosis, and treatment. *J Multidiscip Healthc.* 2014;7:137–146.

56. Yachimski PS, Friedman LS. Gastrointestinal bleeding in the elderly. *Nat Clin Pract Gastroenterol Hepatol.* 2008;5:80–93.

57. National Institute of Diabetes and Digestive and Kidney Diseases: Definition and Facts for Diverticular Disease. Available at: https://www.niddk.nih.gov/health-information/digestive-diseases/diverticulosis-diverticulitis/definition-facts. Accessed July 6, 2021.

58. Diverticular Disease: National Institute of Diabetes and Digestive and Kidney Diseases. Available online at: http://www.niddk.nih.gov/health-information/health-topics/digestive-diseases/diverticular-disease/Pages/facts.aspx. Accessed July 6, 2021.

59. Comparato G, Pilotto A, Franzè A, et al. Diverticular disease in the elderly. *Dig Dis*. 2007;25:151–159. https://doi.org/10.1159/000099480.

60. Shahedi K. Diverticulitis, Medscape. Available online at: http://emedicine.medscape.com/article/173388-overview. Accessed July 5, 2021.

61. Diverticulitis: Mayo Clinic. Available at: https://www.mayoclinic.org/diseases-conditions/diverticulitis/symptoms-causes/syc-20371758. Accessed July 6, 2021.

62. Cleveland Clinic: Diverticulosis and Diverticulitis of the Colon. Available at: https://my.clevelandclinic.org/health/diseases/10352-diverticular-disease#symptoms-and-causes. Accessed July 6, 2021.

63. Medscape: What are the differential diagnoses for Appendicitis? Available at: https://www.medscape.com/answers/773895-18424/what-are-the-differential-diagnoses-for-appendicitis. Accessed July 7, 2021.

64. Knox M, Mortele KJ. Normal anatomy and imaging techniques of the appendix. In: Levy AD, Mortele KJ, Yeh BM, eds. *Gastrointestinal Imaging Cases*. Oxford University Press; 2015:301.

65. Akhavizadegan H. Case report missed appendicitis: mimicking urologic symptoms. *Case Rep Urol*. Dec 2012;2012

66. Odabasi M, Arslan C, Aboglu H, et al. An unusual presentation of perforated appendicitis in epigastric region. *Int J Surg Case Rep*. 2014;5(12):76–78.

67. Adams BD. Pinch-an-inch test for appendicitis. *South Med J*. 2005;98(12):1207–1209.

68. Adams BD. The pinch-an-inch test is more comfortable than rebound tenderness. *Internet J Surg*. 2007;12(2).

69. Ganguly NN, Dutta D, Kasale RJ. Pinch test: a reliable physical sign for management of acute appendicitis. *Int J Med Res Rev*. 2016;4(4):506–511.

70. Vege S. Etiology of acute pancreatitis. UpToDate. Available at: https://www.uptodate.com/contents/etiology-of-acute-pancreatitis. Accessed July 7, 2021.

71. Acute Pancreatitis Causes And Symptoms: National Pancreas Foundation. Available at: https://pancreasfoundation.org/patient-information/acute-pancreatitis/acute-pancreatitis-diagnosis-and-treatment/. Accessed July 7, 2021.

72. Bartel M. Chronic pancreatitis. Merck Manual Consumer Edition. Available at: https://www.merckmanuals.com/home/digestive-disorders/pancreatitis/chronic-pancreatitis. Accessed July 7, 2021.

73. Hamada S, Masamube A, Shimosegawa T. Pancreatic fibrosis. *Pancreapedia: Exocrine Pancreas Knowledge Base*. 2015 Nov 2015.

74. Pannu AK, Saroch A, Sharma N. Cullen's sign & acute pancreatitis, QJM: An. *International Journal of Medicine*. 2017;110(5):315. https://doi.org/10.1093/qjmed/hcx047.

75. Valette X, du Cheyron D. Cullen's and Grey Turner's signs in acute pancreatitis. *NEJM*. 2015;373:e28.

76. Chronic Pancreatitis Causes and Symptoms: The National Pancreas Foundation. Available online at: https://www.pancreasfoundation.org/patient-information/chronic-pancreatitis/causes-and-symptoms/. Accessed July 5, 2021.

77. American Cancer Society: Key Statistics for Pancreatic Cancer. Available at: https://www.cancer.org/cancer/pancreatic-cancer/about/key-statistics.html. Accessed July 8, 2021.

78. Dragonavich T. Pancreatic cancer. Medscape. Available online at: http://emedicine.medscape.com/article/280605-overview. Accessed July 5, 2021.

79. American Cancer Society: Pancreatic Cancer Risk Factors. Available at: Accessed July 8, 2021.

80. American Cancer Society: Can Pancreatic Cancer Be Found Early? Available at: https://www.cancer.org/cancer/pancreatic-cancer/detection-diagnosis-staging/detection.html. Accessed July 8, 2021.

81. Pancreatic Cancer Symptoms: Cancer Research UK. Available online at: http://www.cancerresearchuk.org/about-cancer/type/pancreatic-cancer/about/pancreatic-cancer-symptoms. Accessed July 5, 2021.

82. Rowe WA. Inflammatory bowel disease. *Medscape*. Available online at: http://emedicine.medscape.com/article/179037-overview. Accessed July 5, 2021.

83. Inflammatory Bowel Disease: Mayo Clinic. Available online at: http://www.mayoclinic.org/diseases-conditions/inflammatory-bowel-disease/basics/complications/con-20034908. Accessed July 5, 2021.

84. Crohn's and Colitis Foundation Fact Sheet. *Arthritis and Joint Pain*. Available at: https://www.crohnscolitisfoundation.org/sites/default/files/2020-03/arthritiscomplications.pdf. Accessed July 8, 2021.

85. Mark A Peppercorn, MD, Adam S, et al. Dermatologic and ocular manifestations of inflammatory bowel disease. UpToDate. Available at: https://www.uptodate.com/contents/dermatologic-and-ocular-manifestations-of-inflammatory-bowel-disease. Accessed July 8, 2021.

86. Motta I, Perricone G. Ulcerative pyoderma gangrenosum in inflammatory bowel disease. *Lancet Gastroenterol Hepatol*. June 01, 2019;4(6):488 https://doi.org/10.1016/S2468-1253(19)30038-X. Published:June, 2019.

87. Teitembaum JE. Nutrient deficiencies in inflammatory bowel disease. Up-to-date. Available online at: http://www.uptodate.com/contents/nutrient-deficiencies-in-inflammatory-bowel-disease. Accessed July 5, 2021.

88. The Crohn's and Colitis Foundation: Common Micronutrient Deficiencies in IBD. Available at: https://www.crohnscolitisfoundation.org/sites/default/files/legacy/science-and-professionals/nutrition-resource-/micronutrient-deficiency-fact.pdf. Accessed July 8, 2021.

89. National Institute of Diabetes and Digestive and Kidney Diseases: Definition and Facts for Crohn's Disease. Available at: https://www.niddk.nih.gov/health-information/digestive-diseases/crohns-disease/definition-facts. Accessed July 8, 2021.

90. Rheumatology Network: Here's What You May Not Know about IBD and Arthritis March 22, 2017 Amy Reyes Available at: https://www.rheumatologynetwork.com/view/heres-what-you-may-not-know-about-ibd-and-arthritis. Accessed July 8, 2021.

91. Inflammatory Bowel Disease and Cancer Risk: University of Michigan Health. Available at: https://www.uofmhealth.org/health-library/hw40035. Accessed July 8, 2021.

92. Ulcerative Colitis: National Institute of Diabetes and Digestive and Kidney Diseases. Available online at: http://www.niddk.nih.gov/health-information/health-topics/digestive-diseases/ulcerative-colitis/Pages/facts.aspx#5. Accessed July 4, 2016.

93. International Foundation for Gastrointestinal Disorders: Facts about IBS. Available at: https://aboutibs.org/what-is-ibs/facts-about-ibs/. Accessed July 8, 2021.

94. Jahng J, Kim YS. Irritable Bowel syndrome: is it really a functional disorder? A new perspective on alteration of enteric nervous system. *J Neurogastroenterol Motil*. 2016;22(2):163–165. https://doi.org/10.5056/jnm16043.

95. Sahoo S, Padhy SK. Cross-cultural and psychological issues in irritable bowel syndrome. *J Gastroenterol Hepatol*. 2017;32:1679–1685. https://doi.org/10.1111/jgh.13773.

96. Cleveland Clinic: Irritable Bowel Syndrome. Available at: https://my.clevelandclinic.org/health/diseases/4342-irritable-bowel-syndrome-ibs. Accessed July 8, 2021.

97. Irritable Bowel Syndrome: University of Florida health. Available at: https://ufhealth.org/irritable-bowel-syndrome. Accessed July 8, 2021.

98. Lehrer JK. How are bowel patterns classified by the Rome IV criteria for the diagnosis of irritable bowel (IBS)? Updated: Dec 11, 2019 Medscape. Available at: https://www.medscape.com/answers/180389-10035/how-are-bowel-patterns-classified-by-the-rome-iv-criteria-for-the-diagnosis-of-irritable-bowel-ibs. Accessed July 8, 2021.

99. Lehrer JK. Irritable Bowel Syndrome (IBS). Updated: Dec 11, 2019 Medscape. Available at: https://emedicine.medscape.com/article/180389-overview. Accessed July 8, 2021.

100. Centers for Disease Control and Prevention: Colorectal Cancer Statistics. Available at: https://www.cdc.gov/cancer/colorectal/statistics/index.htm. Accessed July 12, 2021.

101. Key Statistics for Colorectal Cancer: American Cancer Society. Available online at: http://www.cancer.org/cancer/colonandrectumcancer/detailedguide/colorectal-cancer-key-statistics. Accessed July 5, 2021.

102. Siegel RL, Miller KD, Goding Sauer A, et al. Colorectal cancer statistics, 2020. *CA Cancer J Clin.* 2020;70:145–164. https://doi.org/10.3322/caac.21601.

103. American Cancer Society Guidelines for the Early Detection of Cancer American Cancer Society. Available online at: http://www.cancer.org/healthy/findcancerearly/cancerscreening-guidelines/american-cancer-society-guidelines-for-the-early-detection-of-cancer. Accessed July 5, 2021.

104. American Cancer Society: Colorectal Cancer Signs and Symptoms. https://www.cancer.org/cancer/colon-rectal-cancer/detection-diagnosis-staging/signs-and-symptoms.html. Accessed July 12, 2021.

105. Wagner JM. Does this patient have appendicitis? *JAMA.* 1996;276(19):1589–1594.

106. Oberpenning F, Roth S, Leusmann DB, et al. The Alcock syndrome: temporary penile insensitivity due to compression of the pudendal nerve within the Alcock canal. *J Urol.* 1994;151(2):423–425.

107. Chiaramonte R, Pavone P, Vecchio M. Diagnosis, rehabilitation and preventive strategies for pudendal neuropathy in cyclists, a systematic review. *J Funct Morphol Kinesiol.* 2021;6(2):42. https://doi.org/10.3390/jfmk6020042.

108. Rana ALJ, Shah KB. Chapter 7 - Pudendal Neuralgia. In: Pak DJ, Yong RJ, Shah KB, eds. *Interventional Management of Chronic Visceral Pain Syndromes.* Elsevier; 2021:53–61. ISBN 9780323757751. https://doi.org/10.1016/B978-0-323-75775-1.00007-6. https://www.sciencedirect.com/science/article/pii/B9780323757751000076.

Screening for Hepatic and Biliary Disease

Hepatic and biliary organs pertain to the liver, gallbladder and the common bile duct (Fig. 10.1). They could collectively be considered as a unit because of their anatomical proximity. Functionally, there are overlapping features of some diseases that can affect these structures.[1]

The liver has the vital task of maintaining the body's metabolic homeostasis with its 500 separate functions related to the digestive, endocrine, excretory, and hematologic systems.[1,2] While the liver has enormous functional reserve and regenerative capacity, conditions affecting liver function could result in life-threatening consequences.[1]

The gallbladder is a small pouch located under the liver and acts as a reservoir for bile. The arrival of food signals the gallbladder to contract, expelling bile to the duodenum through the common bile duct. Bile assists in fat emulsification, absorption and digestion[2] of fat.

Medical conditions affecting these organs can have presentations that mimic primary musculoskeletal lesions. The musculoskeletal symptoms associated with hepatic and biliary pathologic conditions are generally confined to the midback, scapular, and right shoulder regions. They can occur as the only presenting symptom, or in combination with other systemic signs and symptoms discussed in this chapter.

HEPATIC AND BILIARY SIGNS AND SYMPTOMS

The major causes of acute hepatocellular injury include hepatitis, drug-induced hepatitis, and ingestion of hepatotoxins. The physical therapist is most likely to encounter liver or gallbladder diseases manifested by a variety of signs and symptoms outlined in this section.

Taking a careful history and making close observations of the client's physical condition and appearance can detect telltale signs of hepatic disease. Most of the liver is contained underneath the rib cage and is largely inaccessible (Fig. 10.2). An enlarged liver that is palpable is always a red flag (see Figs. 4.50 and 10.3).[3] Medical diagnosis of liver or gallbladder disease could be made by medical imaging of the abdomen, including the liver. Blood tests may be used to look for signs of infection or obstruction. Laboratory tests useful in the diagnosis and treatment of liver and biliary tract disease are listed on the inside back cover.

Skin and Nail Bed Changes

Skin changes associated with impairment of the hepatic system include jaundice (yellowing of the skin or whites of the eyes), pallor, or orange or green skin in a person with light skin tones. Change in skin tones may be harder to detect in individuals with darker skin tones. In some situations jaundice may be the first and only manifestation of disease. It is first noticeable in people of all skin colors in the sclera of the eye as a yellow hue when bilirubin reaches levels of 2 mg/dL to 3 mg/dL. When the bilirubin level reaches 5 mg/dL to 6 mg/dL, changes in skin color occur (Fig. 10.4).

Other skin changes may include pruritus (itching), bruising, spider angiomas (Fig. 10.5), and palmar erythema (see Fig. 10.6). *Spider angiomas* (arterial spider, spider telangiectasis, vascular spider), branched dilations of the superficial capillaries resembling a spider in appearance, may be vascular manifestations of increased estrogen levels (hyperestrogenism). Spider angiomas and palmar erythema both occur in the presence of liver impairment as a result of increased estrogen levels normally detoxified by the liver.

Palmar erythema, also called liver palms, refers to the reddening of the skin over the palms. This condition is caused by an extensive collection of arteriovenous anastomoses and is especially evident on the hypothenar and thenar eminences and the pulps of the fingers (Fig. 10.6).[4] The person may complain of throbbing, tingling palms and the soles of the feet may be similarly affected (called plantar erythema). Various forms of nail disease have been described in cases of liver impairment, such as the white nails of Terry (Fig. 10.7). Other nail bed changes, such as white bands across the nail plate (leukonychia), clubbed nails (see Fig. 4.36), or koilonychia (see Fig. 4.32), can occur, but these are not specific to liver impairment and can also develop in the presence of other diseases.

Musculoskeletal Pain

Musculoskeletal pain associated with the hepatic and biliary systems includes thoracic pain between the scapulae, right shoulder, right upper trapezius, right interscapular, or right subscapular areas.[5,6] (Table 10.1).

Referred shoulder pain may be the only presenting symptom of hepatic or biliary disease. Afferent pain signals from

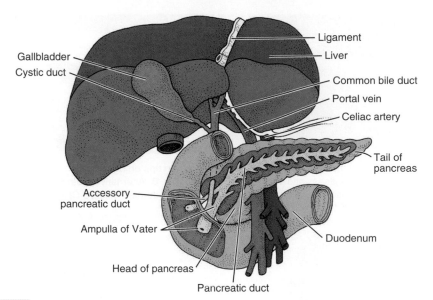

Fig. 10.1   Anatomy of the liver, gallbladder, common bile duct, and pancreas. The pear-shaped *gallbladder* is tucked up under the right side of the liver. The *pancreas* is located behind the stomach anterior to the L1 to L3 vertebral bodies. It is about 6 inches long, wide at one end (the head), then tapered through the body to the narrow end called the tail.

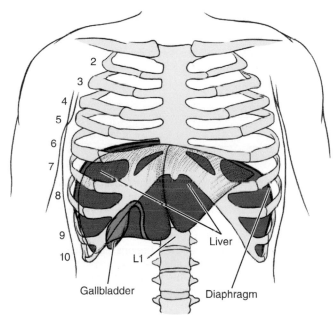

Fig. 10.2   Location of the liver and gallbladder. The *liver* is located just below the respiratory diaphragm, predominately on the right side, but with a portion crossing the midline to the left side. It is a large organ and spans many vertebral levels. The most superior part is the dome of the right lobe. The "peak" of the dome lies at about T8 or T9 during expiration. The inferior border of the left lobe is located just below the level of the left nipple and inclines downward to the right at the tip of the eighth costal margin. The right lobe angles downward to the ninth and tenth costal margins. Posteriorly, the liver is located from approximately T9 to L1 at the midline. This varies from person to person and with inhalation (moves up a level or two) and exhalation (moves down). The fundus (base) of the *gallbladder* usually appears below the edge of the liver in contact with the anterior abdominal wall at the tip of the ninth right costal cartilage.

the superior ligaments of the liver and the superior portion of the liver capsule are transmitted by the phrenic nerves. Sympathetic fibers from the biliary system are connected through the celiac (abdominal) and splanchnic (visceral) plexuses to the hepatic fibers in the region of the dorsal spine (see Fig. 3.3).

The celiac and splanchnic connections account for the intercostal and radiating interscapular pain that accompanies gallbladder disease. Although the innervation is bilateral, most of the biliary fibers reach the cord through the right splanchnic nerves, synapsing with adjacent phrenic nerve fibers innervating the diaphragm and producing pain in the right shoulder (see Fig. 3.4).

Hepatic osteodystrophy, abnormal development of bone, can occur in all forms of cholestasis (bile flow suppression) and hepatocellular disease, especially in individuals who abuse alcohol. Either osteomalacia, or more often, osteoporosis, frequently accompanies bone pain from this condition. Vertebral wedging and kyphosis can be severe. It has been reported from 3% to 18% of individuals with chronic liver disease have osteoporosis.[7]

Pseudofractures, or Looser's zones, are narrow lines of radiolucency (areas of darkness on a radiograph), usually oriented perpendicular to the bone surface. This may represent a stress fracture that is repaired by laying down inadequately mineralized osteoid, or these sites may occur as a result of mechanical erosion caused by arterial pulsations, because arteries frequently overlie sites of pseudofractures.

Osteoporosis associated with primary biliary cirrhosis and primary sclerosing cholangitis parallels the severity of liver disease rather than its duration. Painful osteoarthropathy may develop in the wrists and ankles as a nonspecific complication

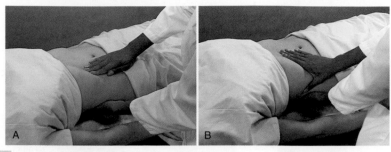

Fig. 10.3 Palpating the liver. **A**, Fingers are extended, with tips on right midclavicular line below the level of liver dullness and pointing toward the head. **B**, Alternative method with the fingers parallel to the costal margin. (From: Ball J, Drains J. Abdomen: *Seidel's Guide to Physical Examination*. Elsevier, 2019. Pp. 393-436.)

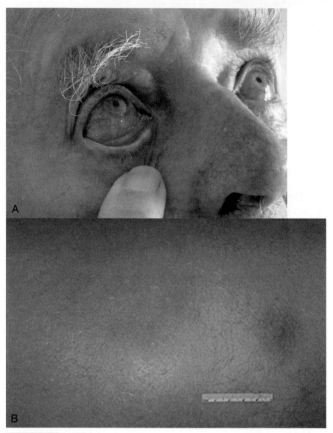

Fig. 10.4 Jaundice condition which causes yellowing of the sclera, *A*, and the skin, *B*, due to high levels of circulating bilirubin, a yellow-orange bile pigment. (From: *A*: Raftery Andrew: *Jaundice. Churchill's Pocketbook of Differential Diagnosis*. Elsevier. 2014, pp. 256-261. *B*, Klatt, EC: *The Liver and Biliary Tract. Robbins and Cotran Atlas of Pathology*. Elsevier, 2021. pp. 225-249.e10.)

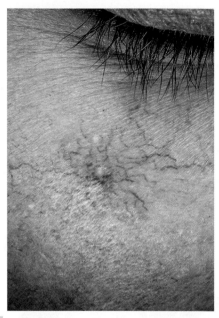

Fig. 10.5 Spider angioma. Permanently enlarged and dilated capillaries visible on the surface of the skin caused by vascular dilation are called *spider angiomas*. These capillary radiations can be flat or raised in the center. Most patients have one or two lesions. They are found most commonly on the face, upper part of the trunk, and backs of the hands. Lesions may occur during pregnancy and resolve months after delivery. Suspect liver disease in patients with many lesions. They do not go away when the underlying lesion is treated; laser therapy is available to remove them for cosmetic reasons. (From Habif PH: *Clinical Dermatology: a Color Guide to Diagnosis and Therapy*, ed 5, St. Louis, 2010, Mosby.)

of chronic liver disease. *Rhabdomyolysis*[5] is a potentially fatal condition is which myoglobin and other muscle tissue contents are released into the bloodstream as a result of muscle tissue disintegration. This could occur with acute trauma (e.g., crush injuries, significant blunt trauma, high-voltage electrical burns, surgery), severe burns, overexertion, or in the case of liver impairment, from alcohol abuse or alcohol poisoning or the use of statins.[8] Most recently, rhabdomyolysis has been noted in the initial presentations of individuals diagnosed with COVID-19 disease.[9,10]

Rhabdomyolysis is characterized by muscle aches, cramps, soreness, and weakness. It may be accompanied by other symptoms of respiratory muscle myopathy (impaired diaphragmatic function)[11] or liver or renal involvement. Laboratory testing will show a creatine kinase (CK) level more than 10 times the upper limit of normal.

Statin-associated myopathy appears to occur more often in people with complex medical problems and/or those who abuse substances such as alcohol, cocaine, and opioids. For additional discussion, see Screening for Side Effects of Statins in Chapter 7.

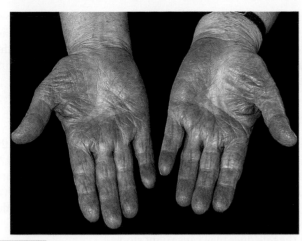

Fig. 10.6 Palmar erythema caused by liver impairment presents as a warm redness of the skin over the palms and soles of the feet in the Caucasian population. Darker skin tones may change from a tan color to a gray appearance. Look for other signs of liver disease such as changes in the nail beds, spider angiomas, liver flap, and bilateral carpal or tarsal tunnel syndrome. Palmar erythema can occur in healthy individuals and in association with nonhepatic diseases. (From Glynn M, Drake WM. *Hutchison's clinical methods: An integrated approach to clinical practice*, ed. 23, 2012, Saunders Ltd.)

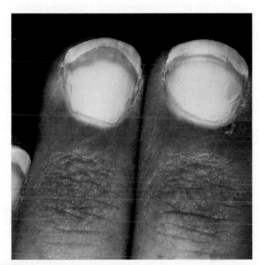

Fig. 10.7 Nails of Terry. Opaque white nails of Terry in a patient with cirrhosis. Various forms of nail disease have been described in patients with cirrhosis. This is an example of the classic white nails of Terry characterized by an opaque nail plate with a narrow line of pink at the distal end instead of the more normal pink nail plate in the Caucasian. Nails of Terry can also present as a result of malnutrition, diabetes mellitus, hyperthyroidism, trauma, and sometimes for unknown reasons (idiopathic). (From Habif, PH: *Clinical Dermatology: A Color Guide to Diagnosis and Therapy*, ed 5, St. Louis, 2010, Mosby.)

Neurologic Symptoms

Neurologic symptoms, such as confusion, sleep disturbances, muscle tremors, hyperreactive reflexes, and asterixis, may occur. When liver dysfunction results in increased serum ammonia and urea levels, peripheral nerve function can be impaired.

TABLE 10.1	Referred Pain Patterns: Liver, Gallbladder, and Common Bile Duct
Systemic Causes	Location (see Fig. 10.11)
Liver disease (abscess, cirrhosis, tumors, hepatitis)	Thoracic spine (T7-T10; midline to the right) Right upper trapezius and shoulder
Gallbladder	Right upper trapezius and shoulder Right interscapular area (T4 or T5-T8) Right subscapular area

Ammonia from the intestine that is produced by protein breakdown, is normally transformed by the liver to urea, glutamine, and asparagine, which are then excreted by the renal system. When the liver does not detoxify ammonia, it is transported to the brain, where it reacts with glutamate, an excitatory neurotransmitter, producing glutamine. This results in the reduction of glutamate concentration in the brain, leading to altered central nervous system (CNS) metabolism and function. Symptoms of poor concentration, fatigue, and other symptoms of encephalopathy can result.

Another outward sign of liver disease producing CNS dysfunction is *asterixis*. Also called *flapping tremors* or *liver flap*, asterixis is described as the inability to maintain wrist extension with forward flexion of the upper extremities. It is tested by asking the client to actively hyperextend the wrist and hand with the rest of the arm supported on a firm surface or with the arms held out in front of the body (Fig. 10.8).[12]

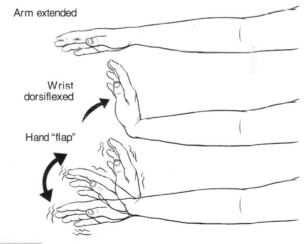

Arm extended

Wrist dorsiflexed

Hand "flap"

Fig. 10.8 To test for asterixis or liver flap, have the client extend the arms, spread the fingers, extend the wrist, and observe for the abnormal "flapping" tremor at the wrist. If a tremor is not readily apparent, ask the client to keep the arms straight while gently hyperextending the client's wrist. There is an alternate method of testing for this phenomenon: have the client relax the legs in the supine position with the knees bent. The feet are flat on the table. As the legs fall to the sides, watch for a flapping or tremoring of the legs at the hip. The knees appear to come back toward the midline repeatedly.[9]

The test is positive if quick, irregular extensions and flexions of the wrist and fingers occur. This condition is caused by an inability of the motor centers of the diencephalon to regulate the tone of the agonistic and antagonistic muscles to maintain correct posture and movement.

There are many potential causes of carpal tunnel syndrome, both musculoskeletal and systemic (see Table 12.2), including liver impairment (Case Example 10.1). Careful examination and evaluation are required; see Box 10.1 for examples of questions to ask or things to look for to evaluate this association.

It is important to generate an accurate history and to closely observe the client to determine if there is a need for medical referral because of possible liver disease. It is not uncommon to observe jaundice in the client postsurgery, but it can be a potentially serious complication of liver damage that follows surgery and anesthesia. Clues to screening for hepatic disease (see Clues to Screening for Hepatic Disease at the end of this chapter) should be taken into consideration when evaluating the clinical history and observations.

Gastrointestinal System

Normally, bilirubin that is excreted in bile and carried to the small intestines is reduced to a form that causes the stool to assume a brown color. Light-colored (almost white) stools and urine the color of tea or cola indicate an inability of the liver or biliary system to excrete bilirubin properly. Gallbladder disease, hepatotoxic medications, or pancreatic cancer blocking the bile duct may cause light stools.

TABLE 10.2	Comparison of Hepatitis A, B and C		
	Hepatitis A	**Hepatitis B**	**Hepatitis C**
Routes of transmission	Fecal-oral route	Percutaneous, mucosal, or noncontact skin exposure to infectious blood, semen and other body fluids. HVB is concentrated most highly in blood, and percutaneous exposure is an efficient mode of transmission.	Direct percutaneous exposure to infected blood. Mucous membrane exposures to blood can also result in transmission, although this route is less efficient
Incubation period	15-50 days (average: 28 days)	60-150 days (average: 90 days)	14-182 days (average range: 14-84 days)
Symptoms of acute infection	Symptoms of all types of viral hepatitis are similar and can include one of more of the following: jaundice, fever, fatigue, loss of appetite, nausea, vomiting, abdominal pain, joint pain, dark urine, clay colored stool, diarrhea (HVA only)		
Potential for Chronic Infection after Acute Infection	None	Chronic infection develops in: • 90% of infants after acute infection at birth • 25-50% of children newly infected at ages 1-5 years • 5% of people newly infected as adults	Chronic infection develops in over 50% of newly infected people.
Severity	• Most people with acute disease recover with no lasting liver damage; death is uncommon but occurs more often among older people and/or those with underlying liver disease	• Most people with acute disease recover with no lasting liver damage; acute illness is rarely fatal • 15%-25% of people with chronic infection develop chronic liver disease, including cirrhosis, liver failure, or liver cancer	• Approximately 5% to 25% of persons with chronic hepatitis C will develop cirrhosis over 10-20 years • People with hepatitis C and cirrhosis have 1%-4% annual risk for hepatocellular carcinoma
Treatment	• No medication available • Best addressed through supportive treatment	• Acute: no medication available; best addressed through supportive treatment • Chronic: regular monitoring for signs of liver disease progression; antiviral drugs are available	• Acute: AASLD/IDSA recommend treatment of acute HCV without a waiting period • Chronic: over 90% of people with hepatitis C can be cured regardless of HCV genotype with 8-12 weeks of oral therapy
Vaccination schedule	• Single-antigen hepatitis vaccine: 2 doses given 6-18 months apart depending on manufacturer • Combination HepA-HepB vaccine: typically 3 doses given over a 6-month period	• Infants and children: 3-4 doses given over a 6- to 18-month period depending on vaccine type and schedule • Adults: 2 doses, 1 month apart or 3 doses over a 6-month period (depending on manufacturer)	• No vaccine available

Excerpts from: Centers of Disease Control. The ABCs of Hepatitis-for Health Professionals. Available at: https://www.cdc.gov/hepatitis/resources/professionals/pdfs/abctable.pdf
Accessed July 25, 2021. More detailed information could be found in the original CDC document.

CASE EXAMPLE 10.1

Carpal Tunnel Syndrome from Liver Impairment

A 45-year-old truck driver was diagnosed by a hand surgeon as having bilateral carpal tunnel syndrome (CTS) and referred to physical therapy. A screening examination was not performed during the evaluation. During the course of treatment, the client commented that he was seeing an acupuncturist, who told him that liver disease was the cause of his bilateral CTS.

The therapist suspected a history of alcohol abuse, which is a risk factor for liver disease. Further questioning at that time indicated the lack of any other associated symptoms to suggest liver or hepatic involvement. However, because his symptoms were bilateral and there is a known correlation between liver disease and CTS, the referring physician was notified of these findings.

The client was referred for evaluation, and a diagnosis of liver cancer was confirmed. Physical therapy for CTS was appropriately discontinued.

BOX 10.1 EVALUATING CARPAL TUNNEL SYNDROME ASSOCIATED WITH LIVER IMPAIRMENT

For any client presenting with bilateral carpal tunnel syndrome:
- Ask about the presence of similar symptoms in the feet
- Ask about a personal history of liver or hepatic disease (e.g., cirrhosis, cancer, hepatitis)
- Look for a history of hepatotoxic drugs (see Box 10.3)
- Look for a history of alcoholism
- Ask about current or previous use of statins (cholesterol-lowering drugs such as Crestor, Lipitor, Mevacor, or Zocor)
- Look for other signs and symptoms associated with liver impairment (see Clinical Signs and Symptoms of Liver Disease)
  - Test for signs of liver disease
  - Skin color changes
  - Spider angiomas
  - Palmar erythema (liver palms)
  - Change in nail beds (e.g., white nails of Terry, white bands, clubbing)
  - Asterixis (liver flap)

CLINICAL SIGNS AND SYMPTOMS

Liver Disease

Gastrointestinal
- Sense of fullness of the abdomen
- Anorexia, nausea, and vomiting

Integumentary
- Change in skin color and nail beds
- Pallor (often linked to cirrhosis or carcinoma)
- Jaundice
- Bruising
- Spider angioma
- Palmar erythema
- White nails of Terry, other nail bed changes may be present

Hepatic
- Dark urine and light-colored or clay-colored stools
- Ascites (Fig. 10.9)
- Edema and oliguria (reduced urine secretion in relation to fluid intake)
- Right upper quadrant (RUQ) abdominal pain

Musculoskeletal
- Musculoskeletal pain, especially right shoulder pain
- Myopathy (rhabdomyolysis in severe cases)

Neurologic
- Confusion
- Sleep disturbances
- Muscle tremors
- Hyperactive reflexes
- Asterixis (motor disturbance resembling body or extremity flapping)
- Bilateral carpal tunnel syndrome (numbness, tingling, burning pain in thumb, index, and middle fingers)
- Bilateral tarsal tunnel (tarsal tunnel characterized by pain around the ankle that extends to the palmar surfaces of the toes, made worse by walking)

Other
- Gynecomastia (enlargement of breast tissue in men)

CLINICAL SIGNS AND SYMPTOMS

Gallbladder Disease

Gastrointestinal
- Right upper abdominal pain
- Indigestion, nausea, feeling of fullness
- Excessive belching, flatulence (intestinal gas)
- Intolerance of fatty foods

Integumentary
- Jaundice (result of blockage of the common bile duct)
- Persistent pruritus (skin itching)

Musculoskeletal
- Sudden, excruciating pain in the mid epigastrium with referral to the back and right shoulder (acute cholecystitis)
- Anterior rib pain (tip of tenth rib; can also affect ribs 11 and 12)

Constitutional
- Low-grade fever, chills

HEPATIC AND BILIARY PATHOPHYSIOLOGY

Liver Diseases

Hepatitis

Hepatitis is an acute or chronic inflammation of the liver. It can be caused by a virus, a chemical, a drug reaction, or alcohol abuse. In addition, hepatitis can be secondary to disease conditions, such as an infection with other viruses (e.g., Epstein-Barr virus or cytomegalovirus).

Viral Hepatitis. Viral hepatitis is an acute infectious inflammation of the liver caused by one of the following identified viruses: hepatitis A (HAV), hepatitis B (HBV), hepatitis C (HCV), hepatitis D (HDV), hepatitis E (HEV), or Hepatitis G (HGV).[13] More than 90% of acute cases of vital hepatitis in the United States is caused by HAV, HBV, and HCV.[13] Table 10.2 lists important characteristics of HAV, HBV, and HCV.

Hepatitis is a major uncontrolled public health problem for many reasons. Not all of the causative agents have been identified, there are limited specific drugs for its treatment, its incidence has increased in relation to illicit drug use, and it can be spread before the appearance of observable clinical symptoms. Viral hepatitis is spread easily to others and usually results in an extended period of convalescence with loss of time from school or work. Many cases are unreported because the persons infected with the disease are either asymptomatic or only have mild symptoms. It is not until these individuals develop cirrhosis of the liver, end-stage liver disease, or hepatocellular carcinoma years or decades after that they find out that hepatitis infection had occurred.

HAV and HEV are transmitted primarily by the fecal-oral route. Common source outbreaks result from contaminated food or water. HAV must also be considered a potential problem in situations where fecal-oral communication along with food handling and/or unsanitary conditions occur. Some examples of potential sources of contact with HAV might include restaurants, day care centers, correctional institutions, sewage plants, and countries where these viruses are endemic.[13]

Hepatitis viruses B, C, D, and G are primarily blood-borne pathogens that can be transmitted from percutaneous or mucosal exposures to blood or other body fluids from an infected person.

HBV is usually transmitted by inoculation of infected blood or blood products or by sexual contact and is also found in body fluids (e.g., spinal, peritoneal, pleural), saliva, semen, and vaginal secretions. HDV must have HBV present to coinfect. Groups at risk include, but are not limited to, health care workers and emergency responders, sexually active heterosexuals with more than one partner in the last 6 months, men who have sex with men, illicit drug users, and residents and workers in correctional facilities.[14] Table 10.3 lists the risk factors for hepatitis.

People with mild to moderate acute hepatitis rarely require hospitalization. The emphasis is on preventing the spread of infectious agents and avoiding further liver damage when the underlying cause is drug-induced or toxic hepatitis. People with fulminant (sudden and severe onset) hepatitis require special management because of the rapid progression of their disease and the potential need for urgent liver transplantation.

TABLE 10.3	Risk Factors for Hepatitis.			
HAV	HBV	HCV	HDV	HEV
Household contacts or sexual contacts of infected persons	Injection drug use	Sharing needles or other equipment to inject drugs; people who use intranasal drugs	Same as B	Same as A
Men who have sex with men	Sex with an infected partner			
Injection/noninjection illegal drug users (regional outbreaks reported)	Incarceration in correctional facilities—adults and youth (drug use, unsafe sexual practices)	Received blood transfusion or organ transplant before July 1992 or blood clotting products made before 1987		
Living in areas with increased rates of HAV (children at greatest risk)	Contact with blood or open sores of an infected person	People with HIV infection		
Travel in areas where HAV is epidemic	Travel to high-risk areas			
Blood clotting factor disorder received prior to 1987	Occupational risk: morticians, dental workers, emergency medical technicians, firefighters, health care workers in contact with body fluid or blood	Occupational risk in health care workers after needle sticks.		
	Liver transplant recipient	Evidence of liver disease		
	Infants born to mothers with HBV	Infants born to HCV-infected mothers		
	Multiple blood product or blood transfusions before July 1992	Chronic kidney dialysis (clients/staff)		
	Sharing items such as razors or toothbrushes with an infected person			

From: Peterson C. The Hepatic, Pancreatic and Biliary Systems. Goodman and Fuller's Pathology: Implications for the Physical Therapist. 5th ed. Elsevier, 2020.

An entire spectrum of rheumatic diseases can occur concomitantly with HBV and HBC, including transient arthralgias, vasculitis, polyarteritis nodosa, rheumatoid arthritis (RA), fibromyalgia, lymphoma, Sjögren's syndrome, and persistent synovitis. Some conditions such as RA and fibromyalgia occur only in association with HCV, whereas others, such as polyarteritis nodosa, are observed in association with both forms of hepatitis.[15,16]

Rheumatic manifestations of hepatitis are varied early in the course of disease and can be indistinguishable from mild RA. The therapist should be suspicious of anyone with risk factors for hepatitis, including injection drug use; previous blood transfusion, especially before 1991; hemodialysis; other

---

BOX 10.2   RISK FACTORS FOR HEPATITIS

- Injection drug use
- Acupuncture
- Tattoo inscription or removal
- Ear or body piercing
- Recent operative procedure
- Liver transplant recipient
- Blood or plasma transfusion before 1991
- Hemodialysis
- Health care worker exposed to blood products or body fluids
- Exposure to certain chemicals or medications
- Unprotected sexual activity
- Severe alcoholism
- Travel to high-risk areas
- Consumption of raw shellfish

CASE EXAMPLE 10.2

Hepatitis C

A 43-year-old man, 1 year following traumatic injury to the right forearm, underwent surgery to transplant his great toe to function as a thumb. The surgery took place in another state, and the man, who had been a client in our facility before surgery, returned for postoperative rehabilitation.

Complaints of hives of the involved forearm, fatigue, depression, and increased perspiration were documented but attributed by his physician to recovery from the traumatic injury and the multiple operations. Medical records from the hospital consisted of therapy notes only.

Eventually, the client developed a yellowing of the sclerae (white outer coat of the eyeballs). Medical referral was requested, and the client was evaluated by an internal medicine specialist.

Hepatitis C was diagnosed, and full medical records then obtained revealed that although the man had donated his own blood in advance for the surgery, he was short by one unit, which he received through a blood bank. The blood donation was attributed as the probable source of contamination.

Continued physical therapy intervention was modified to accommodate liver impairment with particular attention paid to activity level. The therapist also observed the client carefully for signs of fluid shift such as weight gain and orthostasis, dehydration, pneumonia, and vascular problems.

CLINICAL SIGNS AND SYMPTOMS

Hepatitis A

Hepatitis A is often acquired in childhood as a mild infection with symptoms similar to the "flu" and may be misdiagnosed or ignored. It does not usually cause lasting damage to the liver, although the following symptoms may persist for weeks:
- Extreme fatigue
- Anorexia
- Fever
- Arthralgia and myalgia (generalized aching)
- Right upper abdominal pain
- Clay-colored stools
- Dark urine
- Icterus (jaundice)
- Headache
- Pharyngitis
- Alteration in senses of taste and smell
- Loss of desire to smoke cigarettes or drink alcohol
- Low-grade fever
- Indigestion (varying degrees of nausea, heartburn, flatulence)

CLINICAL SIGNS AND SYMPTOMS

Hepatitis B

HBV may be asymptomatic but can include:
- Jaundice (change in skin and eye color)
- Arthralgia
- Rash (over entire body)
- Dark urine
- Anorexia, nausea
- Painful abdominal bloating
- Fever

---

exposure to blood products/body fluids, such as a health care worker (Box 10.2), or a past history of hepatitis that currently appears with arthralgias (Case Example 10.2).

Other red-flag symptoms include joint or muscle pain that is disproportionate to the physical findings, the presence of palmar tendinitis in someone with RA, and positive risk factors for hepatitis.

Chronic Hepatitis. *Chronic hepatitis* is the term used to describe an illness associated with prolonged inflammation of the liver that lasts greater than 6 months.[17] The symptoms and biochemical abnormalities may continue for months or years. It is divided into *chronic active hepatitis* (CAH) and *chronic persistent hepatitis* (CPH) by findings on liver biopsy. Chronic active hepatitis can lead to cirrhosis because of its aggressive process of hepatocellular necrosis and fibrosis.[18] This condition is often a result of HBV, HCV, or HDV infection, autoimmune mechanisms (autoimmune hepatitis) and drugs such as isoniazid, methyldopa, nitrofurantoin, and acetaminophen (rare).[17] Treatment includes antiviral treatments for chronic HBV (entecavir and tenofovir are considered first-line therapies) and interferon-free regimens of direct-acting antivirals for chronic HCV.[17]

CLINICAL SIGNS AND SYMPTOMS
Chronic Active Hepatitis

The clinical signs and symptoms of chronic active hepatitis may range from asymptomatic to the person who is bedridden with cirrhosis and advanced hepatocellular failure. In the latter the prominent signs and symptoms may reflect multisystem involvement, including:
- Fatigue
- Jaundice
- Abdominal pain
- Anorexia
- Arthralgia
- Fever
- Splenomegaly and hepatomegaly
- Weakness
- Ascites (see Fig. 10.9)
- Hepatic encephalopathy

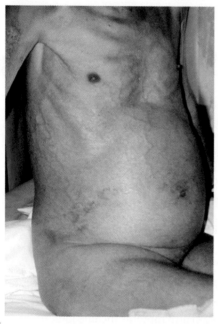

Fig. 10.9 Ascites is an abnormal accumulation of serous (edematous) fluid in the peritoneal cavity associated with liver impairment, especially the portal and hepatic venous hypertension that accompanies cirrhosis of the liver. This condition also may be associated with other disorders such as advanced congestive heart failure, constrictive pericarditis, cancer, chronic hepatitis, and hyperaldosteronism. Any condition affecting the peritoneum by producing increased permeability of the peritoneal capillaries and electrolyte disturbances can result in ascites. (From Little J, Falace D, Miller C, et al.: *Dental Management of the Medically Compromised Patient*, ed 7, St. Louis, 2008, Mosby.)

CLINICAL SIGNS AND SYMPTOMS
Chronic Persistent Hepatitis

- Right upper quadrant (RUQ) pain
- Anorexia
- Mild fatigue
- Malaise

CLINICAL SIGNS AND SYMPTOMS
Toxic and Drug-Induced Hepatitis

These vary with the severity of liver damage and the causative agent. In most individuals symptoms resemble those of acute viral hepatitis:
- Anorexia, nausea, vomiting
- Fatigue and malaise
- Jaundice
- Dark urine
- Clay-colored stools
- Headache, dizziness, drowsiness (carbon tetrachloride poisoning)
- Fever, rash, arthralgias, epigastric or right upper quadrant (RUQ) pain

Metabolic Disease. The most common metabolic diseases that can cause chronic hepatitis and are of interest to a physical therapist are Wilson's disease and hematochromatosis, also termed *hemochromatosis*. Both of these diseases are covered greater detail as metabolic disorders in Chapter 12.

Wilson's disease is an autosomal recessive disorder in which biliary excretion of copper is impaired, and as a consequence, total body copper is progressively increased.[19] There may be mild-to-severe neurologic dysfunction, depending on the rate of hepatocyte injury.[20]

Hemochromatosis is the most common genetic disorder (autosomal recessive defect in iron absorption) causing liver failure. Excessive iron is stored in various parenchymal organs with subsequent development of fibrosis. Arthralgia and arthropathy may develop and are often confused with RA or osteoarthritis.[21,22] The second and third metacarpophalangeal joints are usually involved first. Knees, hips, shoulders, and the low back may be affected. Acute synovitis with pseudogout of the knees has been observed.

Nonviral Hepatitis. Nonviral hepatitis is considered to be a toxic or drug-induced form of liver inflammation. This type of hepatitis occurs secondary to exposure to alcohol, certain chemicals or drugs such as antiinflammatories, anticonvulsants, antibiotics, cytotoxic drugs for the treatment of cancer, antituberculars, radiographic contrast agents for diagnostic testing, antipsychotics, alkaline water products,[23] and antidepressants (Box 10.3).

Acetaminophen, the popular over-the-counter (OTC) pain reliever, has been found to be the most common cause of acute liver failure (ALF) in the United States.[24] The drug is safe when taken properly, but even a small overdose in some people can cause acetaminophen hepatotoxicity that may trigger sudden liver failure. The use of this drug becomes even more dangerous when taken by individuals with an already impaired liver.[25]

Cirrhosis

Cirrhosis is a chronic hepatic disease characterized by the destruction of liver cells and by the replacement of connective tissue by fibrous bands. As the liver becomes more and more scarred (fibrosed), blood and lymph flow become impaired,

BOX 10.3 COMMON HEPATOTOXIC AGENTS

Analgesics
Acetaminophen
Aspirin
Diclofenac

Anesthetics
Halothane
Enflurane
Methoxyflurane
Chloroform

Anticonvulsants
Valproic acid
Phenytoin
Carbamazepine
Lamotrigine

Antidepressants/ antipsychotics
Monoamine oxidase (MAO) inhibitors
Chlorpromazine and other phenothiazines

Antineoplastics
Methotrexate (related to cumulative dose)
Mercaptopurine
L-asparaginase
Carmustine, lomustine
Streptozocin

Antimicrobials
Chloramphenicol
Isoniazid (antitubercular)
Oxacillin
Erythromycin estolate

Novobiocin
Ketoconazole (antifungal)
Nitrofurantoin
Sulfonamides (class)
Minocycline
Tetracyclines (class)
Efavirenz (antiviral)
Nevirapine (antiviral)
Ritonavir (antiviral)

Cardiovascular
Quinidine sulfate
Amiodarone
Methyldopa

Hormonal
Oral contraceptives
Anabolic steroids
Oral hypoglycemics

Recreational Drugs
Alcohol
Cocaine
Ecstasy

Vitamins
Vitamin A (large doses)
Niacin (large doses)

Other
Carbon tetrachloride
Poisonous mushrooms
Heavy metals
Phosphorus
Tannic acid
Propylthiouracil
Diagnostic contrast agents

CLINICAL SIGNS AND SYMPTOMS

Cirrhosis

- Mild right upper quadrant (RUQ) pain (progressive)
- GI symptoms
- Anorexia
- Indigestion
- Weight loss
- Nausea and vomiting
- Diarrhea or constipation
- Dull abdominal ache
- Ease of fatigue (with mild exertion)
- Weakness
- Fever

causing hepatic insufficiency and increased clinical manifestations. The causes of cirrhosis can be varied, although alcohol abuse is the most common cause of liver disease in the United States.

In addition, about 25 of Americans have been reported to have nonalcoholic fatty liver disease (NAFLD),[26,27] defined as fatty infiltration of the liver exceeding 5% to 10% by weight. NAFLD is the most comment form of chronic liver disease, with increasing worldwide prevalence, especially in nations in the western hemisphere. Those with the condition develop liver inflammation, leading to liver scarring and cirrhosis.[27] Disease associated with NAFLD include, but are not limited to the following: high cholesterol, high levels of triglycerides, metabolic syndrome, obesity and type 2 diabetes.[26] Prevention and treatment of diabetes, obesity, and insulin resistance and protection of the liver from medications that cause fatty infiltration and toxins can help to limit the course of this disease.[28]

The activity level of the client with damage from chronic liver impairment is determined by the symptoms. Because hepatic blood flow diminishes with moderate exercise, rest periods are advised and are adjusted according to the level of fatigue experienced by the client both during the exercise and afterward at home.

The person may return to work with medical approval but is advised to avoid straining, such as lifting heavy objects, if portal hypertension and esophageal varices are a problem. Because stress decreases hepatic blood flow, any reduction of stress at home, at work, or during treatment is therapeutic.

Progression of Cirrhosis. As cirrhosis progresses and hepatic insufficiency develops, a series of conditions emerges, including portal hypertension, ascites, and esophageal varices. Late symptoms affecting the entire body develop (Table 10.4).

Portal hypertension refers to elevated pressure in the portal vein (through which blood passes from the GI tract and spleen to the liver) occurring as portal blood meets increased resistance to flow in the fibrotic liver. The blood then backs up into esophageal, stomach, and splenic structures and bypasses the liver through collateral vessels.

Ascites is an abnormal accumulation of fluid containing large amounts of protein and electrolytes in the peritoneal cavity as a result of portal backup and loss of proteins. Cirrhosis of the liver is the most common cause of ascites.[29] The condition presents as a distended abdomen, bulging flanks, and a protruding, displaced umbilicus (see Fig. 10.9).

CLINICAL SIGNS AND SYMPTOMS

Portal Hypertension

- Ascites (see Fig. 10.9)
- Dilated collateral veins
- Esophageal varices (upper GI)
- Hemorrhoids (lower GI)
- Splenomegaly (enlargement of the spleen)
- Thrombocytopenia (decreased number of blood platelets for clotting)

TABLE 10.4	Clinical Manifestations of Cirrhosis
Body System	Clinical Manifestations
Respiratory	Limited thoracic expansion (caused by ascites) Hypoxia • Dyspnea • Cyanosis • Clubbing
Central nervous system (progressive to hepatic coma)	Subtle changes in mental acuity (progressive) Mild memory loss Poor reasoning ability Irritability Paranoia and hallucinations Slurred speech Asterixis (tremor of outstretched hands) Peripheral neuritis Peripheral muscle atrophy
Hematologic	Impaired coagulation/bleeding tendencies • Nosebleeds • Easy bruising • Bleeding gums Anemia (usually caused by GI blood loss from esophageal varices)
Endocrine (caused by liver's inability to metabolize hormones)	Testicular atrophy Menstrual irregularities Gynecomastia (excessive development of breasts in men) Loss of chest and axillary hair
Integument	Severe pruritus (itching) Extreme dryness Poor tissue turgor Abnormal pigmentation Prominent spider angiomas Palmar erythema
Hepatic	Hepatomegaly (enlargement of the liver) Ascites Edema of the legs Hepatic encephalopathy (see Table 10.5)
Gastrointestinal (GI)	Anorexia Nausea Vomiting Diarrhea

CASE EXAMPLE 10.3

Ascites

A 69-year-old man was seen at the Veteran's Administration (VA) Hospital outpatient physical therapy department following a left total hip replacement (THR) 2 weeks ago. The surgery was performed at a civilian hospital, but all his follow-up care has been through the VA. He had a long history of alcohol and tobacco use and medical intervention for heart disease, hypertension, and peripheral vascular disease.

The medical problem list (established by the physician) included:
Liver cirrhosis secondary to alcoholism
   Ascites secondary to portal hypertension
   Coronary artery disease with hypertension
   Peripheral vascular disease (arterial)
   Mild vision loss secondary to macular degeneration
The client was referred to physical therapy for rehabilitation following his THR. During the examination, the client reported various other musculoskeletal aches and pains, including chronic low back pain present off and on for the last 6 months and new onset of groin pain on the left side (just since the THR).

Ascites can be a cause of low back and/or groin pain. How do you screen this client for a medical (vascular, liver) cause of the groin pain?

Past Medical History
Past history of cancer of any kind
Past history of abdominal or inguinal hernia

Clinical Presentation
Ask additional questions about pain pattern as discussed in Chapter 3.
What do you think is causing your groin pain?
Watch for red flags associated with possible vascular involvement: client describes pain as "throbbing."
Pain is worse 5 to 10 minutes after the start of activity involving the lower extremities and relieved by rest (intermittent claudication).
Visual inspection and palpation, including observing for postural components (e.g., lumbar lordosis associated with ascites) as a contributing factor; abdominal or inguinal hernia; liver palpation; and lymph node palpation.
Perform stretching and resistive movements to eliminate, reproduce, or aggravate symptoms; you may be limited in this assessment area because of THR precautions.
Red flag: pain is not altered by stretching or resistive movement; pain cannot be reproduced with palpation.
Assess for trigger points (e.g., adductor magnus), keeping in mind that common systemic perpetuating factors with myofascial pain include anemia and hypothyroidism, as well as vitamin deficiency common with chronic alcohol use. Further screening may require assessing for risk factors and associated signs and symptoms for each of these conditions.

Associated Signs and Symptoms
Ask the client about any other symptoms of any kind that may have developed just before or around the time of the onset of groin pain. As mentioned above, the therapist may have to ask about the presence of signs and symptoms associated with anemia and endocrine disease.

Should you send this client back to the doctor before continuing with physical therapy intervention?
It is very likely that this client will require referral to his physician. Your referral decision will be dependent on your findings, of course. For example, the presence of trigger points may warrant treatment first and reassessment for change in clinical presentation before making a final decision. Given the movement precautions for THR, positional release or stretch positions for trigger points may be contraindicated. You may have to use alternate methods of trigger point release.

Remember true hip pain is often felt in the groin or deep buttock. There could be a problem with the hip implant (e.g., fracture, infection, loosening) causing the groin pain. There will be pain with active or passive motion of the hip joint. The pain increases with weight bearing.[30] If the physician does not know about this new groin pain, medical referral to reevaluate the implant is needed before continuing with a THR rehab protocol.

By continuing the screening process, the therapist can provide the physician with additional information to describe the problem. Communication is an important key element in the referral process. Provide the physician with a *brief* summary of your findings, including a list of any unusual findings (see further discussion regarding physician in Chapter 1).

CLINICAL SIGNS AND SYMPTOMS

Hemorrhage Associated with Esophageal Varices

- Restlessness
- Pallor
- Tachycardia
- Cooling of the skin
- Hypotension

It is the result of free fluid in the peritoneal cavity. For the physical therapist, abdominal hernias and lumbar lordosis observed in clients with ascites may present symptoms that mimic musculoskeletal involvement, such as groin or low back pain (Case Example 10.3).

Esophageal varices are a serious complication of cirrhosis. They are dilated veins of the lower esophagus that occur as a result of portal vein hypertension.[31,32] These varices are thin-walled and can rupture, causing severe hemorrhage and sometimes death.

Hepatic Encephalopathy (Hepatic Coma)

Hepatic encephalopathy (HE) is one of the most debilitating complications of liver disease. This condition occurs as a result of the inability of the liver to detoxify ammonia (produced from protein breakdown) in the intestine. Increased serum levels of ammonia are directly toxic to central and peripheral nervous system function, causing an array of neurologic symptoms. Flapping tremors (asterixis) and numbness/tingling (misinterpreted as carpal/tarsal tunnel syndrome) are common symptoms of this ammonia abnormality.

Clinical Signs and Symptoms. Clinical manifestations of hepatic encephalopathy vary, depending on the severity of neurologic involvement. The condition progressively develops in four stages as the ammonia level increases in the serum, and the accompanying clinical features are presented in Table 10.5.

For the physical therapist, the inpatient with impending hepatic coma has difficulty and unsteadiness in ambulation and may be a fall risk.[33,34] Protection from falling must be taken. In addition, patients with the condition may also present with short attention span, difficulty in concentrating, and cognitive impairment.

Newborn Jaundice

Jaundice affects approximately 60% of newborn infants[35] because liver function is somewhat slow to develop in the first few days of life.[36] In a small percentage of infants, extreme jaundice can occur and if left untreated for too long can result in a condition called kernicterus. Which is a type of brain damage from toxic levels of bilirubin in the blood.[35] This condition may cause athetoid cerebral palsy, hearing loss, vision and teeth abnormalities and intellectual disabilities.[35] It is critically important for all newborns to be screened for the development of this condition. Development of any color

TABLE 10.5	Stages of Hepatic Encephalopathy
Stage	**Symptoms**
Stage I (prodromal stage)	Subtle symptoms may be overlooked Slight personality changes: • Disorientation • Confusion • Euphoria or depression • Forgetfulness • Slurred speech
Stage II (impending stage)	Tremor progresses to asterixis (liver flap) Resistance to passive movement (increased muscle tone) Lethargy Aberrant behavior Apraxia* Ataxia Facial grimacing and blinking
Stage III (stuporous stage)	Client can still be aroused Hyperventilation Marked confusion Abusive and violent Noisy, incoherent speech Asterixis (liver flap) Muscle rigidity Positive Babinski† reflex Hyperactive deep tendon reflexes
Stage IV (comatose stage)	Client cannot be aroused; responds only to painful stimuli No asterixis Positive Babinski reflex Hepatic fetor (musty, sweet odor to the breath caused by the liver's inability to metabolize the amino acid methionine)

*This type of motor apraxia can be best observed by keeping a record of the client's handwriting and drawings of simple shapes such as a circle, square, triangle, and rectangle. Check for progressive deterioration.
†A reflex action of the toes that is normal during infancy but abnormal after 12 to 18 months. It is elicited by a firm stimulus (usually scraping with the handle of a reflex hammer) on the sole of the foot from the heel along the lateral border of the sole to the little toe, across the ball of the foot to the big toe. Normally, such a stimulus causes all the toes to flex downward. A positive Babinski reflex occurs when the great toe flexes upward and the smaller toes fan outward.

change in newborns needs immediate referral and testing for abnormal bilirubin levels.[37,38]

Liver Abscess

Liver abscess is relatively rare but occurs when bacteria (e.g., *Klebsiella pneumoniae* and *Escherichia coli*), fungi (e.g., *Candida albicans*), or ameba (*E. hystolica*) destroy hepatic tissue and produce a cavity that fills with infectious organisms, liquefied liver cells, and leukocytes.[39] Necrotic tissue then isolates the cavity from the rest of the liver. Biliary tract disease (obstruction of bile flow allows for bacterial invasion) is the most frequent cause of liver abscess.

The development of new radiologic techniques, improvement in microbiologic identification, advancement of medical

CLINICAL SIGNS AND SYMPTOMS
Liver Abscess

Clinical signs and symptoms of liver abscess depend on the degree of involvement; some people are acutely ill, others are asymptomatic. Depending on the type of abscess, the onset may be sudden or insidious. The most common signs include:

- Right abdominal pain
- Right shoulder pain
- Weight loss
- Fever, chills, malaise
- Diaphoresis
- Nausea and vomiting, anorexia
- Anemia
- Tender hepatomegaly (with or without a palpable mass)
- Jaundice

treatments, and improved supportive care have decreased mortality rates from 30% to 50% down to 5% to 30%; yet the prevalence of liver abscess has remained relatively unchanged. Untreated, this infection remains uniformly fatal.[39]

Liver Cancer

The incidence of liver cancer has more than tripled since 1980 and deaths have increased at a rate of 2.7% each year.[40] Cancers of the liver and intrahepatic bile duct is expected to account for 30,230 deaths in 2021. Metastatic tumors to the liver occur 20 times more often than primary liver tumors. The liver filters blood coming from the GI tract, making it a primary metastatic site for tumors of the stomach, colorectum, and pancreas. It is also a common site for metastases from other primary cancers such as those of the esophagus, lung, and breast.

Hepatocellular cancer (HCC) is the most common primary liver cancer in adults. This cancer can start as a single tumor that grows larger, spreading to the other parts of the liver in the later stages. It can also start as several small cancer nodules throughout the liver. This type of cancer growth appears to be most commonly noted in individuals with cirrhosis of the liver.[41]

Intrahepatic cholangiocarcinoma is the second most common malignancy coming from the liver.[42] It originates from the epithelium of the small bile ducts within the liver and has many of the same risk factors as HCC, but preexisting biliary disease is the primary risk factor.[41,43]

Several types of benign and malignant hepatic neoplasms can result from the administration of chemical agents. For example, adenoma (a benign tumor) can occur in recipients of oral contraceptives. Regression of the tumor occurs after withdrawal of the drug.[44]

In most instances, interference with liver function does not occur until approximately 80% to 90% of the liver is replaced by metastatic carcinoma or primary carcinoma.[45] Signs of liver impairment are often late in their presentation, making early detection and successful treatment less likely. The alert physical therapist may be the first to identify liver involvement when the neuromuscular or musculoskeletal systems are affected.

GALLBLADDER AND DUCT DISEASES
Cholelithiasis

Gallstones are stone-like masses called *calculi* that form in the gallbladder as a result of an imbalance in the composition of bile.

Cholelithiasis, the presence or formation of gallstones, can be asymptomatic, detected incidentally during medical imaging. Problems arise if a stone leaves the gallbladder and causes obstruction somewhere else in the biliary system, presenting as biliary colic, cholecystitis, or cholangitis.

It has been reported that cholelithiasis affects 10% to 15% of the adult population,[46] and is the leading cause for hospitalization secondary to GI problems. See Box 10.4 for risk factors to watch for in a client's history that correlate with the incidence of gallstones.

CLINICAL SIGNS AND SYMPTOMS
Liver Neoplasm

If clinical signs and symptoms of liver neoplasm do occur (whether of primary or metastatic origin), they may include:
- Jaundice (icterus)
- Progressive failure of health
- Anorexia and weight loss
- Overall muscular weakness
- Epigastric fullness and pain or discomfort
- Constant ache in the epigastrium or midback
- Early satiety (cystic tumors)

BOX 10.4 RISK FACTORS FOR GALLSTONES

- Age: Incidence increases with age
- Sex: Women are affected more than men before age 60 years
- Elevated estrogen levels
  - Pregnancy
  - Oral contraceptives
  - Hormone therapy
  - Multiparity (woman who has had two or more pregnancies resulting in viable offspring)
- Obesity
- Diet: High cholesterol, low fiber
- Diabetes mellitus
- Liver disease
- Rapid weight loss or fasting
- Taking cholesterol-lowering drugs (statins)
- Ethnicity (stronger genetic predisposition in Native Americans, Mexican Americans)
- Genetics (family history of gallstones)

Clients with gallstones may be asymptomatic or may have symptoms of a gallbladder attack described in the next section. The prognosis is usually good with medical treatment, depending on the severity of disease, presence of infection, and response to antibiotics.

Biliary Colic

With biliary colic, the stone gets lodged in the neck of the gallbladder (cystic duct). Pain results as the gallbladder contracts and tries to push the stone through. The classic symptom of this problem is right upper abdominal pain that comes and goes in waves. The pain builds to a peak and then fades away.

Obstructions of the gallbladder can result in biliary stasis, delayed gallbladder emptying, and subsequent mixed stone formation. Stasis and delayed gallbladder emptying can occur with any pathologic condition of the liver, hormonal influence, and pregnancy (usually third trimester when the developing fetus compresses the mother's gallbladder up against the liver).[47]

Cholecystitis

Cholecystitis, the blockage or impaction of gallstones in the cystic duct (Fig. 10.10), leads to infection or inflammation

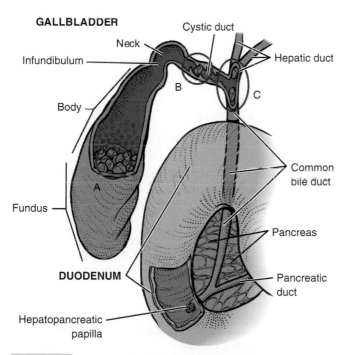

Fig. 10.10 The gallbladder and its divisions: fundus, body, infundibulum, and neck. **A,** Cholelithiasis, the presence or formation of gallstones, can be asymptomatic, detected incidentally during medical imaging. Problems arise if a stone leaves the gallbladder and causes obstruction somewhere else in the biliary system. **B,** If a gallstone enters the cystic duct and becomes lodged there, it can lead to cholecystitis (inflammation of the gallbladder). **C,** Obstruction of either the hepatic or common bile duct by stone or spasm blocks the exit of bile from the liver where it is formed. Jaundice is often the first symptom. If an infection develops and backs up into the liver, a condition called *cholangitis* can occur, a potentially life-threatening problem.

of the gallbladder. This condition may be acute or chronic, causing painful distention of the gallbladder. The affected individual may feel a steady, severe pain that rapidly increases in intensity, lasting several minutes to several hours. Nausea, vomiting, and fever may be present.

Other causes of acute cholecystitis may be bile duct problems, or a malignant tumor obstructing the biliary tract.[48] Whatever the cause of the obstruction, the normal flow of bile is interrupted and the gallbladder becomes distended and ischemic.

Gallstones may also cause chronic cholecystitis (persistent gallbladder inflammation), in which the gallbladder atrophies and becomes fibrotic, adhering to adjacent organs. It is not unusual for affected clients to have repeated episodes before seeking medical attention.

Cholangitis

Gallstones lodged further down in the system in the common bile duct can cause cholangitis. Blocking the flow of bile at this point in the biliary tree can lead to jaundice. Infection can develop here and travel up to the liver, becoming a potentially life-threatening situation.

Clinical Signs and Symptoms

The typical pain of gallbladder disease has been described as colicky pain that occurs in the right upper quadrant (RUQ) of the abdomen after the person has eaten a meal that is high in fat (although food that provokes an attack of pain does not need to be "fatty"). However, the pain is not necessarily limited to the RUQ, and more likely than not, it is constant, not colicky.

Like the stomach, pylorus, and duodenum, the liver and gallbladder can cause spasm of the rectus abdominis muscles above the umbilicus. This occurs when disturbances within the hepatic and biliary systems, as a part of the overall GI system, affect motor reflexes.

These disturbances can be reflected in muscular contractions of the spinal, abdominal, and other muscles supplied by the motor nerves from the anterior horn of the segment innervating the affected viscera.[49]

It looks just like a musculoskeletal problem, but the pain pattern is the result of viscero-somatic reflexes as discussed in Chapter 3. Ask about the timing of symptoms in relation to eating or drinking. Watch for symptoms that are worse immediately after eating (gallbladder inflammation) or pain and nausea 1 to 3 hours after eating (gallstones).

Muscle guarding and tenderness of the spinal musculature in the presence of constitutional symptoms (e.g., fever, sweats, chills, nausea) is another red flag. Ask about a previous history of GI, liver, or gallbladder problems, and review the client's risk factors for hepatic involvement.

In the case of gallbladder disease, it is also possible to get tender points in the soma corresponding to visceral innervation. A gallbladder problem can result in a sore tenth rib tip (right side anteriorly) when messages from the viscera entering the spinal cord at the same level as the innervation of the rib are misinterpreted as a somatic problem.

CASE EXAMPLE 10.4
Gallbladder Pain

A 48-year-old schoolteacher was admitted to the hospital following an episode of intense, sharp pain that started in the epigastric region and radiated around her thorax to the interscapular area. Her gallbladder had been removed 2 years ago, but she remarked that her current symptoms were "exactly like a gallbladder attack." The client was referred to physical therapy for "back care/education" on the day of discharge.

During examination, the client was in acute distress, unable to tolerate a full examination. She had not been able to transfer or ambulate independently. She was instructed in relaxation and breathing techniques to reduce her extreme level of anxiety associated with pain and given supportive reassurance. Instruction and assistance were provided in all transfers to minimize pain and maximize independent function. Given her discharge status, outpatient physical therapy was recommended for follow-up intervention.

She returned to physical therapy as planned and was provided with a back care program. She was also treated locally for scar tissue adhesion at the site of the gallbladder removal. Symptomatic relief was obtained in the first two sessions without recurrence of symptoms.

This case example is included to demonstrate how scar tissue associated with organ removal can reproduce visceral symptoms that are actually of musculoskeletal origin—the opposite concept of what is presented in this text. This may be more of an example of cellular memories sustaining a viscero-somatic reflex via the action of neuropeptides at the cellular level (see discussion of Psychoneuroimmunology in Chapter 3).

The gallbladder has most of its innervation from the right side of the cervical ganglia to the splanchnic nerves, which explains the predominance of right-sided somatic symptoms.

When visceral and cutaneous fibers enter the spinal cord at the same level, the nervous system may respond with sudomotor changes, such as pruritus (itching of the skin) or a sore rib, instead of gallbladder symptoms. The clinical

CLINICAL SIGNS AND SYMPTOMS
Acute Cholecystitis

- Chills, low-grade fever
- Jaundice
- GI symptoms
- Nausea
- Anorexia
- Vomiting
- Tenderness over the gallbladder
- Tenderness on the tip of the tenth rib (right side anteriorly; called a "hot rib"; can also affect eleventh and twelfth ribs (right anterior)
- Severe pain in the right upper quadrant (RUQ) and epigastrium (increases on inspiration and movement)
- Pain radiating into the right shoulder and between the scapulae

CLINICAL SIGNS AND SYMPTOMS
Chronic Cholecystitis

These may be vague or a sense of indigestion and abdominal discomfort after eating, unless a stone leaves the gallbladder and causes obstruction of the common duct (called *choledocholithiasis*), causing:

- Biliary colic: severe, steady pain for 3 to 4 hours in the right upper quadrant (RUQ)
- Pain: may radiate to the midback between the scapulae (caused by splanchnic fibers synapsing with phrenic nerve fibers)
- Nausea (intolerance of fatty foods; decreased bile production results in decreased fat digestion)
- Abdominal fullness
- Heartburn
- Excessive belching
- Constipation and diarrhea

presentation appears as a biomechanical problem, such as a rib dysfunction, instead of nausea and food intolerance normally associated with gallbladder dysfunction.

Likewise, from our understanding of viscerogenic pain patterns based on embryologic development, we know that the visceral pericardium of the heart (see Fig. 7.5) is derived from the same embryologic tissue as the gallbladder. A gallbladder problem can also cause referred pain to the heart and must be ruled out by the physician as a possible cause of chest pain.

Primary Biliary Cirrhosis

Primary biliary cirrhosis (PBC) is a chronic, progressive, autoimmune disease of the liver that involves primarily the intrahepatic bile ducts and results in the impairment of bile secretion. Typical signs include fatigue, pruritus, and dry eyes and mouth, progressing to biochemical evidence of cholestasis.

The cause of PBC is unknown, although various factors are being investigated. Factors being implicated include genetics and infection with organisms of the family Enterobactiriaceae.[50]

CLINICAL SIGNS AND SYMPTOMS
Primary Biliary Cirrhosis

- Pruritus
- Jaundice
- GI bleeding
- Ascites (see Fig. 10.9)
- Fatigue
- Right upper quadrant (RUQ) pain (posterior)
- Osteoporosis (decreased bone mass)
- Osteomalacia (softening of the bones)
- Burning, pins and needles, prickling of the eyes
- Muscle cramping

One of the most significant clinical problems for clients with PBC is metabolic bone disease[51] characterized by impaired osteoblastic activity and accelerated osteoclastic activity. Calcium and vitamin D should be carefully monitored and appropriate replacement instituted. Physical activity following an osteoporosis protocol should be encouraged.

Gallbladder Cancer

Gallbladder cancer, closely associated with gallstone disease, often has a poor outcome because of the delay in diagnosis. The primary associated risk factors include cholelithiasis (especially symptomatic, untreated), obesity, reproductive abnormalities, chronic gallbladder infection, and exposure to radon and certain industrial exposures including cellulose acetate fiber manufacturing. Testing and treatment of symptomatic gallstones is the only preventive measure identified at this time for gallbladder cancer.[52]

PHYSICIAN REFERRAL

A careful history and close observation of the client are important in determining whether a person may need a medical referral for possible hepatic or biliary involvement. Any client with midback, scapular, or right shoulder pain (see Table 10.1) without a history of trauma (e.g., forceful movement of the spine, repetitive movement of the shoulder or back, or easy lifting) should be screened for a possible systemic origin of symptoms.

For the physical therapist, when treating the inpatient population, jaundice in the postoperative individual is not uncommon but can be a potentially serious complication of surgery and anesthesia.

Clinical management of jaundice is complicated by anything that could damage the liver, including physical stress associated with physical therapy intervention. Hypoxemia, blood loss, infection, and administration of multiple drugs can add additional physical stress.

When making the referral, it is important to report to the physician the results of your objective findings, especially when there is a lack of physical evidence to support a musculoskeletal lesion. The Special Questions to Ask at the end of this chapter may assist in assessing the client's overall health status.

Guidelines to Immediate Physician Referral

- New onset of myopathy in any client, but especially in the older adult, with a history of statin use; look for other risk factors, signs, and symptoms of liver or renal impairment.

Guidelines to Physician Referral

- Obvious signs of hepatic disease, especially with a history of previous cancer or risk factors for hepatitis (see Box 10.2)
- Development of arthralgias of unknown cause in anyone with a previous history of hepatitis or risk factors for hepatitis
- Presence of bilateral carpal tunnel syndrome (could be accompanied by bilateral tarsal tunnel syndrome) unknown to the physician; asterixis, or other associated hepatic signs and symptoms
- Presence of sensory neuropathy of unknown cause accompanied by signs and symptoms associated with hepatic system impairment

Clues to Screening for Hepatic Disease

- Right shoulder/scapular and/or upper midback pain of unknown cause (see also Clues to Screening Shoulder Pain in Chapter 19).
- Shoulder motion is not limited by painful symptoms; client is unable to localize or pinpoint pain or tenderness.
- Presence of GI symptoms, especially if there is any correlation between eating and painful symptoms.
- Bilateral carpal/tarsal tunnel syndrome, especially of unknown origin; check for other signs of liver impairment such as liver flap, liver palms, and change in skin or nail beds (see Box 10.1).
- Personal history of cancer, liver, or gallbladder disease.
- Personal history of hepatitis, especially with joint pain associated with rheumatoid arthritis or fibromyalgia accompanied by palmar tendinitis.
- Recent history of statin use (cholesterol-lowering drugs such as Zocor, Lipitor or Crestor) or other hepatotoxic drugs.
- Recent operative procedure (possible postoperative jaundice).
- Recent (within last 6 months) injection drug use, tattoo (received or removed), acupuncture, ear or body piercing, dialysis, blood or plasma transfusion, sexual activity with multiple partners of the same or different sex, consumption of raw shellfish (hepatitis).
- Changes in skin (yellow hue, spider angiomas, palmar erythema) or eye color (jaundice).
- Employment or lifestyle involving alcohol consumption (jaundice).
- Contact with jaundiced persons (health care worker handling blood or body fluids, dialysis clients, injection drug users, sexual activity with multiple partners of the same or different sex).

LIVER/BILIARY PAIN PATTERNS

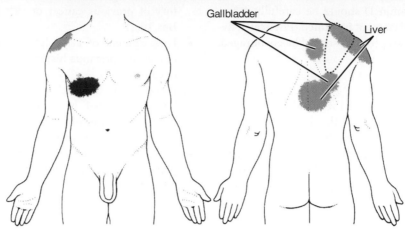

Fig. 10.11 The primary pain pattern from the liver, gallbladder, and common bile duct *(dark red)* presents typically in the midepigastrium or right upper quadrant of the abdomen. Innervation of the liver and biliary system is through the autonomic nervous system from T5 to T11 (see Fig. 3.3). Liver impairment is primarily reflected through the ninth thoracic distribution. Referred pain *(light red)* from the liver occurs in the thoracic spine from approximately T7 to T10 and/or to the right of midline, possibly affecting the right shoulder (right phrenic nerve). Referred pain from the gallbladder can affect the right shoulder by the same mechanism. The gallbladder can also refer pain to the right interscapular (T4 or T5 to T8) or right subscapular area.

LIVER PAIN (FIG. 10.11)

Location:	Pain in the mid epigastrium or right upper quadrant (RUQ) of abdomen
Referral:	Pain over the liver, especially after exercise (hepatitis)
	RUQ pain may be associated with right shoulder pain
	Both RUQ and epigastrium pain may be associated with back pain between the scapulae
	Pain may be referred to the right side of the midline in the interscapular or subscapular area (T7-T10)
Description:	Dull abdominal aching
	Sense of fullness of the abdomen or epigastrium
Intensity:	Mild at first, then increases steadily
Duration:	Constant
Associated signs and symptoms:	Nausea, anorexia (viral hepatitis)
	Early satiety (cystic tumors)
	Aversion to smoking for smokers (viral hepatitis)
	Aversion to alcohol (hepatitis)
	Arthralgias and myalgias (hepatitis A, hepatitis B, or hepatitis C)
	Headaches (hepatitis A, drug-induced hepatitis)
	Dizziness/drowsiness (drug-induced hepatitis)
	Low-grade fever (hepatitis A)
	Pharyngitis (hepatitis A)
	Extreme fatigue (hepatitis A, cirrhosis)
	Alterations in the sense of taste and smell (hepatitis A)
	Rash (hepatitis B)
	Dark urine, light- or clay-colored stools
	Ascites (see Fig. 10.9)
	Edema and oliguria
	Neurologic symptoms (hepatic encephalopathy)
	• Confusion, forgetfulness
	• Muscle tremors
	• Asterixis (liver flap)
	• Slurred speech
	• Impaired handwriting

Continued

LIVER/BILIARY PAIN PATTERNS—cont'd

	Change in skin and nail beds
	Skin pallor (often linked with cirrhosis or carcinoma)
	Jaundice (skin and sclerae changes)
	Spider angiomas
	Palmar erythema (liver palms)
	Nail beds of Terry; leukonychia; digital clubbing; koilonychias
	Bleeding disorders
	• Purpura
	• Ecchymosis
	Diaphoresis (liver abscess)
	Overall muscular weakness (cirrhosis, liver carcinoma)
Possible etiology:	Peripheral neuropathy (chronic liver disease)
	Any liver disease
	• Hepatitis
	• Cirrhosis
	• Metastatic tumor
	Pancreatic carcinoma
	Liver abscess
	Medications: use of hepatotoxic drugs

GALLBLADDER PAIN (SEE FIG. 10.11)

Location:	Pain in the midepigastrium (may be perceived as heartburn)
Referral:	RUQ of abdomen
	RUQ pain may be associated with right shoulder pain
	Both may be associated with back pain between the scapulae; back pain can occur alone as the primary symptom
	Pain may be referred to the right side of the midline in the interscapular or subscapular area
	Anterior rib pain (soreness or tender) at the tip of the tenth rib (less often, can also affect ribs 11 and 12)
Description:	Dull aching
	Deep visceral pain (gallbladder suddenly distends)
	Biliary carcinoma is more persistent and boring
Intensity:	Mild at first, then increases steadily to become severe
Duration:	2–3 hours
Aggravating factors:	Respiratory inspiration
	Eating
	Upper body movement
	Lying down
Associated signs and symptoms:	Dark urine, light stools
	Jaundice
	Skin: green hue (prolonged biliary obstruction)
	Persistent pruritus (cholestatic jaundice)
	Pain and nausea occur 1–3 hours after eating (gallstones)
	Pain immediately after eating (gallbladder inflammation)
	Intolerance of fatty foods or heavy meals
	Indigestion, nausea
	Excessive belching
	Flatulence (excessive intestinal gas)
	Anorexia
	Weight loss (gallbladder cancer)
	Bleeding from skin and mucous membranes (late sign of gallbladder cancer)
	Vomiting
	Feeling of fullness
	Low-grade fever, chills

LIVER/BILIARY PAIN PATTERNS—cont'd

Possible etiology: Gallstones (cholelithiasis)
Gallbladder inflammation (cholecystitis)
Neoplasm
Medications: use of hepatotoxic drugs

COMMON BILE DUCT PAIN (SEE FIG. 10.11)

Location:	Pain in midepigastrium or RUQ of abdomen
Referral:	Epigastrium: heartburn (choledocholithiasis)
	RUQ pain may be associated with right shoulder pain
	Both may be associated with back pain between the scapulae
	Pain may be referred to the right side of the midline in the interscapular or subscapular area
Description:	Dull aching
	Vague discomfort (pressure within common bile duct increasing)
	Severe, steady pain in RUQ (choledocholithiasis)
	Biliary carcinoma is more persistent and boring
Intensity:	Mild at first, increases steadily
Duration:	Constant
	3–4 hours (choledocholithiasis)
Associated signs and symptoms:	Dark urine, light stools
	Jaundice
	Nausea after eating
	Intolerance of fatty foods or heavy meals
	Feeling of abdominal fullness
	Skin: green hue (prolonged biliary obstruction); pruritus (skin itching)
	Low-grade fever, chills
	Excessive belching (choledocholithiasis)
	Constipation and diarrhea (choledocholithiasis)
	Sensory neuropathy (primary biliary cirrhosis)
	Osteomalacia (primary biliary cirrhosis)
	Osteoporosis (primary biliary cirrhosis)
Possible etiology:	Common duct stones
	Common duct stricture (previous gallbladder surgery)
	Pancreatic carcinoma (blocking the bile duct)
	Medications: use of hepatotoxic drugs
	Neoplasm
	Primary biliary cirrhosis
	Choledocholithiasis (obstruction of common duct)

■ Key Points to Remember

1. Primary signs and symptoms of liver diseases vary and can include GI symptoms, edema/ascites, dark urine, light-colored or clay-colored feces, and right upper abdominal pain.
2. Neurologic symptoms, such as confusion, muscle tremors, asterixis, and balance and gait impairments may occur.
3. Skin changes associated with the hepatic system include pruritus, jaundice, pallor, orange or green skin, bruising, spider angiomas, and palmar erythema.
4. Active, intense exercise should be avoided when the liver is compromised (jaundice or other active disease).
5. Antiinflammatory and minor analgesic agents can cause drug-induced hepatitis.

Continued

■ **Key Points to Remember—cont'd**

6. Nonviral hepatitis may occur postoperatively.
7. When liver dysfunction results in increased serum ammonia and urea levels, peripheral nerve function is impaired. Flapping tremors (asterixis) and numbness/tingling (misinterpreted as carpal/tarsal tunnel syndrome) can occur.
8. Musculoskeletal locations of pain associated with the hepatic and biliary systems include thoracic spine between scapulae, right shoulder, right upper trapezius, right interscapular, or right subscapular areas.
9. Referred shoulder pain may be the only presenting symptom of hepatic or biliary disease.
10. Gallbladder impairment can present as a rib dysfunction with tenderness anteriorly over the tip of the tenth rib (occasionally ribs 11 and 12 are also involved).

CLIENT HISTORY AND INTERVIEW

SPECIAL QUESTIONS TO ASK

PAST MEDICAL HISTORY

- Have you ever had an ulcer, gallbladder disease, your spleen removed, or hepatitis/jaundice?
- *If yes* to hepatitis or jaundice: When was this diagnosed? How did you get this?
- Has anyone in your family ever been diagnosed with Wilson's disease (**excessive copper retention**) or hemochromatosis (**excessive iron absorption**)? (**Hereditary**)
- Do you work in a clinical laboratory, operating room, or with clients with dialysis? (**Hepatitis**)
- Have you been out of the United States in the last 6 to 12 months? (**Parasitic infection, country where hepatitis is endemic**)
- Have you worked in any setting that might be high risk for disease transmission such as a day care, correctional setting, or institutional setting? (**Hepatitis**)
- Have you had any recent contact with hepatitis or with a jaundiced person?
- Have you eaten any raw shellfish recently? (**Viral hepatitis**)
- Have you had any recent blood or plasma transfusion, blood tests, acupuncture, ear or body piercing, tattoos (including removal), or dental work done? (**Viral hepatitis**)
- Have you had any kind of injury or trauma to your abdomen? (**Possible liver damage**)
  For women: Are you currently using oral contraceptives? (**Hepatitis, adenoma**)
  For the therapist:
- When asking about drug history, keep in mind that oral contraceptives may cause cholestasis (suppression of bile flow) or liver tumors. Some common OTC drugs (e.g., acetaminophen) and some antibiotics, antitubercular drugs, anticonvulsants, cytotoxic drugs for cancer, antipsychotics, and antidepressants may have hepatotoxic effects. Ask about the use of cholesterol-lowering statins.

- Use questions from Chapter 2 to determine possible consumption of alcohol as a hepatotoxin.

ASSOCIATED SIGNS AND SYMPTOMS

- Have you noticed a recent tendency to bruise or bleed easily? (**Liver disease**)
- Have you noticed any change in the color of your stools or urine? (**Dark urine, the color of cola and light- or clay-colored stools associated with jaundice**)
- Has your weight recently fluctuated 10 to 15 pounds or more without a change in diet? (**Cancer, cirrhosis, ascites, but also congestive heart failure**)
- *If no,* have you noticed your clothes fitting tighter around the waist from abdominal swelling or bloating? (**Ascites**)
- Do you have a feeling of fullness after only one or two bites of food? (**Early satiety: stomach and duodenum, cystic tumors, or gallbladder**)
- Does your stomach feel swollen or bloated after eating? (**Abdominal fullness**)
- Do you have any abdominal pain? (**Abdominal pain may be *visceral* from an internal organ [dull, general, poorly localized], *parietal* from inflammation of overlying peritoneum [sharp, precisely localized, aggravated by movement], or *referred* from a disorder in another site.**)
- How does eating affect your pain? (**When eating aggravates symptoms: gastric ulcer, gallbladder inflammation**)
  - Are there any particular foods you have noticed that aggravate your symptoms?
  - *If yes*, which ones? (**Gallbladder: intolerance to fatty foods**)
- Have you noticed any unusual aversion to odors, food, alcohol, or (for people who smoke) smoking? (**Jaundice**)
- *For clients with only shoulder or back pain:* Have you noticed any association between when you eat and when your symptoms increase or decrease?

CASE STUDY

Hepatitis

REFERRAL

A 29-year-old male law student has come to you (self-referral) with headaches that developed after a motor vehicle accident 12 weeks ago. He was evaluated and treated in the emergency department of the local hospital and is not under the care of a primary care physician.

The headaches occur two to three times each week, starting at the base of the occiput and progressing up the back of his head to localize in the forehead bilaterally. The client has a sedentary lifestyle with no regular exercise, and he describes his stress level as being 6 on a scale of 0 to 10.

The Family/Personal History form (see Fig. 2.2) indicates that he was diagnosed with hepatitis at the time of the accident.

PHYSICAL THERAPY INTERVIEW

What follow-up questions will you ask this client related to the hepatitis?

- I see from your History form that you have hepatitis.
- What type of hepatitis do you have?

Give the client a chance to respond, but you may need to prompt with "type A," "type B," or "types C or D." Remember that hepatitis A is communicable before the appearance of any observable clinical symptoms. If he has been diagnosed, he is probably past this stage.

- Do you know how you initially came in contact with hepatitis? (Depending on the answer to the previous question, you may not need to ask this question.)

Considerations requiring further questioning may include:

- Illicit or recreational drug use
- Inadequate hygiene and poor handwashing in close quarters with travel companion
- Ingestion of contaminated food, water, milk, or seafood
- Recent blood transfusion or contact with blood/blood products
- For type B: modes of sexual transmission

Remember the three stages when trying to determine whether this person may still be contagious. Hepatitis B can persist in body fluids indefinitely, which requires that you practice necessary precautions.

Hepatitis caused by medications or toxins is noninfectious and is not communicable.

Transmissible hepatitis requires handwashing and hygiene precautions, including avoidance of any body fluids on your part through the use of protective gloves. This is especially true when treating a person with diabetes requiring finger stick blood testing, when performing needle electromyograms, or providing open wound care, especially with debridement.

MEDICAL TREATMENT

- Did you receive any medical treatment? (**Immune globulin**)

Immune serum globulin (ISG) is considered most effective in producing passive immunity for 3 to 4 months when administered as soon as possible after exposure to the hepatitis virus, but within 2 weeks after the onset of jaundice. Persons who have been treated with ISG may not develop jaundice, but those who have not received it usually do develop jaundice.

- Are you currently receiving follow-up care for your hepatitis through a local physician?

This information will assist you in determining the appropriate medical source for further information if you need it and in a case like this, assist you with choosing further follow-up questions that may help you determine whether this person requires additional medical follow-up.

Keep in mind that headaches can be a persistent symptom of hepatitis A. If the client is receiving no further medical follow-up (especially if no ISG was administered initially), consider these follow-up questions:

ASSOCIATED SYMPTOMS

- What symptoms did you have with hepatitis?
- Do you have any of those symptoms now?
- Are you experiencing any unusual fatigue or muscle or joint aches and pains?
- Have you noticed any unusual aversion to foods, alcohol, or cigarettes/smoke that you did not have before?
- Have you had any problems with diarrhea, vomiting, or nausea?
- Have you noticed any change in the color of your stools or urine? (1 to 4 days before the icteric stage the urine darkens and the stool lightens)
- Have you noticed any unusual skin rash developing recently?
- When did you notice the headaches developing?

PRACTICE QUESTIONS

1. Referred pain patterns associated with hepatic and biliary pathologic conditions produce musculoskeletal symptoms in the:
   a. Left shoulder
   b. Right shoulder
   c. Midback or upper back, scapular, and right shoulder areas
   d. Thorax, scapulae, right or left shoulder

2. Clients with significant elevations in serum bilirubin levels caused by biliary obstruction will have which of the following associated signs?
   a. Dark urine, clay-colored stools, jaundice
   b. Yellow-tinged sclera
   c. Decreased serum ammonia levels
   d. a and b only

3. Preventing falls and trauma to soft tissues would be of utmost importance in the client with liver failure. Which of the following laboratory parameters would give you the most information about potential tissue injury?
   a. Decrease in serum albumin level
   b. Elevated liver enzyme level
   c. Prolonged coagulation time
   d. Elevated serum bilirubin level

4. Decreased level of consciousness, impaired function of peripheral nerves, and asterixis (flapping tremor) would probably indicate an increase in the level of:
   a. Aspartate aminotransferase (AST)
   b. Alkaline phosphatase
   c. Serum bilirubin
   d. Serum ammonia

5. An inpatient who has had a total hip replacement with a significant history of alcohol use/abuse has a positive test for asterixis. This may signify:
   a. Renal failure
   b. Hepatic encephalopathy
   c. Diabetes
   d. Gallstones obstructing the common bile duct

6. A decrease in serum albumin is common with a pathologic condition of the liver because albumin is produced in the liver. The reduction in serum albumin results in some easily identifiable signs. Which of the following signs might alert the therapist to the condition of decreased albumin?
   a. Increased blood pressure
   b. Peripheral edema and ascites
   c. Decreased level of consciousness
   d. Exertional dyspnea

7. What is the mechanism for referred right shoulder pain from hepatic or biliary disease?

8. Why does someone with liver dysfunction develop numbness and tingling that is sometimes labeled carpal tunnel syndrome?

9. When a client with bilateral carpal tunnel syndrome is being evaluated, how do you screen for the possibility of a pathologic condition of the liver?

10. What is the first most common sign associated with liver disease?

11. You are treating a 53-year-old woman who has had an extensive medical history that includes bilateral kidney disease with kidney removal on one side and transplantation on the other. The client is 10 years post-transplant and has now developed multiple problems as a result of the long-term use of immunosuppressants (cyclosporine) to prevent organ rejection and corticosteroids (prednisone). For example, she is extremely osteoporotic and has been diagnosed with cytomegalovirus and corticosteroid-induced myopathy. The client has fallen and broken her vertebra, ankle, and wrist on separate occasions. You are seeing her at home to implement a strengthening program and to instruct her in a falling prevention program, including home modifications. You notice the sclerae of her eyes are yellow-tinged. How do you tactfully ask her about this?

REFERENCES

1. Kumar V, Abbas AK, Aster JC. *Robbins Basic Pathology*. 9th ed. : Elsevier; 2013.
2. Peterson C. *The Hepatic, Pancreatic and Biliary Systems. Goodman and Fuller's Pathology: Implications for the Physical Therapist*. 5th ed. : Elsevier; 2020.
3. Ball J, Drains J. Abdomen. Palpating the liver. A, Fingers are extended, with tips on right midclavicular line below the level of liver dullness and pointing toward the head. B, Alternative method with the fingers parallel to the costal margin. *Seidel's Guide to Physical Examination*. Elsevier; 2019:393–436.
4. Fernández-Somoza J, Rodríguez I, Tomé S, et al. Diagnostic accuracy of spider naevi for liver disease detection in alcoholics. *Galicia Clin.* 2014;75(1):7–11.
5. Chemmanur AT, Anand BS. Biliary Disease Clinical Presentation. Medscape. http://emedicine.medscape.com/article/171386-clinical. Accessed July 15, 2021.
6. Goodman CC. Screening for gastrointestinal, hepatic/biliary, and renal/urologic disease. *J Hand Ther.* 2010;23(2):140–156.
7. Ehnert S, Aspera-Werz RH, Ruoß M, et al. Hepatic osteodystrophy—molecular mechanisms proposed to favor its development. *Int J Mol Sci.* 2019;20:2555. https://doi.org/10.3390/ijms20102555.
8. Ezad S, Cheema H, Collins N. Statin-induced rhabdomyolysis: a complication of a commonly overlooked drug interaction. *Oxf Med Case Rep.* 2018;2018(3):omx104. https://doi.org/10.1093/omcr/omx104.
9. Valente-Acosta B, Moreno-Sanchez F, Fueyo-Rodriguez O, Palomar-Lever A. Rhabdomyolysis as an initial presentation in a patient diagnosed with COVID-19. *BMJ Case Rep.* 2020;13:e236719..
10. Mukherjee A, Ghosh R, Aftab G. Rhabdomyolysis in a patient with coronavirus disease 2019. *Cureus.* 2020;12(7):e8956. Published 2020 Jul 1. https://doi.org/10.7759/cureus.8956.
11. Parker BA, Capizzi JA, Grimaldi AS, et al. The effect of statins on skeletal muscle function. *Circulation.* 2013;127:96–103.
12. Mendizabal M, Silva MO. Images in clinical medicine. Asterixis. *N Engl J Med.* 2010;363:e14.
13. Samji NS. Medscape. Viral Hepatitis. Updated Jun 12, 2017. https://emedicine.medscape.com/article/775507-overview#a4. Accessed July 26, 2021.

14. High Risk Groups. Hepatitis B Foundation. http://www.hepb. org/professionals/high-risk_groups.htm. Accessed July 15, 2021.

15. Khouqeer RA. Viral Arthritis. Medscape. http://emedicine. medscape.com/article/335692-overview. Accessed July 15, 2021.

16. Xuan D, Yu Y, Shao L, Wang J, Zhang W, Zou H. Hepatitis reactivation in patients with rheumatic diseases after immunosuppressive therapy—a report of long-term follow-up of serial cases and literature review. *Clin Rheumatol.* 2014;33:577–586.

17. Rutherford A. Overview of chronic hepatitis. Merck Manual, Professional Version. http://www.merckmanuals.com/professional/hepatic-and-biliary-disorders/hepatitis/overview-of-chronic-hepatitis. Accessed July 15, 2021.

18. Chronic Hepatitis. University of Pittsburg Medical Center Transplant Pathology Internet Services. http://tpis.upmc.com/ tpislibrary/dlp/Chap3frame.html. Accessed July 15, 2021.

19. Mayo Clinic. Wilson's disease. https://www.mayoclinic.org/ diseases-conditions/wilsons-disease/symptoms-causes/syc-20353251. Accessed July 27, 2021.

20. Bandman O, Weiss KH, Kaler SG. Wilson's disease and other neurological copper disorders. *Lancet Neurol.* 2015;4(1):103–113.

21. Dusek P, Litwin T, Członkowska A. Neurologic impairment in Wilson disease. *Ann Transl Med.* 2019;7(Suppl 2):S64. https:// doi.org/10.21037/atm.2019.02.43.

22. Neek G, Wernitzsch H, Kluter A, et al. Diagnosing hereditary hemochromatosis in the rheumatology practice. *Ann Rheum Dis.* 2014;73:468–469.

23. Centers for Disease Control and Prevention. Investigation of Acute Non-Viral Hepatitis of Unknown Etiology Potentially Associated with an Alkaline Water Product. https://www.cdc. gov/nceh/hsb/chemicals/nonviralhepatitis.htm. Accessed July 27, 2021.

24. Lancaster EM, Hiatt JR, Zarripar A. Acetaminophen hepatotoxicity: an updated review. *Arch Toxicol.* 2015;89(2):193–199.

25. Bunchorntavakul C, Reddy KR. Acetaminophen-related hepatotoxicity. *Clin Liver Dis.* Nov 2013;17(4):587–607.

26. Mayo Clinic. Non alcoholic fatty liver disease. https://www. mayoclinic.org/diseases-conditions/nonalcoholic-fatty-liver-disease/symptoms-causes/syc-20354567. Accessed July 27, 2021.

27. Ahmed M. Non-alcoholic fatty liver disease in 2015. *World J Hepatol Jun.* 2015;7(11):1450–1459.

28. Pasumarthy L, Srour J. Nonalcoholic steatohepatitis: a review of the literature and updates in management. *South Med J.* 2010;103(6):547–550.

29. Cleveland Clinic. Ascites. https://my.clevelandclinic.org/health/ diseases/14792-ascites. Accessed July 27, 2021.

30. Kimbel DL. Hip pain in a 50-year-old woman with RA. *J Musculoskel Med.* 1999;16(11):651–652.

31. Mayo Clinic. Esophageal varices. https://www.mayoclinic.org/ diseases-conditions/esophageal-varices/symptoms-causes/syc-20351538. Accessed July 27, 2021.

32. Tseng Y, Li F, Wang J, Chen S, et al. Spleen and liver stiffness for noninvasive assessment of portal hypertension in cirrhotic patients with large esophageal varices. *J Clin Ultrasound.* 2018;46(7):442–449. SN-0091-2751. https://doi.org/10.1002/ jcu.22635.

33. Cleveland Clinic. Hepatic Encephalopathy. https:// my.clevelandclinic.org/health/diseases/21220-hepatic-encephalopathy. Accessed July 27, 2021.

34. Vilstrup H, Amodio P, Cordoba J, et al. Hepatic encephalopathy in chronic liver disease: 2014 Practice Guideline by the American Association for the Study of Liver Diseases and the European Association for the Study of the Liver. *Hepatology.* 2014;60(2):715–735.

35. Centers of Disease Control and Prevention. What are Jaundice and Kernicterus? https://www.cdc.gov/ncbddd/jaundice/facts. html. Accessed July 27, 2021.

36. Cohen RS. Understanding neonatal jaundice: a perspective on causation. *Pediatr Neonatol.* 2010;51(3):143–148.

37. Lease M, Whalen B. Assessing jaundice in infants of 35-week gestation and greater. *Curr Opin Pediatr.* 2010;22(3):352–365.

38. Mansor N, Hariharan M, Basah SN, Yaacob S. New newborn jaundice monitoring scheme based on combination of preprocessing and color detection method. *Neurocomputing.* 2013;120:258–261.

39. Peralta R. Liver Abscess. Medscape. http://emedicine.medscape. com/article/188802-overview#a7. Accessed July 15, 2021.

40. Liver Cancer Statistics. Cancer.net. https://www.cancer.net/ cancer-types/liver-cancer/statistics. Accessed July 27, 2021.

41. About Liver Cancer? American cancer Society. http://www. cancer.org/acs/groups/cid/documents/webcontent/003114-pdf. pdf. Accessed July 15, 2021.

42. Buettner S, van Vugt JL, IJzermans JN, Groot Koerkamp B. Intrahepatic cholangiocarcinoma: current perspectives. *Onco Targets Ther.* 2017;10:1131–1142. Published 2017 Feb 22. https://doi.org/10.2147/OTT.S93629.

43. Cai H, Kong WT, Chen CB, et al. Cholelithiasis and the risk of intrahepatic cholangiocarcinoma: a meta-analysis of observational studies. *BMC Cancer.* 2015;15:831. Published 2015 Nov 2. https://doi.org/10.1186/s12885-015-1870-0.

44. Whitmer BA. Hepatocellular Adenoma. Medscape. http:// emedicine.medscape.com/article/170205-overview. Accessed July 15, 2021.

45. Cirrhosis. Patient. http://patient.info/doctor/cirrhosis-pro. Accessed July 15, 2021.

46. Gallstones. National Institute of Diabetes and Digestive and Kidney Diseases. https://www.niddk.nih.gov/health-information/digestive-diseases/gallstones/definition-facts. Accessed July 27, 2021.

47. Acute cholecystitis. Medline Plus. US National Library of Medicine. https://www.nlm.nih.gov/medlineplus/ency/article/ 000264.htm. Accessed July 15, 2021.

48. Cholecyctitis. Mayo Clinic. https://www.mayoclinic.org/ diseases-conditions/cholecystitis/symptoms-causes/syc-20364867. Accessed July 27, 2021.

49. Rex L. *Evaluation and Treatment of Somatovisceral Dysfunction of the Gastrointestinal System.* Edmonds, WA: URSA Foundation; 2004.

50. Pyrsopoulos NT. Primary Biliary Cholangitis (Primary Biliary Cirrhosis) Updated: Nov 08, 2017, Medscape. https://emedicine. medscape.com/article/171117-overview#a9. Accessed July 27, 2021.

51. Shibata H, Nakao K. [Bone disease in primary biliary cirrhosis]. *Clin Calcium.* 2015;25(11):1633–1638. Japanese. PMID: 26503867.

52. Mehrotra B. Gallbladder cancer: epidemiology, risk factors, clinical features, and diagnosis. UpToDate. Update March 21, 2021. http://www.uptodate.com/contents/gallbladder-cancer-epidemiology-risk-factors-clinical-features-and-diagnosis. Accessed July 15, 2021.

Screening for Urogenital Disease

Marty Fontenot

The urinary tract consists of the kidneys, ureters, bladder, and urethra (Fig. 11.1). It is an integral component of human functioning that disposes of the body's toxic waste products and unnecessary fluid and expertly regulates extremely complicated metabolic processes. The ureters, bladder, and urethra function primarily as transport vehicles for urine formed in the kidneys. The lower urinary tract is the last area through which urine is passed in its final form for excretion.

Formation and excretion of urine is the primary function of the renal nephron, which is the functional unit of the kidney (Fig. 11.2). Through this process, the kidney is able to maintain a homeostatic environment in the body. Besides the excretory function of the kidney, it plays an integral role in the balance of various essential body functions, including the following:

- Acid-base balance
- Electrolyte balance
- Control of blood pressure with renin
- Formation of red blood cells (RBCs)
- Activation of vitamin D and calcium balance

The failure of the kidney to perform any of these functions causes severe alterations and disruptions in homeostasis, resulting in associated signs and symptoms (Box 11.1).[1-3]

THE URINARY TRACT

The upper urinary tract consists of the kidneys and ureters. The kidneys are located in the posterior upper abdominal cavity in a space behind the peritoneum (retroperitoneal space). Their anatomic position is in front of, and on both sides of, the vertebral column at the level of T11 to L3. The right kidney is usually lower than the left to accommodate the liver.[4]

The upper portion of the kidney is in contact with the diaphragm and moves with respiration. The kidneys are protected anteriorly by the rib cage and abdominal organs (see Fig. 4.49) and posteriorly by the large back muscles and ribs. The lower portions of the kidneys and the ureters extend below the ribs and are separated from the abdominal cavity by the peritoneal membrane.

The lower urinary tract consists of the bladder and urethra. From the renal pelvis, urine is moved by peristalsis to the ureters and into the bladder. The bladder, a muscular,

membranous sac, is located directly behind the symphysis pubis and is used for storage and excretion of urine. The urethra is connected to the bladder and serves as a channel through which urine is passed from the bladder to the outside of the body.

Voluntary control of urinary excretion is based on learned inhibition of reflex pathways from the walls of the bladder. Release of urine from the bladder occurs under voluntary control of the urethral sphincter.

The male genital or reproductive system is made up of the testes, epididymis, vas deferens, seminal vesicles, prostate gland, and penis (Fig. 11.3). These structures are susceptible to inflammatory disorders, neoplasms, and structural defects.

In males, the posterior portion of the urethra is surrounded by the prostate gland, a gland approximately 3.5 cm long by 3 cm wide (about the size of two almonds).[5] Located just below the bladder, this gland can cause severe urethral obstruction when enlarged from a growth or from inflammation, resulting in difficulty starting and continuing a flow of urine, frequency, and/or nocturia.

The prostate gland is commonly divided into five lobes and three zones. Prostate carcinoma usually affects the posterior lobe of the gland; the middle and lateral lobes typically are associated with the nonmalignant process called *benign prostatic hyperplasia* (BPH).

INTRODUCTION TO SCREENING FOR UROGENITAL DISEASE

Complaints of flank pain, low back pain, or pelvic pain may be renal or urologic in origin and should be screened carefully through patient history/interview and tests and measures. Medical referral may be necessary. These symptoms may be secondary to trauma or have an insidious onset. Consider the case of an athletic 40-year-old man who comes to the clinic for an evaluation of back pain that he attributes to a very hard fall on his back while alpine skiing 3 days ago. His chief complaint is a dull, aching costovertebral pain on the left side, which is unrelieved by a change in position or by treatment with ice, heat, or aspirin. He stated that "even the skin on my back hurts." He has no previous history of any medical problems.

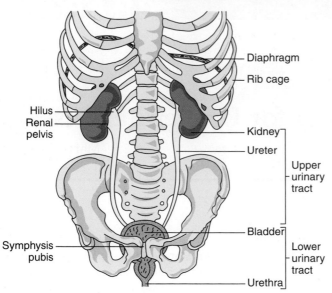

Fig. 11.1   Urinary tract structures. The upper urinary tract is composed of the kidneys and ureters, whereas the lower urinary tract is made up of the bladder and urethra. The upper portion of each kidney is protected by the rib cage, and the bladder is partially protected by the symphysis pubis.

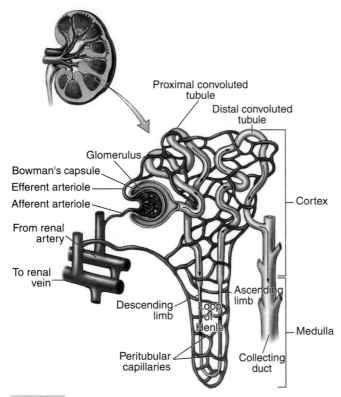

Fig. 11.2   Components of the nephron. The afferent arteriole carries blood to the glomerulus for filtration through Bowman's capsule and the renal tubular system. (From Herlihy B: *The human body in health and illness*, ed 6, St. Louis, MO, 2017, Elsevier Health Sciences.)

BOX 11.1   SIGNS AND SYMPTOMS OF GENITOURINARY DISEASE

Constitutional Symptoms
- Fever, chills
- Fatigue, malaise
- Anorexia, weight loss

Musculoskeletal
- Unilateral costovertebral tenderness
- Low back, flank, inner thigh, or leg pain
- Ipsilateral shoulder pain

Urinary Problems
- Dysuria (painful burning or discomfort with urination)
- Nocturia (getting up more than once at night to urinate)
- Feeling that bladder has not emptied completely but unable to urinate more; straining to start a stream of urine or to empty bladder completely
- Hematuria (blood in urine; pink or red-tinged urine)
- Dribbling at the end of urination
- Frequency (need to urinate or empty bladder more than every 2 hours)
- Hesitancy (weak or interrupted urine stream)
- Proteinuria (protein in urine; urine is foamy)

Other
- Skin hypersensitivity (T10-L1)
- Infertility

Specific to Women
- Abnormal vaginal bleeding
- Painful menstruation (dysmenorrhea)
- Changes in menstrual pattern
- Pelvic masses or lesions
- Vaginal itching or discharge
- Pain during intercourse (dyspareunia)

Specific to Men
- Difficulty starting or continuing a stream of urine
- Discharge from penis
- Penile lesions
- Testicular or penis pain
- Enlargement of scrotal contents
- Swelling or mass in groin
- Sexual dysfunction

After further questioning, the client reveals that inspiratory movements do not aggravate the pain, and he has not noticed any change in the color, odor, or volume of urine output. However, percussion of the costovertebral angle (CVA) (see Fig. 4.54) results in the reproduction of symptoms. This type of symptom complex may suggest renal involvement even without obvious changes in urine.

Urogenital conditions such as inflammatory/infectious conditions, obstructive disorders, chronic kidney disease, and cancers of the urinary tract could have presenting symptoms such as low back pain.[6] In addition, there is a significant association between urinary incontinence (UI) and urinary symptoms and low back pain.[7] It is therefore very critical

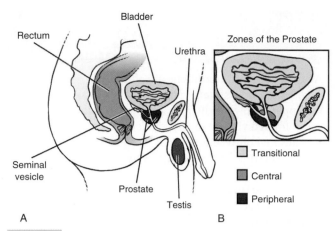

A

B

☐ Transitional

▨ Central

■ Peripheral

Fig. 11.3   **A**, The prostate is located at the base of the bladder, surrounding a part of the urethra. It is innervated by T11-L1 and S2-S4 and can refer pain to the sacrum, low back, and testes (see Fig. 11.10). As the prostate enlarges, the urethra can become obstructed, interfering with the normal flow of urine. **B**, The prostate is composed of three zones. The transitional zone surrounds the urethra as it passes through the prostate. This is a common site for benign prostatic hyperplasia (BPH). The central zone is a cone-shaped section that sits behind the transitional zone. The peripheral zone is the largest portion of the gland and borders the other two zones. This is the most common site for cancer development. Most early tumors do not produce any symptoms because the urethra is not in the peripheral zone. It is not until the tumor grows large enough to obstruct the bladder outlet that symptoms develop. Tumors in the transitional zone, which houses the urethra, may cause symptoms sooner than tumors in other zones.

for physical therapists screen for potential urological conditions to be able to provide the correct physical therapy diagnosis and appropriate patient management. This chapter is intended to guide the physical therapist in understanding the origins and relationships of renal, ureteral, bladder, and urethral symptoms.

SIGNS AND SYMPTOMS OF RENAL AND UROLOGIC DISORDERS

Upper Urinary Tract Pain (Renal/Ureteral)

The kidneys and ureters are innervated by both sympathetic and parasympathetic fibers. The kidneys receive sympathetic innervation from the lesser splanchnic nerves through the renal plexus, which is located next to the renal arteries. Renal vasoconstriction and increased renin release are associated with sympathetic stimulation. Parasympathetic innervation is derived from the vagus nerve, and the function of this innervation is not known.

Renal sensory innervation is not completely understood, even though the capsule (covering of the kidney) and the lower portions of the collecting system seem to cause pain with stretching (distention) or puncture. Information transmitted by renal and ureteral pain receptors is relayed by sympathetic nerves that enter the spinal cord at T10 to L1 (see Fig. 3.3).

Because visceral and cutaneous sensory fibers enter the spinal cord in close proximity and actually converge on some of the same neurons, when visceral pain fibers are stimulated, concurrent stimulation of cutaneous fibers also occurs. The visceral pain is then felt as though it is skin pain (hyperesthesia), similar to the condition of the alpine skier who stated that "even the skin on my back hurts." Renal and ureteral pain can be felt throughout the T10 to L1 dermatomes.

Renal pain (Fig. 11.7) is typically felt in the posterior subcostal and costovertebral regions. To assess the kidney, the test for CVA tenderness can be included in the physical examination (see Fig. 4.54).

Ureteral pain is felt in the groin and genital area (Fig. 11.8). With either renal or ureteral pain, radiation forward and around the flank into the lower abdominal quadrant can occur; abdominal muscle spasms with rebound tenderness on the same side as the source of pain is also possible.

The pain can also be generalized throughout the abdomen. Nausea, vomiting, and impaired intestinal motility (progressing to intestinal paralysis) can occur with severe, acute pain. Nerve fibers from the renal plexus are also in direct communication with the spermatic plexus, and because of this close relationship, testicular pain may also accompany renal pain. Neither renal nor urethral pain is altered by a change in body position.

The typical renal pain sensation is aching and dull in nature but can occasionally be a severe, boring type of pain. The constant dull and aching pain usually accompanies distention or stretching of the renal capsule, pelvis, or collecting system. This stretching can result from intrarenal fluid accumulation such as inflammatory edema, inflamed or bleeding cysts, and bleeding or neoplastic growths. Whenever the renal capsule is punctured, a dull pain can also be felt by the client. Ischemia of renal tissue caused by blockage of blood flow to the kidneys results in a *constant* dull or a *constant* sharp pain.[8-10]

Ureteral obstruction (e.g., from a urinary calculus or "stone" consisting of mineral salts) results in distention of the ureter and causes spasm that produces intermittent or constant severe colicky pain until the stone is passed. Pain of this origin usually starts in the CVA and radiates to the ipsilateral lower abdomen, upper thigh, testis, or labium (Fig. 11.8). Movement of a stone down a ureter can cause *renal colic*, an excruciating pain that radiates to the region just described and usually increases in intensity in waves of colic or spasm.

Chronic ureteral and renal pain tends to be vague, poorly localized, and easily confused with many other problems of abdominal or pelvic origin. There are also areas of *referred pain* related to renal or ureteral lesions. For example, if the diaphragm becomes irritated because of pressure from a renal lesion, shoulder pain may be felt (see Figs. 3.4 and 3.5). If a lesion of the ureter occurs *outside* of the ureter, pain may occur during movement of the adjacent iliopsoas muscle.

Abdominal rebound tenderness results when the adjacent peritoneum becomes inflamed. Active trigger points along the upper rim of the pubis and the lateral half of the inguinal ligament may lie in the lower internal oblique muscle and possibly in the lower rectus abdominis. These trigger points can cause increased irritation and spasm of the detrusor and urinary sphincter muscles, producing urinary frequency, retention of urine, and groin pain.[11,12]

TABLE 11.1	Assessment for Pseudorenal Pain
History	• Trauma (fall, assault, blow, lifting) • History of straining, lifting, accident, or other mechanical injury to thoracic spine
Pain Pattern	• Back and/or flank pain occur at the same level as the kidney • Affected by change in position • Lying on the involved side increases pain • Prolonged sitting increases pain • Symptoms are reproduced with movements of the spine • Costovertebral angle tenderness present on palpation
Associated Signs and Symptoms	• Murphy's percussion (punch) test is negative • Report of bowel and bladder changes unlikely

> ### BOX 11.2 EXTRA-UROLOGIC CONDITIONS CAUSING URINARY TRACT SYMPTOMS
>
> Acute or chronic conditions affecting other viscera outside the urologic system can refer pain and symptoms to the upper or lower urinary tract. These can include:
> - Perforated viscus (any large internal organ)
> - Intestinal obstruction
> - Cholecystitis (inflammation of the gallbladder)
> - Pelvic inflammatory disease
> - Tubo-ovarian abscess
> - Ruptured ectopic pregnancy
> - Twisted ovarian cyst
> - Tumor (benign or malignant)

Pseudorenal Pain

Pseudorenal pain may occur secondary to radiculitis or irritation of the costal nerves caused by mechanical derangements of the costovertebral or costotransverse joints. Disorders of this sort are common in the cervical and thoracic areas, but the most common sites are T10 and T12.[13] Irritation of these nerves causes costovertebral pain that can radiate into the ipsilateral lower abdominal quadrant.

The onset is usually acute with some type of traumatic history such as lifting a heavy object, sustaining a blow to the costovertebral area, or falling from a height onto the buttocks. The pain is affected by body position, and although the client may be awakened at night when assuming a certain position (e.g., side lying on the affected side), the pain is usually absent once awake and increases gradually during the day. It is also aggravated by prolonged periods of sitting, especially when driving on rough roads in the car. It may be relieved by changing to another position (Table 11.1).

Radiculitis may mimic ureteral colic or renal pain, but true renal pain is seldom affected by movements of the shoulder or spine. Exerting pressure over the CVA with the thumb may elicit local tenderness of the involved peripheral nerve at its point of emergence, whereas gentle percussion over the angle may be necessary to elicit renal pain, indicating a deeper, more visceral sensation usually associated with an infectious or inflammatory process such as pyelonephritis, a perinephric abscess, or other kidney problem.

Fig. 4.54 illustrates percussion over the CVA (Murphy's percussion or punch test). Although this test is commonly performed, its diagnostic value has never been validated.

Lower Urinary Tract Pain (Bladder/Urethra)

Bladder innervation occurs through sympathetic, parasympathetic, and sensory nerve pathways. Sympathetic bladder innervation assists in the closure of the bladder neck during seminal emission. Afferent sympathetic fibers also assist in providing awareness of bladder distention, pain, and abdominal distention caused by bladder distention. This input reaches the spinal cord at T9 or higher. Parasympathetic bladder innervation is at S2, S3, and S4 and provides motor coordination for the act of voiding. Afferent parasympathetic fibers assist in sensation of the desire to void, proprioception (position sensation), and perception of pain.

Sensory receptors are present in the mucosa of the bladder and in the muscular bladder walls. These fibers are more plentiful near the bladder neck and the junctional area between the ureters and bladder.

Urethral innervation, also at the S2, S3, and S4 level, occurs through the pudendal nerve. This is a mixed innervation of both sensory and motor nerve fibers. This innervation controls the opening of the external urethral sphincter (motor) and an awareness of the imminence of voiding and heat (thermal) sensation in the urethra.

Bladder or urethral pain is felt above the pubis (suprapubic) or low in the abdomen (Fig. 11.9). The sensation is usually characterized as one of urinary urgency, a sensation to void, and dysuria (painful urination). Irritation of the neck of the bladder or the urethra can result in a burning sensation localized to these areas, probably caused by the urethral thermal receptors. See Box 11.2 for causes of pain outside of the urogenital system that present like upper or lower urinary tract pain of either an acute or chronic nature.

RENAL AND URINARY TRACT PROBLEMS

Pathologic conditions of the upper and lower urinary tract can be categorized according to primary causative factors. Inflammatory/infectious and obstructive disorders are presented in this section along with renal failure and cancers of the urinary tract.

When screening for any condition affecting the kidneys and urinary tract system, keep in mind factors that put people at increased risk for these problems (Case Example 11.1). Early screening and detection is recommended based on the presence of these risk factors.[14]

- Age over 60 years
- Personal or family history of diabetes mellitus or hypertension
- Personal or family history of kidney disease, heart attack, or stroke
- Personal history of kidney stones, urinary tract infections (UTIs), lower urinary tract obstruction, or autoimmune disease

CASE EXAMPLE 11.1

Screening in the Presence of Risk Factors for Kidney Disease

A 66-year-old African-American woman with a personal history of systemic lupus erythematosus (SLE) lost her balance and fell off of the deck at her home. She sustained vertebral and rib fractures at T10 and T11. She is a retired paint factory worker. She reported daily exposure to paint and paint solvents during her 15 years of employment.

She was seen as a walk-in at the local medical clinic where she is a regular patient. She did not see the rheumatologist who was managing her SLE. The attending physician told her the injuries were "probably from the long-term use of prednisone for her lupus." She was referred to physical therapy by the attending physician for postural exercises.

During the interview, when asked, "Are you having any symptoms of any kind anywhere else in your body?" the client admitted to a pink color to her urine and some burning during urination. These symptoms have been present since the day after the fall 3 weeks ago.

There were no other signs or symptoms reported. Blood pressure measured 175/95 on three separate occasions. The client reported her blood pressure was elevated at the time of her visit to the doctor, but she thought it was caused by the stress of the fall.

Question: As you step back and conduct a Review of Systems (ROS), what are the red flags to suggest medical referral is needed? To whom do you refer this client?

Red flags
- Age over 40 years (age over 60 years is a risk factor for kidney disease)
- African-American descent (at risk for diabetes mellitus, kidney disease)
- Long-term use of nonsteroidal antiinflammatory drugs (NSAIDs) (synergistic nephrotoxin in combination with certain chemicals such as paint and paint solvents)
- Elevated blood pressure
- Change in color and pattern of urination

The therapist may not recognize specific factors present that put the client at increased risk for kidney disease, but the obvious changes in urine color and pattern along with changes in blood pressure require medical referral.

Without the medical records, it is impossible to know what (if any) testing was done related to kidney function (e.g., urinalysis, blood test) at the time of the initial injury. A phone call to the referring physician is probably the best place to start. Documentation of the recent events and current red-flag symptoms should be sent to the referring physician, the primary care physician, and the rheumatologist (if different from the primary care doctor).

Physical therapy intervention is still appropriate given her musculoskeletal injuries. Further medical assessment is warranted based on the development of symptoms unknown to the referring physician.

- African, Hispanic, Pacific Island, or Native American descent
- Exposure to chemicals (e.g., paint, glue, degreasing solvents, cleaning solvents), drugs, or environmental conditions
- Low birth weight

TABLE 11.2	**Urinary Tract Infections**
Upper Urinary Tract Infection	Lower Urinary Tract Infection
Renal infections, such as pyelonephritis (renal parenchyma, i.e., kidney tissue) Acute or chronic glomerulonephritis (glomeruli) Renal papillary necrosis Renal tuberculosis	Cystitis (bladder infection) Urethritis (urethra infection)

TABLE 11.3	**Clinical Symptoms of Infectious/ Inflammatory Urinary Tract Problems**
Upper Urinary Tract (Kidney or Ureteral Infection)	Lower Urinary Tract (Cystitis or Urethritis)
Unilateral costovertebral tenderness	Urinary frequency
Flank pain	Urinary urgency
Ipsilateral shoulder pain	Low back pain
Fever and chills	Pelvic/lower abdominal pain
Skin hypersensitivity (hyperesthesia of dermatomes)	Dysuria (discomfort, such as pain or burning during urination)
Hematuria (blood [RBCs] in urine)	Hematuria
Pyuria (pus or white blood cells in urine)	Pyuria
Bacteriuria (bacteria in urine)	Bacteriuria
Nocturia (unusual or increased nighttime need to urinate)	Dyspareunia (painful intercourse)

Inflammatory/Infectious Disorders

Inflammatory disorders of the kidney and urinary tract can be caused by bacterial infection, by change in immune response, and by toxic agents such as drugs and radiation. Common infections of the urinary tract develop in either the upper or lower urinary tract (Table 11.2).

Upper UTIs include kidney or ureteral infections. Lower UTIs include cystitis (bladder infection) or urethritis (urethral infection). Symptoms of UTI depend on the location of the infection in either the upper or lower urinary tract (although rarely, infection could occur in both simultaneously).

Inflammatory/Infectious Disorders of the Upper Urinary Tract

Inflammation or infections of the upper urinary tract (kidney and ureters) are considered to be more serious because these lesions can be a direct threat to renal tissue itself.

The more common conditions include pyelonephritis (inflammation of the renal parenchyma) and acute and chronic glomerulonephritis (inflammation of the glomeruli of both kidneys). Less common conditions include renal papillary necrosis and renal tuberculosis.

Symptoms of upper UTIs and inflammation are shown in Table 11.3. If the diaphragm is irritated, ipsilateral shoulder pain may occur. Signs and symptoms of renal impairment are significant symptoms of impending kidney failure (Table 11.4).

TABLE 11.4	Systemic Manifestations of Chronic Kidney Disease
System	**Manifestation**
General	Fatigue, malaise
Skin and nail beds	Pallor, ecchymosis, pruritus, dry skin and mucous membranes, thin/brittle nail beds, urine odor on skin, uremic frost (white urea crystals) on the face and upper trunk, poor wound healing
Skeletal	Osteomalacia, osteoporosis,* bone pain, myopathy, tendon rupture, fracture, joint pain, dependent edema
Neurologic	*CNS:* recent memory loss, decreased alertness, difficulty concentrating, irritability, lethargy/sleep disturbance, coma, impaired judgment *PNS:* muscle weakness, tremors, and cramping; neuropathies with restless legs syndrome, cramps, carpal tunnel syndrome, paresthesias, burning feet syndrome, pruritus (itching)
Eye, ear, nose, throat	Metallic taste in mouth, nosebleeds, uremic (urine-smelling) breath, pale conjunctiva, visual blurring
Cardiovascular	Hypertension, friction rub, congestive heart failure, pericarditis, cardiomyopathy, arrhythmia, Raynaud's phenomenon
Pulmonary	Dyspnea, pulmonary edema, crackles (rales), pleural effusion
Gastrointestinal	Anorexia, nausea, vomiting, hiccups, gastrointestinal bleeding
Genitourinary	Decreased urine output and other changes in pattern of urination (e.g., nocturia)
Metabolic/endocrine	Dehydration, hyperkalemia, metabolic acidosis, hypocalcemia, hyperphosphatemia, fertility and sexual dysfunction (e.g., impotence, loss of libido, amenorrhea), hyperparathyroidism
Hematologic	Anemia Thrombocytopenia

From Goodman CC, Fuller KS: *Pathology: implications for the physical therapist*, ed 5, St. Louis, 2021, Elsevier.
CNS, Central nervous system; *PNS*, peripheral nervous system.
*Bone demineralization leads to a condition called *renal osteodystrophy*.

Inflammatory/Infectious Disorders of the Lower Urinary Tract

Both the bladder and urine have a number of defense mechanisms against bacterial invasion. These defense mechanisms include voiding, urine acidity, osmolality, and the bladder mucosa itself, which is thought to have antibacterial properties.[15]

Urine in the bladder and kidney is normally sterile, but urine itself is a good medium for bacterial growth. Interferences in the defense mechanisms of the bladder, such as the presence of residual or stagnant urine, changes in urinary pH or concentration, or obstruction of urinary excretion, can promote bacterial growth.

Routes of entry of bacteria into the urinary tract can be *ascending* (most commonly up the urethra into the bladder and then into the ureters and kidney), *bloodborne* (bacterial invasion through the bloodstream), or *lymphatic* (bacterial invasion through the lymph system, the least common route).

A lower UTI occurs most commonly in women because of the short female urethra and the proximity of the urethra to the vagina and rectum. The rate of occurrence increases with age and sexual activity, because intercourse can spread bacteria from the genital area to the urethra. Chronic health problems such as diabetes mellitus, gout, hypertension, obstructive urinary tract problems, and medical procedures requiring urinary catheterization are also predisposing risk factors for the development of these infections.[16-20]

Individuals with diabetes mellitus are prone to complications associated with UTIs. Staphylococcus infection of the urinary tract may be a source of osteomyelitis, an infection of a vertebral body resulting from hematogenous or local spread from an abscess into the vertebra. The infected vertebral body may gradually undergo degeneration and destruction,[21] with collapse and formation of a segmental scoliosis. This condition is suspected from the onset of nonspecific low back pain, unrelated to any specific motion. Local tenderness can be elicited, but the initial x-ray finding is negative. Usually, a low-grade fever is present but undetected, or it develops as the infection progresses. It is therefore important that anyone with low back pain of unknown origin should have his or her temperature taken, even in a physical therapy setting.

Older adults (both men and women) are at increased risk for UTI. They may present with nonspecific symptoms, such as loss of appetite, nausea, and vomiting; abdominal pain; or change in mental health status (e.g., onset of confusion, increased confusion). Watch for predisposing conditions that can put the older client at risk for UTI. These may include diabetes mellitus or other chronic diseases (e.g., Alzheimer's disease, Parkinson's disease), immobility, reduced fluid intake, use of incontinence management products (e.g., pads, briefs, external catheters), indwelling catheterization, and previous history of UTI or kidney stones.

Cystitis

Cystitis (inflammation with infection of the bladder), *interstitial cystitis* (IC; inflammation without infection), and *urethritis* (inflammation and infection of the urethra) appear with a similar symptomatic progression (Case Example 11.2).

According to the Interstitial Cystitis Association (ICA), IC, also known as painful bladder syndrome, is a condition that consists of recurring pelvic pain, pressure, or discomfort in the bladder and pelvic region and affects more than 12 million people in the United States.[22] IC is often associated with urinary frequency and urgency. Men can be affected by this condition, but the majority of people living with IC are women. Several other disorders are associated with IC including allergies, irritable bowel syndrome, sensitive skin, fibromyalgia, systemic lupus erythematosus, and vulvodynia.[23]

CASE EXAMPLE 11.2
Bladder Infection

A 55-year-old woman presents with back pain associated with paraspinal muscle spasms. Pain is of unknown cause (insidious onset) and the client reports that she was "just getting out of bed" when the pain started. The pain is described as a dull aching that is aggravated by movement and relieved by rest (musculoskeletal pattern).

No numbness, tingling, or saddle anesthesia is reported, and the neurologic screening examination is negative. Sacroiliac (SI) testing is negative. Spinal movements are slow and guarded, with muscle spasms noted throughout movement and at rest. Because of her age and the insidious onset of symptoms, further questions are initiated to screen for possible medical pathology.

This client is mid-menopausal and is not taking any hormone replacement therapy (HRT). She had a bladder infection a month ago that was treated with antibiotics; tests for this were negative when she was evaluated and referred by her physician for back pain. Two weeks ago she had an upper respiratory infection (a "cold") and had been "coughing a lot." There was no previous history of cancer.

Local treatment to reduce paraspinal muscle spasms was initiated, but the client did not respond as expected over the course of five treatment sessions. Because of her recent history of upper respiratory and bladder infections, questions were repeated related to the presence of constitutional symptoms and change in bladder function/urine color, force of stream, burning during urination, and so on. Occasional "sweats" (present sometimes during the day, sometimes at night) was the only red flag present. The combination of recent infection, failure to respond to treatment, and the presence of sweats suggested referral to the physician for early reevaluation.

The client did not return to the clinic for further treatment, and a follow-up telephone call indicated that she did indeed have a recurrent bladder infection that was treated successfully with a different antibiotic. Her back pain and muscle spasm were eliminated after only 24 hours of taking this new antibiotic.

Bladder pain associated with IC can be severely painful and incapacitating, and usually accompanied by frequency and urgency.[24] Additional symptoms include pain and discomfort while the bladder fills, and frequent urination, often in small amounts, up to 60 times a day in severe cases.[25]

Clients with any symptoms associated with lower UTI (see Table 11.3) at presentation should be referred promptly to a physician for further diagnostic workup and possible treatment. Infections of the lower urinary tract are potentially very dangerous because of the possibility of upward spread and resultant damage to the renal tissue. Some individuals, however, are asymptomatic, and routine urine culture and microscopic examination are the most reliable methods of detection and diagnosis.

Obstructive Disorders

Urinary tract obstruction can occur at any point in the urinary tract and can be the result of *primary* urinary tract obstructions (obstructions occurring within the urinary tract) or *secondary* urinary tract obstructions (obstructions resulting from disease processes outside of the urinary tract).

A primary obstruction might include problems such as acquired or congenital malformations, strictures, renal or ureteral calculi (stones), polycystic kidney disease, or neoplasms of the urinary tract (e.g., bladder, kidney).

Secondary obstructions produce pressure on the urinary tract from outside and might be related to conditions such as prostatic enlargement (benign or malignant); abdominal aortic aneurysm; gynecologic conditions such as pregnancy, pelvic inflammatory disease, and endometriosis; or neoplasms of the pelvic or abdominal structures.[26]

Obstruction of any portion of the urinary tract results in a backup or collection of urine behind the obstruction. The result is dilation or stretching of the urinary tract structures that are positioned behind the point of blockage.

Muscles near the affected area contract in an attempt to push urine around the obstruction. Pressure accumulates above the point of obstruction and can eventually result in severe dilation of the renal collecting system (hydronephrosis) and renal failure. The greater the intensity and duration of the pressure, the greater is the destruction of renal tissue.

Because urine flow is decreased with obstruction, urinary stagnation and infection or stone formation can result. Stones are formed because urine stasis permits clumping or precipitation of organic matter and minerals.

Lower urinary tract obstruction can also result in constant bladder distention, hypertrophy of bladder muscle fibers, and formation of herniated sacs of bladder mucosa. These herniated sacs result in a large, flaccid bladder that cannot empty completely. In addition, these sacs retain stagnant urine, which causes infection and stone formation.

Obstructive Disorders of the Upper Urinary Tract

Obstruction of the upper urinary tract may be sudden (acute) or slow in development. Tumors of the kidney or ureters may develop slowly enough that symptoms are totally absent or very mild initially, with eventual progression to pain and signs of impairment. *Acute* ureteral or renal blockage by a stone (calculus consisting of mineral salts), for example, may result in excruciating, spasmodic, and radiating pain accompanied by severe nausea and vomiting.

Calculi form primarily in the kidney. This process is called *nephrolithiasis*. The stones can remain in the kidney (renal pelvis) or travel down the urinary tract and lodge at any point in the tract. Strictly speaking, the term *kidney stones* refers to stones that are in the kidney. Once they move into the ureter, they become *ureteral stones*.

Ureteral stones are the ones that cause the most pain. If a stone becomes wedged in the ureter, urine backs up, distending the ureter and causing severe pain. If a stone blocks the flow of urine, urine pressure may build up in the ureter and kidney, causing the kidney to swell (hydronephrosis). Unrecognized hydronephrosis can sometimes cause permanent kidney damage.[27]

The most characteristic symptom of renal or ureteral stones is sudden, sharp, severe pain. If the pain originates deep in the lumbar area and radiates around the side and down toward the testicle in the male and the bladder in the female, it is termed *renal colic*. *Ureteral colic* occurs if the stone becomes trapped in the ureter. Ureteral colic is characterized by radiation of painful symptoms toward the genitalia and thighs (Fig. 11.8). The person with ureteral colic appears in distress, often in constant movement to find a comfortable position. This is in contrast to a person with peritoneal irritation who remains motionless with any movement causing pain.[28]

Because the testicles and ovaries form in utero in the location of the kidneys and then migrate at full term following the pathways of the ureters, kidney stones moving down the pathway of the ureters cause pain in the flank. This pain radiates to the scrotum in males and the labia in females. For the same reason, ovarian or testicular cancer can refer pain to the back at the level of the kidneys.

Renal tumors may also be detected as a flank mass combined with unexplained weight loss, fever, pain, and hematuria. The presence of any amount of blood in the urine always requires referral to a physician for further diagnostic evaluation because this is a primary symptom of urinary tract neoplasm, affecting approximately 80% to 90% of patients.[29]

CLINICAL SIGNS AND SYMPTOMS
Obstruction of the Upper Urinary Tract

- Pain (depends on the rapidity of onset and on the location)
  - Acute, spasmodic, radiating
  - Mild and dull flank pain
  - Lumbar discomfort with some renal diseases or renal back pain with ureteral obstruction
- Hyperesthesia of dermatomes (T10 through L1)
- Nausea and vomiting
- Palpable flank mass
- Hematuria
- Fever and chills
- Urge to urinate frequently
- Abdominal muscle spasms
- Renal impairment indicators (see inside front cover: Renal Blood Studies; see also Table 11.4)

Obstructive Disorders of the Lower Urinary Tract

Common conditions of (mechanical) obstruction of the lower urinary tract are bladder tumors (bladder cancer is the most common site of urinary tract cancer) and prostatic enlargement, either benign (BPH) or malignant (cancer of the prostate). An enlarged prostate gland can occlude the urethra partially or completely.

Mechanical problems of the urinary tract result in difficulty emptying urine from the bladder. Improper emptying of the bladder results in urinary retention and impairment of voluntary bladder control (incontinence). Several possible causes of mechanical bladder dysfunction include pelvic floor dysfunction, UTIs, partial urethral obstruction, trauma, and removal of the prostate gland.

The nerves that carry pain sensation from the prostate do not localize the source of pain very precisely, and therefore it may be difficult for the man to describe exactly where the pain is coming from. Discomfort can be localized in the suprapubic region or in the penis and testicles, or it can be centered in the perineum or rectum (Fig. 11.10).

Prostatitis. Prostatitis is a relatively common inflammation of the prostate causing prostate enlargement. This condition accounts for 25% of male patients presenting with genitourinary symptoms, and accounts for two outpatient treatments per year.[30] Autopsy studies have revealed a histologic prevalence of prostatitis of 64%–86%. It is often disabling, affecting men at any age, but typically found in men aged 40 to 70 years. Acute bacterial prostatitis occurs most often in men under age 35 years.

The National Institutes of Health (NIH) Consensus Classification of Prostatitis[31-34] includes four distinct categories:

Type I	Acute bacterial prostatitis
Type II	Chronic bacterial prostatitis
Type III	Chronic prostatitis/chronic pelvic pain syndrome (CP/CPPS)
	A. Inflammatory
	B. Noninflammatory
Type IV	Asymptomatic inflammatory prostatitis

Type I is an acute prostatic infection with a uropathogen, often with systemic symptoms of fever, chills, and hypotension. The prostate is inflamed and may block urinary flow without treatment. Type II is characterized by recurrent episodes of documented UTIs with the same uropathogen repeatedly and causes pelvic pain, urinary symptoms, and ejaculatory pain. The source of recurrent infections in the lower urinary tract must be identified and treated.

Chronic (type III, nonbacterial) prostatitis is characterized by pelvic pain for more than 3 of the previous 6 months, urinary symptoms, and painful ejaculation without documented UTIs from uropathogens.

The symptoms of CP/CPPS appear to occur as a result of interplay between psychologic factors and dysfunction in the immune, neurologic, and endocrine systems.[35] Studies show a major effect on the quality of life, urinary function, and sexual function along with chronic pain and discomfort (Fig. 11.4).[36]

The pain of prostatitis can be exacerbated by sexual activity, and some men describe pain upon ejaculation. A digital rectal examination (DRE) by the physician will reproduce painful symptoms when the prostate is inflamed or infected (Fig. 11.5).

In men with chronic prostatitis, voiding complaints similar to those caused by BPH are the predominant symptoms. These complaints include urgency, frequency, and nocturia (getting up at nighttime more than once); less frequently, men may complain of difficulty starting the urinary stream or a slow stream.

These symptoms typically differ from symptoms of BPH, in that they are associated with some degree of discomfort before, during, or after voiding. Physical or emotional stress

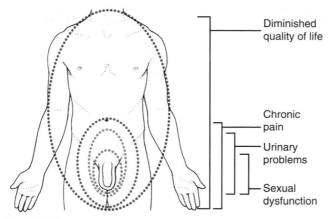

Fig. 11.4 Chronic prostatitis/chronic pelvic pain syndrome (CP/CPPS) can have a serious effect on a man's quality of life as a result of voiding problems, chronic pelvic pain and discomfort, and sexual dysfunction with painful ejaculation, cramping, or discomfort after ejaculation and infertility.

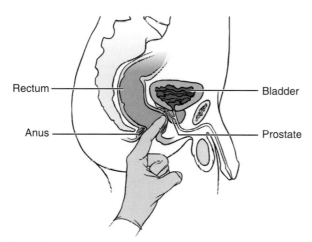

Fig. 11.5 Digital rectal examination performed by a medical doctor or trained health care professional, such as a nurse practitioner or physician's assistant, puts pressure on the inflamed prostate reproducing painful symptoms associated with prostatitis.

and/or irritative components of the diet (e.g., caffeine in coffee, soft drinks) commonly exacerbate chronic prostatitis symptoms.

The causes of prostatitis are unclear. Although it can be the result of a bacterial infection, many men have nonbacterial prostatitis of unknown cause. Risk factors for bacterial prostatitis include some sexually transmitted diseases (e.g., gonorrhea) from unprotected anal and vaginal intercourse, which can allow bacteria to enter the urethra and travel to the prostate.

Other risk factors include bladder outlet obstruction (e.g., stone, tumor, BPH), diabetes mellitus, immunosuppression, and urethral catheterization. Neither prostatitis nor prostate enlargement is known to cause cancer, but men with prostatitis or BPH can develop prostate cancer.

The NIH Chronic Prostatitis Symptom Index (NIH-CPSI) provides a valid outcome measure for men with chronic

(nonbacterial) prostatitis. The index may be useful in clinical practice, as well as research protocols.[37,38]

Anyone with significant symptoms assessed by the NIH-CPSI associated with constitutional symptoms should be rechecked by a physician. Individuals with significant symptoms but no constitutional symptoms and individuals nonresponsive to antibiotics should be assessed by a pelvic floor specialist. The index is available for clinical practice and may be useful for research protocols. It is available online at www.prostatitis.org/symptomindex.html.

A less complete list of questions for screening purposes is most appropriate for men with low back pain and any of the risk factors or symptoms listed for **prostatitis** and may include the following:

? FOLLOW-UP QUESTIONS

- Do you ever have burning pain or discomfort during or right after urination?
- Does it feel like your bladder is not empty when you finish urinating?
- Do you have to go to the bathroom every 2 hours (or more often)?
- Do you ever have pain or discomfort in your testicles, penis, or the area between your rectum and your testicles (perineum)?
- Do you ever have pain in your pubic or bladder area?
- Do you have any discomfort during or after sexual climax (ejaculation)?

The therapist is reminded in asking these questions to offer clients a clear explanation for any questions asked concerning sexual activity, sexual function, or sexual history. There is no way to know when someone will be offended or claim sexual harassment. It is in your own interest to conduct the interview in the most professional manner possible.

There should be no hint of sexual innuendo or humor injected into any of your conversations with clients at any time. The line of sexual impropriety lies where the complainant draws it and includes appearances of misbehavior. This perception differs broadly from client to client.[39]

Prostatitis cannot always be cured but can be managed. Correct diagnosis is the key to the management of prostatitis. Screening men with red-flag symptoms, history, and risk factors can result in early detection and medical referral.

Physical therapy has been shown to have some potential in helping men with chronic prostatitis. Several published studies support the positive effect of physical therapy in decreasing pain and improving function in patients with this diagnosis. Other minimally invasive intervention strategies directed toward reducing pelvic floor muscle tone and improving urinary function include electrostimulation, biofeedback, needle ablation hyperthermia, BOTOX injection, myofascial release, extracorporeal shockwave therapy, and transrectal mobilization of the pelvic ligaments.[40–46]

Benign Prostatic Hyperplasia. BPH (enlarged prostate) is the most common prostate problem in men 50 years or older. Like all cells in the body, cells in the prostate constantly die and are replaced by new cells. As men age, the ratio of new prostate cells to old prostate cells shifts in favor of lower

CLINICAL SIGNS AND SYMPTOMS
Prostatitis

- Sudden moderate-to-high fever
- Chills
- Low back, inner thigh, and perineal pain
- Testicular or penis pain
- Urinary frequency and urgency
- Nocturia (unusual voiding during the night)/sleep disturbance
- Dysuria (painful or difficult urination)
- Weak or interrupted urine stream (hesitancy)
- Unable to completely empty bladder
- Sexual dysfunction (e.g., painful ejaculation, cramping/discomfort after ejaculation, infertility)
- General malaise
- Arthralgia
- Myalgia

CLINICAL SIGNS AND SYMPTOMS
Obstruction of the Lower Urinary Tract (Benign Prostatic Hyperplasia/Prostate Cancer)

Lower urinary tract symptoms of blockage are most commonly related to bladder or urethral pressure (e.g., prostate enlargement). This pressure results in bladder distention and subsequent pain. Common symptoms of lower urinary tract obstruction include:

- Bladder palpable above the symphysis pubis
- Urinary problems
  - Hesitancy: difficulty in initiating urination or an interrupted flow of urine
  - Small amounts of urine with voiding (weak urine stream)
  - Dribbling at the end of urination
  - Frequency: need to urinate often (more than every 2 hours)
  - Nocturia (unusual voiding during the night)/sleep disturbance
- Lower abdominal discomfort with a feeling of the need to void
- Low back and/or hip, upper thigh pain or stiffness
- Suprapubic or pelvic pain
- Difficulty having an erection
- Blood in urine or semen

cell death. With a lower cell turnover, there are more "old" cells than "new" ones and the prostate enlarges, squeezing the urethra and interfering with urination and sexual function. It is unclear why cell replacement is diminished, but it may be related to hormonal changes associated with aging.

Prostate enlargement affects about half of all men between ages 51 and 60 years and close to 90% of men over 80 years.[47] Severity of signs and symptoms varies and less than half of men with prostate enlargement have symptoms of the condition.[48]

Because of the prostate's position around the urethra (Fig. 11.3), enlargement of the prostate quickly interferes with the normal passage of urine from the bladder. Sexual function is not usually affected unless prostate surgery is required and sexual dysfunction occurs as a complication. If the prostate is greatly enlarged, chronic constipation may result.

Urination becomes increasingly difficult, and the bladder never feels completely empty. Straining to empty the bladder can stretch the bladder, making it less elastic. The detrusor becomes less efficient, and urine collecting in the bladder can foster UTIs.

If left untreated, loss of bladder tone and damage to the detrusor may not be reversible. Continued enlargement of the prostate eventually obstructs the bladder completely, and emergency measures become necessary to empty the bladder.

Like prostatitis, BPH cannot be cured, but symptoms can be managed with medical treatment. Anyone with undiagnosed symptoms of BPH should seek medical evaluation as soon as possible. Screening questions for an **enlarged prostate** can include the following:

? FOLLOW-UP QUESTIONS

- Does it feel like your bladder is not empty when you finish urinating?
- Do you have to urinate again less than 2 hours after the last time you emptied your bladder?
- Do you have a weak stream of urine or find you have to start and stop urinating several times when you go to the bathroom?
- Do you have to push or strain to start urinating or to keep the urine flowing?
- Do you have any leaking or dribbling of urine from the penis?
- Do you get up more than once at night to urinate?

Prostate Cancer. Prostate cancer is a slow-growing form of malignancy causing microscopic changes in the prostate; other than skin cancer, prostate cancer is the leading cause of cancer mortality among men of all races.[49] One out of 41 men will die of prostate cancer,[50] with 248,530 new cases and 34,130 deaths estimated in 2021 in the United States to "268,490 new cases and 34,500 deaths estimated in 2022 in the United States.[50]

The number of new diagnosed cases of prostate cancer has increased since the early 1990's, probably as a result of mass screening using a blood test to measure the prostate-specific antigen (PSA). PSA levels rise in men who have any change in the prostate (e.g., tumor, infection, enlargement).[51,52] Despite the many controversies over "normal" levels of PSA, this test has shifted the detection of the majority of prostate cancer cases from late-stage to early-stage disease when prostate cancers are more likely to be curable.[53] Currently, it has been reported that the evidence is insufficient to determine whether screening for prostate cancer (with PSA or DRE) results in a reduced number of deaths. Although screening tests are able to detect the presence of prostate cancer earlier, it is unclear whether early detection and treatment has an effect on progression or outcome.[54] The American Cancer Society has recommendations[55] for prostate cancer early detection that can be found at this link: http://www.cancer.org/cancer/prostatecancer/moreinformation/prostatecancerearlydetection/prostate-cancer-early-detection-acs-recommendations.

Because more men are living longer and the incidence of prostate cancer increases with age, prostate cancer is becoming a significant health issue. Risk factors include advancing age, family history, ethnicity, and diet. Most men with prostate cancer are older than 65 years of age; the disease is rare in men younger than 40 years.[56]

A man's risk of prostate cancer is higher than average if his brother or father had the disease. It is reported that African-American men have a 70% higher risk of developing prostate cancer than non-Hispanic Whites. The 5-year survival rate is high, at 98%, but drops to 30% when the cancer has spread to other parts of the body.[56]

There are no studies reporting that diet and nutrition having a direct cause of development of prostate cancers, but many studies have indicated a possible link.[57] Some studies suggest that a diet high in animal fat or meat may be a risk factor.[58] Other risk factors may include low levels of vitamins or selenium; multiple sex partners[59]; viruses[60,61]; and occupational exposure to chemicals (including farmers exposed to herbicides and pesticides), cadmium, and other metals.[62,63]

Early prostate cancer often does not cause symptoms. However, prostate cancer can cause any of the signs and symptoms listed in Clinical Signs and Symptoms: Obstruction of the Lower Urinary Tract.

It is often diagnosed when the man seeks medical assistance because of symptoms of lower urinary tract obstruction or low back, hip, or leg pain or stiffness (Case Example 11.3). A staging system has been developed by the American Joint Committee on Cancer. Details of the stages can be found at http://www.cancer.org/cancer/prostatecancer/detailedguide/prostate-cancer-staging. There are two types of staging for prostate cancer, namely clinical stage and pathologic stage. Clinical stage is the physician's best estimate of the extent of the disease. The clinical stages are summarized as follows[64]:

- Stage T1: The cancer cannot be felt during a rectal examination. It may be found when surgery is done for another reason, usually for BPH. There is no evidence that the cancer has spread outside of the prostate.
- Stage T2: The tumor is large enough that it can be palpated during a rectal examination or found with a biopsy. There is no evidence that the cancer has spread outside of the prostate.
- Stage T3: The cancer has spread outside of the prostate to nearby tissues.
- Stage T4: The cancer has spread to lymph nodes or to other parts of the body.

Back pain and sciatica can be caused by cancer metastasis via the bloodstream or the lymphatic system to the bones of the pelvis, spine, or femur. Lumbar pain is predominant, but the thoracolumbar pain can be painful as well, depending on the location of metastasis. Prostate cancer is unique in that the bone is often the only clinically detectable site of metastasis. The resulting tumors tend to be osteoblastic (bone forming, causing sclerosis) rather than osteolytic (bone lysing) (see Fig. 11.6; see also Fig. 14.7).[65]

Symptoms of metastatic disease include bone pain, anemia, weight loss, lymphedema of the lower extremities and scrotum, and neurologic changes associated with spinal cord compression when spinal involvement occurs.

Incontinence

UI is the involuntary leakage of urine. It is an underdiagnosed and underreported problem affecting 50% to 84% of older adults in long-term care facilities.[66,67]

UI is not a disease but rather a symptom of other underlying health conditions, including trauma (e.g., childbirth, incest), diabetes mellitus, multiple sclerosis, Parkinson's disease, spinal injury, spina bifida, surgery, hormonal changes, medications, stroke dysfunction, UTIs, neuromuscular conditions, constipation, or even dietary issues, including caffeine intake.

People who are urine incontinent may restrict their activities for fear of urine leak and concerns about odors in public. This reduction in social activity and change in lifestyle can have profound effects on psychologic well-being and health, including depression, skin breakdown, UTIs, and urosepsis. The physical therapist can have an important role in the successful treatment of incontinence. Screening for this symptom is therefore vital and should be a routine part of the health assessment for all adult clients, especially in a primary care setting.

There are four primary types of UI recognized in adults. These are based on the underlying anatomic or physiologic impairments and include stress, urge, mixed (combination of urge and stress), and overflow.

Stress urinary incontinence (SUI) occurs when the support for the bladder or urethra is weak or damaged, but the bladder itself is normal. With stress incontinence, pressure applied to the bladder from coughing, sneezing, laughing, lifting, exercising, or other physical exertion increases abdominal pressure, and the pelvic floor musculature cannot counteract the urethral/bladder pressure.[68] This is one of the most common types of UI and is primarily related to urethral sphincter weakness, pelvic floor weakness, and ligamentous and fascial laxity.

CASE EXAMPLE 11.3
Prostate Cancer

A 66-year-old man with low back pain was evaluated by a female physical therapist but treated by a male physical therapy aide. By the end of the third session, the client reported some improvement in his painful symptoms. During the second week, there was no improvement and even a possible slight setback. During the treatment session, he commented to the aide that he is impotent.

Given this man's age, inconsistent response to therapy, and report of impotency, a medical referral was necessary. A brief note was sent to the physician relating this information and requesting medical follow-up. (The therapist was careful to use the word *follow-up* rather than *medical reevaluation* because the impotency was present at the time of the initial medical evaluation.)

Result: A medical diagnosis of testicular cancer was established and appropriate treatment was initiated. Physical therapy was discontinued until medical treatment was completed and systemic origin of the back pain could be ruled out.

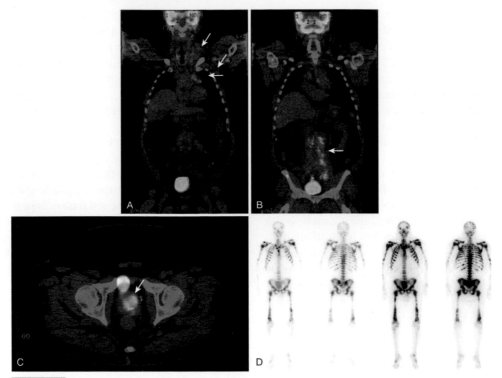

Fig. 11.6 Prostate adenocarcinoma. A 54-year-old man presented with a "lump" in the left lower neck. Outside initial biopsy shows poorly differentiated adenocarcinoma. Further immunohistochemistry shows prostate origin. **A**, Coronal PET/CT shows increased activity in the left lower neck *(top arrow)*, left axillary *(middle arrow)*, and left subpectoral *(bottom arrow)* adenopathy. **B**, Coronal PET/CT scan shows increased activity in the retroperitoneum and pelvis *(arrow)*. **C**, Axial PET/CT scan shows increased activity in the prostate gland *(arrow)*. **D**, Bone scan shows diffuse metastatic disease. (From Silverman P: Oncologic imaging: a multidisciplinary approach, ed 4, Philadelphia, 2012, Saunders.)

Overactive bladder, *also called* **urge incontinence***,* is the involuntary contraction of the detrusor muscle (smooth muscle of the bladder wall) with a strong desire to void (urgency) and loss of urine as soon as the urge is felt without known infection or other pathology.[69] The bladder involuntarily contracts or is unstable, or there may be involuntary sphincter relaxation. Urge incontinence is often idiopathic but can be caused by medications, alcohol, bladder infections, bladder tumor, neurogenic bladder, or bladder outlet obstruction.[70]

Overflow incontinence refers to the overdistention of the bladder, where the bladder cannot empty completely. Urine leaks or dribbles out, so the client does not have any sensation of fullness or emptying.

It may be caused by an acontractile or deficient detrusor muscle, a hypotonic or underactive detrusor muscle secondary to drugs, fecal impaction, diabetes mellitus, lower spinal cord injury, or disruption of the motor innervation of the detrusor muscle (e.g., multiple sclerosis).

In men, overflow incontinence is most often secondary to obstruction caused by prostatic hyperplasia, prostatic carcinoma, or urethral stricture. In women, this type of incontinence occurs as a result of obstruction caused by severe genital prolapse or surgical overcorrection of urethral detachment.

The client with incontinence from overflow will report a feeling that the bladder does not empty completely with an urge to void frequently, including at night. Small amounts of urine are lost involuntarily throughout the day and night. There may be a weak stream or flow sometimes described as "dribbling."

The term ***functional incontinence*** describes another type of UI that occurs when the bladder is normal but the mind and body are not working together. Functional incontinence occurs from mobility and access deficits, such as being confined to a wheelchair or needing a walker to ambulate.[71]

Deficits in dexterity, such as weakness from a stroke or neuropathy and loss of motion from arthritis, may keep the individual from getting their pants unfastened or underwear pulled down in time to avoid an accident. Altered mentation from dementia or Alzheimer's disease can also contribute to untimely urination without a urologic structural problem.

Causes of incontinence can range from urologic/gynecologic to neurologic, psychologic, pharmaceutical, or environmental. Anything that can interfere with neurologic function or produce obstruction can contribute to UI. There is a high prevalence of stress and urge incontinence in female elite athletes. The frequency of UI is significantly higher in athletes with eating disorders.[72]

Risk factors for developing UI are listed in Box 11.3. Chronic constipation at any time, but especially during pregnancy, can lead to increased abdominal pressure, which can cause UI. Any condition leading to an enlarged abdomen

BOX 11.3 RISK FACTORS FOR URINARY INCONTINENCE

- Advancing age
- Alzheimer's disease or dementia
- Arthritis or other musculoskeletal problems
- Overweight/obese
- Chronic cough
- Chronic constipation
- History of recurrent urinary tract infection
- History of sexually transmitted disease
- Enlarged abdomen (e.g., ascites, pregnancy, obesity, tumor)
- Diabetes mellitus
- Neurologic disorder
- Medication
  - Sedatives
  - Diuretics
  - Estrogens
  - Anticholinergics
  - Antibiotics
  - Alpha-adrenergic blockers (antihistamines, decongestants)
  - Calcium channel blockers
  - Antipsychotics
  - Antidepressants
  - Antiparkinsonian drugs
  - Laxatives
  - Opioids
  - Vincristine
  - Angiotensin-converting enzyme (ACE) inhibitors
- Caffeine, alcohol
- Female gender (see below)

Specific to Women
- Pregnancy (multiparity)
- Vaginal or cesarean* birth
- Previous bladder or pelvic surgery
- Pelvic trauma or radiation
- Bladder or bowel prolapse
- Menopause (natural or surgically induced; estrogen deficiency)†
- Tobacco use

Specific to Men
- Enlarged prostate gland
- Prostate or pelvic surgery
- Radiation (acute and late complications), especially when combined with brachytherapy

* Although the abdominal muscles are disrupted with a cesarean section and limit how much the woman can bear down on the bladder, abdominal tone and function are essential for pelvic muscle function.
† Urinary incontinence in middle-aged women may be more closely associated with mechanical factors, such as childbearing, history of urinary tract infections, gynecologic surgery, chronic constipation, obesity, and exertion, than with menopausal transition.[85]

(e.g., ascites, weight gain, pregnancy) with increased pressure on the bladder can contribute to incontinence.

Chemotherapy, radiation, surgery, and medications can cause disruptions in the cycle of micturition (urination) for many different physiologic reasons. For example, chemotherapy can increase fat deposits and decrease muscle mass, which increase the risk of bowel and bladder dysfunction.

External radiation alters tissue viability in the surrounding area, which can affect circulation to the organs and support from muscle, fascia, ligaments, and tendons.[73,74] Radiation can cause fibrosis[75]; if the genitourinary tract is involved, there could be resulting contracted bladder tissue and damaged sphincter, contributing to UI. Surgery to remove tumors, lymph nodes, or the prostate can affect bladder control through alterations of blood and lymphatic circulation, innervation, and fascial support. Edema secondary to lymphatic system compromise can increase bladder (and bowel) dysfunction. Brain, spinal cord, or pelvic surgery can affect nervous control of the bowel and bladder.[76–78]

Incontinence is not a normal part of the aging process. When confronted with UI in an older adult, consider some of the following causes of this disorder: infection, endocrine disorders, atrophic urethritis or vaginitis, restricted mobility, stool impaction (especially in smokers), alcohol or caffeine intake, and medications.

Smoking contributes to constipation and is often accompanied by chronic cough, which stresses the bladder. Some medications can lead to UI or aggravate already existing UI. Medications commonly involved with alterations in urinary continence include oral estrogens, alpha blockers, sedative-hypnotics, antidepressants, antipsychotics, angiotensin-converting enzyme (ACE) inhibitors, loop diuretics, nonsteroidal antiinflammatory drugs (NSAIDs), and calcium channel blockers.[79,80]

With any kind of incontinence, the onset of cervical spine pain at the same time that UI develops is a red flag. These two findings would suggest there is a protrusion pressing on the spinal cord.

If a medical diagnosis for cervical disk protrusion has been established, referral would not be necessary. However, if incontinence is a new development from the time of the medical evaluation, the physician should be made aware of this information. Cervical spinal manipulation is contraindicated.

Many people are embarrassed about having an incontinence problem. It may help to introduce the subject by making a general statement such as, "Many men and women have problems with bladder control. This is an area physical therapists can often help clients with so we routinely ask a few questions about bladder function."

? FOLLOW-UP QUESTIONS

Screening questions for **incontinence** can include:

General Incontinence
- Do you have any problems holding urine or emptying your bladder?
- Do you ever leak urine or have accidents?
- Do you wear pads to protect against urine leaking? Follow-up: How many do you use in a 24-hour period and how wet are they?

- Are your activities limited because of urine leaking?
- If the client answers "yes" to any of these questions, you may want to screen further with the following questions:

For Stress Incontinence

- Do you ever lose urine or wet your pants when you cough, sneeze, or laugh?
- Do you lose urine or wet your pants when getting out of a chair, lifting, or exercising?

For Overactive Bladder (urge incontinence)

- Do you have frequent, strong, or sudden urges to urinate and cannot get to the bathroom in time? For example:
- When arriving home and getting out of the car?
- When using a key to open the door?
- When you hear water running?
- Or when you run water over your hands?
- When you go out into cold weather or put your hands in the freezer?
- Do you get to the toilet and lose urine as you are pulling down your underwear?
- Do you urinate more than eight times a day?
- Do you get up to go more than twice a night?

For Overflow Incontinence

- Do you dribble urine during the day and/or at night?
- Can you urinate with a strong stream or does the urine dribble out slowly?
- Does it feel like your bladder is empty when you are done urinating?

For Functional Incontinence

- Can you get to the toilet easily?
- Do you have trouble getting to the bathroom in time?
- Do you have trouble finding the bathroom or toilet?
- Do you have accidents in the bathroom because you cannot get your pants unfastened or pulled down?

Chronic Kidney Disease

Symptoms of renal failure generally cannot be mistaken for musculoskeletal disorders that are treated by physical or occupational therapists. However, patients/clients with chronic kidney disease leading to kidney failure may receive treatment in both inpatient and outpatient clinics for primary musculoskeletal conditions. Understanding symptoms associated with kidney disease and recognizing complications associated with dialysis shunts are imperative for the therapist.

Kidney failure exists when the kidneys can no longer maintain the homeostatic balances within the body that are necessary for life. Renal failure is classified as acute or chronic in origin and progression. *Acute renal failure* refers to the abrupt cessation of kidney activity, usually occurring over a period of hours to a few days. Acute renal failure is often reversible, with return of kidney function in 3 to 12 months.

Chronic renal failure, or irreversible renal failure (also known as end-stage renal disease [ESRD]), is defined as a state of progressive decrease in the ability of the kidney to filter fluids, metabolites, and electrolytes from the body, resulting in eventual permanent loss of kidney function. ESRD is the final stage (stage 5) of chronic kidney disease. It can develop slowly over a period of years or can result from an episode of acute renal failure that does not resolve.

ESRD is a complex condition with multiple systemic complications. Diabetic nephropathy is the primary cause of ESRD, accounting for approximately 40% of newly diagnosed cases of ESRD.[81] In the United States, 44% of new patients with kidney failure are also diagnosed with diabetes mellitus.[82] Risk factors for ESRD include advancing age, diabetes mellitus, hypertension, chronic urinary tract obstruction and infection (especially glomerulonephritis), and kidney transplantation. Hereditary defects of the kidneys, polycystic kidneys, and glomerular disorders, such as glomerulonephritis, can also lead to renal failure.

Chronic intake of certain medications and over-the-counter (OTC) drugs is also a factor in the development of renal disease. The increasing availability of OTC drugs has led to consumers treating themselves when they may lack the knowledge to do so safely. In the elderly population, hepatotoxicity is related to drug exposure, polypharmacy, and multidrug interactions.[83] Excessive consumption of acetaminophen and NSAIDs can be extremely toxic to the kidneys.[84]

Clinical Signs and Symptoms

Failure of the filtering and regulating mechanisms of the kidney can be either acute (sudden in onset and potentially reversible) or chronic (called *uremia*, which develops gradually and is usually irreversible).

Individuals with diabetes mellitus and ESRD often have autonomic dysfunction and sensorimotor peripheral (uremic) neuropathies affecting the distal extremities. Symptoms tend to be symmetric and more subjective than objective, such as restless legs syndrome, cramps, paresthesias, impaired vibration sense, burning feet syndrome, abnormal Achilles reflex, pruritus (itching of the skin), constipation or diarrhea, abdominal bloating, and decreased sweating. Individuals with either type of renal failure develop signs and symptoms characteristic of impaired fluid and waste excretion and altered renal regulation of other body metabolic processes such as pH regulation, RBC production, and calcium-phosphorus balance.

Signs of renal impairment are shown in Table 11.4. The signs of actual renal failure are the same but more pronounced. In most cases of renal failure, urine volume is significantly decreased or absent. Edema becomes severe and can result in heart failure. Renal anemia is usually associated with extreme fatigue and intolerance to normal daily activities, as well as a marked decrease in exercise capacity.[85]

In addition, the continuous presence of toxic waste products in the bloodstream (urea, creatinine, uric acid) results in damage to many other body systems, including the central nervous system, peripheral nervous system, eyes, gastrointestinal tract, integumentary system, endocrine system, and cardiopulmonary system.

Treatment of renal failure involves several elements designed to replace the lost excretory and metabolic functions of this organ. Treatment options include dialysis, dietary changes, and medications to regulate blood pressure and assist in replacement of lost metabolic functions, such as calcium balance and RBC production.

The choice of treatment options, such as dialysis, transplantation, or conservative treatment depends on many

CLINICAL SIGNS AND SYMPTOMS
Renal Impairment

Symptoms of upper UTI, particularly renal infection, can be categorized according to urinary tract manifestations or systemic manifestations caused by renal impairment (see Table 11.4). Clinical signs and symptoms of urinary tract involvement can include:

- Unilateral costovertebral tenderness
- Flank pain
- Ipsilateral shoulder pain
- Fever and chills
- Skin hypersensitivity
- Hematuria (blood in urine)
- Pyuria (pus in urine)
- Bacteriuria (presence of bacteria in urine)
- Hypertension
- Decreased urinary output
- Dependent edema
- Weakness
- Anorexia (loss of appetite)
- Dyspnea
- Mild headache
- Proteinuria (protein in urine, urine may be foamy)
- Abnormal blood serum level, such as elevated blood urea nitrogen (BUN) and creatinine
- Anemia

CLINICAL SIGNS AND SYMPTOMS
Bladder and Renal Cancer

Bladder Cancer
- Blood in the urine
- Pain during urination
- Urinary urgency

Renal Cancer
- Blood in the urine
- Pain during urination
- Urinary urgency
- Flank or side pain
- Lump or mass in the side or abdomen
- Weight loss
- Fever
- General fatigue; feeling of poor health

factors, including the person's physical and mental condition.[86] Untreated or chronic renal failure eventually results in death.

From a screening perspective, the therapist must be alert to the many complications associated with chronic renal failure and dialysis. Watch for signs and symptoms of fluid and electrolyte imbalances (see Chapter 12), dehydration (see Chapter 12), cardiac arrhythmias (see Chapter 7), and depression (see Chapter 3).

Cancers of the Urinary Tract

Bladder Cancer

Bladder cancer is a common, major public health concern that is strongly linked to cigarette smoking. Half of all bladder cancers in both men and women are caused by smoking. It is the fourth most common cancer in men and the tenth most common in women.[87,88] It has been reported that 9 out of 10 persons with bladder cancer are 55 years of age or older.[89]

The exact cause of bladder cancer is not known, but certain risk factors have been identified that increase the chance of developing this type of cancer.[90,91]

- Age (over 40 years)
- Tobacco use (cigarette, pipe, and cigar)
- Occupation (exposure to workplace carcinogens such as paper, rubber, chemical, dyes, leather industries; hairdressers, machinists, metal workers, dental workers, printers, painters, auto workers, textile workers, truck drivers)
- Infections (parasitic, usually in tropical areas of the world)
- Treatment with cyclophosphamide or arsenic (for other cancers)

- Race (Caucasians highest; Asians lowest)
- Sex (men two to three times more likely than women)
- Previous personal history of bladder cancer
- Family history (slightly increased risk)[92]

Common symptoms of bladder cancer include blood in the urine, pain during urination, and urinary urgency or the feeling of urinary urgency without resulting urination. Measures that have been shown to reduce the risk of developing bladder cancer include cessation of smoking, adequate intake of fluids, intake of cruciferous vegetables, limiting exposure to workplace chemicals, and prompt treatment of bladder infections.

Renal Cancer

Cancer of the kidney (renal cancer) develops most often in people over the age of 40 years and has some associated risk factors. Risk factors for renal cancer include:

- Smoking (two times the risk as nonsmokers)
- Obesity
- Hypertension
- Long-term dialysis
- Von Hippel-Lindau syndrome (genetic, familial syndrome)
- Occupation (coke oven workers in the iron and steel industry; asbestos and cadmium exposure)
- Sex (men twice more likely than women)

Common symptoms of renal cancer are very similar to those of bladder cancer and require immediate referral for follow-up. These symptoms can include blood in the urine, pain in the side that does not go away, a lump or mass in the side or abdomen, weight loss, fever, and general fatigue or feeling of poor health.[93]

Testicular Cancer

The testicles (also called *testes* or *gonads*) are the male sex glands. They are located behind the penis in a pouch of skin called the *scrotum* (Fig. 11.3). The testicles produce and store sperm and serve as the body's main source of male hormones. These hormones control the development of the reproductive organs and other male characteristics such as body and facial hair, low voice, wide shoulders, and sexual function.

Testicular cancer is relatively rare, and the average age at the time of diagnosis is 33 years.[94] It occurs most often in young men between the ages of 15 and 35 years, although any male can be affected at any time.[95] In 2022, it is projected that about 9,910 new cases of testicular cancer will be diagnosed and about 460 men will die of the condition.[94] The cause of most testicular cancer is unknown, but risk factors include an undescended testicle, family history, HIV infection, carcinoma in situ of the testicle, and a previous diagnosis of testicular cancer. Additional risk factors include age (half of the all cases occur between the age of 20 and 34 years), race and ethnicity (Caucasian men have about a four to five times greater risk of developing testicular cancer than African-American or Asian-American men), and body size (several studies have reported that tall men have a somewhat higher risk of testicular cancer).[94]

Clinical Signs and Symptoms

Testicular cancer can be completely asymptomatic. The most common sign is a hard, painless lump in the testicle about the size of a pea. There may be a dull ache in the scrotum and the man may be aware of tender, larger breasts. Other symptoms are listed in the box Clinical Signs and Symptoms: Testicular Cancer.

There are three stages of testicular cancer[95]:
- Stage I: The cancer is confined to the testicle.
- Stage II: The cancer has spread to the retroperitoneal lymph nodes, located in the posterior abdominal cavity below the diaphragm and between the kidneys.
- Stage III: The cancer has spread beyond the lymph nodes to remote sites in the body, including the lungs, brain, or liver.

Testicular cancer is a treatable and curable condition. The American Cancer Society states that some physicians recommend monthly self-examination of the testicles after puberty.[82] Testicular self-examination is an effective way of getting to know this area of the body and thus detecting testicular cancer at a very early, curable stage. The self-examination is best performed once each month during or after a warm bath or shower when the heat has relaxed the scrotum (see Appendix D-8 in the accompanying enhanced eBook version included with print purchase of this textbook).[96]

Men who have been treated for cancer in one testicle have about a 3% to 4% chance of developing cancer in the remaining testicle. If cancer does arise in the second testicle, it is nearly always a new disease rather than metastasis from the first tumor.

Metastases occur via the blood or lymph system. The most common place for the disease to spread is to the lymph nodes in the posterior part of the abdomen. Therefore, low back pain is a frequent symptom of late-stage testicular cancer (Case Example 11.4). If the cancer has spread to the lungs, persistent cough, chest pain, and/or shortness of

breath can occur. Hemoptysis (sputum with blood) may also develop.

Survivors of testicular cancer should be checked regularly by their doctors and should continue to perform monthly testicular self-examinations. Any unusual symptoms should be reported to the doctor immediately. Outcome even after a secondary testicular cancer is still excellent with early detection and treatment.

CASE EXAMPLE 11.4

Testicular Cancer

A 20-year-old track star and college football player developed back, buttock, and posterior thigh pain after a football injury. He was sent to physical therapy by the team physician with a diagnosis of "Sciatica; L4-5 radiculopathy. Please treat using McKenzie exercise program."

During the physical therapy interview, the client reported left low back pain and left buttock pain present for the last 2 weeks after being tackled from the right side in a football game. Symptoms developed approximately 12 hours after the injury. Pain was always present but was worse after sitting and better after standing.

During examination, the client presented with major losses of lumbar spine range of motion in all planes. There was no observable lateral shift and lumbar lordosis was not excessive or reduced. Overall postural assessment was unremarkable.

He was able to lie flat in the prone position and perform a small prone press up without increasing any of his symptoms, but he described feeling a "hard knot in my stomach" while in this position. When asked if he had any symptoms of any kind anywhere else in his body, the client replied that right after the injury, his left testicle swelled up but seemed better now. He denied any blood in the urine or difficulty urinating. Vital signs were within normal limits.

Even though the therapist thought the clinical findings supported a diagnosis of a derangement syndrome according to the McKenzie classification, there were enough red flags to warrant further investigation.

The client was given an appropriate self-treatment program to perform throughout the day with instructions for self-assessment of his condition. In the meantime, the therapist contacted the physician with the following concerns:
- Palpable (nonpulsatile) abdominal mass in the left upper abdominal quadrant (anterior)
- Reported left testicular swelling
- Age
- No imaging studies were done to confirm a disk lesion as the underlying cause of the symptoms

Result: Physician referral was made after a telephone discussion outlining the additional findings listed. An abdominal CT scan showed a 20-cm (5-inch) abdominal mass pressing on the spinal nerves as the cause of the back pain. Further diagnostic testing revealed testicular cancer as the primary diagnosis, with metastases to the abdomen causing the abdominal mass.

Surgery was performed to remove the testicle. The back pain was relieved within 3 days of starting chemotherapy. Physical therapy was discontinued for back pain, but a new plan of care was established for exercise during cancer treatment.

CLINICAL SIGNS AND SYMPTOMS

Testicular Cancer

- A lump in either testicle
- Any enlargement, swelling, or hardness of a testicle
- Significant loss of size in one of the testicles
- Feeling of heaviness in the scrotum and/or lower abdomen
- Dull ache in the lower abdomen or in the groin
- Sudden collection of fluid in the scrotum
- Pain or discomfort in a testicle or in the scrotum
- Enlargement or tenderness of the breasts
- Unexplained fatigue or malaise
- Infertility
- Low back pain (metastases to retroperitoneal lymph nodes)

PHYSICIAN REFERRAL

The proximity of the kidneys, ureters, bladder, and urethra to the ribs, vertebrae, diaphragm, and accompanying muscles and tendinous insertions often can make it difficult to identify the client's problems accurately.

Pain related to a urinary tract problem can be similar to pain felt from an injury to the back, flank, abdomen, or upper thigh. The physical therapist is advised to question the client further whenever any of the signs and symptoms listed in Table 11.3 are reported or observed. Further diagnostic testing and medical examination must be performed by the physician to differentiate urinary tract conditions from musculoskeletal problems.

The physical therapist must be able to recognize the systemic origin of urinary tract symptoms that mimic musculoskeletal pain. Many conditions that produce urinary tract pain also include an elevation in temperature, abnormal urinary constituents, and change in color, odor, or amount of urine.

These types of changes would not be observed or reported with a musculoskeletal condition, and the client may not mention them, thinking these symptoms do not have anything to do with the back, flank, or thigh pain present. The therapist must ask a few screening questions to bring this kind of information to the forefront.

When the physical therapist conducts a Review of Systems, any signs and symptoms associated with renal or urologic impairment should be correlated with the findings of the objective examination and combined with the medical history to provide a comprehensive report at the time of referral to the physician or other health care provider.

Diagnostic Testing

Screening of the composition of the urine is called *urinalysis* (UA), and UA is the commonly used method of determining various properties of urine. This analysis is actually a series of several tests of urinary components and is a valuable aid in the diagnosis of urinary tract or metabolic disorders.

Normal urinary constituents are shown (see inside front cover: Urine Analysis). Urine cultures are also very important studies in the diagnosis of UTIs. Anyone at risk for chronic kidney disease should be tested for markers of kidney damage. This is done by UA for albumin (protein in the urine) and by blood serum for creatinine (waste product of muscle metabolism).

Various *blood studies* can be done to assess renal function (see inside front cover: Renal Blood Studies). These studies examine both the serum and cellular components of the blood for specific changes characteristic of renal performance. Substances that must be examined in the serum are those that are a *direct* reflection of renal function, such as creatinine, and others that are more *indirect* in renal evaluation, such as blood urea nitrogen (BUN), pH-related substances, uric acid, various ions, electrolytes, and cellular components (RBCs). (For a more in-depth discussion of laboratory values, the reader is referred to a more specific source of information.)[97]

Guidelines for Immediate Medical Attention

- The presence of any amount of blood in the urine always requires a referral to a physician. However, the presence of abnormalities in the urine may not be obvious, and a thorough diagnostic analysis of the urine may be needed. Careful questioning of the client regarding urinary tract history, urinary patterns, urinary characteristics, and pain patterns may elicit valuable information relating to potential urinary tract symptoms.
- Presence of cervical spine pain at the same time that UI develops. If a diagnosis of cervical disk prolapse has been made, the physician should be notified of these findings; referral may not be necessary, but communication with the physician to confirm this is necessary.
- Client with bowel/bladder incontinence and/or saddle anesthesia secondary to cauda equina lesion.

Guidelines for Physician Referral

Although immediate (emergency) medical attention is not required, medical referral is needed under the following circumstances:

- When the client has any combination of systemic signs and symptoms presented in this chapter. Damage to the urinary tract structures can occur with accident, injury, assault, or other trauma to the musculoskeletal structures surrounding the kidney and urinary tract and may require medical evaluation if the clinical presentation or response to physical therapy treatment suggests it.

  For example, the alpine skier discussed at the beginning of the chapter had a dull, aching costovertebral pain on the left side that was unrelieved by a change of position or by ice, heat, or aspirin. His pain is related directly to a traumatic episode, and musculoskeletal injury is a definite possibility in his case. He has no medical history of urinary tract problems and denies any changes in urine or pattern of urination. Because the pain is constant and unrelieved by usual measures and the location of the pain is approximate to renal structures, a medical follow-up and UA would be recommended.

- Back or shoulder pain accompanied by abnormal urinary constituents (e.g., change in color, odor, amount, flow of urine)
- Positive Murphy's percussion (punch) test, especially with a recent history of renal or urologic infection

Clues Suggesting Pain of Possible Renal/Urologic Origin

- Men 45 years of age or older
- In men, back pain accompanied by burning during urination, difficulty with urination, or fever may be associated with prostatitis; usually in such a case, there is no limitation of back motion and no muscle spasm (until symptoms progress, causing muscle guarding and splinting)
- Blood in urine
- Change in urinary pattern such as increased or decreased frequency, change in flow of urine stream (weak or dribbling), and increased nocturia

- Presence of constitutional symptoms, especially fever and chills; pain is constant (may be dull or sharp, depending on the cause)
- Pain is unchanged by altering body position; side bending to the involved side and pressure at that level is "more comfortable" (may reduce pain but does not eliminate it)
- Neither renal nor urethral pain is altered by a change in body position; pseudorenal pain from a mechanical cause can be relieved by a change in position
- True renal pain is seldom affected by movements of the spine
- Straight leg–raising test is negative with renal colic appearing as back pain
- Back pain at the level of the kidneys in a woman with previous breast or uterine cancer (ovarian cancer)
- Assessment for pseudorenal pain is negative (see Table 11.1)

RENAL AND UROLOGIC PAIN PATTERNS

KIDNEY (FIG. 11.7)

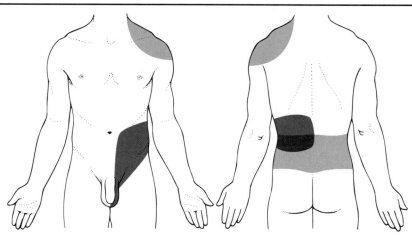

Fig. 11.7 Renal pain is typically felt in the posterior subcostal and costovertebral region *(dark red)*. It can radiate across the low back *(light red)* and/or forward around the flank into the lower abdominal quadrant. Ipsilateral groin and testicular pain may also accompany renal pain. Pressure from the kidney on the diaphragm may cause ipsilateral shoulder pain.

Location:	Posterior subcostal and costovertebral region
	Usually unilateral
Referral:	Radiates forward, around the flank or the side into the lower abdominal quadrant (T11-T12), along the pelvic crest and into the groin
	Pressure from the kidney on the diaphragm may cause ipsilateral shoulder pain
Description:	Dull, aching, boring
Intensity:	Acute: severe, intense
	Chronic: vague and poorly localized
Duration:	Constant
Associated Signs and Symptoms:	Fever, chills
	Increased urinary frequency
	Blood in urine
	Hyperesthesia of associated dermatomes (T9 and T10)
	Ipsilateral or generalized abdominal pain
	Spasm of abdominal muscles
	Nausea and vomiting when severely acute
	Testicular pain may occur in men
	Unrelieved by a change in position

RENAL AND UROLOGIC PAIN PATTERNS—cont'd

URETER (FIG. 11.8)

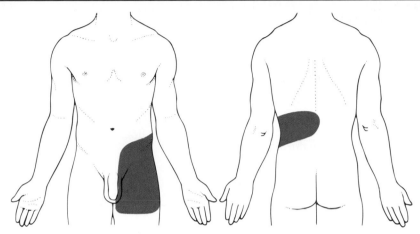

Fig. 11.8 Ureteral pain may begin posteriorly in the costovertebral angle. It may then radiate anteriorly to the ipsilateral lower abdomen, upper thigh, testes, or labium.

Location:	Costovertebral angle
	Unilateral or bilateral
Referral:	Radiates to the lower abdomen, upper thigh, testis, or labium on the same side (groin and genital area)
Description:	Described as crescendo waves of colic
Intensity:	Excruciating, severe (ureteral pain is commonly acute and caused by a kidney stone; lesions outside of the ureter are usually painless until advanced progression of the disease occurs)
Duration:	Ureteral pain caused by calculus is intermittent or constant without relief until treated or until the stone is passed
Associated Signs and Symptoms:	Rectal tenesmus (painful spasm of anal sphincter with urgent desire to evacuate the bowel/bladder; involuntary straining with little passage of urine or feces)
	Nausea, abdominal distention, vomiting
	Hyperesthesia of associated dermatomes (T10-L1)
	Tenderness over the kidney or ureter
	Unrelieved by a change in position
	Movement of iliopsoas may aggravate symptoms associated with a lesion outside of the ureter (see Fig. 8.3)

BLADDER/URETHRA (FIG. 11.9)

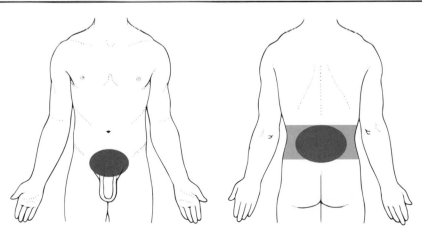

Fig. 11.9 *Left,* Bladder or urethral pain is usually felt suprapubically or ipsilaterally in the lower abdomen. This is the same pattern for gas pain from the lower gastrointestinal (GI) tract for some people. *Right,* Bladder or urethral pain may also be perceived in the low back area (*dark red:* primary pain center; *light red:* referred pain). Low back pain may occur as the first and only symptom associated with bladder/urethral pain, or it may occur along with suprapubic or abdominal pain, or both.

RENAL AND UROLOGIC PAIN PATTERNS—cont'd

Location: Suprapubic or low abdomen, low back

Referral: Pelvis

Can be confused with gas

Description: Sharp, localized

Intensity: Moderate-to-severe

Duration: Intermittent; may be relieved by emptying the bladder

Associated Signs and Symptoms: Great urinary urgency

Tenesmus

Dysuria

Hot or burning sensation during urination

PROSTATE (FIG. 11.10)

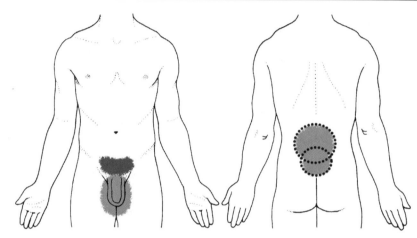

Fig. 11.10   The prostate is segmentally innervated from T11-L1, S2-S4. Prostate problems can be painless. When pain occurs, the primary pain pattern is in the lower abdomen, suprapubic region *(dark red)*, and perineum (between the rectum and testes; not pictured). Pain can be referred to the low back, sacrum, testes, and inner thighs *(light red)*.

Symptoms of prostate involvement vary depending on the underlying cause (e.g., prostatitis versus BPH versus prostate cancer).

Location: May be pain free; lower abdomen, suprapubic region

Referral: Low back, pelvis, sacrum, perineum, inner thighs, testes; thoracolumbar spine with metastases (the latter is not pictured)

Description: Persistent aching pain; pain is reproduced with digital rectal examination

Intensity: Mild-to-severe; varies from person to person and can fluctuate for each individual on any given day

Duration: Varies according to underlying cause

Associated Signs and Symptoms: Chills and fever (prostatitis)

Frequent and/or painful urination

Urgency, hesitancy

Nocturia

Incomplete emptying of bladder

Painful ejaculation

Hematuria

Arthralgia, myalgia

■ Key Points to Remember

1. Renal and urologic pain can be referred to the shoulder or low back.
2. Lesions outside the ureter can cause pain during movement of the adjacent iliopsoas muscle.
3. Radiculitis can mimic ureteral colic or renal pain, but true renal pain is seldom affected by movements of the spine.
4. Inflammatory pain may be relieved by a change in position. Renal colic remains unchanged by a change in position.
5. Change in color, consistency, smell, or reduced volume or flow of urine requires further assessment and change in urgency and frequency, and pain with urination requires further evaluation.
6. Low back, pelvic, or femur pain can be the first symptom of prostate cancer.
7. Change in size, shape, or appearance of testicles or penis with or without urethral discharge requires further assessment.
8. Change in the smell, volume, or consistency of ejaculate with or without pain during intercourse requires further assessment.
9. Urinary incontinence is not a normal part of aging and should be evaluated carefully.
10. With any kind of incontinence, the onset of cervical spine pain at the same time that urinary incontinence develops is a red flag and contraindicates the use of cervical spinal manipulation.
11. Lower thoracic disk herniation can cause groin pain and/or leg pain, mimicking renal pain. The presence of neurologic changes, such as bladder dysfunction, can cause confusion when trying to differentiate a systemic from neuromusculoskeletal cause of symptoms. True renal pain is seldom affected by movements of the spine. Compare the results of palpation and percussion tests.
12. Testicular cancer with metastasis to the lymph system or bone can cause low back pain from pressure on the spinal nerves. Always watch for red flags, even when an injury occurs; this is especially true in the young adult or athlete.
13. Anyone with hypertension and/or diabetes mellitus (and/or other significant risk factors for renal disease) should be monitored carefully and consistently for any systemic signs and symptoms of renal impairment.
14. People with diabetes mellitus are prone to complications associated with UTIs.
15. The sudden onset of nonspecific low back pain, unrelated to any specific motion, may be an indication of osteomyelitis from spread of infection to the spine. Take the client's body temperature and ask him/her to monitor temperature for a few days to uncover the possibility of a low-grade fever associated with osteomyelitis.
16. All the possible pain patterns discussed in this chapter are presented in Figure 11.11.

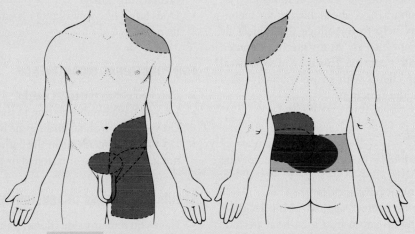

Fig. 11.11 Summary of all pain patterns discussed in this chapter.

CLIENT HISTORY AND INTERVIEW

SPECIAL QUESTIONS TO ASK

Clients may be reluctant to answer the physical therapist's questions concerning bladder and urinary function. The physical therapist is advised to explain the need to rule out possible causes of pain related to the kidneys and bladder and to give the client time to respond if answers seem to be uncertain. For example, the physical therapist may ask the client to observe urinary function over the next 2 days. These questions should be reviewed again at the next appointment.

Continued

CLIENT HISTORY AND INTERVIEW—cont'd

PAST MEDICAL HISTORY

- Have you had any problems with your prostate (for men), kidneys, or bladder? *If so*, describe.
- Have you ever had kidney or bladder stones? *If so*, when? How were these stones treated?
- Have you had an injury to your bladder or kidneys? *If so*, when? How was this treated? (**Be aware of unreported domestic abuse/assault.**)
- Have you had any kidney or bladder infections in the past 6 months? How were these infections treated? Were they related to any specific circumstances (**e.g., pregnancy, intercourse, after strep throat or strep skin infections**)?
- Have you ever had surgery on your bladder or kidneys? *If so*, when and what?
- Have you had any hernias? *If yes*, when and how was this treated?
- Have you ever had cancer of any kind?
- Have you ever had testicular, kidney, bladder, or prostate cancer?
- Have you ever been treated with radiation or chemotherapy?

SPECIAL QUESTIONS TO ASK: BLADDER CONTROL/INCONTINENCE

Begin with a lead-in introduction to these questions such as:

Many people are embarrassed about having an incontinence problem. It may help to introduce the subject by making a general statement such as: "Many men and women have problems with bladder control. This is an area physical therapists can often help clients with so we routinely ask a few questions about bladder function."

GENERAL INCONTINENCE

- Do you have any problems holding urine or emptying your bladder?
- Do you ever leak urine or have accidents?
- Do you wear pads to protect against urine leaking? Follow-up: How many do you use in a 24-hour period? How wet are they?
- Are your activities limited because of urine leaking?

If the male client answers "yes" to any of these questions, you may want to screen further with the following questions. See also Appendix B-30 in the accompanying enhanced eBook version included with print purchase of this textbook

FOR STRESS INCONTINENCE

- Do you ever lose urine or wet your pants when you cough, sneeze, or laugh?

- Do you lose urine or wet your pants when getting out of a chair, lifting, or exercising?

FOR OVERACTIVE BLADDER (URGE INCONTINENCE)

- Do you have frequent, strong, or sudden urges to urinate and cannot get to the bathroom in time? For example:
  - When arriving home and getting out of the car?
  - When using a key to open the door?
  - When you hear water running?
  - Or when you run water over your hands?
  - When you go out into cold weather or put your hands in the freezer?
- Do you get to the toilet and lose urine as you are pulling down your underwear/shorts?
- Do you urinate more than every 2 hours in the daytime?
- Do you get up to go to the bathroom more than once a night?

If yes, does this happen every night? Is it because you drink a large amount of fluids before bedtime?

FOR OVERFLOW INCONTINENCE

- Do you dribble urine during the day and/or at night?
- Can you urinate with a strong stream or does the urine dribble out slowly?
- Does it feel like your bladder is empty when you are done urinating?

FOR FUNCTIONAL INCONTINENCE

- Can you get to the toilet easily?
- Do you have trouble getting to the bathroom in time?
- Do you have trouble finding the bathroom or toilet?
- Do you have accidents in the bathroom because you cannot get your pants unfastened or pulled down?

SPECIAL QUESTIONS TO ASK: URINARY TRACT INFECTION

- Have you had any side (flank) pain (**kidney or ureter**) or pain just above the pubic area (**suprapubic: bladder or urethra, prostate**)?
- *If so*, what relieves this pain? Does a change in position affect it? (**Inflammatory pain** may be relieved by a change in position. **Renal colic** remains unchanged by a change in position.)
- During the last 2 to 3 weeks, have you noticed a change in the amount or number of times you urinate? (**Infection**)
- Do you ever have pain or a burning sensation when you urinate? (**Lower urinary tract irritation; prostatitis; venereal disease**)

CLIENT HISTORY AND INTERVIEW—cont'd

- Does your urine look brown, red, or black? (Change in urine color may be normal with some medications and foods such as beets or rhubarb.)
- Is your urine clear or cloudy? If not clear, describe. How often does this happen? (Could indicate **upper or lower UTI.**)
- Have you noticed an unusual or foul odor coming from your urine? (**Infection, secondary to medication**; may be normal after eating asparagus.)

For Women

- When you urinate, do you have trouble starting or continuing the flow of urine? (**Urethral obstruction**)
- Have you noticed any unusual vaginal discharge during the time that you had pain (pubic, flank, thigh, back, labia)? (**Infection**)
- Have you noticed any change in your sexual activity/function caused by your symptoms?

For Men

- Have you noticed any unusual discharge from your penis during the time that you had pain (especially pain above the pubic area)? (**Infection**)
- Have you noticed any change in your sexual activity/function caused by your symptoms?

SCREENING QUESTIONS TO ASK: PROSTATITIS OR ENLARGED PROSTATE

- Have you ever had any problems with your prostate in the past?
- Do you know if anyone in your family has had any problems with their prostate in the past or currently?

Prostatitis

- Do you ever have burning pain or discomfort during urination?

- Does it feel like your bladder is not empty when you finish urinating?
- Do you have to go to the bathroom every 2 hours (or more often)?
- Do you ever have pain or discomfort in your testicles, penis, or the area between your rectum and your testicles (perineum)?
- Do you ever have pain in your pubic or bladder area?
- Do you have any discomfort during or after sexual climax (ejaculation)?

Enlarged Prostate

- Does it feel like your bladder is not empty when you finish urinating?
- Do you have to urinate again less than 2 hours after you finished going to the bathroom last?
- Do you have a weak stream of urine or find you have to start and stop urinating several times when you go to the bathroom?
- Do you have an urge to go to the bathroom but very little urine comes out?
- Do you have to push or strain to start urinating or to keep the urine flowing?
- Do you have any leaking or dribbling of urine from the penis?
- How often do you get up to urinate at night?

The American Urologic Association recommends using the following scale when asking most of these screening questions. Some questions such as, "How often do you get up at night?" require a single number response. A total score of 7 or more suggests the need for medical evaluation:

0	1	2	3	4	5
Not at all	Less than one time in five	Less than half the time	About half the time	More than half the time	Almost always

CASE STUDY

REFERRAL

The client is self-referred and states that he has been to your hospital-based outpatient clinic in the past. He has a very extensive chart containing his entire medical history for the last 20 years.

BACKGROUND INFORMATION

He is a 44-year-old man who describes his current occupation as "errand boy/gopher," which requires minimal lifting, bending, or strenuous physical activity. His chief complaint today is pain in the lower back, which comes and goes and seems to

Continued

CASE STUDY—cont'd

be aggravated by sitting. The pain is poorly described, and the client is unable to specify any kind of descriptive words for the type of pain, intensity, or duration.

SPECIAL QUESTIONS TO ASK

See Chapter 15 for Special Questions to Ask about the back. The client's answer to any questions related to bowel and bladder function is either "I don't know" or "Well, you know," which makes a complete interview impossible.

EXAMINATION FINDINGS

There are radiating symptoms of numbness down the left leg to the foot. The client denies any saddle anesthesia. Deep tendon reflexes are intact bilaterally, and the client stands with an obvious scoliotic list to one side. He is unable to tell you whether his symptoms are relieved or alleviated when performing a lateral shift to correct the curve. There are no other positive neuromuscular findings or associated systemic symptoms.

RESULT

After 3 days of treatment over the course of 1 week, the client has had no subjective improvement in symptoms. Objectively,

the scoliotic shift has not changed. A second opinion is sought from two other staff members, and the consensus is to refer the client to his physician. The physician performs a rectal examination and confirms a positive diagnosis of prostatitis based on the results of laboratory tests. These tests were consistent with the client's physical findings and previous history of prostate problems 1 year ago. The client was reluctant to discuss bowel or bladder function with the female therapist but readily suggested to his physician that his current symptoms mimicked an earlier episode of prostatitis.

It is not always possible to elicit thorough responses from clients concerning matters of genitourinary function. If the client hesitates or is unable to answer questions satisfactorily, it may be necessary to present the questions again at a later time (e.g., next treatment session), to ask a colleague of the client's sex to confer with the client, or to refer the client to his or her physician for further evaluation. Occasionally, the client will answer negatively to any questions regarding observed changes in urinary function and will then report back at the next session that there was some pathologic condition that was not noted earlier.

In this case, a close review of the extensive medical records may have alerted the physical therapist to the client's previous treatment for the same problem, which he was reluctant to discuss.

PRACTICE QUESTIONS

1. Percussion of the costovertebral angle that results in the reproduction of symptoms:
   a. Signifies radiculitis
   b. Signifies pseudorenal pain
   c. Has no significance
   d. Requires medical referral
2. Renal pain is aggravated by:
   a. Spinal movement
   b. Palpatory pressure over the costovertebral angle
   c. Lying on the involved side
   d. All of the above
   e. None of the above
3. Important functions of the kidney include all the following *except:*
   a. Formation and excretion of urine
   b. Acid-base and electrolyte balance
   c. Stimulation of red blood cell production
   d. Production of glucose

4. What do the following terms mean?
   - Dyspareunia
   - Dysuria
   - Hematuria
   - Urgency
5. Who should be screened for possible renal/urologic involvement?
6. What is the difference between urge incontinence and stress incontinence?
7. What is the significance of "skin pain" over the T9/T10 dermatomes?
8. How do you screen for possible prostate involvement in a man with pelvic/low back pain of unknown cause?
9. Explain why renal/urologic pain can be felt in such a wide range of dermatomes (i.e., from the T9 to L1 dermatomes).
10. What is the mechanism of referral for urologic pain to the shoulder?

REFERENCES

1. Shah A. Introduction to Symptoms of Genitourinary Disorders. Merck Manual Professional Version. https://www.merckmanuals.com/professional/genitourinary-disorders. Accessed April 10, 2021.

2. Urinary Tract Infection-Adults: New York Times. Accessed June 24, 2016.

3. Urinary tract infection (UTI): Mayo Clinic. Updated October 14, 2020. http://www.mayoclinic.org/diseases-conditions/urinary-tract-infection/basics/symptoms/con-20037892. Accessed April 10, 2021.

4. Ball JW, Dains JE, Flynn JA, Solomon BS, Stewart RW. *Seidel's Guide to Physical Examination.* 8 ed. St Louis, MO: Mosby Elsevier; 2015:373.

5. Swartz MH. *Textbook of Physical Diagnosis: History and Examination.* 7th ed. St. Louis, MO: Saunders Elsevier; 2014:473.

6. Paulson JD. Abdominal and urogenital diseases can often be the cause of lower back pain and sciatic-like symptoms. *Pain Manag.* 2012 May;2(3):279–294. https://doi.org/10.2217/pmt.12.14. PMID: 24654670.

7. Welk B, Baverstock R. Is there a link between back pain and urinary symptoms? *Neurourol Urodyn.* 2020;39(2):523–532. https://doi.org/10.1002/nau.24269. Epub 2020 Jan 3. PMID: 31899561.

8. Gill BC. Causes of Flank Pain. Medscape. Updated December 11, 2019. http://emedicine.medscape.com/article/1958746-overview. Accessed April 4, 2021.

9. Goodman CG, Marshall C. *Recognizing and Reporting Red Flags for the Physical Therapist Assistant.* 1st ed. St. Louis, MO: Saunders Elsevier; 2015:125.

10. de la Iglesia F, Asensio P, Díaz A, Darriba M, Nicolás R, Diz-Lois F. Acute renal infarction as a cause of low-back pain. (Case Report). *South Med J.* 2003;96(5):497–499. Accessed 8 June 2021.

11. Simons DG, Travell JG, Simons LS. 2 ed. *Travell & Simons' Myofascial Pain and Dysfunction: The Trigger Point Manual.* vol. 1 Baltimore: Williams & Wilkins; 1999.

12. Gyang A, Hartman M, Lamvu G. Musculoskeletal causes of chronic pelvic pain: what a gynecologist should know. *Obstet Gynecol.* 2013;121:645–650.

13. Hanson K, Quallich S. Assessment of elimination. In: Black JM, Hawks JH, eds. *Medical-Surgical Nursing: Clinical Management for Positive Outcomes.* 8 ed St. Louis, MO: Saunders Elsevier; 2009:662.

14. Stevens PE, Levin A. Kidney Disease: Improving Global Outcomes Chronic Kidney Disease Guideline Development Work Group Members. Evaluation and management of chronic kidney disease: synopsis of the kidney disease: improving global outcomes 2012 clinical practice guideline *Ann Intern Med.* 1582013825–830.

15. Ingersoll MA, Albert ML. From infection to immunotherapy: host immune responses to bacteria at the bladder mucosa. *Mucosal Immunol.* 2013;6(6):1041–1053.

16. Urinary tract infections: Risk Factors. Mayo Clinic. Updated October 14, 2020. http://www.mayoclinic.org/diseases-conditions/urinary-tract-infection/basics/risk-factors/con-20037892. Accessed April 10, 2021.

17. Mehmet NM, Ender O. Effect of urinary stone disease and its treatment on renal function. *World J Nephrol.* 2015;4(2):271–276.

18. Al-Rubeaan KA, Moharram O, Al-Naqeb D, Hassan A, Rafiullah MRM. Prevalence of urinary tract infection and risk factors among Saudi patients with diabetes. *World J Urol.* Jun 2013;31(3):573–578.

19. Urinary tract infections: National Kidney Foundation. https://www.kidney.org/sites/default/files/uti.pdf. Accessed April 10, 2021.

20. Urinary Tract Infections: Diabetes.co.uk. Updated January 15, 2019. http://www.diabetes.co.uk/diabetes-complications/urinary-tract-infections.html. Accessed April 9, 2021.

21. Berbari EF, Kanj SS, Kowalski TJ, et al. Executive summary: 2015 Infectious Diseases Society of America (IDSA) clinical practice guidelines for the diagnosis and treatment of native vertebral osteomyelitis in adults. *Clin Infect Dis.* 2015;61(6):859–863.

22. Interstitial Cystitis Association (ICA): About interstitial cystitis. Revised February 24, 2016. http://www.ichelp.org/. Accessed April 10, 2021.

23. Associated Conditions: Interstitial Cystitis Association. Revised July 7, 2016. http://www.ichelp.org/about-ic/associated-conditions/. Accessed April 10, 2021.

24. Diagnosis of IC: Interstitial Cystitis Association. Revised March 28, 2011. http://www.ichelp.org/diagnosis-treatment/diagnosis-of-ic/. Accessed April 10, 2021.

25. Interstitial cystitis: Mayo Clinic. Updated September 14, 2019. http://www.mayoclinic.org/diseases-conditions/interstitial-cystitis/basics/symptoms/con-20022439. Accessed April 10, 2021.

26. Obstructive Uropathy: Merck Manual, Professional Edition. Updated November 2020. http://www.merckmanuals.com/professional/genitourinary-disorders/obstructive-uropathy/obstructive-uropathy. Accessed April 10, 2021.

27. Obstructive uropathy: Medline Plus. National Institutes of Health, National Library of Medicine. https://www.nlm.nih.gov/medlineplus/medlineplus.html. Accessed April 10, 2021.

28. Patti L, Leslie SW. *Acute Renal Colic. [Updated 2021 Feb 10]. StatPearls [Internet].* Treasure Island (FL): StatPearls Publishing; 2021. January. https://www.ncbi.nlm.nih.gov/books/NBK431091/.

29. Steinberg GD. Bladder cancer. Medscape. Updated February 23, 2021. http://emedicine.medscape.com/article/438262-overview. Accessed April 10, 2021.

30. Turek PJ. Prostatitis. Medscape. Updated November 1, 2019. http://emedicine.medscape.com/article/785418-overview#a6. Accessed April 10, 2021.

31. Nickel JC. Prostatitis. *Can Urol Assoc J.* 2011;5(5):306–315.

32. Nickel JC. A new era in prostatitis research begins. *Rev Urol.* 2002;2(1):16–18.

33. NIH Definition and Classification: Prostatitis Network. http://www.chronicprostatitis.com/nih-definition-of-prostatitis-and-cpps/. Accessed June 28, 2016.

34. Sharp VJ, Powell CR. Prostatitis: diagnosis and treatment. *Am Fam Physician.* https://www.aafp.org/afp/2010/0815/p397.html. Accessed June 7, 2021.

35. Pontari MA. Etiology of chronic prostatitis/chronic pelvic pain syndrome: psychoimmunoneurendocrine dysfunction (PINE syndrome) or just a really bad infection? *World J Urol.* 2013;31(4):725–732.

36. Tripp DA, Nickel JC, Shoskes D, Koljuskov A. A 2-year follow-up of quality of life, pain, and psychosocial factors in patients with chronic prostatitis/chronic pelvic pain syndrome and their spouses. *World J Urol.* 2013;31(4):733–739.

37. Wagenlehner FME, van Till JWO, Magri V, et al. National institutes of health chronic prostatitis symptom index (NIH-CPSI) symptom evaluation in multinational cohorts of patients with chronic prostatitis/chronic pelvic pain syndrome. *Euro Urol.* 2013;63(5):953–959.

38. Lee MH, Seo DH, Lee C, et al. Relationship between the national institutes of health chronic prostatitis symptom index and the international prostate symptom score in middle-aged men according to the presence of chronic prostatitis-like symptoms. *J Men's Health.* 2020;16(1):19–26.

39. Rex L. *Evaluation and Treatment of Somatovisceral Dysfunction of the Gastrointestinal System.* Edmonds, WA: URSA Foundation; 2004.

40. Pontari M, Giusto L. New developments in the diagnosis and treatment of chronic prostatitis/chronic pelvic pain syndrome. *Curr Opin Urol.* 2013;23(6):565–569.

41. Mariotti G, Salciccia S, Innocenzi M, et al. Recovery of urinary continence after radical prostatectomy using early vs late pelvic floor electrical stimulation and biofeedback-associated treatment. *Urol.* 2015;86(1):115–121.

42. Morrison P. Musculoskeletal conditions related to pelvic floor muscle overactivity. In: Padoa A, Rosenbaum TY, eds. *The Overactive Pelvic Floor.* Switzerland: Springer International; 2016:91–111.

43. Anderson RU, Wise D, Sawyer T, Glowe P, Orenberg EK. Six-day intensive treatment protocol for refractory chronic prostatitis/chronic pelvic pain syndrome using myofascial release and paradoxical relaxation training. *J Urol.* 2011;185(4):1294–1299.

44. Gao M, Ding H, Zhong G, et al. The effects of transrectal radio-frequency hyperthermia on patients with chronic prostatitis and the changes of MDA, NO, SOD, and Zn levels in pretreatment and posttreatment. *Urology.* 2012;79(2):391–396.

45. Jhang JF, Kuo HC. Novel treatment of chronic bladder pain syndrome and other pelvic pain disorders by onabotulinumtoxinA injection. *Toxins (Basel).* 2015;7(6):2232–2250.

46. Abdelhameed MA, Nossier AA, Ashm HN, Anwar AMZ. Effect of extracorporeal shockwave therapy, pulsed electromagnetic field therapy and drug therapy on chronic pelvic pain syndrome: a prospective randomized study. *Int J Curr Res Rev.* 2021;13(10):5–10. https://doi.org/10.31782/IJCRR.2021.131001.

47. National Institutes of Health. National Institute of Diabetes and Digestive and Kidney Diseases. Prostate Enlargement: Benign Prostatic Hyperplasia. https://www.niddk.nih.gov/health-information/urologic-diseases/prostate-problems/prostate-enlargement-benign-prostatic-hyperplasia. Accessed April 10, 2021.

48. Enlarged Prostate. The New York Times. http://www.nytimes.com/health/guides/disease/enlarged-prostate/overview.html#Symptoms. Accessed April 10, 2021.

49. Prostate Cancer Statistics. Centers of Disease Control and Prevention. Updated June 8, 2020. https://www.cdc.gov/cancer/prostate/statistics/. Accessed April 10, 2021.

50. Prostate Cancer. American Cancer Society. Revised January 12, 2021. Available online at http://www.cancer.org/cancer/prostatecancer/detailedguide/prostate-cancer-key-statistics. Accessed March 8, 2022.

51. National Cancer Institute. Prostate Specific Antigen Test. https://www.cancer.gov/types/prostate/psa-fact-sheet. Accessed June 8, 2021.

52. Hoffman RM. Screening for prostate cancer. UpToDate. Wolters Kluwer. Updated April 5, 2021. http://www.uptodate.com/contents/screening-for-prostate-cancer. Accessed April 14, 2021.

53. Carroll PR, Nelson WG. Report to the nation on prostate cancer: introduction. Medscape. http://www.medscape.com/viewarticle/489635. Accessed April 14, 2021.

54. National Institutes of Health. National Cancer Institute. Prostate cancer screening. Updated April 10, 2019. http://www.cancer.gov/types/prostate/patient/prostate-screening-pdq. Accessed April 14, 2021.

55. American Cancer Society. American Cancer Society recommendations for prostate cancer early detection. Updated November 17, 2020. http://www.cancer.org/cancer/prostatecancer/moreinformation/prostatecancerearlydetection/prostate-cancer-early-detection-acs-recommendations. Accessed April 14, 2021.

56. Prostate Cancer Statistics. Cancer.net. Approved 02/2021. http://www.cancer.net/cancer-types/prostate-cancer/statistics. Accessed April 14, 2021.

57. Cancer.net Editorial Board. Prostate Cancer: Risk Factors and Prevention. https://www.cancer.net/cancer-types/prostate-cancer/risk-factors-and-prevention. Accessed June 8, 2021.

58. Stefani ED, Boffetta PL, Ronco A, Deneo-Pellegrini H. Meat consumption, related nutrients, obesity and risk of prostate cancer: a case-control study in Uruguay. *APJCP.* 2016;17(4):1937–1945.

59. Spence AR, Rousseau MC, Parent ME. Sexual partners, sexually transmitted infections, and prostate cancer risk. *Cancer Epidemiol.* 2014;38(6):700–707.

60. Caini S, Gandini S, Dudas M, Bremer V, Severi E, Gherasim A. Sexually transmitted infections and prostate cancer risk: a systematic review and meta-analysis. *Cancer Epidemiol.* 2014;38(4):329–338.

61. Lawson JS, Glenn WK. Evidence for a causal role by human papillomaviruses in prostate cancer – a systematic review. *Infect Agents Cancer.* 2020;15:41. https://doi.org/10.1186/s13027-020-00305-8.

62. Houston TJ, Ghosh R. Untangling the association between environmental endocrine disruptive chemicals and the etiology of male genitourinary cancers. *Biochem Pharmacol.* 2020;172:113743 https://doi.org/10.1016/j.bcp.2019.113743. ISSN 0006-2952. (https://www.sciencedirect.com/science/article/pii/S0006295219304423).

63. Parent ME, Siemiatycki J. Occupation and prostate cancer. *Epidemiol Rev.* 2001;23(1):138–143.

64. Prostate Cancer Stages: American Cancer Society. Updated August 1, 2019. http://www.cancer.org/cancer/prostatecancer/detailedguide/prostate-cancer-staging. Accessed April 14, 2021.

65. Bone Metastasis: American Cancer Society. Updated January 22, 2021. http://www.cancer.org/acs/groups/cid/documents/webcontent/003087-pdf.pdf. Accessed April 18, 2021.

66. Vasavada SP. Urinary Incontinence. Medscape.Updated January 22, 2021. http://emedicine.medscape.com/article/452289-overview. Accessed April 18, 2021.

67. Prevalence of Incontinence among Older Americans: Centers for Disease Control and Prevention. http://www.cdc.gov/nchs/data/series/sr_03/sr03_036.pdf. Accessed June 28, 2016.

68. What is Urinary Incontinence? Urology Care Foundation. http://www.urologyhealth.org/urologic-conditions/urinary-incontinence. Accessed April 14, 2021.

69. Nitti VW, Khullar V, van Kerrebroeck P, et al. Mirabegron for the treatment of overactive bladder: a prespecified pooled efficacy analysis and pooled safety analysis of three randomised, double-blind, placebo-controlled, phase III studies. *Int J Clin Pract.* 2013;67(7):619–632.

70. Overactive Bladder: Mayo Clinic. Updated March 20, 2020. http://www.mayoclinic.org/diseases-conditions/overactive-bladder/basics/causes/con-20027632. Accessed April 14, 2021.

71. Functional Incontinence: WebMD. Updated July 23, 2019. http://www.webmd.com/urinary-incontinence-oab/functional-incontinence. Accessed April 14, 2021.

72. Da Roza T, Jorge RN, Mascarenhas T, et al. Urinary incontinence in sport women: from risk factors to treatment – a review. *Curr Womens Health Rev.* 2013;9:77–84.

73. Hulme J. *Regaining Bowel and Bladder Control after Cancer.* Missoula, MT: Phoenix Publishers; 2003.

74. D'Amico AV. Surrogate end point for prostate cancer-specific mortality after radical prostatectomy or radiation therapy. *J Natl Cancer Inst.* 2003;95(18):1376–1383.

75. Hojan K, Milecki P. Opportunities for rehabilitation of patients with radiation fibrosis syndrome. *Rep Pract Oncol Radiother.* 2014;19:1–6.

76. Lamin E, Smith AL. Urologic agents for treatment of bladder dysfunction in neurologic disease. *Curr Treat Opt Neurol.* 2014;16:280.

77. Liu M, Hou C. Classification of and treatment principles for bladder dysfunction caused by spinal cord injury. In: Hou C, ed. *Functional Bladder Reconstruction Following Spinal Cord Injury via Neural Approaches.* : Springer; 2014:17–20.

78. Huber SA, Northington GM, Karp DR. Bowel and bladder dysfunction following surgery within the presacral space: an

overview of neuroanatomy, function, and dysfunction. *Int Urogynecol J*. 2015;26(7):941–946.

79. WebMD. 4 Drugs Linked to Urinary Incontinence. https://www.webmd.com/urinary-incontinence-oab/4-medications-that-cause-or-worsen-incontinence. Accessed June 14, 2021.

80. Panesar K. Drug-induced urinary incontinence. *US Pharmacist*. 2014;39(8):24–29.

81. Burrows NR. Incidence of end-stage renal disease attributed to diabetes among persons with diagnosed diabetes in the United States and Puerto Rico. *MMWR*. 2010;59(42):1361–1366.

82. National Kidney Foundation. Diabetes and Chronic Kidney Disease. https://www.kidney.org/news/newsroom/factsheets/Diabetes-And-CKD. Accessed June 14, 2021.

83. Stine JG, Sateesh P, Lewis JH. Drug-induced liver injury in the elderly. *Curr Gastroenterol Rep*. Jan 2013;15(1):299.

84. Soloman DH. Patient information: Nonsteroidal anti-inflammatory drugs (NSAIDs) (Beyond the Basics). UptoDate. Wolters Kluwer. Updated July 14, 2020. http://www.uptodate.com/contents/nonsteroidal-antiinflammatory-drugs-nsaids-beyond-the-basics. Accessed April 14, 2021.

85. Smart NA, Williams AD, Levinger I, et al. Exercise and Sports Science Australia (ESSA) position statement on exercise and chronic kidney disease. *J Sci Med Sport*. 2013;16(5):406–411.

86. Bling D. Managing and treating chronic kidney disease. Nursing Times, February 9, 2015. http://www.nursingtimes.net/clinical-archive/long-term-conditions/managing-and-treating-chronic-kidney-disease/5081921.fullarticle. Accessed April 14, 2021.

87. Bladder cancer risk factors: American Cancer Society. Updated January 30, 2019. http://www.cancer.org/cancer/bladdercancer/detailedguide/bladder-cancer-risk-factors. Accessed on April 14, 2021.

88. Bladder cancer: University of Iowa Hospitals and Clinics. https://cancer.uiowa.edu/cancer-types/bladder-cancer?gclid=Cj0KCQjwse-DBhC7ARIsAI8YcWIv_LblONXB30fa6NaPeMB 26VzZdnkcoSi0SkPiNgBa6sLxnu1eEYAaAscHEALw_wcB https://www.uihealthcare.org/bladder-cancer/. Accessed April 14, 2021.

89. Key statistics for bladder cancer: American Cancer Society. Updated January 12, 2021. http://www.cancer.org/cancer/bladdercancer/detailedguide/bladder-cancer-key-statistics. Accessed April 14, 2021.

90. Jacobs BL. Bladder cancer in 2010: how far have we come? *CA Cancer J Clin*. 2010;60(4):244–272.

91. Letasiova S, Medvedova A, Dusinska M, et al. Bladder cancer, a review of the environmental risk factors. *Environmental Health*. 2012;11(Suppl 1):S11.

92. National Institutes of Health. National Cancer Institute. What you need to know about bladder cancer. https://www.cancer.gov/types/bladder http://www.cancer.gov/publications/patient-education/wyntk-bladder-cancer. Accessed June 29, 2016.

93. National Institutes of Health: National Cancer Institute. Kidney cancer. https://www.cancer.gov/types/kidney http://www.cancer.gov/publications/patient-education/wyntk-kidney-cancer. Accessed April 14, 2021.

94. American Cancer Society: Testicular cancer. http://www.cancer.org/acs/groups/cid/documents/webcontent/003142-pdf.pdf. Accessed March 8, 2022.

95. National Library of Medicine: Medline Plus. Testicular Cancer. Updated April 2. 2021. https://www.nlm.nih.gov/medlineplus/ency/article/001288.htm. Accessed April 14, 2021.

96. American Cancer Society: Do I have Testicular Cancer? Updated May 17, 2018. http://www.cancer.org/cancer/testicularcancer/do-i-have-testicular-cancer. Accessed April 14, 2021.

97. Tompkins J, Norris T, Levenhagen K. Laboratory tests and values. In: Goodman CG, Fuller K, eds. *Goodman and Fuller's Pathology: Implications for the Physical Therapist*. 5th ed. : Elsevier; 2020.

CHAPTER

12

Screening for Endocrine and Metabolic Disease

Annie Burke-Doe

Endocrinology is the study of the endocrine system and its associated diseases affecting the human body. The function of the endocrine system is to maintain whole body homeostasis through the coordination of chemical messengers (hormones) that relay information and instructions between cells. Hormone signaling pathways regulate cellular activity in target organs throughout the body. The endocrine system works in coordination with the nervous system to regulate metabolism, water and salt balance, blood pressure, response to stress, and sexual reproduction[1]. The nervous system also relies on chemical communication (synapses), but its effects are generally short lived, limited to specific target cells, and are designed to enable you to handle situations requiring split second responses. The endocrine system is slower in response and takes longer to act than the nervous system in transferring biochemical information. Many life processes are not short lived or require long-term maintenance, such as reaching adult stature and reproductive capabilities.

Hormones are the chemical messengers of the endocrine system and are released and transported to their targets by the bloodstream. The pituitary (hypophysis), thyroid, parathyroid, adrenal, and pineal glands make up the endocrine system (Fig. 12.1). The hypothalamus controls pituitary function and thus has an important indirect influence on the other glands of the endocrine system. Positive and negative feedback mechanisms exist in the hypothalamus to keep hormones at normal levels.

The endocrine system meets the nervous system in a complex series of interactions that link behavioral-neural-endocrine-immunologic responses. The hypothalamus, the pituitary and the adrenal gland form an integrated axis (HPA axis) that maintains a set of direct influence and feedback over much of the endocrine system. The discovery and study of this complex axial interface is called psychoneuroimmunology (PNI), which has provided a new understanding of interactive biologic signaling for reactions that are controlled by the HPA axis, such as stress, digestion, immune function,

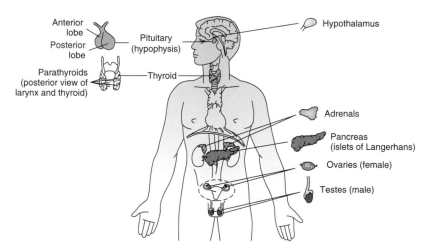

Fig. 12.1 *Location of the nine endocrine glands.* Not shown: adipose tissue (now classified as the largest endocrine gland in the body). Redrawn from Kee JL, Hayes ER, McCuistion LE: *Pharmacology: a patient-centered nursing process approach*, ed 8, St. Louis, Elsevier/Saunders, 2015.

mood, sexuality, energy storage, and expenditure. Defects in signaling pathways of the HPA axis are known to play a role in chronic inflammatory disease such as rheumatoid arthritis,[2] stress-induced immunomodulation in asthma,[3] and the development and progression of cancer.[4] It has been observed in studies that psychological stress can lead to a maladaptive response and breakdown the HPA axis.[5] Stress can be disease-permissive, as in chronic inflammatory diseases, cancer, cardiovascular diseases, acute and chronic viral infections, sepsis, asthma, and others.[4]

ENDOCRINE-ASSOCIATED NEUROMUSCULAR AND MUSCULOSKELETAL SIGNS AND SYMPTOMS[6]

The musculoskeletal system is composed of a variety of connective tissue structures in which normal growth and development are influenced strongly and sometimes controlled by various hormones and metabolic processes. Alterations in these control systems can result in structural changes and altered function of various connective tissues, producing systemic and musculoskeletal signs and symptoms (Table 12.1). Myopathy is observed in endocrine disorders such as hypothyroidism, hyperthyroidism, Cushing syndrome and disease, Addison disease, vitamin D deficiency, and both hyperparathyroidism and hypoparathyroidism.[7]

Muscle Weakness, Myalgia, Cramps, and Fatigue

Muscle weakness, myalgia, cramps, and fatigue may be early manifestations of thyroid or parathyroid disease, acromegaly, diabetes mellitus (DM), Cushing's syndrome, vitamin D deficiency, and osteomalacia. The pattern of weakness

TABLE 12.1	Signs and Symptoms of Endocrine Dysfunction
Neuromusculoskeletal	Systemic
Signs and symptoms associated with rheumatoid arthritis	Excessive or delayed growth
	Polydipsia
Muscle weakness (myopathy)	Polyuria
Muscle atrophy	Mental changes
Myalgia; muscle cramps	(nervousness, confusion, depression)
Fatigue	Changes in hair (quality and distribution)
Carpal tunnel syndrome	
Synovial fluid changes	Changes in skin pigmentation
Periarthritis	
Adhesive capsulitis (diabetes mellitus)	Changes in vital signs (elevated body temperature, pulse rate, increased blood pressure)
Chondrocalcinosis	
Spondyloarthropathy	
Osteoarthritis	Heart palpitations
Hand stiffness	Increased perspiration
Arthralgia	Kussmaul's respirations
Falls	(deep, rapid breathing)
	Dehydration or excessive retention of body water

Adapted from Goodman CC, Fuller KS: *Pathology: implications for the physical therapist*, ed 5, St. Louis, Elsevier, 2021.

in myopathy most commonly involves the proximal upper and/or lower limb muscles symmetrically.[8] Acquired muscle weakness should be investigated for endocrine causes because a significant number of them recover fully with specific treatment.[9]

Bilateral Carpal Tunnel Syndrome

Bilateral carpal tunnel syndrome (CTS), resulting from median nerve compression at the wrist, is a common finding in a variety of systemic and neuromusculoskeletal conditions,[10–12] but especially with certain endocrine and metabolic disorders (Table 12.2).[13] The fact that the majority of persons with CTS are women at or near menopause suggests that the soft tissues about the wrist could be affected in some way by hormones.[14,15]

Thickening of the transverse carpal ligament in certain systemic disorders (e.g., acromegaly, myxedema) may be sufficient to compress the median nerve. Any condition that increases the volume of the contents of the carpal tunnel (e.g., neoplasm, calcium, and gouty tophi deposits) can compress the median nerve.

The signs and symptoms often associated with CTS include paresthesia, tingling, and numbness and/or pain (or burning pain) with cutaneous distribution of the median nerve to the thumb, index, middle, and radial half of the ring finger.[15] Nocturnal paresthesia is a common complaint, and this discomfort causes sleep disruption. It can be partially relieved by shaking of the hand or changing the wrist and hand position. Pain may radiate into the palm and up the forearm and arm.[16]

It should be noted that bilateral tarsal syndrome affecting the feet can also occur either alone or in conjunction with CTS, although the incidence of tarsal tunnel syndrome is not high. Bilateral median nerve neuropathy can be characteristic of many systemic diseases such as inflammatory arthritis, myxedema, amyloidosis, hypothyroidism, DM, and chronic polyarthritis.[17–19]

Whenever a client presents with bilateral symptoms, it represents a red flag, most recently CTS has been linked to early identification of amyloidosis.[20] With bilateral CTS the therapist can screen for medical disease by using the Special Questions to Ask: Bilateral Carpal Tunnel Syndrome section (see Appendix B-4[15] in the accompanying enhanced eBook version included with print purchase of this textbook).

Periarthritis and Calcific Tendinitis

Periarthritis (inflammation of periarticular structures, including the tendons, ligaments, and joint capsule) and calcific tendinitis occur most often in the shoulders of people who have endocrine disease. Those with endocrine disorders of the thyroid and estrogen metabolism may present with tendinitis younger, have longer natural histories, and are more likely to undergo operative treatment.[21] Treatment of the underlying endocrine impairment often improves the clinical picture; ultrasound guided percutaneous treatment with rehabilitation has become more widely used and has been

TABLE 12.2	Causes of Carpal Tunnel Syndrome	
Neuromusculoskeletal	**Systemic**	

Neuromusculoskeletal

IDIOPATHIC

Cause unknown

ANATOMIC (COMPRESSION)

Small carpal canal, anomalous muscles/tendons
Basal joint (thumb) arthritis
Cervical disk lesions
Cervical spondylosis
Congenital anatomic differences or anatomic change in nerve or carpal tunnel (e.g., shape, size, volume of structures; presence of palmaris longus)
History of wrist surgery, especially previous carpal tunnel surgery
Injection: high pressure
Peripheral neuropathy
Poor posture (may also be associated with TOS)
Tendinitis
Trigger points
Tenosynovitis
Thoracic outlet syndrome (TOS)

TRAUMA/EXERTIONAL

Swelling, hemorrhage, scar, wrist fracture, carpal dislocation
Cumulative trauma disorders (CTD)*
Repetitive strain injuries (RSI)*
Vibrational exposure (jackhammer or other manual labor equipment)

Systemic

Chronic kidney disease (fluid imbalance)
Congestive heart failure (fluid imbalance)
Hemochromatosis
Leukemia (tissue infiltration)
Liver disease
Medications
• Nonsteroidal antiinflammatory drugs (NSAIDs)
• Oral contraceptives
• Statins
• Alendronate (Fosamax)
• Lithium
• Beta-blocker
Obesity
Pregnancy (fluid retention)
Tumor (lipoma, hemangioma, ganglia, synovial sarcoma, fibroma, neuroma, neurofibroma)
Use of oral contraceptives
Vitamin deficiency

ENDOCRINE

Acromegaly
Diabetes mellitus
Gout (deposits of tophi and calcium)
Hormonal imbalance (menopause; post-hysterectomy)
Hyperparathyroidism
Hyperthyroidism (Graves' disease)
Hypocalcemia
Hypothyroidism (myxedema)

INFECTIOUS DISEASE

Atypical mycobacterium
Histoplasmosis
Rubella
Sporotrichosis

INFLAMMATORY

Amyloidosis
Arthritis (rheumatoid, gout, polymyalgia rheumatica)
Dermatomyositis
Gout/pseudogout
Scleroderma
Systemic lupus erythematosus

NEUROPATHIC

Alcohol abuse
Chemotherapy (delayed, long-term effect)
Diabetes mellitus
Multiple myeloma (amyloidosis deposits)
Thyroid disease
Vitamin/nutritional deficiency (especially vitamin B_6; folic acid)
Vitamin toxicity

Modified from Goodman CC, Fuller K: *Pathology: implications for the physical therapist*, ed 5, St Louis, 2021, Elsevier.
*The role of repetitive activities and occupational factors (e.g., hand use of any type and keyboard or computer work in particular) has been questioned as a direct cause of carpal tunnel syndrome (CTS) and remains under investigation; sufficient evidence to implicate hand use of any type linked with CTS remains unproven.[9,10]

effective in facilitating prompt shoulder functional recovery and pain relief.[22,–25]

Chondrocalcinosis

Chondrocalcinosis refers to the deposition of calcium pyrophosphate dihydrate (CPPD) crystals in the cartilage chondrocytes of joints.[26] When accompanied by attacks of gout-like symptoms, it is called *pseudogout*. Like gout, pseudogout is a disease in which crystal formation leads to inflammation and mechanical damage.[27] Unlike gout, in which a systemic metabolic derangement promotes crystal deposition, pseudogout usually appears to derive from metabolic abnormalities intrinsic to chondrocytes, resulting in crystal deposition in cartilage.[27] However, the result is similar: innate immune responses to crystals leads to local hyperemia, joint effusion, and neutrophil influx, and the four cardinal signs of inflammation: heat, redness, pain, and swelling.[27] Chondrocalcinosis is commonly seen on x-ray films as calcified hyaline or fibrous cartilage and has a clear association with previous joint trauma.[28] There is an associated underlying endocrine or metabolic disease in approximately 5% to 10% of individuals with chondrocalcinosis (Table 12.3)

Spondyloarthropathy and Osteoarthritis

Spondyloarthropathy (disease of joints of the spine) and osteoarthritis occur in individuals with various metabolic or endocrine diseases, including hemochromatosis (disorder of iron metabolism with excess deposition of iron in the tissues; also known as *bronze diabetes* and *iron storage disease*), ochronosis (metabolic disorder resulting in discoloration of body tissues caused by deposits of alkapton bodies), acromegaly, hypoparathyroidism,[31] and DM.

Hand Stiffness and Hand Pain

Hand stiffness and hand pain, as well as arthralgias of the small joints of the hand, can occur with endocrine and metabolic diseases such as DM.[32,33] Hypothyroidism is often accompanied by CTS; flexor tenosynovitis with stiffness is another common finding.

TABLE 12.3	Endocrine and Metabolic Disorders Associated with Chondrocalcinosis[28–30]
Endocrine	Metabolic
Hypothyroidism	Hemochromatosis
Hyperparathyroidism	Hypomagnesemia
Acromegaly	Hypophosphatasias
Diabetes mellitus	Ochronosis
	Alkaptonuric oxalosis
	Wilson's disease
	Gitelman's syndrome
	Gout
	Hypocalciuric hypercalcemias

ENDOCRINE PATHOPHYSIOLOGY

Disorders of the endocrine glands can be classified as primary (excess or deficiency of secretion of the gland itself), secondary (excess or deficiency of secretion of the pituitary gland), or tertiary (excess or deficiency of secretion by the hypothalamus).[34]

Secondary dysfunction may also occur (iatrogenically) as a result of chemotherapy, surgical removal of the glands, therapy for a nonendocrine disorder (e.g., the use of large doses of corticosteroids resulting in Cushing's syndrome), or excessive therapy for an endocrine disorder.

Pituitary Gland

Diabetes Insipidus

Diabetes insipidus (DI) is caused by a lack of secretion or action of vasopressin (antidiuretic hormone [ADH]). This hormone normally stimulates the distal tubules of the kidneys to reabsorb water. Without ADH, water moving through the kidney is not reabsorbed and is lost in the urine, resulting in severe water loss and dehydration through diuresis.[35]

There are two main types of DI: central DI and nephrogenic DI. Central DI (the inability to synthesize and release vasopressin) is the most common type. It can be idiopathic (primary) or related to other causes (secondary), such as pituitary trauma, head injury (including neurosurgery), infections such as meningitis or encephalitis, pituitary neoplasm, anorexia, and vascular lesions such as aneurysms. Nephrogenic DI (defective hormone or receptor function) occurs as a result of some medications (e.g., lithium, phenytoin, corticosteroids, anticholinergics), alcohol, electrolyte imbalances such as hypercalcemia and hypokalemia, and diseases affecting the renal system (e.g., sarcoidosis, multiple myeloma, pyelonephritis, systemic lupus erythematosus).

If the person with DI is unconscious or confused and is unable to take in necessary fluids to replace those lost, rapid dehydration, shock, and death can occur. Because sleep is interrupted by the persistent need to void (nocturia), fatigue and irritability result.

CLINICAL SIGNS AND SYMPTOMS

Diabetes Insipidus

- Polyuria (increased urination more than 3 L/day in adults)
- Nocturia (a condition in which you wake up at night because you have to urinate)
- Polydipsia (increased thirst, which occurs subsequent to polyuria in response to the loss of fluid)
- Dehydration (dry, cracked lips/skin; fever; orthostatic hypotension; weakness; dizziness; fatigue)
- Decreased urine specific gravity (1.001 to 1.005)
- Fatigue, irritability
- Increased serum sodium (more than 145 mEq/dL; resulting from concentration of serum from water loss)

Syndrome of Inappropriate Secretion of Antidiuretic Hormone

Syndrome of inappropriate secretion of antidiuretic hormone (SIADH) is an excess or inappropriate secretion of vasopressin that results in marked retention of water, resulting in hyponatremia (low sodium in the blood).[35] Urine output decreases dramatically as the body retains large amounts of water. Almost all of the excess water is distributed within body cells, causing intracellular water gain and cellular swelling (water intoxication).

Risk Factors. Risk factors for the development of SIADH include pituitary damage caused by infection, trauma, or neoplasm; secretion of vasopressin-like substances from some types of malignant tumors (particularly pulmonary malignancies); and thoracic pressure changes from compression of pulmonary or cardiac pressure receptors, or both.

Clinical Presentation. Symptoms of SIADH are the clinical opposite of symptoms of DI. They are the result of water retention and the subsequent dilution of sodium in the blood serum (hyponatremia) and body cells. Neurologic and neuromuscular signs and symptoms predominate and are directly related to the swelling of brain tissue and sodium changes within neuromuscular tissues.

CLINICAL SIGNS AND SYMPTOMS

Syndrome of Inappropriate Secretion of Antidiuretic Hormone

- Headache, confusion, lethargy (most significant early indicators)
- Decreased urine output
- Weight gain without visible edema
- Seizure
- Muscle cramping
- Vomiting, diarrhea
- Increased urine specific gravity (greater than 1.03)
- Decreased serum sodium (less than 135 mEq/dL; caused by dilution of serum from water)

Acromegaly

Acromegaly is an abnormal enlargement of the extremities of the skeleton resulting from hypersecretion of growth hormone (GH) from the pituitary gland and consequently insulin-like growth factor 1 (IGF-1).[36] This condition is relatively rare and occurs in adults, most often owing to a tumor of the pituitary gland.[37] In children, overproduction of GH stimulates growth of long bones and results in gigantism, in which the child grows to exaggerated heights. With adults, growth of the long bones has already stopped, so the bones most affected are those of the face, jaw, hands, and feet. Other signs and symptoms include amenorrhea (in women), DM, profuse sweating, and hypertension. The disease also has rheumatologic, cardiovascular, respiratory, neoplastic, neurological, and metabolic manifestations which negatively impact its prognosis and patients' quality of life.[37]

Clinical Presentation. Degenerative arthropathy may be seen in the peripheral joints of a client with acromegaly, most frequently attacking the large joints. On x-ray studies, osteophyte formation may be seen, along with widening of the joint space because of increased cartilage thickness. In late-stage disease, joint spaces become narrowed, and occasionally chondrocalcinosis may be present.

Stiffness of the hand, typically of both hands, is associated with a broad enlargement of the fingers from bony overgrowth and with thickening of the soft tissue. Thickening and widening of the phalangeal tufts are typical x-ray findings in soft tissue. In clients with these x-ray findings, much of the pain and stiffness is believed to be as a result of premature osteoarthritis.

CTS is seen in up to 50% of people with acromegaly. The CTS that occurs with this growth disorder is thought to be caused by compression of the median nerve at the wrist from soft tissue hypertrophy, or bony overgrowth, or by hypertrophy of the median nerve itself.

Proximal myopathy and fibromyalgia in people with acromegaly is commonly reported[36] but poorly understood. Changes in muscle size and strength are associated with acromegaly and are probably multifactorial in origin. Screening individuals with acromegaly for muscle weakness and poor exercise tolerance is now recommended.[38] Exercise has been suggested as a way to improve quality of life, self-esteem, and body image for patients with acromegaly.[39]

About half of the individuals with acromegaly have back pain. X-ray studies demonstrate increased intervertebral disk spaces and large osteophytes along the anterior longitudinal ligament (ALL), mimicking diffuse idiopathic skeletal hyperostosis (DISH).

DISH (also known as *Forestier's disease*) is characterized by abnormal ossification of the ALL, resulting in an x-ray image of large osteophytes seemingly "flowing" along the anterior border of the spine. DISH is particularly common in the thoracic spine and has been reported to be more prevalent among persons with DM than among the nondiabetic population. DISH appears to be an age-related predisposition to ossification of the tendon, joint capsule, and ligamentous attachments. Identification of the presence of DISH syndrome before surgery is important for the prevention of heterotrophic bone formation.[40]

CLINICAL SIGNS AND SYMPTOMS

Acromegaly

- Bony enlargement (face, jaw, hands, feet)
- Amenorrhea
- Diabetes mellitus (DM)
- Profuse sweating (diaphoresis)
- Hypertension
- Carpal tunnel syndrome (CTS)
- Hand pain and stiffness
- Back pain (thoracic and/or lumbar)
- Proximal myopathy and poor exercise tolerance
- Fibromyalgia

Adrenal Glands

The adrenal glands are two small glands located on the upper part of each kidney. Each adrenal gland consists of two relatively discrete parts: an outer cortex and an inner medulla. The outer cortex is responsible for the secretion of mineralocorticoids (steroid hormones that regulate fluid and mineral balance), glucocorticoids (steroid hormones responsible for controlling the metabolism of glucose), and androgens (sex hormones). The centrally located adrenal medulla is derived from neural tissue and secretes epinephrine and norepinephrine. Together, the adrenal cortex and medulla are major factors in the body's response to stress.

Adrenal Insufficiency

Primary Adrenal Insufficiency

Chronic adrenocortical insufficiency (hyposecretion by the adrenal glands) may be primary or secondary. Primary adrenal insufficiency is also referred to as *Addison's disease* (hypofunction),[41] named after the physician who first studied and described the associated symptoms. It can be treated by the administration of exogenous cortisol (one of the adrenocortical hormones).

Primary adrenal insufficiency occurs when a disorder exists within the adrenal gland itself. This adrenal gland disorder results in decreased production of cortisol and aldosterone, two of the primary adrenocortical hormones. The most common cause of primary adrenal insufficiency is an autoimmune process that causes destruction of the adrenal cortex.

The most striking physical finding in the person with primary adrenal insufficiency is the increased pigmentation of the skin and mucous membranes. This discoloration may vary in the white population from a slight tan, or a few black freckles, to an intense generalized pigmentation, which has resulted in persons being mistakenly considered to be of a darker-skinned race. Members of darker-skinned races may develop a slate-gray color that may be obvious only to family members.

Melanin, the major product of the melanocyte, is largely responsible for the coloring of skin. In primary adrenal insufficiency, the increase in pigmentation is initiated by the excessive secretion of melanocyte-stimulating hormone (MSH) that occurs in association with increased secretion of adrenocorticotropic hormone (ACTH). ACTH is increased in an attempt to stimulate the diseased adrenal glands to produce and release more cortisol.

Most commonly, pigmentation is visible over extensor surfaces, such as the backs of the hands; elbows; knees; and creases of the hands, lips, and mouth. Increased pigmentation of scars formed after the onset of the disease is common. However, it is possible for a person with primary adrenal insufficiency to demonstrate no significant increase in pigmentation.

Secondary Adrenal Insufficiency. Secondary adrenal insufficiency refers to a dysfunction of the gland because of insufficient stimulation of the cortex, owing to a lack of pituitary ACTH. Causes of secondary disease include tumors of the hypothalamus or pituitary, removal of the pituitary, or rapid withdrawal of corticosteroid drugs. Clinical manifestations of secondary disease do not occur until the adrenal glands are almost completely nonfunctional and are primarily related to cortisol deficiency only.

CLINICAL SIGNS AND SYMPTOMS
Adrenal Insufficiency

- Dark pigmentation of the skin, especially mouth and scars (occurs only with primary disease; Addison's disease)
- Hypotension (low blood pressure causing orthostatic symptoms)
- Progressive fatigue (improves with rest)
- Hyperkalemia (generalized weakness and muscle flaccidity)
- Gastrointestinal (GI) disturbances
- Anorexia and weight loss
- Nausea and vomiting
- Arthralgias, myalgias (secondary only)
- Tendon calcification
- Hypoglycemia

Cushing's Syndrome

Cushing's syndrome (hyperfunction of the adrenal gland) is a general term for increased secretion of cortisol by the adrenal cortex. When corticosteroids are administered externally, a condition of hypercortisolism called *iatrogenic Cushing's syndrome* occurs, producing a group of associated signs and symptoms. Hypercortisolism caused by excess secretion of ACTH (e.g., from pituitary stimulation) is called *ACTH-dependent Cushing's syndrome.*[42]

Therapists often treat people who have developed Cushing's syndrome after receiving large doses of cortisol (also known as *hydrocortisone*) or cortisol derivatives (e.g., dexamethasone) for a number of inflammatory disorders (Case Example 12.1).

It is important to remember that whenever corticosteroids are administered externally, the increase in serum cortisol levels triggers a negative feedback signal to the anterior pituitary gland to stop adrenal stimulation. Adrenal atrophy occurs during this time, and adrenal insufficiency will result if external corticosteroids are abruptly withdrawn. Corticosteroid medications must be reduced gradually so that normal adrenal function can return.

Because cortisol suppresses the inflammatory response of the body, it can mask early signs of infection. *Any unexplained fever without other symptoms should be a warning to the therapist of the need for medical follow-up.*

CASE EXAMPLE 12.1

Cushing's Syndrome

A 53-year-old woman with Cushing's syndrome resulting from long-term use of cortisol for systemic lupus erythematosus reports the following problems:

- Hair and nail thinning and breaking easily
- Temperature intolerance (always cold)
- Muscle cramps
- Generalized weakness and fatigue

Her primary complaint and reason for referral to physical therapy is for sacroiliac (SI) joint pain as a result of stepping down off of an uneven curb.

You realize the signs and symptoms are of an endocrine origin, but you do not know whether they are a part of the Cushing's syndrome or a separate endocrine problem.

Should you send this client to a physician (or back to the referring physician)?

Not necessarily. This is more a case of a need for additional information. Requesting a copy of the client's most recent physician's notes may answer all of your questions. Reading the physician's systems review portion of the examination may reveal a record of these signs and symptoms with a corresponding medical problem list and plan.

If there is no mention of any of these associated signs and symptoms, a phone call to the physician's office may be the next step. If you speak with the physician directly, identify yourself and your connection with the client by name. Briefly mention why you are seeing this client and make the following observation:

"Mrs. Jones reports muscle cramps and generalized weakness that do not seem consistent with her SI problem. She complains of temperature intolerance and hair and nail bed changes. These symptoms are outside the scope of my practice.

Can you help me understand this? Are they a part of her lupus erythematosus, Cushing's syndrome, or something else?"

CLINICAL SIGNS AND SYMPTOMS

Cushing's Syndrome

- "Moonface" appearance (very round face; Fig. 12.2)
- Buffalo hump at the neck (fatty deposits)
- Protuberant abdomen with accumulation of fatty tissue and stretch marks
- Muscle wasting and weakness
- Decreased density of bones (especially spine)
- Hypertension
- Kyphosis and back pain (secondary to bone loss)
- Easy bruising
- Psychiatric or emotional disturbances
- Impaired reproductive function (e.g., decreased libido and changes in menstrual cycle)
- Diabetes mellitus (DM)
- Slow wound healing
- *For women:* masculinizing effects (e.g., hair growth, breast atrophy, voice changes)

Effects of Cortisol on Connective Tissue. Over production of cortisol or closely related glucocorticoids by abnormal adrenocortical tissue leads to a protein catabolic state. This overproduction causes liberation of amino acids from muscle tissue. The resultant weakened protein structures (muscle and elastic tissue) cause a protuberant abdomen, poor wound healing, generalized muscle weakness, and marked osteoporosis (demineralization of bone causing reduced bone mass), which is made worse by an excessive loss of calcium in the urine.

Excessive glucose resulting from this protein catabolic state is transformed mainly into fat and appears in characteristic sites, such as the abdomen, supraclavicular fat pads, and facial cheeks. The change in facial appearance may not be readily apparent to the client or to the therapist, but pictures of the client taken over a period of years may provide a visual record of those changes.

The effect of increased circulating levels of cortisol on the muscles of clients varies from slight to very marked. There may be so much muscle wasting that the condition simulates muscular dystrophy. Marked weakness of the quadriceps muscle often prevents affected clients from rising out of a chair unassisted. Those with Cushing's syndrome of long duration almost always demonstrate demineralization of bone. In severe cases, this condition may lead to pathologic fractures, but it results more commonly in wedging of the vertebrae, kyphosis, bone pain, and back pain.

Obesity, DM, polycystic ovarian syndrome, and other metabolic/endocrine problems can resemble Cushing's syndrome. It is important to recognize critical indicators of this particular disorder, such as excessive hair growth, moonface, mood disorders, and increased muscle weakness as indicators for further endocrine diagnostic testing.[43]

The poor wound healing that is characteristic of this syndrome becomes a problem when any surgical procedures are required. Inhibition of collagen formation with corticosteroid therapy is responsible for the frequency of wound breakdown in postsurgical clients.

Thyroid Gland

The thyroid gland is located in the anterior portion of the lower neck, below the larynx, on both sides of, and anterior to, the trachea. The chief hormones produced by the thyroid are thyroxine (T_4), triiodothyronine (T_3), and calcitonin. Both T_3 and T_4 regulate the metabolic rate of the body and increase protein synthesis. Calcitonin has a weak physiologic effect on calcium and phosphorus balance in the body.

Genetics plays a role in thyroid disease and a family history of thyroid disease is a risk factor. Age and gender are also factors; most cases occur after 50 years of age. Women are more likely than men to develop thyroid dysfunction.[44] Thyroid function is regulated by the hypothalamus and pituitary feedback controls, as well as by an intrinsic regulator mechanism within the gland itself. Basic thyroid disorders of significance

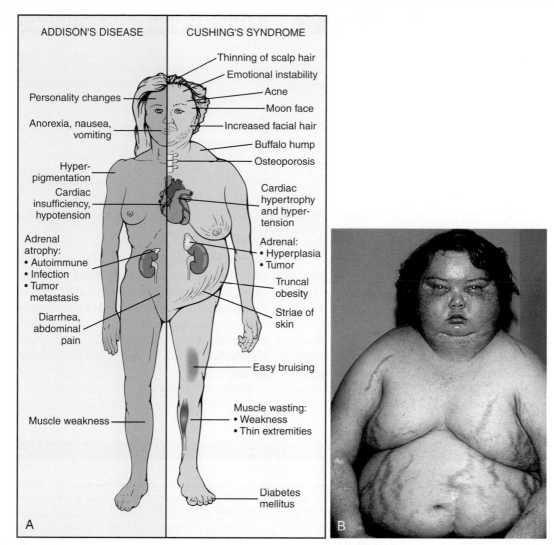

Fig. 12.2   **A,** *Comparison of hyperfunction of the adrenal cortex (Addison's disease) and hypofunction (Cushing's syndrome).* **B,** Individuals treated with corticosteroids can develop clinical features of Cushing's syndrome called *cushingoid features* including "moonface," obesity, and cutaneous striae as shown here. From Damjanov I: *Pathology for the health-related profession,* ed 3, Philadelphia, WB Saunders, 2006. Used with permission.

in physical therapy practice include goiter, hyperthyroidism, hypothyroidism, and cancer. Alterations in thyroid function produce changes in hair, nails, skin, eyes, the gastrointestinal (GI) tract, respiratory tract, heart and blood vessels, nervous tissue, bone, and muscle.

The risk of having thyroid diseases increases with age, but in people older than 60 years of age, it becomes more difficult to detect because it masquerades as other problems such as heart disease, depression, or dementia. Fatigue and weakness may be the first symptoms among older adults, often mistaken or attributed to normal aging. Depression and anxiety syndromes are also symptoms that can indicate thyroid dysfunction.[45]

On the other hand, thyroid dysfunction can mimic signs and symptoms of aging such as hair loss, fatigue, and depression. The therapist may recognize problems early and make a medical referral, minimizing the client's symptoms. A simple and inexpensive blood test called a *thyroid-stimulating hormone* (TSH) *test* is usually recommended

to show whether the thyroid gland is hyperfunctioning or hypofunctioning.

Goiter

Goiter, an enlargement of the thyroid gland, occurs in areas of the world where iodine (necessary for the production of thyroid hormone) is deficient in the diet. It is believed that when factors (e.g., a lack of iodine) inhibit normal thyroid hormone production, hypersecretion of TSH occurs because of a lack of a negative feedback loop. This TSH increase results in an increase in thyroid mass.

Pressure on the trachea and esophagus causes difficulty in breathing, dysphagia, and hoarseness. With the use of iodized salt, this problem has almost been eliminated in the United States. Although the younger population in the United States may be goiter free, older adults may have developed goiter during their childhood or adolescent years and may still have clinical manifestations of this disorder.

Goiter

- Increased neck size
- Pressure on adjacent tissue (e.g., trachea and esophagus)
- Difficulty in breathing
- Dysphagia
- Hoarseness

Thyroiditis

- Painless thyroid enlargement
- Dysphagia, "tight" sensation when swallowing, or choking
- Anterior neck, shoulder, or rib cage pain without biomechanical changes
- Gland sometimes easily palpable over anterior neck (warm, tender, swollen)
- Fatigue, weight gain, dry hair and skin, constipation (these are later symptoms associated with hypothyroidism)

Thyroiditis

Thyroiditis is an inflammation of the thyroid gland. Causes can include infection and autoimmune processes. The most common form of this problem is a chronic thyroiditis called *Hashimoto's thyroiditis*. This condition affects women more frequently than men and is most often seen in the 30- to 50-year-old age group. Destruction of the thyroid gland from this condition can cause eventual hypothyroidism (Case Example 12.2).

Usually, both sides of the gland are enlarged, although one side may be larger than the other. Other symptoms are related to the functional state of the gland itself. Early involvement may cause mild symptoms of hyperthyroidism, whereas later symptoms cause hypothyroidism.

Hyperthyroidism

Hyperthyroidism (hyperfunction), or *thyrotoxicosis*, refers to those disorders in which the thyroid gland secretes excessive amounts of thyroid hormone. Graves' disease is a common type of excessive thyroid activity characterized by a generalized enlargement of the gland (or goiter leading to a swollen neck), and often, protruding eyes (exophthalmos) caused by a retraction of the eyelids and inflammation of the ocular muscles.

Clinical Presentation. Excessive thyroid hormone creates a generalized elevation in body metabolism. The effects of

---

CASE EXAMPLE 12.2

Hashimoto's Thyroiditis

Referral: A 38-year-old woman with right-sided groin pain was referred to physical therapy by her physician. She says that the pain came on suddenly without injury. The pain is worse in the morning and hurts at night, waking her up when she changes position. The woman's symptoms are especially acute when she tries to stand up after sitting, with weight-bearing impossible for the first 5 to 10 minutes.

The woman, who looks athletic, reports that before the onset of this problem she was running 5 miles every other day without difficulty. The x-ray finding is reportedly within normal limits for structural abnormalities. Erythrocyte sedimentation rate (ESR) was 16 mm/hour.* The client has chronic sinusitis and has had two surgeries for that condition in the last 3 years. She is not a smoker and drinks only occasionally, on a social basis.

This client was seen 6 weeks ago by another physical therapist, who tried ultrasound and stretching without improvement in symptoms or function.

Clinical Presentation: The physical therapy evaluation today revealed a positive Thomas test for right hip flexion contracture. However, it was difficult to assess whether there was a true muscle contracture or only loss of motion as a result of muscle splinting and guarding. Patrick's test (FABER) for hip pathology and the iliopsoas test for intraabdominal infection were both negative. Joint accessory motions appeared to be within normal limits, given that the movements were tested in the presence of some residual muscle tension from protective splinting. A neurologic screen failed to demonstrate the presence of any neurologic involvement. Symptoms could be reproduced with deep palpation of the right groin area. There were no active or passive movements that could alter, provoke, change, or eliminate the pain. There were no trigger points in the abdomen or right lower quadrant that could account for the symptomatic presentation.

There was no apparent cause for her movement system impairment. Physical therapy intervention with soft tissue mobilization and proprioceptive neuromuscular facilitation techniques were initiated and used as a diagnostic tool. There was no change in the client's symptoms or clinical presentation as the therapist continued trying a series of physical therapy techniques.

Result: In a young and otherwise healthy adult, a lack of measurable, reportable, or observable progress becomes a red flag for further medical follow-up. The results of the physical therapy examination and lack of response to treatment constitute a valuable medical diagnostic tool.

Further laboratory results revealed a medical diagnosis of Hashimoto's thyroiditis. Treatment with thyroxine (T_4) resulted in resolution of the musculoskeletal symptoms. The correlation between groin pain and loss of hip extension with Hashimoto's remains unclear. Even so, response to the red flag (no change or improvement with intervention) resulted in a correct medical diagnosis.

---

* The ESR (an indication of possible infection or inflammation) was within normal limits for an adult woman.

thyrotoxicosis occur gradually and are manifested in almost every system (Fig. 12.3 and Table 12.4).

In older clients three common signs are tremors, anxiety, palpitations, weight loss, and heat intolerance.[46] In younger clients, clinical signs and symptoms found most often include cold intolerance, weight gain, dry skin, constipation, and mental and physical slowing.[47]

Chronic periarthritis is also associated with hyperthyroidism. Inflammation that involves the periarticular structures, including the tendons, ligaments, and joint capsule, is termed *periarthritis*. The syndrome is associated with pain and a reduced range of motion. Calcification, whether periarticular

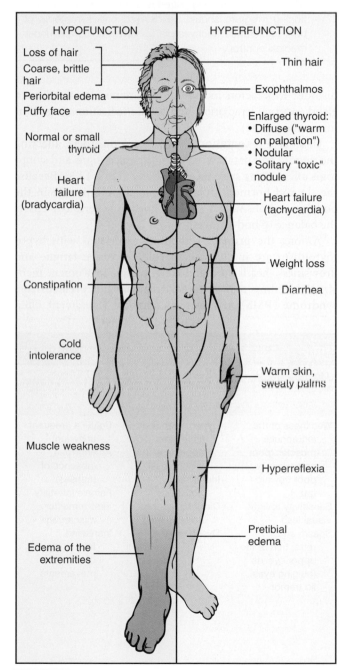

HYPOFUNCTION — HYPERFUNCTION

- Loss of hair
- Coarse, brittle hair
- Periorbital edema
- Puffy face
- Normal or small thyroid
- Heart failure (bradycardia)
- Constipation
- Cold intolerance
- Muscle weakness
- Edema of the extremities

- Thin hair
- Exophthalmos
- Enlarged thyroid:
  - Diffuse ("warm on palpation")
  - Nodular
  - Solitary "toxic" nodule
- Heart failure (tachycardia)
- Weight loss
- Diarrhea
- Warm skin, sweaty palms
- Hyperreflexia
- Pretibial edema

Fig. 12.3 *Comparison of hyperthyroidism and hypothyroidism.*
From Damjanov I: *Pathology for the health-related profession*, ed 3, Philadelphia, WB Saunders, 2006. Used with permission.

or tendinous, may be seen by x-ray studies. Both periarthritis and calcific tendinitis occur most often in the shoulder, and both are common findings in clients who have endocrine disease (Case Example 12.3).

Painful restriction of shoulder motion associated with periarthritis has been widely described among clients of all ages with hyperthyroidism. The involvement can be unilateral or bilateral and can worsen progressively to become adhesive capsulitis (frozen shoulder). Acute calcific tendinitis of the wrist has also been described in such clients. Although anti-inflammatory agents may be needed for the acute symptoms, chronic periarthritis usually responds to treatment of the underlying hyperthyroidism.

There is also a strong relationship between hyperthyroidism and decreased bone mineral density (BMD) and osteoporosis[48] as a result of accelerated bone remodeling.[49,50] A study of women taking thyroid hormone replacement at thyroxine equivalent doses or greater found an association with significant osteopenia at the ultradistal radius, midshaft radius, hip, and lumbar spine.[51] The study also indicated that estrogen use appears to negate thyroid hormone associated loss of bone density in postmenopausal women. With loss of BMD there is an increased risk of fractures.

Proximal muscle weakness (most marked in the pelvic girdle and thigh muscles), accompanied by muscle atrophy known as *myopathy*, occurs in up to 70% of people with hyperthyroidism. Muscle strength returns to normal in about 2 months after medical treatment, whereas muscle wasting resolves more slowly. In severe cases normal strength may not be restored for months.

The incidence of myasthenia gravis is increased in clients with hyperthyroidism, which in turn can aggravate muscle weakness. If the hyperthyroidism is corrected, improvement of myasthenia gravis follows in about two-thirds of clients.

Thyroid Storm. Life-threatening complications with hyperthyroidism are rare but still important for the therapist to recognize. Unrecognized disease, untreated disease, or incorrect treatment can result in a condition called *thyroid storm*. In addition, precipitating factors, such as trauma, infection, or surgery, can turn well-controlled hyperthyroidism into a thyroid storm.

Thyroid storm is characterized by signs and symptoms of hypermetabolism including severe tachycardia with heart failure, shock, and hyperthermia (up to 105.3° F [40.7° C]). Restlessness, agitation, chest pain, abdominal pain, nausea and vomiting, and coma can occur. Immediate medical referral is required to return the client to a normal thyroid state and prevent cardiovascular or hyperthermic collapse. Look for a recent history of the precipitating factors mentioned.

Hypothyroidism

Hypothyroidism (hypofunction) is more common than hyperthyroidism, results from insufficient thyroid hormone, and creates a generalized depression of body metabolism. Hypothyroidism in fetal development and infants is usually

---

CASE EXAMPLE 12.3

Graves' Disease (Hyperthyroidism)

A 73-year-old woman who has rheumatoid arthritis has just joined the Physical Therapy Aquatic Program. Despite the climate-controlled facility, she becomes flushed, demonstrates an increased respiratory rate that is inconsistent with her level of exercise, and begins to perspire profusely. She reports muscle cramping in the arms and legs and sudden onset of headache.

Questions
- How would you handle this situation?
- Can this client resume the aquatic program when her symptoms have resolved?

Result: The client was quickly escorted from the pool. Her vital signs were taken and recorded for future reference. Later, the therapist reviewed the client's health history and noted that the

"thyroid medication" she reported taking was actually an antithyroid medication for Graves' disease.

The heat intolerance associated with her Graves' disease (hyperthermia secondary to accelerated metabolic rate) presents a potential contraindication for aquatic or pool therapy. Heat intolerance contributes to exercise intolerance, and the client was exhibiting signs and symptoms of heat stroke, even when exercising in a climate-controlled facility. The physician was notified of the symptoms and how quickly the onset occurred (after only 5 minutes of warm-up exercises). Strenuous exercise or a conditioning program should be delayed until symptoms of heat intolerance, tachycardia, or arrhythmias are under medical control.

---

a result of absent thyroid tissue and hereditary defects in thyroid hormone synthesis. Untreated congenital hypothyroidism is referred to as *cretinism*.

The condition may be classified as either primary or secondary. *Primary hypothyroidism* results from reduced functional thyroid tissue mass or impaired hormonal synthesis or release (e.g., iodine deficiency, loss of thyroid tissue, autoimmune thyroiditis). *Secondary hypothyroidism* (which accounts for a small percentage of all cases of hypothyroidism) occurs as a result of inadequate stimulation of the gland because of anterior pituitary gland dysfunction.

Risk Factors. Women are 10 times more likely than men to have hypothyroidism. More than 10% of women over age 65 years and 15% over age 70 years are diagnosed with this

disorder. Risk factors include surgical removal of the thyroid gland, external irradiation, and some medications (e.g., lithium, amiodarone).

Clinical Presentation. As with all disorders affecting the thyroid and parathyroid glands, clinical signs and symptoms affect many systems of the body (Table 12.5). Because the thyroid hormones play such an important role in the body's metabolism, lack of these hormones seriously upsets the balance of body processes.

Among the primary symptoms associated with hypothyroidism are intolerance to cold, excessive fatigue and drowsiness, headaches, and weight gain. In women, menstrual bleeding may become irregular, and premenstrual syndrome (PMS) may worsen. Physical assessment often

TABLE 12.4	**Systemic Manifestations of Hyperthyroidism**				
CNS Effects	Cardiovascular and Pulmonary Effects	Joint and Integumentary Effects	Ocular Effects	GI Effects	GU Effects
Tremors Hyperkinesis (abnormally increased motor function or activity) Nervousness, irritability Emotional lability Weakness and muscle atrophy Increased deep tendon reflexes Fatigue	Increased pulse rate/tachycardia/palpitations Arrhythmias (palpitations) Weakness of respiratory muscles (breathlessness, hypoventilation) Increased respiratory rate Low blood pressure Heart failure	Chronic periarthritis Capillary dilation (warm flushed, moist skin) Heat intolerance Onycholysis (separation of the fingernail from the nail bed) Easily broken hair and increased hair loss Hyperpigmentation Hard, purple area over the anterior surface of the tibia with itching, erythema, and occasionally pain	Weakness of the extraocular muscles (poor convergence, poor upward gaze) Sensitivity to light Visual loss Spasm and retraction of the upper eyelids (bulging eyes), lid tremor	Hypermetabolism (increased appetite with weight loss) Increased peristalsis Diarrhea, nausea, and vomiting Dysphagia	Polyuria (frequent urination) Amenorrhea (absence of menses) Female infertility First-trimester miscarriage Increased frequency of bowel movements

CNS, Central nervous system; *GI*, gastrointestinal; *GU*, genitourinary.

reveals dryness of the skin and increasing thinness and brittleness of the hair and nails. There may be nodules or other irregularities of the thyroid palpable during anterior neck examination.

Ichthyosis, or dry scaly skin, may be an inherited dermatologic condition (Fig. 12.4). It may also be the result of a thyroid condition. It must not be assumed that clients who present with this condition are merely in need of better hydration or regular use of skin lotion. A medical referral is needed to rule out underlying pathology.

Myxedema. A characteristic sign of hypothyroidism and more rarely associated with hyperthyroidism (Graves' disease) is *myxedema* (often used synonymously with *hypothyroidism*). Myxedema is a result of an alteration in the composition of the dermis and other tissues, causing connective tissues to be separated by increased amounts of mucopolysaccharides and proteins.

This mucopolysaccharide-protein complex binds with water, causing a nonpitting, boggy edema, especially around the eyes, hands, feet, and in the supraclavicular fossae (Case Example 12.4). The binding of this protein-mucopolysaccharide complex causes thickening of the tongue and the laryngeal and pharyngeal mucous membranes. This results in hoarseness and thick, slurred speech, which are also characteristic of untreated hypothyroidism.

Clients who have myxedematous hypothyroidism may demonstrate synovial fluid that is highly distinctive. The fluid's high viscosity results in a slow fluid wave that creates a sluggish "bulge" sign visible at the knee joint. Often, the fluid

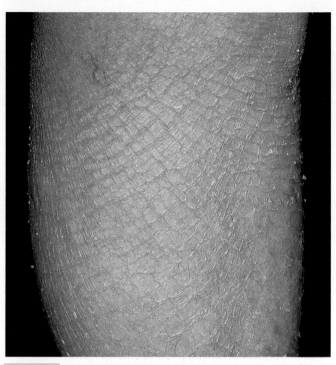

Fig. 12.4 *Dominant ichthyosis vulgaris.* White, translucent, quadrangular scales on the extensor aspects of the arms and legs. From Habif TP: Clinical dermatology: a color guide to diagnosis and therapy, St. Louis, Mosby, 2010.

contains CPPD crystal deposits that may be associated with chondrocalcinosis (deposit of calcium salts in joint cartilage).

TABLE 12.5	Systemic Manifestations of Hypothyroidism							
CNS Effects	Musculoskeletal Effects	Pulmonary Effects	Cardiovascular Effects	Hematologic Effects	Integumentary Effects	GI Effects	GU Effects
Slowed speech and hoarseness Anxiety, depression Slow mental function (loss of interest in daily activities, poor short-term memory) Hearing Impairment Fatigue and increased sleep Headache Cerebellar ataxia	Proximal muscle weakness Myalgia Trigger points Stiffness, cramps Carpal tunnel syndrome Prolonged deep tendon reflexes (especially Achilles) Subjective report of paresthesias without supportive objective findings Muscular and joint edema Back pain Increased bone density Decreased bone formation and resorption	Dyspnea Respiratory muscle weakness Pleural effusion	Bradycardia Congestive heart failure Poor peripheral circulation (pallor, cold skin, intolerance to cold, hypertension) Severe atherosclerosis; hyperlipidemias Angina Elevated blood pressure Increased cholesterol, triglycerides, LDL Cardiomyopathy	Anemia Easy bruising	Myxedema (periorbital and peripheral) Thickened, cool, and dry skin Scaly skin (especially elbows and knees) Carotenosis (yellowing of the skin) Coarse, thinning hair Intolerance to cold Nonpitting edema of hands and feet Poor wound healing Thin, brittle nails	Anorexia Constipation Weight gain disproportionate to caloric intake Decreased absorption of nutrients Decreased protein metabolism (retarded skeletal and soft tissue growth) Delayed glucose uptake Decreased glucose absorption	Infertility Menstrual irregularity Heavy menstrual bleeding

CNS, Central nervous system; *GI*, gastrointestinal; *GU*, genitourinary; *LDL*, low-density lipoprotein.

Thus a finding of a highly viscous, "noninflammatory" joint effusion containing CPPD crystals may suggest to the physician possible underlying hypothyroidism.

When such clients with hypothyroidism have been treated with thyroid replacement, some have experienced attacks of acute pseudogout caused by CPPD crystals remaining in the synovial fluid.

Neuromuscular Symptoms. Neuromuscular symptoms are among the most common manifestations of hypothyroidism. Flexor tenosynovitis with stiffness often accompanies CTS in people with hypothyroidism. CTS can develop before other signs of hypothyroidism become evident. It is thought that this CTS arises from deposition of myxedematous tissue in the carpal tunnel area. Acroparesthesias may occur as a result of median nerve compression at the wrist. The paresthesias are almost always located bilaterally in the hands. Most clients do not require surgical treatment because the symptoms respond to thyroid replacement.

Proximal muscle weakness sometimes accompanied by pain is common in clients who have hypothyroidism. As mentioned earlier, muscle weakness is not always related to either the severity or the duration of hypothyroidism and can be present several months before the diagnosis of hypothyroidism is made. Muscle bulk is usually normal; muscle hypertrophy is rare. Deep tendon reflexes are characterized by slowed muscle contraction and relaxation (prolonged reflex).[7]

There appears to be an association between hypothyroidism and fibromyalgia syndrome (FMS). Individuals with FMS and clients with undiagnosed myofascial symptoms may benefit from a medical referral for evaluation of thyroid function.[52,53]

Neoplasms. Cancer of the thyroid is a relatively uncommon, slow-growing neoplasm that rarely metastasizes. It is often an incidental finding in persons being treated for other disorders (e.g., musculoskeletal disorders involving the head and neck). Primary cancers of other endocrine organs are rare and are not encountered by the clinical therapist very often.

Risk factors for thyroid cancer include female gender, age over 40 years, Caucasian race, iodine deficiency, family history of thyroid cancer, and being exposed to radioactive iodine (I-131), especially as children. In addition, nuclear power plant fallout could expose large numbers of people to I-131 and subsequent thyroid cancer. The use of potassium iodide (KI) can protect the thyroid from the adverse effects of I-131 and is recommended to be made available in areas of the country near nuclear power plants in case of nuclear fallout.[54] The initial manifestation in adults, and especially in children, is a palpable lymph node or nodule in the neck lateral to the sternocleidomastoid muscle in the lower portion of the posterior triangle overlying the scalene muscles[55] (Fig. 12.5).

A physician must evaluate any client with a palpable nodule because a palpable nodule is often clinically indistinguishable from a mass associated with a benign condition. The presence of new-onset hoarseness, hemoptysis, or elevated blood pressure is a red-flag symptom for systemic disease.

CASE EXAMPLE 12.4

Myxedema

Referral: A 36-year-old African American woman with a history of Graves' disease came to an outpatient hand clinic as a self-referral with painless swelling in both hands and feet. She had seen her doctor 6 weeks ago and was told that she did not have rheumatoid arthritis and should see a physical therapist.

Past Medical History: The woman had a 3-year history of Graves' disease, which was treated with thyroid supplementation. She had a family history of thyroid problems, maternal history of diabetes mellitus, and history of early death from heart attack (father). Aside from symptoms of hyperthyroidism, she did not have any other health problems.

Clinical Presentation: There was a mild swelling apparent in the soft tissue of the fingers and toes. Presentation was painless and bilateral, although asymmetric (second and third digits of the right hand were affected; third and fourth digits of the left hand were symptomatic).

The therapist was alerted to the unusual clinical presentation by the following signs:
- Thickening of the skin over the affected digits in the hands and feet
- Clubbing of all digits (fingers and toes)

- Nonpitting edema and thickening of the skin over the front of the lower legs down to the feet

The client did not think these additional symptoms were present at the time she saw her physician 6 weeks ago, but she could not remember exactly.

Result: The therapist was unsure if the symptoms present were normal manifestations of Graves' disease or an indication that the client's thyroid levels were abnormal. The physician was contacted with information about the additional signs and questions about this client's clinical presentation.

The physician requested a return visit from the client, at which time further testing was done. The skin changes and edema of the lower legs are called *pretibial myxedema*. Myxedema is more commonly associated with hypothyroidism. When accompanied by digital clubbing and new bone formation, the condition is called *thyroid acropachy*. This condition is seen most often in individuals who have been treated for hyperthyroidism.

Drug therapy for the thyroid function does not change the acropachy; treatment is palliative for relief of symptoms. Physical therapy intervention can be prescribed but has not been studied to prove effectiveness for this condition.

CLINICAL SIGNS AND SYMPTOMS

Thyroid Carcinoma

- Presence of asymptomatic nodule or mass in thyroid tissue
- Nodule is firm, irregular, painless
- Hoarseness
- Hemoptysis
- Dyspnea
- Elevated blood pressure

Parathyroid Glands

Two parathyroid glands are located on the posterior surface of each lobe of the thyroid gland. These glands secrete parathyroid hormone (PTH), which regulates calcium and phosphorus metabolism. Parathyroid disorders include hyperparathyroidism and hypoparathyroidism.

The therapist may see clients with parathyroid disorders in acute care settings and postoperatively because these disorders can result from diseases and surgical procedures. If damage or removal of these glands occurs, the resulting hypoparathyroidism (temporary or permanent) causes hypocalcemia, which can result in cardiac arrhythmias and neuromuscular irritability (tetany).

Disorders of the parathyroid glands may produce periarthritis and tendinitis. Both types of inflammation may be crystal induced and can be associated with periarticular or tendinous calcification.

Hyperparathyroidism

Hyperparathyroidism (hyperfunction), or the excessive secretion of PTH, disrupts calcium, phosphate, and bone metabolism. The primary function of PTH is to maintain a normal serum calcium level. Elevated PTH causes release of calcium by the bone and accumulation of calcium in the bloodstream.

Symptoms of hyperparathyroidism are related to this release of bone calcium into the bloodstream. This causes demineralization of bone and subsequent loss of bone strength and density. At the same time, the increase of calcium in the bloodstream can cause many other problems within the body, such as renal stones. The incidence of hyperparathyroidism is highest in postmenopausal women.[56]

The major cause of primary hyperparathyroidism is a tumor of a parathyroid gland, which results in the autonomous secretion of PTH. Renal failure, another common cause of hyperparathyroidism, causes hypocalcemia and stimulates PTH production. Hyperplasia of the gland occurs as it attempts to raise the blood serum calcium levels.

Clinical Presentation. Many systems of the body are affected by hyperparathyroidism (Table 12.6). Proximal muscle weakness primarily of the pelvic girdle and thigh muscles and fatigability are common findings and may be secondary to a peripheral neuropathic process. Myopathy of respiratory muscles with associated respiratory involvement often goes unnoticed. Striking reversal of muscle weakness and atrophy occur with successful treatment of the underlying hyperparathyroidism.

Other symptoms associated with hyperparathyroidism are muscle weakness, loss of appetite, weight loss, nausea and vomiting, depression, and increased thirst and urination (Case Example 12.5). Hyperparathyroidism can also cause GI problems, pancreatitis, bone decalcification, and psychotic paranoia (Fig. 12.6).

Bone erosion, resorption, and subsequent destruction from hypercalcemia associated with hyperparathyroidism rarely occurs today. In most cases, hypercalcemia is mild and detected before any significant skeletal disease develops. The classic bone disease *osteitis fibrosa cystica* affects

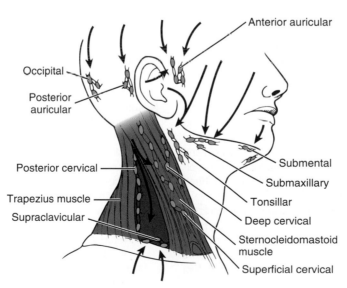

Fig. 12.5 *Lymph node regions of the head and neck.* Palpable nodal disease associated with thyroid carcinoma is commonly located lateral to the sternocleidomastoid muscle in the lower portion of the posterior triangle overlying the scalene muscles *(dark red triangle).* Modified from Swartz MH: *Textbook of physical diagnosis,* Philadelphia, WB Saunders, 1989.

TABLE 12.6	Systemic Manifestations of Hyperparathyroidism		
Early CNS Symptoms	**Musculoskeletal Effects**	**GI Effects**	**GU Effects**
Lethargy, drowsiness, paresthesia	Mild-to-severe proximal muscle weakness of the extremities	Peptic ulcers	Renal colic associated with kidney stones
Slow mentation, poor memory	Muscle atrophy	Pancreatitis	Hypercalcemia (polyuria,
Depression, personality changes	Bone decalcification (bone pain, especially spine; pathologic	Nausea, vomiting, anorexia	polydipsia, constipation)
Easily fatigued	fractures; bone cysts)	Constipation	Kidney infections
Hyperactive deep tendon reflexes	Gout and pseudogout		
Occasionally glove-and-stocking distribution of sensory loss	Arthralgia involving the hands		
	Myalgia and sensation of heaviness in the lower extremities		
	Joint hypermobility		

CNS, Central nervous system; *GI*, gastrointestinal; *GU*, genitourinary.

persons with primary or renal hyperparathyroidism. Bone lesions called *Brown tumors* appear at the end stages of the cystic osteitis fibrosa. There are increasing reports of this condition in hyperparathyroidism secondary to renal failure because of the increasing survival rates of clients receiving hemodialysis.

Currently, skeletal manifestations of primary hyperparathyroidism are more likely to include bone pain secondary to osteopenia, especially diffuse osteopenia of the spine with possible vertebral fractures. In addition, a number of articular and periarticular disorders have been recognized in association with primary hyperparathyroidism. The therapist may encounter cases of ruptured tendons caused by bone resorption in clients with hyperparathyroidism.

Inflammatory erosive polyarthritis may be associated with chondrocalcinosis and CPPD deposits in the synovial fluid. This erosion is called *osteogenic synovitis*. Concurrent illness and surgery (most often parathyroidectomy) are recognized inducers of acute arthritic episodes.

Primary hyperparathyroidism is treated through surgical removal of the parathyroid glands involved, or by pharmacologic management with calcimimetics, hormone replacement therapy, and bisphosphonates.[56]

Hypoparathyroidism

Hypoparathyroidism (hypofunction), or insufficient secretion of PTH, most commonly results from accidental removal or injury of the parathyroid gland during thyroid or anterior neck surgery. A less common form of the disease can occur from genetic autoimmune destruction of the gland. Hypofunction of the parathyroid gland results in insufficient secretion of PTH and subsequent hypocalcemia, hyperphosphatemia, and pronounced neuromuscular and cardiac irritability.

CASE EXAMPLE 12.5

Rheumatoid Arthritis and Hyperparathyroidism

Referral: A 58-year-old man was referred to physical therapy by his primary care physician with a diagnosis of new-onset rheumatoid arthritis. Chief complaint was bilateral sacroiliac (SI) joint pain and pain on palpation of the hands and wrists.

When asked if he had any symptoms of any kind anywhere else in the body, he mentioned constipation, nausea, and loss of appetite. The family took the therapist aside and expressed concerns about personality changes, including apathy, depression, and episodes of paranoia. These additional symptoms were first observed shortly after the hand pain developed.

Past Medical History: The client had a motorcycle accident 2 years ago but reported no major injuries and no apparent residual problems. He had a family history of heart disease and hypertension but was not hypertensive at the time of the physical therapy interview. There was no other contributory personal or family past medical history.

Clinical Presentation: The therapist was unable to account for the SI joint pain. There were no particular movements that made it better or worse, and no objective findings to suggest an underlying movement system impairment.

Other red flags included age, bilateral hand and SI symptoms, gastrointestinal (GI) distress, and psychologic/behavioral changes observed by the family.

Result: The therapist contacted the referring physician with the results of her evaluation. During the telephone conversation, the therapist mentioned the family's concerns about the client's personality change and the fact that the client had bilateral symptoms that could not be provoked or relieved. Additional GI symptoms were also discussed.

At the physician's request, the client completed a short course of physical therapy intervention with an emphasis on posture, core training, and soft tissue mobilization. The client returned to the physician for a follow-up examination 4 weeks later. His symptoms were unchanged.

After additional testing, the client was eventually diagnosed with hyperparathyroidism and treated accordingly. Both his hand and SI pain went away, as well as most of the GI problems.

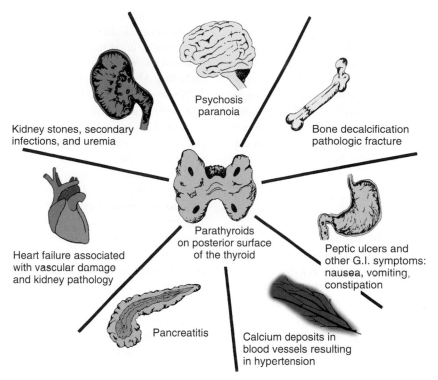

Fig. 12.6 *The pathologic processes of body structures as a result of excess parathyroid hormone.* From Muthe NC: *Endocrinology: a nursing approach*, Boston, 1981, Little, Brown.

Clinical Presentation. Hypocalcemia occurs when the parathyroid glands become inactive. The resultant deficiency of calcium in the blood alters the function of many tissues in the body. These altered functions are described by the systemic manifestations of signs and symptoms associated with hypoparathyroidism (Table 12.7).

The most significant clinical consequence of hypocalcemia is neuromuscular irritability. This irritability results in muscle spasms, paresthesias, tetany, and life-threatening cardiac arrhythmias. Muscle weakness and pain have been reported along with hypocalcemia in clients with hypoparathyroidism.

Hypoparathyroidism is primarily treated through pharmacologic management with intravenous calcium gluconate, oral calcium salts, and vitamin D. Acute hypoparathyroidism is a life-threatening emergency and is treated rapidly with calcium replacement, anticonvulsants, and prevention of airway obstruction.

TABLE 12.7	Systemic Manifestations of Hypoparathyroidism			
CNS Effects	Musculoskeletal Effects*	Cardiovascular Effects*	Integumentary Effects	GI Effects
Personality changes (irritability, agitation, anxiety, depression)	Hypocalcemia (neuromuscular excitability and muscular tetany, especially involving flexion of the upper extremity) Spasm of intercostal muscles and diaphragm compromising breathing Positive Chvostek's sign (twitching of facial muscles with tapping of the facial nerve in front of the ear)	Cardiac arrhythmias Eventual heart failure	Dry, scaly, coarse, pigmented skin Tendency to have skin infections Thinning of hair, including eyebrows and eyelashes Fingernails and toenails become brittle and form ridges	Nausea and vomiting Constipation or diarrhea Neuromuscular stimulation of the intestine (abdominal pain)

CNS, Central nervous system; *GI*, gastrointestinal.

*The most common and important effects for the therapist to be aware of are the musculoskeletal and cardiovascular effects.

Pancreas

The pancreas is a fish-shaped organ that lies behind the stomach. Its head and neck are located in the curve of the duodenum, and its body extends horizontally across the posterior abdominal wall.

The pancreas has dual functions. It acts as both an *endocrine gland*, secreting the hormones insulin and glucagon, and an *exocrine gland*, producing digestive enzymes. Disorders of endocrine function are included in this chapter, whereas disorders of exocrine function affecting digestion are included in Chapter 9.

Diabetes Mellitus

DM is a chronic disorder caused by deficient insulin or defective insulin action in the body. It is characterized by hyperglycemia (excess glucose in the blood) and disruption of the metabolism of carbohydrates, fats, and proteins. Over time, it results in serious small vessel and large vessel vascular complications and neuropathies.

DM is the leading cause of end-stage renal disease (ESRD) (kidney failure requiring dialysis or transplantation), nontraumatic lower extremity amputations, and new cases of blindness among adults in the United States, and is a major cause of heart disease and stroke.[57,58]

Type 1 DM is a condition in which little or no insulin is produced. It occurs in about 10% of all cases and usually occurs in children or young adults. Type 2 DM commonly occurs after age 40 years and is a condition of defective insulin and/or impaired cell receptor binding of insulin. Table 12.8 depicts the major differences between type 1 and type 2 in presentation and treatment. There has been some discussion as to whether Alzheimer's disease is type 3 DM ("brain diabetes"), unique to the brain or if DM is just a risk factor for Alzheimer's disease.[59,60] A relationship between DM and dementia is undeniable, with numerous studies concluding that DM increases the risk of cognitive decline and dementia, including Alzheimer's disease.[61]

Native Americans, Latino Americans, Native Hawaiians, and some Asian Americans and Pacific Islanders have been identified at particularly high risk for type 2 DM and its complications.[62] Lack of exercise and obesity are two major risk factors for type 2 DM. As a result of these lifestyle factors (sedentary lifestyle, obesity), the overall number of persons in the United States with DM has increased from 29.1 million in 2014 to 34.2 million in 2017.[62] New cases have declined from 1.7 million in 2008 to 1.3 million in 2017 with the number of people living with the disease remaining stable with similar trends seen across all ages, racial and ethnic course, sexes, and education levels.[62]

Clinical Presentation. Specific physiologic changes occur when insulin is lacking or ineffective. Normally, the blood glucose level rises after a meal. A large amount of this glucose is taken up by the liver for storage or for use by other tissues such as skeletal muscle and fat. When insulin function is impaired, the glucose in the general circulation is not taken up or removed by these tissues; thus, it continues to accumulate in the blood. Because new glucose has not been "deposited" into the liver, the liver synthesizes more glucose and releases it into the general circulation, which increases the already elevated blood glucose level. With the increase in blood glucose levels, hemoglobin molecules inside of red blood cells become more glycosylated. This serves as a marker for the average blood glucose level over the previous 3 months before the measurement, as this is the lifespan of red blood cells.[63]

TABLE 12.8	Primary Differences Between Type 1 and Type 2 Diabetes Mellitus	
Factors	Type 1	Type 2
Age of onset	Usually younger than 30 years of age	Usually older than 35 years of age (can be younger if history of childhood obesity)
Type of onset	Abrupt	Gradual
Endogenous (own) insulin production	Little or none	Below normal or above normal
Incidence	5%–10%	90%–95%
Ketoacidosis	May occur	Unlikely
Insulin injections	Required	Needed in 20%–30% of clients
Body weight at onset	Normal or thin	80% are obese
Management	Diet, exercise, insulin	Diet, exercise, oral hypoglycemic agents or insulin
Etiology	Possible viral/autoimmune, resulting in destruction of islet cells	Obesity-associated insulin receptor resistance
Hereditary	Yes	Yes
Risk factors	May be autoimmune, environmental, genetic	Insulin resistance syndrome/metabolic syndrome Ethnicity • Native American • Hispanic/Latin • Nativ e Hawaiian, Pacific Islanders

Protein synthesis is also impaired because amino acid transport into cells requires insulin. The metabolism of fats and fatty acids is altered, and instead of fat formation, fat breakdown begins in an attempt to liberate more glucose. The oxidation of these fats causes the formation of ketone bodies. Because the formation of these ketones can be rapid, they can build quickly and reach very high levels in the bloodstream. When the renal threshold for ketones is exceeded, the ketones appear in the urine as acetone (ketonuria).

The accumulation of high levels of glucose in the blood creates a hyperosmotic condition in the blood serum. This highly concentrated blood serum then "pulls" fluid from the interstitial areas, and fluid is lost through the kidneys (osmotic diuresis). Because large quantities of urine are excreted (polyuria), serious fluid loss occurs and the conscious individual becomes extremely thirsty and drinks large amounts of water (polydipsia). In addition, the kidney is unable to resorb all the glucose, so glucose begins to be excreted in the urine (glycosuria).

Certain medications can cause or contribute to hyperglycemia. Corticosteroids taken orally have the greatest glucogenic effect. Any person with DM taking corticosteroid medications must be monitored for changes in blood glucose levels.

Other hormones produced by the body also affect blood glucose levels and can have a direct influence on the severity of diabetic symptoms. Epinephrine, glucocorticoids, and growth hormone can cause significant elevations in blood glucose levels by mobilizing stored glucose to blood glucose during times of physical or psychologic stress.

CLINICAL SIGNS AND SYMPTOMS
Untreated or Uncontrolled Diabetes Mellitus

The classic clinical signs and symptoms of untreated or uncontrolled diabetes mellitus (DM) usually include one or more of the following:

- Polyuria: increased urination caused by osmotic diuresis
- Polydipsia: increased thirst in response to polyuria
- Polyphagia: increased appetite and ingestion of food (usually only in type 1)
- Weight loss in the presence of polyphagia: weight loss caused by improper fat metabolism and breakdown of fat stores (usually only in type 1)
- Hyperglycemia: increased blood glucose level (fasting level greater than 126 mg/dL)[64]
- Glycosylated hemoglobin (A1C levels ≥6.5%)
- Glycosuria: presence of glucose in the urine
- Ketonuria: presence of ketone bodies in the urine (by-product of fat catabolism)
- Fatigue and weakness
- Blurred vision
- Irritability
- Recurring skin, gum, bladder, vaginal, or other infections
- Numbness/tingling in hands and feet
- Cuts/bruises that are difficult and slow to heal

When persons with DM are under stress, such as during surgery, trauma, pregnancy, puberty, or infectious states, blood glucose levels can rise and result in the need for increased amounts of insulin. If these insulin needs cannot be met, a hyperglycemic emergency such as diabetic ketoacidosis can result.

It is essential to remember that clients with DM who are under stress will have increased insulin requirements and may become symptomatic even though their disease is usually well controlled in normal circumstances.

Diagnosis. To be diagnosed with DM, a person must have fasting plasma glucose (FPG) readings of 126 mg/dL or higher on 2 different days. The previous cutoff, set in 1979, was 140 mg/dL. This change occurred as a result of research showing that individuals with readings as low as the mid-120s have already started developing tissue damage from DM. A value greater than 100 mg/dL is a risk factor for future DM and cardiovascular disease. It has been suggested that the term "prediabetes" is no longer used: The person either has DM or does not.[65]

The American Diabetes Association offers consumers a risk test for DM (https://www.diabetes.org/risk-test). All adults should take this risk test; anyone 45 years of age or older should be tested for DM every 3 years. Individuals with elevated FPG values as described should be tested every 1 to 2 years. The therapist can offer at-risk clients information on increased activity and exercise as a means of lowering their risk of developing DM.[66]

Physical Complications. At presentation, the client with DM may have a variety of serious physical problems. Infection and atherosclerosis are the two primary long-term complications of this disease and are the usual causes of severe illness and death in the person with DM.

Blood vessels and nerves sustain major pathologic changes in the person affected by DM. Atherosclerosis in both large vessels (macrovascular changes) and small vessels (microvascular changes) develops at a much earlier age and progresses much faster in the individual with DM. The blood vessel changes result in decreased blood vessel lumen size, compromised blood flow, and resultant tissue ischemia. The pathologic end-products are cerebrovascular disease (CVD), coronary artery disease (CAD), renal artery stenosis, and peripheral vascular disease (PVD).

Microvascular changes, characterized by the thickening of capillaries and damage to the basement membrane, result in diabetic nephropathy (kidney disease) and diabetic retinopathy (disease of the retina). DM is the leading cause of kidney failure and new cases of blindness in the United States as of 2012.[57,67,68]

Poorly controlled DM can lead to various tissue changes that result in impaired wound healing. Decreased circulation to the skin can further delay or diminish healing. Skin eruptions called *xanthomas* (Fig. 12.7) may appear when high lipid levels (e.g., cholesterol and triglycerides) in the blood cause fat deposits in the skin over extensor surfaces such as the elbows, knees, back of the head and neck, and heels. Yellow patches on the eyelids are another sign of hyperlipidemia. Medical referral is required to normalize lipid levels.

Physical Complications of Diabetes Mellitus

- Atherosclerosis
  - Macrovascular disease
    - Cerebrovascular disease (CVD)
    - Coronary artery disease (CAD)
    - Renal artery stenosis
    - Peripheral vascular disease (PVD)
  - Microvascular disease
    - Nephropathy
    - Retinopathy
    - Decreased microcirculation to skin/body organs
- Infection/impaired wound healing
- Neuropathy
  - Autonomic (gastroparesis, diarrhea, incontinence, postural hypotension, decreased heart rate)
  - Peripheral (polyneuropathy, diabetic foot)
  - Diabetic amyotrophy

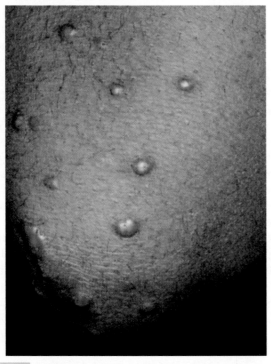

Fig. 12.7 *Multiple eruptive xanthomas over the extensor surface of the elbow in a client with poorly controlled diabetes mellitus (DM).* These lipid-filled nodules characterized by an intracellular accumulation of cholesterol develop in the skin, often around the extensor tendons. Medical referral is required; xanthomas in this population are a sign that the health care team, including the therapist, must work with the client to provide further education about DM, gain better control of their glucose level, and prevent avoidable complications. These skin lesions will go away when the DM is under control. Xanthomas can occur in any condition where there is a disturbance of lipoprotein metabolism (not just DM). From Callen JP, Jorizzo J, Greer KE, et al.: *Dermatological signs of internal disease*, Philadelphia, WB Saunders, 1988. Used with permission.

- Carpal tunnel syndrome (CTS) (mononeuropathy; ischemia of median nerve)
- Charcot's joint (diabetic arthropathy)
- Periarthritis
- Hand stiffness
  - Limited joint mobility (LJM) syndrome
  - Flexor tenosynovitis
  - Dupuytren's contracture
  - Complex regional pain syndrome (CRPS)

Depression. Depression is common in individuals with type 2 DM and is linked with a 1.5-fold increase in mortality in this population.[69] Advances in the understanding of the biologic relationship between depression and diabetes has suggested a bidirectional link between type 2 DM and depression: just as type 2 DM increases the risk for onset of major depression, a major depressive disorder signals increased risk for the onset of type 2 DM.[70,71] Adults with DM and depression are less likely to follow recommendations for nutrition and exercise. They are less likely to check their blood glucose levels routinely and more likely to take drug "holidays" from their other medications (e.g., for hyperlipidemia or hypertension). Clients with DM who are depressed are more likely to miss health care appointments for prevention and intervention.[72,73] Additionally, "diabetes distress" is now recognized as an entity separate from major depressive disorder.[74] This often underrecognized emotional response occurs when individuals are overwhelmed facing lifelong management of a chronic disease. Diabetes distress is thought to be caused by one or more of three interrelated stressors: distress resulting from diabetes and its management (e.g., fears of complications, diabetes burnout), distress resulting from life stressors unrelated to DM (e.g., family, work, financial), and distress resulting from other causes (e.g., personal characteristics, life history, genetics).[74] Failure to recognize diabetes distress will perpetuate poor patient self-management and overall outcomes.[75]

Diabetic Neuropathy. Neuropathy is the most common chronic complication of long-term DM. Neuropathy in the client with DM is thought to be related to the accumulation of sorbitol in the nerve cells, a by-product of improper glucose metabolism. This accumulation then results in abnormal fluid and electrolyte shifts and nerve cell dysfunction. The combination of this metabolic derangement and the diminished vascular perfusion to nerve tissues contributes to the severe problem of diabetic neuropathy.

Risk Factors. Other than glycemic control, there is no curative intervention for diabetic neuropathy. Identifying potentially modifiable risk factors for neuropathy is crucial; the therapist can have a key role in providing risk factor assessment for clients with DM.

Risk factors for the development of diabetic neuropathy include older age, cardiovascular risk factors, the duration and severity of DM, poor long-term glycemic control, elevated triglycerides (dyslipidemia), higher body mass index (BMI), and a history of smoking or hypertension.[76–78]

Clinical Presentation. Neuropathy may affect the central nervous system, peripheral nervous system, or autonomic nervous system. Peripheral neuropathy usually develops first as a sensory impairment of the extremities. Autonomic involvement is more common with long-standing disease.

Most common among the peripheral neuropathies are chronic sensorimotor distal symmetric polyneuropathy (DPN).[79] Polyneuropathy affects peripheral nerves in distal lower extremities, causing burning and numbness in the feet. It can result in muscle weakness, atrophy, and foot drop. Diabetic neuropathy can produce a syndrome of bilateral but asymmetric proximal muscle weakness called *diabetic amyotrophy*. Although the muscle enzyme levels are usually normal, muscle biopsy reveals atrophy of type II muscle fibers.

CTS (mononeuropathy) is also a common finding in persons with DM; it represents one form of diabetic neuropathy. As many as 5% to 16% of people with CTS have underlying DM. The mechanism is thought to be ischemia of the median nerve resulting from DM-related microvascular damage. This ischemia then causes increased sensitivity to even minor pressure exerted in the carpal tunnel area.

Autonomic involvement affects the pace of the heartbeat, blood pressure, sweating, and bladder function and can cause symptoms such as erectile dysfunction and gastroparesis (delayed stomach emptying).[76]

CLINICAL SIGNS AND SYMPTOMS
Diabetic Neuropathy (at least two or more are present)

Peripheral (Motor and Sensory)
- Sensory, vibratory impairment of the extremities
- Burning, stabbing, pain, or numbness in distal lower extremities
- Extreme sensitivity to touch
- Muscle weakness and atrophy (diabetic amyotrophy)
- Absence of distal deep tendon reflexes (knee, ankle)
- Loss of balance
- Carpal tunnel syndrome (CTS)

Autonomic
- Gastroparesis (delayed emptying of the stomach)
- Constipation or diarrhea
- Erectile dysfunction (sex drive unaffected; sexual function decreased)
- Urinary tract infections; urinary incontinence
- Profuse sweating
- Lack of oil production resulting in dry, cracked skin susceptible to bacteria and infection
- Pupillary adjustment restricted (difficulty seeing at night)
- Orthostatic hypotension
- Loss of heart rate variability

Charcot's joint, or neuropathic arthropathy, is a well-known complication of DM. This condition is at least in part caused by the loss of proprioceptive sensation that marks diabetic neuropathy. Severe degenerative arthritis similar to Charcot's joint has been noted in clients with CPPD crystal deposition disease. Shoulder, hand, and foot disorders are very common, and evaluation of clients with DM should include examination of these areas (Case Example 12.6).[80,81]

CLINICAL SIGNS AND SYMPTOMS
Charcot's Joints

- Severe unilateral swelling (bilateral in 20% of cases but not bilateral at the same time)
- Increased skin warmth
- Redness
- Deep pressure sensation, but significantly less pain than anticipated
- Normal x-ray films initially, but change over time
- Joint deformity

The large- and small-vessel changes that occur with DM contribute to the changes seen in the feet of individuals with DM. Sensory neuropathy, which may lead to painless trauma and ulceration, can progress to infection. Neuropathy can result in drying and cracking of the skin, which creates more openings for bacteria to enter. The combination of all these factors can ultimately lead to gangrene and eventually require amputation. Prevention of these problems by meticulous care of the diabetic foot can reduce the need for amputation by 50% to 75%.

An annual foot screen by a health care provider is currently recommended for anyone with DM. This screen includes examination of toenails for length, thickness, and ingrown position. All calluses should be examined because ulceration can occur underneath them. General skin integrity, color, circulation, and structure should also be assessed.[82]

Whether poorly controlled blood glucose is a causative factor in the development of the long-term physical complications of DM is still controversial, but it does seem clear that these complications increase with the duration of the disease. Stable glycemic control (between 80 mg/dL and 110 mg/dL), which prevents the fluctuation of blood glucose levels, has been shown to be helpful in decreasing neuropathic pain (and of course other complications).[83]

Periarthritis. Musculoskeletal disorders of the hand and shoulder, including periarthritis of the shoulder, is five times as common in this group as it is in individuals who do not have DM. The condition most often affects insulin-dependent people, and involvement is typically bilateral.

The mechanism of this association is unclear, but it is believed to be related to fibroblast proliferation in the connective tissue structures around joints or to microangiopathy (disorder involving small blood vessels) involving the tendon sheaths. This periarthritic condition can behave unpredictably: it may regress spontaneously, remain stable, or progress to adhesive capsulitis or frozen shoulder.[84]

CASE EXAMPLE 12.6

Charcot Shoulder (Neuroarthropathy)

Referral: A 44-year-old wheelchair-dependent man with type 2 diabetes mellitus (DM) who was well-known to the physical therapy clinic came in with new symptoms of right shoulder pain. There was no known trauma or injury to account for the change in his shoulder. He had previously been evaluated for an exercise program as a part of his DM management.

Past Medical History: The client was involved in a rock-climbing accident 15 years ago. He has had multiple reconstructive surgeries for broken bones and frostbite of the lower extremities associated with the accident. He was diagnosed with type 2 DM 3 years ago and uses an insulin pump but does not have consistent control of his blood glucose level.

The man remains active and has resumed rock climbing along with many other outdoor activities. This new onset of shoulder pain has limited his activities and impaired his ability to propel his wheelchair.

There is no other significant history to report. The client is a nonsmoker, drinks only occasionally and socially (one or two glasses of wine). He has not had any other symptoms; there have been no constitutional symptoms, loss of appetite, or other gastrointestinal problems.

Clinical Presentation: Cervical spine and elbow were cleared for any loss of motion, weakness, or other problems that might contribute to shoulder pain. Gross examination of motion and strength of the left shoulder revealed no problems. The skin was normal on both sides, no cervical or supraclavicular lymph node changes were observed or palpated, and no other observable changes in the upper quadrant were evident. Range of motion of the right shoulder:

- Active and passive abduction were equal and limited to 60 degrees and painful.

- Active and passive flexion were equal and limited to 65 degrees and painful.
- Biceps and deltoid strength were both 4/5; upper trapezius and triceps strength was normal (5/5).
- Grip strength appeared normal.

Further neurologic screening examination revealed severely decreased proprioception of the entire right upper extremity; no other neurologic changes were observed or reported.

Radial pulses intact and equal bilaterally.

Referral Decision: The therapist decided an x-ray might be helpful before initiating a program of physical therapy intervention. The client was very active and athletic and may have injured the joint or fractured the bone. Given the severity of his diabetic course over the last 3 years, an x-ray might be helpful in revealing any related arthritis that may be present.

The physician agreed with the therapist's assessment, and a radiographic examination was ordered.

Result: X-ray studies revealed destruction of two thirds of the right humeral head with microfractures and fragmentation throughout. The diagnosis of Charcot shoulder or neuroarthropathy was made. In this case the therapist's knowledge of the client's past medical history and awareness of the physical complications possible with DM led to the referral decision before further damage was done to the bone and joint.

It is unusual for someone with this severe of a condition to present with only mild symptoms. His extreme athleticism and stoic attitude may have masked the intensity of his symptoms.

Hand Stiffness. Diabetic stiff hand, LJM syndrome, cheirarthritis (inflammation of the hand and finger joints), and diabetic contractures are common in both types of DM in direct relation to the presence and duration of microvascular complications.

Flexor tenosynovitis, caused by accumulation of excessive dermal collagen in the fingers, results in thickening and induration of the skin around the joints. This condition can lead to sclerodactyly (hardening and shrinking of fingers and toes), which in turn can mimic scleroderma.

Dupuytren's contracture has a strong association with DM.[85] This syndrome is characterized by nodular thickening of the palmar fascia and flexion contracture of the digits. Clients usually have pain in the palm and digits, with decreased mobility and contracture of the fingers. In clients with DM, Dupuytren's contracture must be differentiated from LJM, which may involve the entire hand and is frequently bilateral, and from flexor tenosynovitis, which is marked by trigger finger.

Individuals with DM may develop CRPS (formerly called *reflex sympathetic dystrophy* [RSD] *syndrome*), which is characterized by pain, hyperesthesia, vasomotor and dystrophic skin changes, and tenderness and swelling around the hands and feet.[86]

Intervention

Medical management of the client with DM is directed primarily toward maintenance of blood glucose values within the range of 80 mg/dL to 120 mg/dL. The three primary treatment modalities used in the management of DM are diet, exercise, and medication (insulin and oral hypoglycemic agents; referral).

Recommended preventive care services, such as regular eye and foot examinations, as well as measurements of glycosylated hemoglobin (A1C) are critical in the prevention of diabetic complications such as blindness, amputation, and cardiovascular disease.[87] A1C (also known as *glycated hemoglobin* or *glycohemoglobin*) is an accurate, objective measurement of chronic glycemia in DM.

Most laboratories list the normal reference range as 4% to 6%. A1C equal or greater than 6.5% on two consecutive occasions is diagnostic of DM.[88] The goal is to maintain consistent A1C levels below 7% (American Diabetes Association recommendation),[89] which correlates to an average daily blood glucose below 150 mg/dL to 154 mg/dL. This recommendation (and the plasma glucose level used to diagnose DM) was determined based on the presence of retinopathy at these thresholds.

The guideline for A1C levels applies to the general population; individuals with a history of severe hypoglycemia, limited life expectancy, advanced DM-related complications, and extensive comorbid complications may be advised by their medical doctors to follow levels at or below 7%.[89] The Association of Endocrinologists recommends A1C levels of 6.5% or lower[90] (average blood sugar reading of 135 mg/dL over a 2- to 3-month period). The A1C measurement gives the client and the therapist an indication of how successful diet, exercise, and medication are in controlling their glucose level over time. It can be used as a baseline from which to evaluate results of intervention. An A1C value greater than 10% warrants medical attention (usually insulin treatment) to immediately decrease that value.[91]

For individuals with type 2 DM and the following factors, an A1C goal of less than 8% may be more appropriate than an A1C goal of less than 7%.[92]

- Known cardiovascular disease or high cardiovascular risk
- Inability to recognize and treat hypoglycemia, history of severe hypoglycemia requiring assistance
- Inability to comply with standard goals such as polypharmacy issues
- Limited life expectancy or estimated survival of less than 10 years
- Cognitive impairment
- Extensive comorbid conditions such as renal failure, liver failure, and end-stage disease complications

The therapist can conduct a careful screening examination (Box 12.1). All individuals with type 2 DM should be screened at the time of diagnosis and annually thereafter for diabetic peripheral neuropathies. Individuals with type 1 DM should be screened 5 years after diagnosis and annually thereafter. Screening should include checking knee and ankle reflexes, examining sensory function in the feet, asking about neuropathic symptoms, and examining the distal extremities for ulcers, calluses, and deformities.[79]

Exercise-Related Complications. Any exercise can improve the body's ability to use insulin. Exercise causes a decrease in the amount of insulin the pancreas releases because muscle contractions increase blood glucose uptake. For the person taking insulin, exercise adds to its effects, potentially dropping blood sugar to dangerously low levels. Exercise for the person with DM must be planned and instituted cautiously and monitored carefully because significant complications can result from exercise of higher intensity or longer duration.

Exercise-related complications can be prevented by careful monitoring of the client's blood glucose level before, during, and after strenuous exercise (safe levels are individually determined but usually fall between 100 mg/dL and 250 mg/dL; between 250 mg/dL and 300 mg/dL is considered the "caution zone"). The following recommendations

---

> **BOX 12.1   ROLE OF THE PHYSICAL THERAPIST IN DIABETES MELLITUS SCREENING**
>
> The therapist can provide education and prevention through the screening process, including:
> - Periodic screening for neuropathy
> - Assessment for early signs of neuropathy (e.g., deep tendon reflexes, vibratory and position sense, touch)
> - Education in avoiding late complications of neuropathy (e.g., annual foot and hand screening, preventive foot care; periodic footwear evaluation)
> - Assessment for signs of neuropathic arthropathy (Charcot's joint)
> - Monitoring of blood glucose level in association with exercise
> - Screening for neuromusculoskeletal disorders (e.g., adhesive capsulitis, Dupuytren disease, flexor tenosynovitis, carpal tunnel syndrome, complex regional pain syndrome)
> - Monitoring of vital signs (especially blood pressure)
> - Conducting periodic lower extremity vascular examination (see Box 4.13)
> - Screening for depression and diabetes distress; monitor depression
> - Encouraging/reminding the client to have A1C levels checked periodically
> - Reminding the client about annual eye examination

---

are general guidelines. These are not necessarily "fasting levels" (unless the person has not eaten for the last 12 hours for some reason). Exceptions are common, depending on the type of exercise, training level of the participant, expected glycemic pattern, and whether the individual is using an insulin pump.

If the blood glucose level is between 250 mg/dL and 300 mg/dL at the start of the exercise, the client may be experiencing a state of insulin deficiency and should test urine for ketones, an indication that the body does not have enough insulin to control the blood sugar and is breaking down fat for energy. Exercise is likely to raise blood sugar even more; the exercise session should be postponed until the blood glucose level is under better control. Blood glucose levels of 300 mg/dL or higher indicate the blood sugar level is too high to exercise safely, putting the client at risk for ketoacidosis. Exercise should be postponed until the blood glucose level drops to a safe preexercise range (between 100 mg/dL to 250 mg/dL, possibly up to 300 mg/dL as described).

If the blood glucose level is less than 100 mg/dL, a 10- to 15-g carbohydrate snack should be given and the glucose retested in 15 minutes to ensure an appropriate level.

Clients with active retinopathy and nephropathy should avoid high-intensity exercise that causes significant increases in blood pressure because such increases can cause further damage to the retinas and kidneys. Any exercise that places the head below the waist causing increased intrathoracic and intracranial pressure can also aggravate retinal problems. Screening for neuropathies by testing deep tendon reflexes and vibratory and position sense are also very important in the prevention of exercise-related complications such as ulcerations or fractures.

It is very important to have the client avoid insulin injection to active extremities within 1 hour of exercise because insulin is absorbed much more quickly in an active extremity. It is important to know the type, dose, and time of the client's insulin injections so that exercise is not planned for the peak activity times of the insulin.

Clients with type 1 DM may need to reduce their insulin dose or increase food intake when initiating an exercise program. During prolonged activities, a 10-g to 15-g carbohydrate snack is recommended for each 30 minutes of activity. Activities should be promptly stopped with the development of any symptoms of hypoglycemia, and blood glucose should be tested. In addition, individuals with DM should not exercise alone. Partners, teammates, and coaches must be educated regarding the possibility of hypoglycemia and the way to manage it.

Insulin Pump During Exercise. People with type 1 DM (and some individuals with insulin-requiring type 2 DM) may be using an insulin pump. Continuous subcutaneous insulin infusion (CSII) therapy, known as *insulin pump therapy*, can bring the hormonal and metabolic responses to exercise close to normal for the individual with DM.

Although there are many benefits of pump use for active individuals with DM, there are a few drawbacks as well.[93] Exercise can speed the development of diabetic ketoacidosis (DKA) when there is an interruption in insulin delivery, which can quickly become a life-threatening condition.

Other considerations include the effect of excessive perspiration or water on the infusion set (needle into the skin at the infusion site gets displaced), ambient temperature (insulin degrades under extreme conditions of heat or cold), and the effect of movement or contact at the infusion site (this causes skin irritation).

Insulin pump users who have preexercise blood glucose levels less than 100 mg/dL may not need a carbohydrate snack because they can reduce or suspend base insulin levels during an activity. Insulin reductions and required level of carbohydrate intake needed depend on the intensity and duration of the activity.[93]

The therapist should become familiar with the features of each pump in use by their clients. Knowledge of basic guiding principles for exercise with DM and general recommendations for insulin regimen changes is also helpful.

Severe Hyperglycemic States

The two primary life-threatening metabolic conditions that can develop if uncontrolled or untreated DM progresses to a state of severe hyperglycemia (more than 400 mg/dL) are DKA and hyperglycemic, hyperosmolar, nonketotic coma (HHNC; Table 12.9).

DKA occurs with severe insulin deficiency caused by either undiagnosed DM or a situation in which the insulin needs of the person become greater than usual (e.g., infection, trauma, surgery, emotional stress). It is most often seen in the client with type 1 DM, but can, in rare situations, occur in the client with type 2 DM. Medical treatment is necessary.

HHNC occurs most commonly in the older adult with type 2 DM. This complication is extremely serious and, in many cases, fatal. Factors that can precipitate this crisis are infections (e.g., pneumonia); medications that elevate the blood glucose level (e.g., corticosteroids); and procedures such as dialysis, surgery, or total parenteral nutrition (TPN).

TABLE 12.9	**Clinical Symptoms of Life-Threatening Glycemic States**	
Diabetic Ketoacidosis (DKA)	**Hyperosmolar, Hyperglycemic State (HHS)**	**Hypoglycemia Insulin Shock**
Gradual Onset	Gradual Onset	Sudden Onset
Thirst	Thirst	Sympathetic activity
Hyperventilation	Polyuria leading quickly to decreased urine output	Pallor
Fruity odor to breath	Volume loss from polyuria leading quickly to renal insufficiency	Perspiration
Lethargy/confusion	Severe dehydration	Irritability/nervousness
Coma	Lethargy/confusion	Weakness
Muscle and abdominal cramps (electrolyte loss)	Seizures	Hunger
Polyuria, dehydration	Coma	Shakiness
Flushed face, hot/dry skin	Abdominal pain and distention	CNS activity
Elevated temperature	Blood glucose level >300 mg/dL	Headache
Blood glucose level >300 mg/dL		Double/blurred vision
Serum pH <7.3		Slurred speech
		Fatigue
		Numbness of lips/tongue
		Confusion
		Convulsion/coma
		Blood glucose level <70 mg/dL

There are specific clinical features that identify HHNC. Some of these are similar to those of DKA, such as severe hyperglycemia (1000 mg/dL to 2000 mg/dL) and dehydration. The major differentiating feature between DKA and HHNC, however, is the absence of ketosis in HHNC.

Because it is likely that the therapist will work with clients who have DM, it is imperative that the clinical symptoms of DM and its potentially life-threatening metabolic states are understood. *If anyone with DM arrives for a clinical appointment in a confused or lethargic state or is exhibiting changes in mental function, fingerstick glucose testing should be performed. Immediate physician referral is necessary.*

Hypoglycemia

Hypoglycemia (blood glucose of less than 70 mg/dL) is a major complication of the use of insulin or oral hypoglycemic agents. Hypoglycemia is usually the result of a decrease in food intake or an increase in physical activity in relation to insulin administration. It is a potentially lethal problem. The hypoglycemic state interrupts the oxygen consumption of nervous system tissue. Repeated or prolonged attacks can result in irreversible brain damage and death.

Hypoglycemia Associated With Diabetes Mellitus

Hypoglycemia during or after exercise can be a problem for anyone with DM. This condition results as glucose is used by the working muscles, if the circulating level of injected insulin is too high, or both. The degree of hypoglycemia depends on such factors as preexercise blood glucose levels, duration and intensity of exercise, and blood insulin concentration.

Clinical Presentation. The severity and number of signs and symptoms depend on the individual client and the rapidity of the drop in blood glucose. It is important to note that clients can exhibit signs and symptoms of hypoglycemia when their elevated blood glucose level drops rapidly to a level that is still elevated (e.g., 400 md/dL to 200 mg/dL). The *rapidity* of the drop is the stimulus for sympathetic activity; even though a blood glucose level appears elevated, clients may still have hypoglycemia.

Clients receiving beta-adrenergic blockers (e.g., propranolol) can be at special risk for hypoglycemia by the actions of this medication. These beta-blockers inhibit the normal physiologic response of the body to the hypoglycemic state or block the appearance of the sympathetic manifestations of hypoglycemia. Clients may also have hypoglycemia during nighttime sleep (most often related to the use of intermediate- and long-acting insulin given more than once a day), with the only symptoms being nightmares, sweating, or headache.

Intervention. Hypoglycemia can be treated in the conscious client by immediate administration of sugar. It is always safer to give the sugar, even when there is doubt concerning the origin of symptoms (DKA and HHNC can also have similar central nervous system symptoms at presentation). Most often, 10 g to 15 g of carbohydrate are sufficient to reverse the episode of hypoglycemia. Immediate-acting glucose sources should be kept in every physical therapy department (e.g., half cup of fruit juice or sugared cola, 8 oz of milk, two packets of sugar, a 2-oz tube of honey or cake-decorating gel).

Most people with DM carry a rapid-acting source of carbohydrate, such as readily absorbable glucose tablets, so that it is available for use if a hypoglycemic episode occurs. Some individuals use intramuscular glucagon. If the client loses consciousness, emergency personnel must be notified, and glucose will be administered intravenously.

Any episode or suspected episode of hypoglycemia must be treated promptly and must be reported to the client's physician. It is important to question each client who has DM regarding his or her individual response to hypoglycemia. Information regarding individual symptoms, frequency of episodes, and precipitating factors may be invaluable to the therapist in preventing or minimizing a hypoglycemic attack.

Other Hypoglycemic States

Other conditions that can cause hypoglycemic states are usually related to hormonal deficiencies (e.g., cortisol, glucagon, ACTH) or overproduction of insulin or insulin-like material from tumors.

Reactive hypoglycemia, also known as *functional hypoglycemia,* occurs after the intake of a meal and usually results from stomach or duodenal surgery. This condition involves rapid stomach emptying with rapid rises of glucose levels. Glucose then rapidly falls to below normal levels as an exaggerated response of insulin secretion develops. The cause of reactive hypoglycemia is unknown.

Clinical Presentation. Clinical signs and symptoms of non–DM-related hypoglycemic states are the same as those described earlier for hypoglycemia related to DM. The client is warned to avoid fasting and simple sugars.

INTRODUCTION TO METABOLISM

As noted earlier, the endocrine system works with the nervous system to regulate and integrate the body's metabolic activities. The rate of metabolism can be increased by exercise, elevated body temperature (e.g., high fever), hormonal activity (e.g., thyroxine, insulin, epinephrine), and specific dynamic action that occurs after ingestion of a meal. All metabolic functions require proper fluid and acid-base balance. Although acid-base metabolism is not in itself a sign or a symptom, the consequences of an acid-base metabolism disorder can result in many clinical signs and symptoms.

Therapists are unlikely to evaluate someone with a primary musculoskeletal lesion that reflects an underlying metabolic disorder. However, many inpatients in hospitals and some outpatients may be affected by disturbances in acid-base metabolism and other specific metabolic disorders. Only those conditions that are likely to be encountered by a therapist are included in this text.

Fluid Imbalances

Fluid Deficit/Dehydration

Fluid deficit can occur as a result of two primary types of imbalance. There is either a loss of water without loss of solutes or a loss of both water and solutes.

The loss of body water without solutes results in the excess concentration of body solutes within the interstitial and intravascular compartments. To preserve equilibrium, water will then be forced to shift by osmosis from inside cells to these outside compartments.

If this state persists, large amounts of body water will be shifted and excreted (osmotic diuresis), and severe cellular dehydration will result. This type of imbalance can occur as a result of several conditions:

- Decreased water intake (e.g., unavailability, unconsciousness)
- Water loss without proportionate solute loss (e.g., prolonged hyperventilation, DI)
- Increased solute intake without proportionate water intake (tube feeding)
- Excess accumulation of solutes (e.g., high glucose levels such as in DM)

The second type of fluid imbalance results from a loss of *both* water and solutes. Causes of the loss of both water and solutes include hemorrhage, profuse perspiration (e.g., marathon runners), and loss of GI tract secretions (e.g., vomiting, diarrhea, draining fistulas, ileostomy). Postsurgical patients who have had a joint replacement, hip fracture, multiple traumas, or neurosurgery often lose blood and become hypovolemic despite efforts to maintain their homeostasis through blood transfusion and fluid replacement.

Severe loss of water or solutes (or both) can lead to dehydration and hypovolemic shock. It is important for the therapist to be aware of possible fluid loss or water shift in any client who is already compromised by advanced age or by a situation, such as an ileostomy or tracheostomy, which results in a continuous loss of fluid. Because the response to fluid loss is highly individual, it is important to recognize the early clinical symptoms and to carefully monitor vital signs in clients who are at risk, especially the elderly, the very young, or the chronically ill.[94]

Athletes and normal adults may experience orthostatic hypotension when slightly dehydrated, especially when intense exercise increases the core body temperature. The normal vascular system can accommodate this effectively.

CLINICAL SIGNS AND SYMPTOMS
Dehydration or Fluid Loss

Early clinical signs and symptoms:
- Thirst
- Weight loss

As the condition worsens, other symptoms may include the following:
- Poor skin turgor
- Dryness of the mouth, throat, face
- Absence of sweat
- Increased body temperature
- Low urine output
- Postural hypotension (increased heart rate by 10 bpm and decreased systolic or diastolic blood pressure by 20 mm Hg when moving from a supine to sitting position)
- Dizziness when standing
- Confusion
- Increased haematocrit

Fluid Excess

Fluid excess can occur in two major forms: water intoxication (excess of water without an excess of solutes) or edema (excess of both solutes and water).

Because the etiologic complex, symptoms, and outcomes related to these problems are substantially different, these fluid imbalances are discussed separately.

Water Intoxication. Water intoxication (resulting in hyponatremia) is an excess of extracellular water in relationship to solutes. The extracellular fluid (ECF) becomes diluted, and water must then move into cells to equalize solute concentration on both sides of the cell membrane. High water consumption without solute replacement can result in hyponatremia, a potentially lethal situation.

Water excess can be caused by an accumulation of solute-free fluid. An increase in solute-free fluid usually occurs because of excess ADH (tumors, endocrine disorders) or intake of large amounts of only tap water without balanced solute ingestion. The latter situation occurs most often in older adults who drink additional water after having the flu, with its associated vomiting and diarrhea, or in athletes who have lost a large amount of body fluid during exercise that has been replaced with only water.

Symptoms of water intoxication are largely neurologic because of the shifting of water into the brain tissue and resultant dilution of sodium in the vascular space.

CLINICAL SIGNS AND SYMPTOMS

Water Intoxication

- Decreased mental alertness
  Other accompanying symptoms:
- Sleepiness
- Anorexia
- Poor motor coordination
- Confusion
  In a severe imbalance, other symptoms may include the following:
- Convulsions
- Sudden weight gain
- Hyperventilation
- Warm, moist skin
- Signs of increased intracerebral pressure
  - Slow pulse
  - Increased systolic blood pressure (more than 10 mm Hg)
  - Decreased diastolic blood pressure (more than 10 mm Hg)
- Mild peripheral edema
- Low serum sodium
- Low haematocrit

Edema. An excess of solutes and water is called *isotonic volume excess.* The excess fluid is retained in the extracellular compartment and results in fluid accumulation in the interstitial space *(edema).* Edema can be produced by many different situations, most commonly including vein obstruction, decreased cardiac output, endocrine imbalances, and loss of serum proteins (e.g., burns, liver disease, allergic reactions).

CLINICAL SIGNS AND SYMPTOMS

Edema

- Weight gain (primary symptom)
- Excess fluid (several liters may accumulate before edema is evident)
- Dependent edema (collection of fluid in lower parts of the body)
- Pitting edema (finger pressed into edematous area leaves a persistent indentation in tissue)
- Increased blood pressure
- Neck vein engorgement
- Effusion (pulmonary, pericardial, peritoneal)
- Congestive heart failure

Diuretic medications are used frequently to treat volume excess. Various diuretic medications may be used depending on the underlying cause of the problem and the desired effect of the drug. The most commonly used class are the thiazide diuretics (e.g., chlorothiazide, hydrochlorothiazide). It is important to assess clients who take diuretic therapy for potential fluid loss and dehydration by observing for clinical symptoms of both.

These medications inhibit sodium and water resorption by the kidneys. Potassium is usually also lost with the sodium and water, so continuous replacement of potassium is a major concern for anyone receiving non–potassium-sparing diuretics. It is essential to monitor clients who take diuretics for signs and symptoms of potassium depletion.

It is also very important to check laboratory data for the potassium level in any client taking diuretics, particularly before exercise. Any value below the normal range (less than 3.5 mEq/L) is potentially dangerous and could result in a lethal cardiac arrhythmia, even with moderate cardiovascular exercise.

For clients taking diuretics, the therapist must observe for the appearance of symptoms consistent with dehydration or potassium depletion. Any concerns should be discussed with a physician before physical therapy intervention.

CLINICAL SIGNS AND SYMPTOMS

Potassium Depletion

- Muscle weakness
- Fatigue
- Cardiac arrhythmia
- Abdominal distention
- Nausea and vomiting

Metabolic Disorders

Metabolic Syndrome

Metabolic syndrome[95] is a group of signs and symptoms that are risk factors for coronary heart disease, DM, and stroke.[96] It has been reported that about 34% of adults have this syndrome, and this percentage continues to rise in the United States as a result of the obesity epidemic.[95] The condition is diagnosed when an individual has three or more of the following risk factors:[96]

- Large waistline: waist circumference of 40 inches or above for men and 35 inches or above for women
- High triglyceride level (150 mg/dL or greater)
- Low high-density lipoprotein (HDL) cholesterol (less than 40 mg/dL in men or less than 50 mg/dL in women)
- High blood pressure (130/85 mm Hg or greater)
- High fasting blood sugar (100 mg or greater)

Risk Factors and Red Flags. Serious health complications can be reduced by identifying risk factors early through screening. The dominant underlying risk factors for this syndrome appear to be sedentary lifestyle with little to no physical activity or exercise, abdominal obesity, and insulin resistance.

During all examinations, the therapist should watch for red flags of metabolic syndrome, including a BMI above 30, waist circumference (see Clinical Signs and Symptoms), elevated blood pressure, and signs of insulin resistance (e.g., acanthosis nigricans [Fig. 12.8], fatigue and decreased energy, depression, drowsiness after meals).

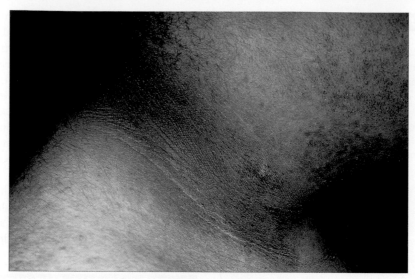

Fig. 12.8 *Acanthosis nigricans is a brown to black hyperpigmentation of the skin with a soft to velvet-like feel to it.* It is usually found in body folds, such as the posterior and lateral folds of the neck, the axilla, groin, umbilicus, forehead, and other areas. Acanthosis nigricans may be genetically inherited, but is also associated with obesity or endocrine disorders such as hypothyroidism or hyperthyroidism, acromegaly, polycystic ovary disease, insulin-resistant diabetes mellitus, or Cushing's disease. From Bolognia JL, Jorizzo JL, Rapini RP: *Dermatology*, ed 2, St. Louis, Mosby, 2007.

TABLE 12.10	Laboratory Values: Metabolic Acidosis and Alkalosis	
	Metabolic Acidosis	Metabolic Alkalosis
Laboratory values	• pH <7.35 • Bicarbonate (HCO_3) decreased <22 mEq/L • $PaCO_2$ decreased <35 mm Hg (compensated)	• pH >7.45 • Bicarbonate (HCO_3) increased >26 mEq/L • $PaCO_2$ increased >45 mm Hg (compensated)
GI effects*	• Loss of appetite (anorexia) • Nausea, vomiting • Abdominal pain, discomfort	• Nausea, vomiting • Diarrhea
CNS effects*	• Weakness • Lethargy • Confusion • Convulsions, coma	• Hyperactive deep tendon reflexes • Muscle weakness, cramping, twitching, tetany • Confusion, seizures • Irritability • Paresthesias
Integumentary effects*	• Warm and flushed	
Cardiovascular effects*	• Peripheral vasodilation • Decreased heart rate • Cardiac dysrhythmias	• Hypotension • Cardiac dysrhythmias
Skeletal system effects*	• Bone disease with chronic acidosis	
Signs of compensation	• Increased respiratory rate and depth • Hyperkalemia • Increased ammonia in urine	• Decreased respiratory rate and depth

CNS, Central nervous system; *GI*, gastrointestinal.
Normal values for pH = 7.35–7.45; $PaCO_2$ = 35–45 mm Hg; and HCO_3 = 22–36 mEq/L
*Signs and symptoms.

Metabolic Alkalosis

Metabolic alkalosis results from metabolic disturbances that cause either an increase in available bases or a loss of nonrespiratory body acids. Blood pH (hydrogen ion concentration in the ECF, a measure of metabolic process function and homeostasis) rises to a level greater than 7.45 (Table 12.10).

Common causes of metabolic alkalosis are usually related to the underlying disorder and include excessive vomiting or upper GI suctioning, diuretic therapy, or ingestion of large quantities of base substances such as antacids.

Decreased respirations may occur as the respiratory system attempts to compensate by buffering the basic environment. The lungs attempt to retain carbon dioxide (CO_2) and thus hydrogen (H) ions.

It is important for the therapist to ask clients about the use of magnesium-containing antacids because symptoms of alkalosis can affect muscular function by causing muscle fasciculation and cramping. Prevention of problems related to alkalosis may be accomplished by education of the client regarding antacid use.

CLINICAL SIGNS AND SYMPTOMS
Metabolic Alkalosis

- Nausea
- Prolonged vomiting
- Diarrhea
- Confusion
- Irritability
- Agitation, restlessness
- Muscle twitching and muscle cramping
- Muscle weakness
- Paresthesias
- Convulsions
- Eventual coma
- Slow, shallow breathing

Metabolic Acidosis

Metabolic or nonrespiratory acidosis is an accumulation of fixed (nonvolatile) acids or a deficit in bases. Blood pH decreases to a level below 7.35 (see Table 12.10). Common causes of metabolic acidosis include DKA, lactic acidosis from a wide range of conditions (e.g., smoke inhalation, sepsis, cardiopulmonary failure, adverse reaction to drugs, alcohol abuse, liver disease, cancer), renal failure, severe diarrhea, and drug (including alcohol) or chemical toxicity.

Ketoacidosis occurs because insufficiency of insulin for the proper use of glucose (or increased insulin requirements) results in increased breakdown of fat. This accelerated fat breakdown produces ketones and other acids, which accumulate to high levels. Although the body attempts to neutralize these increased acids, the plasma bicarbonate (HCO_3) is used up.

Chronic kidney disease with renal failure results in acidosis because the failing kidney not only is unable to rid the body of excess acids, but also cannot produce necessary bicarbonate.

Lactic acidosis occurs as excess lactic acid is produced during strenuous exercise or when oxygen is insufficient for proper use of carbohydrate (CHO), glucose, and water (H_2O).

Intestinal and pancreatic secretions are highly alkaline so that *severe diarrhea* depletes the body of these necessary bases. Metabolic acidosis can result from ingestion of large quantities of acetylsalicylic acid (salicylates); symptoms of possible metabolic acidosis should be carefully assessed in clients undergoing high-dose aspirin therapy.

Hyperventilation may occur as the respiratory system attempts to rid the body of excess acid by increasing the rate and depth of respiration. The result is an increase in the amount of carbon dioxide and hydrogen excreted through the respiratory system.

CLINICAL SIGNS AND SYMPTOMS
Metabolic Acidosis

- Headache
- Fatigue
- Drowsiness, lethargy
- Nausea, vomiting
- Diarrhea
- Muscular twitching
- Convulsions
- Coma (severe)
- Rapid, deep breathing (hyperventilation)

Gout

Primary gout is the manifestation of an inherited inborn error of purine metabolism characterized by an elevated serum uric acid (hyperuricemia). Excess uric acid in the blood can result in the formation of tiny uric acid crystals that collect in the joints, triggering a painful inflammatory response.

Gout affects men predominantly, and the usual form of primary gout is uncommon before the third decade, with its peak incidence in the 40- and 50-year age groups. The frequency of gout in women approaches that in men after menopause when estrogen, which helps clear uric acid from the kidneys, declines dramatically. Risk for gout decreases for those who undergo hormone therapy.[97] Gout may occur as a result of another disorder or of its therapy. This is referred to as *secondary gout*. Secondary gout may be associated with neoplasm, renal disease, or other metabolic disorders such as DM and hyperlipidemia (excess serum lipids).[98]

Risk Factors. Increased serum uric acid levels are associated with middle age, menopause, obesity, white race, stress (including surgery and medical illness), and high dietary intake of purine-rich foods. A variety of medications (e.g., penicillin, insulin, or thiazide diuretics) may increase the serum uric acid level or decrease uric acid excretion, as may a number of acute or chronic disorders other than gout (Table 12.11).

Alcohol consumption, especially beer and hard liquor, is associated with increased risk for gout. Additional dietary factors include meat and seafood consumption, intake of soft drinks sweetened with sugar, consumption of high-fructose products, obesity, and diuretic use.[99-101] Many diseases have a presentation similar to that of acute gouty arthritis. Gout and septic arthritis occasionally occur together. The diagnosis of gout must be based on the demonstration of monosodium urate crystals by synovial fluid analysis rather than on the clinical presentation alone.

Clinical Presentation. Uric acid is usually dissolved in the blood until it is passed through the kidneys into the urine

TABLE 12.11	Causes of Secondary Hyperuricemia
Hematopoietic	Hemolytic anemia Myeloproliferative disorders Polycythemia vera Myeloma
Neoplastic	Leukemia Lymphoma Multiple myeloma
Endocrine	Hypoparathyroidism Hyperparathyroidism Hypothyroidism Diabetes mellitus
Renal	Hemodialysis Renal insufficiency Polycystic kidney disease
Drugs	Low-dose aspirin Diuretics Antineoplastic (cytotoxic) agents Alcohol Vitamin B_{12}
Other	Chondrocalcinosis Psoriasis Sarcoidosis Obesity Hyperlipidemia Starvation, dehydration Toxemia of pregnancy

Adapted from Wade JP, Liang MH: Avoiding common pitfalls in the diagnosis of gout, *J Musculoskel Med* 5(8):16–27, 1988.

and then excreted. In individuals with gout, the uric acid changes to crystals (urate) that deposit in the joints (causing gouty arthritis) and other tissues, such as the kidneys, causing renal disease.

Most renal disease in clients with gout is the result of coexisting conditions such as hypertension or atherosclerosis. Renal dysfunction can occur as a result of urate-related parenchymal damage without the existence of other comorbidities. The most usual symptom of gout is acute monarticular arthritis. The individual may be awakened from sleep with exquisite pain in the affected joint; any pressure (even the touch of clothes or bed sheets) on the joint is intolerable. Redness and swelling occur within a few hours, sometimes accompanied by low-grade fever and chills. Untreated, the attack lasts from 10 days to 2 weeks. Later, episodes may develop more gradually, affecting more than one joint as the disease progresses.

The peripheral joints of the hands and feet are involved, with 90% of gouty clients having attacks in the metatarsophalangeal joint of the great toe. Other typical sites of initial involvement (in order of frequency) are the instep, ankle, heel, knee, and wrist, although any joint may be involved.

In chronic gouty arthritis, periarticular and subcutaneous deposits of sodium urate (or urate salts) form; these are referred to as *tophus (tophi)*. These deposits produce an acute inflammatory response that leads to acute arthritis and later to chronic arthritis. Enlarged tophi in the joints of the hands and feet may erupt and discharge chalky masses of urate crystals.

The formation of tophi is directly related to the elevation of serum urate; the higher the client's serum urate concentration, the higher the rate of urate deposition in soft tissue. Before urate-lowering agents became available, 30% to 50% of people with acute gouty arthritis developed tophi. Today, chronic tophaceous gout is rarely seen.

The therapist should refer anyone taking urate-lowering drugs for gout who is having recurrent symptoms to their physician as it may be necessary to adjust their medication dose. The therapist can reinforce the need for compliance with the management program and provide more education about controlling hypertension and obesity through diet and exercise. Limiting consumption of alcohol, sugary drinks, foods like red meat, organ meat and seafood, and maintaining a healthy weight are other important components of effective management.[102]

CLINICAL SIGNS AND SYMPTOMS
Gout

- Tophi: lumps under the skin, or actual eruptions through the skin, of chalky urate crystals
- Joint pain and swelling (especially first metatarsal joint)
- Fever and chills
- Malaise
- Redness

Pseudogout. Pseudogout is an arthritic condition caused by CPPD crystals. It occurs about one-eighth as often as gout and may be hereditary or secondary to other disease processes (hyperparathyroidism is the most common one; Case Example 12.7). The risk of getting pseudogout also appears to increase with age.[103]

Pseudogout is marked by attacks of gout-like symptoms, usually affecting a single joint (particularly the knee) and is associated with chondrocalcinosis (deposition of calcium salts in joint cartilage). In anyone with pseudogout, routine x-ray studies of the knee and wrist frequently demonstrate cartilage calcification, or chondrocalcinosis. Because these changes are found in up to 10% of older adults, diagnosis must be made through aspiration of synovial fluid to identify the CPPD crystals.

Hemochromatosis

Hemochromatosis, also termed *hematochromatosis*, is a genetic abnormality of iron metabolism. Mutations of the hemochromatosis gene (HFE) are associated with 90% of hemochromatosis cases.[104]

The cardinal defect in hemochromatosis is the lack of regulation of iron absorption, but the exact mechanism is unknown. The intestinal tract absorbs more iron than is required, thus producing an excess with progressive tissue damage in parenchymal organs from iron retention.

CASE EXAMPLE 12.7
Pseudogout

A 69-year-old man in previously good health complained of steadily increasing pain that had developed in his hands over the past several months. There was no history of occupational or accidental trauma.

Although the pain was present bilaterally, the pain in the left hand was more severe than in the right. The gentleman was right-hand dominant. There was a pattern of symptoms of increasing pain (described as deep aching) from morning to evening with a corresponding decrease in function.

Objective findings included reduced wrist range of motion in all directions bilaterally. There was no observed edema, warmth, or redness of the forearms, wrists, or hands. Although there were no reported symptoms at the elbow, left elbow extension and left forearm supination were also decreased by 25% compared with the right side. Grip strength was reduced by 50% bilaterally for age and sex.

Neurologic screening was without significant findings. There were no trigger points corresponding to the pain pattern present.

No constitutional symptoms were reported, and vital signs were unremarkable.

Result: This man was treated by a hand therapist without significant changes in symptoms or function. In fact, he reported an increased inability to write with his right hand. The therapist suggested a medical evaluation with possible inclusion of x-ray examination. Physician assessment resulted in a diagnosis of calcium pyrophosphate dihydrate (CPPD) arthropathy (pseudogout) of unknown cause. Medical treatment included a prescription nonsteroidal antiinflammatory drug (NSAID) and return to physical therapy for continued symptomatic treatment addressing the loss of function.

Although a medical condition existed, physical therapy treatment was still warranted. In this case a medical differential diagnosis provided the client with necessary medical treatment and the physical therapist with information necessary to treat the client more specifically.

Hemochromatosis is found five to ten times more often in men than in women because women lose blood through menstruation and pregnancy. Men seldom have symptoms until after 50 years of age and are rarely symptomatic before 30 years of age. Because of menstrual blood loss, women display symptoms 10 years later than men (median age: 60 years).

Ascorbic acid (vitamin C) and alcohol seem to accelerate the absorption of dietary iron. The high incidence of alcoholism among clients with hemochromatosis (40%) supports this concept.

Clinical Presentation. For many years, hemochromatosis was identified by a classic clinical triad of enlarged liver, skin hyperpigmentation, and DM. The term *bronze diabetes* was used to describe this presentation. Hyperpigmentation is caused by an increased number of melanocytes and a thinning of the epidermis. However, hemochromatosis may have many different signs and symptoms, confusing early diagnosis (Case Example 12.8).

In its early stages, hemochromatosis produces no symptoms because it takes many years of iron accumulation to produce warning signs or symptoms. Unfortunately, when the disease becomes evident, it is often too late because iron accumulation has caused irreversible tissue or end organ damage in the heart, liver, endocrine glands, skin, joints, bone, and pancreas. About half the clients with hemochromatosis will develop arthritis.

Hemochromatosis has a well-known association with chondrocalcinosis (deposition of calcium salts in the cartilage of joints). Acute attacks of synovitis can occur, which may resemble a rheumatoid flare. A biopsy of synovial tissue reveals iron deposition in the cells of the synovial lining that is noninflammatory.

Arthritis may be the presenting symptom of hemochromatosis, but it usually occurs after diagnosis and is more severe in adults older than 50 years of age. Arthritic manifestations are diverse, and joint damage occurs not from iron, but from the deposition of CPPD crystals.

The distribution of joint involvement may resemble rheumatoid arthritis, affecting the metacarpophalangeal (MCP) joints, in particular the second and third MCP joints. However, reduced MCP flexion is not accompanied by ulnar deviation. The arthritis can progress, and large joints may become involved, particularly the hips, knees, and shoulders.

CLINICAL SIGNS AND SYMPTOMS
Hemochromatosis

- Arthropathy
- Arthralgia
- Myalgia
- Progressive weakness
- Bilateral pitting edema (lower extremities)
- Vague abdominal pain
- Hypogonadism (lack of menstrual periods, impotence)
- Congestive heart failure (CHF)
- Hyperpigmentation of the skin (gray/blue to yellow)
- Loss of body hair
- Diabetes mellitus (DM)
- Loss of sex drive[104]
- Erectile dysfunction

Metabolic Bone Disease

Of the numerous metabolic disorders involving connective tissue, only the most commonly occurring diseases that would appear in a physical therapy setting are discussed in this text. These include osteoporosis, osteomalacia, and Paget's disease.

Osteoporosis. Osteoporosis, meaning "porous bone," is defined as a systemic skeletal disease characterized by low

CASE EXAMPLE 12.8
Hemochromatosis

Data from Sokolova Y: Acute shoulder pain and swelling in a 68-year-old man, *J Musculoskel Med* 17(11):699–700, Nov 2000.

A 68-year-old man was admitted to the hospital after sustaining multiple fractures of unknown origin. He was referred to physical therapy for functional mobility, transfers, and active range of motion with prescribed limitations. The admitting physician was a third-year resident on an emergency department rotation.

When the client was seen by the physical therapist, there was obvious swelling and limited range of motion in the right shoulder. The skin was warm and tender over the shoulder joint.

The therapist also observed the following:

- Bony prominences involving the second and third metacarpophalangeal (MCP) joints
- Bony prominences over the wrists, elbows, knees, and ankles
- Palpable and audible crepitus of these same joints
- Gray discoloration to skin throughout the body and axial skeleton
- Very sparse axial hair and an unusual leathery texture to the skin

The client was a poor historian but mentioned a "liver problem" that he experienced years ago. When asked about any other problems anywhere else in the body, the client mentioned difficulty with sexual arousal, erection, and ejaculation over the last 6 months.

The therapist developed a plan of care based on the current medical problem list and physician's orders. She also made it a point to seek out the referring resident to review some of the more unusual findings and ask about the possible cause of these symptoms.

Result: Further testing revealed that this client had a hereditary disease called *hemochromatosis*. The condition is characterized by excessive iron absorption by the small intestine. Individuals with hemochromatosis lack an effective way to remove excess iron, and the iron begins to accumulate in the liver, pancreas, skin, heart, and other organs.

Excess iron accumulation in the body promotes oxidation and causes tissue injury, fatigue, arthralgia or arthritis, and skin changes. Complications can include hepatomegaly, diabetes mellitus, impotence (males), pulmonary involvement, and cardiac myopathy.

Medical treatment for this condition was required to prevent the condition from worsening. Treatment does not improve the associated arthritis in a case like this, but it does keep it from getting worse.

The therapist's careful observations and follow-up made a significant difference in this man's medical outcome.

---

bone mass and microarchitectural deterioration of bone tissue, with a consequent increase in bone fragility and susceptibility to fracture[105] and it is the most prevalent bone disease in the world.

Osteoporosis is classified as *primary* or *secondary*. Primary osteoporosis the most common form is the deterioration of bone mass unassociated with other chronic illnesses or diseases. It is usually related to the aging process, including decreased gonadal function. Idiopathic, postmenopausal, and senile osteoporosis are included in the primary osteoporosis classification.[106] *Postmenopausal osteoporosis* is associated with accelerated bone loss in the perimenopausal and postmenopausal period, accompanied by high fracture rates, particularly involving the vertebrae. *Senile osteoporosis*, or age-related osteoporosis, increases with advancing age; it is caused by the bone loss that normally accompanies aging.

Secondary osteoporosis may accompany various endocrine and metabolic disorders (e.g., hyperthyroidism, hyperparathyroidism, hypogonadism, Cushing's disease, DM) that can produce associated osteopenia conditions (Table 12.12). *Endocrine-mediated bone loss* can produce osteoporosis because numerous endocrine hormones affect skeletal remodeling and hence skeletal mass.

Secondary osteoporosis is associated with other disorders that contribute to accelerated bone loss, such as chronic renal failure, rheumatoid arthritis, a malabsorption syndrome related to GI and hepatic disease, chronic respiratory disease, malignancy, and chronic chemical dependency (e.g., alcoholism).

Transient osteoporosis of the hip, a rare but temporary presentation of spontaneous osteoporosis of the femoral head (and sometimes femoral neck and acetabulum), is discussed in Chapter 17.

TABLE 12.12	Causes of Osteoporosis
Endocrine and Metabolic	**Other**
Diabetes mellitus (type 1)	**MEDICATIONS**
Glucocorticoid excess (hyperadrenocorticism)	
• Iatrogenic Cushing's syndrome	• Immunosuppressants (cyclosporine)
• Hyperadrenalism	• Excess thyroid hormone
Hyperthyroidism (thyrotoxicosis)	• Glucocorticoids
Hyperparathyroidism	• Methotrexate
Hemochromatosis	• Anticonvulsants/seizure medications (e.g., Dilantin, phenobarbital)
Acromegaly	
Testicular insufficiency	**NUTRITIONAL**
	• Anorexia nervosa; any eating disorder
	• Chronic alcohol use
	• Calcium/vitamin D deficiency
	• Chronic liver disease
	• Gastric bypass
	• Malabsorption syndromes (e.g., celiac sprue)
	COLLAGEN/GENETIC DISORDERS
	• Ehlers-Danlos syndrome
	• Marfan syndrome
	• Osteogenesis imperfecta

Risk Factors. Box 12.2 lists the risk factors for osteoporosis.

Comparison of BMD to peak bone mass of women who are at peak bone mass is the designated T-score. T-scores are used as a method of describing severity of risk (Table 12.13). Therapists can be involved in primary prevention and education, encouraging and instructing consumers and clients in risk assessment and risk factor reduction (Fig. 12.9 and Box 12.3).

The World Health Organization (WHO) has developed a computerized tool called the *Fracture Risk Assessment* (FRAX) to calculate the 10-year risk of sustaining a fracture (www.shef.ac.uk/FRAX).[111] It is based on individual patient models that integrate the risks associated with clinical risk factors, as well as BMD at the femoral neck. Medication is recommended for postmenopausal women, and men aged 50 years or older, who have a 3% to 10% risk of incurring a hip fracture or 20% risk of major fracture elsewhere in the body (e.g., wrist, spine, upper arm) according to the test.

The United States Preventive Services Task Force (USPSTF) recommends osteoporosis screening "in women aged 65 years and older and in younger women whose fracture risk is equal to or greater than that of a 65-year-old white woman who has no additional risk factors."[112,113] Chronic heavy alcohol use, particularly during adolescence and young adult years, has been reported to have a negative effect on bone health, thereby increasing the risk of osteoporosis later in life.[114] Also, low calcium and vitamin D levels increase the risk for bone loss, causing osteoporosis.[115] Long-term use of glucocorticoids and several anticonvulsive medications can also increase the risk of osteoporosis.[115]

Although long-term high caffeine use was reported to be associated with a bone density reduction, it did not result in an increased risk for osteoporosis and fractures.[116]

The relationship between cigarette smoking and osteoporosis is complicated because of the presence of other confounding variables that limit a definitive direct association of the risk. However, because tobacco use is associated with risk of fracture and decrease rate of bone healing after fractures, this is another reason for women to quit smoking.[117]

Primary prevention and education begins in childhood and adolescence, which are recognized as critical time periods for the development of normal peak bone mass. Diet and bone-building exercises during this critical period are essential in the development of adequate bone mass.

Men can be affected, especially those who smoke, drink alcohol moderately, fail to maintain a calcium-rich diet, have a sedentary lifestyle, or have a family history of fractures, or those undergoing dialysis or long-term steroid administration. Morbidity and mortality rates related to osteoporosis are higher in men than in women. Moreover, it has been reported that osteoporosis in men is underdiagnosed and therefore untreated.[118]

BOX 12.2 RISK FACTORS FOR OSTEOPOROSIS

Residents in a nursing home, extended care, or skilled nursing facility have a fivefold to tenfold increase in fracture risk compared with community dwellers.[107] Therapists in these work settings have the potential to improve the recognition and management of osteoporosis in these populations, including reducing the number of fractures and falls.

Women

- Caucasian and Asian women are more likely to develop osteoporosis; African American and Hispanic women have a significant risk for developing osteoporosis[108]
- Gender: more common in women than men
- Age: postmenopausal (older than 65 years)
- Early or surgically-induced menopause; menstrual dysfunction (amenorrhea)
- Family history of osteoporosis
- Family history and/or personal history of fractures
- Lifestyle:* cigarette smoking, excessive alcohol intake, inadequate calcium, little or no weight-bearing exercise
- Prolonged exposure to certain medications (more than 6 months):

Thyroid medications, corticosteroids, anti-inflammatories, antiseizure medication, aluminum-containing antacids, lithium, methotrexate, anticoagulants (heparin, warfarin), benzodiazepines (e.g., lorazepam, diazepam), cyclosporine A (immunosuppressant), gonadotropic-releasing hormone agonists, Depo-Provera injections (contraceptives in adolescents)

- Some cancer treatments (oophorectomy, ovarian suppression, chemotherapy-induced ovarian failure, estrogen suppression, bone marrow transplantation)
- Thin, small-boned frame (weight less than or equal to 125 lbs or 57 kg)
- Chronic diseases that affect the kidneys, lungs, stomach, and intestines or alter hormones (especially if treated with corticosteroids); dialysis

Men

- Caucasian
- Gender: increasing incidence among men
- Advancing age
- Lifestyle: same as for women
- Prolonged exposure to medications (same as for women)
- Family history of osteoporosis
- History of prostate cancer with bilateral orchiectomy
- Undiagnosed low levels of testosterone
- Hypogonadism (long-term androgen deprivation therapy [ADT])
- Chronic diseases (as listed for women)

TABLE 12.13	Bone Mineral Density T-Scores	
Status	T-Scores	Interpretation
Normal	−1.0 or above	T-score (BMD) is within (or above) 1 SD of the young adult reference mean
Osteopenia (low bone mass)	−1.0 to −2.5	T-score is 1.0–2.5 SDs below young adult mean for age
Osteoporosis	−2.5 or less	T-score is 2.5 or more SDs below mean for age
Severe osteoporosis	−2.5 or less with one or more fragility fractures	BMD is 2.5 or more SDs below mean for age

Data from World Health Organization: *Criteria for defining bone density*, WHO, 1994. Assessment of fracture risk and its application to screening for postmenopausal osteoporosis, Geneva, World Health Organization. Technical Report Series, No. 843, 1994; Lewiecki EM. Osteoporosis: Clinical Evaluation. [Updated 2018 Apr 23]. In: Feingold KR, Anawalt B, Boyce A, et al., editors. Endotext [Internet]. South Dartmouth (MA): MDText.com, Inc.; 2000-. [Table, Table 1. World Health Organization criteria for classification of patients with bone mineral density measured by dual-energy X-ray absorptiometry (3).]. Available from: https://www.ncbi.nlm.nih.gov/books/NBK279049/table/osteoporosis-clinic.classifica/.

The T-score compares one person's BMD in standard deviations with the average peak BMD in healthy young persons. Sometimes Z-scores are used, which compare one individual's BMD with the mean BMD of persons in the same age group, rather than with the normal values listed for young adults.

The World Health Organization (WHO) has proposed the clinical definition of osteoporosis in the table based on epidemiologic data that link low bone mass with increased fracture risk.

In study populations of Caucasian postmenopausal women, a BMD that was lower than 2.5 SD of normal peak bone mass was associated with a fracture prevalence; 50% of women with bone mass at this level had at least one bone fracture.[109]

On the basis of these data, the WHO defined osteoporosis as BMD 2.5 or more SD below peak bone mass, osteopenia as bone mass between 1.0 and 2.5 SD below peak, and normal as 1.0 SD below normal peak bone mass or higher.

The WHO criteria apply only to Caucasian, postmenopausal women, and not men, premenopausal women, or women of ethnicity other than Caucasian. T-score conversion based on the NHANES database is available for clinically significant low bone mass in other population groups at http://courses.washington.edu/bonephys/opbmdtz.html.

BMD, Bone mineral density; *SD*, standard deviation.

Osteoporosis Screening Evaluation

Name _____ Date _____

	YES	NO
1. Are you 65 years old or older?	☐	☐
2. Is your weight below 57.6 kg (127 pounds)?	☐	☐
3. Are you Caucasian or Asian?	☐	☐
4. Have any of your blood-related family members had osteoporosis?	☐	☐
5. Are you a postmenopausal woman?	☐	☐
6. Do you drink 2 or more ounces of alcohol each day? (1 beer, 1 glass of wine, or 1 cocktail)	☐	☐
7. Do you smoke more than 10 cigarettes each day?	☐	☐
8. Are you physically inactive? (Walking or similar exercise at least three times per week is average.)	☐	☐
9. Have you had both ovaries (with or without a hysterectomy) removed before age 40 years without treatment (hormone replacement)?	☐	☐
10. Have you ever been treated for or told you have rheumatoid arthritis?	☐	☐
11. Have you been taking thyroid medication, antiinflammatories, or seizure medication for more than 6 months?	☐	☐
12. Have you ever broken your hip, spine, rib, or wrist?	☐	☐
13. Do you drink or eat four or more servings of caffeine (carbonated beverages, tea, coffee, chocolate) per day?	☐	☐
14. Is your diet low in dairy products and other sources of calcium? (Three servings of dairy products or two doses of a calcium supplement per day are average.)	☐	☐
15. Are you vegetarian or vegan?	☐	☐

Fig. 12.9 *Osteoporosis Screening Evaluation.* If you answer "yes" to three or more of these questions, you may be at greater risk for developing osteoporosis, or "brittle bone disease," and you should contact your physician for further information.

BOX 12.3 OSTEOPOROSIS RESOURCES

National Osteoporosis Foundation

www.nof.org

Offers information for consumers and professionals about osteoporosis and its prevention. Includes information on bone density testing, risk factor assessment, and a special web link, *Men and Osteoporosis*.

Siteman Cancer Center, Barnes-Jewish Hospital and Washington University School of Medicine http://www.yourdiseaserisk.wustl.edu/

Offers consumers an opportunity to find out their individual risk of developing diseases including cancer, chronic bronchitis, diabetes mellitus, emphysema, heart disease, osteoporosis, and stroke. Also includes tips on prevention for each of these diseases.

WebMD: Medical Tests

http://www.webmd.com/hw/osteoporosis/hw3738.asp

Explains different techniques used to measure bone mineral density, how each one is done, and how to interpret the results.

Johns Hopkins SCORE Screening Quiz

http://www.hopkins-arthritis.org/arthritis-info/osteoporosis/diagnosis.html

The Simple Calculated Osteoporosis Risk Estimation (SCORE) is a six-question screening questionnaire for osteoporosis with 89% sensitivity and 50% specificity in an ambulatory population of postmenopausal women. A score of six or more is an indication that referral for bone density testing is advised.[110]

Fracture Index

An assessment tool for predicting fracture risk. This clinical assessment tool is based on seven risk factors (age, T score, personal or maternal fracture after age 50 years, weight, smoking status, use of arms to stand up from a chair) that can be used to assess a woman's risk of hip, vertebral, and nonvertebral fractures.

From Black DM, Steinbuch M, Palermo L et al.: An assessment tool for predicting fracture risk in postmenopausal women, *Osteoporos Int* 12(7):519–528, 2001.

Clinical Presentation. Osteoporosis is a silent disease with no visible signs or symptoms until bone loss is sufficient to result in fracture. Osteoporosis associated with aging involves fractures of the proximal femur and vertebrae, the hip, pelvis, proximal humerus, distal radius, and the tibia.

Postmenopausal osteoporosis is associated with accelerated bone loss in the perimenopausal period accompanied by high fracture rates, particularly involving the vertebrae. Osteoporotic fracture will affect one in three women over 50 years worldwide.[119] Twenty-five percent of postmenopausal women are diagnosed with compression fracture during their lifetime (Case Example 12.9).[126]

Mild-to-severe back pain and loss of height may be the only early signs observed. Changes in bone density do not show up on x-ray films until there is a 30% loss. The cardinal features of established osteoporosis are bone fracture, pain, and deformity.

More than half of the women in the United States who are 50 years of age or older are likely to have radiologically detectable evidence of abnormally decreased bone mass (osteopenia) in the spine. More than a third of these women develop major orthopedic problems related to osteoporosis. Most fractures sustained by women older than 50 years of age are secondary to osteoporosis.

CLINICAL SIGNS AND SYMPTOMS

Osteoporosis

- Back pain: episodic, acute low thoracic/high lumbar pain
- Compression fracture of the spine (postmenopausal osteoporosis)
- Bone fracture (age-related osteoporosis)
- Decrease in height (more than 1 inch shorter than maximum adult height)
- Kyphosis
- Dowager's hump
- Decreased activity tolerance
- Early satiety

Osteomalacia. Osteomalacia is a softening of the bones caused by a vitamin D deficiency in adults, resulting from impaired mineralization in the bone matrix. This failure in mineralization results in a reduced rate of bone formation.[127] The deficiency may be a result of the lack of exposure to ultraviolet (UV) rays, inadequate intake of vitamin D in the diet, failure to absorb or use vitamin D, increased catabolism of vitamin D, a renal tubular defect, or a pathologically reduced number of vitamin D receptor sites in tissues.

The disease is characterized by decalcification of the bones, particularly those of the spine, pelvis, and lower extremities. X-ray examination reveals transverse, fracture-like lines in the affected bones and areas of demineralization in the matrix of the bone. These pseudofractures, known as *Looser's transformation zones*, are bilateral. The most common sites are the ribs, long bones, the lateral scapular margin, upper femur, and pubic rami. As the bones soften, they become bent, flattened, or otherwise deformed. Looser's zones are believed to result from pressure on the softened bone by the nutrient arteries of its blood supply.

Severe bone pain, skeletal deformities, fractures, and severe muscle weakness and pain are common in people with osteomalacia. Clients typically complain of muscle weakness and pain that sometimes mimics polymyositis or muscular dystrophy.

A similar condition in children, occurring before epiphyseal plate closure, is called *rickets*.[127] In children with rickets, x-ray findings include the well-known bowing of the long bones, in addition to widening, fraying, and clubbing of the areas of active bone growth. These areas especially include the metaphyseal ends of the long bones and the sternal ends of the ribs, the so-called rachitic rosary.

CASE EXAMPLE 12.9

Osteoporosis

Referral: A 77-year-old Caucasian woman was referred to outpatient physical therapy 1 month ago by her primary physician because of her complaint of gradual onset of low back pain (LBP) over the last 2 months. The physician's diagnosis was LBP secondary to osteoarthritis and osteoporosis. A recent radiology report indicated moderate osteoarthritis at L1-L5 and radiolucency of the spine suggesting severe osteoporosis. No fractures or abnormal curvatures were noted.

Past Medical and Social History
- Osteoarthritis
- LBP secondary to L4-L5 herniated disk; status postdiskectomy
- Osteoporosis (2-year history)

The client denied diabetes mellitus, high blood pressure, other heart diseases, or other health concerns.

She is a retired teacher who lives alone in an adult complex and still drives a car. She lost her second son in a motor vehicle accident 3 months ago and appears emotionally stressed from her loss. She has declined any counseling or medication suggested by her physician.

The client is highly motivated to improve so that she can go back to walking about 1 mile every other day; currently her pain level prevents her from this activity.

Medications
- Relafen 500 mg twice daily
- 5% Lidoderm patch applied to the skin once a day for pain
- Norflex 100 mg twice daily to reduce muscle spasms

She has been taking Fosamax 70 mg once a week for 2 years to improve her bone density loss caused by osteoporosis. The client reported little or no change in her pain level with the use of analgesics.

Clinical Presentation: During initial evaluation, LBP was graded as a 7/10 on the Visual Analog Scale (VAS). Pain was localized to the low back without radiation; she described it as worse when getting up in the morning and after sitting or walking for a short period. Pain was progressively worse with walking, and the client stopped walking after 3 or 4 minutes. She denied any urinary or bowel incontinence.

During the examination, the client presented with mild tenderness with palpation of L3-L5 and mild paraspinal muscle spasms with slight loss of lumbar lordosis. There was no sensory loss noted with either the upper or lower extremities or trunk, and no pedal edema.

Range of motion (ROM): ROM was within normal limits (WNL) in both upper and lower extremities. Trunk flexion 0 to 76 degrees, trunk extension 0 to 13 degrees; all other motion: WNL.

Manual muscle test (MMT): Muscle strength for all extremities was grossly 5/5. Trunk extensors and abdominals were graded 4/5.

Straight leg raise (SLR): Negative bilaterally; the client was unable to fully raise both legs because of hamstring tightness.

Normal deep tendon reflex (DTRs) for both quadriceps and Achilles tendons.

Intervention: Physical therapy intervention consisted of education on osteoporosis and its cause, prevention, treatment, and sequelae. Client was instructed in fall prevention and in making her apartment fall-proof.

Moist heat was applied to the low back for 15 minutes to reduce muscle spasm, increase muscle flexibility, and reduce pain associated with osteoarthritis.

Massage/soft tissue mobilization: This has been shown to be effective in reducing LBP when used in conjunction with other treatment modalities.[120]

Therapeutic exercise: Therapeutic exercise has been shown to be effective in the management of LBP.[121] In this case, single and double knee-to-chest exercises were done in the supine position, holding each one for 5 seconds. Single SLR supine and prone (double SLR was avoided because of its tendency to put great pressure on the spine, which may result in fracture in this client).

Walking on a treadmill: During the initial evaluation, the client was able to tolerate only 3.5 minutes on the treadmill at 1.0 mph (zero grade) because of increasing pain. Treadmill walking was used to measure progress because one of the client's goals was to be able to walk up to 1 mile.

All exercises were progressed as the client improved. A written handout was provided with drawings and instructions for each exercise. Precautions were given to stop the exercise if experiencing shortness of breath, palpitation, or increased pain and to report these symptoms to the doctor. Any exercise that increased the pain was to be discontinued until the client checked with the therapist.

Short-term and long-term goals were established; the prognosis was expected to be good.

Outcome: The client showed remarkable improvement with her treatment. She was very diligent in performing her home exercise program (HEP) and following the therapist's instructions. She was highly motivated, attended all scheduled sessions, and was dedicated to achieving her goals.

By the third week of treatment, her pain had reportedly decreased, reduced from 7/10 to 4/10 on the VAS, trunk flexion was 0 to 94 degrees, and she was independent in her home exercise program and she was able to verbalize her fall prevention plan.

At 3 to 4 weeks, the client reported sudden increase in her LBP while getting out of bed. Pain was rated 6/10 and reported as constant but not getting worse. During the examination, there was tenderness over L3-L5, but it was not worse than previously reported.

There were mild low back muscle spasms, but no neurologic signs were noted and no abnormal curvature observed. This appeared to be an exacerbation episode. The primary care physician was notified and the therapist was advised to continue intervention as planned. Treatment was continued as planned for 1 week without much improvement.

Result: The client returned to the physician for reevaluation. X-rays at that time diagnosed a compression fracture at L1. Further physical therapy intervention was placed on hold, pending orthopedic consult. She returned to physical therapy with a recommendation for lumbar corset, rest for 2 weeks, and continued physical therapy intervention.

Continued

Reflections: Compression fracture is a known complication of osteoporosis with or without neurologic deficit.[122] It is accepted that posterior midline tenderness is a red flag for spinal fracture; however, the absence of a posterior midline tenderness does not exclude significant spinal injury without trauma, such as spinal compression fracture.[123] The therapist should remain alert to the possibility of a new vertebral fracture in anyone with osteoporosis who reports a substantial increase in low back pain.[124,125]

Signs and symptoms of compression fracture may be difficult to recognize, especially in a client who is already being treated for chronic LBP 2 years after diskectomy for disk herniation.

It is not uncommon to see occasional flare-ups of pain in physical therapy clients who have been showing good improvement. A typical clinical scenario is the client who increases the frequency, intensity, or duration of activities, even adding activities he or she has been unable to enjoy previously because of back pain.

In some cases, clients overdo the home exercise program or add a new exercise suggested by a friend or seen on TV or at the gym. In some cases, there is no apparent reason for exacerbation of symptoms.

This case study demonstrates how any adverse change in pain level in an individual with osteoporosis undergoing physical therapy for back pain should not be dismissed as insignificant but should be thoroughly investigated, including medical referral when indicated.

From Nubi M: Case report presented in fulfillment of DPT 910, *Institute for Physical Therapy Education*, Widener University, Chester, PA, 2005. Used with permission.

CLINICAL SIGNS AND SYMPTOMS
Osteomalacia

- Bone pain
- Skeletal deformities
- Fractures
- Severe muscle weakness
- Myalgia

Paget's Disease. Paget's disease (osteitis deformans), is a noninflammatory, metabolic, skeletal disorder characterized by localized excessive osteoclastic bone resorption that is followed by compensatory increased osteoblastic activity leading to unstructured, fibroblastic, and biomechanically unstable bone. As a result, there is deformity and enlargement of the bone with a defective and disorganized pattern.[128] The new bone is larger, less compact, more vascular, and more susceptible to fracture than normal bone.

Risk Factors. Paget's disease is the most common skeletal disorder after osteoporosis, affecting men more often than women by a 3:2 ratio. About 1 to 3 million people in the United States are affected by the disorder.[129,130] It is usually diagnosed after age 40 years; incidence increases with advancing age, with the highest prevalence in individuals over 65 years of age. It is reported that around 70% to 90% of persons with this diagnosis are asymptomatic.[129] It is more prevalent in Europe and Australia and in people of Anglo-Saxon descent.

Genetic factors are important in the pathogenesis of Paget's disease. Evidence for a major genetic component is supported by 30% of affected individuals having affected first-degree relatives.[130]

There are no known ways to prevent Paget's disease. Physical therapists can play an important role in optimizing health and well-being of individuals with this condition by educating them on the pathophysiology of the disease, the rehabilitation process, and the importance of carefully graduated and protected weight-bearing activities[129] in postsurgical conditions.

Clinical Presentation. The severity of involvement and associated clinical characteristics vary greatly. Although some people are asymptomatic, with very limited bone involvement, others manifest a disabling, painful form of Paget's disease that is characterized by skeletal pain and bones that are extremely deformed and easily fractured. Bones most commonly involved include (in decreasing order) the pelvis, lumbar spine, sacrum, femur, tibia, skull, shoulders, thoracic spine, cervical spine, and ribs.

Bone pain associated with Paget's disease is described as aching, deep and boring, worse at night, and diminishing but not disappearing with physical activity. Muscular pain may be referred from involved bony structures, or as a result of mechanical changes caused by joint deformities.

Other complications include a variety of nerve compression syndromes, secondary osteoarthritis, and vertebral compression and collapse.

CLINICAL SIGNS AND SYMPTOMS
Paget's Disease

These depend on the location and severity of the bone lesions and may include the following:
- Pain and stiffness
- Fatigue
- Headache and dizziness
- Bone fracture
- Vertebral compression and collapse
- Deformity
- Bowing of long bones
- Increased size and abnormal contour of clavicles
- Osteoarthritis of adjacent joints
- Acetabular protrusion
- Head enlargement
- Periosteal tenderness
- Increased skin temperature over long bones*
- Decreased auditory acuity (if skull is affected)
- Compression neuropathy
- Spinal stenosis
- Paresis
- Paraplegia
- Muscle weakness

*Increased skin temperature over affected long bones is a typical finding and is explained by soft tissue vascularity surrounding the bones.

PHYSICIAN REFERRAL

Disorders of the endocrine and metabolic systems may appear with recognizable clinical signs and symptoms but almost always require a combination of clinical and laboratory findings for accurate identification.

The therapist is encouraged to complete a thorough Family/Personal History form, augmented by the screening interview and careful clinical observations, to provide the physician with pertinent screening information when making a referral. When appropriate, the Osteoporosis Screening Evaluation (see Fig. 12.9; see also Appendix C-6 in the accompanying enhanced eBook version included with print purchase of this textbook) may also be helpful. In most cases, the client who has suffered from an endocrine disorder has already been diagnosed and may have been referred for physical therapy for some other musculoskeletal complaint. Such clients may have musculoskeletal problems that can be affected by symptoms associated with a hormone imbalance (see Tables 12.4 through 12.7).

Diseases of the endocrine-metabolic system, such as DM, obesity, and thyroid abnormalities, account for some of the most common disorders encountered in a physical therapy practice. In recent years, new laboratory techniques have greatly enhanced the physician's ability to diagnose these diseases.

Nevertheless, in many cases, the disorder remains unrecognized until relatively late in their course; signs and symptoms may be attributed to some other disease process or musculoskeletal disorder (e.g., weakness may be the major complaint in Addison's disease). Thus any client who has any of the generalized signs and symptoms associated with the endocrine system without an obvious or already known cause should be further evaluated by a physician.

Guidelines for Immediate Medical Attention

- Any person with DM who is confused, lethargic, exhibiting changes in mental function, profuse sweating (without exercise), or demonstrating signs of DKA should receive medical attention (perform a fingerstick glucose test to help evaluate the situation).
- Likewise, any episode or suspected episode of hypoglycemia must be treated promptly and reported to the client's physician.
- Signs of potassium depletion (e.g., muscle weakness or cramping, fatigue, cardiac arrhythmias, abdominal distention, nausea and vomiting) or fluid dehydration in a client who is taking non–potassium-sparing diuretics requires medical attention. Consultation with the physician is advised before exercising the individual.
- Signs of thyroid storm (tachycardia, elevated core body temperature, restlessness, agitation, abdominal pain, nausea, vomiting); observe clients with known history of hyperthyroidism carefully postoperatively or following trauma or infection.

Guidelines for Physician Referral

- Any unexplained fever without other symptoms in a person taking corticosteroids may be an indication of infection and should be evaluated by a physician.
- Palpable nodules or a palpable mass in the supraclavicular area or the scalene triangle, or both (see Fig. 12.5), especially if accompanied by new-onset hoarseness, hemoptysis, or elevated blood pressure must be evaluated by a physician.
- Any episode (especially a series of episodes) of hypoglycemia in the client with DM should be reported to the physician.
- The presence of multiple eruptive xanthomas on the extensor tendons of anyone with DM may signal uncontrolled glycemia and requires medical referral to normalize lipid levels; exercise remains a key to the management of this condition.
- Signs of fluid loss or dehydration in anyone taking diuretics should be reported to the physician.
- Recurrent arthritic symptoms in a client with gout who is already taking urate-lowering drugs requires medical referral for review of their medication.
- Untreated hypertension (blood pressure >140/90 mm Hg), angina pectoris, previously undetected heart rhythm disturbances, untreated intermittent claudication, fasting hyperglycemia (blood glucose level >16.8 mmol/L, >300 mg/dL), frequent hypoglycemic episodes, untreated wounds in lower extremities, cachexia or sudden body weight loss, untreated autonomic or peripheral neuropathy, or untreated vision disturbances.[131]

Clues to Symptoms of Endocrine or Metabolic Origin

Past Medical History

- Endocrine or metabolic disease has been previously diagnosed. Bilateral CTS, proximal muscle weakness, and periarthritis of the shoulder(s) are common in persons with certain endocrine and metabolic diseases. Look for other associated signs and symptoms of endocrine or metabolic disease (see Box 4.15).
- Long-term use of corticosteroids can result in classic symptoms referred to as *Cushing's syndrome*.

Clinical Presentation

- Identified trigger points are not eliminated or relieved by trigger point therapy. Observe for signs and symptoms of hypothyroidism.
- Palpable lymph node(s) or nodule(s) in the scalene triangle (see Fig. 12.5), especially when accompanied by new-onset hoarseness, hemoptysis, or elevated blood pressure.
- Anyone with muscle weakness and fatigue who is taking diuretics may be experiencing symptoms of potassium depletion. Assess for cardiac arrhythmias and ask about nausea and vomiting.

- Muscle fasciculation and cramping may be associated with antacid use (metabolic alkalosis).

Associated Signs and Symptoms

- Watch for anyone with arthralgias, hand pain and stiffness, or muscle weakness with an accompanying cluster of signs and symptoms of endocrine or metabolic disorders (see Box 4.15).

Clues to Recognizing Osteoporosis

- Pain is usually severe and localized to the site of fracture (usually midthoracic, lower thoracic, and lumbar spine vertebrae).

- Pain may radiate to the abdomen or flanks.
- Aggravating factors: prolonged sitting, standing, bending, or performing Valsalva's maneuver.
- Alleviating factors: sidelying with hips and knees flexed.
- Sitting up from supine requires rolling to the side first.
- Not usually accompanied by sciatica or chronic pain from nerve root impingement
- Tenderness to palpation over the fracture site
- Rib or spinal deformity, Dowager's hump (cervical kyphosis)
- Loss of height

■ Key Points to Remember

1. Clients with a variety of endocrine and metabolic disorders commonly complain of fatigue, muscle weakness, and occasionally muscle or bone pain.
2. Muscle weakness associated with endocrine and metabolic disorders usually involves proximal muscle groups.
3. Periarthritis and calcific tendinitis of the shoulder is common in clients with endocrine issues. Symptoms usually respond to treatment of the underlying endocrine pathologic condition and are not likely to respond to physical therapy treatment.
4. CTS, hand stiffness, and hand pain can occur with endocrine and metabolic diseases.
5. The connection between hypothyroidism and FMS is not clear. Any compromise of muscle energy metabolism aggravates and perpetuates Trigger Points (TrPs). Treatment of the underlying endocrine disorder is necessary to eliminate the TrPs, but myofascial treatment must be part of the recovery process to restore full function.
6. Anyone with DM taking corticosteroid medications must be monitored for changes in blood glucose level because these medications can cause or contribute to hyperglycemia.
7. Exercise for the client with DM must be carefully planned because significant complications can result from strenuous exercise.

8. Clients with DM who are under physical, emotional, or psychologic stress (e.g., hospitalization, pregnancy, personal problems) have increased insulin requirements; symptoms may develop in the person who usually has the disease under control.
9. Exercise for the client with insulin-dependent DM should be coordinated to avoid peak insulin dosage whenever possible. Any client with known DM who appears confused or lethargic must be tested immediately by fingerstick for glucose level. Immediate medical attention may be necessary. Other precautions regarding DM for the therapist are covered in the text.
10. When it is impossible to differentiate between ketoacidosis and hyperglycemia, administration of some source of sugar (glucose) is the immediate action to take.
11. Early osteoporosis has no visible signs and symptoms. History and risk factors are important clues.
12. Cortisol suppresses the body's inflammatory response, masking early signs of infection. Any unexplained fever without other symptoms should be a warning to the therapist of the need for medical follow-up.
13. Excessive use of antacids can result in muscle fasciculation and cramping (see section on Alkalosis).

CLIENT HISTORY AND INTERVIEW

SPECIAL QUESTIONS TO ASK

Endocrine and metabolic disorders may produce subtle symptoms that progress so gradually that the person may be unaware of the significance of such findings. This requires careful interviewing to screen for potential physical and psychologic changes associated with a hormone imbalance or other endocrine or metabolic disorder.

As always, it is important to be aware of client medications (whether over-the-counter or prescribed), the intended purpose of these drugs, and any potential side effects.

Continued

CLIENT HISTORY AND INTERVIEW—cont'd

PAST MEDICAL HISTORY/RISK FACTORS

- Have you ever had head/neck radiation or cranial surgery? **(thyroid cancer, pituitary dysfunction)**
- Have you ever had a head injury? **(pituitary dysfunction)**
- Have you ever been told you have diabetes mellitus or that you have "sugar" in your blood?
- Have you ever been told that you have osteoporosis or brittle bones, fractures, or back problems? **(wasting of bone matrix in Cushing's syndrome, osteoporosis)**
- Have you ever been told that you have Cushing's syndrome?

CLINICAL PRESENTATION

- Have you noticed any decrease in your muscle strength recently? **(growth hormone imbalance, ACTH imbalance, Addison's disease, hyperthyroidism, hypothyroidism)**
- Have you had any muscle cramping or twitching? **(metabolic alkalosis)**
  - *If yes*, do you take antacids with magnesium on a daily basis? How much and how often?
- Do you have any difficulty in going up stairs or getting out of chairs? **(muscle wasting secondary to large doses of cortisol)**

ASSOCIATED SIGNS AND SYMPTOMS

- Have you noticed any change in your vision, such as blurred vision, double vision, loss of peripheral vision, or sensitivity to light? **(thyrotoxicosis, hypoglycemia, diabetes mellitus)**
- Have you had an increase in your thirst or in the number of times you need to urinate? **(adrenal insufficiency, diabetes mellitus, diabetes insipidus)**
- Have you had an increase in your appetite? **(diabetes mellitus, hyperthyroidism)**
- Do you bruise easily? **(Cushing's syndrome, excessive secretion of cortisol causes capillary fragility; small bumps/injuries produce bruising)**
- When you injure yourself, do your wounds heal slowly? **(growth hormone excess, ACTH excess, Cushing's syndrome)**
- Do you frequently have unexplained fatigue? **(hyperparathyroidism, hypothyroidism, growth hormone deficiency, ACTH imbalance, Addison's disease)**

- *If yes*, what activities seem to be too difficult or tiring? (muscle weakness caused by cortisol and aldosterone hypersecretion and adrenocortical insufficiency, hypothyroidism)
- Have you noticed any increase in your collar size (goiter growth), difficulty in breathing or swallowing? **(goiter, Graves' disease, hyperthyroidism)**
  - *To the therapist:* Observe also for hoarseness.
- Have you noticed any changes in skin color? **(Addison's disease, hemochromatosis)** (e.g., overall skin color has become a darker shade of brown or bronze; occurrence of black freckles; darkening of palmar creases, tongue, mucous membranes)

FOR THE CLIENT WITH DIAGNOSED DIABETES MELLITUS

- What type of insulin do you take?
- What is your schedule for taking your insulin?
  - *To the therapist:* Coordinate exercise programs according to the time of peak insulin action. Do not schedule exercise during peak times.
- Do you ever have episodes of hypoglycemia or insulin reaction?
  - *If yes*, describe the symptoms that you experience.
- Do you carry a source of sugar with you in case of an emergency?
  - *If yes*, what is it, and where do you keep it in case I need to retrieve it?
- Have you ever had diabetic ketoacidosis (diabetic coma)?
  - *If yes*, describe any symptoms you may have had that I can recognize if this occurs during therapy.
- Do you use the fingerstick method for testing your own blood glucose level?
  - *To the therapist:* You may want to ask the client to bring the test kit for use before or during exercise.
- Do you have difficulty in maintaining your blood glucose level within an acceptable range (70 mg/dL to 100 mg/dL)?
  - *If yes, to the therapist:* You may want to take a baseline of the blood glucose level before initiating an exercise program.
- Do you ever have burning, numbness, or a loss of sensation in your hands or feet? **(diabetic neuropathy)**

CASE STUDY

REFERRAL

The patient was a 45-year-old client with type 1 diabetes mellitus (DM), has been receiving wound care for a foot ulcer during the last 2 weeks. Today when he came to the clinic, he appeared slightly lethargic and confused. He indicated to you that he has had a "case of the flu" since early yesterday and that he had vomited once or twice the day before and once that morning before coming to the clinic. His wife, who had driven him to the clinic, said that he seemed to be "breathing

Continued

CASE STUDY—cont'd

fast" and urinating more frequently than usual. He has been thirsty, so he has been drinking "7-Up" and water, and those fluids "have stayed down okay."

PHYSICAL THERAPY INTERVIEW

- When did you last take your insulin? (Client may have forgotten because of his illness, forgetfulness, confusion, or just being afraid to take it while feeling sick with the "flu.")
- What type of insulin did you take?
- Do you have a source of sugar with you? If *yes*, where do you keep it? (This question should be asked during the initial physical therapy interview.)
- Have you contacted your physician about your condition?
- Have you done a recent blood glucose level test (fingerstick)? If *yes*, when was the last time that this test was done?

WHAT WERE THE RESULTS?

To his wife: Your husband seems to be confused and is not himself. How long has he been like this? Have you observed any strong breath odor since this "flu" started? (Make your own observations regarding breath odor at this time.)

If possible, have the client perform a fingerstick blood glucose test on himself. This type of client should be sent immediately to his physician without physical therapy intervention. If he is hypoglycemic (unlikely under these circumstances), this condition should be treated immediately. It is more likely that this client is hyperglycemic and may have diabetic ketoacidosis. In either situation, he should not be driving and arrangements should be made for transport to the physician's office.

PRACTICE QUESTIONS

1. Disorders of the endocrine glands can be caused by:
   a. Dysfunction of the gland
   b. External stimulus
   c. Excess or insufficiency of hormonal secretions
   d. a and b
   e. b and c
   f. All the above
2. Clients with diabetes insipidus (DI) would most likely come to the therapist with which of the following clinical symptoms?
   a. Severe dehydration, polydipsia
   b. Headache, confusion, lethargy
   c. Weight gain
   d. Decreased urine output
3. Clients who are taking corticosteroid medications should be monitored for the onset of Cushing's syndrome. You will need to monitor your client for which of the following problems?
   a. Low blood pressure, hypoglycemia
   b. Decreased bone density, muscle wasting
   c. Slow wound healing
   d. b and c
4. Signs and symptoms of Cushing's syndrome in an adult taking oral steroids may include:
   a. Increased thirst, decreased urination, and decreased appetite
   b. Low white blood cell count and reduced platelet count
   c. High blood pressure, tachycardia, and palpitations
   d. Hypertension, slow wound healing, easy bruising
5. Parathyroid hormone (PTH) secretion is particularly important in the metabolism of bone. The client with an oversecreting parathyroid gland would most likely have:
   a. Increased blood pressure
   b. Pathologic fractures
   c. Decreased blood pressure
   d. Increased thirst and urination

6. Which glycosylated hemoglobin (A1C) value is within the recommended range?
   a. 6%
   b. 8%
   c. 10%
   d. 12%
7. A 38-year-old man comes to the clinic for low back pain. He has a new diagnosis of Graves' disease. When asked if there are any other symptoms of any kind, he replies, "increased appetite and excessive sweating." When you perform a neurologic screening examination, what might be present that would be associated with the Graves' disease?
   a. Hyporeflexia, but no change in strength
   b. Hyporeflexia with decreased muscle strength
   c. Hyperreflexia, but no change in strength
   d. Hyperreflexia with decreased muscle strength
8. All of the following are common signs or symptoms of insulin resistance except:
   a. Acanthosis nigricans
   b. Drowsiness after meals
   c. Fatigue
   d. Oliguria
9. List three of the most common symptoms of diabetes mellitus (DM).
10. What is the primary difference between the two hyperglycemic states: diabetic ketoacidosis (DKA) and hyperglycemic, hyperosmolar, nonketotic coma (HHNC)?
11. Is it safe to administer a source of sugar to a lethargic or unconscious person with diabetes mellitus (DM)?
12. What are the most common musculoskeletal symptoms associated with endocrine disorders?
13. What systemic conditions can cause carpal tunnel syndrome (CTS)?
14. What are the mechanisms by which carpal tunnel syndrome (CTS) occurs?

REFERENCES

1. Hall JE, Guyton AC. *Guyton and Hall Textbook of Medical Physiology*. ed 14. Philadelphia: Elsevier; 2021.
2. Altcn R, Wiebe E. Hypothalamic-pituitary-adrenal axis function in patients with rheumatoid arthritis treated with different glucocorticoid approaches. *Neuroimmunomodulation*. 2015;22(1-2):83–88. https://doi.org/10.1159/000362731. Published online September 12, 2014.
3. Miyasaka T, Dobashi-Okuyama K, Takahashi T, et al. The interplay between neuroendocrine activity and psychological stress-induced exacerbation of allergic asthma. *Allergol Int*. 2018;67(1):32–42. https://doi.org/10.1016/j.alit.2017.04.013. Published online May 20, 2017.
4. Straub RH, Cutolo M. Psychoneuroimmunology-developments in stress research. *Wien Med Wochenschr*. 2018;168(3-4):76–84. https://doi.org/10.1007/s10354-017-0574-2. Published online June 9, 2017.
5. J Orthop Sports Phys Ther 49(5):CPG1-CPG85, 2019. doi:10.2519/jospt.2019.0301
6. Diseases of Muscle Accessed November 24. In: Ropper AH, Samuels MA, Klein JP, Prasad S, eds. *Adams and Victor's Principles of Neurology, 11e*. : McGraw-Hill; 2020.
7. Douglas VC, Aminoff MJ. Myopathic Disorders. In: Papadakis MA, McPhee SJ, Rabow MW, eds. *Current Medical Diagnosis & Treatment*. : McGraw-Hill; 2021.
8. Yeter HH. Endocrine myopathies: clinical review. *Endocrinol Metab Synd*. 2015;4:178.
9. Sharma V, Borah P, Basumatary L, et al. Myopathies of endocrine disorders: a prospective clinical and biochemical study. *Ann Indian Acad Neurol*. Jul-Sept 2014;17(3):298–302.
10. Schnetzler KA. Acute carpal tunnel syndrome. *J Am Acad Orthop Surg*. 2008;16:276–282.
11. Palmer KT. Carpal tunnel syndrome and its relation to occupation: a systematic literature review. *Occup Med*. 2007;57:57–66.
12. Bickel KD. Carpal tunnel syndrome. *J Hand Surg*. 2010;35A:147–152.
13. Lozano-Calderon S. The quality and strength of evidence for etiology: example of carpal tunnel syndrome. *J Hand Surg*. 2008;33A(4):525–538.
14. Song CH, Gong HS, Bae KJ, et al. Evaluation of female hormone-related symptoms in women undergoing carpal tunnel release. *J Hand Surg Eur*. Feb 2014;39(2):155–160.
15. Erickson M, Lawrence M, Jansen CWS, et al. Hand Pain and Sensory Deficits: Carpal Tunnel Syndrome. *J Orthop Sports Phys Ther*. 2019;49(5):CPG1–CPG85. https://doi.org/10.2519/jospt.2019.0301. PMID: 31039690.
16. Michlovitz S. Conservative interventions for carpal tunnel syndrome. *J Orthop Sports Phys Ther*. 2004;34(10):591–598.
17. Ghasemi-rad M, Nosair E, Vegh A, et al. A handy review of carpal tunnel syndrome: from anatomy to diagnosis and treatment. *World J Radiol*. 2014;6(6):284–300.
18. Kodaira M, et al. Non-senile wild-type transthyretin systemic amyloidosis presenting as bilateral carpal tunnel syndrome. *J Peripher Nerv Syst*. 2008;13:148–150.
19. Karadag O, Kalyoncu U, Akdogan A, et al. Sonographic assessment of carpal tunnel syndrome in rheumatoid arthritis: prevalence and correlation with disease activity. *Rheumatol Int*. 2012;32(8):2313–2319.
20. Donnelly JP, Hanna M, Sperry BW, et al. Carpal Tunnel Syndrome: A Potential Early, Red-Flag Sign of Amyloidosis. *J Hand Surg Am*. 2019;44(10):868–876. https://doi.org/10.1016/j.jhsa.2019.06.016. Published online August 7, 2019.
21. Harvie P, Pollard TC, Carr AJ. Calcific tendinitis: natural history and association with endocrine disorders. *J Shoulder Elbow Surg*. 2007;16(2):169–173.
22. Pasquotti G, Faccinetto A, Marchioro U, et al. US-guided percutaneous treatment and physical therapy in rotator cuff calcific

tendinopathy of the shoulder: outcome at 3 and 12 months. *Eur Radiol*. 2016;26(8):2819–2827.
23. Silvestri E, Barile A, Albano D, et al. Interventional therapeutic procedures in the musculoskeletal system: an Italian survey by the Italian College of Musculoskeletal Radiology. *La Radiologia Medica*. 2018;123(4):314–321. https://doi.org/10.1007/s11547-017-0842-7.
24. Serafini G, Sconfienza LM, Lacelli F, et al. Rotator cuff calcific tendonitis: short-term and 10-year outcomes after two-needle us-guided percutaneous treatment--nonrandomized controlled trial. *Radiology*. 2009;252(1):157–164. https://doi.org/10.1148/radiol.2521081816.
25. Albano D, Gambino A, Messina C, et al. Ultrasound-Guided Percutaneous Irrigation of Rotator Cuff Calcific Tendinopathy (US-PICT): Patient Experience. *Biomed Res Int*. 2020:3086395 https://doi.org/10.1155/2020/3086395. PMID: 32596294; PMCID: PMC7303755.
26. Krishnan Y, Grodzinsky AJ. Cartilage diseases. *Matrix Biol*. 2018;71-72:51–69. https://doi.org/10.1016/j.matbio.2018.05.005. Published online May 24, 2018.
27. Keenan RT, Krasnokutsky S, Pillinger MH. Gout, Pseudogout, and Osteoarthritis. In: McKean SC, Ross JJ, Dressler DD, Scheurer DB, eds. *Principles and Practice of Hospital Medicine, 2e*. : McGraw-Hill; 2017.
28. Macmullan P, McCarthy G. Treatment and management of pseudogout: insights for the clinician. *Ther Adv Musculoskelet Dis*. 2012;4(2):121–131. https://doi.org/10.1177/1759720X11432559.
29. Becker M.A.: Patient Information: Pseudogout: Beyond the Basic. UptoDate. Available online at http://www.uptodate.com/contents/pseudogout-beyond-the-basics. Accessed December 29, 2020.
30. Anbari K.K.: Pseudogout Cases. Arthritis-health. Available online at http://www.arthritis-health.com/types/pseudogout-cppd/pseudogout-causes. Accessed December 29, 2020.
31. John DR, Pokhraj P. Radiologic features of hypoparathyroidism. *Pol J Rad*. 2016;81:42–45.
32. Kiani J, Goharifar H, Moghimbeigi A, et al. Prevalence and risk factors of five most common upper extremity disorders in diabetics. *J Res Health Sci*. 2014;14(1):92–95.
33. Magnusson K, Bech Holte K, Juel NG, et al. Long term type 1 diabetes is associated with hand pain, disability and stiffness but not with structural hand osteoarthritis features - The Dialong hand study. *PLoS One 16*. 2017;12(5):e0177118.
34. Barrett KE, Barman SM, Boitano S, et al. General principles and energy production in medical physiology. In: Barrett KE, Barman SM, Boitano S, eds. *Ganong's Review of Medical Physiology*. ed 26 New York, NY: McGraw-Hill; 2019.
35. Else T, Hammer GD. Disorders of the Hypothalamus & Pituitary Gland. In: Hammer GD, McPhee SJ, eds. *Pathophysiology of Disease: An Introduction to Clinical Medicine, 8e*. : McGraw-Hill; 2019.
36. Killinger Z, Kužma M, Sterančáková L, et al. Osteoarticular changes in acromegaly. *Int J Endocrinol*. 2012:2012.
37. Vilar L, Vilar CF, Lyra R, et al. Acromegaly: clinical features at diagnosis. *Pituitary*. 2017;20(1):22–32. https://doi.org/10.1007/s11102-016-0772-8. PMID: 27812777.
38. McNab T, Khandwala H. Acromegaly as an endocrine form of myopathy: a case report and review of the literature. *Endocr Prac*. 2005;11(1):18–22.
39. Alcalar N, Camliguney AF, et al. Impact of exercise on quality of life and body-self perception of patients with acromegaly. *Pituitary*. 2014;17(1):38–43.
40. Mader R, Verlaan JJ, Buskila D. Diffuse idiopathic skeletal hyperostosis: clinical features and pathogenic mechanisms. *Nature Reviews Rheumatology*. 2013;9:741–750.
41. Husebye ES, Allolio B, Arlt W, Badenhoop K, et al. Consensus statement on the diagnosis, treatment and follow-up of patients with primary adrenal insufficiency. *J Intern Med*.

2014;275(2):104–115. https://doi.org/10.1111/joim.12162. Epub 2013 Dec 16. PMID: 24330030.

42. Cam H.: Endogenous Cushing Syndrome. Medscape. Available online at http://emedicine.medscape.com/article/2233083-overview. Accessed December 29, 2020.

43. Holcomb SS. Detecting thyroid disease. *Nursing*. 2005;35(10):S4–S9. 2005.

44. The thyroid and you: coping with a common condition: NIH Medicine Plus, *Spring*, 2012. Available online at https://medlineplus.gov/magazine/issues/spring12/articles/spring12pg22-23.html. Accessed December 29, 2020.

45. Ittermann T, Völzke H, Baumeister SE, et al. Diagnosed thyroid disorders are associated with depression and anxiety. *Soc Psychiatry Psychiatr Epidemiol*. 2015;50:1417.

46. Papaleontiou M, Haymart MR. Approach to and treatment of thyroid disorders in the elderly. *Med Clin N Am*. 2012;96(2):297–310.

47. Rehman S, Cope DW, Senseney AD, et al. Thyroid disorders in elderly patients. *South Med J*. 2005;98(5):543–549.

48. González-Rodríguez LA, Felici-Giovanini ME, Haddock L. Thyroid dysfunction in an adult female population: a population-based study of Latin American vertebral osteoporosis study (LAVOS) - Puerto Rico site. *Hypothyroidism P R Health Sci J*. June 2013;32(2):57–62.

49. Linde J, Friis T. Osteoporosis in hyperthyroidism estimated by photon absorptiometry. *Acta Endocrinol*. 1979;91(3):437–448.

50. Eriksen EF. Normal and pathological remodeling of human trabecular bone: three-dimensional reconstruction of the remodeling sequence in normals and in metabolic bone disease. *Endocr Rev*. 1986;7(4):379–408.

51. Schneider D, Barrett-Connor EL, Morton DJ. Thyroid hormone use and bone mineral density in elderly women effects of estrogen. *JAMA*. 1994;271(16):1245–1249.

52. Bilge M, Adas M, Yanmaz MN, et al. Fibromyalgia in patients with euthyroid Hashimoto's thyroiditis. *Ann Rheum Dis*. 2015;74:310.

53. Bazzichi L, Rossi A, Zirafa C, et al. Thyroid autoimmunity may represent a predisposition for the development of fibromyalgia? *Rheumatol Int*. 2012;32:335.

54. Potassium Iodide (KI). Radiation Emergency Medical Management. Available online at https://www.remm.nlm.gov/potassiumiodide.htm. Accessed December 29, 2020.

55. Gagel RF, Goepfert H, Callender DL. Changing concepts in the pathogenesis and management of thyroid carcinoma. *CA Cancer J Clin*. 1996;46(5):261–283.

56. MacKenzie-Feder J, Sirrs S, Anderson D, et al. Primary hyperparathyroidism: an overview. *Int J Endocrinol*. 2011:2011.

57. Burrows NR. Incidence of end-stage renal disease attributed to diabetes among persons with diagnosed diabetes in the United States and Puerto Rico. *MMWR*. 2010;59(42):1361–1366.

58. Centers for Disease Control and Prevention November is American diabetes month. *MMWR*. 2010;59(42):1361.

59. Nguyen TT, Ta QTH, Nguyen TKO, et al. Type 3 Diabetes and Its Role Implications in Alzheimer's Disease. *Int J Mol Sci*. 2020;21(9):3165 https://doi.org/10.3390/ijms21093165. Published online April 30, 2020.

60. de la Monte SM, Wands JR. Alzheimer's disease is type 3 diabetes-evidence reviewed. *J Diabetes Sci Technol*. 2008;2(6):1101–1113. https://doi.org/10.1177/193229680800200619.

61. Wood L, Setter SM. Type 3 diabetes: brain diabetes? *US Pharm*. 2010;35(5):36–41.

62. Diabetes: National Diabetes Fact Sheet for the United States. Available online at http://www.cdc.gov/diabetes/statistics/index.htm. December 29, 2020.

63. Choi SH, Kim TH, Lim S, et al. Hemoglobin A_{1c} as a diagnostic tool for diabetes screening and new-onset diabetes prediction: a 6-year community-based prospective study. *Diabetes Care*. Apr 2011;34(4):944–949.

64. International Expert Committee International Expert Committee report on the role of the A1C assay in the diagnosis of diabetes. *Diabetes Care*. 2009;32(7):1327–1334.

65. Centers for Disease Control and Prevention (CDC) Number of Americans with diabetes projected to double or triple by 2050. *Older, more diverse populations and longer lifespans contribute to increase*. October 22, 2010 Available online at. http://www.cdc.gov/media/pressrel/2010/r101022.html. Accessed December 29, 2020.

66. Dempsey PD, Owen N, Biddle SJH, et al. Managing sedentary behavior to reduce the risk of diabetes and cardiovascular disease. *Curr Diabetes Rep*. Sept 2014;14:522.

67. U.S. Renal Data System *USRDS 2014 annual data report: Atlas of chronic kidney disease and end-stage renal disease in the United States. National Institutes of Health, National Institute of Diabetes and Digestive and Kidney Diseases*. MD: Bethesda; 2014.

68. Villarivera C, Wolcott J, Jain A, et al. The US Preventive Services Task Force Should Consider A Broader Evidence Base In Updating Its Diabetes Screening Guidelines. *Health Aff*. 2012;31(1):35–42. http://content.healthaffairs.org/content/31/1/35.abstract.

69. van Dooren FEP, Nefs G, Schram MT, et al. Depression and risk of mortality in people with diabetes mellitus: a systematic review and meta-analysis. *PLoS ONE*. 2013;8(3):e57058.

70. Alzoubi A, Abunaser R, Khassawneh A, et al. The Bidirectional Relationship between Diabetes and Depression: A Literature Review. *Korean J Fam Med*. 2018;39(3):137–146. https://doi.org/10.4082/kjfm.2018.39.3.137.

71. Ducat L, Philipson LH, Anderson BJ. The mental health comorbidities of diabetes. *JAMA 20*. 2014;312(7):691–692. https://doi.org/10.1001/jama.2014.8040. PMID: 25010529; PMCID: PMC4439400.

72. Ciechanowski P, Russo J, Katon W, et al. Where is the patient? The association of psychosocial factors and missed primary care appointments in patients with diabetes. *Gen Hosp Psychiatry*. 2006;28(1):9–17.

73. Katon W, Cantrell CR, Sokol MC, et al. Impact of antidepressant drug adherence on comorbid medication use and resource utilization. *Arch Intern Med*. 2005;165(21):2497–2503.

74. Fisher L, Gonzalez JS, Polonsky WH. The confusing tale of depression and distress in patients with diabetes: a call for greater clarity and precision. *Diabet Med*. 2014;31(7):764–772. https://doi.org/10.1111/dme.12428.

75. Fisher L, Mullan JT, Arean P, et al. Diabetes distress but not clinical depression or depressive symptoms is associated with glycemic control in both cross-sectional and longitudinal analyses. *Diabetes Care*. 2010;33(1):23–28.

76. Barclay L. Modifiable Risk Factors May Be Linked to Risk of Developing Diabetic Neuropathy, *Medscape*, 2005. Available online at http://www.medscape.org/viewarticle/498185. Accessed July 29, 2016.

77. Tesfaye S, Chaturvedi N, Eaton SE, et al. Vascular risk factors and diabetic neuropathy. *N Engl J Med*. 2005;352(4):341–350.

78. Jaiswal M, Divers J, Dabelea D, et al. Prevalence of and risk factors for diabetic peripheral neuropathy in youth with type 1 and type 2 diabetes: SEARCH for Diabetes in Youth Study. *Diabetes Care*. 2017;40:1226–1232.

79. Said G. Diabetic neuropathy—a review. *Nat Clin Pract Neurol*. 2007;3(6):331–340.

80. Cagliero E, Apruzzese W, Perlmutter GS. Watch for hand, shoulder disorders in patients with diabetes. *Am J Med*. 2002;112:487–490.

81. Cullen A, Ofloglu O, Donthineni R. Neuropathic arthropathy of the shoulder, Charcot shoulder. *Medscape*. 2005;7(1).

82. Silva NCM, Chaves ECL, Carvalho EC, et al. Instrument for assessing tissue integrity of the feet of patients with diabetes mellitus. *Acta Paul Enferm*. 2013;26(6):535–541.

83. Gibbons CH, Freeman R. Treatment induced diabetic neuropathy—a reversible painful autonomic neuropathy. *Ann Neurol.* 2010;67(4):534–541.

84. Garcilazo C, Cavallasca JA, Musuruana JL. Shoulder manifestations of diabetes mellitus. *Curr Diabetes Rev.* 2010;6(5):334–340.

85. Melling M, Reihsner R, Pfeiler W, et al. Comparison of palmar aponeuroses from individuals with diabetes mellitus and Dupuytren's contracture. *Anat Rec.* 1999;255(4):401–406. doi: 10.1002/(SICI)1097_0185(19990801)255:4<401::AID_AR6> 3.0.CO;2_D. PMID: 10409813.

86. Choi JH, Yu KP, Yoon YS. Relationship Between HbA1c and Complex Regional Pain Syndrome in Stroke Patients With Type 2 Diabetes Mellitus. *Ann Rehabil Med.* 2016;40(5):779–785. https://doi.org/10.5535/arm.2016.40.5.779.

87. American Diabetes Association Standards of medical care in diabetes—2014. *Diabetes Care.* 2014;37(Suppl 1):S14–S80.

88. Type 2 diabetes. Mayo Clinic. Available online at http://www.mayoclinic.org/diseases-conditions/type-2-diabetes/diagnosis-treatment/diagnosis/dxc-20169894. Accessed December 29, 2020.

89. American Diabetes Association's Standards of Medical Care in Diabetes—2020. *Diabetes Care.* 2020;43(Suppl. 1):S1–S212.

90. Handelsman Y, Bloomgarden ZT, Grunberger G, et al. American association of clinical endocrinologists and American college of endocrinology—clinical practice guidelines for developing a diabetes mellitus comprehensive care plan – 2015. *Endocr Pract.* 2015;21 (Suppl 1(Suppl 1):1–87. https://doi.org/10.4158/EP15672.GL.

91. Pearson T.L. Initiating Insulin in the Type 2 Diabetes Patient. Medscape. Available online at http://www.medscape.org/viewarticle/567952. Accessed July 29, 2013.

92. Redmon B., Caccamo D., Flavin P. et al. Institute for Clinical Systems Improvement. Diagnosis and Management of Type 2 Diabetes Mellitus in Adults. Updated July 2014. Available online at https://www.icsi.org/_asset/3rrm36/Diabetes.pdf. Accessed July 29, 2016.

93. Colberg S. Exercising With an Insulin Pump. Diabetes Self-Management. Available online at http://www.diabetes-selfmanagement.com/nutrition-exercise/exercise/exercising-with-an-insulin-pump/. Accessed December 29, 2020.

94. Dehydration. Mayo Clinic. Available online at http://www.mayoclinic.org/diseases-conditions/dehydration/basics/definition/con-20030056. Accessed December 29, 2020.

95. What is Metabolic Syndrome? National Heart, Lung, and Blood Institute. Available online at http://www.nhlbi.nih.gov/health/health-topics/topics/ms. Accessed December 29, 2020.

96. About Metabolic Syndrome. American Heart Association. Available online at https://www.heart.org/HEARTORG/Conditions/More/MetabolicSyndrome/About-Metabolic-Syndrome_UCM_301920_Article.jsp. Accessed December 29, 2020.

97. Hak EA, Curham GC, Grodtein F, et al. Menopause, postmenopausal hormone use and risk of incident gout. *Ann Rheum Dis.* 2010;69(7):1305–1309.

98. Kurakula PC, Keenan RT. Diagnosis and management of gout: an update. *J Musculoskel Med.* 2010;27(Suppl):S13–S19.

99. Choi HK. A prescription for lifestyle change in patients with hyperuricemia and gout. *Curr Opin Rheumatol.* 2010;22(2): 165–172.

100. Gout: Centers for Disease Control and Prevention. http://www.cdc.gov/arthritis/basics/gout.html. Accessed December 29, 2020.

101. Singh JA, Reddy SG, Kundukulam J. Risk factors for gout and prevention: a systematic review of the literature. *Curr Opin Rheumatol.* Mar 2011;23(2):192–202.

102. Gout: Mayo Clinic. Available online at http://www.mayoclinic.org/diseases-conditions/gout/basics/treatment/con-20019400. Accessed December 29, 2020.

103. Pseudogout: Mayo Clinic. Available online at http://www.mayoclinic.org/diseases-conditions/pseudogout/basics/definition/con-20028152. Accessed December 29, 2020.

104. Hemochromatosis: National Institute of Diabetes and Digestive and Kidney Diseases. Available online at https://www.niddk. nih.gov/health-information/health-topics/liver-disease/hemochromatosis/Pages/facts.aspx. Accessed December 29, 2020.

105. Consensus Development Conference Diagnosis, prophylaxis, and treatment of osteoporosis. *Am J Med.* 1993;94:646–650.

106. Dobbs MB, Buckwalter J, Saltzman C. Osteoporosis: the increasing role of the orthopaedist. *Iowa Orthop J.* 1999;19:43–52.

107. Elliott ME, Drinka PJ, Krause P, et al. Osteoporosis assessment strategies for male nursing home residents. *Maturitas.* 2004;48(3):225–233.

108. National Osteoporosis Foundation (NOF): What women need to know. Available online at https://www.nof.org/prevention/general-facts/what-women-need-to-know/. Accessed December 29, 2020.

109. The WHO Study Group *Assessment of fracture risk and its application to screening for postmenopausal osteoporosis.* Geneva: WHO Technical Report Series 843, World Health Organization; 1994.

110. Lydick E, Cook K, Turpin J, et al. Development and validation of a simple questionnaire to facilitate identification of women likely to have low bone density. *Am J Man Care.* 1998;4:37–48.

111. WHO Fracture Risk Assessment: World Health Organization. Available online at http://www.shef.ac.uk/FRAX/. Accessed December 29, 2020.

112. Osteoporosis: Screening. United States Preventive Services Task Force. Available online at http://www.uspreventiveservicestask-force.org/Page/Document/UpdateSummaryFinal/osteoporosis-screening?ds=1&s=osteoporosis. Accessed December 29, 2020.

113. Curry S.J., Krist A.H., Owens D.K. et al.: Screening for Osteoporosis to Prevent Fractures: US Preventive Services Task Force Recommendation Statement, *JAMA* 26;319(24):2521-2531, 2018. doi: 10.1001/jama.2018.7498. PMID: 29946735.

114. Osteoporosis Health Care: WebMD. Available online at http://www.webmd.com/osteoporosis/features/alcohol. Accessed December 29, 2020.

115. Osteoporosis Overview: National Institute of Health Osteoporosis and Related Bone Diseases National Resource Center. Available online at http://www.niams.nih.gov/health_info/bone/osteoporosis/overview.asp. Accessed December 29, 2020.

116. Hallstrom H, Byberg L, Glynn A, et al. Long-term coffee consumption in relation to fracture risk and bone mineral density in women. *Am J Epidemiol.* 2013;178(6):898–909.

117. Smoking and Bone Health: National Institute of Health Osteoporosis and Related Bone Diseases National Resource Center. Available online at http://www.niams.nih.gov/health_info/bone/Osteoporosis/conditions_Behaviors/bone_smoking.asp#b. Accessed December 29, 2020.

118. Rao S.S.: Osteoporosis in Men. American Family Physician. Available online at http://www.aafp.org/afp/2010/0901/p503. html. Accessed December 29, 2020.

119. Facts and Statistics: International Osteoporosis Foundation. Available online at https://www.iofbonehealth.org/facts-statistics. Accessed December 29, 2020.

120. Antony LA, Iyer LS. Effectiveness of integrated soft tissue mobilization on the functional outcome in chronic low back pain patients. *J Exer Sci Physiother.* 2013;9(1):57–68.

121. Hayden JA, Van Tulder MW, Malmivaara AV, et al. Meta-analysis: exercise therapy for non-specific low back pain. *Ann Intern Med.* 2005;142(9):765–775.

122. Heggeness MH. Spinal fracture with neurological deficit in osteoporosis. *Osteoporos Int.* 1993;3(4):215–221.

123. D'Costa H, George G, Parry M, et al. Pitfalls in the clinical diagnosis of vertebral fractures: a case series in which posterior midline tenderness was absent. *Emerg Med J.* 2005;22:330–332.

124. Nevitt MC, Ettinger B, Black DM, et al. The association of radiographically detected vertebral fractures with back pain and function: a prospective study. *Ann Intern Med.* 1998;128(10):793–800.

125. Fink HA, Milaetz DL, Palermo L, et al. What proportion of incident radiographic vertebral deformities is clinically diagnosed and vice versa? *J Bone Miner Res.* 2005;20(7):1216–1222.

126. Alexandru D, So W. Evaluation and management of vertebral compression fractures. *Permanente J.* 2012;4(16):46–51.

127. Uday S, Högler W. Nutritional Rickets and Osteomalacia in the Twenty-first Century: Revised Concepts, Public Health, and Prevention Strategies. *Curr Osteoporos Rep.* 2017 Aug;15(4):293–302. https://doi.org/10.1007/s11914-017-0383-y. Erratum in: Curr Osteoporos Rep. 2017 Aug 14;: PMID: 28612338; PMCID: PMC5532418.

128. Nebot Valenzuela E, Pietschmann P. Epidemiology and pathology of Paget's disease of bone - a review. Epidemiologie und Pathologie des Morbus Paget – ein Überblick. *Wien Med Wochenschr.* 2017;167(1-2):2–8. https://doi.org/10.1007/s10354-016-0496-4.

129. Alikhan M.: Paget Disease. Medscape. Available online at http://emedicine.medscape.com/article/334607-overview. Accessed December 29, 2020.

130. Paget's Disease of the Bone: American College of Rheumatology. Available online at http://www.rheumatology.org/I-Am-A/Patient-Caregiver/Diseases-Conditions/Pagets-Disease-of-Bone. Accessed December 29, 2020.

131. Hansen D, Peeters S, Zwaenepoel B, et al. Exercise assessment and prescription in patients with type 2 diabetes in the private and home care setting: clinical recommendations from AXXON (Belgian Physical Therapy Association. *Phys Ther.* 2013;93(5):597–610. https://doi.org/10.2522/ptj.20120400. Epub 2013 Feb 7. PMID: 23392184.

CHAPTER

13

Screening for Immunologic Disease

Erin Green and William Garcia

Immunology, one of the few disciplines with a full range of involvement in all aspects of health and disease, is one of the most rapidly expanding fields in medicine. Staying current is difficult at best, considering the volume of new immunologic information generated by clinical researchers each year. The information presented here is a simplistic representation of the immune system, with the main focus on screening for immune-induced signs and symptoms mimicking neuromuscular or musculoskeletal dysfunction.

Immunity denotes protection against infectious organisms. The immune system is a complex network of specialized organs and cells that has evolved to defend the body against attacks by "foreign" invaders. Immunity is provided by lymphoid cells residing in the immune system. This system consists of central and peripheral lymphoid organs (Fig. 13.1).

By circulating its component cells and substances, the immune system maintains an early warning defense system against both exogenous microorganisms (infections produced by bacteria, viruses, parasites, and fungi) and endogenous cells that have become neoplastic.

The immune system includes both the innate or nonspecific immunity, which consists of external barriers such as skin and mucosal membranes, and the adaptive immunity. Immunologic responses by adaptive immunity in humans can be divided into two broad categories: humoral immunity, which takes place in the body fluids (extracellular) and is concerned with antibody and complement activities, and cell-mediated or cellular immunity, primarily intracellular, which involves a variety of activities designed to destroy, or at least contain, cells that are recognized by the body as being alien and harmful. Both types of responses are initiated by lymphocytes and are discussed in the context of lymphocytic function.

USING THE SCREENING MODEL

As always, in the screening evaluation of any client, the medical history is the most important variable, followed by any red flags in the clinical presentation and an assessment of associated signs and symptoms. Many immune system disorders have a unique chronology or sequence of events that define them. When the immune system may be involved, some important questions to ask include the following:

- How long have you had this problem? (acute versus chronic)
- Has the problem gone away and then recurred?
- Have additional symptoms developed or have other areas become symptomatic over time?
- How is/has this condition been previously managed? Are you currently receiving treatment?

PAST MEDICAL HISTORY

As mentioned, the environmental and family history is important when assessing the role of the immune system in presenting signs and symptoms. For example, persons with firbromyalgia or chronic widespread pain may have a history of sleep disorders, anxiety and depression, other musculoskeletal disorder, or other medical disorders such as gastrointestinal (GI) disorders.[17]

Clients with systemic inflammatory disorders may have a family history of an identical or related disorder such as rheumatoid arthritis (RA), systemic lupus erythematosus (SLE), autoimmune thyroid disease, multiple sclerosis (MS), or myasthenia gravis (MG). Other rheumatic diseases that are often genetically linked include seronegative spondyloarthritis.

There is an increased rate of disease in twins and first-degree relatives with seronegative spondyloarthrititis.[1] The seronegative spondyloarthritides include a wide range of diseases linked by common characteristics such as inflammatory spine involvement (e.g., sacroiliitis, spondylitis), asymmetric peripheral arthritis, enthesopathy, inflammatory eye disease, and musculoskeletal and cutaneous features. All of these changes occur in the absence of serum rheumatoid factor (RF), which is present in about 80% of people with RA.[2] This group of diseases includes ankylosing spondylitis (AS), reactive arthritis (ReA), psoriatic arthritis (PsA), and arthritis associated with inflammatory bowel disease (IBD; such as Crohn's disease or ulcerative colitis). A recent history of surgery may be indicative of bacterial or ReA, which requires immediate medical evaluation.

RISK FACTOR ASSESSMENT

The cause and risk factors for many conditions related to immune system dysfunction remain unknown. Past medical history with a positive family history for systemic inflammatory or related disorders may be the only available red flag in this area.

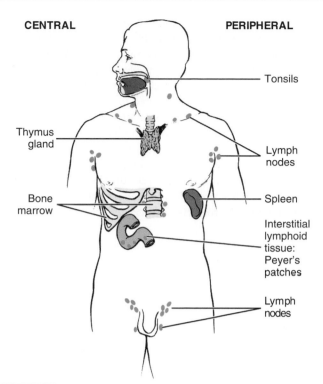

CENTRAL   **PERIPHERAL**

Tonsils

Thymus gland

Lymph nodes

Bone marrow

Spleen

Interstitial lymphoid tissue: Peyer's patches

Lymph nodes

Fig. 13.1 Major organs of the immune system. Two thirds of the immune system resides in the intestines (intestinal lymphoid tissue), emphasizing the importance of diet and nutrition on immune function.

CLINICAL PRESENTATION

Symptoms of rheumatic disorders often include soft tissue and/or joint pain, stiffness, swelling, weakness, constitutional symptoms, Raynaud's phenomenon, and sleep disturbances. Inflammatory disorders, such as RA and polymyalgia rheumatica (PMR), are marked by prolonged *stiffness* in the morning lasting more than 1 hour. This stiffness is relieved with activity, but it recurs after the person sits down and subsequently attempts to resume activity. This is referred to as the *gel phenomenon.*

Specific arthropathies have a predilection for involving specific joint areas. For example, involvement of the wrists and proximal small joints of the hands and feet is a typical feature of RA. RA tends to involve joint groups symmetrically, whereas the seronegative spondyloarthritides tend to be asymmetric. PsA often involves the distal joints of the hands and feet.[3]

In anyone with *swelling*, especially single-joint swelling, it is necessary to distinguish whether this swelling is articular (as in arthritis), periarticular (as in tenosynovitis), involves an entire limb (as with lymphedema), or occurs in another area (such as with lipoma or palpable tumors). The physical therapist will need to assess whether the swelling is intermittent, persistent, symmetric, or asymmetric and whether the swelling is minimal in the morning but worse during the day (as with dependent edema).

Generalized *weakness* is a common symptom of individuals with immune system disorders in the absence of muscle disease. If the weakness involves one limb without evidence of weakness elsewhere, a neurologic disorder may be present. Anyone having trouble performing tasks with the arms raised above the head, difficulty climbing stairs, or problems arising from a low chair may have muscle disease.

Nail bed changes are especially indicative of underlying inflammatory disease. For example, small infarctions or splinter hemorrhages (see Fig. 4.34) occur in endocarditis and systemic vasculitis. Characteristics of systemic sclerosis and limited scleroderma include atrophy of the fingertips, calcific nodules, digital cyanosis, and sclerodactyly (tightening of the skin). Dystrophic nail changes are characteristic of psoriasis. Spongy synovial thickening or bony hypertrophic changes (Bouchard's nodes) are present with RA and other hand deformities.

ASSOCIATED SIGNS AND SYMPTOMS

With few risk factors and only the family history to rely upon, the clinical presentation is very important. Most of the immune system conditions and diseases are accompanied by a variety of associated signs and symptoms. Disease progression is common with different clinical signs and symptoms during the early phase of illness compared with the advanced phase.

REVIEW OF SYSTEMS

With many problems affecting the immune system, taking a step back and reviewing each part of the screening model (history, risk factors, clinical presentation, associated signs and symptoms) may be the only way to identify the source of the underlying problem. Remember to review Box 4.15 during this process.

For anyone with new onset of joint pain, a review of systems should include questions about symptoms or diagnoses involving other organ systems. In particular, the presence of dry, red, or irritated and itching eyes; chest pain with dyspnea; urethral or vaginal discharge; skin rash or photosensitivity; hair loss; diarrhea; or dysphagia should be assessed.

IMMUNE SYSTEM PATHOPHYSIOLOGY

Immune disorders involve dysfunction of the immune response mechanism, causing over responsiveness or blocked, misdirected, or limited responsiveness to antigens. These disorders may result from an unknown cause, developmental defect, infection, malignancy, trauma, metabolic disorder, or drug use. Immunologic disorders may be classified as one of the following:

- Immunodeficiency disorder
- Hypersensitivity disorder
- Autoimmune disorder
- Immunoproliferative disorder

Immunodeficiency Disorders

When the immune system is underactive or hypoactive, it is referred to as being *immunodeficient* or *immunocompromised,* such as occurs in the case of anyone undergoing cancer chemotherapy or taking immunosuppressive drugs after organ transplantation.

Human Immunodeficiency Syndrome

Human immunodeficiency virus (HIV) is a cytopathogenic virus that causes acquired immunodeficiency syndrome (AIDS) and has severe implications for both humoral and cellular immunity. HIV has been identified as the causative agent, its genes have been mapped and analyzed, drugs that act against it have been found and tested, and vaccines against the HIV infection have been under development. The advanced stage of HIV infection is known as AIDS.

Acquired refers to the fact that the disease is not inherited or genetic but develops as a result of a virus. *Immuno* refers to the body's immunologic system and *deficiency* indicates that the immune system is under functioning, resulting in a group of signs or symptoms that occur together called a *syndrome*.

People who are infected with HIV are vulnerable to serious illnesses called *opportunistic* infections or diseases, so named because they use the opportunity of lowered resistance to infect and destroy. These infections and diseases would not be a threat to most individuals whose immune systems function normally. *Pneumocystis carinii* pneumonia continues to be a major cause of morbidity and mortality in the AIDS population.

It is estimated that there are 1.1 million persons living with HIV (PLWH) in the United States, and there were 15,815 deaths of adults and adolescent diagnosed with HIV in 2019 (though it is important to note these deaths can be from any cause). Mortality rates have dramatically reduced since 1996 with the introduction of antiretroviral (ARV) medications, specifically the ARV therapy (ART). Combination ART regimens have not only allowed PLWH to lead healthy lives but also prevent transmission to others, limit opportunistic infection, and reduce viral load count to almost undetectable levels. However, despite a 9% decline in new HIV diagnoses between 2015 and 2019, Black/African-American and Hispanic/Latino people continue to be disproportionately affected by HIV/AIDS compared with other ethnic groups. In 2019, adult and adolescent Black/African-American accounted for 42% of new HIV diagnoses and Hispanic/Latino people accounted for 29% of new HIV diagnoses, but each group accounts for only 13% and 18% percent of the population, respectively. Further, HIV diagnoses are not evenly distributed across regions of the United States. In 2019, the southern states accounted for higher rates of new infection though the mortality rate have decreased in that region compared to previous years. The annual number of infections was decreased in people aged 13–24 and 45–54 years between 2015 and 2019, and has remained stable in people aged 25–34 years.[4] Increased HIV vulnerability is often associated with socioeconomic factors which impact exposure to high-risk situations and access barriers to healthcare.[5]

Risk Factors. Population groups at greatest risk include men having sex with men, people who inject drugs (PWID), people who have sex for money or nonmonetary items and their clients, transgender people, blood recipients, dialysis recipients, organ transplant recipients, fetuses of mothers with HIV infection or babies being breastfed by a mother with HIV infection, and people with sexually transmitted diseases.[6] Though the aforementioned groups have an increased risk of transmission, it should be noted that condomless intercourse (vaginal or anal) is the most common mode of transmission worldwide.[7] In addition, the prevalence rate of people living in urban poverty area is higher (2.1%), and researchers have identified that these prevalence rates are inversely related to socioeconomic status, i.e., lower socioeconomic status is attributed to higher HIV prevalence. Authors recommended both community-level and systemic interventions are necessary to address infection rates in urban areas of poverty in the United States.[8]

Transmission. Transmission occurs through either *horizontal* (from either sexual contact or parenteral exposure to blood and blood products) or *vertical* transmission (from mother with HIV infection to infant). HIV is not transmitted through casual contact, such as the shared use of food, towels, cups, razors, or toothbrushes, or even by kissing. Despite substantial advances in the treatment of HIV, the number of new HIV infections has leveled off at approximately 39,000 infections per year since 2013, but the annual number of new diagnoses has decreased by 9% between 2015 and 2019.[4,8] Prevention of infection transmission by reduction of behaviors that might transmit HIV to others is critical.[9]

Transmission always involves exposure to some body fluid from an infected client. The greatest concentrations of virus have been found in blood, semen, cerebrospinal fluid, and cervical/vaginal secretions. HIV has been found in low concentrations in tears, saliva, and urine, but no cases have been transmitted by these routes. The probability for acquiring HIV from an infected source is highest for blood transfusion, then through receptive anal intercourse, needle sharing during injection drug use, and percutaneous transmission (needle stick)[10] (Table 13.1).

Any injectable drug, legal or illegal, can be associated with HIV transmission. It is not injection drug use that spreads HIV, but the sharing of HIV-infected intravenous (IV) drug needles among individuals. Despite the perception that only IV injection is dangerous, HIV can also be transmitted through subcutaneous and intramuscular injection. Use of needles contaminated with blood for tattooing or body piercing is included in this category.

PWID who sterilize their drug paraphernalia with a 1:10 solution of bleach to water before passing the needles are less likely to spread HIV. Despite the high infection rate among

TABLE 13.1	Risk of HIV Exposure According to Type
Type of Exposure From an HIV-Infected Source (Patel)	Risk per 10,000 Exposures
Blood transfusion	9250
Receptive anal intercourse	138
Needle sharing during injection drug use	63
Percutaneous (needle stick)	23
Insertive anal intercourse	11
Receptive penile-vaginal intercourse	8
Insertive penile-vaginal intercourse	4

PWIDs, the overall rate of new infection in this group was down by 31% in 2018.[11] The increase in the number of comprehensive community-based prevention and intervention programs, also known as Syringe Service Programs, have reduced HIV and other bloodborne infections like hepatitis C virus by an estimated 50%.[12] For further information regarding this or other HIV/AIDS-related questions, contact the CDC-INFO (formerly the CDC National AIDS Hotline) 24 hours/day, 7 days a week, at 1-800-CDC-INFO (1-800-232-4636).

Vertical transmission through maternal-to-child transmission (MCT), can occur during pregnancy, labor, delivery, or breast milk.[13] In the United States, the rate of MCT is < 1% due to routine prenatal HIV testing, rapid testing upon labor and delivery, maternal ART, infant retroviral prophylaxis, use of cesarean section, and formula feeding. Women who are adherent to ART regimens prior to and during pregnancy have very low rates of MCT.[14] Worldwide efforts to reduce MCT are directed toward improved access to ART.[15,16] Unfortunately, prompt HIV diagnosis, disease awareness, adequate prenatal care, and access to ART therapies are not universal, and the rate of MCT can be up to 15%–45% in the untreated population.[17] High MCT rates disproportionately affect non-Caucasian populations.[18] Breastfeeding for HIV-infected women is contraindicated in industrialized nations like the United States. Despite the Centers for Disease Control and Prevention (CDC) recommendations to use formula for feeding, many women, including those in the United States, continue to breastfeed either because of limited access to formula or other social influences. Particularly in resource-poor settings, the reduction of HIV transmission through breast milk remains a significant challenge.[19] However, without intervention, 15% to 30% of infants may become vertically infected, a number which increases to 20% to 45% if breastfeeding is continued.[20] Exclusive breastfeeding for HIV-infected women, even in the absence of ART, is still recommended for infants in low-resource or high-risk areas where contaminated water sources prevent safe use of formula.[18]

Blood and Blood Products. Parenteral transmission occurs when there is direct blood-to-blood contact with a PLWH. This can occur through sharing of contaminated needles and drug paraphernalia, through transfusion of blood or blood products, by accidental needlestick injury to a health care worker, or from blood exposure to non-intact skin or mucous membranes. Health care workers who have contact with individuals with HIV or AIDS and who follow routine instructions for self-protection are a very low-risk group.

Almost all persons with hemophilia born before 1985 have been infected with HIV. Heat-treated factor concentrates, involving a method of chemical and physical processes that completely inactivate HIV, became available in 1985, effectively eliminating the transmission of HIV to anyone with a clotting disorder who is receiving blood or blood products. The risk for acquiring HIV infection through blood transfusion today is estimated conservatively to be less than one in 1 million.[21]

TABLE 13.2	Clinical Signs and Symptoms of HIV
Stage	**Clinical Signs and Symptoms**

Stage 1: Acute HIV infection	– Onset of flu-like symptoms within 2–4 weeks after infection with HIV
	  • Fever
	  • Diarrhea
	  • Malaise and/or fatigue
	  • Myalgias
	– High viral load and very contagious
	– May be unaware of infection

Stage 2: Clinical latency (HIV inactivity or dormancy)	– HIV active but replicating a very low levels – May expressed periods of generalized lymphadenopathy – PLWH may remain in this stage for decades or indefinitely with ART medication – PLWH without ART medication may remain in this stage for a decade or longer or may progress more quickly through this stage – End of this phase marked by increased viral load and decreased CD4 count

Stage 3. Advanced HIV infection (AIDS)	– CD4 count < 200 cells/μL
	– Vulnerable to opportunistic infection and ADC
	– Symptoms include:
	  • HIV-related wasting or dementia
	  • Weight loss or gain
	  • Fatigue
	  • Night sweats
	  • Fever
	  • Thrush or yeast infections
	  • Prolonged recovery from illness

ADC, AIDS-defining cancer; *AIDS*, acquired immunodeficiency syndrome; *ART*, antiretroviral therapy; *HIV*, human immunodeficiency virus; *PLWH*, people living with HIV.

Clinical Signs and Symptoms. Symptoms of HIV vary and are depending on the stage of the infection. There are three stages of infection recognized by the CDC: stage 1, acute HIV infection; stage 2, clinical latency; and stage 3, advanced HIV infection (AIDS)[22,23] (Table 13.2). Early stage 1 symptoms associated with initial HIV viremia may include flu-like symptoms. Many individuals with HIV infection remain asymptomatic for years in stage 2, with a mean time of approximately 10 years between exposure and development of AIDS, and 16% to 18% of PLWH may be unaware of their infection.[24,25] Additionally, over 90% of newly acquired infections were transmitted from people who either were unaware of their infection or not retained in medical care.[25] If untreated, a PLWH can remain in the dormant or chronic phase for variable time periods. Overtime, the viral load will increase and CD4 white cell count will decrease. As CD4 cell count decreases and the immune system is progressively weakened, PLWH may develop other systemic complaints, opportunistic infections, cardiac diseases, brain disease, pulmonary diseases, and/or cancers. With ART, PLWH can remain virally suppressed indefinitely but still may incur complications related to the HIV infection itself or drug treatment toxicity.[6]

Systemic complaints, such as weight loss, fevers, and night sweats, are common. Cough or shortness of breath may occur with HIV-related pulmonary disease. GI complaints include changes in bowel function, especially diarrhea.

Cutaneous complaints are common and include dry skin, new rashes, and nail bed changes. Because virtually all of these findings may be seen with other diseases, a combination of complaints is more suggestive of HIV infection than any one symptom.

Chronic pain occurs in 39% to 85% of PLWH compared with 20% to 30% of the general population.[26] Sources of chronic pain in this population can include musculoskeletal and/or neuropathic. High prevalence of chronic pain in PLWH may be due to HIV itself causing peripheral neuropathic pain; exposure to older HIV medication which can cause peripheral neuropathy (PN); shared risk factors for HIV and chronic pain such as substance abuse and mental illness; and biological mechanisms that may contribute to non-neuropathic chronic pain.[27] Low bone mineral density (BMD), such as osteopenia, osteoporosis, and osteonecrosis, has a higher prevalence in PLWH (people living with HIV). Risk factors may be associated with the HIV disease process and treatment as well as traditional risk factors such as menopause and low body mass index and behavioral risk factors such as smoking, alcohol intake, and sedentary lifestyle.[28] Evidence suggests that PLWH who engage in moderate to vigorous physical activity (≥150 minutes/week) demonstrate increased BMD compared with those who do not engage in the recommended physical activity levels.[29] Physical therapists should conduct a risk factor assessment for bone loss in anyone with a known HIV diagnosis and educate regarding possible prevention strategies.

Any woman at risk for AIDS should be aware of the possibility that recurrent or stubborn cases of vaginal candidiasis may be an early sign of infection with HIV. Pregnancy, diabetes, oral contraceptives, and antibiotics are more commonly linked to these fungal infections.

Side Effects of Medication. Although ART medications provide vital life-long management for PLWH, continual monitoring for adverse drug reactions and risk factors such as other illnesses are required to improve care and safety outcomes.[30] The physical therapist should review the potential side effects and ARV toxicity. Delayed toxicity with long-term treatment of HIV-1 infection with ART occurs in a substantial number of affected individuals.[31,32] The more commonly occurring symptoms include rash, nausea, headaches, dizziness, muscle pain, weakness, fatigue, and insomnia. Symptoms of drug toxicity can also include: electrocardiographic abnormalities, clinical jaundice, central nervous system (CNS) toxicity and mental illness, severe skin hypersensitivity, pancreatitis, gynaecomastia, dyslipidemia, and convulsions.[33] Hepatotoxicity is a common complication; the therapist should be alert for carpal tunnel syndrome, liver palms, asterixis, and other signs of liver impairment (see Chapter 10).

Body fat redistribution to the abdomen, upper body, and breasts occurs as a part of a condition called *lipodystrophy* associated with ART. Other metabolic abnormalities, such as dysregulation of glucose metabolism (e.g., insulin resistance, diabetes), combined with lipodystrophy are labeled lipodystrophic syndrome (LDS). LDS contributes to problems with body image and increases the risk of cardiovascular complications.[34–37]

AIDS and Other Diseases

When left untreated, HIV infection progressively compromises the immune system and PLWH become susceptible to opportunistic infection. The virus results in the destruction of CD4 white blood cells (WBCs). When CD4 counts fall below 200 cell/μL, the immune system is severely compromised and the individual has progressed into stage 3, or AIDS. A person with AIDS has a very high risk for contracting opportunistic infections. AIDS is a unique disease—no other known infectious disease causes its damage through a direct attack on the human immune system. Because the immune system is the final mediator of human host–infectious agent interactions, it was anticipated early that HIV infection would complicate the course of other serious human diseases.

This has proved to be the case, particularly for tuberculosis (TB) and certain sexually transmitted infections such as syphilis and the genital herpes virus. Cancer has been linked to AIDS since 1981; this link was discovered with the increased appearance of a highly unusual malignancy, Kaposi's sarcoma (KS). Since then, HIV infection has been associated with other malignancies, including both AIDS-defining cancers (ADCs) such as KS, non-Hodgkin's lymphoma (NHL), and cervical cancer and non-AIDs defining cancers like anal, liver, and lung cancers.[38] Research is currently unclear as to why these cancers have increased, but there are known associations with other viral infections including the human papilloma virus, hepatitis B, hepatitis C, and Epstein-Barr virus. Since ART was introduced, the rate of ADCs has decreased but remain higher than that of the general population.[39,40] However, due to the increased incidence of cancer in this population, adequate screening during the physical therapist examination is of great importance. Finally, in addition to TB, syphilis, and herpes simplex virus 1, other opportunistic infections can include: bacterial pneumonia, GI disorders, skin infections, salmonella, toxoplasmosis, and bacterial lymphadenopathy.[41,42]

Kaposi's Sarcoma. Classic KS was first recognized as a malignant tumor of the inner walls of the heart, veins, and arteries in 1873 in Vienna, Austria. Before the AIDS epidemic, KS was a rare tumor that primarily affected older people of Mediterranean and Jewish origin.

Clinically, KS in HIV-infected immunodeficient persons occurs more often as purplish-red lesions of the feet, trunk, and head (Fig. 13.2). The lesion is not painful or contagious. It can be flat or raised and over time frequently progresses to a nodule. The mouth and many internal organs (especially those of the GI and respiratory tracts) may be involved either symptomatically or subclinically.

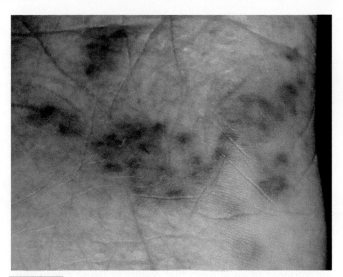

Fig. 13.2 AIDS-related Kaposi's sarcoma. The early lesions appear most commonly on the toes or soles as reddish or bluish-black macules and patches that spread and coalesce to form nodules or plaques. Lesions can appear anywhere on the body including the tongue and genitals. (From James WD, Andrews' Diseases of the Skin: Clinical Dermatology. 10th ed. WB Saunders: Philadelphia; 2006.)

Prognosis depends on the status of the individual's immune system. People who die of AIDS usually succumb to opportunistic infections rather than to KS.

Non-Hodgkin's Lymphoma. People diagnosed with HIV have an increased incidence of NHL, particularly the AIDS-defining subtypes: Burkitt's lymphoma, diffuse large B-cell lymphoma, and primary lymphomas of the CNS.[43] The incidence of NHL increases with age and as the immune system weakens. The lifetime risks for people with HIV developing NHL is roughly about 1 in 25.[44]

These malignancies are difficult to treat because clients often cannot tolerate the further immunosuppression that treatment causes. As with KS, prognosis depends largely on the initial level of immunity. Clients with an adequate immune reserve may tolerate therapy and respond reasonably well. However, in people with severe immunodeficiency, survival is only 4 to 7 months on average. Clients diagnosed with HIV-related brain lymphomas have a very poor prognosis.

Tuberculosis. TB was considered a stable, endemic health problem, but now, in association with the HIV/AIDS pandemic, TB is resurgent.[45] The recent emergence of multi-drug-resistant TB bacteria, which has reached epidemic proportions in New York City, has created a serious and growing threat to the capacity of TB control programs.

In urban areas of the United States, the present upsurge in TB cases is occurring among young (aged 25–44 years) PWIDs, ethnic minorities, prisoners and prison staff (because of poorly ventilated and overcrowded prison systems), homeless people, and immigrants from countries with a high prevalence of TB. Since the peak of the TB resurgence in 1992 until 2018, the number of reported TB cases in the United States has decreased annually by 66%.[46] In the United States, foreign-born people are disproportionately affected by TB

to constitute 70.2% of the total cases identified, with people immigrating from Mexico, the Philippines, India, Vietnam, and China being the most frequently found to have TB.[47]

The first major interaction between HIV and TB occurs as a result of the weakening of the immune system in association with progressive HIV infection. The great majority of individuals exposed to TB are infected but not clinically ill. Their subclinical TB infection is kept in check by an active, healthy immune system. However, when a person with TB infection becomes infected with HIV, the immune system begins to decline, and at a certain level of immunocompromise due to HIV, the TB bacteria become active, resulting in clinical pulmonary TB. Globally, TB is thought to be the leading cause of HIV/AIDS-related deaths,[48] and is the only opportunistic infection associated with AIDS/HIV that is directly transmissible to household and other contacts. Therefore, each individual case of active TB is a threat to community health.

Pulmonary TB is the most common manifestation of TB disease in HIV-positive clients. When TB precedes the diagnosis of AIDS, disease is usually confined to the lung, whereas when TB is diagnosed after the onset of AIDS, the majority of clients also have extrapulmonary TB, most commonly involving the bone marrow or lymph nodes.[49] Fever, night sweats, wasting, cough, and dyspnea occur in the majority of clients (see further discussion of TB in Chapter 8).

HIV-Associated Neurologic Disease. HIV-associated neurologic disease may be the presenting symptom of HIV infection and can involve the CNS and peripheral nervous system (PNS). HIV is a neurotropic virus and can affect neurologic tissues from the initial stages of infection. In the early course of the infection, the virus can cause demyelination of CNS and PNS tissues.[50] HIV-associated neurocognitive disorders (HAND) describes the variety of neurocognitive deficits associated with the HIV infection.[51] Signs and symptoms range from mild sensory polyneuropathy to seizures, hemiparesis, paraplegia, and dementia. HIV replication and inflammation can persist in the brain despite viral suppression, and less severe forms of HAND can remain in PLWH treated with ART.[51,52]

Central Nervous System. CNS disease in HIV-infected clients can be divided into intracerebral space–occupying lesions, encephalopathy, meningitis, and spinal cord processes. The spectrum of HAND neurocognitive disorders is divided into the following subgroups: asymptomatic neurocognitive impairment (ANI), mild neurocognitive disorder, and HIV-associated dementia (HAD).[51,6] Currently, ANI is the most prevalent and accounts for 70% of all forms of HAND.[52] HAND presents with memory and executive function deficits as well as motor impairment, i.e., bradykinesia, coordination impairments, and gait dysfunction.[51] Risk factors for the development of HAND include: age, low CD4 count, use of illicit drugs, hepatitis C co-infection, cerebrovascular disease (CVD) risk factors, sleep disorders, and psychiatric co-morbidities.[51]

Prior to ART, HAD was the most common neurologic complication and the most common cause of mental status changes in HIV-infected clients. It is characterized by cognitive, motor, and behavioral dysfunction. This disorder is similar to Alzheimer's dementia but has less effect on memory loss and a greater effect on time-related skills (i.e., psychomotor skills learned over time, such as playing piano or reading).

In addition to HAND, immunosuppressed patients are vulnerable to other diseases affecting the brain such as toxoplasmosis, TB, cryptococcosis, John Cunningham virus (more commonly known as JC virus) virus encephalitis, and pneumococcal meningitis. Toxoplasmosis is the most common space-occupying lesion in HIV-infected clients. Presenting symptoms may include headache, focal neurologic deficits, seizures, or an altered mental status. Progressive multifocal leukoencephalopathy due to JC virus, which produces localized lesions within the brain, causes demyelination of the oligodendrocytes in the brain and leads to death within a few months.

In addition to the brain, neurologic disorders related to AIDS and HIV may affect the spinal cord, appearing as myelopathies. A vacuolar myelopathy often appears in the thoracic spine and causes gradual weakness, painless gait disturbance characterized by spasticity, and ataxia in the lower extremities that progresses to include weakness of the upper extremities.

Structural and inflammatory abnormalities in the muscles of people with HIV have been reported to impair the muscle's ability to extract or utilize oxygen during exercise. Clinical manifestations of HIV-associated myopathies include proximal weakness, myalgia, abnormal electromyogram activity, elevated creatine kinase, and decreased functioning of the muscle.[53]

Peripheral Nervous System. PN is a common complication of the HIV infection. While the introduction of ART has reduced prevalence of more severe forms of HAND and CNS opportunistic infections, the prevalence of HIV-associated PN remains high and is estimated to be 31% to 50% in PLWH, compared with 0.1% to 12.6% in the overall population.[54,55] PNS syndromes include inflammatory polyneuropathies, sensory neuropathies, and mononeuropathies. An inflammatory demyelinating polyneuropathy similar to Guillain-Barré syndrome (GBS) can occur in PLWH. Cytomegalovirus, a highly host-specific herpes virus that infects the nerve roots, may result in an ascending polyradiculopathy characterized by lower extremity weakness progressing to flaccid paralysis.

Most commonly, PLWH develop distal sensory polyneuropathies characterized by numbness, burning, tingling, or weakness starting distally in the feet and hands and ascending proximally into the legs and arms, respectively. The most prevalent sign of PLWH who were clinically diagnosed with PN is decreased or absent Achilles reflexes, and the most common symptom is numbness of the feet and legs.[56] Immobility caused by painful neuropathies can result in deconditioning and eventual cardiopulmonary decline. Decreased sensation associated with PN can result in increased fall risk.

Hypersensitivity Disorders

The immune system primarily protects the body from antigens such as viruses, bacteria, fungi, and toxins; however, an excessive response from the immune system can lead to undesirable reactions and chronic disease states. This increased immune response is referred to as a hypersensitivity reaction. Hypersensitivity designates an increased immune response to the presence of an antigen that results in tissue destruction. Hypersensitivity disorders also include autoimmune diseases where the immune response identifies self-antigens as foreign antigens or there is an excessive response to foreign antigens.[57]

The classification of hypersensitivity reactions was established by Gell and Coombs[58] and remains the most widely accepted classification of hypersensitivity reactions. The Gell and Coombs classification consists of four subtypes (I–IV) which are based on the type of immune response[57,59] (Table 13.3).

Type I Immediate Reactions

Immediate reactions are mediated by the antibody immunoglobulin E (IgE), and are commonly associated with allergies. Type I reactions require an individual to be sensitized by a specific allergen by either ingesting or inhaling the antigen. The IgE antibodies bound to mast cells then bind to the antigen resulting in a release of histamine and inflammatory cytokines.[57,60] Examples of type I immediate reactions include hay fever, allergic asthma, allergic rhino conjunctivitis, and anaphylaxis.[57,60] In atopic persons, allergen-specific IgE antibodies may develop in response to allergens in the environment, foods, or drugs.[59]

CLINICAL SIGNS AND SYMPTOMS

HIV Neurologic Disease

- Difficulty with concentration and memory
- Change in personality (depression, withdrawal, apathy)
- Headache
- Seizure
- Paralysis (hemiparesis, paraplegia)
- Motor dysfunction (balance and coordination)
- Gradual weakness of extremities
- Numbness and tingling (peripheral neuropathy)
- Radiculopathy

TABLE 13.3	Gell and Coombs Classification	
Classification	Type of Reaction	Clinical Presentation
Type I	Immediate: IgE mediated	Urticaria (hives), asthma, allergic rhinitis, anaphylaxis
Type II	Cytotoxic: IgG/IgM mediated	Chronic idiopathic urticarial, Graves' disease, anemia
Type III	Immune complex: IgG/IgM mediated	Vasculitis, arthritis, immune complex disease; e.g., systemic lupus erythematosus
Type IV	Delayed: T-cell mediated	Contact dermatitis, persistent asthma, allergic rhinitis

Adapted from Uzzamen et al. 2012 and Rajan TV 2003 reactions.

Atopy refers to a genetic predisposition to produce large quantities of IgE, resulting in hypersensitivity. The reaction between the allergen and the susceptible person (i.e., atopic individual) results in the development of a number of typical signs and symptoms usually involving the GI tract, respiratory tract, or skin.

Clinical Signs and Symptoms of Type I Immediate Hypersensitivity. Clinical signs and symptoms vary from one client to another according to the allergies present. The family/personal history form should be utilized to identify any known allergies and specific reactions to the allergen. The physical therapist can then be alerted to any of the clients signs or symptoms during treatment and take necessary measures, from grading exercise to the client's tolerance, controlling the room temperature, or ensuring the patient is appropriately using prescribed medications.

Anaphylaxis. Anaphylaxis is a sudden-onset type I hypersensitivity that can be fatal. Immunologic anaphylaxis is mediated via IgE antibodies and can be due to food allergies, insect stings or bites, medications (e.g., penicillin), and latex.[61] The common foods that can result in anaphylaxis in children include eggs, milk, peanuts, soy, shellfish, tree nuts, wheat, and fish. The common food allergens in adults include peanuts, tree nuts, shellfish, and fish.

Diagnostic criteria have been established for identifying anaphylaxis in the emergency department (ED).[62] Fig. 13.3 provides the National Institute of Allergy and Infectious Disease/Food Allergy and Anaphylaxis Network diagnostic criteria and has been found to be useful in the ED for

diagnosis.[63] The reported sensitivity and specificity at a 95% confidence interval was 96.7% and 82.45%, respectively, while the positive likelihood ratio and negative likelihood ratio at a 95% confidence interval was 5.48 and 0.04, respectively.[63]

Clients with previous anaphylactic reactions (and the specific signs and symptoms of that individual's reaction) should be identified using the Family/Personal History form. Identification information should be worn at all times by individuals who have had previous anaphylactic reactions. For identified and unidentified clients, immediate action is required if they have a severe reaction. In such situations, the therapist is advised to call for emergency assistance.

Type II Cytotoxic Hypersensitivity

A type II hypersensitivity reaction is caused by the abnormal production of IgG or IgM which targets normal tissue antigens or a response to foreign antigens.[57] Type II reactions are often referred to as antigen-antibody interactions and have the following mechanisms: (1) IgG or IgM antibodies can coat or opsonize cells, or activate complement proteins. Once the complement system is activated, cells are phagocytosed and removed by leukocytes.[57,59] (2) The membrane attack complex attacks the cell by opening the cell membrane, this results in cell lysis. (3) Antibody-dependent cell-mediated cytotoxicity occurs when IgG antibodies bind to natural killer cells and macrophages. This complex results in cell death via apoptosis.[59] Examples of type II hypersensitivities include blood transfusion reactions, hemolytic anemia, idiopathic

Anaphylaxis is highly likely when any one of the following 3 criteria is fulfilled:
1. Acute onset of an illness (minutes to several hours) with involvement of the skin, mucosal tissue, or both (eg, generalized hives, pruritus or flushing, swollen lips-tongue-uvula)
AND AT LEAST ONE OF THE FOLLOWING
a. Respiratory compromise (eg, dyspnea, wheeze-bronchospasm, stridor, reduced PEF, hypoxemia)
b. Reduced BP or associated symptoms of end-organ dysfunction (eg, hypotonia [collapse], syncope, incontinence)
2. Two or more of the following that occur rapidly after exposure to a likely allergen for that patient (minutes to several hours):
a. Involvement of the skin-mucosal tissue (eg, generalized hives, itch-flush, swollen lips-tongue-uvula)
b. Respiratory compromise (eg, dyspnea, wheeze-bronchospasm, stridor, reduced PEF, hypoxemia)
c. Reduced BP or associated symptoms (eg, hypotonia [collapse], syncope, incontinence)
d. Persistent gastrointestinal symptoms (eg, crampy abdominal pain, vomiting)
3. Reduced BP after exposure to known allergen for that patient (minutes to several hours):
a. Infants and children: low systolic BP (age specific) or greater than 30% decrease in systolic BP*
b. Adults: systolic BP of less than 90 mm Hg or greater than 30% decrease from that person's baseline
PEF, Peak expiratory flow; BP, blood pressure.
*Low systolic blood pressure for children is defined as less than 70 mm Hg from 1 month to 1 year, less than (70 mm Hg + [2 x age]) from 1 to 10 years, and less than 90 mm Hg from 11 to 17 years.
Modified from Sampson, et al.[6] Used with permission.

Fig. 13.3 National Institute of Allergy and Infectious Disease/Food Allergy and Anaphylaxis Network diagnostic criteria. (From Cambell RL, Hagan JB. Evaluation of National Institute of Allergy and Infectious Diseases/Food Allergy and Anaphylaxis Network criteria for the diagnosis of anaphylaxis in emergency department patients. J Allergy Clin Immunol 2012;129:748-752.)
PEF: peak expiratory flow BP = blood pressure mmHg = millimeters of mercury x = times

thrombocytopenic purpura, and antibody produced against acetylcholine receptors in MG resulting in muscular weakness or drug-induced anemia.[57] In general, type II hypersensitivity reactions are tissue specific, antibody mediated, and cytotoxic.

Type III Immune Complex Reactions

Immune complex reactions are the result of antigen-antibody complexes in the blood, which are then deposited in tissues.[60] Antigen-antibody complexes are deposited in small vessels of the skin, renal glomeruli, alveoli of the lungs, and synovial joints.[59] This results in symptoms affecting the skin (vasculitis), the kidneys (nephritis), allergic alveolitis, and joint arthritis.[59]

The mechanisms of type III reactions are similar to type II and they can overlap. The time for type II and III reactions to develop is slower than type I, taking 3–6 hours to develop after antigen exposure.[64] Serum sickness is another example of a type II and III hypersensitivity that develops after injection such as penicillin. Systemic lupus erythematous is an autoimmune disease (discussed in detail later in this chapter) and is an example of a type III hypersensitivity resulting in a chronic condition.[57]

Serum sickness is another type III hypersensitivity response that develops 6 to 14 days after injection of a foreign serum (e.g., penicillin, sulfonamides, streptomycin, thiouracils, hydantoin compounds). Deposition of complexes on vessel walls causes complement activation with resultant edema, fever, inflammation of blood vessels and joints, and urticaria.

Type IV Delayed-Type Hypersensitivity or T-Cell Mediated

Type IV hypersensitivity reactions are considered delayed-type, due to symptoms taking 24–48 hours to develop after exposure to an antigen.[64] Type IV reactions are T-cell mediated, resulting in cytokine and growth factor release which can lead to tissue fibrosis and contact dermatitis.[59,64]

With the first exposure, no reaction occurs; however, antigens are formed. If subsequent exposure occurs, hypersensitivity reactions are triggered, which leads to itching, erythema, and vesicular lesions. Contact dermatitis is a type IV reaction that occurs after sensitization to an allergen, commonly a cosmetic, adhesive, topical medication, drug additive (e.g., lanolin added to lotions, ultrasound gels, or other preparations used in massage or soft tissue mobilization), or plant toxin (e.g., poison ivy).

Anyone with a known type IV hypersensitivity such as contact dermatitis (identified through the Family/Personal History form) should have a small area of skin tested before use of large amounts of topical agents in the physical therapy clinic. Careful observation and communication throughout the episode of care is essential.

Being aware of the presence of hypersensitivity disorders is useful for the clinician to respond appropriately if a patient were to experience a reaction and to prevent undo exposure to a patient in the case of contact dermatitis. While the Gell-Coombs classification system is older, it is the most accepted classification system for differentiating immediate to delayed hypersensitivity reactions. The clinician should keep in mind the majority of clients will present with a known history of a hypersensitivity. If changes in the client's history are present or they experience a change in their condition, the clinician should question the patient on the following: Is their physician aware? and Has the situation changed since last MD visit?

Autoimmune Disorders

Fibromyalgia Syndrome

Fibromyalgia syndrome (FMS) is a noninflammatory condition appearing with generalized musculoskeletal pain in conjunction with tenderness to touch in a large number of specific areas of the body and a wide array of associated symptoms, including fatigue, sleep disturbance, and cognitive dysfunction.[65] The prevalence of FMS in the United States ranges from 2% to 8% of the population and is dependent on the diagnostic criteria utilized.[66-68] Women are more likely to have FMS than men, with the newer diagnostic criteria indicating the female to male ratio is 2:1.[68] FMS is two to five times more common than RA and occurs in age groups ranging from preadolescents to early postmenopausal women.[69] The condition is less common in older adults. People with FMS who are of a lower socioeconomic status have been noted to have greater severity of symptoms and functional impairment.[70]

Controversy exists over the exact nature of FMS including debate over whether FMS is an organic disease with abnormal biochemical or immunological pathologic aspects. Some theories suggest that it is a genetically predisposed condition with dysregulation of the neurohormonal and autonomic nervous systems.[71] It may be triggered by viral infection, a traumatic event, or stress. The role of inadequate thyroid hormone regulation as a main mechanism of FMS has been proposed and is under investigation.[72,73] Environmental factors are also likely to contribute to the development of FMS.[74] Fibromyalgia cannot be classified as an autoimmune disorder; however, FMS is common in individuals with autoimmune diseases. Conditions such as osteoarthritis, SLE, and RA often have a concomitant diagnosis of FMS.[68]

More recent research suggests that chronic pain related to FMS is *centrally mediated* (central sensitization) indicating the pain associated with FMS is less likely due to nociceptive input. Central sensitization refers to amplification of neural signals within the CNS, resulting in pain hypersensitivity.[75] Peripheral nociception may play a small role; however, the widespread pain/symptoms and hypersensitivity indicates a centrally mediated process versus a focal problem in the tissues (e.g., low back, hips, or wrists). Central sensitization may also play a role in the symptoms of fatigue, sleep disturbance, changes in mood, and memory issues.[68]

Functional magnetic resonance imaging (MRI) studies of the brain have demonstrated increased activity in areas of the brain involved in pain processing when mild pressure or heat is applied to symptomatic areas of the body.[76] Neuroimaging studies have consistently demonstrated abnormal responses to painful and nonpainful stimuli in individuals with FMS compared with healthy age-matched controls. The abnormal responses consist of increased metabolic activity and resting state connectivity in areas of the brain identified with pain processing.[77]

The initial diagnostic criteria created by the American College of Rheumatology (ACR) criteria in 1990 was based on the presentation of widespread symmetrical pain in addition to 18 specific symmetrical tender points.[78] Initially, individuals needed to have 11 of 18 areas positive for tenderness; however, the initial criteria has been identified as problematic due to tenderness to palpation being common regardless of the presence of FMS.[79,80] The Symptom Intensity Scale was subsequently developed and validated by Wolfe et al.[81–83] to help differentiate FMS from other rheumatologic conditions (e.g., SLE or PMR) that may present with widespread pain.

In 2010, Wolfe et al. created diagnostic criteria, which focused on measuring symptom severity rather than relying on the tender point examination.[84,85] The new criteria use a clinician-queried checklist of painful sites and a symptom severity scale (SSS) that focuses on fatigue, cognitive dysfunction, and sleep disturbance.[85] Based on the 2016 revision of the fibromyalgia diagnostic criteria,[86] individuals are considered to have a diagnosis of FMS if the following criteria are met: (1) presence of generalized pain, in > 4 of 5 defined regions; (2) symptoms present at a similar level for at least 3 months; (3) widespread pain index (WPI) >7 and SSS score > 5 or WPI of 4–6 and SSS score > 9; and (4) a diagnosis of fibromyalgia is valid irrespective of other diagnoses (Fig. 13.4).[86]

FMS has been differentiated from myofascial pain in that FMS is considered a systemic problem with multiple tender points as one of the key symptoms; there is usually a cluster of associated signs and symptoms. Myofascial pain is a localized condition specific to a muscle (trigger point [TrP]) and may involve as few as one or several areas without associated signs and symptoms.

The hallmark of myofascial pain syndrome is the TrP, as opposed to tender points in FMS. Both disorders cause myalgia with aching pain and tenderness and exhibit similar local histologic changes in the muscle. Painful symptoms in both conditions are increased with activity, although FMS involves more generalized aching, whereas myofascial pain is more direct and localized (Table 13.4).

FMS has striking similarities to chronic fatigue syndrome (CFS), with a mix of overlapping symptoms (about 70%) that have some common biologic denominator. Diagnostic criteria for CFS focus on fatigue, whereas the criteria for FMS focus on pain, the two most prominent symptoms of these syndromes. Studies have shown that CFS and FMS are characterized by greater similarities than differences and both involve the CNS and PNS as well as the body tissues themselves.[87–89]

Risk Factors. Numerous studies have implicated a genetic predisposition related to brain and/or body chemistry; however, psychosocial issues such as a history of childhood trauma, family stressors, and/or physical/sexual abuse

TABLE 13.4	Differentiating Myofascial Pain Syndrome from Fibromyalgia Syndrome	
Myofascial Pain Syndrome	**Fibromyalgia Syndrome**	
Trigger points (pain with deep pressure); often radiates locally	Tender points (pain with light touch); no radiation	
Localized musculoskeletal condition	Systemic condition	
Palpable taut band found in muscle; no associated signs and symptoms	No palpable or visible local abnormality; wide array of associated signs and symptoms	
Etiology: Overuse, repetitive motions; reduced muscle activity (e.g., casting or prolonged splinting)	Etiology: Neurohormonal imbalance; autonomic nervous system dysfunction	
Risk factors: Immobilization, repetitive use	Risk factors: Trauma, psychosocial stress, mood (or other psychologic) disorders; other medical conditions	
Pathophysiology: Unknown, possibly muscle spindle dysfunction	Pathophysiology: Sensitization of spinal neurons from excitatory nerve messenger substances	
Prognosis: Excellent	Prognosis: Good with early diagnosis and intervention, variable with delayed diagnosis; often a chronic condition	

Data from Lowe JC, Yellin JG. The Metabolic Treatment of Fibromyalgia. Utica, Kentucky: McDowell Publications; 2000.

are significant risk factors for developing FMS.[90] Anxiety, depression, and posttraumatic stress disorder are also linked with FMS.[91,92] Having a bipolar illness increases the risk of developing FMS dramatically.[93]

Clinical Signs and Symptoms. The core features of FMS include symptoms lasting more than 3 months, widespread pain identified on the WPI, and response to the SSS (see Fig. 13.4). Primary musculoskeletal symptoms most frequently reported are (1) aches and pains; (2) stiffness; (3) swelling in soft tissue; (4) tender points; and (5) muscle spasms or nodules. Fatigue, cognitive changes, and sleep disturbance with waking unrefreshed may be present, and comprise the diagnostic criteria (see Fig. 13.4).[86,94]

Nontender control points (such as mid-forehead and anterior thigh) have been included in the examination by some clinicians. These control points may be useful in distinguishing FMS from a conversion reaction, referred to as *psychogenic rheumatism*, or central sensitization due to persistent pain (not related to FMS), in which wide spread tenderness may be present. However, evidence suggests that individuals with FMS may have a generalized lowered threshold for pain on palpation and the control points may also be tender on occasion. There is also an increased sensitivity to sensory stimulation such as pressure stimuli, heat, noise, odors, and bright lights.[95]

Fibromyalgia criteria-2016 revision

Criteria

A patient satisfies modified 2016 fibromyalgia if the following 3 conditions are met:

(1) Widespread pain index (WPI) $\geq$ 7 and symptom severity scale (SSS) score $\geq$ 5 OR WPI of 4-6 and SSS score $\geq$ 9.
(2) Generalized pain, defined as pain in at least 4 of 5 regions, must be preasent. Jaw,chest, and abdominal pain are not incluedeed in generalized pain definition.
(3) Symptoms have been generally present for at least 3 months.
(4) A diagnosis of fibromyalgia is vaild irres pective of other diagnoses. A diagnosis of fibromyalgia does not exclude the presence of other clinically important illnesses.

Ascertainment

(1) **WPI**: note the number of areas in which the patient the patient has had pain over the last week. In how many areas has the patient had pain? Score will be between 0 and 19

Left upper region (Region 1)	**Left upper region (Region 2)**	**Axial region (Region 5)**
Jaw, left[2]	Jaw, right[2]	Neck
Shoulder girdle, left	Shoulder girdle, right	Upper back
Upper arm, left	Upper arm, right	Lower back
Lower arm, left	Lower arm, right	Chest[3]
		Abdomen[3]

Left lower region (region 3)	**Right lower region (region 3)**	
Hip (buttock,trochanter), left	Hip (buttock,trochanter), right	
Upper leg, left	Upper leg, right	
Lower leg, left	Lower leg, right	

(2) Symptom severity scale (SSS) score

Fatigue
Walking unrefershed
Cognitive symptoms

For the each of the 3 symptoms above, indicate the level of severity over the past week using the following scale:

  0 = No problem
  1 = Slight or mild problems, generally mild or intermittent
  2 = Moderate, considerable problems, often present and/or at a moderate level
  3 = Severe: pervasive, continuous, life-disturbing problems

The symptom severity scale (SSS) score: is the of the severity scores of the 3 symptoms (fatigue, waking unrefreshed, and cognitive symptoms) (0-9) plus the sum
  (0-3) of the number of the following symptoms the patient has been brothered by that occurred during the previous 6 months:

(1) Headaches (0-1)
(2) Pain or cramps in lower abdomen (0-1)
(3) And depression (0-1)

The final symptom severity score is between 0 and 12
The fibromyalgia severity (FS) scale is the sum of the WPI ans SSS

Fig. 13.4   Fibromyalgia criteria. (From Wolfe F, et al. 2016 Revisions to the 2010/2011 fibromyalgia diagnostic criteria. Seminars Arthritis Rheum 2016; 46:319-329. https://doi.org/10.1016/j.semarthrit.2016.08.012)

CLINICAL SIGNS AND SYMPTOMS

Fibromyalgia Syndrome

- Myalgia (generalized aching)
- Fatigue (mental and physical)
- Sleep disturbances, nocturnal myoclonus, nocturnal bruxism
- Tender points of palpation
- Chest wall pain mimicking angina pectoris
- Tendinitis, bursitis
- Temperature dysregulation
  - Raynaud's phenomenon; cold-induced vasospasm (hypersensitivity to cold)
  - Hypothermia (mild decrease in core body temperature)
- Dyspnea, dizziness, syncope
- Headache (migraine or tension type)
- Paresthesia (numbness and tingling)
- Gastrointestinal system disorders: Irritable bowel syndrome, gastroesophageal reflux (GERD)
- Depression/anxiety
- Cognitive difficulties (e.g., short-term memory loss, decreased attention span; sometimes referred to as *fibro fog*)
- Pelvic pain
- Premenstrual syndrome (PMS)
- Weight gain from physical inactivity due to pain and fatigue

Symptoms are aggravated by cold, stress, excessive or no exercise, and physical activity, including overstretching, and may be improved by warmth or heat, rest, and exercise, including gentle stretching. Smoking has been linked with increased pain intensity and more severe FMS symptoms, but not necessarily a higher number of tender points. Exposure to tobacco products may be a risk factor for the development of FMS, but this has not been investigated fully or proven.[96]

DIFFERENTIAL DIAGNOSIS

Fibromyalgia

The following disorders are commonly part of the differential diagnosis for fibromyalgia:

- Hypothyroidism, hyperparathyroidism
- Adult growth hormone deficiency
- Polymyalgia rheumatica/giant cell arteritis
- Rheumatoid arthritis (RA), seronegative
- Polymyositis/dermatomyositis
- Systemic lupus erythematosus (SLE)
- Multiple sclerosis
- Myofascial pain syndrome
- Metabolic myopathy (e.g., alcohol)
- Lyme disease
- Neurosis (depression/anxiety)

- Metastatic cancer
- Chronic fatigue syndrome
- Myalgia due to medication adverse reactions (e.g., statins)
- Parasitic infection
- Depression, anxiety

A multidisciplinary or interdisciplinary team approach to this condition requires medical evaluation and treatment as a part of the intervention strategy for FMS. Physical therapists should refer clients suspected of having FMS for further medical follow-up while continuing to treat activity limitations and participation restrictions.

Rheumatoid Arthritis

RA is an autoimmune systemic inflammatory disease that predominantly involves the synovial membrane of diarthrodial joints and results in bony degradation. Joints of the wrist, hands, and feet are most commonly impacted first with a bilateral and symmetric presentation.[97] In addition to synovium and bony degradation, RA can impact organs resulting in cardiovascular disease and interstitial lung disease.[97] RA impacts physical function due to pain and musculoskeletal deficits.[98]

The prevalence of RA is about 0.5%–1.0% of the worldwide population, with Native American Indian populations presenting with higher rates than China and Japan. Women are affected by RA two to three times more often than men.[99] Although it may occur at any age, RA is most common in persons between the fourth and sixth decades of life.

Pathophysiology. As discussed earlier, RA is a chronic autoimmune disease with an unknown cause. The manifestation of RA is a result of immune system dysfunction along with genetic and environmental factors.[97] One gene in particular (HLA-DRB1 on chromosome 6) has been identified in determining susceptibility. A genetically susceptible person encountering an unidentified agent (e.g., virus, self-antigen), which then results in an immunopathologic response may be susceptible to RA.[100,101] It has been hypothesized that an infection could trigger an immune reaction that is mediated through multiple complex genetic mechanisms and continues clinically even if the organism is eradicated from the body. The complex immune activity occurs when the synovial membrane of joints is infiltrated by T cells, B cells, and monocytes. Synovial fibroblast-like and macrophage-like cells are activated which invade the periarticular bone resulting in bony erosion and cartilage degradation.[97] Additionally, prostaglandins and matrix metalloproteinases are induced by proinflammatory cytokines which perpetuate signs and symptoms of pain, swelling, and degradation of cartilage and bone.[97]

Environmental factors such as smoking, hormones, infection, and microbiota have been linked to the development of RA.[102] Smoking and cigarette exposure is a very strong risk factor associated with RA.[102] Additionally, individuals who have first-degree relatives with a smoking history of > 10 pack/years and younger than 50 years of age are at a higher risk of developing inflammatory joint signs.[103] Environmental and occupational causes, such as chemicals (e.g., hair dyes, industrial pollutants), minerals, mineral oil, organic solvents, silica, toxins, medications, food allergies, and stress remain under investigation as possible triggers for those individuals who are genetically susceptible to RA.[104] Many systemic disorders can express themselves through the musculoskeletal system, often presenting first with rheumatic manifestations.[105]

Clinical Signs and Symptoms. Clinical features of RA vary between individuals, as well as over the course of the disease. In the early stages, autoantibodies form prior to individuals experiencing signs or symptoms of RA. The term for this is "pre-RA" and can be present for < 1 year to > 10 years.[106] Some individuals in the "pre-RA" stage may present with subtle inflammatory changes. Early presentations range from mild arthritis with only a few joints involved to severe polyarticular disease.[97] The multidimensional aspects of RA pain can be assessed quantitatively using the Rheumatoid Arthritis Pain Scale.[107] The Arthritis Impact Measurement Scales (AIMS/AIMS2) is an outcome measure for arthritis and assesses the physical, social, and emotional well-being of the patient.[108]

Symptoms of RA include the spontaneous onset pain and swelling of the metacarpophalangeal (MCP) or metatarsophalangeal joints (MTP); and morning stiffness lasting longer than 30 minutes to several hours. Inactivity, such as sleep or prolonged sitting, is commonly followed by stiffness. "Morning" stiffness occurs when the person arises in the morning or after prolonged inactivity. Clients should be asked: "After you wake up in the morning and get out of bed, how long does it take until you are feeling the best you will feel for the day?" Physical function such as a person's ability to walk, climb stairs, open doors, perform other activities of daily living, and work can be impacted by RA. If not treated early and sufficiently, 80% of patients can develop malalignment of the joints (e.g., MCP or MTP) and 40% will be unable to work within 10 years from disease onset.[97]

Current evidence suggests that cartilage damage is more related to irreversible disability than bony damage.[109] Individuals with RA are also likely to have significant joint erosion as evidenced on x ray within 2 years of disease onet.[110] Early diagnosis and treatment is estimated to prevent progression of joint destruction by 90% in early RA.[111] Therefore, it is important that clinicians recognize potential RA early and facilitate medical referral. Awareness of the group of symptoms that suggest inflammatory arthritis is critical. It is recommended that the criteria for referral of a person with early inflammatory symptoms include significant discomfort on the compression of the MCP and MTP joints, the presence of three or more swollen joints, and a report of morning stiffness lasting longer than 60 minutes.[112]

Shoulder. Chronic synovitis of the elbows, shoulders, hips, knees, and/or ankles creates special secondary disorders. When the shoulder is involved, limitation of shoulder mobility, dislocation, and spontaneous tears of the rotator cuff result in chronic pain and adhesive capsulitis.

Elbow. Destruction of the elbow articulations can lead to flexion contracture, loss of supination and pronation, and subluxation. Compressive ulnar nerve neuropathies may develop related to elbow synovitis. Symptoms include paresthesia of the fourth and fifth fingers and weakness in the flexor muscle of the little finger.

Wrists. The joints of the wrist are frequently affected in RA, with variable tenosynovitis of the dorsa of the wrists and, ultimately, interosseous muscle atrophy and diminished movement owing to articular destruction or bony ankylosis. Volar synovitis can lead to carpal tunnel syndrome.

Hands and Feet. Forefoot pain may be the only small-joint complaint and is often the first one. Subluxation of the heads of the MTP joints and shortening of the extensor tendons give rise to "hammer toe" or "cock up" deformities. A similar process in the hands results in volar subluxation of the MCP joints and ulnar deviation of the fingers. An exaggerated inflammatory response of an extensor tendon can result in a spontaneous, often asymptomatic rupture. Hyperextension of a proximal interphalangeal (PIP) joint and flexion of the distal interphalangeal (DIP) joint produce a swan neck deformity. The boutonnière deformity is a fixed flexion contracture of a PIP joint and extension of a DIP joint. The dynamic nature of RA results in progressive damage and deformity of the joints resulting in malalignment over time (Fig. 13.5). Swelling of the MCP or MTP joints is "soft" due to synovitis and effusion compared with "hard" or bony swelling of osteoarthritis.[97] Finger swelling in RA will present with specific joint swelling

(fusiform) versus the whole finger ("sausage finger") presentation with PsA.

Cervical Spine. Involvement of the cervical spine by RA tends to occur late in more advanced disease. Clinical manifestations of early disease consist primarily of neck stiffness that is perceived through the entire arc of motion. Inflammation of the supporting ligaments of C1-C2 eventually produces laxity, sometimes giving rise to atlantoaxial subluxation. Spinal cord compression can result from anterior dislocation of C1 or from vertical subluxation of the odontoid process of C2 into the foramen magnum.

Extraarticular. Extraarticular features, such as rheumatoid nodules, atherosclerosis, arteritis, anemia, neuropathy, scleritis, pericarditis, lymphadenopathy, and splenomegaly, occur with considerable frequency (Table 13.5). Once thought to be complications of RA, they are now recognized as being integral parts of the disease and serve to emphasize its systemic nature. A consequence of chronic inflammation over time is cardiovascular disease. Cardiovascular disease often results in the primary cause of death in individuals with RA. Interstitial lung disease in individuals with RA can be a manifestation of the disease or complication of treatment with methotrexate and leflunomide.[97]

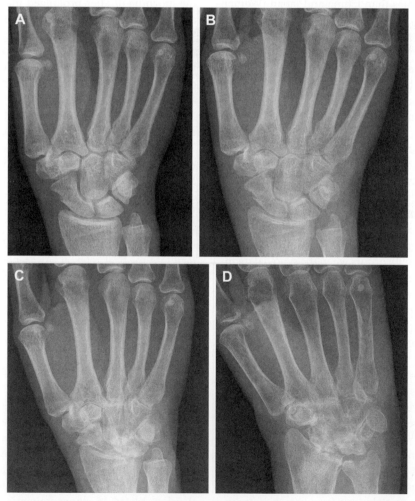

Fig. 13.5 Cartilage loss and progressive destruction of wrist due to RA. (A) Early stage plain film; (B) periarticular osteoporosis is visible with minimal loss of joint space; (C) carpal collapse beginning to show and joint space is significantly decreased; (D) collapse of the carpal bones. (From Llopis E, Herman M. Conventional radiology in rheumatoid arthritis. Radiol Clin N Am 2017; 55(5):917-941.)

TABLE 13.5	Extraarticular Manifestations of Rheumatoid Arthritis
Organ System	Extraarticular Manifestations
Skin	Cutaneous vasculitis
	Rheumatoid nodules
	Ecchymoses/petechiae (drug-induced)
Eye	Episcleritis
	Scleritis
	Scleromalacia perforans
	Corneal ulcers/perforation
	Uveitis
	Retinitis
	Glaucoma
	Cataract
Lung	Pleuritis
	Diffuse interstitial fibrosis
	Vasculitis
	Rheumatoid nodules
	Caplan's syndrome
	Pulmonary hypertension
Heart and	Pericarditis
blood vessels	Myocarditis
	Coronary arteritis
	Valvular insufficiency
	Conduction defects
	Vasculitis
	Felty's syndrome
Nervous	Mononeuritis multiplex
system	Distal sensory neuropathy
	Cervical spine instability (spinal cord compression)

Modified from Andreoli TE, Benjamin I, Griggs RC, et al. Andreoli and Carpenter's Cecil Essentials of Medicine. 8th ed. Philadelphia: Saunders; 2010.

Juvenile Idiopathic Arthritis. Juvenile idiopathic arthritis (JIA) replaces the term juvenile RA. JIA is a chronic inflammatory disorder that occurs during childhood and is made up of a heterogeneous group of diseases that share synovitis as a common feature. There are seven subcategories of JIA[113]:

- Oligoarthritis JIA
- Polyarthritis JIA (positive RF)
- Polyarthritis JIA (negative RF)
- Systemic onset JIA
- Psoriatic JIA
- Enthesitis-related arthritis
- Other arthritis

CLINICAL SIGNS AND SYMPTOMS
Rheumatoid Arthritis

- Swelling in one or more joints, typically symmetrical and bilateral
- Morning stiffness lasting several hours
- Recurring pain or tenderness in any joint
- Obvious redness and warmth in a joint
- Unexplained weight loss, fever, or weakness combined with joint pain
- Symptoms such as these that last for more than 2 weeks
- See also Table 13.5

Early recognition of JIA is key to timely initiation of treatment. For a diagnosis of JIA to be made, arthritis (defined as motion loss of the joint, swelling, heat, pain, or tenderness) must be seen in one or more joints for at least 6 weeks in children younger than 16 years.[113] Children should be screened for an array of symptoms, depending on the appropriate subcategory of disease. The number of joints involved, involvement of small joints, symmetry of joint involvement, uveitis risk, systemic features, and family history are important parts of this screening. It is important to educate parents regarding symptoms of JIA since parents are often the first line of communication between children and health care professionals.

Diagnosis. The presence of joint involvement in one or more joints (evidence of swelling, pain, or tenosynovitis) and the presence of RF measured by laboratory studies are two indicators of RA. Currently, a set of diagnostic criteria is lacking; however, the ACR and European League Against Rheumatism (EULAR) established classification criteria in 2010 that is widely accepted.[114] It was primarily established for creating homogenous groups for research and has a specificity of 0.61 and sensitivity of 0.82.[115]

The ACR/EULAR classification criteria of RA (Table 13.6) is difficult in the early course of the disease, when articular symptoms are accompanied only by constitutional symptoms such as

TABLE 13.6	American College of Rheumatology and European League Against Rheumatism Classification Criteria for Rheumatoid Arthritis

Population to be tested: Patients with the following:
1. At least 1 joint with swelling
2. Presence of synovitis not explained by another disease

Rheumatoid Arthritis classification criteria (add score of categories A–D; score of > 6/10 needed to define condition as RA)	Score
A. Joints involved	
1 large joint	0
2–10 large joints	1
1–3 small joints (with or without large joint involvement)	2
4–10 small joints (with or without large joint involvement)	3
>10 joints (at least 1 small joint)	5
B. Serology (at least 1 test result is needed)	
Negative RF and negative ACPA	0
Low-positive RF or low-positive ACPA	2
High-positive RF or high-positive ACPA	3
C. Acute-phase reactants (at least 1 test result is needed for classification)	
Normal CRP and normal ESR	0
Abnormal CRP or abnormal ESR	1
D. Duration of symptoms	
<6 weeks	0
> 6weeks	1

ACPA, Anticitrullinated protein antibody; *CRP*, C-reactive protein; *ESR*, erythrocyte sedimentation rate; *RF*, rheumatoid factor.
Modified from Aletaha D, et al. Rheumatoid arthritis classification criteria: An American college of rheumatology/European league against rheumatism collaborative initiative. Arthritis Rheum 2010;62(9):2569-2581.

fatigue or loss of appetite, which are common to a number of chronic diseases. The following must be present to establish a diagnosis of RA; the presence of at least 1 clinically swollen joint and at least 6 of 10 points from the ACR/EULAR criteria.

Additional laboratory tests of significance in the diagnosis and management of RA include WBC count, erythrocyte sedimentation rate (ESR), hemoglobin and hematocrit, urinalysis, antinuclear antibodies (ANA), and anticyclic citrullinated peptide antibody (anti-CCP). The elevation of C-reactive protein (CRP) has been discovered in significant levels within 2 years preceding a confirmed diagnosis of RA. Increased levels of CRP signal a steady, low-grade inflammation that may be an early predictor of later symptomatic inflammation.[116,117]

The presence of RF is helpful in diagnosing RA, but about 15% of patients with RA do not have a positive RF test. This test has been found to be 69% sensitive and 85% specific. Due to the number of false positives, the anti-CCP test is the preferred test with a 67% sensitivity and 95% specificity.[118]

The number of WBCs will increase in the presence of joint inflammation, as will the ESR. Anemia may be present along with an elevated RF in clients with active RA. If the client's urinalysis reveals any protein, blood cells, or casts, SLE should be suspected. This type of abnormal urinalysis would necessitate further diagnostic evaluation and immediate physician referral (Case Example 13.1).

Treatment. Early treatment to decrease the inflammatory process has been proven to decrease long-term joint destruction.[112] Aggressive treatment of early RA with new medications has shown marked improvement in outcome.[119] RA is classically treated by a class of drugs called disease-modifying antirheumatic drugs (DMARDs). The more common of these medications are methotrexate, sulfasalazine, hydroxychloroquine, and leflunomide.

The emergence of therapeutic biologic DMARDSs such as antitumor necrosis factor (TNF) and biologic response modifiers has led to treatments that combine DMARDs such as methotrexate with a biologic when treatment with a traditional DMARD alone is not effective.[98] These medications have both immunosuppressive and biologic side effects that must be monitored. Side effects and safety concerns are critical in the prevention of serious side effect–related problems, including the following:

- Congestive heart failure
- Serious infections as a result of immunosuppression (e.g., TB, *Listeria monocytogenes*, coccidioidomycosis, histoplasmosis, viral hepatitis)
- Skin reactions (erythema, pruritus, rashes, urticaria, infection, eczema)
- New-onset symptoms of MS, optic neuritis, and transverse myelitis

CASE EXAMPLE 13.1
Rheumatoid Arthritis

History: A 67-year-old woman with a 13-year history of rheumatoid arthritis (RA) requiring gold and methotrexate fell and fractured her right acetabulum, requiring a total hip replacement. She was referred to physical therapy through a home health agency for "aggressive rehabilitation." After 10 weeks, she was walking unassisted after having progressed from a walker to a cane and participating in a swimming program sponsored by the local arthritis organization. She was discharged with a home program to continue working on strength and balance activities.

About 6 weeks later, the physical therapist received a telephone call from the client's husband, who reported that there had been a gradual decline in her walking and asked the physical therapist for a reevaluation. The woman came into the outpatient clinic and was examined with the following findings.

Clinical Presentation: The client had resumed the use of a cane, and her gait was characterized by wide-based stance, shortened steps, and trunk instability. She frequently took a few steps forward before tottering backward without falling. The client was unable to stand from a sitting position without assistance. When moving from a standing to a sitting position, she consistently fell backward.

When asked about the new onset of any other symptoms, the client noted urinary urge incontinence, and her husband commented that she had just started having difficulty remembering the dates of their children's birthdays and the names of their grandchildren.

The physical therapist performed both an orthopedic and a neurologic screening examination and measured vital signs. The client's blood pressure was 135/78 mm Hg, resting pulse was 78 bpm, and body temperature was considered normal. The

orthopedic examination was consistent with a total hip replacement 6 months ago, with mild hip flexor weakness and mild loss of hip motion on the left (compared with the right). However, the neurologic examination raised some red flags.

Muscle tone was increased in the lower extremities, with proprioception and deep tendon reflexes decreased in both feet (right more than left). Pinprick, light-touch, and two-point discrimination were normal. Romberg's sign was absent, but a test for dysmetria of the upper extremities revealed mild cogwheeling. There was an observable tremor when the client's arms were stretched out in front of her trunk.

Result: Given the history of a progressive gait disturbance, new onset of urge incontinence, and positive findings on a neurologic screening examination, this client was referred to her family physician for a medical evaluation. The physical therapist explained to the client and her husband that these findings were not typical of someone who has had a total hip replacement or someone with RA.

The client was examined by her family physician and referred to a neurologist. A magnetic resonance imaging (MRI) study was ordered, and a diagnosis of basilar impression was made. *Basilar impression* is the term used when the odontoid peg of C2 pushes up into the foramen magnum.

RA is a classic cause of this via atlantoaxial dislocation. The destructive inflammatory process of RA weakens ligaments that attach the odontoid to the atlas into the skull. The subsequent dislocation of the atlas on the axis can remain mobile, producing intermittent problems, or it can become fixed, producing persistent symptoms.

Modified from Williams ME, Richman J, Scatliff J. A 67-year-old woman with a progressive gait disturbance. J Am Geriatr Soc 1996;44(7):843-84.

- Hematologic abnormalities such as aplastic anemia, pancytopenia
- Increased risk of lymphomas

Polymyalgia Rheumatica

PMR is a systemic rheumatic inflammatory disorder with an unknown cause; however, genetic and environmental factors may play a role.[120]

Risk Factors. PMR is considered the most common form of inflammatory rheumatic disease in the elderly population.[121] It occurs in people over 50 years of age, with the mean age of onset being 73 years, and predominantly affects the Caucasian population.[122,123] The prevalence in individuals over the age of 50 has been estimated to be 1:200 persons.[121]

Clinical Signs and Symptoms. PMR is characterized by bilateral aching and stiffness primarily in the muscles, as opposed to the joints. Symmetrical shoulder girdle pain and stiffness are the most common symptoms, reported in 70% to 95% of patients.[123] The neck and hip girdle may also be involved in some individuals with PMR.[121] Onset is usually very sudden and insidious. Additional clinical features may include morning stiffness that lasts longer than 30 minutes, distal musculoskeletal manifestations such as arthralgias of the hands, pitting edema, and carpal tunnel. Low-grade fever, malaise, and anorexia can be present.[121] The diagnosis of PMR is made on the basis of age, clinical presentation, and a very high ESR. The ESR measures the total inflammation in the body (Case Example 13.2).

PMR is closely linked with giant cell or temporal arteritis. Giant cell arteritis (GCA) primarily affects the medium-sized muscular arteries, such as the cranial and extracranial branches of the carotid artery that pass over the temples in the scalp.[124] The temporal arteries become inflamed, subjecting them to damage. In GCA, the most common symptom is a severe headache on one or both sides of the head, that is a new-onset headache.[120] The head pain presentation typically spans the temporal or occipital areas; however, clinicians should keep in mind that the head pain symptoms can localize to any portion of the head.[120] The pain in individuals with headache due to GCA is typically constant during the day and can disrupt normal sleep patterns. Headache symptoms due to GCA do not completely respond to analgesic medications.[120]

The ophthalmic arteries can be affected in individuals with GCA. Visual loss that is either permanent, partial, or complete in one or both eyes, occurs in approximately 20% of individuals. Early diagnosis and treatment of GCA is critical to prevent blindness. Treatment for GCA typically involves glucocorticosteroids with dosing adjusted to quickly address the clinical presentation.[120]

PMR is self-limiting, typically lasting 2 to 3 years. In some cases, it goes away for reasons unknown. However, some persons may have a longer course of disease, requiring low-dose steroids for much longer; a few have PMR for less than a year. Oral corticosteroids (especially prednisone) are used to suppress the inflammation, treat the symptoms, and provide remission, but do not cure the illness.[125,126] These drugs

---

CASE EXAMPLE 13.2

Polymyalgia Rheumatica

Current Complaint: The client was a 51-year-old female referred to physical therapy by her primary care physician for evaluation and treatment of persistent shoulder girdle pain and stiffness. The client reports that she had 1 or 2 days of fever and flu-like symptoms associated with neck stiffness. The problem did not go away after the fever passed, and the symptoms gradually worsened.

A month later, both shoulders were particularly worse in the morning when she was waking up. It usually took her 3 to 4 hours before she was able to function properly. Her best moment in the day was late afternoon. Symptoms were persisting and also waking her up at night when she was trying to change positions. She tried to exercise and take nonsteroidal antiinflammatory drugs (NSAIDs) in order to overcome the symptoms, but this did not help.

She saw her primary care physician for an annual physical but did not put much emphasis on these symptoms. She was given a prescription NSAID, which only minimally improved the symptoms. She again got in touch with her doctor, who referred her to physical therapy for evaluation of shoulder girdle pain.

Past Medical History: The client is postmenopausal and is no longer taking hormone replacement therapy (HRT). She has hypertension, which is controlled by medication. She had a cesarean section for delivery of twins in 1992 but no other surgeries. Family history reveals that her mother had Alzheimer's disease and passed away in December 2003. Her father had a stroke in 1991, which left him aphasic; he has hypertension and a history

of coronary artery disease with coronary artery bypass graft surgery in 1975. There was no family history of cancer.

The client is married, has three children, and works full-time in health care. Her desired outcome is to decrease the pain and stiffness in the shoulder area and get back to her full activities.

Current medications included atenolol/chlorthalidone 50/25 daily for blood pressure management; potassium 10 mEq/L daily; aspirin 81 mg daily; calcium 1000 mg daily. She was prescribed 10 mg prednisone by her primary care physician. There are no known allergies.

Evaluation
Examination: Tests and Measures

Cardiovascular/pulmonary: During the initial evaluation at 3 p.m., the patient's blood pressure was 120/80 mm Hg and resting pulse was 68 bpm. The client routinely exercises using the treadmill and performs aerobic exercises three times per week. Lungs were clear to auscultation. There was no history of angina, dyspnea, or chronic cough. In the mornings, there is some pain when coughing and during deep breathing.

Pain: Using a Visual Analog Scale, from 0 (no pain) to 10 (worst pain imaginable), pain was rated as 8/10 in the shoulder girdle area.

Posture: Mild kyphosis and a mild forward head (possible sign of osteoporosis), but otherwise unremarkable.

Gait: Gait examination revealed an antalgic gait as a result of pain. She was not using any assistive devices or orthotics.

CASE EXAMPLE 13.2—cont'd

Range of motion (ROM) and strength: Full active and passive shoulder ROM with moderate stiffness/pain during movement. There were no gross deformities or evidence of impingement. Hands, wrists, and elbows present painless full ROM. Lower extremity evaluation revealed a prominent first left metatarsophalangeal (MTP) joint, but tibiotalar joints were fully mobile without pain. Knee and hip ROM were normal during examination. There was no effusion or instability noted.

Neurologic examination: There was no focal or diffuse muscle strength deficit. Deep tendon reflexes were normal bilaterally. Cranial nerves and sensation were intact.

Work, community, and leisure: Client has reported she has had difficulty getting out of bed in the morning and difficulty with sleep because it is very painful when she changes positions at night. Lack of sleep has been affecting her work.

Red Flags

- Age: over 50 years
- Postmenopausal
- Persistent symptoms of shoulder girdle stiffness and pain for the last 3 months despite medication use
- The musculoskeletal examination of the upper quadrant is not consistent with rheumatoid arthritis (RA) or other musculoskeletal problems.
- No apparent red flags suggestive of cardiopulmonary involvement

Result: The physical therapist contacted the physician by phone to discuss findings and concerns. A written report was faxed to the physician's office before the phone call. The physician ordered blood tests that showed the following results:

	Client's Value	Reference Range (female)
WBC	7.7	4.5–11.0/mm^3
Hemoglobin	11.6	12-15 g/dL
Hematocrit	33.6	35%–47%
Platelets	410	150-400/mm^3
Sedimentation rate	71*	1–25 mm/hr
Rheumatoid factor	36.3	Less than 60 µ/mL (units per milliliter)

*Outside normal range.

Client was diagnosed with polymyalgia rheumatica (PMR) with a recommendation for continued physical therapy intervention. Because of her prednisone use and the fact that she is postmenopausal, attention to management of the potential for osteoporosis must be included in the treatment plan. Client was advised to have a baseline dual-energy x-ray absorptiometry (DEXA) scan to determine bone mineral density, given her postmenopausal status and the fact that she is likely going to be taking corticosteroids for some time.

Even though the client was seen by the physician before referral to physical therapy, there were enough red flags to warrant consultation before beginning physical therapy intervention. Early diagnosis can be important with PMR to prevent permanent disability, including visual loss when giant cell arteritis is present.

From Anita Bemis-Dougherty, PT, MAS. Case report presented in fulfillment of DPT 910. Institute for Physical Therapy Education, Widener University: Chester, PA; 2005.

---

usually afford prompt relief of symptoms, providing further diagnostic confirmation that PMR is the underlying problem.[127] The physical therapist must remain alert to the possibility of steroid-induced osteopenia and diabetes.

With medical intervention, most people with PMR (with or without GCA) do not have lasting disability. However, in GCA, if one or both eyes are affected before treatment, some form of blindness may be permanent.

Systemic Lupus Erythematosus

SLE is an autoimmune disease that is complex and has a heterogeneous presentation. It is a chronic, systemic, inflammatory disease characterized by injury to the skin, joints, kidneys, nervous system, and mucous membranes.[128]

CLINICAL SIGNS AND SYMPTOMS

Polymyalgia Rheumatica

- Muscle pain or aching (proximal muscle groups: neck, shoulder, and hip girdle)
- Stiffness upon arising in the morning lasting > 30 minutes
- Fatigue, malaise, anorexia
- Low-grade fever

Lupus comes from the Latin word for wolf, referring to the belief in the 1800s that the rash of this disease was caused by a wolf bite. The characteristic malar (butterfly rash across the checks and nose) rash of lupus is red (Fig. 13.6), leading to the term *erythematosus.*

There are four forms of lupus: SLE, cutaneous lupus erythematosus, drug-induced lupus erythematosus (DIL), and neonatal lupus. Cutaneous lupus refers to primary skin involvement and can result in various rashes or sores. *Discoid lupus* is a form of cutaneous lupus presenting as coin-shaped lesions, which are raised, red, and scaly; however, they are not itchy (see Fig. 13.6).[128] The classic malar rash is an example of cutaneous lupus; however, additional rashes can appear on the face, neck, or scalp. These areas are more susceptible due to sunlight or fluorescent light exposure.[128] Alopecia, skin pigment changes, and sores in the mouth, nose, or vagina can also occur with cutaneous lupus. DIL presents with symptoms similar to SLE (Table 13.7); however, the symptoms are reactions to specific prescription medications. Prescription drugs associated with a high risk of DIL include procainamide and hydralazine, with frequencies reported at 15%–20% and 7%–13%, respectively.[129] Penicillamine, carbamazepine, methyl-dopa, sulfasalazine, isoniazid, among others are considered low-risk drugs.[129] DIL incidence is variable and the symptoms typically resolve

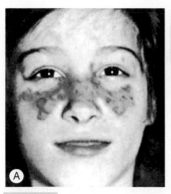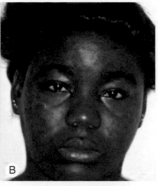

Fig. 13.6 Example of malar rash (A) and discoid lupus rash in a malar distribution (B). (From Sadum R, Ardioin S, Schamber L. Systemic Lupus Erythematosus. Nelson Textbook of Pediatrics, Philadelphia, PA: Elsevier Inc; 2020.)

upon stopping the insulting prescription drug. The male-to-female ratio is closer to 1:1 in DIL; however, females taking TNF-α due to RA have been shown to have a higher ratio than men.[179] This may also be due to the epidemiology of RA. Neonatal lupus is a rare condition that is not a true form of lupus. Infants of mothers who have lupus can demonstrate a rash at birth along with, liver issues, or low blood counts.[128] The symptoms are present for a few months after birth without residual effects.

SLE is the most common form and varies in its presentation and disease severity. Symptoms can affect almost any organ or system of the body. Some clients will have skin and joints involvement with others, can develop issues in the lungs, kidneys, blood, or other organs.[130] The variability in presentation and level of disease involvement makes the diagnosis of SLE difficult.

Epidemiology. The exact cause of SLE is unknown, it is a complex autoimmune disease that is multisystemic. The diverse manifestation of SLE can be due to an interplay of genetic, epigenetic, environmental, hormonal, and immunoregulatory factors.[131] Worldwide incidence rates for SLE vary from approximately 0.3 to 23.7 per 100,000 person-years, and the worldwide prevalence ranges from 6.5 to 178.0 per 100,000.[132]

Environmental factors that may trigger SLE include infections (e.g., Epstein-Barr virus), antibiotics (especially those in the sulfa and penicillin groups) exposure to ultraviolet (sun) light, smoking, occupational exposure to silica dust and hazardous waste, air pollution, psychosocial stress.[131,132]

SLE is more common in African-American, African Caribbean, Hispanic American, American-Indian, and Asian persons than in the Caucasian population.[128,133] Women are more likely to have SLE than men with an approximate 9:1 ratio.[132] It is more common to be diagnosed in persons between the ages of 15 and 40 years old. It is possible that hormones contribute to the increased prevalence in women, however the mechanism is unknown. In women who are pregnant, SLE symptoms can become aggravated and create a clinical challenge requiring a team of specialists for appropriate management during pregnancy.

TABLE 13.7	Main Demographic and Clinical Manifestations of Drug-Induced Lupus (DIL) and Idiopathic Systemic Lupus Erythematosus (SLE)	
	DIL	Idiopathic SLE
F:M	1:1	Up to 9:1
Symptom onset	Gradual, but can also be abrupt drug-dependent, tends to be older than in idiopathic SLF	Usually gradual
Age at onset		20–40 years
Fever/malaise	40%–50%	40%–85%
Arthralgia/arthritis	80%–95%	75%–95%
Rash (*all*)	10%–30%	50%–70%
Rash (*malar/acute cutaneous*)	2%	42%
Raynaud's phenomenon	<25%	35%–50%
Pleuritis/pleural effusion	10%–50% (procainamide)	16%–60%
Lung infiltrates	5%–40% (procainamide)	0%–10%
Renal involvement	<5%	30%–50%
CNS involvement	<2%	20%–70%
Hematologic involvement	Rare	Common

From Vaglio A, Grayson P, et al. Drug-induced lupus: Traditional and new concepts. Autoimmu Rev 2018; 912-918.

The role of genes in SLE is evolving. Genes that likely contribute to lupus have been found in studies of whole-genome scans of families with multiple members diagnosed with SLE.[134] Studies have linked the major histocompatibility complex (MHC) genes (HLA-A1, B8, and DR3) to SLE.[134] Certain MHC genes have been associated with an increased risk of the immune system responding to self-antigens resulting in diseases such as lupus.

The immunoregulatory impact on lupus is complex and beyond the scope of this text to discuss in great detail. Individuals with SLE present with altered T-cell and B-cell antigen receptor-mediated activation. This altered activation is partially responsible for disease expression. B cells appear to produce autoantibodies which contribute to tissue damage and have been shown to present antigens and autoantigens to T cells.[131] This process results in additional tissue damage and disease expression. In addition to altered B-cell and T-cell activation, immune complexes are involved. ANA bind to nuclear material in blood and tissues. This accumulation of immune complexes in the blood or tissues is not cleared in large part due to deficient complement (specifically C3 and C4).[131] The kidney is a good example of immune complexes accumulating in the subendothelial and mesangial regions, resulting in nephritis.[131] Lastly, some individuals with SLE will have antiphospholipid syndrome, where antiphospholipid antibodies disrupt coagulation. Individuals with antiphospholipid syndrome are susceptible to thrombolytic events; therefore, they are often treated with blood thinner therapies.[131]

Clinical Signs and Symptoms. A common clinical pattern of symptoms in individuals with SLE does not exist. Clients may differ dramatically in the relative severity and pattern of organ involvement. Given the heterogeneity of SLE presentation, clients can present with a wide variety of symptoms and organ involvement. The most common areas involved include the integument, kidney, hematologic, and musculoskeletal. Given the variability in presentation, the diagnosis of SLE can be a challenge. Diagnostic criteria have been established in an attempt to improve the accuracy of ruling in or ruling out SLE.[135,136]

Diagnostic Criteria. The ACR classification criteria for SLE has been the most widely utilized criteria. The ACR criteria were first established in 1971 and have undergone revisions in 1982 and 1997. The most recent classification criteria for SLE was established by the EULAR and the ACR.[135] This updated classification has an entry criterion of a positive ANA test followed by 10 domains with weighted clinical criteria in each domain. The 10 domains include the following potential clinical signs/symptoms: constitutional, hematologic, neuropsychiatric, mucocutaneous, serosal, musculoskeletal, renal, antiphospholipid antibody test results, complement protein levels (specifically C3 and C4), and SLE-specific antibody test results. If a client has a positive ANA test and > 10 points from the 10 domains, they are considered to have a diagnosis of SLE[135] (Fig. 13.7). Validation of the EULAR/ACR classification criteria demonstrated at a 95% confidence interval a specificity of 0.93 (0.91–0.95) and sensitivity of 0.96 (0.95–0.98).[135] This updated clinical criteria for ruling in or ruling out SLE identifies the various clinical features that clients may present with. Clinically, if a client presents with a new onset of unexplained fever, arthralgias, and recent onset of a rash or oral ulcers, a referral to their primary care provider is warranted for further workup.

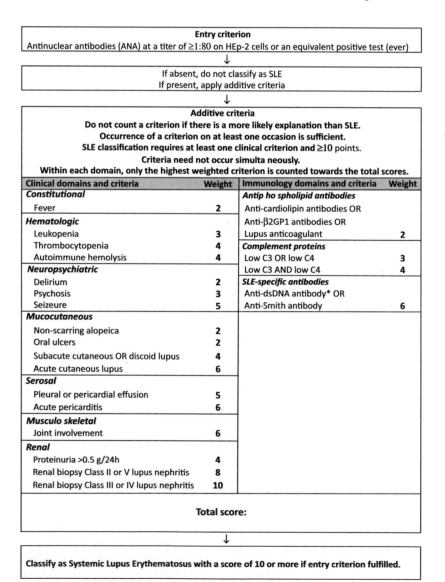

Fig. 13.7 Classification of systemic lupus erythematosus. (From Aringer M, Costenbader K, et al. 2019 European league against rheumatism/American College of Rheumatology classification criteria for systemic lupus erythematosus. Arthritis Rheumatol 2019; 71(9):1400-1412.)

Integumentary Changes. The classic malar or butterfly rash associated with SLE often appears on the cheeks, bridge of the nose, forehead, chin, and V-area of the neck (see Fig. 13.6). Photosensitivity is common for a malar rash; however, it is typically nonscarring.[137] Facial involvement is usually symmetric, and the nasolabial folds are typically spared. Skin rash can also appear over the extensor surfaces of the arms, forearms, and hands/fingers. Discoid lupus discussed earlier is distinctly different in presentation than the integument changes associated with SLE. Flare up of SLE can occur in individuals susceptible to photosensitivity; therefore, it is recommended they utilize sunscreen for appropriate skin coverage, and avoid midday sun exposure.[137]

Musculoskeletal Changes. Arthralgia and arthritis are common presenting manifestations of SLE. Acute migratory or persistent nonerosive arthritis may involve any joint, but typically the small joints of the hands and feet, and knees are symmetrically involved.[137] Lupus does not directly affect the spine, but syndromes, such as costochondritis and cervical myofascial syndrome associated with SLE, are commonly treated in physical therapy practice. Avascular necrosis has been detected in adults with SLE (femoral head is the most common). This is considered a complication of treatment with corticosteroid therapies.[137,138]

Myositis can also be present in SLE which may be due to the disease process or a drug-related reaction. Proximal muscle weakness may be present in clients with SLE. If this is a new onset and unknown to the client's medical provider, it is recommended the client be assessed for potential muscle enzyme elevation or steroid myopathy.[137]

Neuropsychiatric Manifestations. Individuals with SLE are at increased risk of several neuropsychiatric manifestations; these manifestations can be focal or diffuse and are difficult to manage. CNS and PNS changes have been identified along with psychiatric disorders. It appears CNS changes are more common and may present as psychosis, depression, stroke, or transverse myelitis. Neuropsychiatric manifestations of SLE include CVD, seizures, severe depression, acute confusional state, psychosis, neuropathy (cranial, mono, and poly), and movement disorders.[139] Mood disorders in SLE such as depressive disorders have a reported prevalence range of 6% to 44% and anxiety disorders range from 13% to 27%.[139] In adults with SLE, the prevalence of headache ranges 39%–61%, seizures 8%–18%, CVD 2%–8%, cranial neuropathy 1.5%–2.1%, and movement disorders 1%.[115]

Peripheral Neuropathy. PN is considered a neuropsychiatric manifestation of SLE and can present as a motor, sensory (stocking-glove distribution), or mixed motor and sensory polyneuropathy. These may develop subacutely in the lower extremities and progress to the upper extremities. PN in clients with SLE will often present with additional neuropsychiatric manifestations and is typically diagnosed via electromyography and nerve conduction studies.[140] Touch, vibration, and position sense are most prominently affected, and the distal limb reflexes are depressed (Case Example 13.3).

CASE EXAMPLE 13.3
Systemic Lupus Erythematosus

Current Complaint: A 33-year-old woman with a known diagnosis of systemic lupus erythematosus (SLE) came to the physical therapy clinic with the following report: "About 3 weeks ago, I was carrying a heavy briefcase with a strap around my shoulder. I put weight on my right leg and felt my hip joint slip in the back with immediate pain, and I was unable to put any weight on that leg. I moved my hip around in the socket and was able to get immediate relief from the pain, but it felt like it could catch at any time." The client also reported that "it feels like my left hip is 2 inches higher than my right."

Past Medical History: The client reported prolonged (over 7 years) use of prednisone and a past medical history of proteinuria and compromised kidney function. Muscle weakness 2 years ago resulted in a muscle biopsy and a diagnosis of "abnormal" muscle tissue of unknown cause. The client developed a staph infection from the biopsy, which resolved very slowly.

Other past medical history included a motor vehicle accident 2 years ago, at which time her knees went through the dashboard, which left both knees "numb" for a year after the accident.

Clinical Presentation: Aggravating and relieving factors from this visit fit a musculoskeletal pattern of symptoms, and objective examination was consistent with lumbar/sacroiliac mechanical dysfunction with a multitude of other compounding factors, including bilateral posterior cruciate ligament laxity, poor posture, obesity, and emotional lability.

Physical therapy treatment was initiated, but a week later, when the client woke up at night to go to the bathroom, she swung her legs over the edge of her bed and experienced immediate hip and diffuse low back pain and lower extremity weakness.

She went to the emergency department by ambulance and later was admitted to the hospital. She was evaluated by a neurologist (results unknown), recovered from her symptoms within 24 hours, and was released after a 3-day hospitalization. She was directed by her primary care physician to continue outpatient physical therapy services.

Result: After consulting with this client's physician, conservative symptomatic treatment was planned. Within 2 weeks, she experienced another middle-of-the-night acute exacerbation of symptoms. A subsequent magnetic resonance image (MRI) resulted in a diagnosis of disk extrusion (annulus fibrosus perforated with diskal material in the epidural space) at two levels (L4-L5 and L5-S1).

This case example is included to point out the complexity of treating a musculoskeletal condition in a client with a long-term chronic inflammatory disease process requiring years of steroidal antiinflammatory medications. Before including any resistive exercises, muscle energy techniques, or joint or self-mobilization techniques, the physical therapist must be aware of any clinically significant changes in bone density and the presence of developing osteoporosis.

Scleroderma

Scleroderma, one of the lesser-known chronic multisystem diseases in the family of rheumatic diseases, is characterized by inflammation and fibrosis of many parts of the body, including the skin, blood vessels, synovium, skeletal muscle, and certain internal organs such as the kidneys, lungs, heart, and GI tract.

There are two categories of scleroderma: localized scleroderma and systemic. Localized scleroderma is subcategorized into morphea and linear scleroderma.[141] Systemic scleroderma (SSc) is subcategorized into limited and diffuse.[141]

Localized scleroderma typically presents benign, confined to the skin or underlying tissue, and is benign. Morphea is most commonly associated with localized scleroderma that results in sclerotic changes in the skin due to increased quantities of collagen.[142] Multiple subtypes of morphea exist, each of which has unique presentations. Localized scleroderma is a rare condition that can impact adults and children with an incidence of approximately 0.3 to 3 cases per 100,000 inhabitants/year. Caucasian women are more at risk for developing localized scleroderma at a rate of 2–4 women versus 1 man.[142] In adults, the peak incidence occurs in the fifth decade and children are more likely to be diagnosed between ages 2–14.[142] The generalized form of morphea includes plaques identified in more than two body sites. Typically, the plaques are slightly inflamed, pigmented, ill-defined, and adhered to deep planes, fascia, and muscle. The plaques are predominately identified on the trunk and extremities. Generalized morphea may also result in sclerosis of the fingers (without ulcerations) and flexion contractures of joints are common.[142] Pulmonary, esophageal, renal, and cardiac involvement can develop in generalized morphea; however, it is less common.

CLINICAL SIGNS AND SYMPTOMS
Systemic Lupus Erythematosus

Although lupus can affect any part of the body, most people experience symptoms in only a few organs. The most common symptoms associated with lupus are listed.
- Constitutional symptoms (especially low-grade fever and fatigue)
- Achy joints (arthralgia)
- Arthritis (swollen joints)
- Arthralgia
- Skin rashes (malar)
- Pulmonary involvement (e.g., pleurisy, pleural effusion: chest pain, difficulty breathing, cough)
- Anemia
- Kidney involvement (e.g., lupus nephritis)
- Sun or light sensitivity (photosensitivity)
- Hair loss
- Raynaud's phenomenon (fingers turning white or blue in the cold)
- Nervous system involvement:
  - Seizures
  - Headache
  - Peripheral neuropathy
  - Cranial neuropathy
  - Cerebral vascular accidents
  - Organic brain syndrome
  - Psychosis
- Mouth, nose, or vaginal ulcers

Children affected by juvenile localized scleroderma develop multiple extracutaneous manifestations including joint, neurologic (e.g., epilepsy, PN, headache), vascular, and ocular changes. These manifestations are often unrelated to the site of the skin lesions and can be associated with multiple organ involvement. Despite these extracutaneous manifestations, the risk of developing SSc is very low.[141]

SSc is an uncommon disease, with a high mortality rate and multiorgan involvement.[143] Raynaud's phenomenon and gastroesophageal reflux are early clinical signs of SSc. Additionally, patients may present with inflammation of the skin, puffy and swollen fingers, and musculoskeletal inflammation.[143] Constitutional symptoms such as fatigue may be present along with internal organ manifestations, including GI effects and pulmonary fibrosis, as well as severe life-threatening involvement of the heart and kidneys.[143,144]

Clinical Signs and Symptoms

Skin. Raynaud's phenomenon and tight skin are the hallmarks of SSc. The majority of individuals with SSc have Raynaud's phenomenon, which is defined as episodic pallor of the digits following exposure to cold or stress associated with cyanosis, followed by erythema, tingling, and pain. Raynaud's phenomenon primarily affects the hands and feet and less commonly the ears, nose, and tongue.

As discussed earlier, systemic sclerosis can be subdivided into two subsets: diffuse or limited. Both diffuse and limited systemic sclerosis have unique cutaneous presentations that distinguish between the two subsets. Diffuse SSc presents with proximal involvement including a loss of hand function and severe digital ulcers (Fig. 13.8).[145] Restrictions involving the extremities distal to the elbows or knees, with or without facial involvement are consistent with limited SSc (Fig. 13.9).

Musculoskeletal. Involvement of the musculoskeletal system can often be overlooked in individuals with SSc, given the complications of the internal organs. Musculoskeletal presentations can include arthralgia, inflammatory polyarthritis, small and large joint contractures, subcutaneous calcinosis, and tendon friction rubs.[145] Tendon friction rubs are not well understood; however, they may be due to fibrin deposits in the tendon's synovial sheath.[146] Presence of tendon friction rubs have been estimated to be present in 20% of individual's with SSc and are related to disease activity.[146]

Viscera. Skin changes, Raynaud's phenomenon, and involvement of the GI tract are the most common manifestation of SSc. Changes in the small intestine can result in reduced motility causing intermittent diarrhea, bloating, cramping, malabsorption, and weight loss. Inflammation and fibrosis can also affect the lungs, resulting in interstitial lung disease, a restrictive lung disease.[147,148]

The overall course of scleroderma is highly variable. Once remission occurs, relapse is uncommon. The diffuse form generally has a worse prognosis due to the potential for cardiac involvement, such as cardiomyopathy, pericarditis, pericardial effusion, or arrhythmia.

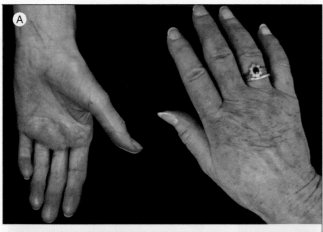

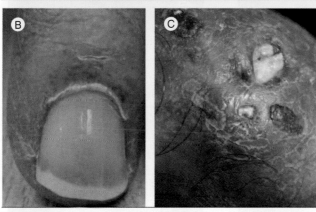

Fig. 13.8 Diffuse systemic sclerosis presents with proximal involvement including a loss of hand function (A) and severe digital ulcers (B and C). (From Denton CP, Khanna D. Systemic sclerosis. Lancet. 2017; 390:1685–1699.)

CLINICAL SIGNS AND SYMPTOMS

Scleroderma

Localized Scleroderma
- Circumscribed sclerotic plaques with ivory-colored center
- Widespread skin involvement with multiple plaques and hyperpigmentation
- Muscle atrophy
- Sclerodactyly (chronic hardening and shrinking of fingers and toes)
- Telangiectasia (spider-like hemangiomas formed by dilation of a group of small blood vessels; occurs most commonly on the face and hands)

Systemic Scleroderma: Diffuse
- Short history of Raynaud's phenomenon
- Proximal limb or trunk involvement, with skin sclerosis
- Increased risk of renal crisis
- Increased risk of cardiac involvement
- Severe lung fibrosis

Systemic Scleroderma: Limited
- Long history of Raynaud's phenomenon
- Distal skin sclerosis (distal to elbows or knees)
- Pulmonary arterial hypertension
- Severe gut disease

Spondyloarthritis

Spondyloarthropathy/spondyloarthritis (SpA) is an interrelated group of noninfectious, inflammatory, and erosive rheumatic conditions that target not only spinal and peripheral joints but also have extraarticular manifestations such as enthesitis (attachments of ligaments and tendons to bones), uveitis (eye inflammation), dactylitis (inflammation of the fingers and/or toes), psoriasis, and inflammation of the GI tract (see discussion in Chapter 9; see Box 13.1). This group of diseases is currently divided into two major categories: axial SpA and predominantly peripheral SpA.[148–150] Patients with SpA may have concurrent prominent peripheral and axial SpA or successive manifestations of either. SpA includes Ankylosing Spondylitis (AS), Psoriatic arthritis (PsA), Reactive Arthritis (ReA), and Inflammatory Bowel Disease (IBD)-related arthritis.

Classification of SpA has evolved over time to represent the complex relationship between these associated yet heterogeneous disorders (Fig. 13.10). The Assessment of Spondyloarthritis International Society (ASAS) has offered updated classification criteria which seek to classify patients based on interrelated clinical manifestations to capture patients earlier in the disease process. Since early intervention with TNF-α can retard the disease progression, expeditious recognition of clinical manifestations and timely diagnosis could facilitate patient outcomes.[151–152] However, some argue whether these conditions should be "lumped" together according to similar clinical manifestations or should be "split" into specific subcategories.[154] For the purposes of this text, the current ASAS criteria as well as the characteristics of the classic classifications of SpA will be discussed (Fig. 13.11).

Individuals with SpA are not seropositive for RF, and the progressive joint fibrosis present is associated with the genetic marker human leukocyte antigen (HLA-B27). The estimated absolute risk of SpA in persons with HLA B27 is 2%–10% but increases if a first-degree relative also has the disease.[155] Spondyloarthritis is more common in men, who by gender have a familial tendency toward the development of this type of disease.

Axial Spondyloarthritis. Axial spondyloarthritis (AxSpA) is a chronic, progressive inflammatory disease, and the term is used to describe both nonradiographic AxSpA and radiographic AxSpA, or AS.[156] The prevalence of AxSpA is estimated to be 0.9%–1.4% in the United States.[157] The terminology related to this condition has been updated to identify patients in the early stages of AxSpA who may have evidence of sacroilial inflammation on MRI and features of AxSpA but do not yet demonstrate radiographic changes of the sacroiliac (SI) joints, which can take years to develop.[158] Patients with nonradiographic AxSpA may or may not progress to radiographic AxSpa, or AS.[159] It is important to note that AxSpA and peripheral SpA can overlap and exist together.[158] Other musculoskeletal features of AxSpA include asymmetrical arthritis affecting a few joints predominantly in the lower extremities and most notably the hips and enthesitis as well as the extraarticular manifestations (see Box 13.1).[148]

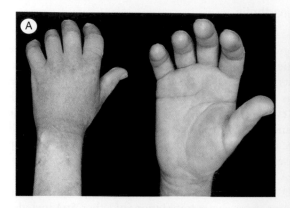

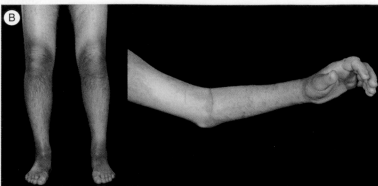

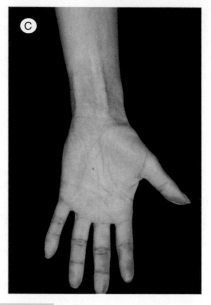

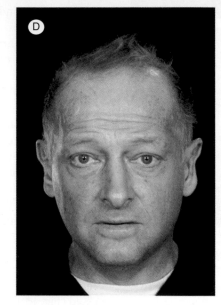

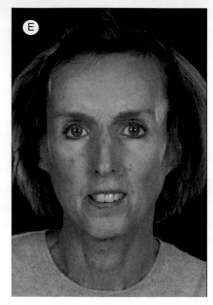

Fig. 13.9 Restrictions involving the extremities distal to the elbows or knees (A, B, and C), with or without facial involvement (D and E) are consistent with limited Systemic Sclerosis. (From Denton CP, Khanna D. Systemic sclerosis. Lancet. 2017; 390:1685-1699.)

BOX 13.1 EXTRAARTICULAR FEATURES OF SPA

- Anterior uveitis
- Conjunctivitis
- Enthesitis
- Psoriasis
- Inflammatory bowel disease
- Osteoporosis
- Cardiovascular involvement, e.g., aortic regurgitation, atrioventricular block
- Pulmonary involvement
- Renal involvement, e.g., secondary amyloidosis, IgA nephropathy

(Taurog, 2016; Pereira, 2012)

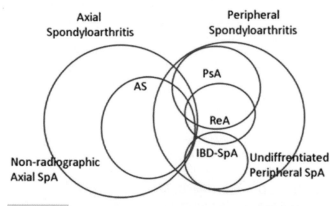

Fig. 13.10 Classification of spondyloarthritis. (From Raychaudhuri SP, Deodhar A. The classification and diagnostic criteria for ankylosing spondylitis. J Autoimmun 2014; 48-49:128–133.)

There are no clear diagnostic criteria for AS, but the modified New York Criteria remain the "gold standard" (see Box 13.2). However, these criteria require radiological evidence of sacroiliitis which, as mentioned previously, can take years to develop.[148] Diagnosis may be delayed or inappropriate when reliance is only on x-ray films because disease progression over time is required for a confirmed diagnosis. New diagnostic criteria using MRI have helped improve rates of early diagnosis.[160] The ASAS classification criteria were developed to provide greater specificity for clinical research purposes though these criteria are not without limitations (see Fig. 13.11).[152,157]

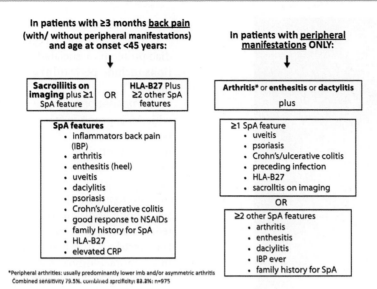

In patients with ≥3 months <u>back pain</u>
(with/ without peripheral manifestations)
and age at onset <45 years:

In patients with <u>peripheral</u>
<u>manifestations</u> ONLY:

| **Sacroiliitis on imaging** plus ≥1 SpA feature | OR | **HLA-B27** Plus ≥2 other SpA features |

Arthritis* or **enthesitis** or **dactylitis**
plus

SpA features
- inflammators back pain (IBP)
- arthritis
- enthesitis (heel)
- uveitis
- daciylitis
- psoriasis
- Crohn's/ulcerative colitis
- good response to NSAIDs
- family history for SpA
- HLA-B27
- elevated CRP

≥1 SpA feature
- uveitis
- psoriasis
- Crohn's/ulcerative colitis
- preceding infection
- HLA-B27
- sacrolitis on imaging

OR

≥2 other SpA features
- arthritis
- enthesitis
- daciylitis
- IBP ever
- family history for SpA

*Peripheral arthrities: usually predominantly lower imb and/or asymmetric arthritis
Combined sensitivity 79.5%. combined sprcificity: 83.3%; n=975

Fig. 13.11 Criteria for axial and peripheral spondyloarthritis. (From Rudwaleit M, van der Heijde D, Landewé R, et al. The assessment of Spondyloarthritis International Society classification criteria for peripheral spondyloarthritis and for spondyloarthritis in general. Ann Rheum Dis. 2011;70(1):25–31.)

BOX 13.2   MODIFIED NEW YORK CRITERIA

1 Radiological criterion

Bilateral sacroiliitis grade ≥ II or unilateral sacroiliitis grade Ill to IV

2 Clinical criteria

(a) Low back pain and stiffness of at least 3 months duration improved by exercise and not relieved by rest

(b) Limitation of motion of the lumbar spine in both the sagittal and the frontal planes

(c) Limitation of chest expansion relative to values normal for age and sex

Definite AS is diagnosed if the radiological criterion plus 2 of the 3 clinical criteria are present.

(From van der Linden S, Valkenburg HA, Cats A. Evaluation of diagnostic criteria for ankylosing spondylitis. A proposal for modification of the New York criteria. Arthritis Rheum. 1984;27(4):361–368.)

Risk Factors. The prevalence of AS is 31.9 people per 10,000 in North America.[94] Although 90% of patients with AS are HLA-B27 positive, it appears that additional factors (e.g., environmental) are needed for the condition to appear.[161]

Clinical Signs and Symptoms. The classic presentation of AS is insidious onset of inflammatory middle and low back pain and stiffness for more than 3 months in a person (usually male) under 40 years of age. Inflammatory back pain is characterized by prolonged morning stiffness (lasting > 1 hour), and symptoms worse with rest and at night (typically 2 AM to 5 AM), and improved with movement and exercise[149,162]. Patients may note achy or sharp ("jolting") pain, typically localized to the pelvis, buttocks, and hips; this pain can be confused with sciatica. A neurologic examination will be within normal limits.

Paravertebral muscle spasm, aching, and stiffness are common, but some clients may have slow progressive limitation of motion with no pain at all. Most clients have sacroiliitis as the earliest feature seen on x-ray films before clinical involvement extends to the lumbar spine. MRI can demonstrate acute and chronic changes of sacroiliitis, osteitis, discovertebral lesions, disk calcifications and ossification, arthropathic (joint) lesions, and complications such as fracture and cauda equina syndrome.[163]

During the physical examination, decreased mobility in the anteroposterior and lateral planes will be symmetric. Reduction in lumbar flexion is an early sign of AS. Schober's test (and modified Schober's test, which is now more commonly used) is used to confirm reduction in spinal motion associated with AS[164] The SI joint is rarely tender by direct palpation; however, provocative testing of the SI joint may reproduce symptoms though it should be noted that the specificity of these tests is low.[156] As the disease progresses, the inflamed ligaments and tendons around the vertebrae ossify (turn to bone), causing a rigid spine and the loss of lumbar lordosis. In the most severe cases, the spine becomes so completely fused that the person may be locked in a rigid upright position or in a stooped position, unable to move the neck or back in any direction. Peripheral joint involvement usually (but not always) occurs after involvement of the spine. Typical extraspinal sites include the manubriosternal joint, symphysis pubis, shoulder, and hip joints. If the ligaments that attach the ribs to the spine become ossified, diminished chest expansion (<2 cm) occurs, making it difficult to take a deep breath. Chest wall stiffness seldom leads to respiratory disability as long as diaphragmatic movement is intact. This process of vertebral and costovertebral fusion results in the formation of syndesmophytes (Fig. 13.12). This reparative process also

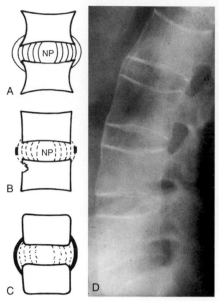

Fig. 13.12 Pathogenesis of the syndesmophyte. The syndesmophyte, along with destruction of the sacroiliac (SI) joint, is the hallmark of inflammatory spondyloarthropathies such as ankylosing spondylitis (AS). It should be distinguished from the osteophyte, which is characteristic of degenerative spondylosis. (A) Normal intervertebral disk. The inner fibers of the annulus fibrosus are next to the nucleus pulposus (NP). The outer fibers insert into the periosteum of the vertebral body at least one third the distance toward the next end-plate. (B) With early inflammation, the corners of the bodies are reabsorbed and appear to be square or even eroded. Fine deposits of amorphous apatite (calcium phosphate, a mineral constituent of bone) first appear in radiographs as thin, delicate calcification in the outer fibers of the mid-annulus. (C) and (D) The process progresses to bridging calcification, with the syndesmophyte extending from one midbody to the next. Thus, the spine takes on its bamboo-like appearance in radiographs. (A to C, From Hadler NM. Medical Management of the Regional Musculoskeletal Diseases. Grune & Stratton: Orlando, FL, 1984:5; D, From Bullough PG. Bullough and Vigorita's Orthopaedic Pathology. 3rd ed. London: Mosby-Wolfe; 1987:68.)

forms linear bone ossification along the outer fibers of the annulus fibrosis of the disk.

This bridging of the vertebrae is most prominent along the anterior longitudinal ligament and occurs earliest in the thoracolumbar region. Destructive changes of the upper and lower corners of the vertebrae (at the insertion of the annulus fibrosis of the disk) are responsible for the vertebral squaring. Late in the disease, the vertebral column takes on an appearance that is referred to as *bamboo spine.*

A physical exam of the eyes, skin, and cardiopulmonary systems may reveal extraarticular features which occur in 25% of patients and is unrelated to the severity of the joint disease.[156,163] As with other forms of SpA, enthesitis, especially of the Achilles tendon and proximal attachment of the plantar fascia, is common in patients with AS (Fig. 13.13).[149] Ocular symptoms may precede spinal symptoms by several weeks or years. Pulmonary changes (chronic infiltrative or fibrotic bullous changes of the upper lobes) occur in 1% to 3% of persons with AS and may be confused with TB. Conduction abnormalities, particularly atrioventricular

node, are the most common cardiac complications related to AS. Aoritis and aortic regurgitation are other common cardiac problems associated with AS. Less common manifestations include pericarditis, cardiomyopathy, and mitral valve disease.[149]

Complications. The very stiff osteoporotic spine of clients with AS is prone to fracture from even minor trauma. It has been estimated that the incidence of thoracolumbar fractures in AS is four times higher than that of the general population.[165] The most common site of fracture is the lower cervical spine. Risk of neurologic damage may be compounded by the development of epidural hematoma from lacerated vessels. Spondylodiscitis (erosive and destructive lesions of vertebral bodies) is seen in clients with long-standing disease. Intervertebral disk lesions occur at multiple levels, especially in the thoracolumbar region.[149,167]

Patients with AS may present with symptomatic or asymptomatic atlantoaxial subluxation (AAS). The estimated prevalence of AAS in patients with AS is 14.1%.[168] Severe neck or occipital pain possibly referring to the retro-orbital or frontal area can be a presenting symptom of AAS. This underappreciated entity may be either an early or a late manifestation, but it is frequently seen in clients with persistent peripheral arthritis, longer duration of AS, higher levels of disease activity (increased levels of CRP), and failure to respond to conventional nonsteroidal antiinflammatory drugs (NSAIDs). Careful monitoring for this complication is warranted due to its association with spinal cord and vascular compression.[168] The diagnosis of AAS is usually made from lateral x-ray views of the cervical spine in flexion and extension.

Neurological complications related to AS can arise due to fracture, AAS, or cauda equina syndrome. Cauda equina syndrome is a late (rare) manifestation of the disease. The initial deficit is loss of sensation of the lower extremities, along with urinary and rectal sphincter disturbances and/or perineal pain and weakness or saddle anesthesia and potentially complaints of neurogenic pain in the rectum and/or lower quarter.[149] Anyone with a known diagnosis of AS and a history of incontinence (bowel or bladder) or neurologic deficit should be evaluated for surgical intervention. Spinal stenosis occurs as a result of bony overgrowth of the spinal ligaments and facet joints. Symptoms consistent with neurogenic claudication, such as pain and numbness of the lower extremities brought on by walking and relieved by rest, can occur is the presence of spinal stenosis.

Reactive Arthritis. ReA was formerly known as Reiter's syndrome. Reiter described a triad of arthritis, conjunctivitis, and nonspecific urethritis in soldiers during the First World War, but the disease has been described since the 1500 s.[168] ReA typically presents after a triggering bacterial infection of the GI or urogenital tract.[169] Only a third of patients with ReA demonstrate the classic triad of symptoms and manifestations can vary based on the triggering event, the individual's genetic makeup, and the sequential reaction.[149] ReA can occur in men, women, and children; however, it more commonly occurs in adults than in children.

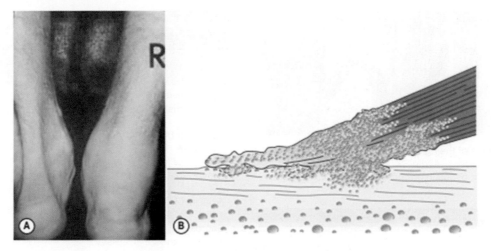

Fig. 13.13   Enthesitis (schematic diagram in B), especially of the Achilles tendon (A) and proximal attachment of the plantar fascia, is common in patients with ankylosing spondulosis. (From Reveille J. Spondyloarthritis. In: Rich R, Fleisher T, Shearer W, Schroeder H, Frew A, Weyand C. Clinical immunology: Principles and Practice. 5th edition. New York: Elsevier; 2019:769–787.)

Relative risk is higher in women after an enteric infection, but men are more affected after a venereal infection.[170,172] Most commonly inciting pathogens for ReA are *Chlamydia trachomatis, Salmonella, Shigella, Campylobacter jenjuni,* and *Yersinia.*[172] The initial infection is generally resolved before the onset of ReA-associated signs and symptoms,[172] and the onset of ReA may be abrupt, occurring over several days or more gradually over several weeks after the triggering infection.[172]

Risk Factors. HLA-B27, present in a high-frequency pattern, supports a genetic predisposition for the development of this syndrome after a person is exposed to certain bacterial infections. Having HLA-B27 does not necessarily mean that the person will develop this syndrome, but indicates that the person will have a greater chance of developing ReA than persons without this marker.[170]

ReA can be differentiated from AS by the presence of urethritis and conjunctivitis, the prominent involvement of distal joints, and the presence of asymmetric radiologic changes in the SI joints and spine.

Clinical Signs and Symptoms. ReA often occurs precipitously and frequently affects the knees and ankles, lasting weeks to months. The distribution of the arthritis typically follows that of peripheral SpA and begins in the weight-bearing joints, especially of the lower extremities, but patients can also present with arthritis of the upper extremities and axial skeleton.[169]

The arthritis may vary in severity from absence to extreme joint destruction. Involvement of the feet and spine is most common and is associated with HLA-B27 positivity. Affected joints are usually warm, tender, and edematous, with pain during active and passive movement. A dusky-blue discoloration or frank erythema accompanied by exquisite tenderness is a sign of a septic joint. Although the joints usually begin to improve after 2 or 3 weeks, many people continue to have pain, especially in the heels and back.

Low back and buttock pain are common in ReA; such pain is caused by SI joint or other spinal joint involvement.

SI changes seen by x-ray films are usually asymmetric and similar to those of AS. Small joint involvement, especially in the feet, is more common in ReA than in AS and is often asymmetric.

In addition to arthritis, dactylitis and enthesitis is common (Figs. 13.13 and 13.14).[170] Enthesitis most commonly occurs at the insertions of the plantar aponeurosis and Achilles tendon, on the calcaneus, leading to heel pain—one of the most frequent, distinctive, and disabling manifestations of the disease. Other common sites for enthesitis include ischial tuberosities, iliac crests, tibial tuberosities, and ribs, with associated musculoskeletal pain at sites other than the joints (Case Example 13.4).

The *conjunctivitis* of ReA is mild and characterized by irritation with redness, tearing, and burning usually lasting a few days (or less commonly as long as several weeks). The process is ordinarily self-limiting.

Urethritis manifested by burning and urinary frequency is often the earliest symptom. A profuse and watery diarrhea can precede the onset of urethritis in ReA.

Psoriatic Arthritis. PsA is a form of peripheral SpA with multiple, heterogenous musculoskeletal and dermatological characteristics. It is not just a variant of RA but is a distinct disease that combines features of both RA (e.g., joint pain, erythema, swelling, stiffness) and SpA (e.g., enthesopathy: inflammation at insertion points of tendon, ligament, capsule; iritis) (Table 13.8). There are no validated diagnostic criteria for PsA; however, the 2006 Classification for Psoriatic Arthritis (CASPAR) criteria are most used as a means of selecting patients for clinical trials and guiding clinicians.[174] Psoriasis is quite common, affecting 1% to 3% of the general population. This arthritis occurs in one third of clients with psoriasis.[175]

In contrast to RA, there is no sex predilection in PsA. Both sexes are affected equally, although women tend to develop symmetric polyarthritis, and spinal involvement is more common in men. PsA can occur at any age, although it usually occurs between the ages of 20 and 30 years. The onset of

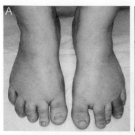
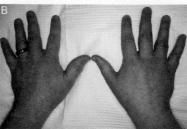

Fig. 13.14 Dactylitis of the right fourth toe (A) and left thumb (B). (From Kaeley GS, Eder L, Aydin SZ, Gutierrez M, Bakewell C. Dactylitis: A hallmark of psoriatic arthritis. *Semin Arthritis Rheum.* 2018;48(2):263–273.)

CASE EXAMPLE 13.4

Reactive Arthritis

Past Medical History: At presentation, a 22-year-old man had left heel pain that had developed 3 weeks before his appointment in physical therapy. He could not attribute any trauma to the foot and was not involved in any sports or athletic activities. Previous medical history was minimal, except for an appendectomy when he was 18 years old.

Clinical Presentation: The client reported that his pain was worst when he first got out of bed in the morning but improved with stretching and taking aspirin. He did not wear any orthotics or special shoes. The physical therapist did not ask about the presence of associated signs or symptoms.

No obvious gait abnormalities were observed. During palpation of the foot, there was no warmth, bruising, or redness in the area of the plantar fascia or calcaneus. Tenderness was reported along the plantar fascia, with a painful response to palpation of the tendinous attachment to the calcaneus. Ankle range of motion and muscle strength of the left lower leg were within normal limits. There was no tenderness of the surrounding bones, tendons, or muscles. A neurologic screen was also considered normal.

Intervention: The physical therapist treated this client by using a treatment protocol for plantar fasciitis, including ultrasound, deep friction massage, and stretching exercises. Symptoms subsided, and the client was discharged. He returned 6 weeks later with recurrence of the original symptoms and new onset of low back pain.

The physical therapist reevaluated the client, including an in-depth evaluation of postural components and performance of a back screening examination, but again did not ask any questions related to associated signs and symptoms. Before his next appointment, the client called and canceled further physical therapy treatment.

Result: A follow-up call determined that this young man had developed other symptoms, such as fever, red and itching eyes, and frequent urination. He went to a walk-in clinic, was referred to an internist, and received a diagnosis of reactive arthritis (ReA).

Whenever a client has musculoskeletal pain or symptoms of unknown cause, a series of questions must be posed to screen for medical disease. This is especially important when symptoms do not respond to treatment, when symptoms recur, or when new musculoskeletal symptoms develop.

Although joint pain, heel pain, or back pain usually occurs after the development of conjunctivitis, enteritis, or urethritis in ReA, this young man developed musculoskeletal symptoms first. At the time of the initial physical therapy evaluation, he was experiencing fatigue, low-grade fever, and malaise that he did not report. Asking the question "Are there any other symptoms of any kind anywhere in your body?" or additional questions as part of a systems review might have elicited the early red flag–associated signs and symptoms of an infection.

TABLE 13.8	Comparison of Features of Psoriatic Arthritis and Rheumatoid Arthritis	
	Psoriatic Arthritis	Rheumatoid Arthritis
Age of onset	36	20–40
Male: Female ratio	1:1	1:2–3
Joint distributions at onset	Asymmetric	Symmetric
Number of joints involved	Any joint, including distal interphalangeal joints	Usually distal interphalangeal joints spared
Axial involvement	Axial spondylarthritis phenotype common	Erosive cervical spine disease
Sacroiliitis	Common	Absent
Sites of hands/ feet involved	Distal	Proximal
Enthesitis	Typically present, (60%–80%)	Not typical
Dactylitis	Common (40%)	Not typical

Data from: Ritchlin CT, Colbert RA, Gladman DD. Psoriatic arthritis [published correction appears in N Engl J Med. 2017 May 25;376(21):2097]. N Engl J Med. 2017;376(10):957-970 and Coates LC, Helliwell PS. Psoriatic arthritis: State of the art review. Clin Med (London) 2017;17(1):65-70.

the arthritis may be acute or insidious and is usually preceded by the skin disease.[174]

Risk Factors The cause of psoriasis and any risk factors for PsA are unknown. PsA is a complex, multifactorial disease; multiple genes are likely to influence disease susceptibility and severity.[176] The presence of the histocompatibility complex marker HLA-B27 and other HLA antigens is not uncommon, and they occur in clients with peripheral arthritis and spondylitis.

The presence of these genetic markers may be associated with an increased susceptibility to unknown infectious or environmental agents or to primary abnormal autoimmune phenomena. There is some evidence to support dysregulated angiogenesis as a primary pathogenic mechanism in PsA.[178]

Clinical Signs and Symptoms. *Skin lesions* that characterize psoriasis are readily recognized as piles of well-defined, dry, erythematous, often overlapping silver-scaled papules and plaques. These may appear in small, easily overlooked patches or may run together and cover wide areas. The scalp, extensor surfaces of the elbows and knees, back, and buttocks are common sites. The lesions, which do not usually itch, come and go and may be present for years (typically 5 to 10 years) before the onset of arthritis.

Nail lesions, including pitting, ridging (transverse grooves), cracking, onycholysis (loosening or separation of the nail; see Fig. 4.31), brown-yellow discoloration, and destruction of the nail, are the only clinical features that may identify clients with psoriasis in whom arthritis is likely to develop. The nail changes may be mistaken for those produced by a fungal infection.

Arthritis appears as an early and severe sign in a symmetric distal distribution (DIP joints of fingers and toes before involvement of MCP and MTP joints) in half of all clients with PsA, which distinguishes it from RA. Severe erosive disease may lead to marked deformity of the hands and feet, called arthritis mutilans. Wrists, ankles, knees, and elbows can also be involved.

Clients report pain and stiffness in the inflamed joints, with morning stiffness that lasts more than 30 minutes. Other evidence of inflammation includes pain if stressing the joint, tenderness at the joint line, and the presence of effusion. Painful symptoms are aggravated by prolonged immobility and are reduced by physical activity.

Marked vertebral involvement can result in *ankylosis of the spine*. This differs from AS in a number of respects, most notably in the tendency for many of the syndesmophytes to arise not at the margins of the vertebral bodies, but from the lateral and anterior surfaces of the bodies. Asymmetric spondylitis, including erosions, sclerosis, and ankylosis similar to that in ReA, occur in up to 40% clients with PsA.[178]

Soft-tissue involvement, similar to clinical manifestations of spondyloarthritis, occurs often in PsA. Enthesitis, or inflammation at the site of tendon insertion or muscle attachment to bone, is frequently observed at the Achilles tendon, plantar fascia, and pelvic bones (see Fig. 13.13). Also common is tenosynovitis of the flexor tendons of the hands, extensor carpi ulnaris, and other sites.

Dactylitis, which occurs in more than 16%–69% of PsA clients, is marked by diffuse swelling of the whole finger.[179] Inflammation in this typical "sausage finger" extends to the tendon sheaths and adjacent joints (see Fig. 13.14).

Extraarticular features similar to those seen in clients with other seronegative spondyloarthritides are frequently seen. These extraarticular lesions include uveitis, mouth ulcers, urethritis, and, less commonly, colitis and aortic valve disease. Patients with PsA have also been found to have a higher prevalence of hypertension, dyslipidemia, and diabetes mellitus.[181]

Early recognition of this disorder is important because medical intervention with newer biologic agents can help prevent long-term complications such as permanent joint destruction and disability.[180]

Lyme Disease

In the early 1970s, a mysterious clustering of juvenile arthritis occurred among children in Lyme, Connecticut, and in surrounding towns. Medical researchers soon recognized the illness as a distinct disease, which they called Lyme disease. They were able to identify the deer tick infected with a spiral bacterium or spirochete (later named *Borrelia burgdorferi*) as the key to its spread.

The number of reported cases of Lyme disease, as well as the number of geographic areas in which it is found, has been increasing. Most cases are concentrated in the coastal northeast, the mid-Atlantic states, Wisconsin, Minnesota, Oregon, and northern California. Children may be more susceptible than adults simply because they spend more time outdoors and are more likely to be exposed to ticks.

Clinical Signs and Symptoms. About 70% to 80% of individuals with Lyme disease will first develop a red rash, known as *erythema migrans*, which starts as a small red spot that expands forming a circular, triangular, or oval rash (Fig. 13.15). The rash will typically have a delayed onset 7 days after a bite, on average, but onset can be between 3 to 30

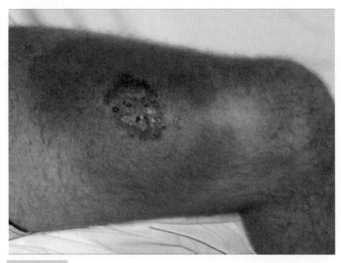

Fig. 13.15 Erythema migrans in lyme disease. (From Wetter D, Ruff C, Erythema migrans in Lyme disease. Canadian Med Assoc J 183(11):1281–1281.)

days after the bite. Sometimes the rash resembles a bull's-eye because it appears as a red ring surrounding a central clear area. The rash can range in size from that of a dime to the entire width of a person's back, and usually at the site of the bite, which is often the axilla or groin. As infection spreads, several rashes can appear at different sites on the body.[181]

Erythema migrans is often accompanied by flu-like symptoms such as fever, headache, stiff neck, body aches, and fatigue. Although these symptoms resemble those of common viral infections, Lyme disease symptoms tend to persist or may occur intermittently over a period of several weeks to months.

Arthritis appears several months after infection with *B. burgdorferi*. Slightly more than half of the people who are not treated with antibiotics develop recurrent attacks of painful and swollen joints that last a few days to a few months. About 10% to 20% of untreated clients will go on to develop chronic arthritis.[182]

In most clients, Lyme arthritis is monoarticular or oligoarticular (few joints), most commonly affecting the knee, but the arthritis can shift from one joint to another. Other large joints, such as the hip, shoulder, and elbow, are also commonly affected.[183] Involvement of the hands and feet is uncommon, and it is these features that help differentiate Lyme arthritis from RA.[184]

Neurologic symptoms (including cognitive dysfunction referred to as *neurocognitive symptoms*) may appear because Lyme disease can affect the nervous system. Symptoms include stiff neck; severe headache associated with meningitis; Bell's palsy; numbness, pain, or weakness in the limbs; radiculopathy; or poor motor coordination. Memory loss, difficulty in concentrating, mood changes, and sleep disturbances have also been associated with Lyme disease. Nervous system involvement can develop several weeks, months, or even years following an untreated infection. These symptoms last for weeks or months and may recur.

Cardiac involvement occurs in less than 1% of the people affected by Lyme disease. Symptoms of irregular heartbeat, dizziness, and dyspnea occur several weeks after the infection and rarely last more than a few days or weeks. Recovery is usually complete.

Finally, although Lyme disease can be divided into early and later stages, each with a different set of complications, these stages may vary in duration, may overlap, or may even be absent.

Lyme disease is still mistaken for other ailments, including GBS, MS, and FMS, and can be difficult to diagnose. The only distinctive hallmark unique to Lyme disease, the erythema migrans rash, is absent in at least one fourth of those who become infected. Many people are unaware that they have been bitten by a tick (Case Example 13.5).

In general, the sooner treatment is initiated, the quicker and more complete the recovery, with less chance for the development of subsequent symptoms of arthritis and neurologic problems. Following treatment for Lyme disease, some persons still have persistent fatigue and achiness, which can take months to subside.

Unfortunately, having had Lyme disease once is no guarantee that the illness will be prevented in the future. The disease can strike more than once in the same individual if they are reinfected with the Lyme disease bacterium.

Autoimmune-Mediated Neurologic Disorders

There are neurologic disorders encountered by therapists that whose manifestation is in part due to dysfunction of the immune system. Such diseases include MS, GBS, and MG. Other dysfunctions, such as amyotrophic lateral sclerosis and acute disseminated encephalomyelitis, also associated with

immunologic dysfunction but less often encountered by therapists, are not discussed.

Multiple Sclerosis

MS is an inflammatory demyelinating disease of the CNS, affecting areas of the brain, spinal cord, and optic nerve. The PNS is spared in MS. MS is the most common inflammatory condition effecting the CNS and one of the most common sources of nontraumatic disability in younger individuals and adults.[185] Diagnosis usually occurs between 20 and 50 years of age, with a peak onset of age 31.[185] MS is typically divided into four disease courses: clinically isolated syndrome (CIS), relapsing-remitting (RRMS), primary progressive (PPMS), and secondary progressive (SPMS).[186]

Risk Factors. Women are 1.5 to 2.5 times more affected than men.[187] Men with MS typically experience a more aggressive progression of the disease and a worse prognosis.[188] Caucasians of Northern European descent have a higher incident of MS than individuals of Asian, African, or Hispanic ancestry. MS is more prevalent in the temperate (colder) climates of North America and Europe than in tropical areas, even among people with similar genetic backgrounds. This may be due to a lack of vitamin D, given the reduced sun exposure for those living further from the equator. Vitamin D appears to have a role in neuroprotection and myelin repair, and lack of vitamin D is under investigation as a potential contributing factor for developing MS.[189] Additional environmental risk factors for MS, include cigarette smoking, obesity, and exposure to infections (Epstein-Barr virus and infectious mononucleosis).[190,191] MS is identified as an autoimmune disease; however, the actual cause remains unknown. A virus or other infectious agents, toxins, vaccinations, and surgery are all thought to be possible triggers for the immune-mediated response, which is believed to destroy the CNS myelin.[107] Activated T and B cells in response to a virus, toxin, or stressor become involved in the degradation of myelin which along with proinflammatory mediators results in demyelination, axonal injury, and loss of oligodendrocytes.

The disease is characterized by inflammatory demyelinating (destructive removal or loss) lesions that later form scars known as plaques, which are scattered throughout the CNS white matter of the cerebrum, spinal cord, and optic nerves. Initially considered a disease that impacted only the white matter, the gray matter is also involved resulting in neuron cell body degradation. When edema and inflammation subside, some remyelination occurs, but it is often incomplete. Axonal injury may cause permanent neurologic dysfunction and ultimately a decline in function.

The progression of MS is difficult to predict and depends on several factors, including the person's age and the intensity of onset, the neurologic status at 5 years after the onset, and the course of exacerbation and remission. The survival rate after the onset of symptoms is typically favorable; however, at least 50% of patients die of MS-related causes. Mean ages at death vary slightly between PPMS (76.3 years) and RRMS

CASE EXAMPLE 13.5

Lyme Disease

A 54-year-old business executive developed searing neck and back pain and was diagnosed as having a cervical disk protrusion. He was sent to physical therapy but had a very busy travel schedule and was unable to make even half of his scheduled appointments.

He chose to discontinue physical therapy, but his symptoms worsened and the pain became so intense that he was unable to go to work some mornings. He also started experiencing numbness in his right arm along the ulnar nerve distribution. He returned to physical therapy, but there was no discernible improvement subjectively, by client report, or objectively, as measured by functional improvement.

Anterior cervical discectomy was performed to remove the fifth cervical disk but with no change in symptoms postoperatively. There was significant right extremity paresis, with maximal functional loss of the right hand and continued neck and back pain.

This client was eventually discharged from further physical therapy services and underwent a second surgical procedure, with no improvement in his condition. A year later, he telephoned the physical therapist to report that he had been diagnosed with Lyme disease. This man spent his vacations in the woods of Connecticut and Long Island, but this important piece of information was never gleaned from his past medical history.

Despite the lengthy time before diagnosis, the client was almost entirely recovered and ready to return to work after completing a course of antibiotics.

CLINICAL SIGNS AND SYMPTOMS
Lyme Disease

Early Infection (one or more may be present at different times during infection):
- Red rash (erythema migrans)
- Flu-like symptoms (fever, headache, stiff neck, fatigue)
- Migratory musculoskeletal pain (joints, bursae, tendons, muscle, or bone)
- Neurologic symptoms:
  - Severe headache (meningitis)
  - Numbness, pain, weakness of extremities or radiculopathy
  - Poor motor coordination
  - Cognitive dysfunction: memory loss, difficulty in concentrating, mood changes, sleep disturbances

Less Common Symptoms
- Eye problems such as conjunctivitis
- Heart abnormalities and myocarditis

Late Infection (months to years)
- Arthritis, intermittent or chronic
- Encephalopathy (mood and sleep disturbances)
- Neurocognitive dysfunction
- Peripheral neuropathy

(76.9 years), but there is a correlation between an accelerated mortality from the onset of disease in individuals with PPMS.[192]

Clinical Signs and Symptoms. Clinically, MS is characterized by multiple and varying signs and symptoms and by unpredictable and fluctuating periods of remission and exacerbation. Symptoms are variable based on the area or areas of the CNS affected. Symptoms can develop rapidly over a course of minutes or hours.[193] The onset may be insidious, occurring during a period of weeks or months, although 80% to 90% of patients will present with an acute episode known as a CIS.[194]

Motor Symptoms. Many persons with MS experience weakness in the extremities, leading to difficulty with ambulation, coordination, and balance. Ataxia or tremor may be present if plaques develop in the cerebellum. Spasticity and hyperreflexia are common causes of disability with severe, uncontrollable spasms of the extremities. Profound fatigue, the most common symptom, occurs in 80% of people with MS,[195] and along with dysmetria (intention tremor), can contribute to motor impairment.[196]

Dysphagia, difficulty with chewing, and dysarthria can occur if the brainstem or cranial nerves are affected. Urinary frequency, urgency, incontinence, retention, or hesitancy commonly characterizes motor and/or sensory bowel/bladder dysfunction.

Sensory Symptoms. Unilateral visual impairment (e.g., double vision, visual loss, red-green color blindness) that comes and goes as a result of optic neuritis is often the first indication of a problem. Optic neuritis occurs in about 20% of persons initially presenting with MS, although 40% may present with optic neuritis during the course of their disease.[197] Extreme sensitivity to temperature changes is evident in more than 60%–80% of people diagnosed with MS.[198] Elevated temperature shortens the duration of nerve impulses and worsens symptoms, whereas cooler temperatures actually restore conduction in blocked nerves and improve symptoms.

Paresthesia (numbness and tingling) accompanied by burning in the extremities can result in injury to the hands or feet. Lhermitte's sign (electric shock-like sensation down the spine, radiating to the extremities; initiated by neck flexion) can be suggestive of MS; however, clinicians need to rule out cervical spine dysfunction which can also be a source of symptoms with neck flexion.

Other Symptoms. Sleep and seizure disorders can have severe effects on a person's life and have been shown to have higher incidence and prevalence in persons with MS than in the general population.[199]

Guillain-Barré Syndrome (Acute Idiopathic Polyneuritis)

GBS is an acute, acquired autoimmune disorder that involves the demyelination of the PNS (specifically nerve roots and peripheral nerves) and is characterized by an abrupt onset of paralysis.[200] The disease has four main subtypes[201]:
- Acute inflammatory demyelinating polyradiculoneuropathy (AIDP)
- Acute motor axonal neuropathy (AMAN)
- Acute motor and sensory axonal neuropathy (AMSAN)
- Miller-Fisher syndrome

The disease affects all age groups, and incidence is not related to race or sex. Global incidence of the disease is 1 to 4 cases per 100,000 persons,[202] with the incidence lower in children at 0.62 cases per 100,000 between the ages of 0–9 years.[200,203]

Risk Factors. The exact cause of the disease is unknown, but it frequently occurs after an infection or triggering event.

CLINICAL SIGNS AND SYMPTOMS
Multiple Sclerosis

Symptoms
- Unilateral visual impairment
- Paresthesia
- Complaints of unsteadiness
- Vertigo (sensation of rotation of self or surroundings)
- Fatigue
- Muscle weakness
- Bowel/bladder dysfunction:
  - Frequency
  - Urgency
  - Incontinence
  - Retention
  - Hesitancy
- Speech impairment (slow, slurred speech)

Signs
- Optic neuritis
- Nystagmus
- Spasticity or hyperreflexia
- Ataxia
- Babinski's sign
- Absent abdominal reflexes
- Dysmetria or intention tremor
- Labile or change in mood
- Lhermitte's sign

Upper respiratory infections, influenza, vaccinations, or viral infections such as measles, hepatitis, or mononucleosis commonly precede acute idiopathic polyneuritis by 1 to 3 weeks.[204] The immune system's complement system is activated and facilitates a breakdown of myelin (AIDP) or specific damage to axons of spinal roots or peripheral nerves (AMAN).[205] Individuals who received the H1N1 vaccination were found to have lower incidence of GBS, suggesting a possible protective effect of the vaccination.[206] The Zika virus may also be associated with an onset of GBS in adults.[207]

Clinical Signs and Symptoms. The onset of GBS is generally characterized by a rapidly progressive weakness and fatigue over a period of 1–2 weeks. It is usually symmetric, involving first the lower extremities, then the upper extremities, followed by the respiratory musculature. Weakness and paralysis are frequently preceded by paresthesia and numbness of the limbs, but actual objective sensory loss is usually mild and transient.[205]

Although muscular weakness is usually described as bilateral, progressing from the legs upward toward the arms, this syndrome may be missed when the client has unilateral symptoms that do not progress proximally. Oculomotor changes, along with ataxia and areflexia, are typical of the Miller-Fisher subtype.[201]

Muscular weakness of the chest may appear early in the disease process as respiratory compromise. Respiratory involvement as such may be unnoticed until the person develops more severe symptoms associated with GBS.

The progression of paralysis varies from one client to another, often with full recovery from the paralysis. Usually symptoms develop over a period of 1 to 2 weeks, and the progression of paralysis may stop at any point. Once the weakness reaches a maximum (usually during the second week), the client's condition plateaus for days or even weeks before spontaneous improvement and eventual recovery begins, extending over a period of 6 to 9 months.

Cranial nerves, most commonly the facial nerve, can be involved. Deep tendon reflexes are decreased or lost early in the course of the illness. The incidence of residual neurologic deficits is higher than was previously recognized, and deficits may occur in as many as 50% of all cases.

CLINICAL SIGNS AND SYMPTOMS

Guillain-Barré Syndrome (Acute Idiopathic Polyneuritis)

- Muscular weakness (bilateral, progressing from the legs to the arms to the chest and neck)
- Diminished deep tendon reflexes
- Paresthesia (without loss of sensation)
- Pain
- Absence of fever at onset of symptoms; may have experienced recent flu-like illness
- Oculomotor dysfunction (Miller-Fisher subtype)
- Ataxia (Miller-Fisher subtype)
- Areflexia (Miller-Fisher subtype)

Treatment. There is no immediate cure for this disease, but medical support is vital during the progression of symptoms, particularly in the acute phase when respiratory function may be compromised. Physical therapy is initiated at an early stage to maintain joint range of motion (ROM) and to monitor muscle strength until active exercise can be initiated.

The usual precautions for clients immobilized in bed are required to prevent complications during the acute phase. A major precaution is to provide active exercise at a level consistent with the client's muscle strength. Overstretching and overuse of painful muscles may result in a prolonged recovery period, or a lack of recovery (Case Example 13.6).

Myasthenia Gravis

MG is an autoimmune disease that impacts the neuromuscular junction resulting in muscle weakness and fatigue.[208] Antibodies acting on acetylcholine receptors at the neuromuscular junction result in transmission failure and fatigue.[208] Different MG syndromes are categorized by where the muscle weakness occurs, what type of antibody defect exists, the age of onset, and the degree of thymus pathology.[209]

MG may begin at any time in life, including newborn infants, but there are two major peaks of onset. Early-onset MG occurs from age 20 to 30 years, with women more often

CASE EXAMPLE 13.6

Guillain Barré Syndrome

A 67-year-old retired aeronautics engineer was referred to physical therapy by his physician for electrotherapy and therapeutic exercise. The physician's diagnosis was right-sided Bell's palsy. Past medical history was significant for an upper respiratory infection 2 weeks before the onset of his first symptoms.

The client reported difficulty in closing his eyes, chewing, and drinking, and he was unable to smile. There were no changes in sensation or hearing. During the neurologic examination, the client was unable to raise his eyebrows or close his eyes, and there was obvious facial drooping on both sides. A gross manual muscle test revealed full (5/5) muscle strength in all four extremities, but muscle stretch reflexes were absent in all four extremities.

Result: The physical therapist recognized three red-flag symptoms in this case: (1) recent upper respiratory infection followed by the development of neurologic symptoms; (2) progressive development of symptoms from right-sided to bilateral between the time the client was evaluated by the physician and went to the physical therapist; and (3) absent deep tendon reflexes, an inconsistent finding for Bell's palsy.

The therapist contacted the physician by telephone to relay this information and confirm the treatment plan given this new information. The physician requested that the client return for further medical testing, and a revised diagnosis of Guillain-Barré syndrome was made.

The client's clinical status stabilized and he returned to the physical therapist. The treatment plan was modified accordingly. This case again demonstrates the importance of performing a careful examination, including screening for systemic disease, and recognizing red-flag symptoms.

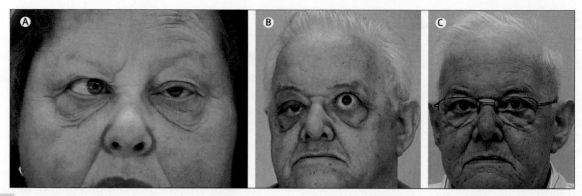

Fig. 13.16 External eye weakness (A–C) in myasthenia gravis. (From Gilhus NE, Vershuuren JJ. Myasthenia gravis: Subgroup classification and therapeutic strategies. Lancet Neurol. 2015;14:1023–1036.)

affected than men. Late-onset MG occurs after age 50 years, with men being more affected than women. The incidence of MG in older individuals (>50 years old) is rising and is not just because of improved disease recognition; however, additional etiologic factors remain unclear.[210]

Clinical Signs and Symptoms. Clinically, the disease is characterized by muscle weakness, most commonly in the muscles controlling eye movement, chewing, swallowing, and facial expressions. Weakness of the limb and axial muscles may be present as well. External eye muscle weakness is commonly symmetrical (Fig. 13.16), whereas limb weakness is symmetrical and occurs more proximal compared with distal musculature.[211] In approximately 60% of patients, ptosis or diplopia is present (or both).[211] MG localized to the ocular involvement occurs in 20% of individuals, referred to as ocular MG.[211]

Symptoms show a fluctuation[212] in intensity and are more severe late in the day or after prolonged activity. Speech may become unintelligible after prolonged periods of talking. Fluctuations also occur with superimposed illness, menses, and air temperature (worse with warming, improved with cold). Common comorbid conditions include thymoma and hyperthyroidism.

Fatigable and rapidly fluctuating asymmetric ptosis is a hallmark of the problem, because ocular muscle dysfunction is usually one of the first symptoms. The ice pack test, rest test, sleep tests, and peek sign are all useful in confirming the presence of MG (Box 13.3).[213]

Due to proximal muscles being more affected than distal, the clinician can expect clients to experience difficulty in climbing stairs, rising from chairs, combing their hair, or even holding up their head. Cranial, neck, respiratory, and proximal limb muscles are the primary areas of involvement. Neurologic findings are normal except for muscle weakness. There is no muscular atrophy or loss of sensation. Muscular weakness ranges from mild to life-threatening (when involving respiratory muscles). Pain is a common complaint, along with difficulty sleeping. Sleep disturbances may be a result of abnormal breathing at night, despite the possibility of wake-time breathing appearing normal.[214]

BOX 13.3 ELICITING SIGNS AND SYMPTOMS OF MYASTHENIA GRAVIS

The characteristic finding in myasthenia gravis (MG) is decreased muscle strength that becomes worse with repetition and improves with rest. Asymmetric drooping of the eyelids (ptosis) is one of the first signs and can be identified using the following tests:

The client sits and fixes his or her gaze on a distant object without blinking. The frontalis muscle should be relaxed, although this may be difficult. The eye with the most noticeable ptosis is tested.

The Ice Pack Test

Place a latex-free glove filled with crushed ice over the eyelid for 2 minutes.

The Rest Test

Place a cotton-filled latex-free glove (rest) over the eyelid while holding the eyes closed for 2 minutes.

The Sleep Test

Client is placed in a dark room with eyes closed for 30 minutes.

Key: Evaluate response to these tests immediately following timed period. A positive response is defined as complete or almost complete resolution of the ptosis. Improvement may be greater with the ice test than with the rest test.[129] Medical referral is required.

(Data from Scherer K, Bedlack RS, Simel L. Does this patient have myasthenia gravis? JAMA 2005;293(15):1906–1914.)

There are four main medical MG treatment options including use of medications to increase the amount of neuromuscular acetylcholine, plasma exchange, immunosuppression using corticosteroids, and thymectomy. Each of these treatment options has the goal of increasing muscle function; however, they have various timelines of effectiveness and do not have an effect on the actual disease itself.[214]

CLINICAL SIGNS AND SYMPTOMS
Myasthenia Gravis

- Muscle fatigability and proximal muscle weakness aggravated by exertion
- Ptosis (extraocular muscle weakness resulting in drooping of the upper eyelid)
- Diplopia (double vision)
- Dysarthria (slurred speech)
- Bulbar involvement
- Alteration in voice quality
- Dysphagia (difficulty swallowing)
- Nasal regurgitation
- Choking, difficulty in chewing
- Pain
- Respiratory failure from progressive involvement of respiratory muscles

Immunoproliferative Disorders

Immunoproliferative disorders are characterized by the abnormal proliferation of the primary cells of the immune systems, such as B cells, T cells, and overproduction of immunoglobulins. Immunoproliferative disorders include lymphoproliferative disorders such as lymphoma, leukemia, and multiple myeloma, among several others. Several of these disorders have been covered in other parts of this text and are not discussed further in this chapter.

PHYSICIAN REFERRAL

In most immunologic disorders, physicians must rely on the client's history and clinical findings in association with supportive information from diagnostic tests to make a differential diagnosis. Often, there are no definitive diagnostic tests, such as in the case of MS. The physician instead relies on objectively measured CNS abnormalities, a history of episodic exacerbation, and remission of symptoms with progressive worsening of symptoms over time.

In the early stages of treating disorders such as MS, GBS, and myositis, factors such as the effect of fatigue on the client's progress and fragile muscle fibers necessitate that the physical therapist keep close contact with the physician, who will use a physical examination and laboratory tests to determine the most opportune time to initiate physical therapy treatment. Although the physician is monitoring serum enzyme levels and the overall medical status of the client, the physical therapist will continue to provide the physician with essential feedback regarding objective findings such as muscle tenderness, muscle strength, overall physical endurance, and improvements in activity limitations and participation restrictions.

A careful history and close clinical observation may elicit an indication that the client is demonstrating signs and symptoms unrelated to a musculoskeletal disorder. Because the immune system can implicate many of the body's systems, the physical therapist should not hesitate to relay to the physician any unusual findings reported or observed.

Guidelines for Immediate Medical Attention

- Anyone exhibiting signs and symptoms of anaphylactic shock, especially vocal hoarseness, difficulty breathing, and chest discomfort or tightness
- New onset of joint pain with a recent history of surgery **(bacterial or ReA)**
- A dusky blue discoloration or erythema accompanied by exquisite tenderness is a sign of a septic (infected) joint; ask about a recent history of infection of any kind anywhere in the body; medical referral is advised

Guidelines for Physician Referral

- New onset of joint pain within 6 weeks of surgery, especially when accompanied by constitutional symptoms, rash, or skin lesions
- Symmetric swelling and pain in peripheral joints may be an early sign of RA; early medical intervention is critical to prevent erosive joint disease and disability[60]
- Development of progressive neurologic symptoms within 1 to 3 weeks of a previous infection or recent vaccination
- Evidence of spinal cord compression in anyone with cervical RA who has progressed from generalized stiffness to new onset of cervical laxity (C1-C2 subluxation or dislocation)
- Presence of incontinence (bowel or bladder) in anyone with AS requires medical referral; surgical treatment of the underlying dural ectasia may be helpful[87]
- Positive ptosis tests for MG (ice pack, rest test, sleep tests)

Clues to Immune System Dysfunction

- Client with a history of RA taking DMARDs who develops symptoms of drug toxicity (e.g., rash, petechiae/ecchymosis, photosensitivity, dyspnea, nausea/vomiting, lymph node swelling, edema, oral ulcers, diarrhea)
- Long-term use of NSAIDs or other antiinflammatory drugs, especially with new onset of GI symptoms; back or shoulder pain of unknown cause
- Long-term use of immunosuppressive drugs or corticosteroids with onset of constitutional symptoms, especially fever
- Insidious onset of episodic back pain in a person younger than 40 years of age who has a family history of SpA
- Joint pain preceded or accompanied by burning and urinary frequency (urethritis) and/or accompanied by eye irritation, crusting, redness, tearing, or burning usually lasting only a few days **(conjunctivitis; ReA)**
- Joint pain preceded or accompanied by skin rash or lesions **(PsA; Lyme disease; rheumatic fever)**
- New onset of inflammatory joint pain (especially monoarticular joint involvement) postoperatively, especially accompanied by extraarticular signs or symptoms such as rash, diarrhea, urethritis **(ReA or bacterial arthritis)**; mouth ulcers **(ReA, SLE)**; raised skin patches **(PsA)**
- Development of neurologic symptoms 1 to 3 weeks after an infection **(GBS)**

■ Key Points to Remember

1. Pain in the knees, hands, wrists, or elbows may indicate an autoimmune disorder; aching in the bones can be caused by expanding bone marrow.
2. True arthritis produces pain and limitation during both active and passive ROM. Limitation from tendinitis is typically worse during active ROM.
3. Any change in cough, pain, or fever and any change or new presentation of symptoms should be reported to the physician.
4. Be alert to any warning signs of hypersensitivity response (allergic reaction) during therapy and be prepared to take necessary measures (e.g., graded exercise to client tolerance, control of room temperature, client use of medications).

5. Immediate emergency procedures are required when a client has a severe allergic reaction (anaphylactic shock).
6. For the client with GBS, active exercise must be at a level consistent with the client's muscle strength. Overstretching and overuse of painful muscles may result in a prolonged, or lack of, recovery.
7. For the client with MS, treatment should take place in the coolest (temperature) setting possible.
8. For the client with RA or AS, the risk of fracture from the development of atlantoaxial subluxation necessitates the use of extreme caution in treatment procedures. The most common site of fracture is the lower cervical spine.

CLIENT HISTORY AND INTERVIEW

SPECIAL QUESTIONS TO ASK

Signs and symptoms of immune disorders can appear in any body system. A thorough review of the Family/Personal History form, patient/client interview, and appropriate follow-up questions will help the physical therapist identify signs and symptoms that are not consistent with a musculoskeletal pattern. Special attention should be given to the question on the Family/Personal History form concerning general health. Clients with immune disorders or immunocompromised clients often have poor general health or history of recurrent infections.

When the immune system is involved, some important questions to ask include the following:

- How long have you had this problem? (acute versus chronic)
- Has the problem gone away and then recurred?
- Have additional symptoms developed or have other areas become symptomatic over time?
- How is/has this condition been previously managed? Are you currently receiving treatment?

PAST MEDICAL HISTORY

- Have you ever been told that you had/have an immune disorder, autoimmune disease, or cancer? (predisposes the person to other diseases)
- Have you ever had radiation treatment? (diminishes blood cell production, predisposes to infection)
- Have you ever had an organ transplant (especially kidney) or removal of your thymus? (**MG**)

ASSOCIATED SIGNS AND SYMPTOMS

- Do you have difficulty with combing your hair; raising your arms; getting out of the bathtub, bed, or chair; or climbing stairs? (**MG**)

- Do you have difficulty when raising your head from the pillow when you are lying down on your back? (**MG**)
- Do you have difficulty with swallowing, or have you noticed any change in your voice? (**MG**)
- Have you noticed any change in your skin texture or pigmentation? Do you have any skin rashes? (**scleroderma, allergic reactions, SLE, RA, dermatomyositis, PsA, AIDS, Lyme disease**)
  - *If yes*, have you noticed any association between the development of the skin rash and pain or swelling in any of your joints (or other symptoms)?
  - Do these other symptoms go away when the skin rash clears up?
  - Have you been exposed to ticks? For example, have you been out walking in the woods or in tall grass or in contact with pets? (**Lyme disease**)
- Have you had any recent vision problems? (**MS**)
- Have you had any body tattooing or ear/body piercing done in the last 6 weeks to 6 months? (**AIDS, hepatitis**)
- Have you had any difficulty with urination—for example, a change in appearance of urine, incontinence, or increased frequency? (**MS, MG, ReA**)

For the Person with Known Allergies (check the Family/ Personal History form)

- What are the usual symptoms that you experience in association with your allergies?
- Describe a typical allergic reaction for you.
- Do the symptoms relate to physical changes (e.g., cold, heat, or dampness)?
- Do the symptoms occur in association with activities (e.g., exercise)?
- Do you take medication for your allergies?

For the Client Reporting Fatigue and Weakness

For the Client with Fever (fevers recurring every few days, fevers that rise and fall within 24 hours, and fevers

CLIENT HISTORY AND INTERVIEW—cont'd

that recur frequently should be documented and reported to the physician)

- Do you feel tired all the time or only after exertion?
- Do you get short of breath after mild exercise or at rest?
- How much sleep do you get at night?
- Do you take naps during the day?
- Have you ever been told by a physician that you are anemic?
- How long have you had this weakness?
- Does it come and go, or is it persistent (there all the time)?
- Are you able to perform your usual daily activities without stopping to rest or nap?

   For the Client with Sudden Onset of Joint Pain (ReA; see also Appendix B-18 in the accompanying enhanced eBook version included with print purchase of this textbook)

- Have you recently noticed any crusting, redness, or burning of your eyes?
- Have you noticed any burning when you urinate?
- Have you noticed an increase in the number of times you urinate?
- Have you had any bouts of diarrhea over the last 1 to 3 weeks (before the onset of joint pain)?
  - *If yes* to any of these questions, have you ever been told you have a sexually transmitted infection such as herpes, genital warts, reactive arthritis, or other disease?
- When did you first notice this fever?
- Is it constant, or does it come and go?
- Does your temperature fluctuate?
  - *If yes,* over what period of time does this occur?

CASE STUDY

REFERRAL

A 28-year-old male has come to physical therapy for an evaluation without a medical referral. He has seen no medical practitioner for his current symptoms, consisting of an unusual gait pattern and weakness of the lower extremities, which he noticed during the last 2 days. His Personal/Family History form (see example in Fig. 2.2) indicates no previous or current health or medical problems of any kind. He does note that he has had influenza in the last 3 weeks but that he is fully recovered now.

PHYSICAL THERAPY INTERVIEW

Using the format outlined in the chapter on Interviewing as a Screening Tool (see Chapter 2), begin with an open-ended question and follow up with additional appropriate questions incorporating the following:

CURRENT SYMPTOMS

- Tell me why you are here (open-ended question). Or, you may prefer to say, "I notice from your intake form that you have had some weakness in your legs and a change in the way you walk. What can you tell me about this?"
- When did you first notice these changes?
- What did you notice that made you think something was happening?
- Just before the development of these symptoms, did you injure yourself in any way that you can remember?
- Did you have a car accident, fall down, or twist your trunk or hips in any unusual way?
- Do you have any pain in your back, hips, or legs? *If yes,* use Fig. 3.6 to elicit a further description.

ASSOCIATED SYMPTOMS

- Have you had any numbness or tingling in your back, buttocks, hips, or down your legs?
- Have you had any other change in sensation in these areas, such as a burning or prickling feeling?
- Besides the flu, have you had any other infection recently (e.g., head cold, upper respiratory infection, urinary tract infection)?
- Have you had a fever or elevated temperature in the last 48 hours?
- Do you think that you have a temperature right now?
- Have you noticed any other symptoms that I should know about?

Give the client time to answer this last question. Prompt him or her if necessary with various suggestions (include any others that seem appropriate to the information and responses already given by the client; a similar checklist is provided in Fig. 3.6) such as the following:

- Nausea or dizziness
- Diarrhea or constipation
- Unusual fatigue
- Choking, difficulty with chewing
- Recent headache
- Vomiting
- Cold sweats during the day or night
- Change in vision or speech
- Skin rash
- Joint pain
- Shortness of breath with mild exertion (e.g., walking to the car or even at rest)
- Have you noticed any other respiratory, lung, or breathing problems?

Continued

CASE STUDY—cont'd

FINAL QUESTION

Is there anything else you think that I should know about your current condition or general health that I have not asked yet?

PROCEDURES TO CARRY OUT DURING THE FIRST SESSION

Given the client's report of lower extremity weakness and antalgic gait of sudden onset without precipitating cause, the following possible problems should be assessed during the examination:

- Neurologic disease or disorder (immunologically based or otherwise), such as:
  - Discogenic lesion
  - Tumor
  - Myasthenia gravis (MG) (unlikely because of the man's age)
  - Guillain-Barré syndrome (recent history of the "flu")
  - Multiple sclerosis (MS)
- AIDS dementia (unlikely, given the way the history was presented)
- Psychogenic disorder (e.g., hysteria, anxiety, alcoholism, or drug addiction)

OBSERVATION/INSPECTION

- Take the client's vital signs.
- Note any obvious changes such as muscle atrophy, difficulty with breathing or swallowing, facial paralysis, intention tremor.
- Describe the gait pattern: observe for ataxia, incoordination, positive Trendelenburg position, balance, patterns of muscular weakness or imbalance, and other gait deviations.

Neurologic Screening Examination

- All deep tendon reflexes
- Manual muscle testing of proximal-to-distal large muscle groups, looking for a pattern of weakness
- Babinski sign and clonus
- Gross sensory screen, looking for any differences in perceived sensation, proprioception, or vibration from one side to the other
- Test for dysmetria, balance, and coordination

Orthopedic Assessment

- Lower extremity range of motion (ROM): active and passive
- Lumbar spine and lower quadrant evaluation protocol[124]

Testing Results

In the case of this client, the interview revealed very little additional information because he denied any other associated (systemic) signs or symptoms and denied bowel/bladder dysfunction, precipitating injury or trauma, and neurologic indications such as numbness, tingling, or paresthesia. Subjectively, he did not appear to be feigning illness or physical disablement or a hysterical/anxious individual.

The client's gait pattern could best be described as ataxic. His lower extremities would not support him fully, and he frequently lost his balance and fell down, although he denied any pain or warning that he was about to fall.

Objective findings revealed inconsistent results of muscle testing. The proximal muscles were more involved than the distal muscles (difference of one grade: proximal muscles = fair grade; distal muscles = good grade), but repeated tests elicited alternately strong, weak, or cogwheel responses, as if the muscles were moving in a ratcheting motion against resistance through the ROM.

The only other positive findings were slightly diminished deep tendon reflexes of the lower extremities compared with the upper extremities, but, again, these findings were inconsistent when tested over time.

Final Results

Because the patient history, interview, and tests and measures were so inconsistent and puzzling, the physical therapist asked another physical therapist to briefly examine this client. In turn, the second physical therapist decided to ask the client to return either at the end of the day or for the first appointment of the next day to reexamine him for any changes in the pattern of his symptoms. It was more convenient for him to return the next day, and he did.

At that time, the patient demonstrated slurred speech pattern compared to his previous visit. His gait remained unchanged, but the muscle strength of the proximal pelvic muscles was consistently weak over several trials spread out during the therapy session, which lasted for 1 hour.

This time the physical therapist checked the muscles of his upper extremities and found that the scapular muscles were also unable to move against any manual resistance. Deep tendon reflexes of the upper extremities were inconsistently diminished, and reflexes of the lower extremities were now consistently diminished.

The client was referred to a physician for further follow-up and was not treated at the physical therapy clinic that day. He was examined by his family physician, who referred him to a neurologist. A diagnosis of Guillain-Barré syndrome was confirmed when the client's symptoms progressed dramatically, requiring hospitalization.

PRACTICE QUESTIONS

1. Fibromyalgia syndrome (FMS) is a:
   a. Musculoskeletal disorder and primarily due to nerve root irritation
   b. Psychosomatic disorder and primarily nociceptive
   c. Neurosomatic disorder and primarily nociceptive
   d. Noninflammatory rheumatic disorder and primarily due to central sensitization

2. Which of the following best describes the pattern of rheumatic arthritis?
   a. Pain and stiffness in the morning for several hours that gradually improves with gentle activity and movement during the day.
   b. Pain and stiffness accelerate during the day and are worse in the evening.
   c. Night pain is frequently associated with advanced structural damage seen in x-ray films.
   d. Pain is brought on by activity and resolves predictably with rest.

3. Match the following skin lesions with the associated underlying disorder:
   a. Raised, scaly patches   _____ Psoriatic arthritis
   b. Flat or slightly raised   _____ Systemic lupus
      malar on the face   erythematosus
   c. Petechiae   _____ HIV infection
   d. Tightening of the skin   _____ Scleroderma
   e. Kaposi's sarcoma   _____ Allergic reaction
   f. Erythema migrans   _____ Lyme disease
   g. Hives   _____ Thrombocytopenia

4. A new client has come to you with a primary report of new onset of knee pain and swelling. Name three clues that this client might give from his medical history that should alert you to the possibility of immunologic disease.

5. A positive Schober's test is a sign of:
   a. Reactive arthritis
   b. Infectious arthritis
   c. Ankylosing spondylitis
   d. Juvenile idiopathic arthritis

6. What is Lhermitte's sign, and what does it signify?

7. Proximal muscle weakness may be a sign of:
   a. Paraneoplastic syndrome
   b. Neurologic disorder
   c. Myasthenia gravis
   d. Scleroderma
   e. b, c, and d
   f. All of the above

8. Which of the following skin assessment findings in the patient with HIV infection occurs with Kaposi's sarcoma?
   a. Darkening of the nail beds
   b. Purple-red blotches or bumps on the trunk and head
   c. Cyanosis of the lips and mucous membranes
   d. Painful blistered lesions of the face and neck

9. Which is the most prevalent form of HIV-associated neurological disorders?
   a. Meningitis
   b. HIV-associated dementia
   c. Space-occupying lesions
   d. Asymptomatic neurocognitive impairment

10. Symptoms of anaphylaxis that would necessitate immediate medical treatment or referral are:
    a. Hives and itching
    b. Vocal hoarseness, sneezing, and chest tightness
    c. Periorbital edema
    d. Nausea and abdominal cramping

REFERENCES

1. Duba AS, Mathew SD. The seronegative spondyloar-thropathies. *Prim Care*. 2018;45(2):271–287. https://doi.org/10.1016/j.pop.2018.02.005.
2. Shiel WC. Rheumatoid Factor. WebMD-MedicineNet.com. http://www.medicinenet.com/rheumatoid_factor/article.htm. Accessed June 30, 2016.
3. Klippel JH, ed. *Primer on the Rheumatic Diseases*. 13 ed. Arthritis Foundation, Atlanta: Springer; 2008.
4. Centers for Disease Control and Prevention. New HIV Diagnoses and People with Diagnosed HIV in the US and Dependent Areas by Area of Residence, 2019. https://www.cdc.gov/hiv/basics/statistics.html. Accessed 8/12/2021.
5. WHO. HIV/AIDS Fact Sheets. https://www.who.int/newsroom/fact-sheets/detail/hiv-aids. Accessed 5/25/2020.
6. Lucas S, Nelson AM. HIV and the spectrum of human disease. *J Pathol*. 2015;235(2):229–241. https://doi.org/10.1002/path.4449.
7. Askew I, Berer M. The contribution of sexual and reproductive health services to the fight against HIV/AIDS: a review. *Reprod Health Matters*. 2003;11(22):51–73. https://doi.org/10.1016/s0968-8080(03)22101-7.
8. Denning P, DiNenno E. Communities in crisis: is there a generalized HIV epidemic in impoverished urban areas of the United States. InXVIII international AIDS conference 2010 Jul 18 (Vol. 1).
9. Centers for Disease Control and Prevention. HIV Prevention. https://www.cdc.gov/hiv/basics/prevention.html. Accessed on 5/25/2020.
10. Patel P, Borkowf CB, Brooks JT, Lasry A, Lansky A, Mermin J. Estimating per-act HIV transmission risk: a systematic review. *AIDS*. 2014;28(10):1509–1519.
11. Centers for Disease Control and Prevention. HIV and People Who Inject Drugs. https://www.cdc.gov/hiv/group/hiv-idu.html.
12. Source: Platt L, Minozzi S, Reed J, et al. Needle syringe programmes and opioid substitution therapy for preventing hepatitis C transmission in people who inject drugs. *Cochrane Database Syst Rev* 2017;9:CD012021. doi:10.1002/14651858.CD012021.pub2. Found on https://www.cdc.gov/ssp/syringe-services-programs-factsheet.html.
13. Lynch NG, Alexandra KJ. "Congenital HIV: Prevention of maternal to child transmission." Advances in Neonatal Care 18.5 (2018):330–340.
14. Uthman OA, Nachega JB, Anderson J, et al. Timing of initiation of antiretroviral therapy and adverse pregnancy outcomes: a systematic review and meta-analysis.

Lancet HIV. 2017;4(1):e21–e30. https://doi.org/10.1016/S2352-3018(16)30195-3.

15. Lamorde M, Schapiro JM, Burger D, Back DJ. Antiretroviral drugs for prevention of mother-to-child transmission: pharmacologic considerations for a public health approach. *AIDS.* 2014;28(17):2551–2563.

16. Centers for Disease and Control. HIV and Pregnant Women, Infants, and Children. https://www.cdc.gov/hiv/group/gender/pregnantwomen/index.html. Accessed 5/25/2020.

17. Creed F. A review of the incidence of risk factors for fibromyalgia and chronic widespread pain in population based studies. *Pain.* 2020; 161(6): 1169–1176.

18. Lynch NG, Johnson AK. Congenital HIV: prevention of maternal to child transmission. *Adv Neonatal Care.* 2018;18(5):330–340. https://doi.org/10.1097/ANC.0000000000000559.

19. Levison J, Weber S, Cohan D. Breastfeeding and HIV-infected women in the United States: harm reduction counseling strategies. *Clin Infect Dis.* 2014;59(2):304–309.

20. Zunza M, Mercer G, Thabane L, Esser M, Cotton MF. Effects of postnatal interventions for the reduction of vertical HIV transmission on infant growth and non-HIV infections: a systematic review. *J Int AIDS Soc.* 2013;16:18865.

21. National Institutes of Health, National Heart, Lung, and Blood Institute: What are the Risks of a Blood Transfusion? http://www.nhlbi.nih.gov/health/health-topics/topics/bt/risks. Accessed 5/25/2020. https://wwwn.cdc.gov/hivrisk/what_is/stages_hiv_infection.html

22. Centers for Disease Control and Prevention. HIV Risk and Stages of Infection. Accessed 06/01/2020.

23. Sowers K, Galantino ML, Kietrys DM. Chapter 34: Human immunodeficiency virus: living with a chronic illness. In: Umphred DA, ed. *Umphred's neurological rehabilitation.* St. Louis, Mo: Elsevier/Mosby; 2013.

24. Graham CS. HIV and hepatitis C virus infection in the United States: whom and how to test? *Clin Infect Dis.* 2014;59(6):875–882.

25. Skarbinski J, Rosenberg E, Paz-Bailey G, et al. Human immunodeficiency virus transmission at each step of the care continuum in the United States. *JAMA Intern Med.* 2015;175(4):588–596.

26. Merlin JS. Chronic pain in patients with HIV infection: what clinicians need to know. *Top Antivir Med.* 2015;23(3):120–124.

27. Merlin JS, Long D, Becker WC, et al. Brief report: the association of chronic pain and long-term opioid therapy with HIV treatment outcomes. *J Acquir Immune Defic Syndr.* 2018;79(1):77–82. https://doi.org/10.1097/QAI.0000000000001741.

28. Carr A, Grund B, Neuhaus J, et al. Prevalence of and risk factors for low bone mineral density in untreated HIV infection: a substudy of the INSIGHT Strategic Timing of AntiRetroviral Treatment (START) trial. *HIV Med.* 2015;16(Suppl 1(01)):137–146. https://doi.org/10.1111/hiv.12242.

29. Perazzo JD, Webel AR, Alam SMK, Sattar A, McComsey GA. Relationships between physical activity and bone density in people living with HIV: results from the SATURN-HIV study. *J Assoc Nurses AIDS Care.* 2018;29(4):528–537. https://doi.org/10.1016/j.jana.2018.03.004.

30. WHO: Implementation Tool For Monitoring The Toxicity of New Antiretroviral adn Antiviral Medicines in HIV and Viral Hepatitis Programmes. July 2018. Accessed 05/25/2020.

31. De La Torre-Lima J, Aguilar A, Santos J, et al. Durability of the first antiretroviral treatment regimen and reasons for change in patients with HIV infection. *HIV Clin Trials.* 2014;14(1):25–35.

32. Jones M, Nunez M. Liver toxicity of antiretroviral drugs. *Semin Liver Dis.* 2012;32(02):167–176.

33. WHO: The Use of Antiretroviral Drugs For Treating and Prevention HIV Infection. 2nd Edition, 2016. Accessed 05/25/2020.

34. Troll JG. Approach to dyslipidemia, lipodystrophy, and cardiovascular risk in patients with HIV infection. *Curr Atheroscler Rep.* 2011;13(1):51–56.

35. Malita FM, Karelis AD, Toma E, Rabasa-Lhoret R. Effects of different types of exercise on body composition and fat distribution in HIV-infected patients: a brief review. *Can J Appl Physiol.* 2005;30(2):233–245.

36. Magkos F. Body fat redistribution and metabolic abnormalities in HIV-infected patients on highly active antiretroviral therapy. *Metabolism.* 2011;60(6):749–753.

37. Sweet DE. Metabolic complications of antiretroviral therapy. *Top HIV Med.* 2005;13(2):70–74.

38. Shiels MS, Engels EA. Evolving epidemiology of HIV-associated malignancies. *Curr Opin HIV AIDS.* 2017;12(1):6–11. https://doi.org/10.1097/COH.0000000000000327.

39. Rubinstein PG, Aboulagia DM, Zloza A. Malignancies in HIV/AIDS: from epidemiology to therapeutic challenges. *AIDS.* 2014;28(4):435–465.

40. Mitsuyasu RT. Non-AIDS-defining cancers. *Top Antiviral Rev.* 2014;22(3):660–665.

41. Khademi F, Yousefi-Avarvand A, Sahebkar A, Ghanbari F, Vaez H. Bacterial co-infections in HIV/AIDS-positive subjects: a systematic review and meta-analysis. *Folia Med (Plovdiv).* 2018;60(3):339–350. https://doi.org/10.2478/folmed-2018-0007.

42. https://www.cdc.gov/hiv/basics/livingwithhiv/opportunisticinfections.html

43. Gibson TM, Morton LM, Shiels MS, Clarke CA, Engels EA. Risk of non-Hodgkin lymphoma subtypes in HIV-infected people during the HAART era: a population-based study. *AIDS.* 2014;28(15):2313–2318. https://doi.org/10.1097/QAD.0000000000000428.

44. Silverberg MJ, Lau B, Achenbach CJ, et al. Cumulative incidence of cancer among HIV-infected individuals in North America. *Ann Intern Med.* 2015;163(7):507–518.

45. Centers for Disease Control and Prevention: Trends in tuberculosis—United States, 2010. MMWR 2011;60(11):333-337.

46. Centers for Disease and Control. TB Incidence in the United States, 1953–2020. https://www.cdc.gov/tb/statistics/tbcases.htm Accessed 05/25/2020.

47. Centers for Disease and Control. TB Incidence in the United States, 1953-2020. https://www.cdc.gov/tb/publications/factsheets/statistics/tbtrends.htm 2018. Accessed 5/25/2020/.

48. Gupta RK, Lucas SB, Fielding KL, Lawn SD. Prevalence of tuberculosis in post-mortem studies of HIV-infected adults and children in resource-limited settings: a systematic review and meta-analysis. *AIDS.* 2015;29(15):1987–2002.

49. Gopalan N, Chandrasekaran P, Swaminathan S, Tripathy S. Current trends and intricacies in the management of HIV-associated pulmonary tuberculosis. *AIDS Res Ther.* 2016;13:34 https://doi.org/10.1186/s12981-016-0118-7. Published 2016 Sep 26.

50. Deshpande AK, Patnaik M. Nonopportunistic neurologic manifestations of the human immunodeficiency virus: an Indian study. Medscape. http://www.medscape.com/viewarticle/511865. Accessed June 30, 2016.

51. Saylor D, Dickens AM, Sacktor N, et al. HIV-associated neurocognitive disorder--pathogenesis and prospects for treatment [published correction appears in Nat Rev Neurol. 2016 May;12(5):309]. *Nat Rev Neurol.* 2016;12(4):234–248.

52. Heaton RK, Clifford DB, Franklin DR, Woods SP, Ake C, Vaida F, Ellis RJ, Letendre SL, Marcotte TD, Atkinson JH, Rivera-Mindt M. HIV-associated neurocognitive disorders persist in the era of potent antiretroviral therapy: CHARTER Study. Neurology. 2010 Dec 7;75(23):2087–96.

53. Chawla J. Stepwise approach to myopathy in systemic disease. *Front Neurol.* 2011;2(49):1–10.

54. Ghosh S, Chandran A, Jansen JP. Epidemiology of HIV-related neuropathy: a systematic literature review. *AIDS Res Hum Retrovir.* 2012;28(1):36–48.

55. Hanewinckel R, van Oijen M, Ikram MA, van Doorn PA. The epidemiology and risk factors of chronic polyneuropathy. *Eur J Epidemiol.* 2016;31(1):5–20.

56. Benevides MLACSE, Filho SB, Debona R, Bergamaschi ENC, Nunes JC. Prevalence of Peripheral Neuropathy and associated factors in HIV-infected patients. *J Neurol Sci.* 2017;375:316–320. https://doi.org/10.1016/j.jns.2017.02.011.

57. Munoz-Carrillo JL, Castro-García FP, Chávez-Rubalcaba F, et al. Immune System Disorders: Hypersensitivity and Autoimmunity. 2018. https://doi.org/10.5772/intechopen.75794

58. Gell PGH, Coombs RRA. The classification of allergic reactions underlying disease. Clinical Aspects of Immunology 1963 Blackwell Science.

59. Uzzaman A, Cho SH. Classification of hypersensitivity reactions. *Allergy Asthma Proc.* 2012;33:S96–S99. https://doi.org/10.2500/aap.2012.33.3561.

60. Rajan TV. The Gell-Coombs classification of hypersensitivity reactions: a re-interpretation. *Trends Immunol.* 2003;24(7):376–379.

61. Greenberg PA, Ditto AM. Anaphylaxis. *Allergy Asthma Proc.* 2012;33:S80–S83. https://doi.org/10.2500/aap.2012.33.3557.

62. Sampson HA, Munoz-Fulong A, Campbell RL, et al. Second symposium on the definition and management of anaphylaxis: summary report- Second National Institute of Allergy and Infectious Disease/Food Allergy and Anaphylaxis network symposium. *J Allergy Clin Immunol.* 2006;117:391–397.

63. Cambell RL, Hagan JB. Evaluation of National Institute of Allergy and Infectious Diseases/Food Allergy and Anaphylaxis Network criteria for the diagnosis of anaphylaxis in emergency department patients. *J Allergy Clin Immunol.* 2012;129:748–752.

64. Sheldon J, Wheeler R, Riches P. Ch. 30 Immunology for clinical biochemists. https://doi.org/10.1016/B978-0-7020-5140-1.00030-4

65. Katz RS, Wolfe F, Michaud K. Fibromyalgia Diagnosis: a comparison of clinical, survey, and American college of rheumatology criteria. *Arthritis Rheum.* 2006;54(1):169–176.

66. Vincent A, Lahr B, Wolfe F, et al. Prevalence of fibromyalgia: a population-based study in Olmsted county, Minnesota, utilizing the Rochester epidemiology project. *Arthritis Care Res.* 2013;65:786–792.

67. Lawrence RC, Felson DT, Helmick CG, et al. Estimates of the prevalence of arthritis and other rheumatic conditions in the United States. Part II. *Arthritis Rheum.* 2008;58(1):26–35.

68. Clauw DJ. Fibromyalgia a clinical review. *JAMA.* 2014;311(15):1547–1555.

69. Queiroz LP. Worldwide epidemiology of fibromyalgia. *Curr Pain Headache Rep.* 2013;17(8):356.

70. Fitzcharles MA, Rampakakis E, Ste-Marie PA, et al. The association of socioeconomic status and symptom severity in persons with fibromyalgia. *J Rheumatol.* Jul 2014;41(7):1398–1404.

71. Williams DA, Clauw DJ. Understanding fibromyalgia: lessons from the broader pain research community. *J Pain.* 2009;10(8):777–791.

72. Lowe JC, Yellin J. Inadequate thyroid hormone regulation as the main mechanism of fibromyalgia: a review of the evidence. *Thyroid Sci.* 2008;3(6):R1–R14.

73. Friedman M. Fibromyalgia, thyroid dysfunction and treatment modalities. *J Restor Med.* 2013;2(1):60–69.

74. Buskila D, Atzeni F, Sarzi-Puttini P. Etiology of fibromyalgia: the possible role of infection and vaccination. *Autoimmun Rev.* 2008;8:41–43. https://doi.org/10.1016/j.autrev.2008.07.023.

75. Smart KM. Mechanisms-based classifications of musculoskeletal pain: part 1 of 3: symptoms and signs of central sensitization in patients with low back (+ leg) pain. *Man Ther.* 2012;17:336–344.

76. Cook DB, Lange G. Functional imaging of pain in patients with primary fibromyalgia. *J Rheumatol.* 2004;31(2):364–378.

77. Lopez-Sola M, Woo C-W, Pujol J, et al. Toward a neurophysiological signature of fibromyalgia. *Pain.* 2017;158(1):34–47.

78. Khanis A. Diagnosing fibromyalgia: moving away from tender points. *J Musculoskel Med.* 2010;27(4):155–162.

79. Garg N, Deodhar A. New and Modified Fibromyalgia Diagnostic Criteria. Rheumatology Network. http://www.rheumatologynetwork.com/fibromyalgia/new-and-modified-fibromyalgia-diagnostic-criteria. Accessed June 01, 2020.

80. Wolfe F. Stop using the American College of Rheumatology criteria in the clinic. *J Rheumatol.* 2003;30(8):1671–1672.

81. Wolfe F, Rasker JJ. The symptom intensity scale, fibromyalgia, and the meaning of fibromyalgia-like symptoms. *J Rheumatol.* 2006;22:2291–2299.

82. Wolfe F. Pain extent and diagnosis: development and validation of the regional pain scale in 12,799 patients with rheumatic disease. *J Rheumatol.* 2003;30:369–378.

83. Magrey MN, Antonelli M, James N, Khan MA. High frequency of fibromyalgia in patients with psoriatic arthritis: a pilot study. *Arthritis.* 2013;2013:762921.

84. Wolfe F. The American College of Rheumatology preliminary diagnostic criteria for fibromyalgia and measurement of symptom severity. *Arthritis Care Res.* 2010;62:600–610.

85. Bernstein C, Marcus D. Fibromyalgia: current concepts in diagnosis, pathogenesis, and treatment. *Pain Medicine News.* Dec 2008;6(9):8–19.

86. Wolfe F, Claw DJ, Fitzcharles M-A, et al. 2016 Revisions to the 2010/2011 fibromyalgia diagnostic criteria. *Semin Arthritis Rheum.* 2016;46:319–329. https://doi.org/10.1016/j.semarthrit.2016.08.012.

87. Yasui M, Yoshimura T, Takeuchi S, et al. A chronic fatigue syndrome model demonstrates mechanical allodynia and muscular hyperalgesia via spinal microglial activation. *Glia.* 2014;62:1407–1417.

88. Thompson D. The common threads of fibromyalgia and chronic fatigue syndrome in everyday health. http://www.everydayhealth.com/fibromyalgia/fibromyalgia-and-chronic-fatigue-syndrome.aspx. Accessed June 30, 2016.

89. American Association for Chronic Fatigue Syndrome CFS conference highlights: the merging of two syndromes. *Fibromyalgia Network.* 2003;61:4–70.

90. Low L, Schweinhardt P. Early life adversity as a risk factor for fibromyalgia in later life. *Pain Res Treat.* 2012:2012.

91. Puente CP, Furlong LV, Gallardo CE, Cigarán Méndez M, McKenney K. Anxiety, depression and alexithymia in fibromyalgia: are there any differences according to age? *J Women Aging.* 2013;25(4):305–320.

92. Häuser W, Galek A, Erbslöh-Möller B, et al. Posttraumatic stress disorder in fibromyalgia syndrome: prevalence, temporal relationship between posttraumatic stress and fibromyalgia symptoms, and impact on clinical outcome. *Pain.* Aug 2013;154(8):1216–1223.

93. Wallace DJ. Hypothesis: bipolar illness with complaints of chronic musculoskeletal pain is a form of pseudofibromyalgia. *Semin Arthritis Rheum.* 2008;37:256–259.

94. Leventhal L, Bouali H. Fibromyalgia: 20 clinical pearls. *J Musculoskel Med.* 2003;20(2):59–65.

95. Wilbarger JL, Cook D. Multisensory hypersensitivity in women with fibromyalgia: implications for well being and intervention. *Arch Phys Med Rehabil.* Apr 2011;92(4):653–656.

96. Weingarten TN. Impact of tobacco use in patients presenting to a multidisciplinary outpatient treatment program for fibromyalgia. *Clin J Pain.* 2009;25(1):39–43.

97. Aletaha D, Smolen JS. Diagnosis and management of rheumatoid arthritis: a review. *JAMA*. 2018;320(13):1360–1372. https://jama.jamanetwork.com/article.aspx?doi=10.1001/jama.2018.13103&utm_campaign=articlePDF%26utm_medium=articlePDFlink%26utm_source=articlePDF%26utm_content=jama.2018.13103.

98. Fazal SA, Khan M, Nishi SE, et al. A clinical update and global economic burden of rheumatoid arthritis. *Endocr Metab Immune Disord Drug Targets*. 2018;18:98–109.

99. Cross M, Smith E, Hoy D, et al. The global burden of rheumatoid arthritis: estimates from the global burden of disease 2010 study. *Ann Rheum Dis*. 2014;73(7):1316–1322.

100. Koch A. Targeting cytokines and growth factors in RA. *J Musculoskel Med*. 2005;22(3):130–136.

101. Yuksel-Konuk Baltaci V. Current advances in the genetic basis of rheumatoid arthritis. *Turk J Rheumatol*. 2009;24:218–221.

102. Angelotti F, Parma A, Cafaro G, Capecchi R, Alunno A, Puxeddu I. One year in review 2017: pathogenesis of rheumatoid arthritis. *Clin Exp Rheumatol*. 2017;35:368–378.

103. Sparks JA, Chang SC, Deane KD, et al. Associations of smoking and age with inflammatory joint signs among unaffected first-degree relatives of rheumatoid arthritis patients: results from studies of the etiology of rheumatoid arthritis. *Arthritis Rheumatol*. 2016;68(8):1828–1838.

104. Yavari N. What role do occupational exposures play in RA? *J Musculoskel Med*. 2008;25(3):130–136.

105. Andreoli TE, Benjamin I, Griggs RC, et al. *Andreoli and Carpenter's Cecil Essentials of Medicine*. 8 ed. Philadelphia: WB Saunders; 2010.

106. Nielen MM, van Shaardenburg D, Reesink HW, et al. Specific autoantibodies precede the symptoms of rheumatoid arthritis: a study of serial measurements in blood donors. *Arthritis Rheum*. 2004;50(2):380–386. https://doi.org/10.1002/art.20018.

107. Burckhardt CS, Jones KD. Adult measures of pain: the McGill pain questionnaire (MPQ), rheumatoid arthritis pain scale (RAPS), short-form McGill pain questionnaire (SF-MPQ), verbal descriptive scale (VDS), visual analog scale (VAS), and West Haven-Yale multidisciplinary pain inventory (WHYMPI). *Arthr Care Res*. 2003;49(S5):S96–S104.

108. American College of Rheumatology: Arthritis Impact Measurement Scales (AIMS/AIMS2). http://www.rheumatology.org/I-Am-A/Rheumatologist/Research/Clinician-Researchers/Arthritis-Impact-Measurement-Scales-AIMS. Accessed June 30, 2016.

109. Aletaha D, Funovits J, Smolen JS. Physical disability in rheumatoid arthritis is associated with cartilage damage rather than bone destruction. *Ann Rheum Dis*. 2011;70:733–739.

110. Freeston J, Keenan AM, Emery P. Spotting the early warning signs of aggressive RA. *J Musculoskel Med*. 2008;25(3):110–115.

111. Goekoop-Ruiterman YPM, de Vries-Bouwstra JK, Allaart CF, et al. Clinical and radiographic outcomes of four different treatment strategies in patients with early rheumatoid arthritis (the BeSt Study). *Arthritis Rheum*. 2005;52(11):3381–3390.

112. Bykerk V, Keystone E. RA in primary care: 20 clinical pearls. *J Musculoskel Med*. 2004;21(3):133–146.

113. Weiss JE, Ilowite NT. Juvenile Idiopathic Arthritis. *Rheumatic Dis Clin North Am*. 2007;33(3):441–470.

114. Aletaha D, Neogi T, Silman AJ, et al. 2010 Rheumatoid Arthritis Classification Criteria: An American college of rheumatology/European league against rheumatism collaborative initiative. *Arthritis Rheum*. 2010;62(9):2569–2581.

115. Radner H, Neogi T, Smolen JS, Aletaha D. Performance of the 2010 ACR/EULAR classification criteria for rheumatoid arthritis: a systematic literature review. *Ann Rheum Dis*. 2014;73(1):114–123.

116. Smolen JS, Van Der Heijde DM, St. Clair EW, et al. Predictors of joint damage in patients with early rheumatoid arthritis treated with high-dose methotrexate with or without concomitant infliximab: results from the ASPIRE trial. *Arthritis Rheum*. 2006;54(3):702–710.

117. Marnell M, Mold C, Du Clos TW. C-reactive protein: ligands, receptors and role in inflammation. *Clin Immunol*. 2005;117(2):104–111.

118. Nishimura K, Sugiyama D, Kogata Y, et al. Meta-analysis: diagnostic accuracy of anti-cyclic citrullinated peptide antibody and rheumatoid factor for rheumatoid arthritis. *Ann Intern Med*. 2007;146(11):797–808.

119. Olson NY, Lindsley CB. Advances in pediatric rheumatology paving the way to better care. *J Musculoskel Med*. 2008;25:505–512.

120. Salvarani C, Cantini F, Hunder GG. Polymyalgia rheumatica and giant-cell arteritis. *Lancet*. 2008;372:234–245. https://doi.org/10.1016/S0140-6736(08)61077-6.

121. Nesher G. Polymyalgia rheumatic- Diagnosis and classification. 2014;48-49:76-78. https://doi.org/10.1016/j.jaut.2014.01.016

122. Polymyalgia Rheumatica: American College of Rheumatology. http://www.rheumatology.org/I-Am-A/Patient-Caregiver/Diseases-Conditions/Polymyalgia-Rheumatica. Accessed June 01, 2020.

123. Polyarthralgia Rheumatica and Giant Cell Arteritis: Cleveland Clinic Disease management. http://www.clevelandclinicmeded.com/medicalpubs/diseasemanagement/rheumatology/polymyalgia-rheumatica-and-giant-cell-arteritis/. Accessed June 01, 2020.

124. Gota CE. Giant Cell Arteritis. Merck Manual, Professional Edition. http://www.merckmanuals.com/professional/musculoskeletal-and-connective-tissue-disorders/vasculitis/giant-cell-arteritis. Accessed June 01, 2020.

125. Reiter S. Giant cell arteritis misdiagnosed as temporomandibular disorder: a case report and review of the literature. *J Orofac Pain*. 2009;23(4):360–365.

126. Corticosteroids for Polymyalgia Rheumatica or Giant Cell Arteritis: WebMD. http://www.webmd.com/arthritis/corticosteroids-for-polymyalgia-rheumatica-or-giant-cell-arteritis. Accessed June 03, 2020.

127. Hernandez-Rodriguez J. Medical management of polymyalgia rheumatica. *Expert Opin Pharmacother*. 2010;11(7):1077–1087.

128. Lupus Foundation of America (LFA): Understanding lupus. One of five patient education booklets available online at www.lupus.org. Accessed May 28, 2020.

129. Vaglio A, Grayson P, Fenaroli P, et al. Drug-induced lupus: traditional and new concepts. *Autoimmun Rev*. 2018;17:912–918.

130. Grau RH. Cutaneous cues to diagnosis of lupus. *J Musculoskel Med*. 2007;24(6):247–263.

131. Tsokos G. Mechanisms of disease. *N Engl J Med*. 2011;365:2110–2121.

132. Pons-Estel GJ, Ugarte-Gil MF, et al. Epidemiology of systemic lupus erythematosus. *Expert Rev Clin Immunol*. 2017;13:799–814. https://doi.org/10.1080/1744666X.2017.1327352.

133. Pons-Estel GJ, Alarcon GS, Scofield L, Reinlib L, Cooper GS. Understanding the epidemiology and progress of systemic lupus erythematosus. *Semin Arthritis Rheum*. 2010;39(4):257–268.

134. Rahman A, Isenberg D. Mechanisms of disease: systemic lupus erythematosus. *N Engl J Med*. 2008;358:929–939.

135. Aringer M, Costenbader K, Daikh D, et al. 2019 European League Against Rheumatism/American College of Rheumatology Classification Criteria for Systemic Lupus Erythematosus. *Arthritis Rheumatol*. 2019;71(9):1400–1412.

136. Yu C, Gershwin ME, Chang C. Diagnostic Criteria for systemic lupus erythematosus: a critical review. *J Autoimmun*. 2014;48-49:10–13. https://doi.org/10.1016/j.jaut.2014.01.004.

137. https://doi.org/10.1016/B978-0-444-63596-9.00008-6

138. Sayarlioglu M, Yuzbasioglu N, Inanc M, et al. Risk factors for avascular bone necrosis in patients with systemic lupus erythematosus. *Rheumatol Int*. Jan 2012;32(1):177–182.

139. Sciascia S, Bertolaccini ML. Central nervous system involvement in systemic lupus erythematosus: overview on

classification criteria. *Autoimmun Rev.* 2013;12:426–429. https://doi.org/10.1016/j.autrev.2012.08.014.

140. Bertsias GK. EULAR recommendations for the management of systemic lupus erythematosus with neuropsychiatric manifestations. Report of a task force of the EULAR standing committee for clinical affairs. *Ann Rheum Dis.* 2010;69(12):2074–2082.

141. Zulian F, Vallongo C, Woo P, et al. Localized scleroderma in childhood is not just a skin disease. *Arthritis Rheum.* 2005;52(9):2873–2881.

142. Careta MF, Romiti R. Localized scleroderma: clinical spectrum and therapeutic update. *An Bras Dermatol.* 2015;90(1):62–73. https://doi.org/10.1590/abd1806-4841.20152890.

143. Denton CP, Khanna D. Systemic sclerosis. *Lancet.* 2017;390:1685–1699.

144. What is Scleroderma? Scleroderma Foundation. http://www.scleroderma.org/site/PageNavigator/patients_whatis.html#.V3WBl_krLcc. Accessed June 01, 2020.

145. Stoenoiu MS, Houssiau FA, Lecouvet FE. Tendon friction rubs in systemic sclerosis: a possible explanation- an ultrasound and magnetic resonance imaging study. *Rheumatology.* 2013;52:529–533.

146. Highland KB, Silver RM. New developments in scleroderma interstitial lung disease. *Curr Opin Rheumatol.* 2005;17(6):737–745.

147. Hassoun M. Lung involvement in systemic sclerosis. *Presse Med.* 2010;40(1 Pt 2):e3–e17.

148. Reveille J. Spondyloarthritis. In: Rich R, Fleisher T, Shearer W, Schroeder H, Frew A, Weyand C, eds. *Clinical immunology: principles and practice.* 5th ed. : Elsevier; 2019:769–787.

149. Rudwaleit M, van der Heijde D, Landewé R, et al. The Assessment of SpondyloArthritis International Society classification criteria for peripheral spondyloarthritis and for spondyloarthritis in general. *Ann Rheum Dis.* 2011;70(1):25–31. https://doi.org/10.1136/ard.2010.133645.

150. Pereira IA, Neves FS, Castro GRW. Extra-articular manifestations of spondyloarthritis are common and should be screened. *Rheumatol Curr Res.* 2012;2(3). https://doi.org/10.4172/2161-1149.1000111.

151. Lipton S. Deodhar. The new ASAS classification criteria for axial and peripheral spondyloarthritis: promises and pitfalls. *Int J Clin Rheumatol.* 2012;7(6):675–682.

152. Zeidler H, Amor B. The Assessment in Spondyloarthritis International Society (ASAS) classification criteria for peripheral spondyloarthritis and for spondyloarthritis in general: the spondyloarthritis concept in progress. *Ann Rheum Dis.* 2011;70(1):1–3. https://doi.org/10.1136/ard.2010.135889.

153. Rudwaleit M, van der Heijde D, Landewé R, et al. The development of Assessment of SpondyloArthritis international Society classification criteria for axial spondyloarthritis (part II): validation and final selection [published correction appears in Ann Rheum Dis. 2019 Jun;78(6):e59]. *Ann Rheum Dis.* 2009;68(6):777–783. https://doi.org/10.1136/ard.2009.108233.

154. Garg N, van den Bosch F, Deodhar A. The concept of spondyloarthritis: where are we now? *Best Pract Res Clin Rheumatol.* 2014;28(5):663–672. https://doi.org/10.1016/j.berh.2014.10.007.

155. Taurog JD, Chhabra A, Colbert RA. Ankylosing spondylitis and axial spondyloarthritis. *N Engl J Med.* 2016;374(26):2563–2574. https://doi.org/10.1056/NEJMra1406182.

156. Raychaudhuri SP, Deodhar A. The classification and diagnostic criteria of ankylosing spondylitis. *J Autoimmun.* 2014;48-49:128–133. https://doi.org/10.1016/j.jaut.2014.01.015.

157. Reveille JD, Witter JP, Weissman MH. Prevalence of axial spondyloarthritis in the United States: estimates from a cross-sectional survey. *Arthritis Care Res.* 2012;64:905–910.

158. Sieper J, Poddubnyy D. Axial spondyloarthritis. *Lancet.* 2017;390(10089):73–84. https://doi.org/10.1016/S0140-6736(16)31591-4.

159. Wang R, Gabriel SE, Ward MM. Progression of patients with non-radiographic axial spondyloarthritis to ankylosing spondylitis: a population-based cohort study. *Arthritis Rheumatol.* 2016;68:1415–1421.

160. Toussirot E. Late-onset ankylosing spondylitis and spondylarthritis: an update on clinical manifestations, differential diagnosis, and pharmacological therapies. *Drugs Aging.* 2010;27(7):523–531.

161. Shiel WC. Ankylosing Spondylitis. MedisineNet.com. http://www.medicinenet.com/ankylosing_spondylitis/page2.htm. Accessed June 30, 2016.

162. Curtis JR, Harrold LR, Asgari MM, et al. Diagnostic prevalence of ankylosing spondylitis using computerized Health Care Data, 1996 to 2009: Underrecognition in a US Health Care Setting. *Perm J.* 2016;20(4):15–151. https://doi.org/10.7812/TPP/15-151.

163. Østergaard M, Lambert RGW. Imaging in ankylosing spondylitis. *Ther Adv Musculoskelet Dis.* 2012;4(4):301–311.

164. Francis R, Dheerendra S, Natali C, et al. Schober's test: revisited. *Orthopedic Proceedings.* 2012;92-B(Suppl IV-563).

165. Chaudhary SB, Hullinger H, Vives MJ. Management of acute spinal fractures in ankylosing spondylitis. *ISRN Rheumatol.* 2011;2011:150484.

166. Mitra D, Elvins DM, Speden DJ, Collins AJ. The prevalence of vertebral fractures in mild ankylosing spondylitis and their relationship to bone mineral density. *Rheumatology (Oxford).* 2000;39(1):85–89. https://doi.org/10.1093/rheumatology/39.1.85.

167. Lee JS, Lee S, Bang SY, et al. Prevalence and risk factors of anterior atlantoaxial subluxation in ankylosing spondylitis. *J Rheumatol.* 2012;39(12):2321–2326. https://doi.org/10.3899/jrheum.120260.

168. Lu DW, Katz KA. Declining use of the eponym "Reiter's syndrome" in the medical literature, 1998-2003. *J Am Acad Dermatol.* 2005;53(4):720–723. https://doi.org/10.1016/j.jaad.2005.06.048.

169. Carter JD, Hudson AP. Reactive arthritis: clinical features and treatment. In: Espinoza L, ed. *Infections and the Rheumatic Diseases.* Cham: Springer; 2019.

170. Townes JM, Deodhar AA, Laine ES, et al. Reactive arthritis following culture-confirmed infections with bacterial enteric pathogens in Minnesota and Oregon: a population-based study. *Ann Rheum Dis.* 2008;67(12):1689–1696. https://doi.org/10.1136/ard.2007.083451.

171. Carter JD. Reactive arthritis: defined etiologies, emerging pathophysiology, and unresolved treatment. *Infect Dis Clin North Am.* 2006;20(4):827–847. https://doi.org/10.1016/j.idc.2006.09.004.

172. Schmitt SK. Reactive arthritis. *Infect Dis Clin North Am.* 2017;31(2):265–277. https://doi.org/10.1016/j.idc.2017.01.002.

173. Taylor W, Gladman D, Helliwell P, et al. Classification criteria for psoriatic arthritis: development of new criteria from a large international study. *Arthritis Rheum.* 2006;54(8):2665–2673. https://doi.org/10.1002/art.21972.

174. Ritchlin CT, Colbert RA, Gladman DD. Psoriatic Arthritis [published correction appears in N Engl J Med. 2017 May 25;376(21):2097]. *N Engl J Med.* 2017;376(10):957–970. https://doi.org/10.1056/NEJMra1505557.

175. Raychaudhuri SP, Wilken R, Sukhov AC, Raychaudhuri SK, Maverakis E. Management of psoriatic arthritis: early diagnosis, monitoring of disease severity and cutting edge therapies. *J Autoimmun.* 2017;76:21–37. https://doi.org/10.1016/j.jaut.2016.10.009.

176. Korendowych E, McHugh N. Genetic factors in psoriatic arthritis. *Curr Rheumatol Rep.* 2005;7(4):306–312.

177. Raychaudhuri SP. A cutting edge overview: psoriatic disease. *Clin Rev Aller Immunol.* 2013;44(2):109–113.

178. Gladman DD, Antoni C, Mease P, Clegg DO, Nash P. Psoriatic arthritis: epidemiology, clinical features, course, and outcome. *Ann Rheum Dis.* 2005;64(Suppl 2(Suppl 2)):ii14–ii17. https://doi.org/10.1136/ard.2004.032482.

179. Kaeley GS, Eder L, Aydin SZ, Gutierrez M, Bakewell C. Dactylitis: A hallmark of psoriatic arthritis. *Semin Arthritis Rheum.* 2018;48(2):263–273. https://doi.org/10.1016/j.semarthrit.2018.02.002.

180. Tam LS, Tomlinson B, Chu TT, et al. Cardiovascular risk profile of patients with psoriatic arthritis compared to controls – the role of inflammation. *Rheumatology.* 2008;47(5):718–723.

181. CDC: Signs and Symptoms of Untreated Lyme Disease. http://www.cdc.gov/lyme/signs_symptoms/index.html, August 13, 2020. Accessed 27 May 2020.

182. Milewski MD. Lyme arthritis in children presenting with joint effusions. *J Bone Joint Surg.* 2011;93A(2):252–260.

183. Smith BG. Lyme disease and the orthopaedic implications of Lyme arthritis. *J Am Acad Orthop Surg.* 2011;19(2):91–100.

184. Venables MA, Maini RN. Diagnosis and differential diagnosis of rheumatoid arthritis. UpToDate. Wolters Kluwer. http://www.uptodate.com/contents/diagnosis-and-differential-diagnosis-of-rheumatoid-arthritis. Accessed 25 May 2020.

185. Kister I, Chamot E, Salter AR, Cutter GR, Bacon TE, Herbert J. Disability in multiple sclerosis. a reference for patients and clinicians. *Neurology.* 2013;80(11):1018–1024.

186. Types of MS. National Multiple Sclerosis Society. http://www.nationalmssociety.org/What-is-MS/Types-of-MS. Accessed June 03, 2020.

187. Munger KL, Ascherio A. Epidemiology of multiple sclerosis: from risk factors to prevention- an update. *Semin Neurol.* 2016;36(2):103–114.

188. Courtney AM, Treadway K, Remington G, Frohman E. Multiple sclerosis. *Med Clin North Am.* 2009;93:451–476.

189. Sundström P, Salzer J. Vitamin D and multiple sclerosis- from epidemiology to prevention. *Acta Neurol Scand.* 2015;132(199):56–61.

190. Ascherio A, Munger KL. Environmental risk factors for multiple sclerosis. Part II: noninfectious factors. *Ann Neurol.* 2007;61(6):504–513.

191. Handel AE, Williamson AJ, Disanto G, Handunnetthi L, Giovannoni G, Ramagopalan SV. An updated meta-analysis of risk of multiple sclerosis following infectious mononucleosis. *PLoS One.* 2010;5(9):e12496.

192. Haslam C. Managing bladder symptoms in people with multiple sclerosis. *Nursing Times.* 2005;101(2):48–52.

193. Scalfari A, Knappertz V, Cutter G. Mortality in patients with multiple sclerosis. *Neurol.* 2013;81(2):184–192.

194. Maroney M, Hunter SF. Implications for multiple sclerosis in the era of the affordable care act: a clinical overview. *Am J Manag Care.* 2014;20(Suppl 11):S220–S227.

195. MS Symptoms: National Multiple Sclerosis Society. http://www.nationalmssociety.org/Symptoms-Diagnosis/MS-Symptoms. Accessed June 03, 2020.

196. Winser S, Smith CM, Hale LA, et al. Balance assessment in multiple sclerosis and cerebellar ataxia: rationale, protocol and demographic data. *Physical Med Rehabil Int.* 2014;5(4):1–6.

197. Costello F. Neuro-Ophthalmologic Manifestations of Multiple Sclerosis. Updated Jan 22, 2016. http://emedicine.medscape.com/article/1214270-overview. Accessed June 03, 2020.

198. Christogianni A, Bibb R, Davis SL, et al. Temperature sensitivity in multiple sclerosis: an overview of its impact on sensory and cognitive symptoms. *Temperature.* 2018;5(3):208–223.

199. Marrie RA, Reider N, Cohen J. A systematic review of the incidence and prevalence of sleep disorders and seizure disorders in multiple sclerosis. *Mult Scler.* 2015;21(3):342–349.

200. Ramchandren S. The immunopathogenesis of Guillain-Barré syndrome. *Clin Adv Hematol Oncol.* 2010;8(3):203–206.

201. McGrogan A, Madle GC, Seaman HE. The epidemiology of Guillain-Barré syndrome worldwide. *Neuroepidemiol.* 2009;32(2):150–163.

202. Sudulagunta SR, Sodalagunta MB, Sepehrar S. Guillain-Barré syndrome: clinical profile and management. *Ger Med Sci.* 2015:13.

203. Sejvar JJ, Baughman AL, Wise M, Morgan OW. Population incidence of Guillain-Barré syndrome: a systematic review and meta-analysis. *Neuroepidemiology.* 2011;36:123–133.

204. Lehmann HC. Guillain-Barré syndrome after exposure to influenza virus. *Lancet Infect Dis.* 2010;10(9):643–651.

205. van den Berg B, Walgaard C, Drenthen J, Fokke C, Jacobs BC, van Doorn PA. Guillan-Barré syndrome: pathogenesis, diagnosis, treatment and prognosis. *Nat Rev Neurol.* 2014;10:469–482.

206. Vellozzi C, Iqbal S, Steward B. Cumulative risk of Guillain-Barré syndrome among vaccinated and unvaccinated populations during the 2009 H1N1 influenza pandemic. *Am J Public Health.* 2014;104(4):696–701.

207. Pan American Health Organization: World Health Organization. Zika: Epidemiological Update. http://www.paho.org/hq/index.php?option=com_docman&task=doc_view&Itemid=270&gid=34906&lang=en, June 2, 2016. Accessed June 03, 2020.

208. McGrogan A, Sneedon S, de Vries CS. The incidence of Myasthenia Gravis: a systematic literature review. *Neuroepidemiology.* 2010;34:171–183.

209. Wu X, Shen D, Li T. Distinct clinical characteristics of pediatric Guillain-Barré syndrome: a comparative study between children and adults in Northeast China. *PLoS One.* 2016;11(3):e0151611.

210. Sieb JP. Myasthenia gravis: an update for the clinician. *Clin Exp Immunol.* 2014;175(3):408–418.

211. Farrugia ME, Vincent A. Autoimmune mediated neuromuscular junction defects. *Curr Opin Neurol.* 2010;23(5):489–495.

212. Gilhus NE, Vershuuren JJ. Myasthenia gravis: subgroup classification and therapeutic strategies. *Lancet Neurol.* 2015;14:1023–1036.

213. Angelini C. Diagnosis and management of autoimmune myasthenia gravis. *Clin Drug Investig.* 2011;31(1):1–14.

214. Scherer K, Bedlack RS, Simel L. Does this patient have myasthenia gravis? *JAMA.* 2005;293(15):1906–1914.

215. Magee DJ. *Orthopedic Physical Assessment.* 6 ed Philadelphia: WB Saunders; 2014.

Screening for Cancer

Jeannette Lee

A 56-year-old man has come to you for an evaluation without a referral. He has not seen any type of physician for at least 3 years. He is seeking an examination at the insistence of his wife, who has noticed that his collar size has increased two sizes in the last year and that his neck looks "puffy." He has no complaints of any kind (including pain or discomfort), and he denies any known trauma; however, his wife insists that she has observed that he has limited ability in turning his head when backing the car out of the driveway.

- What questions would be appropriate for your first physical therapy interview with this client?
- What test procedures will you carry out during the first session?
- If you suggest to this man that he should see his physician, how would you make that recommendation? (See the Case Study at the end of this chapter.)

A large part of the screening process is identifying red-flag histories and red-flag signs and symptoms. Advancing age and previous history of any kind of cancer are two of the most important risk factors for cancer. Following the screening model presented in Chapters 1 and 2, the therapist should use past medical history, clinical presentation, and associated signs and symptoms as the basic tools to screen for cancer.

The client history with interview is the number one tool for cancer screening. Take the client's history, looking for the presence of any risk factors for cancer. Cancer in its early stages is often asymptomatic. Survival rates are increased with early detection and screening, making this element of client management extremely important.

Keep in mind that some cancers, such as malignant melanoma (MM) (skin cancer), do not currently have a highly effective treatment. Early detection and referral may make a life and death difference in the final outcome. Morbidity can be reduced and quality of life and function improved with early intervention.

Whether primary cancer, cancer that has recurred locally, or cancer that has metastasized, clinical manifestations can mimic neuromuscular or musculoskeletal dysfunction. The physical therapist's task is to identify abnormal tissue, not diagnose the lesion.

CANCER STATISTICS

Cancer accounts for more deaths than heart disease in the United States in persons between 45 to 79 years of age. There are more than 1.8 million new cases of cancer in the United States each year; more than 600,000 people will die of cancer this year. One in four deaths in the United States is attributed to cancer.[1]

Predicting lifetime risk of cancer is based on present rates of cancer. Using today's epidemiologic data, 41% of all men and 39% of all women will develop cancer in their lifetime.[1] It is estimated that by 2030, 20% of the U.S. population will be 65 years old or older, accounting for 70% of all cancers and approximately 80% of all cancer-related mortality.[2]

In the past, certain types of cancer were invariably fatal. Today, however, death rates continue to decline for most cancers, and there continues to be a reported reduced mortality from cancer, by about an average of 1.5% per year overall, decreasing slightly more rapidly among men (by 1.8% per year) than among women (1.4% per year). The percentage of people who have survived longer than 5 years after cancer diagnosis has increased over the past two decades.[3]

Fig. 14.1 summarizes current U.S. figures for cancer incidence and deaths by site and sex. Although prostate and breast cancers are the most common malignancies in men and women, respectively, the cancer that most commonly causes death is lung cancer.[1]

Carcinoma in situ is not included in the statistics related to invasive carcinoma or sarcoma as reported by the American Cancer Society (ACS) or the National Cancer Institute (NCI). Carcinoma in situ is considered a premalignant cancer that is localized to the organ of origin. As noted, it is reported separately and primarily relative to breast and skin cancer. Carcinoma in situ of the breast accounted for about 38,000 new cases, and in situ melanoma accounted for about 96,000 new cases in the most recent report.[1]

Cancer Cure and Recurrence

Cancer is considered cured or in remission when evidence of the disease cannot be found in the individual's body. Early diagnosis and aggressive intervention can help people obtain

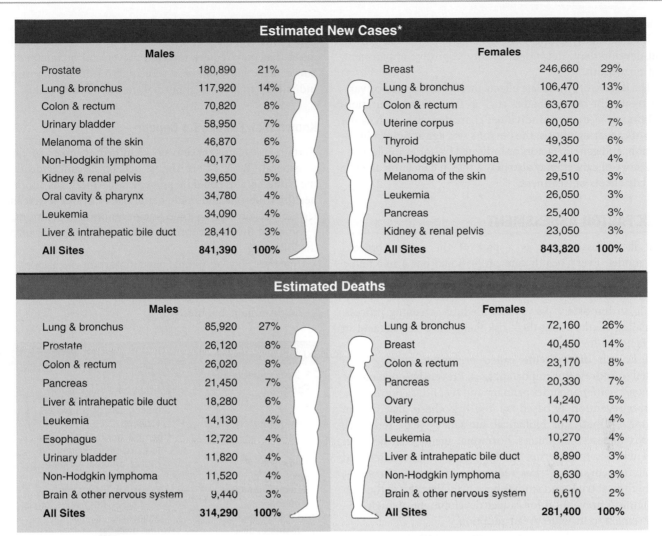

Estimated New Cases*

Males				Females		
Prostate	180,890	21%		Breast	246,660	29%
Lung & bronchus	117,920	14%		Lung & bronchus	106,470	13%
Colon & rectum	70,820	8%		Colon & rectum	63,670	8%
Urinary bladder	58,950	7%		Uterine corpus	60,050	7%
Melanoma of the skin	46,870	6%		Thyroid	49,350	6%
Non-Hodgkin lymphoma	40,170	5%		Non-Hodgkin lymphoma	32,410	4%
Kidney & renal pelvis	39,650	5%		Melanoma of the skin	29,510	3%
Oral cavity & pharynx	34,780	4%		Leukemia	26,050	3%
Leukemia	34,090	4%		Pancreas	25,400	3%
Liver & intrahepatic bile duct	28,410	3%		Kidney & renal pelvis	23,050	3%
All Sites	**841,390**	**100%**		**All Sites**	**843,820**	**100%**

Estimated Deaths

Males				Females		
Lung & bronchus	85,920	27%		Lung & bronchus	72,160	26%
Prostate	26,120	8%		Breast	40,450	14%
Colon & rectum	26,020	8%		Colon & rectum	23,170	8%
Pancreas	21,450	7%		Pancreas	20,330	7%
Liver & intrahepatic bile duct	18,280	6%		Ovary	14,240	5%
Leukemia	14,130	4%		Uterine corpus	10,470	4%
Esophagus	12,720	4%		Leukemia	10,270	4%
Urinary bladder	11,820	4%		Liver & intrahepatic bile duct	8,890	3%
Non-Hodgkin lymphoma	11,520	4%		Non-Hodgkin lymphoma	8,630	3%
Brain & other nervous system	9,440	3%		Brain & other nervous system	6,610	2%
All Sites	**314,290**	**100%**		**All Sites**	**281,400**	**100%**

Fig. 14.1   Estimated new cases of cancer and cancer deaths by site for men and women. *Estimates are rounded to the nearest 10 and exclude basal and squamous cell skin cancers and in situ carcinoma, except urinary bladder carcinoma. (Redrawn from Siegel RL, Miller KD, Jemal A. Cancer statistics, 2020. *CA: A Cancer J Clin* 2020;70(1):7-30. doi:10.3322/caac.21590)

positive outcomes. In general, individuals with no evidence of cancer are considered to have the same life expectancy as those who never had cancer. However, late and/or long-term physical and psychosocial complications of the disease and treatment are being increasingly recognized and addressed.[4]

Cancer recurrence or a new cancer can occur in some individuals with a previous personal history of cancer. Some causes of cancer recurrence include inadequate surgical margins, skip metastases, tumor thrombus, and lymph node metastasis.

Additionally, many of the antineoplastic strategies (e.g., chemotherapy, hormone therapy, radiation therapy) mutate cells further and can initiate or stimulate new malignant tumors. Besides secondary malignancies, these treatments can come with many unintended long-term problems and adverse consequences (e.g., fibrosis, lymphedema, occlusive coronary artery disease and cardiotoxicity, impaired motion and strength). The therapist should consider it a red flag any time a client has a previous history of cancer or cancer treatment.

Childhood Cancers

Cancer is the second leading cause of death in children between the ages of 1 and 14, surpassed only by accidents. The most frequently occurring cancers in children are leukemia (primarily acute lymphocytic leukemia and acute myeloid leukemia), brain and other nervous system cancers, soft tissue sarcomas, lymphomas (Hodgkin's and non-Hodgkin's) and renal (Wilms') tumors.[5]

Survival rates for childhood cancer have increased to 84% because of improvements in the treatment for many types over the past two decades.[1,5] The result is an increasing population of long-term cancer survivors (or "overcomers" or "thrivers" as some "survivors" prefer to call themselves). Currently, 1 in 530 young adults is a childhood cancer survivor. Long-term health problems related to the effects of cancer therapy are a major focus of this population group.[6,7]

It has been shown that, to varying degrees, long-term survivors of childhood cancer are at risk of developing secondary cancers and of experiencing late effects of cancer treatment, such as cardiomyopathy, joint dysfunction, reduced growth and development, decreased fertility, cognitive impairment, and early death.[8,9]

The degree of risk of late effects may be influenced by various treatment-related factors such as the intensity, duration, and timing of therapy. Individual characteristics, such as the type of cancer diagnosis, the person's sex, age at time of intervention, and genetic factors as indicated by, for example, family history of cancer, may also play a role in cancer recurrence and late effects of treatment.[9,10]

RISK FACTOR ASSESSMENT

Risk factor assessment is a part of the cancer prevention model. Every health care professional has a role and a responsibility to help clients identify risk factors for disease. Knowing the various risk factors for different kinds of cancers is an important part of the medical screening process. Educating clients about their risk factors is a key element in risk factor reduction.

A branch of medicine called *preventive oncology* was started to address this important area. Preventive oncology or *chemoprevention* includes primary and secondary prevention. Chemoprevention is based on the hypothesis that certain natural, synthetic, or biological substances (e.g., retinoids, cyclooxygenase-2 inhibitors, hormonal agents) can be given preventatively to interrupt the biological processes involved in carcinogenesis and thus reduce its incidence. Currently, many clinical trials and studies have been devoted to the idea of chemical prevention for cancer development, though barriers remain to its widespread adoption.[11]

Therapists can have an active role in both primary and secondary prevention through screening and education. Primary prevention involves stopping the processes that lead to the formation of cancer in the first place. According to the *Guide to Physical Therapist Practice* (the *Guide*), physical therapists are involved in primary prevention by "preventing a target condition in a susceptible or potentially susceptible population through such specific measures as general health promotion efforts."[12] Risk factor assessment and risk reduction fall under this category.

Secondary prevention involves regular screening for early detection of cancer and the prevention of progression of known premalignant lesions such as skin and colon lesions. This does not prevent cancer but improves the outcome. The *Guide* outlines the physical therapist's role in secondary prevention as "decreasing duration of illness, severity of disease, and number of sequelae through early diagnosis and prompt intervention."[12]

Another way to look at this is through the use of screening and surveillance. *Screening* is a method for detecting disease or body dysfunction before an individual would normally seek medical care. Medical screening tests are usually administered to individuals who do not have current symptoms but who may be at high risk for certain adverse health outcomes.

Surveillance is the analysis of health information (e.g., patient history, diagnosis) to identify problems at the earliest onset that may require targeted prevention or intervention. Surveillance has often used screening results from groups of individuals to look for abnormal trends in health status.

Known Risk Factors for Cancer

Certain risk factors have been identified as linked to cancer in general (Table 14.1). Almost half of all cancer deaths in the United States could be prevented if Americans adopted a healthier lifestyle and made better use of available screening tests, especially among lower socioeconomic populations.[13]

Some of the most common risk factors for cancer include the following:

- Age over 50 years (single most important risk factor)
- Ethnicity
- Family history (first generation)
- Environment and lifestyle

TABLE 14.1	Risk Factors for Cancer	
Nonmodifiable Risk Factors	**Modifiable Risk Factors**
Age	Smoking, use of smokeless tobacco
Previous history of cancer	Chemical or other exposure (e.g., paint, cadmium, dye, rubber, arsenic, asbestos, radon, benzene, ionizing radiation, Agent Orange, pesticides, herbicides, organic amines)
Ethnicity	
Skin color	
Sex	
Heredity (identified oncogenes)	
Age of menarche, menopause	Urban dwelling
Adenomatous polyps	Alcohol consumption (more than 1–2 drinks per day)
Inflammatory bowel disease	Sedentary lifestyle; lack of exercise
Fat distribution patterns	Obesity; diet high in animal fat
Congenital immunodeficiencies	Insulin resistance (elevated serum insulin)
Congenital diseases	Radiation/chemotherapy treatment
Long-term *Helicobacter* infection	Estrogen replacement therapy
	Sexually transmitted diseases
	Ionizing radiation
	HTLV-1 (virus, rare in United States)
	Previous lung scarring
	Organ transplantation (immunosuppression)
	HIV infection
	Chronic exposure to UV rays
	Geographic location
	Smoked foods, salted fish, and meat (nitrates and nitrites)
	Tamoxifen use
	Nulliparity (never having children)
	Vitamin B12 deficiency
	Lack of access to or use of health care and screening tests

HIV, Human immunodeficiency virus; *HTLV-1*, human T-lymphotropic virus type 1; *UV*, ultraviolet.

Age

The majority of cancer incidence and mortality occurs in individuals aged 65 and older.[14] With estimates from the U.S. Census Bureau predicting a rapid rise in the number of people aged 65 years and older, the therapist must pay close attention to the client's age, especially in correlation with a personal or family history of cancer. Many cancers, such as prostate, colon, ovarian, and some types of chronic leukemia, have an increased incidence in older adults. The incidence of cancer doubles after 25 years of age and increases with every 5-year increase in age until the mid-80s, when cancer incidence and mortality reach a plateau and even decline slightly.

Other cancers occur within very narrow age ranges. Testicular cancer is often diagnosed in men from about 20 to 40 years of age. Breast cancer shows a sharp increase after the age of 45 years. Ovarian cancer is more common in women older than 55 years. A number of cancers, such as Ewing's sarcoma, acute leukemia, Wilms' tumor, and retinoblastoma, occur mainly in childhood.

Screening for age is discussed more completely in Chapter 2. Please refer to this section for information on screening for this red flag or risk factor.

Ethnicity

Racial or ethnic minorities account for a disproportionate number of newly diagnosed cancers. African Americans have a 10% higher incidence rate than Whites and a 30% higher death rate from all cancers combined than Whites.[1,15]

African Americans have the highest mortality and worst survival of any population for most cancers, and diagnosis occurs at a later stage.[1,15] Even when studies have shown that equal treatment yields equal outcomes among individuals with equal disease, cancer death rates have been historically higher for African Americans than for Whites, though that gap has been narrowing in the past few years. The overall cancer mortality rate is dropping faster in Blacks than in Whites, particularly in lung, colorectal, and prostate cancers.[16-18]

Compared with the general population, African Americans die of cancer at a 40% greater rate (they are 30% more likely to die of heart disease). The Institute of Medicine (IOM) document, *Unequal Treatment, Confronting Racial and Ethnic Disparities in Health Care*, suggests that care providers may be a part of the problem.[19] Though this document prompted the IOM to add equity to its list of aims for the U.S. health care system,[20] there is still much work to be done to address ethnic and racial disparities in health care.[21]

In terms of risk assessment, therapists must keep these figures in mind when examining and evaluating clients of African-American descent. For any ethnic group, the therapist is advised to be aware of cancer and disease demographics and epidemiology for that particular group.

Cancer statistics for Hispanic Americans compared with non-Hispanic Americans are becoming more available.[1,22] The rates of incidence and mortality from the four major cancer killers (breast, prostate, lung, colorectal) are lower, but cancer with an infectious etiology (stomach, liver, uterine, cervix, gallbladder) occurs at a higher rate.

The use of early detection cancer screening tests has been increasing among this group. Mammography among Hispanic women exceeds the national average, but screening for colorectal, cervical, and prostate cancers remain below average.

Cancer statistics and epidemiology in this group are problematic. Hispanic people originate from 23 different countries and have enormous diversity among themselves. They are one of the poorest minority groups in the United States and have the highest uninsured rate of all groups.[23] The uninsured are less likely to have preventive care, such as cancer screening.

The most common cancer among Hispanic women is breast cancer; second is lung cancer. Men are more likely to have prostate cancer but die more often of lung cancer. Hispanics have twice the incidence rate and a 70% higher death rate from liver cancer compared with non-Hispanics. This type of cancer is on the rise in Hispanic women. Cancer is typically diagnosed in Hispanics at a later stage than in non-Hispanic white Americans. Consequently, they have lower cure or remission rates.

Therapists can offer health care education and cancer screening to this unique group of people. This will be increasingly common in our practice as our health care delivery system moves from an illness-based system to a health promotion–based system. For all groups, high-quality prevention and early detection and intervention can reduce cancer incidence and mortality.[3] Screening for ethnicity is discussed more completely in Chapter 2. Please refer to this section for information on screening for this important red-flag/risk factor.

Family History and Genetics

Family history is often an important factor in the development of some cancers. This usually includes only first-generation family members, including parents, siblings, and children.

Hereditary cancer syndromes account for approximately 5% of breast, ovarian, and colon cancers. Both clients and providers are becoming aware of the potential therapeutic advantages of early identification of hereditary cancer risk.[24,25]

The hereditary syndromes most frequently identified are hereditary breast and ovarian cancer (HBOC) syndrome as a result of mutations in BRCA1 and BRCA2 genes; hereditary colon cancer (HCC), specifically, familial adenomatous polyposis (FAP); and hereditary nonpolyposis colorectal cancer.

The small percentage of people who may be suspected of a hereditary cancer syndrome can be screened regarding personal and family medical history. Critical details, such as the cancer site and age at diagnosis, are needed for risk assessment. The following are some basic hallmarks of families who could have a hereditary cancer syndrome[26-30]:

- Diagnosis of cancer in two or more relatives in a family
- Diagnosis of cancer in a family member under the age of 50 years
- Occurrence of the same type of cancer in several members of a family
- Occurrence of more than one type of cancer in one person

BOX 14.1 CANCERS LINKED TO OBESITY, DIET, AND NUTRITION[31]

Mouth, pharynx, esophagus	Colon, rectum
Larynx	Breast
Lung	Ovary
Stomach	Endometrium
Pancreas	Cervix
Gallbladder	Prostate
Liver	Kidney
Uterus	Bladder

- Occurrence of a rare type of cancer in one or more members of a family

Environment and Lifestyle Factors

It is now apparent that, although genetic predisposition varies, the two key factors determining whether people develop cancer are environment and lifestyle. The most important way to reduce cancer risk is to avoid cancer-causing agents.

Obesity, diet, sedentary lifestyle, sexual practices, and the use of tobacco, alcohol, and/or other drugs make up the largest percentage of modifiable risk factors for cancer. Current data support the findings that obesity, inappropriate diet, and excess weight cause around one third of all cancer deaths (Box 14.1).[32] Increased body weight and obesity (as measured by body mass index [BMI], an approximation of body adiposity) are associated with increased death rates for all cancers and for cancers at specific sites, especially when combined with a sedentary lifestyle.[33,41]

Obesity and being overweight has been reported to account for 20% of all cancer deaths in U.S. women and 14% in U.S. men over the last 25 years; however, these rates may be underestimated as the average weight has continued to increase worldwide over the same time. It is estimated that over 90,000 cancer deaths could be prevented each year if Americans maintained a healthy body weight.[40] Excess body weight increases amounts of circulating hormones, such as estrogens, androgens, and insulin,[42,43] all of which are associated with cellular and tumor growth. It has also been shown that physical activity reduces the risk of breast and colon cancers and may reduce the risk of several other types of cancer by decreasing excess body weight and by actually decreasing the circulation of some of the growth-related hormones.[44]

An estimated 7.8 million premature deaths could be prevented if everyone ate at least 10 fruits and vegetables each day. Even just two to three portions of fruits and vegetables, about 200 g (each serving defined as 80 g), reduced cancer mortality from 3%–10% compared to those who ate none.[45] Numerous resources on nutrition and its influence in preventing and treating cancer are available.[31,46–50]

Dietary guidelines were updated to 10 servings a day (equal to 5 cups) for overall health and chemoprevention in 2015 by the U.S. Department of Health and Human Services (HHS) in the publication *Dietary Guidelines for Americans 2015-2020*.[51] The *Guidelines* provide authoritative advice for people aged 2 years and older about how good dietary habits can promote health and reduce risks of major chronic diseases. The number of avoidable cancers through avoidance of excess weight are substantial.[52] The 2020–2025 Dietary Guidelines for Americans was just released. Overall the focus of the guidelines is on healthy dietary habits rather than individual foods or nutrients in isolation.[53]

Specific factors associated with individual cancer types are known in some cases. For example, inadequate hydration is known to increase the risks of colon and bladder cancers. Alcohol consumption is linked with breast, head or neck, and gastrointestinal (GI) cancers. High dietary animal fat intake and tobacco use increase prostate cancer risk. Current smoking is an additive risk factor when combined with obesity for esophageal squamous cell carcinoma and lung and pancreatic cancers. Adenomatous polyps in the colon are known precursors of colorectal cancer.[54]

Sexually Transmitted Infections. Sexually transmitted diseases (STDs) or sexually transmitted infections (STIs) have been positively identified as a risk factor for cancer. Not all STIs are linked with cancer, but studies have confirmed that human papillomavirus (HPV) is the primary cause of cervical cancer. With current technology, high-risk HPV DNA can be detected in cervical specimens.[55] HPV is the leading viral STI in the United States. More than 200 types of HPV have been identified; more than 40 types are transmitted sexually, 13 types of which are associated with cervical cancer. Infection with one of these viruses does not predict cancer but increases the risk of cancer, particularly for cervical, anal, and oropharyngeal cancers.[56]

Incidence and prevalence estimates suggest that young people aged 15–24 years acquire about half of all new STIs and that one in four sexually active adolescent females has an STI, such as chlamydia or HPV. Compared with older adults, sexually active adolescents aged 15–19 years and young adults aged 20–24 years are at higher risk of acquiring STIs for a variety of reasons.[57] While the prevalence of genital herpes decreased steadily in the United States among individuals aged 14–49 years, the decline has not been equal across all races/ethnicities, in particular among non-Hispanic Blacks.[58] In the United States, the HPV vaccine that protects against the most common types (i.e., HPV 6, HPV 11, HPV 16, and HPV 18) has been licensed for use in females since 2006, and in males since 2011. The HPV vaccine has been recommended for use in previously unvaccinated females aged 11 to 12 years through 26 years, and in previously unvaccinated males aged 11 to 12 years through 21 years of age.[59] Current available data show, however, that HPV vaccine uptake is lower than the 80% coverage goal in Healthy People 2020, with < 40% for girls and < 15% for boys completing the three-dose series in the HPV vaccine series.[60]

Tobacco Use. Tobacco and tobacco products are known carcinogens, not just for lung cancer but also for leukemia and cancers of the cervix, kidney, pancreas, stomach, bladder, esophagus, and oropharyngeal and laryngeal structures. This includes second-hand smoke, pipes, cigars, cigarettes, and chewing (smokeless) tobacco. Combining tobacco with caffeine and/or alcohol brings on additional problems. More people die of tobacco use than from use of alcohol and all the other addictive agents combined.

In any physical therapy practice, clients should be screened for the use of tobacco products. Client education includes a review of the physiologic effects of tobacco (for a more complete discussion of screening for tobacco use, see Chapter 2).

If the client indicates a desire to quit smoking or using tobacco, the therapist must be prepared to help him or her explore options for smoking cessation. Pamphlets and other reading material should be available for any client interested in tobacco cessation. Referral to medical doctors who specialize in smoking cessation may be appropriate for some clients.

Occupation and Local Environment. Well-defined problems occur in people engaging in specific occupations, especially involving exposure to chemicals and gases. Exposure to carcinogens in the air, water, and our food sources may be linked to cancer.[61]

Reactions can be delayed up to 30 years, making client history an extremely important tool in identifying potential risk factors. People may or may not even remember past exposures to chemicals or gases. Some may not be aware of childhood exposures. Taking a work or military history may be important (see Chapter 2 and Appendix B-14 in the accompanying enhanced eBook version included with print purchase of this textbook).

The industrial chemicals people are exposed to vary across the country and will depend on where the individual has lived or where the client lives now. Each state in the United States has its own unique environmental issues. For example, in Montana, there has been a significant chlorine spill, exposure to agricultural chemicals, vermiculite mining, and many other forms of mining.

In New York, Love Canal was the focus of concern in the 1980s and 1990s, when the effects of hazardous wastes dumped in the area were discovered. Alaskan oil spills, air pollution in Los Angeles, and hazardous and radioactive nuclear waste in Washington state burial grounds are a few more examples.

In Utah, Nevada, and Arizona, the Radiation Exposure Compensation Act (RECA) was passed by Congress in 1990 after studies showed a possible link between hundreds of above-ground nuclear tests in the late 1950s and early 1960s and various cancers and primary organ diseases.[62] Groundwater wells at old open-pit copper mines in various states have tested positive for uranium up to 40 times higher than legal limits. Hundreds of active wells tap into groundwater within 5 miles of these sites.

Wherever the therapist practices, it is important to be aware of local environmental issues and the effect these may have on people in the vicinity.

Ionizing Radiation. Exposure to ionizing radiation is potentially harmful. Ionizing radiation is the result of electromagnetic waves entering the body and acting on neutral atoms or molecules with sufficient force to remove electrons, creating an ion. The most common sources of ionizing radiation exposure in humans are accidental environmental exposure and medical, therapeutic, or diagnostic irradiation.

Nonionizing radiation is electromagnetic radiation that includes radio waves, microwaves, infrared light, and visible light. Nonionizing radiation does not have enough energy to ionize (i.e., break up) atoms. Electronic devices, such as laser scanners, high-intensity lamps, and electronic antitheft surveillance devices, can expose people to nonionizing radiation. There is no proven link between exposure to nonionizing radiation and cancer, but there is considerable debate that long-term exposure to electromagnetic fields may be correlated with the development of various illnesses and diseases.[63,64]

Some studies have reported the possibility of increased cancer risk, especially of leukemia and brain cancers, for electrical or utility workers and others whose jobs require them to be around electrical equipment. Additional risk factors, however, such as exposure to cancer-initiating agents, may also be involved.

Some researchers have looked at possible associations between electromagnetic exposure and breast cancer, miscarriage, depression, suicide, Alzheimer's disease, and amyotrophic lateral sclerosis (ALS, or Lou Gehrig's disease), but the general scientific consensus is that the evidence is not yet conclusive.[65]

Ultraviolet radiation (UVR), sometimes also called UV light, is invisible electromagnetic radiation of the same nature as visible light but having shorter wavelengths and higher energies. The main source of natural UVR is the sun. UVR is conventionally divided into three bands in order of increasing energy: UVA, UVB, and UVC.

In the electromagnetic spectrum, UVR extends between the blue end of the visible spectrum and low-energy x-rays, straddling the boundary between ionizing and nonionizing radiation (which is conventionally set at 100 nm). Because of the different wavelengths and energies, each of the three bands has distinct effects on biologic tissue.

The highest-energy band, UVC, can damage DNA and other molecules and is used in hospitals for sterilization. UVC is rapidly attenuated in air, and therefore it is not found in ground-level solar radiation. Exposure to UVC, however, can take place close to sources such as welding arcs or germicidal lamps.

UVB is the most effective UV band in causing a tan and sunburn (erythema), and it can affect the immune system. UVA penetrates deeper in the skin because of its longer wavelength and plays a role in skin photoaging. UVA can also affect the immune system. Exposure to UVA and UVB has been implicated in the development of skin cancer.

Tanning lamps emit mostly UVA radiation with a few percentage content of UVB. Use of tanning lamps and beds can lead to significant exposure to UVA radiation. An important study published by the International Agency for Cancer Research examined the link between indoor tanning and melanoma. The risk of melanoma reportedly increases 75% when the first exposure to indoor tanning starts before the age of 35 years.[66]

The greater the frequency and intensity of exposure, the greater the risk. The risk is even higher for individuals using high-intensity or high-pressure devices. Despite known negative health effects from the use of indoor tanning devices, this practice is fairly popular in the United States and Europe.[67]

Therapists have a role in client education, especially concerning reducing modifiable risk factors such as outdoor exposure to the sun without protection, exposure to sun lamps, and indoor tanning.

Military Workers. Survivors of recent wars who have been exposed to chemical agents may be at risk for the development of soft tissue sarcoma, non-Hodgkin's lymphoma (NHL), Hodgkin's disease, respiratory and prostate cancers, skin diseases, and many more problems in themselves and their offspring.

Three million Americans served in the armed forces in Vietnam during the 1960s and early 1970s. Large quantities of defoliant agents, such as Agent Orange, were used to remove forest cover, destroy crops, and clear vegetation from around U.S. military bases.

At least half of the 3 million Americans in Vietnam were there during the heaviest spraying. Many of our military personnel were exposed to this toxic substance. Exposure could occur through inhalation, ingestion, and skin or eye absorption.

In early 2003, the military acknowledged that exposure to Agent Orange is associated with chronic lymphocytic leukemia among surviving veterans. There is also sufficient evidence of an association between Agent Orange and soft tissue sarcoma and NHL.[68-72]

Taking an environmental, occupational, or military history may be appropriate when a client has a history of asthma, allergies, or autoimmune disease, along with puzzling, nonspecific symptoms such as myalgia, arthralgia, headache, back pain, sleep disturbance, loss of appetite, loss of sexual interest, and recurrent upper respiratory symptoms.

The affected individual often presents with an unusual combination of multiorgan signs and symptoms. A medical diagnosis of chronic fatigue syndrome, fibromyalgia, or another more nonspecific disorder is a yellow flag. When and how to take the history and how to interpret the findings are discussed in Chapter 2. The mnemonic CH2OPD2 (Community, Home, Hobbies, Occupation, Personal habits, Diet, and Drugs) can be used as a tool to identify a client's history of exposure to potentially toxic environmental contaminants.[73]

Risk Factors for Cancer Recurrence

As cancer survivors live longer, the chance of recurring cancer increases. Positive lymph nodes, tumor size greater than 2 cm, and a high-grade histopathologic designation increase a client's risk of cancer recurrence. Recurrence can occur at the original location of the first cancer, in local or distant lymph nodes, or in metastatic sites such as the bone or lung tissues.

Each type of cancer has its own risk factors for cancer recurrence. For example, increased numbers of positive lymph nodes and negative estrogen/progesterone receptor (ER/PGR) status for breast cancer survivors are risk factors (Case Example 14.1). A positive ER/PGR status lowers the risk of breast cancer recurrence because it allows the woman to receive treatment for prevention of recurrence according to age and stage of cancer.

CASE EXAMPLE 14.1
Risk Factors for Cancer Recurrence

A 46-year-old woman presented with midthoracic back pain, which she has had for the past 2 weeks. She described the pain as sharp and rated it as a 7 on the numeric rating scale. The pain was increased when she raised her arms overhead and relieved when she put her arms down. There were no other aggravating or relieving factors.

The client also noted occasional shoulder pain, sometimes with back pain and sometimes by itself. There were no other reported symptoms of any kind.

Past medical history included breast cancer diagnosed and treated 8 years ago with no cancer recurrence. The client had 17 nodes removed (12 were positive) and a mastectomy, followed by chemotherapy (short-term) and tamoxifen (long-term). The client was estrogen negative.

The clinical presentation was consistent with a posterior rib dysfunction, but there was no identified trauma or cause attributed to the onset of the back pain. The therapist's judgment was that there were enough risk factors in the history for cancer recurrence combined with additional red flags (e.g., age over 40 years, pain level, insidious onset) to warrant medical evaluation before a plan of care was established.

Results: Client was diagnosed with cancer metastases to the thoracic vertebrae at T4-T6. The physician called the therapist to ask what tipped her off to the need for medical referral. Knowing the risk factors for cancer AND for cancer recurrence made a difference in this case.

CANCER PREVENTION

Cancer prevention begins with risk factor assessment and risk reduction. The key to cancer prevention lies in minimizing as many of the individual modifiable risk factors as possible. The American Institute for Cancer Research estimates that recommended diets, together with maintenance of physical activity and appropriate body mass, can in time reduce cancer incidence by 30% to 40%. At current rates, on a global basis, this represents about 3 to 4 million cases of cancer per year that could be prevented by dietary and associated means.[32]

There are some simple steps to take in starting this process. The first is to assess personal/family health history. Note any cancers present in first-generation family members. Some helpful tools are available for assessing cancer risk. The Washington University School of Medicine, Public Health Sciences Division, offers an interactive tool to estimate an individual's risk of cancer and other major diseases such as cardiovascular disease, osteoporosis, and stroke, as well as offering prevention strategies. It is available online at https://publichealthsciences.wustl.edu/community-focus/your-disease-risk-assessment-tool/. Cancer screening is available and widely recommended for the following types of cancer: colorectal, breast, cervix (women), and prostate (men). Early detection at a localized stage is linked with less morbidity and lower mortality.

For example, 90% of colon cancer cases and deaths can be prevented. The ACS provides a summary of risk factors and early detection screening tests for many types of cancer, including colon cancer. (This information is available at the following link: http://www.cancer.org/cancer/colonandrectumcancer/detailedguide/colorectal-cancer-risk-factors.) The NCI provides a quick tool for assessing personal risk for breast cancer. It is available at: https://bcrisktool.cancer.gov/.

As health care educators, therapists can make use of this information to promote cancer prevention for themselves, their families, and their clients.

Genomics and Cancer Prevention

The Human Genome Project, with the goal of determining the DNA sequence of the entire euchromatic human genome, was declared complete in April 2003. Along with this significant milestone has come the development of a new biology of genetics called genomics. Understanding gene–environment interaction will be a major focus of genomics-based public health.[74,75]

There are many known or suspected carcinogens that increase an individual's risk of cancer. Different people respond to carcinogens differently. It is still not clear why one person develops cancer and another does not when both have the same risk factors.

Toxicogenomics, the development of molecular signatures for the effects of specific hazardous chemical agents, will bring to our understanding ways to track multiple sources of the same agent, multiple media and pathways of exposures, multiple effects or risks from the same agent, and multiple agents that cause similar effects.[76]

Defects may occur in one or more genes. Damage may occur in genes that involve the metabolism of carcinogens or in genes that deal with the DNA repair process.[77] An important discovery in the area of gene identification related to cancer suppression is discovery of the p53 tumor-suppressor gene. The p53 gene encodes a protein with cancer-inhibiting properties. Loss of p53 activity predisposes cells to become unstable and more likely to take on mutations. Mutation of the p53 gene is the most common genetic alteration in human cancers.[78]

It is possible that genetic mutations combined with lifestyle or environmental factors may contribute to the development of cancer. For example, there is a known increase in risk of breast cancer in American women born after 1940 who have a BRCA1 or BRCA2 mutation. This suggests that changes in the environment or lifestyle may increase the risk already conferred by these genes.[79]

Air pollution is moderately associated with increased lung cancer, but when combined with exposure to tobacco smoke, the risk increases dramatically. About 50% of all people lack the GSTM1 metabolic gene that can detoxify tobacco smoke and air pollution. People who have this genetic defect and who have heavy exposure to pollution may have a higher risk of developing lung cancer.[80]

Once it is understood how genes and the environment work to contribute to cancer development, this knowledge can be applied to intervention. Anyone with genes that lead to a higher risk of cancer may benefit from chemoprevention.

MAJOR TYPES OF CANCER

From a histological standpoint, there are six major types of cancer: carcinoma, sarcoma, myeloma, bloodborne cancers such as lymphomas and leukemias, and mixed-type cancers.[81]

Carcinoma is a malignant tumor that comprises epithelial tissue and accounts for 80% to 90% of all cancers. Carcinomas affect structures such as the skin, large intestine, stomach, breast, and lungs. These can be fast-growing tumors because they are derived from the epithelial lining of the organ, which grows rapidly and replaces itself frequently.

Carcinomas spread by invading local tissue and by metastasis. Generally, carcinomas tend to metastasize via the lymphatics, whereas sarcomas are more likely to metastasize hematogenously.

Sarcoma is a fleshy growth and refers to a large variety of tumors arising in the connective tissues that are grouped together because of similarities in pathologic appearance and clinical presentation.

Tissues affected include connective tissue such as bone and cartilage (discussed subsequently under Bone Tumors), muscle, fibrous tissue, fat, and synovium. The different types of sarcomas are named for the specific tissues affected (e.g., fibrosarcomas are tumors of the fibrous connective tissue; osteosarcomas are tumors of the bone; and chondrosarcomas are tumors arising in cartilage) (Table 14.2).

As a general category, sarcoma differs from carcinoma in the origin of cells composing the tumor (Table 14.3). As mentioned, sarcomas arise in the connective tissue (embryologic mesoderm), whereas carcinomas arise in the epithelial tissue (embryologic ectoderm) (i.e., cellular structures covering or lining surfaces of body cavities, small vessels, or visceral organs).

Myelomas are cancers that originate in the plasma cells of the bone marrow. *Leukemias* and *lymphomas* arise from the blood and lymphatic system. Metastasis is hematogenous. Leukemias are often associated with overproduction of immature or defective white blood cells (WBCs), although it can also affect red blood cells (RBCs). Examples of leukemias include myelogenous leukemia, lymphoblastic leukemia, and polycythemia vera. Lymphomas often arise in the glands or nodes of the lymphatic system, and may occur in specific organs such as the stomach or thymus. Lymphomas are typically subclassified into two subgroups: Hodgkin's lymphoma and NHL, distinguished from each other by the presence of Reed-Sternberg cells in Hodgkin's lymphoma. *Mixed-type* cancers have components from different categories of cancers.

RESOURCES

Although there are many websites related to cancer, we recommend what the physicians use: the well-known and respected National Comprehensive Cancer Network (NCCN). The

TABLE 14.2	Classification of Soft Tissue and Bone Tumors[82–84]	
Tissue of Origin	Benign Tumor	Malignant Tumor
CONNECTIVE TISSUE		
Fibrous	Fibroma	Fibrosarcoma
Cartilage	Chondroma Enchondroma Chondroblastoma	Chondrosarcoma
Bone	Osteoma	Osteosarcoma
Bone marrow		Leukemia Multiple myeloma Ewing family of tumors (EFT)
Adipose (fat)	Lipoma	Liposarcoma
Synovial	Ganglion, giant cell of tendon sheath	Synovial sarcoma
MUSCLE		
Smooth muscle	Leiomyoma	Leiomyosarcoma
Striated muscle	Rhabdomyoma	Rhabdomyosarcoma
ENDOTHELIUM (VASCULAR/LYMPHATIC)		
Lymph vessels	Lymphangioma	Lymphangiosarcoma Kaposi's sarcoma
Lymphoid tissue		Lymphosarcoma (lymphoma) Lymphatic leukemia
Blood vessels	Hemangioma	Hemangiosarcoma
NEURAL TISSUE		
Nerve fibers and sheaths	Neurofibroma Neuroma Neurinoma (neurilemmoma/ schwannoma)	Neurofibrosarcoma Neurogenic sarcoma
Glial tissue Epithelium	Gliosis	Glioma
Skin and mucous membrane	Papilloma	Squamous cell carcinoma
	Polyp	Basal cell carcinoma
Glandular epithelium	Adenoma	Adenocarcinoma

TABLE 14.3	Subcategories of Malignancy by Cell Type of Origin
Subcategory	Cell Type of Origin
Carcinomas	Arise from epithelial cells: • Breast • Colon • Pancreas • Skin • Large intestine • Lung • Stomach • Metastasize via lymphatics
Sarcomas	Develop from connective tissues: • Fat • Muscle • Bone • Cartilage • Synovium • Fibrous tissue • Metastasize hematogenously • Local invasion
Lymphomas	Originate in lymphoid tissues: • Lymph nodes • Spleen • Intestinal lining • Spread by infiltration
Leukemias	Cancers of the hematologic system: • Bone marrow • Invasion and infiltration

NCCN Clinical Practice Guidelines in Oncology are recognized by clinicians around the world as the standard for oncology care. The NCCN now has consumer versions of its clinical practice guidelines (www.nccn.com).

Other reliable sites include Abramson Cancer Center of the University of Pennsylvania at www.oncolink.org or www.oncolink.com and the NCI (www.cancer.gov/).

METASTASES

Neoplasms can be divided into three categories: benign, invasive, and metastatic. Benign neoplasms are noncancerous tumors that are localized, encapsulated, slow growing, and unable to move or metastasize to other sites.

Invasive carcinoma is a malignant cancer that has invaded the surrounding tissue. The spread of cancer cells from the primary site to secondary sites is called *metastasis*. A regional metastasis is the local arrest, growth, and development of a malignant lesion to regional lymph nodes (RLNs).

A distal or distant metastasis is the distant arrest, growth, and development of a malignant lesion to another organ (e.g., lung, liver, brain). Within the categories of invasive and metastatic tumors, four large subcategories of malignancy have been identified and classified according to the cell type of origin (see Table 14.3).

For the therapist, primary cancers arising from specific body structures are not as likely to present with musculoskeletal signs and symptoms. It is more likely that recurrence of a previously treated cancer will have metastasized from another part of the body (secondary neoplasm) with subsequent bone, joint, or muscular presentation.

Metastatic spread can occur as late as 15 to 20 years after initial diagnosis and medical intervention. As many as 70% of people who die of cancer have been shown by autopsy to have spinal metastases; up to 14% exhibit clinical symptomatic disease before death.[85] For these reasons, the therapist must take care to conduct a screening interview during the examination, including past medical history of cancer or cancer treatment (e.g., chemotherapy, radiation).

Use the Personal/Family History form in Chapter 2 to assess for a personal or first-degree family history of cancer. When asked about a past medical history of cancer, clients

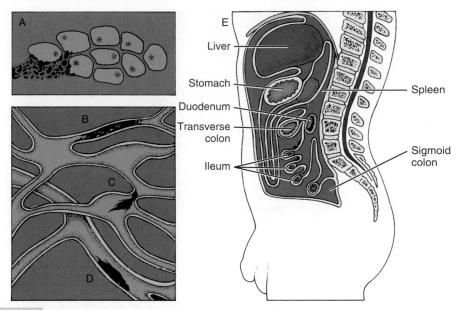

Fig. 14.2 Some modes of dissemination of cancer. **A**, Direct extension into neighboring tissue. **B**, Permeation along lymphatic vessels. **C**, Embolism via lymphatic vessels to the lymph nodes. **D**, Embolism via blood vessels (hematogenous spread). **E**, Invasion of a body cavity by diffusion. (Modified from Monahan FD, Sand JK, Neighbors M, Marek JF, Green CJ. Phipps' Medical-Surgical Nursing: Health and Illness Perspective. 8th ed. St. Louis: Mosby; 2007.)

may say "No," even in the presence of a personal history of cancer. This is especially common in those clients who have reached and/or passed the 5-year survival mark.

Always link these two questions together:

? FOLLOW-UP QUESTIONS

- Have you ever had any kind of cancer?
- If no, have you ever had chemotherapy, radiation therapy, or immunotherapy of any kind?

Mechanisms and Modes of Metastasis

Cancer cells can spread throughout the body through the bloodstream (hematogenous or vascular dissemination), via the lymphatic system, or by direct extension into the neighboring tissue or body cavities (Fig. 14.2). Once a primary tumor is initiated and starts to move by local invasion, tumor angiogenesis occurs (blood vessels from surrounding tissue grow into the solid tumor). Tumor cells then invade host blood vessels and are discharged into the venous drainage.

Many individuals develop multiple sites of metastatic disease because of the potential of cancers to spread. A metastatic colony is the end result of a complicated series of tumor–host interactions called the *metastatic cascade.*

Metastasis requires a good deal of coordination between cancer cells and the body. Fortunately, many early metastases die in transit for a number of reasons such as blood vessel turbulence and genes that normally suppress the growth of micrometastases in new environments. Even so, some metastatic cells do survive and move on to other sites. At secondary sites, the malignant cells continue to reproduce, and new tumors or lesions develop.

Some clients with newly diagnosed cancers have clinically detectable metastases; remaining clients who are clinically free of metastases may harbor occult metastases.

The usual mode of spread and eventual location of metastases vary with the type of cancer and the tissue from which the cancer arises. Early clinical observations led to the idea that carcinomas spread by the lymphatic route and mesenchymal tumors, such as melanoma, spread through the bloodstream. We now know that both the lymphatic and vascular systems have many interconnections that allow tumor cells to pass from one system to the other.

During invasion, tumor cells can easily penetrate small lymphatic vessels and are then transported via the lymph. Tumor emboli may be trapped in the first draining lymph node, or they may bypass these RLNs to form noncontinuous and distant nodal metastases called "skip metastasis."

The relatively high incidence of anatomic skip metastasis can be attributed to aberrant distribution of lymph nodes.[86,87] Multiple interconnections between the lymphatic and hematogenous systems may also allow transport of tumor cells via the arterial or venous blood supply, bypassing some lymph nodes but reaching other more distant ones.[88]

Patterns of blood flow, regional venous drainage, and lymphatic channels determine the distribution pattern of most metastases. For example, breast cancer spreads via the *lymphatics* and via the vertebral venous system to bones in the shoulder, hip, ribs, vertebrae, lungs, and liver.

Primary bone cancer, such as osteogenic sarcoma, initially metastasizes via the *blood* to the lungs. Prostate cancer spreads via the *lymphatics* to the pelvic and vertebral bones, sometimes appearing as low back and/or pelvic pain radiating down the leg. The more common cancers and their metastatic pathways are provided in Table 14.4.

TABLE 14.4	Pathways of Cancer Metastases*	
Primary Cancer	Mode of Dissemination	Location of Primary Metastasis
Breast	Lymphatics	Bone (shoulder, hips, sacrum, ribs, vertebrae); CNS (brain, spinal fluid, brachial plexus)
	Blood (vascular or hematogenous)	Lung, pleural cavity, liver, bone
Bone	Blood	Lungs, liver, bone, then CNS
Cervical (cervix)	Local extension and lymphatics	Retroperitoneal lymph nodes, bladder, rectum; paracervical, parametrial lymphatics
	Blood	CNS (brain), lungs, bones, liver
Chordoma	Direct extension	Neighboring soft tissues, spine
	Blood	Liver, lungs, heart, brain, spine
	Lymphatics	Lymph nodes, peritoneum
Colorectal	Direct extension	Bone (vertebrae, hip, sacrum)
	Peritoneal seeding	Peritoneum
	Blood	Liver, lung
Ewing sarcoma	Blood	Lung, bone, bone marrow
Giant cell tumor of bone	Blood	Lung
Kidney	Lymph	Pelvis, groin
	Blood	Lungs, pleural cavity, bone, liver, brain
Leukemia		Does not really "metastasize" as it is present throughout the body and therefore causes symptoms throughout body
Liver	Blood	CNS (brain)
Lung (bronchogenic sarcoma)	Blood	CNS (brain, spinal cord)
	Blood	Bone (ribs, sacrum, vertebrae)
	Direct extension, lymphatics	Mediastinum (tissue and organs between the sternum and vertebrae such as the heart, blood vessels, trachea, esophagus, thymus, lymph nodes)
Lung (apical or Pancoast's tumors)	Direct extension	Eighth cervical and first and second thoracic nerves within the brachial plexus
	Blood	CNS (brain, spinal cord), bone
Lung (small cell)	Blood	CNS (brain, spinal fluid)
Lymphomas	Blood	CNS (spinal cord, spinal fluid), bone
	Lymphatics	Can occur anywhere, including skin, visceral organs, especially liver
Malignant melanoma	No typical pattern	Metastasis can occur anywhere; skin and subcutaneous tissue; lungs; CNS (brain, spinal fluid); liver; gastrointestinal tract; bone
Multiple myeloma	Blood	Bone (sacrum)
Nonmelanoma skin cancer	Usually remain local without metastases; local invasion	Bones underlying involved skin; brain
Osteogenic sarcoma (osteosarcoma)	Blood	Lungs, CNS (brain)
	Lymphatics	Lymph nodes, lungs, bone, kidneys
Ovarian	Direct extension into abdominal cavity	Nearby organs (bladder, colon, rectum, uterus, fallopian tubes); spread beyond abdomen is rare
	Lymphatics, peritoneal fluid through the abdomen	Liver, lungs; regional and distant
Pancreatic	Blood	Liver
Prostate	Lymphatics	Pelvic, sacrum, and vertebral bones, sacral plexus
		Bladder, rectum
		Distant organs (lung, liver, brain)
Soft tissue sarcoma	Blood; lymphatics (rare)	Lung (first) but also bone, brain, liver, soft tissue (distant)
Spinal cord	Local invasion; dissemination through the intervertebral foramina	CNS (brain, spinal cord)
Stomach, gastric	Blood	Liver, vertebrae, abdominal cavity (intraperitoneum)
	Local invasion	
Testes	Local invasion	Bone (pelvis, lumbar spine, hip)
	Blood, lymphatics	Lung
Thyroid	Direct extension	Bone; nearby tissues of neck
	Lymphatics	Regional lymph nodes (neck, upper chest, mediastinum)
	Blood	Distant (lung, bone, brain)

*Use this table to identify the most likely location of symptoms associated with cancer recurrence/metastasis. If the new symptoms match areas of common metastasis for the client's primary cancer, further screening and/or consult or referral are indicated.
CNS, Central nervous system; *Mets,* metastases.

The high proportion of bone metastases in breast, prostate, and lung cancers is an example of selective movement of tumor cells to a specific organ. For example, in breast cancer, it is thought that the continuous remodeling of bone by osteoclasts and osteoblasts predisposes bone to metastatic lesions.[89] For some cancers, such as MM, no typical pattern exists, and metastases may occur anywhere.

Increased tumor contact with the circulatory system provides tumors with a mechanism to enter the general circulation and colonize at distant sites. Both vascular endothelial growth factor (VEGF) and fibroblast growth factor (FGF) stimulate proliferation of vascular cells and even allow the newly formed blood vessels to be easily invaded by the cancer cells that are adjacent to them.[90] Resection of tumors without clear margins has the potential to provide remaining tumor cells with a means of metastasizing, as new blood vessels form during the healing process.

Benign Mechanical Transport

Mechanical transport rather than metastasis may be another mechanism of cancer spread. Two potential modes of benign mechanical transport (BMT) have been detected in breast cancer: lymphatic transport of epithelial cells displaced by biopsy of the primary tumor, and breast massage–assisted sentinel lymph node (SLN) localization.[91]

Samples of malignant tissues should be carefully excised by surgeons who are expert in biopsy of malignant tissues. The risk of local recurrence is increased when intralesional curettage is performed.[92] Recurrence along the surgical pathway has been reported for some tumors following needle biopsy.[93] It is hypothesized that this recurrence is the result of intraoperative seeding. Poorly planned biopsies or incomplete tumor resection increases the risk of local recurrence and metastasis. The biopsy tract should be excised when complete tumor removal occurs.[94]

A second mode of BMT may be the pre-SLN breast massage used to facilitate the localization of SLNs during breast cancer staging. Mechanical transport of epithelial cells to SLNs has been verified. The significance of small epithelial clusters in SLN is unknown; further research and refinement of techniques would be beneficial for biopsy and SLN-localizing practices.[91]

The bottom line for the therapist is this: Anyone who has had a recent biopsy (within the past 6 months) must be followed carefully for any signs of local cancer recurrence.

CLINICAL MANIFESTATIONS OF MALIGNANCY

The therapist may be the first to see clinical manifestations of primary cancer but is more likely to see signs and symptoms of cancer recurrence or cancer metastasis. In general, the five most common sites of cancer metastasis are the bone, lymph nodes, lung, liver, and brain. However, the therapist is most likely to observe signs and symptoms affecting one of the following systems:

- Integumentary
- Pulmonary
- Neurologic
- Musculoskeletal
- Hepatic

Each of these systems has a core group of most commonly observed signs and symptoms that will be discussed throughout this section (Table 14.5).

Early Warning Signs

For many years, the ACS has publicized the seven warning signs of cancer, the appearance of which could indicate the presence of cancer and the need for medical evaluation. The mnemonic in Box 14.2 is often used as a helpful reminder of these warning signs.

Other early warning signs can include rapid, unintentional weight loss in a short period of time (e.g., 10% of the person's body weight in 2 weeks), an unusual change in vital signs, frequent infection (e.g., respiratory or urinary), and night pain. Bleeding is an important sign of cancer, but a cancer is generally well established by the time bleeding occurs. Bleeding develops secondary to ulcerations in the central areas of the tumor or by pressure on, or rupture of, local blood vessels. As the tumor continues to grow, it may enlarge beyond its capacity to obtain necessary nutrients, resulting in revitalization of portions of the tumor.

This process of invading and compressing the local tissue, shutting off blood supply to normal cells, is called *necrosis*. Tissue necrosis leads ultimately to secondary infection, severe hemorrhage, and the development of pain when regional sensory nerves become involved. Other symptoms can include pathologic fractures, anemia, and thrombus formation.

Awareness of these signals is useful, but it is generally agreed that these symptoms do not always reflect early curable cancer nor does this list include all possible signs for the different types of cancer.

Lumps, Lesions, and Lymph Nodes

The therapist should take special note of "T," which is *thickening or lump in breast or elsewhere*. Clients often point out a subcutaneous lesion (often a benign lipoma) and ask us to identify what it is. Baseline examination of a lump or lesion is important. Palpation of skin lesions and lymph nodes is presented in Chapter 4.

Whenever examining a lump or lesion, one should use the mnemonic in Fig. 4.6 to document and report findings on location, size, shape, consistency, mobility or fixation, and signs of tenderness. A clinically detectable tumor of the size of a small pea already contains billions of cells. Most therapists will be able to palpate a lesion below the skin when it is half that size.[95]

Review Appendix B-21 in the accompanying enhanced eBook version included with print purchase of this textbook for appropriate follow-up questions. Keep in mind that the therapist cannot know what the underlying pathology may be when lymph nodes are palpable and questionable.

TABLE 14.5	Signs and Symptoms of Metastasis*			
Integumentary	Musculoskeletal	Neurologic (CNS)	Pulmonary	Hepatic
Any skin lesion or observable/palpable skin changes	May present as an asymptomatic soft tissue mass	Drowsiness, lethargy	Pleural pain	Abdominal pain and tenderness
Any observable or palpable change in nail beds (fingers or toes)	Bone pain	Headache	Dyspnea	Jaundice
Unusual mole (use ABCDE method of assessment)	• Deep or localized	Nausea, vomiting	New onset of wheezing	Ascites (see Fig. 9.8)
Cluster mole formation	• Increased with activity	Depression	Productive cough with rust, green, or yellow-tinged sputum	Distended abdomen
Bleeding or discharge from mole, skin lesion, scar, or nipple	• Decreased tolerance to weight-bearing; antalgic gait	Increased sleeping		Dilated upper abdominal veins
Tenderness and soreness around a mole; sore that does not heal	• Does not respond to physical agents	Irritability, personality change		Peripheral edema
	Soft tissue swelling	Confusion, increased confusion		General malaise and fatigue
	Pathologic fractures	Change in mental status, memory loss, difficulty concentrating		Bilateral carpal/tarsal tunnel syndrome
	Hypercalcemia (see Table 14.7)	Vision changes (blurring, blind spots, double vision)		Asterixis (liver flap) (see Fig. 9.7)
	• CNS	Numbness, tingling		Palmar erythema (liver palms) (see Fig. 9.5)
	• Musculoskeletal	Balance/coordination problems		Spider angiomas (over the abdomen) (see Fig. 9.3)
	• Cardiovascular	Changes in deep tendon reflexes		Nail beds of Terry (see Fig. 9.6)
	• Gastrointestinal	Change in muscle tone for individual with previously diagnosed neurologic condition		Right shoulder pain
	Back or rib pain	Positive Babinski reflex		
		Clonus (ankle or wrist)		
		Changes in bowel and bladder function		
		Myotomal weakness pattern		
		Paraneoplastic syndrome (see text)		

*Seen most often in a physical therapy practice.
ABCDE, Asymmetry, border, color, diameter, evolving; *CNS*, Central nervous system.

BOX 14.2   EARLY WARNING SIGNS OF CANCER

Changes in bowel or bladder habits
A sore that does not heal in 6 weeks
Unusual bleeding or discharge
Thickening or lump in breast or elsewhere
Indigestion or difficulty in swallowing
Obvious change in a wart or mole
Nagging cough or hoarseness
Supplemental signs and symptoms (rapid unintentional weight loss, change in vital signs, frequent infections, night pain, pathologic fracture, proximal muscle weakness, change in deep tendon reflexes)
  For the physical therapist:
Change in vital signs
Proximal muscle weakness
Change in deep tendon reflexes

Performing a baseline assessment and reporting the findings are important outcomes of the assessment. All suspicious lymph nodes should be evaluated by a physician (Case Example 14.2).

Supraclavicular lymph nodes that are easily palpable during the examination may indicate possible metastatic disease. Any lymph nodes that are hard, immovable, and nontender raise the suspicion of cancer, especially in the presence of a previous history of cancer.

Keep in mind that lymph nodes can fluctuate over the course of 10 to 14 days. When making the medical referral, look for a cluster of signs and symptoms, recent trauma (including recent biopsy), or a past history of chronic fatigue syndrome, mononucleosis, and allergies. Record and report all findings.

Proximal Muscle Weakness

For the therapist, idiopathic proximal muscle weakness may be an early sign of cancer (Fig. 14.3). This syndrome of proximal muscle weakness is referred to as *carcinomatous neuromyopathy*. The most common neuromuscular manifestation is difficulty walking or going up stairs. It is accompanied by changes in two or more deep tendon reflexes (DTRs; ankle jerk usually remains intact). Muscle weakness may occur secondary to cachexia, nonspecific effects of the neoplasm, or hypercalcemia, which occurs as an indirect humoral effect on bone (see the later discussion on Paraneoplastic Syndrome in this chapter). Clients with advanced cancer, multiple myeloma, or breast or lung cancer are affected most often by hypercalcemia.

Screening for muscle weakness is not always a straightforward process. Sometimes questions must be directed toward function to find out this information. If a client is asked whether he or she has any muscle weakness, difficulty getting up from sitting, trouble climbing stairs, or shortness of breath, the answer may very well be "No" on all accounts. Consider using the following flow of questions:

CASE EXAMPLE 14.2
Palpable and Observable Lymph Nodes

A 73-year-old woman was referred to a physical therapy clinic by her oncologist with a diagnosis of cervical radiculopathy. She had a history of uterine cancer 20 years ago and a history of breast cancer 10 years ago.

Treatment included a hysterectomy, left radical mastectomy, radiation therapy, and chemotherapy. She has been cancer-free for almost 10 years. Her family physician, oncologist, and neurologist all evaluated her before she was referred to the physical therapist.

Examination by a physical therapist revealed obvious lymphadenopathy of the left cervical and axillary lymph nodes. When asked if the referring physician (or other physicians) saw the "swelling," she told the therapist that she had not disrobed during her medical evaluation and consultation.

The question for us as physical therapists in a situation like this one is how to proceed?

Several steps must be taken. First, the therapist must document all findings. If possible, photographs of the chest, neck, and axilla should be obtained.

Second, the therapist must ascertain whether or not the physician is already aware of the problem and has requested physical therapy as a palliative measure. Requesting the physician's dictation or notes from the examination is essential.

Contact with the physician will be important soon after the records are obtained, either to confirm the request as palliative therapy or to report your findings and confirm the need for medical reevaluation.

If it turns out that the physician is, indeed, unaware of these physical findings, it is best to send a problem list identified as "outside the scope of a physical therapist" when returning the client to the physician. Be careful to avoid making any statements that could be misconstrued as a medical diagnosis.

We recommend writing a brief letter with the pertinent findings and ending with one of two one-liners:

What do you think?

Please advise.

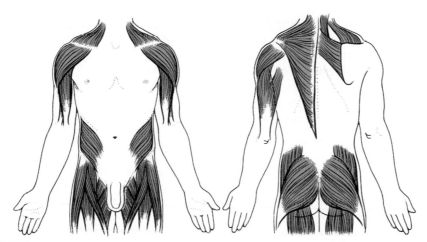

Fig. 14.3 Proximal muscle weakness can be observed clinically as a positive Trendelenburg test (usually present bilaterally) and abnormal manual muscle testing. It can also be observed functionally when the client has difficulty getting up from sitting or climbing stairs. As the weakness progresses, the client may have trouble getting into and out of a vehicle and/or the bathtub. Respiratory muscle weakness may be seen as shortness of breath or reported as altered activity to avoid dyspnea.

? FOLLOW-UP QUESTIONS

- Do you have any muscle weakness in your arms, legs, back, or chest?
- Do you have any trouble getting in and out of a chair?
- Are there any activities you would like to be able to do that you currently cannot do?
- Are there any activities you used to be able to do that you cannot do now?
- Are there activities you can do now that used to be much easier?
- Do you have any trouble going up and down stairs without stopping?
- Can you do all your grocery shopping without sitting down or stopping?
- Are you able to complete your household chores (e.g., make a meal, wash and dry clothes) without stopping?

Pain

Pain is rarely an early warning sign of cancer, even in the presence of unexplained bleeding. Night pain that is constant and intense (often rated 7 or higher on the numeric rating scale) is a red-flag symptom of primary or recurring cancer, though not all people with musculoskeletal cancers may experience night pain.

Pain is usually the result of destruction of tissue or pressure on the tissue as a result of the presence of a tumor or lesion. The lesion, or lesions, must be of significant size or location to create pressure and/or occlusion of normal structures; pain will be dependent on the area of the body affected.

Acute and chronic cancer-related pain syndromes can occur in association with diagnostic and therapeutic interventions such as bone marrow biopsy, lumbar puncture, colonoscopy, percutaneous biopsy, and thoracentesis. Chemotherapy and radiation toxicity can result in painful peripheral neuropathies.

Likewise, many different chronic pain syndromes (e.g., tumor-related radiculopathy, phantom breast pain, postsurgical pelvic or abdominal pain, burning perineum syndrome, postradiation pain syndrome) can occur as a result of tumors or cancer therapy. See further discussion under Oncologic Pain in this chapter.

Change in One or More Deep Tendon Reflexes

When a neurologic screening examination is performed, testing of DTRs is usually included. Some individuals have very brisk reflexes under normal circumstances; others are much more hyporeflexive.

Tumors (whether benign or malignant) can also press on the spinal nerve root, mimicking a disk problem. A lesion that is small enough can put just enough pressure to irritate the nerve root, resulting in a hyperreflexive DTR. A large tumor can obliterate the reflex arc, resulting in diminished or absent reflexes.

Either way, changes in DTRs must be considered a red-flag sign (possibly of cancer) that should be documented and further investigated. For example, a hyporesponsive patellar tendon reflex that is unchanged with distraction or repeated testing and is accompanied by back, hip, or thigh pain, along with a past history of prostate cancer, presents a different clinical picture altogether. Guidelines for assessing reflexes are discussed in Chapter 4.

Integumentary Manifestations

Internal cancers can invade the skin through vascular dissemination or direct extension. Metastases to the skin may be the first sign of malignancy, especially for breast or upper respiratory tract cancer. Integumentary carcinomatous metastases often present as asymmetrical, firm, skin-colored, red, purple, or blue nodules near the site of the primary tumor.

Distant cutaneous metastasis can result from lymphoma, multiple myeloma, and stomach/colon, ovarian, pancreatic, kidney, and breast cancer (Case Example 14.3). The scalp is a common site for such lesions, which are sometimes accompanied by hair loss called *alopecia neoplastica*.

The integumentary screening examination, including the assessment of common skin lesions and the nail beds, is presented in Chapter 4. Cancer-related skin lesions (e.g., pinch purpura, renal nodule, local cancer recurrence, Kaposi's sarcoma, xanthomas) are also included in Chapter 4.

During observation and inspection, the therapist should be alert to any potential signs of primary skin cancer or integumentary metastases. When a suspicious skin lesion is noted, the therapist should conduct a risk factor assessment and ask three questions:

- How long have you had this area of skin discoloration/mole/spot (use whatever brief description seems most appropriate)?

CASE EXAMPLE 14.3
Cancer-Related Skin Rash

A 42-year-old woman with a previous history of breast cancer and breast lumpectomy asked a fellow clinician to examine her scar for any sign of cancer recurrence. She had just had her 6-month cancer check-up and was not scheduled to see her oncologist for another 6 months.

In the meantime, she had developed a skin rash over the upper chest wall and axilla of the involved side (upper back and left thigh) (Figs. 14.4 and 14.5). When asked if there were any other symptoms present, she reported feeling feverish and a bit nauseous, and noted slight muscle aching. During the examination, the client's vital signs were taken. (See Chapter 2 about the importance of vital signs in the screening process; see also discussion of constitutional symptoms.)

All vital signs were within normal limits for the client's age, except body temperature, which was 102.2° F. The client reported that her normal body temperature was usually 98° F. She was not aware of an elevated body temperature, although she stated she had awakened in the night feeling feverish and took some Tylenol.

Upper quadrant examination was unremarkable, except for skin rash and the presence of bilateral anterior cervical adenopathy. There was a fullness of lymph node tissue without firmness or distinct nodes palpated in the axilla on the involved side. The clinician was unable to palpate as far into the zone II space as would be expected.

Results: This client had three red flags: recent history of cancer, skin rash, and a constitutional symptom (fever). Even though there was no external sign of local cancer recurrence and even though she was just seen by her oncologist, these new findings warranted a return visit to her physician.

The skin rash turned out to be Sweet's syndrome, a disorder usually associated with significant constitutional symptoms and involvement of the lungs and joints. Most cases are idiopathic, but some have been associated with malignancies.[96,97]

In this case no further findings were made despite laboratory and medical tests performed. The use of systemic corticosteroids is usually recommended for Sweet's syndrome, but the client declined and opted to use vitamin supplements, as her symptoms were resolving by that time. She was followed more closely for any cancer recurrence with more frequent testing thereafter.

- Has it changed in the past 6 weeks to 6 months?
- Has your physician examined this area?

No matter what the therapist's own cultural background, as a health care professional, his or her responsibility to screen skin lesions is clear. *How* questions are posed is just as important as *what* is said.

The therapist may want to introduce the subject by saying that as health care professionals, we are trained to observe many body parts (skin, joints, posture, and so on). You notice that the client has an unusual mole (or rash or whatever has been observed), and you wonder whether this is something that has been there for years. Has it changed in the past 6 weeks to 6 months? Has the client ever shown it to the doctor?

A client with a past medical history of cancer now presenting with a suspicious skin lesion that has not been evaluated by a physician must be advised to have it evaluated as soon as possible.

For any client with a previous history of cancer with surgical removal, it is always a good idea to look at the surgical site(s) for any sign of local cancer recurrence. Start by asking the client if he or she has noticed any changes in the scar. Continue by asking the following:

? FOLLOW-UP QUESTIONS

- Would you have any objections if I looked at (or examined) the scar tissue?

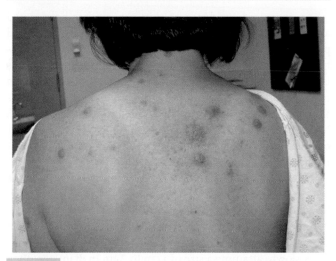

Fig. 14.4 Day 1. Skin rash on upper back associated with Sweet's syndrome (acute febrile neutrophilic dermatosis), a disorder usually associated with significant constitutional symptoms and involvement of the lungs and joints. Red, tender papules, plaques, or nodules appear on the face, extremities, and upper trunk. The surface appears vesicular and may produce pustules. Most cases are idiopathic, associated with inflammatory bowel disease, or preceding upper respiratory tract infection, but some have been associated with malignancy. (Courtesy Flaig IP. University of Minnesota Medical Center, Fairview, MN; 2003.)

Any suspicious scab or tissue granulation, redness, or discoloration must be noted (photographed, if possible). Again, three screening questions apply in this situation. The therapist has a responsibility to report these findings to the appropriate health care professional and to make every effort to ensure client compliance with follow-up.

Skin Cancers

Skin cancers are the most common of all types of cancer and are usually classified as nonmelanoma skin cancer (NMSC) or melanoma. Most skin cancers are classified as NMSCs and are slow growing, easy to recognize, and responsive to intervention, if found early. NMSCs are further classified as basal cell or squamous cell, depending on the tissue affected. They rarely metastasize to other parts of the body and have a nearly 100% rate of cure.

Melanoma, the most serious of the skin cancers, has a 92% 5-year survival rate if localized, but only a 25% 5-year survival if it is invasive or has spread to other parts of the body.[98] Melanoma accounts for less than 1% of skin cancer cases, but the vast majority of skin cancer deaths. The primary warning sign for melanoma is a flat, colored, irregularly shaped lesion that can be mottled with light brown to black colors. It may turn various shades of red, blue, or white or crust on the surface and bleed. A changing mole, the appearance of a new mole, or a mole that is different or growing requires prompt medical attention.[99] The Skin Cancer Foundation advocates use of the ABCDE (asymmetry, border irregularity, color variegation, a diameter of 6 mm or greater, and an evolution or change in size, shape, color or any other trait) method of early detection of melanoma and dysplastic (abnormal in size or shape) moles (see discussion, Chapter 4).

Actinic keratosis is a common premalignant form of skin cancer. With actinic keratosis, overexposure to sunlight results in abnormal cell growth, causing a well-defined, crusty patch or bump on sun-exposed parts of the body.

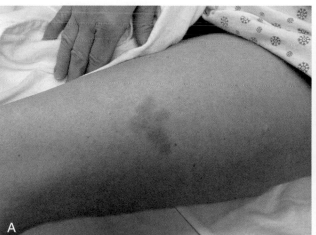
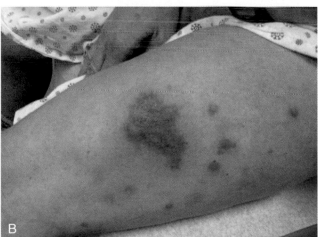

Fig. 14.5 **A**, Day 1 (same client as in Fig. 14.4). Skin rash on upper thigh associated with Sweet's syndrome. **B**, Day 5. Rash progressed quickly to cover larger areas of the left thigh. (Courtesy Flaig IP. University of Minnesota Medical Center, Fairview, MN; 2003.)

BOX 14.3 RISK FACTOR ASSESSMENT FOR SKIN CANCER

- Older age
- Personal or family history of skin cancer (particularly melanoma)
- Moles with any of the ABCDE features, or moles that are changing in any way
- Complexion that is fair or light with green, blue, or gray eyes
- Skin that sunburns easily; skin that never tans
- History of painful sunburns with blistering during childhood or the adolescent years
- Use of tanning beds or lamps
- Short, intense episodes of sun exposure: the indoor worker who spends the weekend out in the sun without skin protection (or any sporadic exposure to strong sunshine of normally covered skin)
- Transplant recipient

Clients often point out skin lesions or ask the therapist about various lumps and bumps. In addition, the therapist may observe changes in skin, skin lesions, or aberrant tissue during the visual inspection and palpation portion of the examination (see Chapter 4) that need further medical investigation. Mortality is reduced when lesions are found early and treated promptly. Therapists can and should be a part of the screening process for skin cancer.

The cause of skin cancer is well known. Prolonged or intermittent exposure to UVR from the sun, especially when it results in sunburn and blistering, damages DNA. The majority of all NMSCs occur on parts of the body unprotected by clothing (i.e., face, neck, forearms, and backs of hands) and in persons who have received considerable exposure to sunlight.

Risk Factor Assessment. All adults, regardless of skin tone and hair color, are at risk for skin cancer; however, some people are at much greater risk than others (Box 14.3). In general, individuals with red, blonde, or light brown hair with light complexion and maybe freckles, many of Celtic or Scandinavian origin, are most susceptible; persons of African or Asian origin are least susceptible.

The most severely affected people usually have a history of long-term occupational or recreational sun exposure. Australia and New Zealand have the highest incidence of melanoma in the world. New Zealand has nearly five times the amount of skin cancer that occurs in the United States.[50]

Melanoma occurs in every part of the North American continent. In the United States, the five states with the highest predicted rates of melanoma are Utah, Vermont, New Hampshire, Minnesota, and Arizona. Men are more likely than women to develop nonmelanoma and melanoma skin cancers. The rate of melanoma is 10 times higher for Caucasians than African Americans because African Americans have the protective effects of skin pigment.[100]

Many older adults assume that skin changes are a "normal" sign of aging and do not see a physician when lesions first appear. Early detection and referral is always the key to a better prognosis. In asking the three important questions, the therapist plays an instrumental part in the cancer screening process.

❓ FOLLOW-UP QUESTIONS

- How long have you had this?
- Has it changed in the past 6 weeks to 6 months?
- Has your physician seen it?

An increased incidence of skin cancers has been noted after solid organ transplantation, especially heart, lung, and pancreas transplants. In the United States, skin cancer mortality was nearly nine times higher in transplant recipients than in the general population.[101] Skin cancers developing in transplant recipients are more aggressive, making early detection and intervention imperative. Renal transplant recipients have a cumulative increase that corresponds with the number of years post-transplantation (e.g., 7% after 1 year of immunosuppression, 45% after 11 years, 70% after 20 years).[102]

Basal Cell Carcinoma. Basal cell carcinoma involves the bottom layer of the epidermis and occurs mainly on any hair-bearing area exposed to the sun (e.g., face, neck, head, ears, hands). Occasionally, basal cell carcinoma may appear on the trunk, especially the upper back and chest. These lesions grow slowly, attaining a size of 1 cm to 2 cm in diameter, often after years of growth. Metastases almost never occurs, but neglected lesions may ulcerate and produce great destruction, ultimately invading vital structures.

There are a number of common forms of basal cell carcinoma:

- Pearly papule, 2–3 mm in diameter and covered by tightly stretched epidermis laced with small, delicate, branching vessels (telangiectasia)
- Pearly papule with a small crater in the center
- Scaly, red, sharply outlined plaque
- Ill-defined pale, tough, scar-like tumor

Squamous Cell Carcinoma. Squamous cell carcinoma arises from the top of the epidermis and is found on areas often exposed to the sun, which are typically the rim of the ear, the face, lips and mouth, and the dorsa of the hands. These lesions appear as small, red, hard nodules with a smooth or warty surface. The central portion may be scaly, ulcerated, or crusted. Premalignant lesions include sun-damaged skin or dysplasias (whitish-discolored areas), scars, radiation-induced keratosis, actinic keratosis (rough, scaly spots), and chronic ulcers.

Metastases are uncommon but much more likely to occur in lesions arising from chronic leg ulcers, burn scars, and areas of prior x-ray exposure. Although these tumors do not usually metastasize, they are potentially dangerous. They may infiltrate surrounding structures and metastasize to lymph nodes and eventually to distant sites, including the bone, brain, and lungs to become fatal. Invasive tumors are firm and increase in elevation and diameter. The surface may be granular and may bleed easily.

Malignant Melanoma. MM is the most serious form of skin cancer. It arises from pigmented cells in the skin called *melanocytes*. In contrast to basal and squamous cell carcinomas, the majority of MMs appear to be associated with the intensity rather than the duration of sunlight exposure.

Overall, the lifetime risk of getting melanoma is about 2.6% (1 in 38) for Whites, 0.1% (1 in 1,000) for Blacks, and 0.6% (1 in 167) for Hispanics.[103] An individual's risk is much greater if any of the risk factors listed in Box 14.3 are present.

Melanoma can appear anywhere on the body, not just on sun-exposed areas. The clinical characteristics of early MM are similar, regardless of anatomic site. Unlike benign pigmented lesions, which are generally round and symmetric, the shape of an early MM is often asymmetric.

Whereas benign pigmented lesions tend to have regular margins, the borders of early MM are often irregular. Round, symmetric skin lesions, such as common moles, freckles, and birthmarks, are considered "normal." If an existing mole or other skin lesion starts to change and a line drawn down the middle shows two different halves, medical evaluation is needed.

Compared with benign pigmented lesions, which are more uniform in color, MMs are usually variegated, ranging from various hues of tan and brown to black, sometimes intermingled with red and white. The diameters of MM are often 6 mm or larger when first identified.

The most common sites of distant metastasis associated with MM are the skin and subcutaneous tissue, lungs, and surrounding visceral pleura, although any anatomic site may be involved. In-transit metastases (unique malignancies that have spread from the primary tumor but may not have reached the RLNs) typically develop multiple bulky tumors on an arm or leg. Often, these tumors cause pain, swelling, bleeding, ulceration, and decreased mobility.[104]

Other signs that may be important include irritation and itching; tenderness, soreness, or new moles developing around the mole in question; or a sore that keeps crusting and does not heal within 6 weeks. Benign moles tend to be flat, hairless, round or oval, and less than 6 mm in diameter. Pigmentation is generally even. Although there may be color variations, especially in shades of brown, benign moles, freckles, "liver spots," and other benign skin changes are usually of a single color (most often, a single shade of brown or tan). A single lesion with more than one shade of black, brown, or blue may be a sign of MM.

Adolescents frequently have nevi with irregular borders, multiple shades of pigment, or both. Most are normal variations of benign nevi, but a physician should examine any lesion that arouses clinical suspicion or is of concern to the client.

If any of these signs and symptoms are present in a client whose skin lesion has not been examined by a physician, a medical referral is recommended. If the client is planning a follow-up visit with the physician within the next 2 to 4 weeks, the client is advised to point out the mole or skin

CLINICAL SIGNS AND SYMPTOMS

Early Melanoma

A = Asymmetry: uneven edges, lopsided in shape, one half unlike the other half

B = Border: irregularity, irregular edges, scalloped or poorly defined edges

C = Color: black, shades of brown, red, white, occasionally blue

D = Diameter: larger than a pencil eraser

E = Evolving: mole or skin lesion that looks different from the rest or is changing in size, shape, or color

The ABCDE criteria have been verified in multiple studies, documenting the effectiveness and diagnostic accuracy of this screening technique. Their efficacy has been confirmed with digital imaging analysis. When the criteria is used individually, sensitivity ranges from 57% to 90% and specificity from 59% to 90%; however, when criteria are used in combination, sensitivity and specificity increases to 89.3% and 65.2% for two criteria, and 65.5% and 81% for three criteria.[105]

changes at that time. If no appointment is pending, the client is encouraged to make a specific visit either to the family/personal physician or to a dermatologist.

Resources. The Skin Cancer Foundation (www.skincancer.org) has many public education materials available to help the therapist identify suspicious skin lesions. In addition to its website, the Skin Cancer Foundation has posters, brochures, videos, and other materials available for use in the clinic. It is highly recommended that these types of education materials be available in waiting rooms as a part of a nationwide primary prevention program.

Other websites, such as the Melanoma Education Foundation at http://www.skincheck.org/, provide additional photos of suspicious lesions with additional screening guidelines. For information on ratings of sunscreen sold in the United States, see the Environmental Working Group's Sunscreen Guide at https://www.ewg.org/sunscreen/.

The therapist must become as familiar as possible with what suspicious skin aberrations may look like in order to refer as early as possible. Prognosis in melanoma is directly related to the depth of the neoplasm. Melanoma typically starts to grow horizontally within the epidermis (in situ), but then becomes invasive as tumor cells penetrate into the dermis. The vertical depth of the melanoma correlates with prognosis.[106] That is why early detection and referral is so important. See also the discussion on Examining a Mass or Skin Lesion in Chapter 4.

Pulmonary Manifestations

Pulmonary metastases are the most common of all metastatic tumors because venous drainage of most areas of the body passes through the superior and inferior venae cavae into the heart, making the lungs the first organ to filter malignant cells. *Primary* bone tumors (e.g., osteogenic sarcoma) metastasize first to the lungs.

Pleural pain and dyspnea may be the first two symptoms experienced by the person (Case Example 14.4). When

CASE EXAMPLE 14.4

Lung Cancer

A 69-year-old man with a recent total hip replacement (THR) was referred to home health for physical therapy. He did not have a good postoperative recovery and has been slow to regain range of motion, strength, and function.

He experienced dyspnea and chest pain within the first 10 feet of ambulation. He has a past medical history of cancer.

What are the red flags here? How should you proceed?

Red Flags

Age (>40 years old)

Past medical history of cancer

Cardiopulmonary symptoms: shortness of breath and chest pain

How to Proceed: Ask the client how long he has had these symptoms. Take all vital signs as discussed in Chapter 2.

Your next steps may depend, in part, on any procedural instructions you have received from your home health agency. If there is a case manager, contact him or her with your concerns. Ask for a copy of the medical file. Contact the physician's office with your findings.

Difficulty in referral arises when a client has been seen by an orthopedic surgeon but is demonstrating signs and symptoms of possible systemic disease. Diplomacy and communication are the keys to success here.

Document your findings and make sure these are sent to the primary care physician AND the orthopedic surgeon. The medical record may already indicate awareness of these red flags with no further follow-up being needed.

If not, then a brief cover letter with your full report should be sent to the physician. The letter should contain the usual "thank you for the referral" kind of introduction with a paragraph about physical therapy intervention.

Then, include a medical problem list such as:

Patient reports shortness of breath and chest pain within the first 3 minutes of ambulation. This has just started in the last few days. His vital signs are: [list these].

Given the patient's age, past medical history of cancer, and new onset of cardiopulmonary symptoms, we would like medical clearance before progressing his exercise and rehab program. Please advise if there are any contraindications for exercise at this time. Thank you.

Make sure you call the physician's office and alert the staff of your concerns and that this letter/fax is on its way. Make telephone contact again within 3 days (sooner if the information is faxed or emailed to the doctor's office).

Results: The orthopedic surgeon advised the client to see his primary care physician for follow-up of this problem. After medical examination and testing, the final diagnosis was lung cancer. The medical doctor surmised that the stress of the surgery was enough to advance the cancer from subclinical to clinical status with new onset of symptoms that were not present before the orthopedic surgery.

up are indicative of pulmonary impairment and must be reported to the physician.

Symptoms may not occur until tumor cells have expanded and become large enough or invasive enough to reach the parietal pleura, where pain fibers are stimulated. The lining surrounding the lungs allows no pain perception, so it is not until the tumor is large enough to press on other nearby structures or against the chest wall that symptoms may first appear.

Lung cancer is the most common primary tumor to metastasize to the brain. Tumor cells from the lung, embolizing via the pulmonary veins and carotid artery, can result in metastases to the central nervous system (CNS). Anyone with a history of lung cancer should be screened for neurologic involvement.[107]

Neurologic Manifestations

As just mentioned, cancer metastases to the CNS is a common problem. Secondary metastases to the brain are 10 times more common than primary brain tumors. In all, about 20% to 25% of individuals with primary sites outside of the CNS will develop brain metastases.[108] The most common primary cancers with metastases to the brain are lung, colon, kidney, skin (melanoma), and breast cancer (Case Example 14.5).

Tumor cells can easily embolize via the pulmonary veins and carotid artery to the brain. The blood–brain barrier does not prevent invasion of the brain parenchyma by circulating metastatic cells. Metastatic brain tumors can increase intracranial pressure, obstruct the normal flow of cerebrospinal fluid, change mentation, and reduce sensory and motor function.

Whether the pressure-causing lesion is a primary cancer of the brain or spinal cord, or whether it is a cancer that has metastasized to the CNS, clinical signs and symptoms of pressure will be the same because in both cases, the same system is affected.

Primary tumors can also cause peripheral nervous system (PNS) problems when tumors compress, impinge, or infiltrate any of the nerve plexuses. No matter where neural compression occurs, the primary sign is unrelenting pain (worse at night) followed by development of weakness. Watch for focal sensory disturbances or weakness in the distribution of the affected plexus or spinal cord segment involved. Brachial plexopathy most commonly occurs in carcinoma of the breast and lung; lumbosacral plexopathy is most common with colorectal and gynecologic tumors, sarcomas, and lymphomas.[109,110]

Clinical Signs and Symptoms

Brain tumors can be asymptomatic. When symptoms do occur, they are usually general or focal, depending on the size and location of the lesion. For example, if a tumor is growing in the motor cortex, the client may develop isolated extremity weakness or hemiparesis. If the tumor is developing in the cerebellum, coordination may be affected with ataxia as an observable sign.

either or both of these pulmonary symptoms occur, look for increased symptoms with deep breathing and activity. Ask about a productive cough with bloody or rust-colored sputum. Ask about new onset of wheezing at any time or difficulty breathing at night. Symptoms that are relieved by sitting

CASE EXAMPLE 14.5

Bone Metastases and Wrist Sprain

A 75-year-old woman fell and sprained her wrist. Her family doctor sent her to physical therapy. After the interview, her daughter took the therapist aside and commented that her mother seems confused. Other family members are wondering if her fall had anything to do with mental deterioration.

There is a positive personal history for breast cancer. Past medical history included breast cancer, diverticulosis, gallbladder removal, and hysterectomy. There were no current health concerns expressed by the client or her family. She is not taking any medication (prescription or over-the-counter).

Because the wrist was obviously not broken, no x-rays were taken.

What are the red flags in this case? Because she just came to physical therapy from a medical doctor, is follow-up medical attention needed?

Red Flags: Age, confusion, past medical history of cancer, recent loss of balance and fall, lack of diagnostics.

This client actually presents with a cluster of four significant red flags in the screening process. The therapist should carry out a balance and vestibular function screening examination and neurologic screening examination (see Chapter 5). Additional key information may be obtained from this testing.

The next step is to inquire of the client or family member if the doctor is aware of the past history of cancer. Older adults moving closer to family members may give up their lifelong family provider. The new physician may not have all the history compiled. This is especially true when patients visit a "Doc-in-a-Box" at the local mall or convenience care facility.

Likewise, check with the family to see whether the physician has been notified of the client's new onset of confusion.

This is the number one sign of nervous system impairment in older adults.

The therapist is advised to document these findings and report them to the physician. As always, a letter of appreciation for the referral is a good idea. State the physical therapy diagnosis in terms of the human movement system (see the *Guide to Physical Therapist Practice* and discussion of physical therapy diagnosis in Chapter 1 of this text).

Include a follow-up paragraph with this information:

I am concerned that the combination of the patient's age, new onset of confusion as described by her family, and recent history of falls resulting in this episode of care may be an indication of significant underlying pathology.

What do you think? I will treat the musculoskeletal impairment, but please advise if any further follow-up is needed.

Results: Given the client's past history of cancer, and knowing that confusion is not a "normal" sign of aging, and that any neurologic sign can be an indicator of cancer, the physical therapist suggested that the family also talk with the referring physician about these observations.

The client progressed well with the wrist rehabilitation program. The family reported that the physician did not seem concerned about the developing confusion or recent falls. No further medical testing was recommended. Six weeks later, the client fell and broke her hip. At that time, she was given a diagnosis of metastases to the bone and brain (central nervous system [CNS]).

Two of the most common clinical manifestations of a brain tumor are headache and personality change, but personality change is often attributed to depression, delaying the diagnosis of a brain tumor. Tumors that affect the frontal lobes are most likely to produce personality changes. Seizures occur in approximately one third of persons with metastatic brain tumors.

Headaches occur in 30% to 50% of persons with a brain tumor and are usually bioccipital or bifrontal.[111] They are usually intermittent and of increasing duration and may be intensified by a change in posture or by straining.

The headache is characteristically worse when awakening because of differences in CNS drainage in the supine and prone positions; it usually disappears soon after the person arises. It may be intensified or precipitated by any activity that increases intracranial pressure, such as straining during a bowel movement, stooping, lifting heavy objects, or coughing.

Often, the pain can be relieved by taking aspirin, acetaminophen, or other moderate painkillers. Vomiting with or without nausea (unrelated to food) occurs in about 25% to 30% of people with brain tumors and often accompanies headaches when there is an increase in intracranial pressure. If the tumor invades the meninges, the headaches will be more severe.

Focal manifestations of a space-occupying brain lesion are caused by the local compression or destruction of the brain tissue, as well as by compression secondary to edema. Papilledema (edema and hyperemia of the optic disc) may be the first sign of intracranial tumors. Visual changes do not occur until prolonged papilledema causes optic atrophy.

Nerve and Cord Compression

Symptoms of nerve and/or cord compression may occur when tumors invade and impinge directly on the spinal cord, thecal sac, or nerve root.[112] Severe destructive osteolytic lesions of the vertebral bodies from metastases can lead to pathologic fracture, fragility, and subsequent deformity of one or more vertebral bodies. Bone collapse can occur spontaneously or following trivial injury, sometimes with bone fragments adding to the compression.

Compressive pathologies affecting the spinal cord and nerve roots affect 5% to 10% of all people with cancer.[113] The thoracic spine is affected most often (70% of all cases), usually secondary to metastatic lung and breast cancer. Twenty percent develop in the lumbosacral region as a result of metastases from prostate and GI cancers or melanoma. A small number of cases (10%) arise in the cervical region of the vertebral column.[114]

Other (more rare) cancer-related causes of spinal cord compression include radiation myelopathy, malignant plexopathy, and paraneoplastic disorders. Chronic progressive radiation myelopathy can occur in anyone who has received irradiation to the spine or nearby structures. Localized spinal cord dysfunction within the area of the radiation port occurs with numbness and upper motor neuron findings.[115,116]

Whether from a primary cord tumor or a metastasis, compression of the cord can be the first symptom of cancer.

Prostate, lung, and breast cancers are the most common tumors to metastasize to the spine, leading to epidural spinal cord compression, but lymphoma, multiple myeloma, carcinomas of the colon or kidney, and sarcomas can also result in spinal cord and nerve root compression.[117]

Individuals with lymphoma or retroperitoneal tumors may suffer cord compression from tumors that grow through the intervertebral foramen and compress the cord without involving the vertebra. Cord compression is becoming increasingly common, as individuals affected by cancer survive longer with medical treatment.

Signs and Symptoms of Cord Compression. Spinal cord compression with resultant quadriplegia, paraplegia, and possible death is the most common pathologic feature of all tumors within the spinal column. Pain and sensory symptoms usually occur in the body below the level of the tumor but not necessarily at predictable levels. For example, 54% of individuals with T1-T6 compression have reported lumbosacral pain, and a similar number with lumbosacral compression have thoracic pain.[118]

The location of the metastasis is proportionate to the volume or mass of bone in each region: 60% of metastases occur in the thoracic spine, 30% in the lumbosacral spine, and 10% in the cervical spine.[119] Compression at the level of the cauda equina is relatively rare.[120] The therapist must observe carefully for subtle objective neurologic deficits (e.g., decreased sensory function, decreased but useful motor function, change in reflexes) that might otherwise be interpreted as side effects of medication.

Breast and lung cancers typically cause thoracic lesions, whereas colon and pelvic carcinomas are more likely to affect the lumbosacral spine. In some individuals, spinal cord compression may occur at multiple sites.[117,121]

Early characteristics of spinal cord compression include pain, sensory loss, muscle weakness, and muscle atrophy. Back pain at the level of the spinal cord lesion occurs in up to 95% of cases, presenting hours to months before the compression is diagnosed.

Pain is caused by the expanding tumor in the bone, bone collapse, and/or nerve damage. Pain is usually described as sharp, shooting, deep, or burning and may be aggravated by lying down, weight-bearing, bending, sneezing, or coughing.[117,121]

Discomfort may occur as thoracolumbar back pain in a belt-like distribution; the pain may extend to the groin or the legs. The pain may be constant or intermittent and occur most often at rest; pain occurring at night can awaken an individual from sleep; the person reports that it is impossible to go back to sleep.

Symptoms of severe pain preceding the onset of motor weakness generally correlate with epidural compression, whereas muscle weakness and bowel/bladder sphincter dysfunction with very little pain may indicate intramedullary metastasis.[112]

Weakness in an individual with cancer may be incorrectly attributed to fatigue, anemia, pain medication, or metabolic derangement. The therapist must remain alert to any subtle signs and symptoms of spinal cord compression as the underlying etiology and report these to the physician immediately.[114]

Over half of individuals present with sensory changes, either starting in the toes and moving caudally in a stocking-like pattern to the level of the lesion or starting one to five levels below the level of the actual cord compression.[122]

Less commonly, chest or abdominal pain may occur, caused by nerve root compression from epidural tumor(s). Progressive cord compression is manifested by spastic weakness below the level of the lesion, decreased sensation, and increased weakness. Bowel and bladder dysfunction are late findings.

Cauda Equina Syndrome. Cauda equina syndrome is defined as a constellation of symptoms that result from damage to the cauda equina, the portion of the nervous system below the conus medullaris (i.e., lumbar and sacral spinal nerves descending from the conus medullaris). Although tumors are the focus here, other causes of cauda equina syndrome include acute lumbar disk herniation, spinal stenosis, spinal infection, epidural hematoma, and spinal fracture or dislocation. This syndrome involves peripheral nerves (sensory and motor) within the spinal canal and thecal sac.

Individuals with cauda equina syndrome present differently from those with spinal cord compression. The three most common symptoms of cauda equina syndrome include saddle anesthesia, bowel or bladder dysfunction, and lower extremity weakness.[123]

Diminished sensation over the buttocks and posterior-superior thighs is also common.

Decreased anal (rectal) sphincter tone occurs in 60% to 80% of patients at the time of diagnosis. This results in urinary retention and overflow incontinence and about half of all clients need urinary catheters.[124]

Individuals with cauda equina syndrome caused by neoplasm may present with a long history of back pain and paresthesia; urinary difficulties are very common.[125] The

---

CLINICAL SIGNS AND SYMPTOMS
Cauda Equina Syndrome

- Low back pain
- Sciatica
- Saddle and/or perianal hypersthesia or anesthesia
- Change or dysfunction in bowel and/or bladder (e.g., difficulty initiating flow of urine, urine retention, urinary or fecal incontinence, constipation, decreased rectal tone and sensation)
- Lower extremity weakness (variable); gait disturbance
- Sexual dysfunction:
- Men: erectile dysfunction (inability to attain or sustain an erection)
- Women: dyspareunia (painful intercourse)
- Decreased rectal tone
- Decreased perineal reflexes
- Diminished or absent lower extremity reflexes (patellar, Achilles)

presentation may mimic a discogenic source, causing a delay in diagnosis, especially in the young adult with a primary tumor.

Associated signs and symptoms of primary or metastatic tumors causing cauda equina syndrome may include abnormal weight loss, hematuria, hemoptysis, melena, and/or constipation. The medical diagnosis of cauda equina syndrome is not always straightforward. Abnormal rectal tone may be delayed in individuals presenting with cauda equina syndrome.[126] This is because sensory nerves are smaller and more sensitive than motor nerves; even so, some people present with abnormal rectal tone (motor) without saddle anesthesia.

Peripheral Neuropathy. Peripheral neuropathy with loss of vibratory sense, proprioception, and DTRs is most often chemotherapy-related (e.g., cisplatin, Taxol, vincristine). Numbness, tingling, burning pain in the hands and feet, loss of balance, and difficulties with mobility are common with this problem.[127] It is important to differentiate the type and etiology of peripheral neuropathy before planning treatment intervention.

For example, chemotherapy-induced peripheral neuropathy (CIPN) may not be as likely to respond to lymph drainage and compression bandaging, whereas good results have been seen when this treatment intervention is used for weakness and paresthesias from lymphedema-induced nerve compression (e.g., breast cancer, ovarian cancer, testicular cancer).

In other words, resolution of neuropathy symptoms utilizing principles of manual lymphatic drainage may confirm subclinical lymphedema as the major etiologic factor in some clients.

Paraneoplastic Syndromes

Other neurologic problems occur frequently in individuals with cancer. These may be nonmetastatic and associated with cancer-related opportunistic infections, metabolic disturbances, vascular complications, treatment neurotoxicity, and paraneoplastic syndromes.

When tumors produce signs and symptoms at a distance from the tumor or its metastasized site(s), these "remote effects" of malignancy are collectively referred to as *paraneoplastic syndromes*. This can be the first sign of malignancy and may show up months (even years) before the cancer is detected. They are usually caused by one of three phenomena:
- Tumor metastasis to the brain
- Endocrine, fluid, and electrolyte abnormalities
- Remote effects of tumors on the CNS

The causes of these syndromes are not well understood. In contrast to the hormone syndromes in which the cancer directly produces a substance that circulates within blood to produce symptoms, the neurologic syndromes are a group of syndromes mediated by the immune response.

Tumors involved in this type of syndrome stimulate the production of immunologically active nervous system proteins. These immune responses are frequently associated with antineuronal antibodies that can be used as diagnostic markers of paraneoplastic disorders. As a result of these immune responses, discrete or multifocal areas of nervous system degeneration can occur, causing diverse symptoms and deficits.[128]

These are not direct effects of either the tumor or its metastases. Cancer cells can acquire new cellular functions uncharacteristic of the originating tissue. Many of these syndromes involve ectopic hormone production by tumor cells. These hormones are distributed by the circulation and act on target organs at a site other than the location of the tumor. Some tumor cells secrete biochemically active substances that can also cause metabolic abnormalities.

The reported frequency of paraneoplastic syndromes ranges from 10% to 15% to 2% to 20% of malignancies. However, these could be underestimates. Neurologic paraneoplastic syndromes are estimated to occur in less than 1% of patients with cancer.[129]

The neuromusculoskeletal system is often affected and the clinical presentation is unusual. The clinical manifestation of paraneoplastic syndrome depends on the tumor effects. The therapist is often the first health care professional to see and/or recognize the incongruence of the signs and symptoms.

In fact, the presentation may confound the medical staff. When the client fails to respond to palliative treatment, physical therapy is recommended. The alert therapist will recognize the unusual presentation and will follow up with a screening examination.

The paraneoplastic syndromes are of considerable importance because they may accompany relatively limited neoplastic growth and provide an early clue to the presence of certain types of cancer (e.g., osteoarthropathy caused by bronchogenic carcinoma, hypercalcemia from osteolytic skeletal metastases). The most common cancer associated with paraneoplastic syndromes is small cell cancer of the lungs (produces adrenocorticotrophic hormone [ACTH] and causes Cushing's syndrome).

Clinical Signs and Symptoms of Paraneoplastic Syndromes. Clinical findings of paraneoplastic syndromes may resemble those of primary endocrine, metabolic, hematologic, or neuromuscular disorders. Depending on which system is compromised, symptoms can include rheumatologic, renal, GI, vascular, hematologic, cutaneous, metabolic, endocrine, neurologic, and/or neuromuscular physical findings.[130-133]

For example, the Lambert-Eaton myasthenic syndrome (LEMS), often secondary to small cell lung carcinoma, results in muscle weakness when autoantibodies directed against the presynaptic calcium channels at the neuromuscular junction cause impaired release of acetylcholine from presynaptic nerve terminals. The clinical presentation is distinct from myasthenia gravis (MG), with lower limb muscle fatigability and autonomic symptoms appearing first in the paraneoplastic form.[134]

Gradual, progressive muscle weakness during a period of weeks to months (especially of the pelvic girdle muscles) may occur. Proximal muscles are most likely to be involved (see Fig. 14.3). The weakness does stabilize. Reflexes of the involved extremities are present but diminished. The weakness often improves and DTRs may return with exercise.

In clients who develop myopathies, such as dermatomyositis (DM) or polymyositis (PM), the myositis may precede, follow, or arise concurrently with the malignancy. No particular type of cancer has been found to predominate in such cases, but the clients affected are generally older and respond poorly to medical treatment for the myositis.

The course of the paraneoplastic syndrome usually parallels that of the tumor. Therefore, effective medical intervention (rather than physical therapy) should result in resolution of the syndrome. A paraneoplastic syndrome may be the first sign of a malignancy or recurrence of cancer that may be cured if detected early. Paraneoplastic syndromes with musculoskeletal manifestations are listed in Table 14.6.

Even nonspecific symptoms such as anorexia, malaise, weight loss, and fever are truly neoplastic and are probably caused by the production of specific factors by the tumor itself. For example, anorexia is a common symptom in clients with cancer that is attributed to tumor production of the protein tumor necrosis factor (TNF), also called *cachectin*. Fever may be seen in clients with cancer in the absence of infection

TABLE 14.6	Paraneoplastic Syndromes Having Musculoskeletal Manifestations[135]	
Malignancy	Rheumatic Disease	Clinical Features
Lymphoproliferative disease (leukemia, lymphomas)	Vasculitis	Necrotizing vasculitis
Plasma cell dyscrasia	Polyarthritis	Polymyalgia, swelling
Hodgkin's disease	Cryoglobulinemia	Vasculitis;
Ovarian cancer	Immune complex disease	Raynaud's
Carcinoid syndrome (breast, uterus, lung cancers)	Reflex sympathetic dystrophy	phenomenon; arthralgia; neurologic
Colon cancer	Scleroderma	symptoms
Mesenchymal tumors	Pyogenic arthritis	Nephrotic
Renal cell cancer (and other tumors)	Osteogenic osteomalacia	syndrome
Pancreatic cancer	Severe Raynaud's phenomenon	Palmar fasciitis and
Lung cancers	Panniculitis	polyarthritis
	Hypertrophic osteoarthropathy	Scleroderma-like changes; anterior tibia
		Enteric bacteria cultured from joint
		Bone pain; stress fractures
		Digital necrosis
		Subcutaneous nodules, especially in males
		Digital clubbing, excess bone formation

Data from Santacroce L. Paraneoplastic syndromes, eMedicine. El-Deiry,WS (ed). https://emedicine.medscape.com/article/280744-overview. Accessed Dec. 15, 2020.

> ### CLINICAL SIGNS AND SYMPTOMS
> #### *Paraneoplastic Syndromes*
>
> **Constitutional Symptoms**
> - Fever
> - Fatigue
> - Anorexia, malaise, weight loss, cachexia
> - Confusion (also a neurologic symptom)
>
> **Cardiovascular**
> - Hypertension
> - Thrombophlebitis
> - Endocarditis
>
> **Integument**
> - Skin rash, skin flushing, pigmentation changes
> - Clubbing of the fingers or toes
> - Itching, ichthyosis (dry, flaking skin)
> - Alopecia (hair loss)
> - Herpes zoster
> - Acanthosis nigricans
>
> **Rheumatic**
> - Arthralgia, polyarthritis
> - Palmar fasciitis
> - Bone pain
>
> **Neurologic**
> - Proximal muscle weakness
> - Change in DTRs (most often hyporeflexia)
> - Sensory neuropathy (progressive sensory loss of hands and feet; may or may not be symmetric)
> - CNS (cerebellar degeneration): gait difficulties, dizziness, nausea, diplopia (double vision), ataxia, dysphagia
>
> **Hematologic**
> - Anemia
> - Polycythemia
> - Signs and symptoms of hypercalcemia (Table 14.7)
> - Thrombocytosis (platelet count greater than 500,000/dL)
>
> **GI**
> - Diarrhea (malabsorption, electrolyte imbalance)
>
> **Renal/Urologic**
> - Nephropathy

when it is produced by tumor induction of pyrogen formation by host WBC or by direct tumor production of a pyrogen.

Rheumatologic Manifestations. Cancer can be associated with arthritis and can present as a paraneoplastic syndrome called *carcinoma polyarthritis.* Paraneoplastic rheumatic disorders of this type are induced by the malignancy through hormones, peptides, autocrine and paracrine mediators, antibodies, and cytotoxic lymphocytes. Polyarthritis has been reported in adults 43 to 80 years of age when associated with solid tumors and in individuals from 12 to 65 years old with hematologic malignancies.[136]

Cancer-associated rheumatic syndromes are characterized by a relatively short interval between the appearance of the rheumatic disorder and diagnosis of its associated neoplasm (usually less than 2 years).[136,137]

Rheumatic disorders caused by cancer have been associated most often with breast and lung cancers. Palmar fasciitis and polyarthritis have been reported in association with metastatic ovarian carcinoma (Case Example 14.6).[138] Even though cancer polyarthritis is a fairly uncommon occurrence, the therapist is more likely than most other health care professionals to see this. Timely recognition can reduce morbidity and mortality.

The medical diagnosis can be missed or delayed without careful evaluation. Sometimes, the diagnosis of polymyalgia rheumatica is made in error. Anyone with a sudden onset of rheumatic disease that is seronegative and monoarticular and occurs in the presence of a past history of cancer may be demonstrating signs of metastatic cancer or an occult malignancy.

Rheumatologic complaints have a sudden onset and may spare the small joints of the hands and wrists. Clinical features of carcinoma polyarthritis primarily affect asymmetric joints of the lower extremities, often the result of metastasis to the joint or periarticular bone.

Other rheumatologic conditions and muscular disorders can be associated with malignancy (Box 14.4). These conditions often disappear after successful treatment of the underlying malignancy.[139]

There is also a link between longstanding rheumatic disorders and cancer. The risk of malignant transformation during the course of chronic rheumatic disorders, including rheumatoid arthritis, Sjögren's syndrome, and systemic sclerosis, is well-known. The underlying mechanism is likely the result of immune dysregulation.[140]

Digital Clubbing. Digital clubbing is another possible sign of paraneoplastic syndrome, especially when associated with pulmonary malignancy. Clubbing of the fingers and toes is seen most often with chronic conditions such as congenital heart disease with cyanosis, cystic fibrosis, or chronic obstructive pulmonary disease (COPD). It can also develop with paraneoplastic syndromes and typically within 10 days of acute systemic illness, such as acute pulmonary abscess, heart disease, and ulcerative colitis.

Digital clubbing occurs in the distal phalanx and causes the ends of the digits to become round and wide, like "little clubs." The thumb and index finger are affected first and can be assessed by the Schamroth method.

Look for recent onset of other signs and symptoms (e.g., pulmonary, hepatic, cardiac, GI). For example, digital clubbing accompanied by a recent, unexplained weight loss, hemoptysis, and a significant smoking history may be a red-flag sign associated with lung cancer.

Skeletal Manifestations

Primary bone cancer is uncommon; primary cancers of the musculoskeletal system are discussed later in this chapter. The skeleton is, however, the most common organ affected by metastatic cancer. Tumors arising from the breast, prostate, thyroid, lung, and kidney possess a special propensity to spread to bone.

Tumor cells commonly metastasize to the most heavily vascularized parts of the skeleton, particularly the red bone marrow of the axial skeleton and the proximal ends of the

---

CASE EXAMPLE 14.6
Arthritis Associated with Ovarian Carcinoma

A 56-year-old woman was sent to physical therapy by a hand surgeon with a provisional diagnosis of rheumatoid arthritis, pending results of laboratory studies. She described a 3-month history of bilateral finger stiffness with swelling and pain. Most recently, she developed nodules at the proximal interphalangeal joints (PIPs) and thickening of the palms with erythema, both bilaterally.

At the time of her first physical therapy visit, she also reported new onset of right shoulder pain and loss of motion. When asked if she had noticed any symptoms or changes of any kind anywhere else in the body, she mentioned pain and a sense of "fullness" in the left lower abdominal quadrant. She denied having any hip pain on that side or any gastrointestinal (GI) or genitourinary (GU) signs and symptoms.

There was no previous history of any significance. When asked about birth histories and deliveries, she reported never being married and never being pregnant. She had her last menstrual period 3 years ago. Her last Papanicolaou (PAP) smear and clinical breast examination were performed 2 years ago, and results were reportedly within normal limits.

During a screening physical examination, the therapist noted visible asymmetry of the lower abdominal quadrant with distention observed on the left side compared with the right. There was no warmth or tenderness to abdominal palpation, but an unidentified mass could be felt just to the midline of the left anterior superior iliac spine (ASIS). Because the client was postmenopausal, there was no need to screen for possible pregnancy.

How would you proceed in a situation like this? Do you suggest the client call and report new onset of shoulder pain and "fullness" to the referring physician? Or should you suggest she go to her gynecologist for a pelvic examination and updated PAP smear?

The new onset of shoulder pain is important information, given the physician's "provisional diagnosis" while waiting for laboratory results. Although the apparent pelvic mass is not usually of interest to a hand surgeon, it will be up to the referring physician to decide what further medical testing is needed.

The therapist should provide the physician with the new and additional information obtained, present a plan for physical therapy intervention, and request approval before proceeding, given the new signs and symptoms present. Until a final medical diagnosis is made and cancer ruled out, ultrasound should not be used.

Results: Laboratory tests revealed a normal complete blood count (CBC), erythrocyte sedimentation rate (ESR), and routine chemistry results. Special tests for markers to indicate rheumatoid arthritis (rheumatoid factor, antinuclear antibody) were normal.

When this additional information was presented, further tests were ordered. A diagnosis of ovarian cancer (stage IV) was made, indicating distant metastases. Physical therapy intervention was put on hold until medical treatment (i.e., surgery and chemotherapy) could be completed. She received occupational therapy as an inpatient for home adaptive aids and stretching exercises. Her hand symptoms resolved with medical treatment of the carcinoma.

BOX 14.4 MUSCULAR DISORDERS ASSOCIATED WITH MALIGNANCY

Dermatomyositis and polymyositis
Type II muscle atrophy
Myasthenia gravis (MG)
Lambert-Eaton myasthenic syndrome (LEMS)
Metabolic myopathies
Primary neuropathic diseases
Amyotrophic lateral sclerosis (ALS)
Amyloidosis

Adapted from Gilkeson GS, Caldwell DS. Rheumatologic associations with malignancy. J Musculoskel Med 1990;7:70.

BOX 14.5 MOST COMMON SITES OF BONE METASTASES (IN ORDER OF FREQUENCY)[141]

- Vertebrae (thoracic 60%/lumbosacral 30%)
- Pelvis
- Ribs (posterior)
- Skull
- Femur (proximal)
- Others: sternum, cervical spine

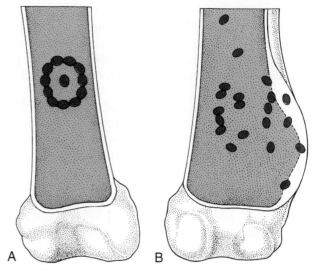

Fig. 14.6 **A**, Benign bone tumors have a characteristic sclerotic rim around the periphery of the lesion. The lesion is usually well defined and there is no evidence of erosion of the cortex or of a soft tissue mass. **B**, Malignant bone tumors can have lytic or sclerotic components. It is frequently difficult to know the extent of the lesion within the bone because there is no well-defined sclerotic rim around the tumor. The destructive process is diffuse within the medullary cavity of the bone, and the tumor may break through the cortex of the bone, producing Codman's triangle. Frequently, an associated soft tissue mass is present. Medical differential diagnosis of this lesion is between an osteogenic sarcoma and a chondrosarcoma.

long bones (humerus and femur), and the vertebral column, pelvis, and ribs (Box 14.5).

Occasionally, a growing bone mass is the first sign of disease. Diagnosis is made by x-ray study and surgical biopsy, requiring immediate attention to suspicious symptoms by referral to the client's physician.

Local swelling can be detected when the lesion protrudes beyond the normal confines of the bone. The swelling of a benign lesion is usually firm and nontender. In the presence of a rapidly growing malignant neoplasm, however, the swelling is more diffuse and frequently tender (Fig. 14.6).

The overlying skin may be warm because of the highly vascularized nature of neoplasms. If the lesion is close to a joint, function in that joint may be disturbed, with painful and restricted range of motion.

Bone Pain

Bone pain, resulting from structural damage, rate of bone resorption, periosteal irritation, and nerve entrapment, is the most common complication of metastatic disease to the skeletal system. A history of sudden onset of severe pain usually indicates the complication of a pathologic fracture (a break in an already weakened bone). Pathologic fractures are the result of metastatic disease of primary cancers most often affecting the lung, prostate, and breast.

Pathologic fractures tend to affect the vertebral body at both the thoracic and lumbar levels. Kyphotic deformity can occur with compression of the cord or cauda equina (see further discussion on Cauda Equina Syndrome in this chapter).

Bone pain is usually deep, intractable, and poorly localized, sometimes described as burning or aching and accompanied by episodes of stabbing discomfort (Case Example 14.7). The pain may be cyclic and progressive until it becomes constant. The pain is made worse by activity, especially weight-bearing. The pain is often associated with trauma during a game or exercise and may be dismissed in children as "growing pains."

It is often worse at night, awakening the person; neither sleep nor lying down provides relief. Pain at night that is unrelieved by rest or change in position is a red flag. Assessing night pain is discussed in detail in Chapter 3 in Night Pain and Cancer.

Beware of the client who reports disproportionate (excessive) pain relief with aspirin, as this may be a sign of a particular bone cancer called *osteoid osteoma*. Pain subsiding with aspirin (contains salicylates) is the hallmark of this entity. Salicylates inhibit the prostaglandins that are produced by osteoid osteomas.

Bone pain associated with skeletal metastasis can often be reproduced with a heel strike when an undiagnosed fracture is present in the lower extremities. Watch for pain on weight-bearing with a positive heel strike test or reproduced symptoms when hopping on one leg (in the younger client; this is not a likely test to use in the older adult). Perform translational/rotational tests for stress fracture.

The pain typically does not respond to physical agents or physical therapy intervention. Sometimes the client has some relief after the first few sessions of physical therapy, but pain

CASE EXAMPLE 14.7

Uterine Cancer With Bone Metastasis

A 44-year-old slender, athletic woman with isolated left knee pain of unknown cause was referred to physical therapy by her physician for a "strengthening program." She was actively involved in a variety of physical activities, including a coed baseball team, a hiking club, and church basketball intramurals, but could not recall any specific injury, fall, or other impact to her leg. She had a pair of shoe orthotics prescribed by a podiatrist 5 years ago "to compensate for my excessive Q-angle."

The physical therapy examination was unremarkable for any joint swelling, redness, or palpable warmth. There was point tenderness along the medial joint line and a palpable, though asymptomatic, plica. Joint integrity was intact and all special tests were negative.

A neurologic screening examination was also considered within normal limits, although muscle strength for the quadriceps and hamstrings was diminished by pain. Pain was present during weight-bearing activities, but did not prevent the woman from participating in all activities. There was no reported night pain, fever, or other associated signs and symptoms.

Without a definitive physical therapy diagnosis, a treatment plan was outlined to include modalities for pain and a stretching and strengthening program. Within a week's time, this client's pain level escalated on the numeric rating scale (NRS) from 3 to 10 (on a scale of 1 to 10) with constant pain that kept her awake at night for hours. When she returned to the physical therapy clinic, she was using crutches and was not bearing weight on the left leg.

Results: Therapists should be careful about assuming that physical therapy treatment has exacerbated a client's symptoms and instituting a change in program. If the treating therapist decided to continue physical therapy, with the use of some other approach, the physician should have been notified of the change in status.

Given the insidious onset of this joint pain and the rapidly progressive nature of the symptoms, this client was immediately sent back to her physician. A diagnosis of bone metastasis was made, with early stage endometrial carcinoma appearing as an unusual, isolated skeletal lesion.

She was treated with aggressive multidisciplinary therapy, including limb salvage and physical therapy as part of her rehabilitation program. The early referral most likely contributed to her favorable prognosis and cancer-free status 2 years later.

returns and may even be worse than before. The therapist may think the chosen intervention has been unsuccessful and is at fault. Consider it a red flag whenever a client fails to improve or improves and then gets worse. Further investigation and screening is advised under these circumstances.

Pain may occur around joints because of mechanical, chemical, or bony change; pain and the rate of bone resorption appear to be linked. There is often disturbance of the highly innervated periosteum, giving bone pain its neurogenic-like qualities, especially its unrelenting, intractable quality.

Fracture

Pathologic fractures (e.g., vertebrae, long bones) occur in half of all people with osteolytic metastases. In fact, this may be the presenting sign of bone cancer. An injury with subsequent medical evaluation reveals the fracture and the cancer simultaneously.

Back Pain

Neoplastic disease can cause backache, particularly in older adults, or shoulder pain in the presence of breast cancer. Although primary neoplasms of the spine are rare, myeloma and metastatic disease are more common. Malignancy as a cause of low back pain in primary care clients is quite rare, but early detection of spinal malignancy could prevent the further spread of metastatic disease.[142]

In anyone with a known cancer, the onset of back pain could suggest spinal metastasis. An insidious onset of waist-level or midback pain that becomes progressively more severe and more persistent often occurs. The pain is usually unrelieved by lying down and frequently becomes worse at night. Unexplained weight loss with severe back pain aggravated by rest may point to metastatic carcinoma of the spine. Other bone-related cancers, such as multiple myeloma, can cause severe, unremitting backaches that are present at rest and become worse when lying down.

Cancer causing low back pain can be ruled out with 100% sensitivity if the client is less than 50 years old, has not experienced unexplained or unintentional weight loss, has never had cancer before, and has responded to the physical therapist's intervention within 1 month. Referral to a spine specialist may not be needed if radiographs have not been taken yet and/or laboratory tests have not been ordered to complete a simple screening strategy.[143] If the therapist is not in a setting that allows these next steps to be generated from within the department, then referral may be advised.

Hypercalcemia from Skeletal Metastases

Hypercalcemia (greater than normal amounts of calcium in the blood) occurs frequently in clients with metastatic bone disease who have osteolytic lesions (Fig. 14.7). Normal serum calcium levels range between 8.2 mg/dL and 10.2 mg/dL. Mild hypercalcemia occurs when this level drops to around 12 mg/dL; severe hypercalcemia is defined by serum calcium at 14 mg/dL or more.

Hypercalcemia is very common in cases of breast cancer and myeloma, primarily because of an increase in bone resorption, which is caused in turn by tumor cell production of parathyroid hormone–related protein that stimulates osteoclastic bone resorption.[119,144]

Other tumors associated with hypercalcemia may include carcinomas of the lung (most commonly, small cell lung cancers), squamous cell carcinoma of the head and neck, renal cell cancer, prostate cancer, lymphoma and leukemia, thyroid cancer, and parathyroid carcinoma (rare). In most cases, hypercalcemia is an indication of progression of disease. Hypercalcemia associated with metastatic breast cancer involving bone may occur with hormone therapy.

Hypercalcemia is characterized by musculoskeletal, nervous system, cardiovascular/pulmonary, and GI symptoms (see Table 14.7). The therapist may see the first signs and

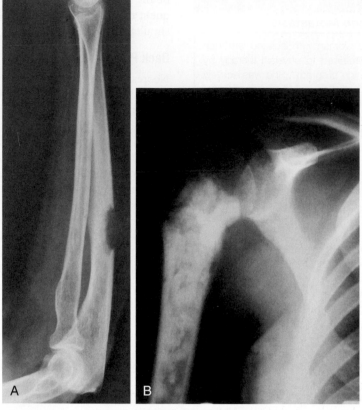

Fig. 14.7　Lytic versus blastic bone. **A**, A lytic bone lesion from breast cancer. Notice how the bone has distinct punched-out segments. This is characteristic of a lytic lesion. **B**, Blastic bone lesions from osteosarcoma. The blastic form of bone cancer is a more diffuse pattern of degeneration. (From Dorfman HD, Czerniak B. Bone Tumors. St. Louis: Mosby; 1998.)

TABLE 14.7	Hypercalcemia
System	Symptom
Central nervous system (CNS)	Drowsiness, lethargy, coma
	Irritability, personality change
	Confusion, increased confusion
	Headache
	Depression, memory loss, difficulty concentrating
	Visual disturbance
	Balance/coordination problems
	Changes in deep tendon reflexes (hyporeflexive or hyperreflexive)
	Change in muscle tone for individual with neurologic condition
	Positive Babinski and/or clonus reflex
	Changes in bowel/bladder function
Musculoskeletal	Muscle pain or tenderness and weakness
	Muscle spasms
	Bone pain (worse at night and when weight-bearing)
	Pathologic fracture
Cardiovascular	Hypertension
	Arrhythmia
	Cardiac arrest
Gastrointestinal	Anorexia (loss of appetite)
	Nausea
	Vomiting
	Constipation
	Dehydration
	Thirst

symptoms of hypercalcemia in the musculoskeletal system but should watch for others as well.

Signs and symptoms of CNS-related hypercalcemia are similar to other causes of CNS problems and include confusion, drowsiness, lethargy, headache, depression, and irritability. Hypercalcemia can also affect the GI system. The most common hypercalcemia-induced GI signs and symptoms are anorexia, nausea, vomiting, constipation, dehydration, and thirst.

Finally, in the clinical practice of a therapist, hypercalcemia secondary to bone cancer or metastasis to the bone may affect the cardiac system. These clients are usually inpatients or are known to have cancer. Hypertension may be the only outward sign of hypercalcemia-induced cardiovascular changes. Vital sign assessment may help identify early signs of cardiac involvement. However, cardiac arrest may present as the first sign of a problem.

Bisphosphonates (bone resorption inhibitors, such as alendronate [Fosamax], risedronate [Actonel], raloxifene [Evista], and calcitonin-salmon [Miacalcin]) are drugs used to control hypercalcemia and limit or prevent bone loss. In emergent or predictable situations, intravenous use of bisphosphonates (e.g., pamidronate, zoledronic acid) can be used to stabilize and/or prevent hypercalcemia. With their use, health care professionals expect to see fewer cases of hypercalcemia than in the past. These drugs also reduce bone pain, delay skeletally related events (SREs), reduce the number of pathologic fractures, and in some cases, prolong survival.

Hepatic Manifestations

Liver metastases are among the most ominous signs of advanced cancer. The liver filters blood coming in from the GI tract, making it a primary metastatic site for tumors of the stomach, colorectum, and pancreas.

Symptoms observed in a physical therapy practice include bilateral carpal/tarsal tunnel syndrome, possibly accompanied by abdominal pain and tenderness with general malaise and fatigue. Right upper quadrant pain with possible referral to the right shoulder may also occur with or without carpal tunnel syndrome (CTS; see Table 14.5).

Carpal Tunnel Syndrome

CTS can be caused by a wide range of both neuromusculoskeletal and systemic conditions and illnesses. Whenever anyone presents with *bilateral* symptoms of any kind, it is considered a "red-flag" symptom. In Chapter 2 of this text, we discussed the various bilateral symptoms the therapist might encounter in a clinical practice.

A common systemic cause of CTS involves the hepatic system (see Chapter 9 for an explanation). Briefly, liver dysfunction results in increased serum ammonia and urea levels. When these toxins are no longer absorbed into the portal vein and removed from the body, they pass directly to the brain.

Ammonia transported to the brain reacts with glutamate (an excitatory neurotransmitter), producing glutamine. The reduction of brain glutamate impairs neurotransmission. This leads to altered CNS metabolism and function. As the blood ammonia level rises, many unusual compounds (e.g., octopamine) form and serve as false neurotransmitters in the CNS. Asterixis (also known as liver flap) and numbness/tingling occur as a result of this ammonia abnormality, causing intrinsic nerve pathology. This can be misinterpreted as CTS (or tarsal tunnel syndrome) (Case Example 14.8).

When screening for bilateral CTS as a result of liver impairment, always ask about the presence of similar symptoms in the feet. Look for a history of alcoholism, cirrhosis, previous cancer, other liver disease, and the use of statins (cholesterol-lowering drugs such as simvastatin [Zocor] and atorvastatin calcium [Lipitor]; liver damage occurs in some people taking these medications).

Ask about the presence of other GI signs and symptoms. A client presenting with shoulder or upper back pain may not think nausea and abdominal bloating are related in any way to the symptoms in the wrists and hands. Perform a quick liver screen and look for signs of liver disease (see Box 10.1 or Appendix B-4 in the accompanying enhanced eBook version included with print purchase of this textbook).

ONCOLOGIC PAIN

As mentioned earlier, pain is rarely an early warning sign of cancer and is uncommon in some cancers such as leukemia. However, pain occurs in 45% to 65% of clients receiving

---

CASE EXAMPLE 14.8

Carpal Tunnel Syndrome Associated With Liver Cancer

A 52-year-old male who was employed as an over-the-road (OTR) trucker was referred by a hand surgeon for bilateral carpal tunnel syndrome (CTS). The client did not want surgery and opted for a more conservative, nonoperative approach.

He was hostile and verbally abusive, refusing to even sit down for his treatment. His wife reported a history of alcohol use/abuse. He was not screened for medical disease, just treated with the CTS protocol in a hand clinic.

During a treatment session, he commented that he had just seen an acupuncturist who told him he has liver disease. Because symptoms of bilateral numbness and tingling in the hands and feet can be a sign of liver impairment, a screening examination was performed.

The client was tested for liver flap and was observed for palmar erythema and nail bed and skin changes. Liver flap was not present, but tremoring of the hands was observed along with palmar erythema. No obvious ascites or angiomas were present.

The client was later given a medical diagnosis of liver cancer.

What are the red flags in this case? How do you return the client to the referring physician for further follow-up?

Red Flags

Age over 50 years

Reported history of alcohol use/abuse

Bilateral symptoms

Liver impairment diagnosis by acupuncturist

Palmar erythema, motor tremor

Physician Referral: This may depend on the therapist's relationship with the physician. It may be possible to telephone the physician with exactly what happened and what the therapist sees as "red flags."

If that is not feasible, then a letter (brief and to the point) with a quick summary of the findings and an open-ended question should be faxed or sent. For example,

Date (very important for documentation)

Dear Dr. Lowell,

Thank you for your recent referral of Mr. Smith for hand therapy. We are following our usual protocol for CTS. Something has come up that concerns me. Mr. Smith saw Dr. Jyn, the local acupuncturist, who mentioned liver impairment.

Given his age, drinking history, and bilateral CTS, I am wondering if there is something else going on. I noticed a fine tremor in both hands (present at rest and with activity) and color change of the skin on his hands, suggestive of palmar erythema.

We will continue treating him, but perhaps an appointment with you sooner than his scheduled 4-week follow-up is in order. What do you think? (Alternate: Please advise.)

Signature, etc.

---

cancer treatment, and 60% to 80% of clients with advanced disease.[145] This pain syndrome has multiple causes, and the therapist must always keep in mind common patterns of referred pain (see Chapter 3). Some pain is caused by pressure on the peripheral nerves or displacement of these nerves. Pain may also result from interference with blood supply or from blockage within hollow organs.

A common cause of cancer pain is metastasis of cancer to the bone. This type of pain can occur as a result of pathologic fracture with resultant muscle spasms; if the spine is involved, nerves may be affected. Pain may also result from iatrogenic causes such as surgery, radiation therapy, and chemotherapy. Immobility and inflammation also can lead to pain.

Signs and Symptoms Associated with Levels of Pain

The severity of pain varies from one client to another, but certain signs and symptoms are characteristic of particular levels of pain. For example, in *mild-to-moderate superficial pain*, a sympathetic nervous system response is usually elicited with hypertension, tachycardia, and tachypnea (rapid, shallow breathing).

In *severe* or *visceral pain*, a parasympathetic nervous system response is more characteristic, with hypotension, bradycardia, nausea, vomiting, tachypnea, weakness, or fainting. Depression and anxiety may increase the client's perception of pain, requiring additional psychologic and emotional support.

Biologic Mechanisms

Five biologic mechanisms have been implicated in the development of chronic cancer pain. The characteristics of the pain depend on tissue structure and the mechanisms involved.

Bone Destruction

Bone destruction secondary to infiltration by malignant cells or resulting from metastatic lesions is the first and most common of the biologic mechanisms causing chronic cancer pain. Bone metastases cause an increased release of prostaglandins and subsequent bone breakdown and resorption.

The client's pain threshold is reduced through sensitization of free nerve endings. Bone pain may be mild to intense. Maladaptive outcomes of bone destruction may include sharp, continuous pain that increases during movement or ambulation. The rich supply of nerves and tension or pressure on the sensitive periosteum or endosteum may cause bone pain.

Other factors contributing to the intense discomfort reported by clients include limited space for relief of pressure, altered local metabolism, weakening of the bone structure, and pathologic fractures ranging in size from microscopic to large.

Visceral Obstruction

Obstruction of a hollow visceral organ and ducts, such as the bowel, stomach, or ureters, is a second physiologic factor in the development of chronic cancer pain.

Viscus obstruction is often caused by the obstruction of an organ lumen by tumor growth. In the GI or genitourinary (GU) tract, obstruction results in either a severe, colicky, crampy pain or true visceral pain that is dull, diffuse, boring, and poorly localized.

If a vein, artery, or lymphatic channel is obstructed, venous engorgement, arterial ischemia, or edema, respectively, will result. In these cases, pain is described as dull, diffuse, burning, and aching. Obstruction of the ducts leading from the gallbladder and pancreas is common in cancer of these organs, although jaundice is more frequently an earlier symptom than pain. Cancer of the throat or esophagus can obstruct these organs, leading to difficulties with eating or speaking.

Nerve Compression

Infiltration or compression of peripheral nerves is the third physiologic factor that produces chronic cancer pain and discomfort. Pressure on the nerves from adjacent tumor masses and microscopic infiltration of nerves by tumor cells results in continuous, sharp, stabbing pain that generally follows the pattern of nerve distribution. The invading cells affect the conduction of impulses by the nervous system and sometimes result in constant, dull, poorly localized pain and altered sensation.

Blockage of the blood in arteries and veins, again both by pressure from tumor masses nearby and by infiltration, can decrease oxygen and nutrient supply to tissues. This deficiency can be perceived as pain that is similar in origin and character to cardiac pain or angina pectoris, which is chest pain from an insufficient supply of oxygen to the heart. Hyperesthesia or paresthesia may result.

Skin or Tissue Distention

Infiltration or distention of the integument (skin) or tissue is the fourth physiologic phenomenon resulting in chronic, severe cancer pain. This type of pain is secondary to the painful stretching of skin or tissue because of underlying tumor growth. This stretching produces severe, dull, aching, and localized pain, with severity of pain increasing concurrently with tumor size.

Pain associated with headache secondary to brain tumor is thought to be caused by traction on the pain-sensitive intracranial structures.

Tissue Inflammation, Infection, and Necrosis

Inflammation, infection, and necrosis of tissue may be another cause of cancer pain. Inflammation, with its accompanying symptoms of redness, edema, pain, heat, and loss of function, may progress to infection, necrosis, and sloughing of tissue.

If the inflammatory process alone is present, the pain is characterized by a sensitive tenderness. If, however, necrosis and tissue sloughing have occurred, pain may be excruciating.

SIDE EFFECTS OF CANCER TREATMENT

Conventional cancer treatment has many side effects because the goal of treatment is to remove or to kill certain tissues. In any situation, healthy tissue also is usually sacrificed. It is not always possible to differentiate between cancer recurrence and the acute or long-term effects of cancer treatment. For this reason, knowledge of both immediate and delayed side effects of cancer treatment is helpful.

For many years, three basic modalities of cancer treatment have been used, either alone or in combination: surgery, radiation therapy, and chemotherapy. In recent years, immunotherapies involving the use of cells of the immune system to prompt a tumor-killing response have been developed. Immunotherapy may be most effective when combined with conventional treatments, such as chemotherapy and radiation, to improve the success of treatment and decrease the side effects of conventional modalities.

The pharmaceuticals used in chemotherapy are cytotoxic (destructive) and are designed to kill dividing cells selectively by blocking the ability of DNA and RNA to reproduce and by lysing cell membranes. All types of rapidly dividing cells, not just cancer cells, are affected. Damage to otherwise healthy tissue, such as bone marrow, hair follicles, and mucosal cells in the mouth, digestive tract, and reproductive system, is the cause of most side effects.

In addition, a combination of drugs (each causing cell death through different pharmacologic mechanisms) is traditionally used for greater efficacy in the systemic treatment of some cancers (e.g., breast cancer). Hence, an overlap of toxicities may result in greater side effects.

Common Physical Effects

The effects of treatment for cancer can be debilitating physiologically, physically, and psychologically. Common physical side effects include bone marrow suppression, severe mucositis, mouth sores, nausea and vomiting, fluid retention, pulmonary edema, cough, headache, CNS effects, peripheral neuropathies, malaise, fatigue, dyspnea, and loss of hair. Emotional and psychologic side effects are present but less evident (Table 14.8).

Bone marrow suppression (myelosuppression) is a common and serious side effect of many chemotherapeutic agents and can be a side effect of radiation therapy in some instances. This condition may lead to a significant decrease in production of WBCs (leukopenia), RBCs (anemia), and, in some cases, platelets (thrombocytopenia).

Leukopenia (neutropenia) and resultant opportunistic infections have been shown to result in dose reductions, treatment delays, and hospitalizations. People at risk for leukopenia are taught infection prevention techniques and are often supportively or emergently treated with injections of colony-stimulating factors, such as granulocyte colony-stimulating factor (GCSF) or a newer version colony-stimulating factor, pegfilgrastim (Neulasta), to stimulate increased production of needed WBCs.[146]

TABLE 14.8	Side Effects of Cancer Treatment

The health care professional must remember that some of the delayed effects of radiation, such as cerebral injury, pericarditis, pulmonary fibrosis, hepatitis, intestinal stenosis, other GI disturbances, and nephritis, may also be signs of recurring cancer. The physician must be notified by the affected individual of any new symptoms, change in symptoms, or increase in symptoms.

Surgery	Radiation	Chemotherapy	Biotherapy	Hormonal Therapy	Transplant (Bone Marrow, Stem Cell)
Fatigue	Fatigue	Fatigue	Fatigue	Nausea	Severe bone
Disfigurement	Radiation sickness	GI effects	Fever	Vomiting	marrow
Loss of	Immunosuppression	Anorexia	Chills	Hypertension	suppression
function	Decreased platelets	Nausea	Nausea	Steroid-induced	Mucositis
Infection	Decreased WBCs	Vomiting	Vomiting	diabetes	Nausea and
Increased pain	Infection	Diarrhea	Anorexia	Myopathy	vomiting
Deformity	Fibrosis	Ulcers	Fluid retention	(steroid-	Graft versus
Scar tissue	Mucositis	Constipation	CNS effects	induced)	host disease
Fibrosis	Diarrhea	Hemorrhage	Anemia	Bone loss,	(allogenic only)
Hemorrhage,	Edema	Bone marrow	Leukopenia	fractures	Delayed wound
bleeding	Hair loss	suppression	Altered taste/	Weight gain	healing
	Delayed wound	Anemia	sensation	Altered mental	Veno-occlusive
	healing	Leukopenia		status	disease
	PNS/CNS effects	Neutropenia		Hot flashes	Infertility
	Malignancy	Thrombocytopenia		Sweating	Cataract
	Osteonecrosis	Skin rashes		Decreased	formation
	(mandible, clavicle,	Neuropathies		libido, sexual	Thyroid
	humerus, femur)	Hair loss		dysfunction	dysfunction
	Radiation recall	Infertility, sexual		Morning stiffness	Growth hormone
		dysfunction		Arthralgia, myalgia	deficiency
		Phlebitis		Vaginal dryness	Osteoporosis
		Anxiety, depression			Secondary
		Weight gain/loss			malignancy

Adapted from Goodman CC, Fuller KS. Pathology: Implications for the Physical Therapist. 5th ed. Elsevier; 2020.
CNS, central nervous system; *GI*, gastrointestinal; *PNS*, peripheral nervous system; *WBC*, white blood cell.

Another relatively common treatment associated with toxicity to the bone marrow is *anemia*. A drop in the production of RBCs and associated hemoglobin levels causes a loss of oxygenation to many body tissues and results in the many associated symptoms of anemia such as severe fatigue, muscle weakness, dizziness, dyspnea, pallor, and tachycardia.

RBC transfusions and/or the use of injectable epoetin alfa (Epogen), the recombinant form of human erythropoietin, or darbepoetin (Aranesp), a newer version of Epogen, is very useful in the treatment of anemia.

Closely related to anemia is *fatigue*. Cancer-related fatigue is a frequent, difficult, and often debilitating problem. It differs from fatigue of healthy people because it happens independently of rest and activity patterns, and is not relieved by rest.[147] Factors contributing to fatigue can include many physical and emotional components of cancer such as anemia, poor nutrition, infection, low thyroid output, tumor breakdown by-products, depression, pain, and medications.

Fatigue has been identified as a major determinant of perceived quality of life; it may be temporary, may persist throughout the episode of care, and may even continue many months after treatment has concluded. Adequate hydration, exercise, dietary measures, and treatment of anemia and depression, and addressing barriers to exercise are all measures used to help with the treatment of patients with cancer-related fatigue.[147-149]

Aggressive chemotherapeutic agents and chest irradiation can cause *cardiopulmonary dysfunction*, especially in the treatment of Hodgkin's disease and breast and lung cancers. High-dose radiation can result in pericardial fibrosis (scarring of the pericardium) and constrictive pericarditis (inflammation of the pericardium). These conditions are usually asymptomatic until the client starts to exercise, and then, exertional *dyspnea* is the first symptom.

Other causes of dyspnea include deconditioning, anemia, peripheral arterial disease, and increased physiologic demand for oxygen because of fever or infection. During radiation therapy, the client may be more tired than usual. Resting throughout exercise is important, as are adequate nutrition and hydration.

The skin in the irradiated area may become red or dry and should be exposed to the air but protected from the sun and tight clothing. Gels, lotions, oils, or other topical agents should not be used over the irradiated skin without a physician's approval. Clients may have other side effects depending on the areas treated; for example, radiation to the low back may cause nausea, vomiting, or diarrhea because the lower digestive tract is exposed to the radiation.

Radiation recall is a severe skin reaction that can occur when certain chemotherapy drugs (e.g., actinomycin, doxorubicin, methotrexate, fluorouracil, hydroxyurea, paclitaxel, liposomal doxorubicin) are given during or soon after radiation treatment.

The skin reaction appears like a severe sunburn or rash on the area of skin where the radiation was previously administered. It can appear weeks to months after the last dose of radiation. It is very important that this reaction be immediately reported because symptoms may be severe enough that chemotherapy must be delayed until the skin has healed.

Bone necrosis and demineralization *(radiation osteonecrosis)* can also result from radiation therapy and are usually not reversible. Individuals with this problem have an increased likelihood of pathologic fractures and need to be carefully handled by the therapist. Any activities, including weight-bearing activities and range of motion, should be addressed before the initiation of therapeutic exercise.[150]

Monitoring Laboratory Values

It is very important to review hematologic values in clients receiving these treatment modalities before any type of vigorous physical therapy is initiated. A guideline still used by some physical therapy exercise programs is the Winningham Contraindications for Aerobic Exercise. According to these guidelines, aerobic exercise is contraindicated in chemotherapy clients when laboratory values are as follows[151]:

Platelet count	<50,000/mm^3
Hemoglobin	<10 g/dL
White blood cell count	<3000/mm^3
Absolute granulocytes	<2500/mm^3

These guideline values have not been tested under today's patient or treatment parameters and may not be considered valid or reliable. More specific exercise guidelines for all diseases are available that may emphasize clinical reasoning to formulate patient-centered treatment decisions rather than using lab values per se.[152] In addition, the Academy of Acute Care Physical Therapy of the American Physical Therapy Association published guidelines regarding interpretation of laboratory values and additional resources. It is common practice that treatment facilities (and even individual physicians within the center) establish their own parameters and protocols. Many centers use hemoglobin levels exclusively because hematocrit is linked with hydration and may not provide the information needed. Currently, it does not appear that there is an "industry standard" for these measures.

In an outpatient setting without the benefit of laboratory values for guidance, the therapist is advised to use vital signs as discussed in Chapter 3, along with rate of perceived exertion (RPE) during exercise. Observe for clinical signs and symptoms of infection and fever, thrombocytopenia, deep vein thrombosis, dehydration, and electrolyte imbalance.

Late and Long-Term Physical Effects

Today, more than 10 million individuals treated for various types of cancers are surviving disease-free (but not "free of their disease") for many years following surgery, chemotherapy, immunotherapy, stem cell transplantation, and/or radiation. Many treatments are not highly specific and put normal cells, organs, and systems (especially the nervous system) at risk. Adjunctive medications, such as corticosteroids, antiepileptic medications, immunosuppressive agents, opioids, hypnotics, and antiemetics, contribute to impaired cognition.

Late effects from treatment, recurrence, secondary malignancies, and issues related to body image and quality of life are often a part of the survivorship experience. Any body system can be affected with long-term sequelae determined by the specific treatment received (Box 14.6). Therapists are increasingly becoming a part of cancer rehabilitation and survivorship care and will need to be aware of the potential issues they are faced with.[153] These may include fatigue, lymphedema, endocrine and fertility effects in male survivors, reproductive and hormonal changes in women, sleep disturbances, impaired cognitive function, osteoporosis, spiritual issues, financial problems, poor quality of life, pain, disfigurement, neuropathy, sexuality and body image, and dental changes. There can be functional decline, poor quality of life, and psychosocial stress and difficulty coping.[154-156]

Primary muscle shortening and secondary loss of muscle activity may produce movement disorders. Radiation-induced changes in vascular networks resulting in ischemia may affect muscle contractility. Magnetic resonance imaging (MRI) studies have shown radiation-induced muscle morbidity in several cancers including cervical, prostate, and breast cancers.[157]

The existence of *chemobrain* is widely accepted though the details behind the concept remains controversial. The term is often used to describe mental fogginess experienced by some people during the course of chemotherapy. However, this type of cognitive function is reported to persist well after treatment has ended. Memory lapses, difficulty concentrating or staying focused on a task, trouble remembering details (e.g., names, dates, phone numbers), and difficulty with word retrieval are just a few examples of the specific experiences represented by chemobrain. Depression, insomnia, and difficulty doing two things at once (e.g., talking on the phone and cleaning or cooking while carrying on a conversation) are also typical of people with chemobrain.[158,159]

CANCERS OF THE MUSCULOSKELETAL SYSTEM

In addition to increasing age as a red flag and risk factor for cancer, we now add "young age" as a possible red-flag factor. Primary bone cancer is more likely to occur in the population under the age of 25 years. Both primary bone cancer and cancer that has metastasized to the bone present with the same subset of clinical signs and symptoms, because in both cases, the same system (skeletal) is affected.

Sarcoma

Malignant neoplasms or new growths that develop as *primary* lesions in the musculoskeletal tissues are relatively rare, representing less than 1% of malignant disease in all age groups and 15% of annual pediatric malignancies.[160]

BOX 14.6 LATE AND LONG-TERM EFFECTS OF CANCER TREATMENT

Cardiovascular
Cardiomyopathy
Pericarditis
Coronary artery disease
Congestive heart failure
Valvular heart disease
Sinus node dysfunction

Lymphatic
Lymphedema

Pulmonary
Fibrosis

Neurologic/sensory
Hearing loss
Visual impairment
Vestibular impairment (balance loss)
Neuropathy*/plexopathy
Postsurgical pain syndrome
Thoracic outlet syndrome

Musculoskeletal
Muscle and joint pain
Raynaud's phenomenon
Avascular necrosis
Altered muscle activity/movement disorder syndromes/ mobility decline
Bone loss, pathologic fractures

Integument
Radiation recall

Gastrointestinal
Malabsorption
Bowel dysfunction, chronic pain (scarring, fibrosis, ischemia)
Increased risk of second malignancy (e.g., radiation for prostate cancer)
Fecal incontinence

Rheumatologic (various arthritic conditions)

Renal (chronic kidney disease)

Endocrine/Metabolic
Thyroid impairment
Diabetes mellitus
Diabetes insipidus
Adrenal insufficiency
Osteoporosis

*Referred to as chemotherapy-induced peripheral neuropathy (CIPN).
Data from Miller KD, Triano LR. Medical issues in cancer survivors—a review. Cancer J 2008;14(6):375–387.

Secondary neoplasms that develop in the connective tissues as metastases from a primary neoplasm elsewhere (especially metastatic carcinoma) are common. Fibrosarcoma occurring after radiotherapy can occur usually after a significant latent period (4 years or longer).[161]

High grade (higher grade represents greater likelihood of metastasis based on measures of cell differentiation and growth) and evidence of metastasis are associated with a poor prognosis for all neoplasms of bone or soft tissue. The prognosis for clients with soft tissue sarcoma depends on several factors. Factors associated with a poorer prognosis include age older than 60 years, tumors larger than 5 cm, and histology of high grade.[162]

Soft Tissue Tumors

Soft tissue sarcomas make up a group of relatively rare malignancies. Little is known about important epidemiologic or etiologic factors in clients with soft tissue sarcomas. There is no proven genetic predisposition to the development of soft tissue sarcomas, but studies do indicate that workers exposed to phenoxyacetic acid in herbicides and chlorophenols in wood preservatives and persons who had radiation to the tonsils, adenoids, and thymus may have an increased risk of developing soft tissue sarcoma. There are two peaks of incidence in human sarcoma development: early adolescence and the middle decades.

Soft tissue sarcomas can arise anywhere in the body. In adults, most soft tissue sarcomas arise in the extremities (usually the lower extremity, at or below the knee), followed by the trunk and the retroperitoneum. In their early stages, these sarcomas do not usually cause symptoms because soft tissue is relatively elastic, allowing tumors to grow rather large before they are felt or seen.

In contrast, the overwhelming majority of childhood soft tissue sarcomas are rhabdomyosarcomas, and the anatomic distribution of these lesions is entirely different. In adults, rhabdomyosarcoma tends to be seen in the extremities, GU tract, and head and neck.[163] Many of the primary sites in children (e.g., orbit of the eye, paratesticular region, prostate) are not the primary sites for soft tissue sarcoma in adults.

Risk Factors. Soft tissue sarcomas occur more frequently in persons who have one of the following conditions:
- von Recklinghausen's disease
- Gardner's syndrome
- Werner's syndrome
- Tuberous sclerosis
- Basal cell nevus syndrome
- Li-Fraumeni syndrome (p53 suppressor-gene mutations)
- Exposure to radiation, herbicides, wood preservatives, vinyl chloride
- Acquired immunodeficiency syndrome (AIDS; Kaposi's sarcoma)

Metastases. In children, tumors of the extremities tend to behave relatively aggressively, with a high incidence of nodal spread and distant metastases. In adults, soft tissue sarcomas rarely spread to RLNs, instead invading aggressively into surrounding tissues with early hematogenous dissemination, usually to the lungs and to the liver.

Even with pulmonary metastases, the survival rate has greatly improved over the past decade with an interprofessional approach that includes multiagent chemotherapy and limb-sparing surgery.[164] However, as more people survive for increasingly longer periods, serious and potentially life-threatening complications of such therapy can develop months to years later.

Clinical Signs and Symptoms. Soft tissue sarcomas most often appear as asymptomatic soft tissue masses. Because these lesions arise in compressible tissues and are often far from vital organs, symptoms are few, unless they are located close to a major nerve or in a confined anatomic space.

The most common manifestations of these neoplasms are swelling and pain. Pelvic sarcomas may appear with swelling of the leg or pain in the distribution of the femoral or sciatic nerve. Some people attribute swelling to a minor injury, reporting a misleading cause of onset to the therapist. The therapist must always keep this in mind when evaluating a client of any age.

More often, the neoplasm goes unnoticed until some trauma or injury requires medical attention and an x-ray study reveals the lesion. When pain is the most significant symptom, it is usually mild and intermittent, progressively becoming more severe and more constant with rapidly growing neoplasms.

No reliable physical signs are present to distinguish between benign and malignant soft tissue lesions. Consequently, all soft tissue lumps that persist or grow should be reported immediately to the physician.

CLINICAL SIGNS AND SYMPTOMS
Soft Tissue Sarcoma

- Persistent swelling or lump in a muscle (most common finding)
- Pain
- Pathologic fracture
- Local swelling
- Warmth of overlying skin

Bone Tumors

Malignant (primary) bone tumors are relatively rare, accounting for 1% of total deaths from cancer. Excluding multiple myeloma, the ratio of benign to malignant bone tumors is approximately 7:1.

Primary bone cancer affects children and young adults most commonly, whereas secondary bone tumors or metastatic neoplasms occur in adults with primary cancer (e.g., cancer of the prostate, breast, lungs, kidneys, thyroid).

Symptoms are not necessarily different between primary and secondary bone cancer, but the *history* is very different. Medical screening with possible referral is essential for anyone with clinical manifestations discussed in this chapter (see Clinical Manifestations of Malignancy: Skeletal) who also has a past medical history of any kind of cancer.

This text is limited to the most common forms of bone tumors. The two most common childhood sarcomas of the bone are osteosarcoma (osteogenic sarcoma) and Ewing family of tumors (EFT).

Osteosarcoma. Osteosarcoma (also known as osteogenic sarcoma) is the most common type of bone cancer, occurring between the ages of 10 and 30 years, with teens being the most commonly affected age group. It is slightly more common in boys, and about 1 in 10 osteosarcomas occur in people older than age 60 years.[165]

Although it can involve any bone in the body, because it arises from osteoblasts, the usual site is the epiphyses of the long bones, where active growth takes place (e.g., lower end of the femur, upper end of the tibia or fibula, upper end of the humerus).

In general, 80% to 90% of osteosarcomas occur in the long bones; the axial skeleton is rarely affected. The growth spurt of adolescence is a peak time for the development of osteosarcoma. Half of all osteosarcomas are located in the upper leg above the knee, where the most active epiphyseal growth occurs.

Risk Factors. There appears to be an association between rapid bone growth and risk of tumor formation. Young people previously treated with radiation for an earlier cancer have an increased risk of developing osteosarcoma later.

With chemotherapy given before and after surgical removal, many people can now be cured of osteosarcoma. Survival decreases if metastases are present. Limb-sparing surgery rather than amputation is effective in the majority of people.[160]

Metastases. Bone tumors, unlike carcinomas, disseminate almost exclusively through the blood; bones lack a lymphatic system. Metastases to the lungs, pleura, lymph nodes, kidneys, brain, and other bones are common and occur early in the disease process.

Hematogenous spread occurs to the lungs first and to other bones second. In some cases, surgery can be attempted to remove pulmonary metastases, but survival decreases if metastatic sites are present.

Clinical Signs and Symptoms. Osteosarcoma usually appears with pain in a lesioned area, usually around the knee in clients with femur or tibia involvement. The pain is initially mild and intermittent but becomes progressive and more severe and more constant over time.

CLINICAL SIGNS AND SYMPTOMS
Osteosarcoma

- Pain and swelling of the involved body part
- Loss of motion and functional movement of adjacent joints
- Tender lump
- Pathologic fracture
- Occasional weight loss
- Malaise
- Fatigue

Most lesions produce pain as the tumor starts to expand the bony cortex and stretch the periosteum. A tender lump may develop and a bone weakened by erosion of the metaphyseal cortex may break with little or no stress. This pathologic fracture often brings the person into the medical system, at which time a diagnosis is established by x-ray study and surgical biopsy. This neoplasm is highly vascularized so that the overlying skin is usually warm.

Ewing Sarcoma. Four percent of all childhood tumors are in the EFT. In the United States, approximately 200 children and adolescents are diagnosed with a Ewing tumor each year. Although rare, it is the third most frequent primary sarcoma of bone after osteosarcoma and chondrosarcoma. Almost any bone can be involved, but typically, the pelvis, femur, tibia, ulna, and metatarsus are most common. Soft tissue involvement is rare.[166]

Risk Factors. Ewing sarcoma is most common between the ages of 5 and 16 years, with a slightly greater incidence in boys than in girls. Anyone of any age can develop Ewing sarcoma, but most people who have Ewing tumors are in the second decade of life and Caucasian, either Hispanic or non-Hispanic. This tumor is rare in other racial groups. A spontaneous (rather than environmentally or trauma-induced) gene translocation in chromosome 22 has been found with EFT, and there is study in this area. No other risk factors have been identified in the development of EFTs.[166]

Metastases. Metastases are predominantly hematogenous (to lungs and bone), although lymph node involvement may occur. Metastases usually occur late in the disease process, but aggressive chemotherapy has increased 5-year survival rates from 10% to 70%.

Clinical Signs and Symptoms. Ewing sarcoma is a rapidly growing tumor that often outgrows its blood supply and quickly erodes the bone cortex, producing a painful, soft, tender, palpable mass. Intramedullary tumors that erode into the periosteum often result in an "onion skin" appearance as the periosteum is elevated and replaced by a new periosteal bone.

The most common symptom of EFT, bone pain, appears in about 85% of people with bone tumors. The pain may be caused by periosteal erosion from a break or fracture of a bone weakened by the tumor. The pain may be intermittent and may not be accompanied by swelling, resulting in a physical therapy referral. Systemic symptoms, such as fatigue, weight loss, and intermittent fever, may be present, especially in clients with metastatic disease. Fever may occur when products of bone degeneration enter the bloodstream. In addition, the blood supply to local areas of bone may be compromised, with resultant avascular necrosis of bone.

Ewing sarcoma occurs most frequently in the long bones and the pelvis, the most common site being the distal metaphysis and the diaphysis of the femur. The next most common sites are the pelvis, tibia, fibula, and humerus (Case Example 14.9). About 30% of the time, the bone tumor may be soft and warm to the touch and the child may have a fever.

Less common presentations of Ewing sarcoma include primary rib tumor associated with a pleural effusion and respiratory symptoms, mandibular lesions presenting with chin and

CASE EXAMPLE 14.9

Back Pain Associated with Ewing Sarcoma

A 17-year-old male high school athlete noted low back pain 6 weeks ago. He was unable to identify a specific traumatic event or injury but noted that he had been "training pretty hard" the last 2 weeks. Spinal motions were all within normal limits with no apparent step suggestive of spondylolisthesis. There were no obvious postural changes such as a scoliotic shift or unusual kyphosis/lordosis of the spinal curves.

The only positive evaluation findings included a mild left foot drop and an absent left ankle jerk. Pain was intensified during weight-bearing and movement of any kind. Pain was not relieved by rest or aspirin.

There was no fever or recent history of sore throat, upper respiratory or ear infection, and so on. After 1 week in physical therapy, pain began radiating into the posterior aspect of the left thigh. The client had also noted, for the first time, paresthesias along the lateral side of the left leg. The pain had increased rather markedly over the past 2 weeks.

The therapist might assume that the physical therapy intervention aggravated this client's condition, causing increased symptoms. However, given the unknown cause of pain, symptoms inconsistent with musculoskeletal conditions (e.g., unrelieved by rest), combined with the recent change in symptoms and the presence of positive neurologic symptoms, this client was returned to the physician before continuing further therapy.

Results: A blood test performed at that time indicated that the WBC count was 10,000/mm³ (normal range = 4300/mm³ to 10,800/mm³). Further testing, including x-ray studies, resulted in a diagnosis of Ewing sarcoma.

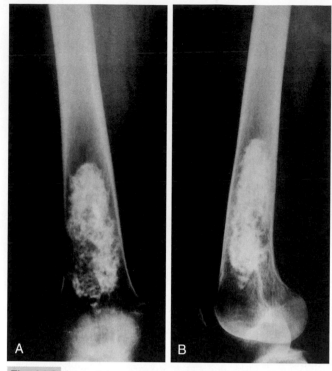

Fig. 14.8 Large intramedullary calcified lesion diagnosed as a low-grade chondrosarcoma of the femur. **A**, Anteroposterior radiograph. **B**, Lateral view. (From Dorfman HD, Czerniak B. Bone Tumors. St. Louis: Mosby; 1998.)

lip paresthesias, primary vertebral (cervical, lumbar) tumor with symptoms of nerve root or spinal cord compression, primary sacral tumor with neurogenic bladder, and pelvic tumor with pain and bowel/bladder disturbance. Neurologic symptoms may occur secondary to nerve entrapment by the tumor, and misdiagnosis as lumbar disk disease can occur.[167] If the tumor has spread, the child may feel very tired or may lose weight.

Chondrosarcoma. Chondrosarcoma, the most common malignant cartilage tumor (and second most common sarcoma of bone after osteosarcoma), occurs most often in adults older than 40 years. However, when it does occur in a younger age group, it tends to be a higher grade of malignancy and capable of metastasis.

CLINICAL SIGNS AND SYMPTOMS

Ewing Family of Tumors

- Increasing and persistent pain
- Increasing and persistent swelling over a bone (localized over the area of tumor)
- Decrease in movement if a limb bone is involved
- Fever
- Fatigue
- Weight loss
- Bowel and/or bladder disturbance

It occurs most commonly in some part of the pelvic or shoulder girdles or long bones of the axial skeleton such as the femurs (Fig. 14.8). It is rarely seen in the hands and feet.[168]

Chondrosarcoma is usually a relatively slow-growing malignant neoplasm that arises either spontaneously in previously normal bone or as a result of malignant change in a preexisting benign bone tumor (osteochondromas and enchondromas or chondromas). The latter are referred to as *secondary* chondrosarcomas, which are composed entirely of cartilaginous tissue and usually represent a low-grade malignancy.[169]

Risk Factors. See information related to soft tissue sarcomas.

Metastases. Although slow growing, chondrosarcoma has a high tendency for thrombus formation in the tumor blood vessels, with an increased risk for pulmonary embolism and metastatic spread to the lungs. Metastases develop late, so the prognosis of chondrosarcoma is considerably better than that of osteosarcoma.

Clinical Signs and Symptoms. Clinical presentation of chondrosarcoma varies. *Peripheral chondrosarcomas* (arising from bone surface) grow slowly and may be undetected and quite large. Local symptoms develop only because of mechanical irritation; otherwise, pain is not a prominent symptom.

Pelvic chondrosarcomas are often large and appear with pain referred to the back or thigh, sciatica caused by sacral plexus irritation, urinary symptoms from bladder neck involvement, or unilateral edema caused by iliac vein obstruction.

Conversely, *central chondrosarcomas* (arising within bone) appear with dull pain, and a mass is rare. Pain, which indicates active growth, is an ominous sign of a central cartilage lesion.

CLINICAL SIGNS AND SYMPTOMS

Chondrosarcoma

- Palpable mass
- Back, pelvis, or thigh pain
- Sciatica
- Bladder symptoms
- Unilateral edema

Osteoid Osteoma. Osteoid osteoma is a noncancerous osteoblastic tumor that accounts for approximately 12% of benign bone tumors. It occurs predominantly in children and young adults between the ages of 7 and 25 years, affecting males two to three times more often than females.[170]

Osteoid osteoma is a noncancerous lesion with distinct histologic features, consisting of a central core of vascular osteoid tissue and a peripheral zone of sclerotic bone (Fig. 14.9). This type of tumor commonly occurs in the diaphysis of long bones such as the proximal femur, accounting for more than half of all cases; less often, the hands and feet and posterior elements of the spine are involved.

In x-ray films, the lesion is seen as a translucent area representing the nidus, usually measuring less than 1 cm, and is surrounded by bone sclerosis. The nidus may be uniformly radiolucent or may contain variable amounts of calcification. Computed tomography (CT) images will show a well-circumscribed small area of low attenuation, representing the nidus, surrounded by a larger area of higher attenuation, representing the reactive bone formation.

Clinical Signs and Symptoms. The clinical presentation typically consists of pain, which is often worse at night,

increased skin temperature, sweating, and tenderness in the affected region. In many cases, pain is completely relieved by aspirin (a salicylate compound), which is a hallmark finding for this particular type of bone cancer.[170]

The pathogenesis of this pain may be related to the production of prostaglandins by the tumor cells. Prostaglandins can cause changes in vascular pressure, which result in local stimulation of sensory nerve endings. Salicylates in the aspirin inhibit the prostaglandins, reducing painful symptoms.

CLINICAL SIGNS AND SYMPTOMS

Osteoid Osteoma

- Bone pain (femur, 50% of cases), worse at night; relieved by aspirin
- Warmth and tenderness over the involved site

PRIMARY CENTRAL NERVOUS SYSTEM TUMORS

Primary tumors of the CNS once thought to be rare are now recognized as a significant problem in the United States. Malignant primary brain tumors are the leading cause of death from solid tumors in children and the third leading cause of death from cancer in adolescents and adults aged 15 to 34 years, although the majority of people who develop primary brain tumors are over the age of 40 years.[171]

CNS neoplasms include tumors that lie within the spinal cord (intramedullary), within the dura mater (extramedullary), or outside the dura mater (extradurally). About 80% of CNS tumors occur intracranially, and 20% affect the spinal cord and peripheral nerves. Of the intracranial lesions, about 60% are primary; the remaining 40% are metastatic lesions, often multiple and most commonly from the lung, breast, kidney, and GI tract.

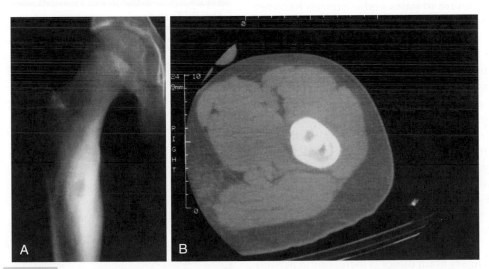

Fig. 14.9 Osteoid osteoma. **A,** A 15-year-old boy whose pain was worse at night and relieved by aspirin was found to have a well-defined lytic intracortical lesion in the proximal femoral shaft. Note the thickening around, and extending above and below, the nidus. **B,** Computed tomography (CT) imaging of the same osteoid osteoma shows marked sclerosis of the bone around the nidus. (From Dorfman HD, Czerniak B. Bone Tumors. St. Louis: Mosby; 1998.)

More common benign tumors are meningiomas (from meninges) and schwannomas (from nerve sheaths), both arising from tissues of origin. These tumors are considered noncancerous histologically, but sometimes malignant by location, meaning that they can be located in an area where tumor removal is difficult and deficit and death can result.

Any CNS tumor, even if well differentiated and histologically benign, is potentially dangerous because of the lethal effects of increased intracranial pressure and tumor location near critical structures. For example, a small, well-differentiated lesion in the pons or medulla may be more rapidly fatal than a massive liver cancer.

Primary CNS tumors rarely metastasize outside the CNS; there is no lymphatic drainage available, and hematogenous spread is also unlikely. In most cases, CNS spread is contained within the cerebrospinal axis, involving local invasion or CNS seeding through the subarachnoid space and the ventricles.

Whether from primary CNS tumors or cancer that has metastasized to the CNS from some other source, the effects are the same. Clinical manifestations of CNS involvement were discussed earlier in this chapter.

Risk Factors

The incidence of primary CNS lymphoma is increasing among older adults who are immunocompetent and even more so among aging adults who are immunodeficient. The etiology of most primary brain tumors is unknown, although ionizing radiation has been implicated most often.

Children with a history of cranial radiation therapy, such as low-dose radiation of the scalp for fungal infection, are at a significantly greater risk of developing primary brain tumors. However, most radiation-induced brain tumors are caused by radiation to the head used for the treatment of other types of cancer.[172]

Occupational exposure to gases and chemicals has been proposed to be a risk factor. Several congenital genetic disorders are directly linked with an increased risk of primary brain tumors (e.g., neurofibromatosis, Turcot syndrome, tuberous sclerosis). Other potential environmental risk factors, such as exposure to vinyl chloride and petroleum products, have shown inconclusive results. Current preliminary evidence has shown altered brain activity with exposure to electromagnetic fields from cell phones or other wireless devices. Whether this effect on the brain is neutral, positive, or negative remains under investigation, especially as electromagnetic frequency ranges keep widening because of the various types of electrical and wireless devices in use.[173]

Brain Tumors

The incidence of primary brain tumor is increasing in persons of all ages; in children, it is second only to leukemia as a cause of death. Although the causes for this overall increase remain unknown, it is clear that it is not simply a matter of better diagnostic techniques. Adding the number of people who survive other primary cancers but later develop metastatic brain tumors increases the overall incidence dramatically.

Individuals with mental disorders are more likely to be diagnosed with brain tumors and at younger ages than people without mental illness. This increased risk for brain tumors may reflect the early presence of mental symptoms, or there may be a true association between the two conditions. The exact relationship remains unknown at this time.[174]

Primary Malignant Brain Tumors

The most common primary malignant brain tumors are astrocytomas. Low-grade astrocytomas (Grade I), such as juvenile pilocytic astrocytomas, have an excellent prognosis after surgical excision.

At the other extreme is the Grade IV glioma such as glioblastoma multiforme, which is an aggressive, high-grade tumor with a very poor prognosis (usually less than 12 months). There are intermediate histologic grades (II, III) with intermediate survival statistics. Low-grade tumors are more common in children than adults.[175]

Metastatic Brain Tumors

Cancer can spread through bloodborne metastasis or via cerebrospinal fluid pathways. Therefore, the brain is a common site of metastasis. In fact, metastatic brain tumors are probably the most common form of malignant brain tumors.

The cerebrum is the most common site of metastasis. Cerebellar metastases are less frequent; brain stem metastases are the least common. Approximately two thirds of people with brain metastasis will present with multiple metastases.

Up to 50% of individuals affected by some type of cancer develop neurologic symptoms resulting from a brain metastasis. Headache, seizures, loss of motor function, and cerebellar signs are the most common early symptoms.

CLINICAL SIGNS AND SYMPTOMS
Brain Tumor

- Increased intracranial pressure
- Headache, especially retroorbital; sometimes worse upon awakening, improves during the day
- Vomiting (with or without nausea)
- Change in vision (blurring, blind spots, diplopia, abnormal eye movement)
- Change in mentation (impaired thinking, difficulty concentrating or reading, memory, or speech)
- Change in personality, irritability
- Unusual drowsiness, increased sleeping
- Seizures (without previous history)
- Sensory changes
- Muscle weakness or hemiparesis
- Bladder dysfunction
- Increased lower extremity reflexes compared with upper extremity
- Decreased coordination, change in gait, ataxia
- Positive Babinski reflex
- Clonus (ankle or wrist)
- Vertigo, head tilt

As mentioned previously, any neurologic sign can be the silent presentation of cancer metastasized to the CNS. The most common sources of brain metastases are cancers of the lung, breast, metastases from melanomas, and cancers of the colon and kidney.

Spinal Cord Tumors

Spinal tumors are similar in nature and origin to intracranial tumors, but occur much less often. They are most common in young and middle-aged adults, occurring most often in the thoracic spine because of its length, proximity to the mediastinum, and likelihood of direct metastatic extension from lymph nodes involved with lymphoma, breast cancer, or lung cancer.

Metastases

Most metastasis is disseminated by local invasion. Spinal cord tumors account for less than 15% of brain tumors. As mentioned, 10% of spinal tumors are themselves metastasized neoplasms from the brain.

One other means of dissemination is through the intervertebral foramina. The extradural space communicates through the intervertebral foramina with adjacent extraspinal compartments such as the mediastinum and retroperitoneal space.

In most cases, extradural tumors are metastatic, reaching the extradural space and then the adjacent extraspinal spaces through this foraminal connection. Tumors within the spinal cord (intramedullary) or outside of the spinal cord (extramedullary) may metastasize to the dural tube to become intradural tumors.

Clinical manifestations of spinal tumors vary according to their location. See previous discussion in this chapter on Clinical Manifestations of Malignancy: Neurologic. Pain associated with *extramedullary tumors* can be located primarily at the site of the lesion or may refer down the ipsilateral extremity, with radicular involvement from nerve root compression, irritation, or occlusion of blood vessels supplying the cord. Progressive cord compression is manifested by spastic weakness below the level of the lesion, decreased sensation, and increased weakness.

Intramedullary tumors produce more variable signs and symptoms. High cervical cord involvement causes spastic quadriplegia and sensory changes. Tumors in descending

---

CLINICAL SIGNS AND SYMPTOMS

Spinal Cord Tumors

- Pain
- Decreased sensation
- Spastic muscle weakness
- Progressive muscle weakness
- Muscle atrophy
- Paraplegia or quadriplegia
- Thoracolumbar pain
- Unilateral groin or leg pain
- Pain at rest and/or night
- Bowel/bladder dysfunction (late finding)

---

areas of the spinal cord produce motor and sensory changes appropriate to functions of that level.

CANCERS OF THE BLOOD AND LYMPH SYSTEM

Cancers arising from the bone marrow include acute leukemia, chronic leukemia, multiple myeloma, and some types of lymphoma. These cancers are characterized by the uncontrolled growth of blood cells.

The major lymphoid organs of the body are the lymph nodes and the spleen. Cancers arising from these organs are called *malignant lymphomas* and are categorized as either Hodgkin's disease or NHL.

Leukemia

Leukemia, a malignant disease of the blood-forming organs, is the most common malignancy in children and young adults. About half of all leukemias are classified as *acute*, with rapid onset and progression of disease resulting in 100% mortality within days to months without appropriate therapy.

Acute leukemias are most common in children from 2 to 4 years of age, with a peak incidence again at age 65 years and older. The remaining leukemias are classified as *chronic*, which have a slower course and occur in persons between the ages of 25 and 60 years. From these two broad categories, leukemias are further classified according to specific malignant cell line (Table 14.9).

Leukemia develops in the bone marrow and is characterized by abnormal multiplication and release of WBC precursors. The disease process originates during WBC development in the bone marrow or lymphoid tissue. In effect, leukemic cells become arrested in "infancy," with most of the clinical manifestations of the disease being related to the absence of functional "adult" cells, which are products of normal differentiation.

With rapid proliferation of leukemic cells, the bone marrow becomes overcrowded with immature WBCs, which then spill over into the peripheral circulation. Crowding of the bone marrow by leukemic cells inhibits normal blood cell production.

Decreased RBC (erythrocyte) production results in anemia and reduced tissue oxygenation. Decreased platelet production results in thrombocytopenia and risk of hemorrhage. Decreased production of normal WBCs results in increased vulnerability to infection, especially because leukemic cells are functionally unable to defend the body against pathogens.

Leukemic cells may invade and infiltrate vital organs such as the liver, kidneys, lung, heart, or brain.

Risk Factors

Several predisposing factors for the development of leukemia have been identified. Exposure to ionizing radiation remains the most conclusively identified causative factor in humans. Prior drug therapies, such as chloramphenicol, phenylbutazone, chemotherapy alkylating agents, and benzene, have been implicated in the development of acute leukemia.

TABLE 14.9	Overview of Leukemia[176]*			
	Acute Lymphoblastic Leukemia (ALL)	Acute Myeloid Leukemia (AML)	Chronic Lymphocytic Leukemia (CLL)	Chronic Myelogenous Leukemia (CML)
INCIDENCE				
Percentage of all leukemias	20%	20%	25%–40%	15%–20%
Adults	20%	85%	100%	95%–100%
Children	80%–85%	10%–20%	—	3%
AGE	Peak: 3–7 years 65+ (older adults)	15–40 years Incidence increases with age from 40–80+	50+	25–60 years
ETIOLOGY	Unknown Chromosomal abnormality Environmental factors Down syndrome (high incidence)	Benzene Alkylating agents Radiation Myeloproliferative disorders Aplastic anemia	Chromosomal abnormalities Slow accumulation of CLL lymphocytes	Philadelphia chromosome; BCR-ABL gene Radiation exposure
PROGNOSIS	Adult: Poor Child: 66% with aggressive treatment; 90.8% under age 5	Poor even with treatment 10%–15% survival	2–10 years survival Median survival: 6 years	Poor; 2–8 years Median survival: 3–4 years

*There are many alternate names for these four main types of leukemia. For further details, see the Leukemia and Lymphoma Society website online at www.lls.org.
From Leukemia and Lymphoma Society. Facts and statistics. Available at https://www.lls.org/facts-and-statistics/facts-and-statistics-overview/facts-and-statistics. Accessed Dec. 15, 2020.

Hereditary syndromes associated with development of leukemia include Bloom syndrome, Down syndrome, Klinefelter's syndrome, and neurofibromatosis. In addition, viruses and immunodeficiency disorders have been associated as causative factors.[177]

Clinical Signs and Symptoms

Most of the clinical findings in acute leukemia are as a result of bone marrow failure, which results from replacement of normal bone marrow elements by malignant cells. Infections are caused by a depletion of competent WBCs needed to fight infection. Abnormal bleeding is caused by a lack of blood platelets required for clotting, and severe fatigue is from a lack of RBCs. The most common symptoms of leukemia include infection, fever, pallor, fatigue, anorexia, bleeding, anemia, neutropenia, and thrombocytopenia.

For women, the abnormal bleeding may be prolonged menstruation leading to anemia. The Special Questions for Women (see Appendix B-32A and B in the accompanying enhanced eBook version included with print purchase of this textbook) may elicit this kind of valuable information, which would then require medical referral. Less common manifestations include direct organ infiltration; clients may experience easy bruising of the skin or abnormal bleeding from the nose, urinary tract, or rectum.

The appearance of a painless, enlarged lymph node or skin lesion is followed by weakness, fever, and weight loss. A history of chronic immunosuppression (e.g., antirejection drugs for organ transplants, chronic use of immunosuppressant drugs for inflammatory or autoimmune diseases, cancer treatment) in the presence of this clinical presentation is a major red flag.

Clients taking immunosuppressants do not usually have an elevated body temperature, so the presence of a fever is a red flag for this group. Significant weight loss with inactivity secondary to pain is another red flag; most inactive individuals experience weight gain, not weight loss. A good rule of thumb to use in recognizing significant weight loss is 10% of the individual's total body weight in 10 to 14 days without trying.

Lymphoproliferative malignancies, such as leukemia and lymphoma, may also involve extramedullary areas and can present with localized or generalized symptoms such as an enlarged liver and spleen, bone and joint pain, bone fracture, and parotid gland and testicular infiltration.

CLINICAL SIGNS AND SYMPTOMS

Acute and Chronic Leukemias

- Infections, fever
- Abnormal bleeding
- Easy bruising of the skin
- Petechiae
- Epistaxis (nosebleeds) and/or bleeding gums
- Hematuria (blood in the urine)
- Rectal bleeding
- Weakness
- Easily fatigued
- Enlarged lymph nodes
- Bone and joint pain
- Weight loss
- Loss of appetite
- Pain or enlargement in the left upper abdomen (enlarged spleen)

Involvement of the synovium may lead to symptoms suggestive of rheumatic disease. A possible presentation in a child with acute lymphoblastic leukemia (ALL) can be joint pain and swelling that mimics juvenile idiopathic arthritis (JIA; formerly JRA). Leukemic arthritis is present in about 5% of leukemia cases. Acute leukemia can cause joint pain that is severe, episodic, and disproportionately severe in comparison to the minimal heat and swelling that are present.[178]

Arthritic symptoms in such a child may be a consequence of leukemic synovial infiltration, hemorrhage into the joint, synovial reaction to an adjacent tumor mass, or crystal-induced synovitis.

Multiple Myeloma

Multiple myeloma is a cancer caused by uncontrolled growth of plasma cells in the bone marrow. Excessive growth of plasma cells originating in the bone marrow destroys bone tissue and is associated with widespread osteolytic lesions (decreased areas of bone density). Plasma cells are part of the immune system, and in multiple myeloma, they grow uncontrolled, forming tumors in the bone marrow.

Bone lesions and hypercalcemia can occur in some hematologic malignancies such as multiple myeloma. Multiple myeloma to date is an incurable disease, but the prognosis has improved, with lengthy remissions possible with treatment.

Risk Factors

There are no clear predisposing factors, other than age or exposure to ionizing radiation. This disease can develop at any age from young adulthood to advanced age but peaks among persons between the ages of 50 and 70 years. It is more common in men and African Americans. Molecular genetic abnormalities have been identified in the etiologic complex of this disease. There has been data to suggest that a virus (Kaposi-associated herpes virus, HHV-8) may be implicated in AIDS-related cases, although recent evidence has refuted this.[179,180]

Clinical Signs and Symptoms

Multiple myeloma causes symptoms in many areas of the body. It normally originates in the bone marrow and then causes difficulties in other organs. The onset of multiple myeloma is usually gradual and insidious. Most clients pass through a long presymptomatic period that lasts 5 to 20 years.

Early symptoms involve the skeletal system, particularly the pelvis, spine, and ribs. Some clients have backache or bone pain that worsens with movement (Case Example 14.10). Bone disease is the most common complication and results in severe bone pain, pathologic fractures, hypercalcemia, and spinal cord compression. Renal failure, anemia, cardiac failure, and infection are serious and may be fatal complications of this process.[181]

Bone Destruction. Bone pain is the most common symptom of myeloma. It is caused by infiltration of the plasma cells into the marrow with subsequent destruction of bone. Initially, the skeletal pain may be mild and intermittent,

CLINICAL SIGNS AND SYMPTOMS

Multiple Myeloma

- Recurrent bacterial infections (especially pneumococcal pneumonias)
- Anemia with weakness and fatigue
- Bleeding tendency

Bone Destruction
- Skeletal/bone pain (especially pelvis, spine, and ribs)
- Spontaneous fracture
- Osteoporosis
- Hypercalcemia (confusion, increased urination, loss of appetite, abdominal pain, vomiting, and constipation)

Renal Involvement
- Kidney stones
- Renal insufficiency

Neurologic Abnormalities
- CTS
- Back pain with radicular symptoms
- Spinal cord compression (motor or sensory loss, bowel/bladder dysfunction, paraplegia)

or it may develop suddenly as severe pain in the back, rib, leg, or arm, often the result of an abrupt movement or effort that has caused a spontaneous (pathologic) bone fracture.

The pain is often radicular and sharply cutting to one or both sides and is aggravated by movement. As the disease progresses, more and more areas of bone destruction and hypercalcemia develop. Symptoms associated with bone pain usually subside within days to weeks after initiation of antiresorptive agents. If left untreated, this disease will result in skeletal deformities, particularly of the ribs, sternum, and spine.

Hypercalcemia. Bone fractures are a result of osteoclast activity and bone destruction. This process results in calcium release from the bone and hypercalcemia. Hypercalcemia is considered an oncologic emergency. To rid the body of excess calcium (hypercalcemia), the kidneys increase the output of urine, which can lead to serious dehydration if there is an inadequate intake of fluids. Vomiting may compound this dehydration. Clients who have symptoms of hypercalcemia (see Table 14.7) should seek immediate medical care because this condition can be life-threatening.

Renal Effects. Drainage of calcium and phosphorus from damaged bones eventually leads to the development of renal stones, particularly in immobilized clients. Renal insufficiency is the second most common cause of death, after infection, in clients with multiple myeloma.

In addition to bone destruction, multiple myeloma is characterized by disruption of RBC, leukocyte, and platelet production, which results from plasma cells crowding the bone marrow. Impaired production of these cell forms causes anemia, increased vulnerability to infection, and bleeding tendencies.

Neurologic Complications. Approximately 10% of persons with myeloma have amyloidosis, deposits of insoluble

CASE EXAMPLE 14.10
Rib Metastases Associated with Multiple Myeloma

At presentation, a 57-year-old man had rib pain that began 1 month ago. He could not think of any possible cause and denied any repetitive motions, recent trauma, forceful coughing, or history of tobacco use.

Past medical history was significant for hepatitis A (10 years ago) and benign prostatic hyperplasia (BPH). The BPH is reportedly well controlled with medication, but he noticed a decreased need to urinate and mentioned that he has been meaning to have a recheck of this problem.

During the examination, there was bilateral point tenderness over the posterior seventh and eighth ribs. Symptoms were not increased by respiratory movements, trunk movements, position, or palpation of the intercostal spaces. Trunk and extremity movements were considered within normal limits and a neurologic screening examination was unremarkable.

The therapist could not account for the client's symptoms given the history and clinical presentation. Further screening revealed that the client had noticed progressive fatigue and generalized aching over the previous 2 weeks that he attributed to the "flu." He had lost about 10 lbs during the week that he experienced vomiting and diarrhea. Vital signs were taken and were within normal limits. There were no other red-flag symptoms to suggest a systemic origin of symptoms.

Results: Without a proper physical therapy diagnosis on which to base treatment, the therapist did not have a clear plan of care. There was no well-defined musculoskeletal problem, but a variety of systemic variables were present (e.g., sudden weight loss and constitutional symptoms accounted for by the "flu," oliguria attributed to BPH, insidious onset of rib pain).

The therapist decided to treat the client for 7 to 10 days and reassess at that time. Intervention consisted of stretching, manual therapy, postural exercises, and Feldenkrais techniques. At the end of the prescribed time, there was no change in clinical presentation.

The therapist asked a colleague in the same clinic for a second opinion at no charge to the client. Ultrasound imaging for possible rib fracture was performed and was considered negative. No new findings were uncovered and it was agreed collaboratively (including the client) to request a medical evaluation of the problem from the client's family physician. The client was subsequently given a diagnosis of multiple myeloma and was treated medically.

NOTE: The use of ultrasound over the painful rib is contraindicated in the presence of bone metastases.

---

fragments of a monoclonal protein resembling starch. These deposits cause tissues to become waxy and immobile and may affect the nerves, muscles, tendons, and ligaments, especially the carpal tunnel area of the wrist. CTS with pain, numbness, or tingling of the hands and fingers may develop. Excess immunoglobulins, caused by multiple myeloma, can cause a hyperviscosity syndrome characterized by changes in mental status, vision, fatigue, angina, and bleeding disorders.

More serious neurologic complications may occur in 10% to 15% of clients with multiple myeloma. Spinal cord compression is usually observed early or in the late relapse phase of disease. Back pain is usually present as the initial symptom, with radicular pain that is aggravated by coughing or sneezing. Motor or sensory loss and bowel/bladder dysfunction are signs of more extensive compression. Paraplegia is a later, irreversible event.

Hodgkin's Disease

Hodgkin's disease (or Hodgkin's lymphoma) is a chronic, progressive, neoplastic disorder of lymphatic tissue characterized by the painless enlargement of lymph nodes with progression to extralymphatic sites such as the spleen and liver. Hodgkin's lymphoma is marked by the presence of Reed-Sternberg cells, which are not present in NHL.

In industrialized countries, Hodgkin's disease demonstrates constant incidence rates, with a first peak occurring in adolescents and young adults and a second peak occurring in older adults. Men are affected more often than women.[182]

Epidemiologic and clinical-pathologic features of Hodgkin's disease suggest that an infectious agent may be involved in this disorder. Recently accumulated data provide direct evidence supporting a causal role of Epstein-Barr virus (EBV) in a significant portion of cases, and a greater incidence of Hodgkin's disease has been observed in young individuals who previously had infectious mononucleosis.

Risk Factors

Infection with EBV and infectious mononucleosis has been associated with Hodgkin's lymphoma. No other risk factors have been identified.

Metastases

The exact mechanism of growth and spread of Hodgkin's disease remains unknown. The disease may progress by extension to adjacent structures or via the lymphatics because lymphoreticular cells inhabit all tissues of the body except the CNS. Hematologic spread may also occur, possibly by means of direct infiltration of blood vessels.

Clinical Signs and Symptoms

Hodgkin's disease usually appears as a painless, enlarged lymph node, often in the neck, underarm, or groin. The therapist may palpate these nodes during a cervical spine, shoulder, or hip examination.

Lymph nodes are evaluated on the basis of size, consistency, mobility, and tenderness. Lymph nodes up to 1 cm in diameter of soft-to-firm consistency that move freely and easily without tenderness are considered within normal limits. Lymph nodes more than 1 cm in diameter that are firm and rubbery in consistency or tender are considered suspicious.

Enlarged lymph nodes associated with infection are more likely to be tender, soft, and movable than the slow-growing nodes associated with cancer. Lymph nodes enlarged in response to infections throughout the body require referral to a physician, especially in someone with a current or previous history of cancer. The physician should be notified of these findings and the client should be advised to have the lymph nodes checked at their next follow-up visit, if not sooner, depending on the client's particular circumstances.

As always, *change* in size, shape, tenderness, and consistency raise a red flag. Supraclavicular nodes are common metastatic sites for occult lung and breast cancers, whereas inguinal nodes implicate tumors arising in the legs, perineum, prostate, or gonads.

Other early symptoms may include unexplained fevers, night sweats, weight loss, and pruritus (itching). The itching occurs more intensely at night and may result in severe scratches because the client is unaware of scratching during the sleep state. Fever typically peaks in the late afternoon, and night sweats occur when the fever breaks during sleep. Fatigue, malaise, and anorexia may accompany progressive anemia. Some clients with Hodgkin's disease experience pain over the involved nodes after ingesting alcohol.

Symptoms may arise when enlarged lymph nodes obstruct or compress adjacent structures, causing edema of the face, neck, or right arm secondary to superior vena cava compression or causing renal failure secondary to urethral obstruction.

Obstruction of bile ducts as a result of liver damage causes bilirubin to accumulate in the blood and discolor the skin. Mediastinal lymph node enlargement with involvement of lung parenchyma and invasion of the pulmonary pleura progressing to the parietal pleura may result in pulmonary symptoms, including nonproductive cough, dyspnea, chest pain, and cyanosis.

Dissemination of disease from the lymph nodes to bone may cause compression of the spinal cord, leading to paraplegia. Compression of nerve roots of the brachial, lumbar, or sacral plexus can cause nerve root pain.

CLINICAL SIGNS AND SYMPTOMS
Hodgkin's Disease/Hodgkin's Lymphoma

- Painless, progressive enlargement of unilateral lymph nodes, often in the neck
- Pruritus (itching) over entire body
- Unexplained fevers, night sweats
- Anorexia and weight loss
- Anemia, fatigue, malaise
- Jaundice
- Edema
- Nonproductive cough, dyspnea, chest pain, cyanosis
- Nerve root pain
- Paraplegia

Non-Hodgkin's Lymphoma

NHL is a group of lymphomas affecting the lymphoid tissue and occurring in persons of all ages. It is more common in adults in their middle and older years (40 to 60 years of age).

Risk Factors

Males are affected more often than females and individuals with congenital or acquired immunodeficiencies (e.g., those undergoing organ transplantation and anyone with autoimmune diseases are all at increased risk for development of NHL). In addition, some people who have been exposed to large levels of radiation (e.g., nuclear reactor accidents) or extensive radiation and chemotherapy for a different cancer site may be at increased risk for lymphoma.[183]

Individuals infected with the human immunodeficiency virus (HIV) are at increased risk for developing NHL and to a lesser extent, Hodgkin's disease as well. AIDS-related lymphoma (ARL) is now the second most common cancer associated with HIV after Kaposi's sarcoma. The relative risk of developing lymphoma within 3 years of an AIDS diagnosis is increased by 165-fold compared with people without AIDS.[184]

Several possible etiologic mechanisms are hypothesized for NHL. Immunosuppression, possibly in combination with viruses or exposure to certain infectious agents, could be the primary cause. Chemicals, UV light, blood transfusion, acquired and congenital immune deficiency, and autoimmune disorders increase the risk for NHL.[185]

Other studies link the disease to widespread environmental contaminants such as benzene found in cigarette smoke, gasoline, automobile emissions, and industrial pollution.

Clinical Signs and Symptoms

NHL presents a clinical picture broadly similar to that of Hodgkin's disease, except that the disease is usually initially more widespread and less predictable. The disease starts in the lymph nodes, although early involvement of the oropharyngeal lymphoid tissue or the bone marrow is common, as is abdominal mass or GI involvement with complaints of vague back or abdominal discomfort.[185]

The most common manifestation is painless enlargement of one or more peripheral lymph nodes. Systemic symptoms are not as commonly associated with NHL as with Hodgkin's disease. Clients with NHLs often have remarkably few symptoms, even though many node areas or extranodal sites are involved.

Most NHLs fall into two broad categories related to their clinical activity: indolent and aggressive. Indolent disease may be minimally active and treatable for many years. However, the disease is frequently disseminated at the time of diagnosis. Surgery is usually used only for staging or debulking purposes. Combination chemotherapy, biotherapy (targeted monoclonal antibodies), and radiation therapies are now used as treatment for NHL. Radioactive isotope

CLINICAL SIGNS AND SYMPTOMS
Non-Hodgkin's Lymphoma

- Enlarged lymph nodes
- Fever
- Night sweats
- Weight loss
- Bleeding
- Infection
- Red skin and generalized itching of unknown origin

combinations with monoclonal antibodies are also in use for some types of NHL.[186]

Acquired Immunodeficiency Syndrome–Non-Hodgkin's Lymphoma

AIDS-NHL has emerged as a major sequela of HIV infection. It now occurs frequently in clients who survive other consequences of AIDS.

The etiologic basis of AIDS-NHL is still under investigation; profound cellular immunodeficiency plays a central role in lymphoma genesis. The molecular pathogenesis is a complex process involving both host factors and genetic alterations.

Nearly 95% of all HIV-associated malignancies are either NHL or Kaposi's sarcoma. People with CNS lymphoma usually have advanced AIDS, are severely debilitated, and are usually thought to be at terminal stages of the disease.[187]

EBV often accompanies NHL. It is generally accepted that EBV acts in the pathogenesis of lymphoma owing to the alteration in balance between host and latent EBV infection in immunodeficiency states, with increased activity of the virus.

Risk Factors

Infection with HIV and related immunodeficiencies resulting from HIV are the primary risk factors for this disease. NHL is more likely to develop among clients who have Kaposi's sarcoma, a history of herpes simplex infection, and a lower neutrophil count.

Clinical Signs and Symptoms

The most common presentations of HIV-related NHL are systemic B symptoms (which may suggest an infectious process), a rapidly enlarging mass lesion, or both. At the time of diagnosis, approximately 75% of clients will have advanced disease. Extranodal disease frequently involves any part of the body, with the most common locations being the CNS, bone marrow, GI tract, and liver.

Diagnosis of NHL in areas of the body other than the CNS is complicated by a history of fevers, night sweats, and weight loss and loss of appetite, which are also common symptoms related to HIV infection and AIDS.

Although musculoskeletal lesions are not reported as commonly as pulmonary or CNS abnormalities in HIV-positive individuals, a wide variety of osseous and soft tissue changes are seen in this group. Diffuse adenopathy, lower extremity pain and swelling, subcutaneous nodules, and lytic lesions of the extremities are common.

CLINICAL SIGNS AND SYMPTOMS

AIDS-NHL

- Painless, enlarged mass
- Subcutaneous nodules
- Constitutional symptoms (fever, night sweats, weight loss)
- Musculoskeletal lesions (lytic bone, pain, swelling)

PHYSICIAN REFERRAL

Early detection of cancer can save a person's life. Any suspicious sign or symptom discussed in this chapter should be investigated immediately by a physician. This is true especially in the presence of a positive family history of cancer, a previous personal history of cancer, and environmental risk factors, and/or in the absence of medical or dental (oral) evaluation during the previous year.

The therapist is not responsible for diagnosing cancer. The primary goal in screening for cancer is to make sure the client's problem is within the scope of a physical therapist's practice. In this regard, documentation of key findings and communication with the physician are both very important.

When trying to sort out neurologic findings, remember to look for changes in DTRs, a myotomal weakness pattern, and changes in bowel/bladder function. These findings will not give you a definitive diagnosis but will provide you with valuable information to offer the physician if further medical testing is advised.

Pain while weight-bearing that is unrelieved by rest or change in position and does not respond to treatment, unremitting pain at night, and a history of cancer are all red flags indicating that medical evaluation is needed.

Any recently discovered lumps or nodules must be examined by a physician. Any suspicious finding by report, during observation, or by palpation should be checked by a physician.

If any signs of skin lesions are described by the client or if they are observed by the therapist and the client has not been examined by a physician, a medical referral is recommended.

If the client is planning a follow-up visit with the physician within the next 2 to 4 weeks, that client is advised to indicate the mole or skin changes at that time. If no appointment is pending, the client is encouraged to make a specific visit either to the family/personal physician or to a dermatologist.

Guidelines for Immediate Physician Referral

- Presence of recently discovered lumps or nodules or changes in previously present lumps, nodules, or moles, especially in the presence of a previous history of cancer or when accompanied by carpal tunnel or other neurologic symptoms.
- Detection of palpable, fixed, irregular mass in the breast, axilla, or elsewhere requires medical referral or a recommendation to the client to contact a physician for evaluation of the mass. Suspicious lymph node enlargement or lymph node changes; generalized lymphadenopathy.
- Recurrent cancer can appear as a single lump, a pale or red nodule just below the skin surface, a swelling, a dimpling of the skin, or a red rash. Report any of these changes to a physician immediately.
- Notify physician of any suspicious changes in lymph nodes; note the presence of lymphadenopathy and describe the location and any observed or palpable characteristics.
- Presence of any of the early warning signs of cancer, including idiopathic muscle weakness accompanied by decreased DTRs.

- Any unexplained bleeding from any area (e.g., rectum, blood in urine or stool, unusual or unexpected vaginal bleeding, breast, penis, nose, ears, mouth, mole, skin, or scar).
- Any sign or symptom of metastasis in someone with a previous history of cancer (see individual cancer types for specific clinical signs and symptoms; see also Clues to Screening for Cancer).
- Any man with pelvic, groin, sacroiliac, or low back pain accompanied by sciatica and a past history of prostate cancer.

Clues to Screening for Cancer

- Age older than 50 years
- Previous personal history of any cancer, especially in the presence of bilateral carpal tunnel symptoms, back pain, shoulder pain, or joint pain of unknown or rheumatic cause at presentation
- Previous history of cancer treatment (late physical complications and psychosocial complications of disease and treatment can present in a somatic presentation)
- Any woman with chest, breast, axillary, or shoulder pain of unknown cause, especially with a previous history of cancer and/or over the age of 40 years
- Anyone with back, pelvic, groin, or hip pain accompanied by abdominal complaints, palpable mass
- *For women:* Prolonged or excessive menstrual bleeding (or in the case of the postmenopausal woman who is not taking hormone replacement, breakthrough bleeding)
- *For men:* Additional presence of sciatica and past history of prostate cancer
- Recent weight loss of 10% of total body weight (or more) within a 2-week to 1-month period of time without trying; weight gain is more typical with true musculoskeletal dysfunction because pain has limited physical activities

- Musculoskeletal symptoms are made better or worse by eating or drinking (GI involvement)
- Shoulder, back, hip, pelvic, or sacral pain accompanied by changes in bowel and/or bladder function or changes in stool or urine
- Hip or groin pain is reproduced by heel strike/hopping test or translational/rotational stress (bone fracture from metastases)
- When a back "injury" is not improving as expected or if symptoms are increasing
- Early warning signs, including proximal muscle weakness and changes in DTRs
- Constant pain (unrelieved by rest or change in position); remember to assess constancy by asking, "Do you have that pain right now?"
- Intense pain present at night (rated 7 or higher on a numeric scale from 0 for "no pain" to 10 for "worst pain")
- Signs of nerve root compression must be screened for cancer as a possible cause
- Development of new neurologic deficits (e.g., weakness, sensory loss, reflex change, bowel or bladder dysfunction)
- Change in size, shape, tenderness, and consistency of lymph nodes, especially painless, hard, rubbery lymph nodes present in more than one location
- A growing mass, whether painless or painful, is assumed to be a tumor unless diagnosed otherwise by a physician; a hematoma should decrease in size over time, not increase
- Disproportionate pain relieved with aspirin may be a sign of bone cancer (osteoid osteoma)
- Signs or symptoms seem out of proportion to the injury and persist longer than expected for physiologic healing of that type of injury; no position is comfortable (remember to conduct a screening examination for emotional overlay)
- Change in the status of a client currently being treated for cancer

CANCER PRESENCE AND PAIN

METASTASES (MOST COMMONLY SEEN IN A PHYSICAL THERAPY SETTING)

Location:	Integumentary system
	Pulmonary system
	Neurologic system
	Musculoskeletal
	Hepatic
Referral:	See Table 14.5

SKIN (MELANOMA ONLY)

Location:	Anywhere on the body
	Women: arms, legs, back, face
	Men: head, trunk
	African Americans: palms, soles, under the nails
Referral:	None

CANCER PRESENCE AND PAIN—cont'd

Description:	Usually painless; see ABCDE method of detection
	Sore that does not heal
	Irritation and itching
	Cluster mole formation
	Tenderness and soreness around a mole
Intensity:	Mild
Duration:	Constant
Associated Signs and Symptoms:	None

PARANEOPLASTIC SYNDROMES

Location:	Remote sites from primary neoplasm
Referral:	Organ dependent
Description:	Asymmetric joint involvement
	Lower extremities primarily
	Concurrent arthritis and malignancy
	Explosive onset at late age
	See Table 14.6 and Box 14.4
Intensity:	Symptom dependent
Duration:	Symptom dependent
Associated Signs and Symptoms:	Fever
	Skin rash
	Clubbing of the fingers
	Pigmentation disorders
	Arthralgia
	Paresthesia
	Thrombophlebitis
	Proximal muscle weakness
	Anorexia, malaise, weight loss
	Rheumatologic complaints

ONCOLOGIC (CANCER) PAIN

Location:	Localized bone pain; referred pain
Referral:	May follow nerve distribution
Description:	Bone pain: sharp, intense, constant
	Viscera: colicky, cramping, dull, diffuse, boring, poorly localized
	Vein, artery, lymphatic channel: dull, diffuse, burning, aching
	Nerve compression: sharp, stabbing; follows nerve distribution or dull, poorly localized
	Inflammation: sensitive tenderness
Intensity:	Varies from mild to severe or excruciating
	Bone pain: increases during movement or weight-bearing
Duration:	Usually constant; may be worse at night
Associated Signs and Symptoms:	With mild-to-moderate superficial pain: sympathetic nervous system response (e.g., hypertension, tachycardia, tachypnea)
	With severe or visceral pain: parasympathetic nervous system response (e.g., hypotension, tachypnea, weakness, fainting)
	Organ dependent (e.g., esophagus: difficulty eating or speaking; gallbladder: jaundice, nausea; nerve involvement: altered sensation, paresthesia; see individual visceral cancers)

Continued

CANCER PRESENCE AND PAIN—cont'd

SOFT TISSUE TUMORS

Location:	Any connective tissue (e.g., tendon muscle, cartilage, fat, synovium, fibrous tissue)
Referral:	According to the tissue involved
Description:	Persistent swelling or lump, especially in the muscle
Intensity:	Mild, increases progressively to severe
Duration:	Intermittent, increases progressively to constant
Associated Signs and Symptoms:	Local swelling with tenderness and skin warmth Pathologic fracture

BONE TUMORS

Location:	Can affect any bone in the body, depending on the specific type of bone cancer
Referral:	According to pattern and location of metastases
Description:	Sharp, knife-like, aching bone pain Occurs during movement and weight-bearing, with pathologic fractures Pain at night, preventing sleep
Intensity:	Initially mild, progressing to severe
Duration:	Usually intermittent, progressing to constant
Associated Signs and Symptoms:	Fatigue and malaise Significant unintentional weight loss Swelling and warmth over localized areas of tumor Soft, tender palpable mass over bone Loss of range of motion and joint function if limb bone is involved Fever Sciatica Unilateral edema

PRIMARY CENTRAL NERVOUS SYSTEM: BRAIN TUMORS

Location:	Intracranial
Referral:	Specific symptoms depend on tumor location Headache
Description:	Bioccipital or bifrontal headache
Intensity:	Mild to severe
Duration:	Worse in morning when awakening Diminishes or disappears soon after rising
Aggravating Factors:	Activity that increases intracranial pressure (e.g., straining during bowel movements, stooping, lifting heavy objects, coughing, bending over) Prone/supine position at night during sleep
Relieving Factors:	Pain medications, including aspirin or acetaminophen

Associated Signs and Symptoms:	Papilledema
	Altered mentation:
	    Increased sleeping
	    Difficulty in concentrating
	    Memory loss
	    Increased irritability
	    Poor judgment
	    Vomiting unrelated to food, accompanies headaches
	    Seizures

CANCER PRESENCE AND PAIN—cont'd

Neurologic findings:
  Positive Babinski reflex
  Clonus (ankle or wrist)
  Sensory changes
  Decreased coordination
  Ataxia
  Muscle weakness
  Increased lower extremity deep tendon reflexes
  Transient paralysis

PRIMARY CENTRAL NERVOUS SYSTEM: SPINAL CORD TUMORS

Location:	Intramedullary (within the spinal cord)
	Extramedullary (within the dura mater)
	Extradural (outside the dura mater)
Referral:	Back pain at the level of the spinal cord lesion
	Pain may extend to the groin or legs
Description:	Dull ache; sharp, knife-like sensation
Intensity:	Mild to severe, progressive; night pain
Duration:	Intermittent, progressing to constant, or constant
Aggravating Factors:	(Back pain) Lying down/rest
	Weight-bearing
	Sneezing or coughing
Associated Signs and Symptoms:	Muscle weakness
	Muscle atrophy
	Sensory loss
	Paraplegia/quadriplegia
	Chest or abdominal pain
	Bowel/bladder dysfunction (late findings)

LEUKEMIA

Location:	Usually painless; may have pain in the left abdomen; bone and joint pain possible
Referral:	None
Description:	Dull pain in the abdomen; may occur only during palpation
Intensity:	Mild to moderate
Duration:	Intermittent (with applied pressure)
Associated Signs and Symptoms:	Enlarged lymph nodes
	Unusual bleeding from the nose or rectum, or blood in urine
	Prolonged menstruation
	Easy bruising of the skin
	Fatigue
	Dyspnea
	Weight loss, loss of appetite
	Fevers and sweats

Continued

CANCER PRESENCE AND PAIN—cont'd

MULTIPLE MYELOMA

Location:	Skeletal pain, especially in the spine, sternum, rib, leg, or arm
Referral:	According to the location of the tumor
Description:	Sharp, knife-like
Intensity:	Moderate to severe
Duration:	Intermittent, progressing to constant
Associated Signs and Symptoms:	Hypercalcemia: dehydration (vomiting), polyuria, confusion, loss of appetite, constipation Bone destruction with spontaneous bone fracture Neurologic: CTS; back pain with radicular symptoms; spinal cord compression (motor or sensory loss, bowel/bladder dysfunction, paraplegia)

HODGKIN'S DISEASE

Location:	Lymph nodes, usually unilateral neck or groin
Referral:	According to the location of the metastasis
Description:	Usually painless, progressive enlargement of lymph nodes
Intensity:	Not applicable
Duration:	Not applicable
Associated Signs and Symptoms:	Fever peaks in the late afternoon, night sweats Anorexia and weight loss Severe itching over the entire body Anemia, fatigue, malaise Jaundice Edema Nonproductive cough, dyspnea, chest pain, cyanosis

NON-HODGKIN'S LYMPHOMA (INCLUDING AIDS-NHL)

Location:	Peripheral lymph nodes
Referral:	Not applicable
Description:	Usually painless enlargement
Intensity:	Not applicable
Duration:	Not applicable
Associated Signs and Symptoms:	Constitutional symptoms (fever, night sweats, weight loss) Bleeding Generalized itching and reddened skin AIDS-NHL: musculoskeletal lesions, subcutaneous nodules

■ **Key Points to Remember**

1. When put to the task of screening for cancer, always remember our three basic clues:
   - Past Medical History
   - Clinical Presentation
   - Associated Signs and Symptoms
2. Any suspicious lesions or red-flag symptoms, especially in the presence of a past medical history of cancer or risk factors for cancer, should be investigated further. With the increasing number of people diagnosed with cancer, recognizing hallmark findings of cancer is important.
3. Knowing the systems most often affected by cancer metastasis and the corresponding clinical manifestations is a good starting point. Any time a client reports a past medical history of cancer, we must be alert for signs or indications of cancer recurrence (locally or via metastasis).
4. Knowing the most common risk factors for cancer in general and risk factors for specific cancers is the next step. Risk factor assessment and cancer prevention are a part of every health care professional's role as an educator and in primary prevention.
5. Whether you are working in an oncology setting or in a general practice with an occasional client, good resource information is available. An example of a web resource with thorough, reliable, and up-to-date information about specific types of cancer, cancer treatments, and recent breakthroughs in cancer research is https://www. oncolink.org/, affiliated with The Abramson Cancer Center of the University of Pennsylvania (Philadelphia).
6. Spinal malignancy involves the lumbar spine more often than the cervical spine and is usually metastatic rather than primary.
7. Spinal cord compression from metastases may appear as back pain, leg weakness, and bowel/bladder symptoms.
8. Fifty percent of clients with back pain from a malignancy have an identifiable preceding trauma or injury to account for the pain or symptoms. Always remember that clients may erroneously attribute symptoms to an event.
9. Back pain may precede the development of neurologic signs and symptoms in any person with cancer.
10. The presence of jaundice in association with any atypical presentation of back pain may indicate liver metastasis.
11. Signs of nerve root compression may be the first indication of cancer, in particular, lymphoma, multiple myeloma, or cancer of the lung, breast, prostate, or kidney.
12. The five most common sites of metastasis are the lymph nodes, liver, lung, bone, and brain.
13. Lung, breast, prostate, thyroid, and the lymphatics are the primary sites responsible for most metastatic bone disease.
14. Monitoring physiologic responses (vital signs) to exercise is important in the immunosuppressed population. Watch closely for early signs (dyspnea, pallor, sweating, and fatigue) of cardiopulmonary complications of cancer treatment.
15. To determine appropriate exercise levels for clients who are immunosuppressed, review blood test results (WBCs, RBCs, hematocrit, platelets). When these are not available, monitor vital signs and use RPE as a guideline. However, do not use blood test results as the sole parameter for exercise prescription.
16. Besides the seven early warning signs of cancer, the therapist should watch for idiopathic muscle weakness accompanied by decreased DTRs.
17. Change in size, shape, tenderness, and consistency of lymph nodes raises a red flag. Supraclavicular nodes and inguinal nodes are common metastatic sites for cancer.
18. No reliable physical signs distinguish between benign and malignant soft tissue lesions. All soft tissue lumps that persist or grow should be reported immediately to the physician.
19. Malignancy is always a possibility in children with musculoskeletal symptoms.

CLIENT HISTORY AND INTERVIEW

SPECIAL QUESTIONS TO ASK

Special questions to ask will vary with each client and the clinical signs and symptoms presented at the time of evaluation. The therapist should refer to the specific chapter representing the client's current complaints. The case study provided here is one example of how to follow up with necessary questions to rule out a systemic origin of musculoskeletal findings.

A previous history of drug therapy and current drug use may be important information to obtain because prolonged use of drugs such as phenytoin (Dilantin) or immunosuppressive drugs such as azathioprine (Imuran) and cyclosporine may lead to cancer. Postmenopausal use of estrogens has been linked with breast cancer.[188]

Past Medical History

A previous personal/family history of cancer may be significant, especially any history of breast, colorectal, or lung cancer that demonstrates genetic susceptibility.

CLIENT HISTORY AND INTERVIEW—cont'd

- Have you ever had cancer or do you have cancer now?
  If no, have you ever received chemotherapy, hormone therapy, or radiation therapy?
  If yes, what was the treatment for?
  If yes to previous history of cancer, ask about type of cancer, date of diagnosis, stage (if known), treatment, and date of most recent follow-up visit with oncologist or other cancer specialist.
- Has your physician said that you are cancer-free?
- Have you ever been exposed to chemical agents or irritants, such as asbestos, asphalt, aniline dyes, benzene, herbicides, fertilizers, wood dust, or others? (**Environmental causes of cancer;** see complete environmental/occupational screening survey in Chapter 2 and Appendix B-14 in the accompanying enhanced eBook version included with print purchase of this textbook)

Clinical Presentation: Early Warning Signs

When using the seven early warning signs of cancer as a basis for screening (see Box 14.2), one or all of the following questions may be appropriate:

- Have you noticed any change in your bowel movement or in the flow of urination?
  - *If yes*, ask pertinent follow-up questions as suggested in Chapter 10; see also Appendix B-5 in the accompanying enhanced eBook version included with print purchase of this textbook.
  - *If the client answers no*, it may be necessary to provide prompts or examples of what changes you are referring to (e.g., difficulty in starting or continuing the flow of urine, numbness or tingling in the groin or pelvis).
- Have you noticed any sores that have not healed properly?
  - *If yes*, where are they located? How long has the sore been present? Has your physician examined this area?
- Have you noticed any unusual bleeding (*for women:* including prolonged menstruation or *any* bleeding for the postmenopausal woman who is not taking hormone replacement) or prolonged discharge from any part of your body?
  - *If yes*, where? How long has this been present? Has your physician examined this area?
- Have you noticed any thickening or lump of any muscle, tendon, bone, breast, or anywhere else?
  - *If yes*, where? How long has this been present? Has your physician examined this area?*
  - *If no (for women):* Do you examine your own breasts? How often do you examine yourself?
- When was the last time you did a breast self-examination (see Appendix D-6 in the accompanying enhanced eBook version included with print purchase of this textbook)?

- Do you have any pain, swelling, or unusual tenderness in the breasts? (**Pain can be a symptom of cancer; cyclic pain is common with normal breasts, use of oral contraceptives, and fibrocystic disease.**)
  - *If yes*, is this pain brought on by strenuous activity? (**Spontaneous/systemic or related to specific musculoskeletal cause** [e.g., use of one arm])
- Have you noticed any rash on the breast or discharge from the nipple? (**Medications such as oral contraceptives, phenothiazines, diuretics, digitalis, tricyclic tranquilizers, reserpine, methyldopa, and steroids can cause clear discharge from the nipple; blood-tinged discharge is always significant.**)
- Have you noticed any difficulty in eating or swallowing? Have you had a chronic cough, recurrent laryngitis, hoarseness, or any difficulty with speaking?
  - *If yes*, how long has this been happening? Have you discussed this with your physician?
- Have you had any change in your digestive pattern? Have you had increasing indigestion or unusual constipation?
  - *If yes*, how long has this been happening? Have you discussed this with your physician?
- Have you had a recent, sudden weight loss without dieting? (**10% of client's total body weight in 10 days to 2 weeks is significant.**)
- Have you noticed any obvious change in color, shape, or size of a wart or mole?
  - *If yes*, what have you noticed? How long has this wart or mole been present? Have you discussed this problem with your physician?
- Have you had any unusual headaches or change in vision?
  - *If yes*, please describe. (**Brain tumors: bioccipital or bifrontal**)
  - Can you attribute these to anything in particular?
  - Do you vomit (unrelated to food) when your headache occurs? (**Brain tumors**)
- Have you been more tired than usual or experienced persistent fatigue during the last month?
- Can you think of any time during the past week when you may have bumped yourself, fallen, or injured yourself in any way? (Ask when in the presence of local swelling and tenderness.) (**Bone tumors**)
- Have you noticed any bone pain or problems with any of your bones? Is the pain affected by movement? (**Fractures cause sharp pain that increases with movement. Bone pain from systemic causes usually feels dull and deep and is unrelated to movement.**)

Associated Signs and Symptoms

- Are you having any symptoms of any kind anywhere else in your body?

---

* An asymptomatic mass that has been present for years and causes only cosmetic concern is usually benign, whereas a painful mass of short duration that has caused a decrease in function may be malignant.

CASE STUDY

REFERRAL

A 56-year-old man has come to you for an evaluation without referral. He has not been examined by a physician of any kind for at least 3 years. He is seeking an evaluation on the insistence of his wife, who has noticed that his collar size has increased two sizes in the last year and that his neck looks "puffy." He has no complaints of any kind (including pain or discomfort), and he denies any known trauma, but his wife insists that he has limited ability in turning his head when backing the car out of the driveway.

PHYSICAL THERAPY SCREENING INTERVIEW

First, read the client's Family/Personal History form with particular interest in his personal or family history of cancer, presence of allergies or asthma, use of medications or over-the-counter drugs, previous surgeries, available x-ray studies of the neck or spine, and/or history of cigarette smoking (or other tobacco use).

An appropriate lead-in to the following series of questions may be: "Because you have not seen a physician before your appointment with me, I will ask you a series of questions to find out if your symptoms require examination by a physician rather than treatment in this office."

CURRENT SYMPTOMS

- What have you noticed different about your neck that brings you here today?
- When did you first notice that your neck was changing (in size or shape)?
- Can you remember having any accidents, falls, twists, or any other kind of potential trauma at that time?
- Do you ever notice any pain, stiffness, soreness, or discomfort in your neck or shoulders?
- If *yes*, please describe (as per the outline in the Core Interview, Chapter 2).
- Does this or any pain ever awaken you at night or keep you awake? (**Night pain associated with cancer**)
  - If *yes*, follow-up with appropriate questions (see the Core Interview, Chapter 2).

ASSOCIATED SYMPTOMS

- Have you noticed any numbness or tingling in your arms or hands?
- Have you noticed any swollen glands, lumps, or thickened areas of skin or muscle in your neck, armpits, or groin? (**Cancer screen**)
- Do you have any difficulty in swallowing? Do you have recurrent hoarseness, flu-like symptoms, or a persistent cough or cold that never seems to go away? (**Cancer screen**)
- Have you noticed any low-grade fevers or night sweats? (**Systemic disease**)
- Have you had any recent unexplained weight gain or loss? (You may need to explain that you mean a gain or loss of 10 lbs to 15 lbs in as many days without dieting.) Have you had a loss of appetite? (**Cancer screen or other systemic disease**)
- Do you ever have any difficulty with breathing or find yourself short of breath at rest or after minimal exercise? (**Dyspnea**)
- Do you have frequent headaches, or do you experience any dizziness, nausea, or vomiting? (**Systemic disease, carotid artery affected**)

FUNCTIONAL CAPACITY

- What kind of work do you do?
- Do you have any limitations caused by this condition that affects you in any way at work or at home? (**Occupational disease, limitations of activities of daily living [ADL] skills**)

FINAL QUESTIONS

- How would you describe your general health?
- Have you ever been diagnosed with cancer of any kind?
- Is there anything that you would like to tell me that you think is important about your neck or your health in general?

FIRST VISIT: ASSESSING THE MUSCULOSKELETAL SYSTEM

- Observation/Inspection
- Observe for the presence of swelling anywhere, tender or swollen lymph nodes (cervical, supraclavicular, and axillary), changes in skin temperature, and unusual moles or warts. Perform a brief posture screen (general postural observations may be made while you are interviewing the client). Palpate for carotid artery and upper extremity pulses. Check vital signs and **take the client's temperature!**
- Cervical active range of motion (AROM)/passive range of motion (PROM)
- Assess for muscle tightness, loss of joint motion (including accessory movements, if indicated by a loss of passive motion). Assess for compromise of the vertebral artery, and if negative, clear the cervical spine by using a quadrant test with overpressure (e.g., Spurling's test) and assess accessory movements of the cervical spine. Perform tests for thoracic outlet syndrome. Palpate the anterior cervical spine for pathologic protrusion while the client swallows.

CASE STUDY—cont'd

- Temporomandibular joint (TMJ) screen
- Clear the joint above (i.e., TMJ) using AROM, observation, and palpation specific to the TMJ.
- Shoulder screen
- Clear the joint below (i.e., shoulder) by using a screening examination (e.g., AROM/PROM and quadrant testing).
- Neurologic screen (see Chapter 4)

DTRs, sensory screen (e.g., gross sensory testing for light touch), manual muscle test (MMT) screening using break testing of the upper quadrant, grip strength. If the test(s) is abnormal, consider further neurologic testing (e.g., balance, coordination, stereognosis, in-depth sensory examination, dysmetria). Ask about the presence of recent change in vision, headache, numbness, or tingling into the jaw or down the arm(s).

It is always recommended that the therapist give the client ongoing verbal feedback during the examination regarding evaluation results, such as: "I notice you cannot turn your head to the right as much as you can to the left—from checking your muscles and joints, it looks like muscle tightness, not any loss of joint movement." or "I notice your reflexes on each side are not the same (your right arm reacts more strongly than the left)—let me see if we can find out why."

RECOMMENDATION FOR PHYSICIAN VISIT

- I noticed on your intake form that you have not listed the name of a personal or family physician. Do you have a physician?
- If *yes*, when was the last time you saw your physician? Have you seen your physician for this current problem?

Give the client a brief summary of your findings while making your recommendations, for example, "Mr. X, I noticed today that although you do not have any ongoing neck pain, the lymph nodes in your neck and armpit are enlarged but not particularly tender. Otherwise, all of my findings are negative. Your loss of motion while turning your head is not unusual

for a person your age and certainly would not cause your neck to increase in size or shape. Given the fact that you have not seen a physician for almost 3 years, I strongly recommend that you see a physician of your choice, or I can give you the names of several to choose from. In either case, I think some medical tests are necessary to rule out any underlying medical problem. For instance, a neck x-ray examination would be recommended before physical therapy treatment is started."

If the client has indicated a positive family history of cancer, it might be appropriate to suggest, "Given your positive family history of previous medical illnesses, the 3 years since you have seen a physician, and the lack of musculoskeletal findings, I strongly recommend …" It is important to provide the client with all the information available to you but without causing undue alarm and emotional stress, which could actually prevent the client from seeking further testing.

If the client does give the name of a physician, you may ask for written permission (disclosure release) to send a copy of your results to the physician. If the client does not have a physician and requests recommendations from you, you may offer to send a copy of your results to the physician with whom the client makes an appointment.

If you think that a problem may be potentially serious and you want this person to receive adequate follow-up without causing alarm, you may offer to let him make the appointment from your office, suggest that your administrative assistant or receptionist make the appointment for him, or even offer to make the initial telephone contact yourself.

RESULTS

This client did comply with the therapist's suggestion to see a physician and was diagnosed with Hodgkin's disease (a cancer of the lymph system) without constitutional symptoms (i.e., without evidence of weight loss, fever, or night sweats). Medical intervention was initiated and physical therapy treatment was not warranted.

PRACTICE QUESTIONS

1. Name three predisposing factors to cancer that the therapist must watch for during the interview process as red flags.
2. How do you monitor exercise levels in the oncology patient without laboratory values?
3. Complete the following mnemonic:
   C
   A
   U
   T
   I
   O
   N
   S
4. Whenever a therapist observes, palpates, or receives a client report of a lump or nodule, what three questions must be asked?
5. Give a general *description* and *explanation* of the changes seen in deep tendon reflexes associated with cancer.
6. Why is weight loss a significant red-flag sign in a physical therapy practice?

7. When tumors produce signs and symptoms at a site distant from the tumor or its metastasized sites, these "remote effects" of malignancy are called:
   a. Bone metastases
   b. Vitiligo
   c. Paraneoplastic syndrome
   d. Ichthyosis

8. A suspicious skin lesion requiring medical evaluation has:
   a. Round, symmetric borders
   b. Notched edges
   c. Matching halves when a line is drawn down the middle
   d. A single color of brown or tan

9. What is the significance of Beau's lines in a client treated with chemotherapy for leukemia?
   a. Impaired nail formation from death of cells
   b. Temporary longitudinal groove or ridge through the nail
   c. Increased production of the nail by the matrix as a sign of healing
   d. A sign of local trauma

10. A 16-year-old boy was hurt in a soccer game. He presents with exquisite right ankle pain while weight-bearing but reports no pain at night. Upon further questioning, you find he is taking ibuprofen at night before bed, which may be masking his pain. What other screening examination procedures are warranted?
    a. Perform a heel strike test.
    b. Review response to treatment.
    c. Assess for signs of fracture (edema, exquisite tenderness to palpation, warmth over the painful site).
    d. All of the above.

11. When is it advised to take a work or military history?
    a. Anyone with head and/or neck pain who uses a cell phone more than 8 hours/day
    b. Anyone over the age of 50 years
    c. Anyone presenting with joint pain of unknown cause accompanied by multiple other signs and symptoms
    d. This is outside the scope of a physical therapist's practice

12. A 70-year-old man came to outpatient physical therapy with a complaint of pain and weakness of his fingers and morning stiffness lasting about an hour. He presented with bilateral swelling of the metacarpophalangeal (MCP) joints of the index and ring fingers. He saw his family doctor 4 weeks ago and was given diclofenac, which has not changed his symptoms. Now he wants to try physical therapy. Since he last saw his physician, he has developed additional joint pain in the left knee and right shoulder. How can you tell if this is cancer, polyarthritis, or a paraneoplastic disorder?
    a. Ask about a previous history of cancer and recent onset of skin rash.
    b. You cannot. This requires a medical evaluation.
    c. Look for signs of digital clubbing, cellulitis, or proximal muscle weakness.
    d. Assess vital signs.

13. A 49-year-old man was treated by you for bilateral synovitis of the proximal interphalangeal (PIP) joints in the second, third, and fourth fingers. His symptoms went away with treatment, and he was discharged. Six weeks later, he returned with the same symptoms. There was obvious soft tissue swelling with morning stiffness worse than before. He also reports problems with his bowels but is not able to tell you exactly what is wrong. There are no other changes in his health. He is not taking any medications or over-the-counter drugs and does not want to see a doctor. Are there enough red flags to warrant medical evaluation before resumption of physical therapy intervention?
    a. Yes; age, bilateral symptoms, progression of symptoms, report of GI distress.
    b. No; treatment was effective before—it is likely that he has done something to exacerbate his symptoms and needs further education about joint protection.

14. A client with a past medical history of kidney transplantation (10 years ago) has been referred to you for a diagnosis of rheumatoid arthritis. His medications include tacrolimus, methotrexate, Fosamax, and Wellbutrin. During the examination, you notice a painless lump under the skin in the right upper anterior chest. There is a loss of hair over the area. What other symptoms should you look for as red-flag signs and symptoms in a client with this history?
    a. Fever, muscle weakness, weight loss
    b. Change in deep tendon reflexes, bone pain
    c. Productive cough, pain during inspiration
    d. Nosebleeds or other signs of excessive bleeding

15. A 55-year-old man with a left shoulder impingement also has palpable axillary lymph nodes on both sides. They are firm but movable, about the size of an almond. What steps should you take?
    a. Examine other areas where lymph nodes can be palpated.
    b. Ask about history of cancer, allergies, or infections.
    c. Document your findings and contact the physician with your concerns.
    d. All of the above.

REFERENCES

1. Siegel RL, Miller KD, Jemal A. Cancer statistics, 2020. *CA: A Cancer J Clin.* 2020;70(1):7–30. https://doi.org/10.3322/caac.21590.
2. National Comprehensive Cancer Network. NCCN Practice Guidelines in Oncology. Older Adult Oncology (Version 1.2020). https://www.nccn.org/professionals/physician_gls/pdf/senior.pdf. Accessed August 27, 2020.
3. Henley SJ, Ward EM, Scott S, et al. Annual report to the nation on the status of cancer, part I: National cancer statistics. *Cancer.* 2020;126:2225–2249. https://doi.org/10.1002/cncr.32802.
4. National Comprehensive Cancer Network. NCCN Practice Guidelines in Oncology. Survivorship (Version 2.2020). https://www.nccn.org/professionals/physician_gls/pdf/survivorship.pdf. Accessed August 27, 2020.
5. Howlader N, Noone AM, Krapcho M, et al. (eds). SEER Cancer Statistics Review, 1975-2017. Bethesda, MD: National Cancer Institute. https://seer.cancer.gov/csr/1975_2017/, posted to the SEER web site, April 2020. Accessed August 27, 2020.
6. Oeffinger KC, Mertens AC, Hudson MM, et al. Health care of young adult survivors of childhood cancer: a report from the Childhood Cancer Survivor Study. *Ann Fam Med.* 2004;2:61–70.
7. Robison LL, Hudson MM. Survivors of childhood and adolescent cancer: life-long risks and responsibilities. *Nat Rev Cancer.* 2014;14(1):61–70. https://doi.org/10.1038/nrc3634.
8. St. Jude Children's Research Hospital. The Childhood Cancer Survivor Study (CCSS). https://ccss.stjude.org/ Accessed August 27, 2020.
9. PDQ® Pediatric Treatment Editorial Board. *PDQ Late Effects of Treatment for Childhood Cancer.* Bethesda, MD: National

Cancer Institute. Updated 08/11/2020. https://www.cancer.gov/types/childhood-cancers/late-effects-hp-pdq. Accessed August 27, 2020. [PMID: 26389273]

10. Galligan AJ. Childhood cancer survivorship and long-term outcomes. *Adv Pediatr.* 2017;64(1):133–169. https://doi.org/10.1016/j.yapd.2017.03.014.

11. Penny LK, Wallace HM. The challenges for cancer chemoprevention. *Chem Soc Rev.* 2015;44(24):8836–8847. https://doi.org/10.1039/c5cs00705d.

12. Guide to Physical Therapist Practice 3.0. Alexandria, VA: American Physical Therapy Association; 2015. http://guidetoptpractice.apta.org/. Accessed August 27, 2020.

13. American Cancer Society *Cancer Prevention & Early Detection Facts & Figures 2019-2020.* Atlanta: American Cancer Society; 2019.

14. Pilleron S, Sarfati D, Janssen-Heijnen M, et al. Global cancer incidence in older adults, 2012 and 2035: a population-based study. *Int J Cancer.* 2019;144:49–58. https://doi.org/10.1002/ijc.31664.

15. American Cancer Society *Cancer Facts and Figures for African Americans 2019-2021.* Atlanta: American Cancer Society; 2019.

16. DeSantis CE, Miller KD, Goding Sauer A, Jemal A, Siegel RL. Cancer statistics for African Americans, 2019. *CA Cancer J Clin.* 2019;69:211–233. https://doi.org/10.3322/caac.21555.

17. Rhoads KF, Patel MI, Ma Y, Schmidt LA. How do integrated health care systems address racial and ethnic disparities in colon cancer? *J Clin Oncol.* 2015;33(8):854–860. https://doi.org/10.1200/JCO.2014.56.8642.

18. Collins Y, Holcomb K, Chapman-Davis E, Khabele D, Farley JH. Gynecologic cancer disparities: a report from the health disparities taskforce of the society of gynecologic oncology. *Gynecol Oncol.* 2014;133:353–361. https://doi.org/10.1016/j.ygyno.2013.12.039.

19. Institute of Medicine (IOM) *Unequal Treatment, Confronting Racial and Ethnic Disparities in Health Care.* Washington DC: IOM; 2003. https://www.nationalacademies.org/hmd/~/media/Files/Report%20Files/2003/Unequal-Treatment-Confronting-Racial-and-Ethnic-Disparities-in-Health-Care/Disparitieshcproviders8pgFINAL.pdf. Accessed July 31, 2016.

20. Six Domains of Health Care Quality. Agency for Healthcare Research and Quality, Rockville, MD. https://www.ahrq.gov/talkingquality/measures/six-domains.html. Accessed 12/15/2020.

21. IOM (Institute of Medicine) *How Far have we Come in Reducing Health Disparities? Progress Since 2000: Workshop Summary.* Washington DC: The National Academies Press; 2012.

22. Miller KD, Sauer AG, Ortiz AP, et al. Cancer statistics for Hispanics/ Latinos, 2018. *CA: A Cancer J Clin.* 2018;68:425–445.

23. Uninsured Rates for the Non-elderly by Race/Ethnicity. State Health Facts. Kaiser Family Foundation. https://www.kff.org/uninsured/state-indicator/nonelderly-uninsured-rate-by-race ethnicity/?currentTimeframe=0&sortModel=%7B%22colId%22:%22Location%22,%22sort%22:%22asc%22%7D. Accessed December 15, 2020.

24. Ziogas A. Clinically relevant changes in family history of cancer over time. *JAMA.* 2011;306:172–178.

25. Drake I, Dias JA, Teleka S, Stocks T, Orho-Melander M. Lifestyle and cancer incidence and mortality risk depending on family history of cancer in two prospective cohorts. *Int J Cancer.* 2020;146(5):1198–1207. http://doi.org/10.1002/ijc.32397. Epub 2019 May 21. PMID: 31077359.

26. Sifri R, Gangadharappa S, Acheson L. Identifying and testing for hereditary susceptibility to common cancers. *CA Cancer J Clin.* 2004;54:309–326.

27. Rahner N, Steinke V. Hereditary cancer syndromes. *Dtsch Arztebl.* 2008;105(41):706–714.

28. Hereditary cancer syndromes and risk assessment: ACOG COMMITTEE OPINION, Number 793. *Obstet Gynecol* 2019;134(6):e143–e149. https://doi.org/10.1097/AOG.0000000000003562. PMID: 31764758.

29. Kulkarni A, Carley H. Advances in the recognition and management of hereditary cancer. *Br Med Bull.* 2016;120(1):123–138. https://doi.org/10.1093/bmb/ldw046. Epub 2016 Nov 23. PMID: 27941041.

30. PDQ® Cancer Genetics Editorial Board. PDQ cancer genetics risk assessment and counseling. Bethesda, MD: National Cancer Institute. Updated <MM/DD/YYYY>. https://www.cancer.gov/about-cancer/causes-prevention/genetics/risk-assessment-pdq. Accessed December 15, 2020Fbox. [PMID: 26389258].

31. World Cancer Research Fund/American Institute for Cancer Research. diet, nutrition, physical activity and cancer: a global perspective. Continuous Expert Project Report 2018. https://www.wcrf.org/dietandcancer. Accessed December 15, 2020.

32. Cancer Prevention. Arlington, VA: American Institute for Cancer Research. https://www.aicr.org/cancer-prevention/. Accessed December 15, 2020.

33. Calle EE, Rodriquez C, Walker-Thurmond K, Thun MJ. Overweight, obesity, and mortality from cancer in a prospectively studied cohort of U.S. adults. *N Engl J Med.* 2003;348:1625–1638.

34. Harriss DJ. Lifestyle factors and colorectal cancer risk: systematic review and meta-analysis of associations with mass index. *Colorectal Dis.* 2009;11(6):547–563.

35. Roberts DL. Biological mechanisms linking obesity and cancer risk: new perspectives. *Ann Rev Med.* 2010;61:301–316.

36. Key TJ, Schatzkin A, Willett WC, Allen NE, Spencer EA, Travis RC. Diet, nutrition, and the prevention of cancer. *Public Health Nutr.* 2004;7:187–200.

37. Patel AV, Rodriquez C, Bernstein L, Chao A, Thun MJ, Calle EE. Obesity, recreational physical activity, and risk of pancreatic cancer in a large U.S. cohort. *Cancer Epidemiol Biomarkers Prev.* 2005;14:459–466.

38. Lauby-Secretan B, Scoccianti C, Loomis D, et al. Body fatness and cancer: viewpoint of the IARC working group. *N Engl J Med.* 2016;375:794–798. https://doi.org/10.1056/NEJMsr1606602.

39. Avgerinos KI, Spyrou N, Mantzoros CS, Dalamaga M. Obesity and cancer risk: Emerging biological mechanisms and perspectives. *Metabolism.* 2019;92:121–135. https://doi.org/10.1016/j.metabol.2018.11.001. Epub 2018 Nov 13. PMID: 30445141.

40. De Pergola G, Silvestris F. Obesity as a major risk factor for cancer. *J Obes.* 2013;2013:291546 https://doi.org/10.1155/2013/291546. Epub 2013 Aug 29. PMID: 24073332; PMCID: PMC3773450.

41. Grosso G, Bella F, Godos J, et al. Possible role of diet in cancer: systematic review and multiple meta-analyses of dietary patterns, lifestyle factors, and cancer risk. *Nutr Rev.* 2017;75(6):405–419. https://doi.org/10.1093/nutrit/nux012. PMID: 28969358.

42. Hopkins BD, Goncalves MD, Cantley LC. Obesity and cancer mechanisms: cancer metabolism. *J Clin Oncol.* 2016;34(35):4277–4283. https://doi.org/10.1200/JCO.2016.67.9712. Epub 2016 Nov 7. PMID: 27903152; PMCID: PMC5562429.

43. Nimptsch K, Pischon T. Obesity biomarkers, metabolism and risk of cancer: an epidemiological perspective. *Recent Results Cancer Res.* 2016;208:199–217. https://doi.org/10.1007/978-3-319-42542-9_11. PMID: 27909909.

44. Kohler LN, Garcia DO, Harris RB, Oren E, Roe DJ, Jacobs ET. Adherence to diet and physical activity cancer prevention guidelines and cancer outcomes: a systematic review. *Cancer Epidemiol Biomarkers Prev.* 2016;25(7):1018–1028. https://doi.org/10.1158/1055-9965.EPI-16-0121. Epub 2016 Jun 23. PMID: 27340121; PMCID: PMC4940193.

45. Aune D, Giovannucci E, Boffetta P, et al. Fruit and vegetable intake and the risk of cardiovascular disease, total cancer and all-cause mortality-a systematic review and dose-response meta-analysis of prospective studies. *Int J Epidemiol.* 2017;46(3):1029–1056. https://doi.org/10.1093/ije/dyw319. PMID: 28338764; PMCID: PMC5837313.

46. National Cancer Institute (NCI). Nutrition in Cancer Care 2010. http://www.cancer.gov/about-cancer/treatment/side-effects/appetite-loss/nutrition-pdq#section/all. Accessed July 31, 2016.

47. American Institute for Cancer Research. Diet and Cancer Materials. Food, Nutrition, Physical Activity and the Prevention of Cancer. http://www.aicr.org/assets/docs/pdf/reports/Second_Expert_Report.pdf. Accessed July 31, 2016.

48. American Cancer Society. Nutrition for People with Cancer. http://www.cancer.org/treatment/survivorshipduringandaftertreatment/nutritionforpeoplewithcancer/index?sitearea=M. Accessed July 31, 2016.

49. PDQ® Supportive and Palliative Care Editorial Board. *PDQ Nutrition in Cancer Care.* Bethesda, MD: National Cancer Institute. Updated 05 May 2020. https://www.cancer.gov/about-cancer/treatment/side-effects/appetite-loss/nutrition-hp-pdq. Accessed December 15, 2020. [PMID: 26389293].

50. American Cancer Society Nutrition for People with Cancer. Atlanta, GA: American Cancer Society. https://www.cancer.org/treatment/survivorship-during-and-after-treatment/staying-active/nutrition.html?sitearea=M. Accessed December 15, 2020.

51. U.S. Department of Health and Human Services and U.S. Department of Agriculture. 2015–2020 Dietary Guidelines for Americans. 8 ed. December 2015. http://health.gov/dietaryguidelines/2015/guidelines/. Accessed December 9, 2016.

52. Renehan AG. Interpreting the epidemiological evidence linking obesity and cancer. *Eur J Cancer.* 2010;46(145):2581–2592.

53. U.S. Department of Health and Human Services and U.S. Department of Agriculture. 2020-2025 Dietary Guidelines for Americans. https://www.dietaryguidelines.gov/work-underway. Accessed December 15, 2020.

54. Islami F, Goding Sauer A, Miller KD, et al. Proportion and number of cancer cases and deaths attributable to potentially modifiable risk factors in the United States. *CA Cancer J Clin.* 2018;68(1):31–54. https://doi.org/10.3322/caac.21440. Epub 2017 Nov 21. PMID: 29160902.

55. Drolet M, Bénard É, Boily MC, et al. Population-level impact and herd effects following human papillomavirus vaccination programmes: a systematic review and meta-analysis. *Lancet Infect Dis.* 2015;15(5):565–580. https://doi.org/10.1016/S1473-3099(14)71073-4. Epub 2015 Mar 3. PMID: 25744474; PMCID: PMC5144106.

56. National Cancer Institute. Cancer causes and prevention. HPV and cancer. https://www.cancer.gov/about-cancer/causes-prevention/risk/infectious-agents/hpv-and-cancer. Updated Jan. 10, 2020. Accessed December 15, 2020.

57. Centers for Disease Control and Prevention. Sexually transmitted disease surveillance 2018. Special Focus Profiles. STDs in Adolescents and Young Adults. CDC, Atlanta, GA. Available at https://www.cdc.gov/std/stats18/adolescents.htm#ref2 Accessed December 15, 2020.

58. Fanfair RN, Zaidi A, Taylor LD, Xu F, Gottlieb S, Markowitz L. Trends in seroprevalence of herpes simplex virus type 2 among non-Hispanic blacks and non-Hispanic whites aged 14 to 49 years—United States, 1988–2010. *Sex Transm Dis.* 2013;40(11):860–864.

59. Meites E, Szilagyi PG, Chesson HW, Unger ER, Romero JR, Markowitz LE. Human papillomavirus vaccination for adults: updated recommendations of the advisory committee on immunization practices. *MMWR Morb Mortal Wkly Rep.* 2019;68:698–702. https://doi.org/10.15585/mmwr.mm6832a3external icon.

60. National Vaccine Advisory Committee Overcoming barriers to low HPV vaccine uptake in the united states: recommendations from the national vaccine advisory committee: approved by the national vaccine advisory committee on June 9, 2015. *Public Health Rep.* 2016;131(1):17–25. https://doi.org/10.1177/003335491613100106.

61. NTP (National Toxicology Program) *Report on Carcinogens.* 4th ed. Research Triangle Park, NC: U.S. Department of Health and Human Services, Public Health Service; 2016. https://ntp.niehs.nih.gov/go/roc14. Accessed December 15, 2020.

62. US Justice Department: Radiation Exposure Compensation Program. https://www.justice.gov/civil/common/reca. Accessed December 15, 2020.

63. International Agency for Research on Cancer *Non-ionizing Radiation, Part 2: Radiofrequency Electromagnetic Field.* Lyon, France: IARC; 2013. IARC monographs on the evaluation of carcinogenic risks to humans, Volume 102.

64. National Cancer Institute. Cancer causes and prevention. electromagnetic fields and cancer. NCI, Bethesda, MD. https://www.cancer.gov/about-cancer/causes-prevention/risk/radiation/electromagnetic-fields-fact-sheet#:~:text=Several%20studies%20conducted%20in%20the,leukemia%2C%20brain%20tumors%2C%20and%20male. Updated Jan. 3, 2019. Accessed December 15 2020.

65. Carpenter DO. Human disease resulting from exposure to electromagnetic fields. *Rev Environ Health.* 2013;28(4):159–172. https://doi.org/10.1515/reveh-2013-0016. PMID: 24280284.

66. IARC International Agency for Research on Cancer Working Group on artificial ultraviolet light and skin cancer The association of use of sunbeds with cutaneous malignant melanoma and other skin cancers: a systematic review. *Int J Cancer.* 2007;120:1116–1122.

67. Wehner MR, Chren MM, Nameth D, et al. International prevalence of indoor tanning: a systematic review and meta-analysis. *JAMA Dermatol.* 2014;150(4):390–400. https://doi.org/10.1001/jamadermatol.2013.6896. Erratum in: JAMA Dermatol. 2014 May;150(5):577. PMID: 24477278; PMCID: PMC4117411.

68. Veterans and Agent Orange: Update 2014. http://www.nationalacademies.org/hmd/Reports/2016/Veterans-and-Agent-Orange-Update-2014.aspx. Accessed July 31, 2016.

69. Air Force Health Study (Ranch Hand) Research Assets. http://www.nationalacademies.org/hmd/Activities/Veterans/AirForceHealthStudyResearchAssets.aspx. Accessed July 31, 2016.

70. Jayakody N, Harris EC, Coggon D. Phenoxy herbicides, soft-tissue sarcoma and non-Hodgkin lymphoma: a systematic review of evidence from cohort and case–control studies. *Brit Med Bull.* 2015;114:75–94.

71. National Academies of Sciences, Engineering, and Medicine *Veterans and Agent Orange: Update 11 (2018).* Washington, DC: The National Academies Press; 2018. https://doi.org/10.17226/25137.

72. Committee on the management of the air force health study data and specimens—report to congress; board on the health of select populations; institute of medicine. The Air Force Health Study Assets Research Program. Washington (DC): National Academies Press (US); 2015 Apr 9. 2, The Air Force Health Study.

73. Kreisberg J. Preventive medicine: taking an environmental history. *Integr Med.* 2009;8(5):58–59.

74. National human genome research institute. The Human Genome Project. https://www.genome.gov/human-genome-project. Updated Sept. 16, 2020. Accessed December 15, 2020.

75. Molster CM, Bowman FL, Bilkey GA, et al. The evolution of public health genomics: exploring its past, present, and future.

Front Public Health. 2018;6:247 https://doi.org/10.3389/fpubh.2018.00247. Published 2018 Sep 4.

76. Liu Z, Huang R, Roberts R, Tong W. Toxicogenomics: a 2020 vision. *Trends Pharmacol Sci.* 2019;40(2):92–103. https://doi.org/10.1016/j.tips.2018.12.001. Epub 2018 Dec 26. PMID: 30594306.

77. Basu AK. DNA damage, mutagenesis and cancer. *Int J Mol Sci.* 2018;19(4):970 https://doi.org/10.3390/ijms19040970. Published 2018 Mar 23.

78. Hashimoto N, Nagano H, Tanaka T. The role of tumor suppressor p53 in metabolism and energy regulation, and its implication in cancer and lifestyle-related diseases. *Endocr J.* 2019;66(6):485–496. https://doi.org/10.1507/endocrj.EJ18-0565. Epub 2019 May 18. PMID: 31105124.

79. Winters S, Martin C, Murphy D, Shokar NK. Breast cancer epidemiology, prevention, and screening. *Prog Mol Biol Transl Sci.* 2017;151:1–32. https://doi.org/10.1016/bs.pmbts.2017.07.002. . Epub 2017 Oct 10. PMID: 29096890.

80. Li W, Song LQ, Tan J. Combined effects of CYP1A1 MspI and GSTM1 genetic polymorphisms on risk of lung cancer: an updated meta-analysis. *Tumour Biol.* 2014;35:9281–9290.

81. Classification: National Cancer Institute–SEER. https://training.seer.cancer.gov/disease/categories/classification.html. Accessed December 15, 2020.

82. Monahan F, Sand JK, Neighbors M, Marek JF, Green CJ. *Phipps' Medical-Surgical Nursing: health and illness perspectives (Medical Surgical Nursing: Concepts & Clinical Practice (Phipps)).* 8th ed. St. Louis MO: Mosby; 2006.

83. American Cancer Society. Soft Tissue Sarcoma. What is a soft tissue sarcoma. ACS, Atlanta, GA. Updated May 8, 2019. https://www.cancer.org/cancer/soft-tissue-sarcoma/about/soft-tissue-sarcoma.html. Accessed December 15, 2020.

84. National Cancer Institute. SEER Training Modules. Categories of Cancer. NCI, Bethesda, MD. https://training.seer.cancer.gov/disease/categories/tissues.html. Accessed December 15, 2020.

85. Rose PS, Buchowski JM. Metastatic disease in the thoracic and lumbar spine: evaluation and management. *J Am Acad Orthop Surg.* 2011;19(1):37–48.

86. Ji RC. Lymph nodes and cancer metastasis: new perspectives on the role of intranodal lymphatic sinuses. *Int J Mol Sci.* 2016;18(1):51 https://doi.org/10.3390/ijms18010051. Published 2016 Dec 28.

87. Harrison BT, Brock JE. Contemporary evaluation of breast lymph nodes in anatomic pathology. *Am J Clin Pathol.* 2018;150(1):4–17. https://doi.org/10.1093/ajcp/aqy024.

88. Baldawa P, Shirol P, Alur J, Kulkarni VV. Metastasis: to and fro. *J Oral Maxillofac Pathol.* 2017;21(3):463–464. https://doi.org/10.4103/jomfp.JOMFP_158_17.

89. Hardy E, Fernandez-Patron C. Destroy to rebuild: the connection between bone tissue remodeling and matrix metalloproteinases. *Front Physiol.* 2020;11:47. https://doi.org/10.3389/fphys.2020.00047.

90. Schaaf MB, Garg AD, Agostinis P. Defining the role of the tumor vasculature in antitumor immunity and immunotherapy. *Cell Death Dis.* 2018;9:115. https://doi.org/10.1038/s41419-017-0061-0.

91. Diaz NM, Vrcel V, Centeno BA, Muro-Cacho C. Modes of benign mechanical transport of breast epithelial cells to axillary lymph nodes. *Adv Anat Pathol.* 2005;12:7–9.

92. Saikia KC, Bhattacharyya TD, Bhuyan SK, Bordoloi B, Durgia B, Ahmed F. Local recurrences after curettage and cementing in long bone giant cell tumor. *Indian J Orthop.* 2011;45(2):168–173. https://doi.org/10.4103/0019-5413.77138.

93. Barrientos-Ruiz I, Ortiz-Cruz EJ, Serrano-Montilla J, Bernabeu-Taboada D, Pozo-Kreilinger JJ. Are biopsy tracts a concern for seeding and local recurrence in sarcomas? *Clin Orthop Relat Res.* 2017;475(2):511–518. https://doi.org/10.1007/s11999-016-5090-y.

94. Okada K. Points to notice during the diagnosis of soft tissue tumors according to the "clinical practice guideline on the diagnosis and treatment of soft tissue tumors". *J Orthop Sci.* 2016;21(6):705–712. https://doi.org/10.1016/j.jos.2016.06.012.

95. Cancer Rehabilitation . In: Stubblefield M, ed. *Principles and Practice.* 2 ed. New York: Demos Medical Publishing; 2018.

96. Sweet's syndrome: Mayo Clinic. https://www.mayoclinic.org/diseases-conditions/sweets-syndrome/symptoms-causes/syc-20351117. Accessed December 15, 2020.

97. Villarreal-Villarreal CD, Ocampo-Candiani J, Villarreal-Martínez A. Sweet syndrome: a review and update. *Actas Dermosifiliogr.* 2016;107(5):369–378. English, Spanish. https://doi.org/10.1016/j.ad.2015.12.001. Epub 2016 Jan 27. PMID: 26826881.

98. American Society of Clinical Oncology. Cancer.net. Melanoma: Statistics. Updated Aug. 2020. https://www.cancer.net/cancer-types/melanoma/statistics. Accessed December 15, 2020.

99. American Cancer Society: How to spot skin cancer. https://www.cancer.org/latest-news/how-to-spot-skin-cancer.html. Accessed December 15, 2020.

100. Centers for Disease Control and Prevention. Skin cancer. Melanoma of the skin statistics. Atlanta, GA: CDC. Updated June 8, 2020. https://www.cdc.gov/cancer/skin/statistics/index.htm. Accessed December 15, 2020.

101. Garrett GG, Lowenstein SE, Singer JP, He SY, Arron ST. Trends of skin cancer mortality after transplantation in the United States: 1987–2013. *J Am Acad Dermatol.* 2016;75(1):106–112.

102. Sprangers B, Nair V, Launay-Vacher V, Riella LV, Jhaveri KD. Risk factors associated with post-kidney transplant malignancies: an article from the cancer-kidney international network. *Clin Kidney J.* 2018;11(3):315–329. https://doi.org/10.1093/ckj/sfx122.

103. American Cancer Society. Melanoma skin cancer. key statistics for melanoma skin cancer. Atlanta, GA: ACS. Updated Jan 8, 2020. https://www.cancer.org/cancer/melanoma-skin-cancer/about/key-statistics.html. Accessed December 15, 2020.

104. Coping with symptoms of advanced melanoma: Cancer Research UK. http://www.cancerresearchuk.org/about-cancer/type/melanoma/living/advanced/coping-with-the-symptoms-of-advanced-melanoma. Accessed July 31, 2016.

105. Tsao H, Olazagasti JM, Cordero KM, et al. Early detection of melanoma: reviewing the ABCDEs. *J Am Acad Dermatol.* 2015;72.717–723.

106. National Cancer Institute: SEER Training module. Melanoma Staging. https://training.seer.cancer.gov/melanoma/abstract-code-stage/staging.html. Accessed December 15, 2020.

107. Enders F, Geisenberger C, Jungk C, et al. Prognostic factors and long-term survival in surgically-treated brain metastasis from non-small cell lung cancer. *Clin Neurol Neurosurg.* 2016;142:72–80.

108. Saha A, Ghosh SK, Roy C, Choudhury KB, Chakrabarty B, Sarkar R. Demographic and clinical profile of patients with brain metastases: a retrospective study. *Asian J Neurosurg.* 2013;8(3):157–161. https://doi.org/10.4103/1793-5482.121688.

109. Stubblefield MD, Keole N. Upper body pain and functional disorders in patients with breast cancer. *PM R.* 2014;6:170–183.

110. Jaeckle KA. Neurologic manifestations of neoplastic and radiation-induced plexopathies. *Semin Neurol.* 2014;30:254–262.

111. Comelli I, Lippi G, Campana V, Servadei F, Cervellin G. Clinical presentation and epidemiology of brain tumors firstly diagnosed in adults in the emergency department: a 10-year, single center retrospective study. *Ann Transl Med.* 2017;5(13):269. https://doi.org/10.21037/atm.2017.06.12.

112. Raj VS, Lofton L. Rehabilitation and treatment of spinal cord tumors. *J Spinal Cord Med.* 2013;36(1):4–11. https://doi.org/10.1179/2045772312Y.0000000015.

113. Robson P. Metastatic spinal cord compression: a rare but important complication of cancer. *Clin Med (Lond).*

2014;14(5):542–545. https://doi.org/10.7861/clinmedicine. 14-5-542.

114. Morris GS. Oncologic emergencies. *Acute Care Perspectives*. 2007;16(4). 1, 3-7.

115. Schiff D. Peer viewpoint. *J Support Oncol*. 2004;2(398):401.

116. Wong CS, Fehlings MG, Sahgal A. Pathobiology of radiation myelopathy and strategies to mitigate injury. *Spinal Cord*. 2015;53(8):574–580. https://doi.org/10.1038/sc.2015.43. Epub 2015 Mar 24. PMID: 25800695.

117. Lawton AJ, Lee KA, Cheville AL, et al. Assessment and management of patients with metastatic spinal cord compression: a multidisciplinary review. *J Clin Oncol*. 2019;37(1):61–71. https://doi.org/10.1200/JCO.2018.78.1211. Epub 2018 Nov 5. PMID: 30395488.

118. Levack P, Graham J, Collie D, et al. Don't wait for a sensory level—listen to the symptoms: a prospective audit of the delays in diagnosis of malignant cord compression. *Clin Oncol (R Coll Radiol)*. 2002;14:472–480.

119. Tatu B. Physical therapy intervention with oncological emergencies. *Rehabil Oncol*. 2005;23:4–6.

120. Liu Y, Wang B, Qian Y, Di D, Wang M, Zhang X. Cauda equina syndrome as the primary symptom of leptomeningeal metastases from lung cancer: a case report and review of literature. *Onco Targets Ther*. 2018;11:5009–5013. https://doi. org/10.2147/OTT.S165299.

121. Abrahm JL. Assessment and treatment of patients with malignant spinal cord compression. *J Support Oncol*. 2004;2:377–401.

122. Boussios S, Cooke D, Hayward C, et al. Metastatic spinal cord compression: unraveling the diagnostic and therapeutic challenges. *Anticancer Res*. 2018;38(9):4987–4997. https://doi. org/10.21873/anticanres.12817. PMID: 30194142.

123. Rider LS, Marra EM. *Cauda Equina And Conus Medullaris Syndromes. [Updated 2020 Aug 10]. StatPearls [Internet]*. Treasure Island (FL): StatPearls Publishing; 2020 Jan. https:// www.ncbi.nlm.nih.gov/books/NBK537200/.

124. Della-Gustina D, Goldflam K. *Orthopedic Emergencies, an Issue of Emergency Medicine Clinics of North America*. St. Louis: Elsevier; 2015:322.

125. Uchiyama T, Sakakibara R, Hattori T, Yamanishi T. Lower urinary tract dysfunctions in patients with spinal cord tumors. *Neurourol Urodyn*. 2002;23:68–75.

126. Hazelwood JE, Hoeritzauer I, Pronin S, Demetriades AK. An assessment of patient-reported long-term outcomes following surgery for cauda equina syndrome. *Acta Neurochir*. 2019;161:1887–1894. https://doi.org/10.1007/ s00701-019-03973-7.

127. Park SB, Goldstein D, Krishnan AV, et al. Chemotherapy-induced peripheral neurotoxicity: a critical analysis. *CA Cancer J Clin*. 2013;63(6):419–437. https://doi.org/10.3322/ caac.21204. PMID: 24590861.

128. Galli J, Greenlee J. Paraneoplastic diseases of the central nervous system. *F1000Res*. 2020;9 https://doi.org/10.12688/ f1000research.21309.1. F1000 Faculty Rev-167. Published 2020 Mar 6.

129. Kannoth S. Paraneoplastic neurologic syndrome: a practical approach. *Ann Indian Acad Neurol*. 2012;15(1):6–12. https:// doi.org/10.4103/0972-2327.93267.

130. Berzero G, Psimaras D. Neurological paraneoplastic syndromes: an update. *Curr Opin Oncol*. 2018;30(6):359–367. https://doi.org/10.1097/CCO.0000000000000479. PMID: 30124520.

131. Popławska-Domaszewicz K, Florczak-Wyspiańska J, Kozubski W, Michalak S. Paraneoplastic movement disorders. *Rev Neurosci*. 2018;29(7):745–755. https://doi.org/10.1515/rev-neuro-2017-0081. PMID: 29561731.

132. Ikuerowo SO, Ojewuyi OO, Omisanjo OA, Abolarinwa AA, Bioku MJ, Doherty AF. Paraneoplastic syndromes and oncological outcomes in renal cancer. *Niger J Clin*

Pract. 2019;22(9):1271–1275. https://doi.org/10.4103/njcp. njcp_35_19. PMID: 31489865.

133. Owen CE. Cutaneous manifestations of lung cancer. *Semin Oncol*. 2016;43(3):366–369. https://doi.org/10.1053/j.semi-noncol.2016.02.025. Epub 2016 Feb 23. PMID: 27178690.

134. Bukhari S, Soomro R, Fawwad S, Alvarez C, Wallach S. Adenocarcinoma of lung presenting as lambert-eaton myasthenic syndrome. *J Investig Med High Impact Case Rep*. 2017;5(3). https://doi.org/10.1177/2324709617721251. 2324709617721251. Published 2017 Jul 14.

135. Pelosof LC, Gerber DE. Paraneoplastic syndromes: an approach to diagnosis and treatment. *Mayo Clin Proc*. 2010;85(9):838–854. https://doi.org/10.4065/mcp.2010.0099. Erratum in: Mayo Clin Proc. 2011 Apr;86(4):364. Dosage error in article text. PMID: 20810794; PMCID: PMC2931619.

136. Wen J, Ouyang H, Yang R, et al. Malignancy dominated with rheumatic manifestations: a retrospective single-center analysis. *Sci Rep*. 2018;8:1786. https://doi.org/10.1038/ s41598-018-20167-w.

137. Naschitz JE, Rosner I. Musculoskeletal syndromes associated with malignancy (excluding hypertrophic osteoarthropathy). *Curr Opin Rheumatol*. 2008;20(1):100–105.

138. Martorell EA, Murray PM, Peterson JJ, Menke DM, Calamia KT. Palmar fasciitis and arthritis syndrome associated with metastatic ovarian carcinoma: a report of four cases. *J Hand Surg*. 2004;29(4):654–660.

139. Azar L, Khasnis A. Paraneoplastic rheumatologic syndromes. *Curr Opin Rheumatol*. 2013;25(1):44–49. https://doi. org/10.1097/BOR.0b013e328359e780.

140. Klippel JH. *Primer on the Rheumatic Diseases*. 13 ed. Arthritis Foundation, New York: Springer Science Media; 2008.

141. Macedo F, Ladeira K, Pinho F, et al. Bone metastases: an overview. *Oncol Rev*. 2017;11(1):321 https://doi.org/10.4081/ oncol.2017.321. Published 2017 May 9.

142. Downie A, Williams CM, Henschke N, et al. Red flags to screen for malignancy and fracture in patients with low back pain: systematic review. *BMJ*. 2013;347:f7095.

143. Mabry LM, Ross MD, Tonarelli JM. Metastatic cancer mimicking mechanical low back pain: a case report. *J Man Manip Ther*. 2014;22(3):162–169. https://doi.org/10.1179/20426186 13Y.0000000056.

144. Zagzag J, Hu MI, Fisher SB, Perrier ND. Hypercalcemia and cancer: Differential diagnosis and treatment. *CA Cancer J Clin*. 2018;68(5):377–386. https://doi.org/10.3322/caac.21489. Epub 2018 Sep 21. PMID: 30240520.

145. van den Beuken-van Everdingen MH, Hochstenbach LM, Joosten EA, Tjan-Heijnen VC, Janssen DJ. Update on prevalence of pain in patients with cancer: systematic review and meta-analysis. *J Pain Symptom Manage*. 2016;51(6). 1070–1090.e9. https://doi.org/10.1016/j.jpainsymman.2015.12.340. Epub 2016 Apr 23. PMID: 27112310.

146. Lustberg MB. Management of neutropenia in cancer patients. *Clin Adv Hematol Oncol*. 2012;10(12):825–826.

147. National Comprehensive Cancer Network. Cancer-related fatigue (version 1.2021) https://www.nccn.org/professionals/ physician_gls/pdf/fatigue.pdf. Accessed December 15, 2020.

148. Hilfiker R, Meichtry A, Eicher M, et al. Exercise and other non-pharmaceutical interventions for cancer-related fatigue in patients during or after cancer treatment: a systematic review incorporating an indirect-comparisons meta-analysis. *Br J Sports Med*. 2018;52(10):651–658. https://doi.org/10.1136/ bjsports-2016-096422. Epub 2017 May 13. PMID: 28501804; PMCID: PMC5931245.

149. Mustian KM, Alfano CM, Heckler C, et al. Comparison of pharmaceutical, psychological, and exercise treatments for cancer-related fatigue: a meta-analysis. *JAMA Oncol*. 2017; 3(7):961–968. https://doi.org/10.1001/jamaoncol.2016.6914. PMID: 28253393; PMCID: PMC5557289.

150. Volk K, Wruble E. Irradiation side effects and their impact on physical therapy. *Acute Care Perspect.* 2001;10:11–13.

151. Winningham ML, McVicar M, Burke C. Exercise for cancer patients: guidelines and precautions. *Phys Sportsmed.* 1986;14:121–134.

152. Campbell KL, Winters-Stone KM, Wiskemann J, et al. Exercise Guidelines for Cancer Survivors: Consensus Statement from International Multidisciplinary Roundtable. *Med Sci Sports Exerc.* 2019;51(11):2375–2390. https://doi.org/10.1249/MSS.0000000000002116. . PMID: 31626055.

153. Smith SR, Zheng JY, Silver J, Haig AJ, Cheville A. Cancer rehabilitation as an essential component of quality care and survivorship from an international perspective. *Disabil Rehabil.* 2020;42(1):8–13. https://doi.org/10.1080/09638288.2018.1514662. Epub 2018 Dec 21. PMID: 30574818.

154. Han TS, Gleeson HK. Long-term and late treatment consequences: endocrine and metabolic effects. *Curr Opin Support Palliat Care.* 2017;11(3):205–213. https://doi.org/10.1097/SPC.0000000000000289. PMID: 28661901.

155. Kiserud CE, Dahl AA, Fosså SD. Cancer survivorship in adults. *Recent Results Cancer Res.* 2018;210:123–143. https://doi.org/10.1007/978-3-319-64310-6_8. PMID: 28924683.

156. Treanor C, Donnelly M. Late effects of cancer and cancer treatment–the perspective of the patient. *Support Care Cancer.* 2016;24(1):337–346. https://doi.org/10.1007/s00520-015-2796-4. Epub 2015 Jun 13. PMID: 26066051.

157. Straub JM, New J, Hamilton CD, Lominska C, Shnayder Y, Thomas SM. Radiation-induced fibrosis: mechanisms and implications for therapy. *J Cancer Res Clin Oncol.* 2015;141(11):1985–1994. https://doi.org/10.1007/s00432-015-1974-6.

158. Li M, Caeyenberghs K. Longitudinal assessment of chemotherapy-induced changes in brain and cognitive functioning: a systematic review. *Neurosci Biobehav Rev.* 2018;92:304–317. https://doi.org/10.1016/j.neubiorev.2018.05.019. Epub 2018 May 20. PMID: 29791867.

159. Bompaire F, Durand T, Léger-Hardy I, Psimaras D, Ricard D. Chemotherapy-related cognitive impairment or « chemobrain »: concept and state of art. *Geriatr Psychol Neuropsychiatr Vieil.* 2017;15(1):89–98. English. https://doi.org/10.1684/pnv.2017.0659. PMID: 28266346.

160. Durfee RA, Mohammed M, Luu HH. Review of osteosarcoma and current management. *Rheumatol Ther.* 2016;3:221–243. https://doi.org/10.1007/s40744-016-0046-y.

161. Falavigna A, da Silva PG, Teixeira W. Radiotherapy-induced tumors of the spine, peripheral nerve and spinal cord: case report and literature review. *Surg Neurol Int.* 2016;7(suppl 4):S108–S115.

162. National Cancer Institute. Adult Soft Tissue Sarcoma Treatment (PDQ®)–Health Professional Version. Bethesda, MD: National cancer Institute. Updated Feb. 4, 2020. https://www.cancer.gov/types/soft-tissue-sarcoma/hp/adult-soft-tissue-treatment-pdq Accessed December 15, 2020.

163. Khosla D, Sapkota S, Kapoor R, Kumar R, Sharma SC. Adult rhabdomyosarcoma: Clinical presentation, treatment, and outcome. *J Can Res Ther.* 2015;11:830–834.

164. Cirstoiu C, Cretu B, Serban B, Panti Z, Nica M. Current review of surgical management options for extremity bone sarcomas. *EFORT Open Rev.* 2019;4(5):174–182. https://doi.org/10.1302/2058-5241.4.180048. Published 2019 May 10.

165. American Cancer Society. Osteosarcoma. key statistics about osteosarcoma. Atlanta, GA: ACS. Updated Oct 8, 2020. https://www.cancer.org/cancer/osteosarcoma/about/key-statistics.html. Accessed December 15, 2020.

166. American Cancer Society. Ewing Tumors. Atlanta, GA: ACS. Updated May 31, 2018. https://www.cancer.org/cancer/ewing-tumor/about/what-is-ewing-family-tumors.html. Accessed December 15, 2020.

167. Gopalakrishnan CV, Shrivastava A, Easwer HV, Nair S. Primary Ewing's sarcoma of the spine presenting as acute paraplegia. *J Pediatr Neurosci.* 2012;7(1):64–66. https://doi.org/10.4103/1817-1745.97630.

168. Limaiem F, Davis DD, Sticco KL. *Chondrosarcoma. [Updated 2020 Dec 2]. StatPearls.* Treasure Island (FL): StatPearls Publishing; 2020 Jan. https://www.ncbi.nlm.nih.gov/books/NBK538132/.

169. Tsuda Y, Gregory JJ, Fujiwara T, Abudu S. Secondary chondrosarcoma arising from osteochondroma: outcomes and prognostic factors. *Bone Joint J.* 2019;101-B(10):1313–1320. https://doi.org/10.1302/0301-620X.101B9.BJJ-2019-0190.R1. PMID: 31564158.

170. de Ga K, Bateni C, Darrow M, McGahan J, Randall RL, Chen D. Polyostotic osteoid osteoma: a case report. *Radiol Case Rep.* 2020;15(4):411–415. https://doi.org/10.1016/j.radcr.2020.01.012. ISSN 1930-0433.

171. McNeill KA. Epidemiology of brain tumors. *Neurol Clin.* 2016;34(4):981–998. https://doi.org/10.1016/j.ncl.2016.06.014. PMID: 27720005.

172. American Cancer Society. *Brain and Spinal Cord Tumors in Adults. Risk Factors for Brain and Spinal Cord Tumors.* Atlanta, GA: ACS. Updated May 5, 2020. https://www.cancer.org/cancer/brain-spinal-cord-tumors-adults/causes-risks-prevention/risk-factors.html. Accessed December 15, 2020.

173. Kim JH, Lee JK, Kim HG, Kim KB, Kim HR. Possible effects of radiofrequency electromagnetic field exposure on central nerve system. *Biomol Ther (Seoul).* 2019;27(3):265–275. https://doi.org/10.4062/biomolther.2018.152.

174. Sartorius N, Holt RIG, Maj M, eds. *Comorbidity of Mental and Physical Disorders. Key Issues Ment Health.* 179. Basel: Karger; 2015:88–98. https://doi.org/10.1159/000365541.

175. American Association of Neurological Surgeons. AANS/CNS Section on Tumors. Classification of brain tumors. AANS Rolling Meadows, IL. https://www.aans.org/en/Media/Classifications of Brain-Tumors. Accessed December 15, 2020.

176. National Cancer Institute's Surveillance, Epidemiology and End Results (SEER) Program, Cancer Statistics Review (CSR) 1975-2016 (published online in April 2019, www.seer.cancer.gov). Accessed December 15, 2020.

177. Hong WK, Holland JF, Frei E. *Holland-Frei Cancer Medicine.* Shelton, CT: Peoples Medical Publishing House; 2010.

178. Puckett Y, Chan O. *Acute Lymphocytic Leukemia. [Updated 2020 Nov 18]. StatPearls [Internet].* Treasure Island (FL): StatPearls Publishing; 2020 Jan. https://www.ncbi.nlm.nih.gov/books/NBK459149/.

179. Sadeghian MH, Avval MM, Ayatollahi H, et al. Is there any relationship between human herpesvirus-8 and multiple myeloma? *Lymphoma.* 2013:5 Article ID 123297. https://doi.org/10.1155/2013/123297.

180. Kahouli S, Zahid H, Benkirane M, Messaoudi N. Sarcome de kaposi et myélome multiple: s'agit-il d'une association causée par le HHV-8? [Association between Kaposi's sarcoma and multiple myeloma: is it caused by HHV-8?]. *Pan Afr Med J.* 2020;36:85 French. https://doi.org/10.11604/pamj.2020.36.85.22407. PMID: 32774644; PMCID: PMC7392862.

181. Kyle RA, Rajkumar SV. Treatment of multiple myeloma: a comprehensive review. *Clin Lymphoma Myeloma.* 2009;9(4):278–288.

182. Wang HW, Balakrishna JP, Pittaluga S, Jaffe ES. Diagnosis of hodgkin lymphoma in the modern era. *Br J Haematol.* 2019;184(1):45–59. https://doi.org/10.1111/bjh.15614. Epub 2018 Nov 8. PMID: 30407610; PMCID: PMC6310079.

183. Chihara D, Nastoupil LJ, Williams JN, Lee P, Koff JL, Flowers CR. New insights into the epidemiology of non-Hodgkin lymphoma and implications for therapy. *Expert Rev Anticancer*

Ther. 2015;15(5):531–544. https://doi.org/10.1586/14737140.2015.1023712.

184. Borges AH, Dubrow R, Silverberg MJ. Factors contributing to risk for cancer among HIV-infected individuals, and evidence that earlier combination antiretroviral therapy will alter this risk. Curr Opin. *HIV AIDS*. 2014;9(1):34–40. https://doi.org/10.1097/COH.0000000000000025.

185. Chiu BC, Hou N. Epidemiology and etiology of non-hodgkin lymphoma. *Cancer Treat Res*. 2015;165:1–25. https://doi.org/10.1007/978-3-319-13150-4_1.

186. Shankland KR, Armitage JO, Hancock BW. Non-Hodgkin lymphoma. *Lancet*. 2012;380(9844):848–857. https://doi.org/10.1016/S0140-6736(12)60605-9. Epub 2012 Jul 25. PMID: 22835603.

187. Noy A. Optimizing treatment of HIV-associated lymphoma. *Blood*. 2019;134(17):1385–1394. https://doi.org/10.1182/blood-2018-01-791400. PMID: 30992269; PMCID: PMC7493463.

188. Collaborative Group on Hormonal Factors in Breast Cancer Type and timing of menopausal hormone therapy and breast cancer risk: individual participant meta-analysis of the worldwide epidemiological evidence. *Lancet*. 2019;394(10204):1159–1168. https://doi.org/10.1016/S0140-6736(19)31709-X. Epub 2019 Aug 29. PMID: 31474332; PMCID: PMC6891893.

189. Howlader N, Noone AM, Krapcho M, et al. *SEER Cancer Statistics Review*. Bethesda, MD: National Cancer Institute; 1975–2013. http://seer.cancer.gov/csr/1975_2013/. Accessed May 26, 2016.

190. Bach PB, Schrag D, Brawley OW, Galaznik A, Yakren S, Begg CB. Survival of blacks and whites after a cancer diagnosis. *JAMA*. 2002;287:2106–2113.

191. National Society of Genetic Counselors (NSGC). Your Genetic health: Patient Information. http://nsgc.org/p/cm/ld/fid=52. Accessed August 3, 2016.

192. Mai V, Kant AK, Flood A, Lacey Jr JV, Schairer C, Schatzkin A. Diet quality and subsequent cancer incidence and mortality in a prospective cohort of women. *Int J Epidemiol*. 2005;34:54–60.

193. Kabat GC, Kim M, Caan BJ, et al. Repeated measures of serum glucose and insulin in relationship to postmenopausal breast cancer. *Int J Cancer*. 2009;125(11):2704–2710.

194. Duggan C, Irwin ML, Xiao L, et al. Associations of insulin resistance and adiponectin with mortality in women with breast cancer. *J Clin Oncol*. 2011;29(1):32–39.

195. Eyre H, Kahn R, Robertson RM. ACS/ADA/AHA Collaborative Writing Committee. Preventing cancer, cardiovascular disease and diabetes: a common agenda for the ACS, American Diabetes Association, American Heart Association. *CA Cancer J Clin*. 2004;54:190–207.

196. Vineis P, Perera F. Molecular epidemiology and biomarkers in etiologic cancer research: the new in light of the old. *Cancer Epidemiol Biomarkers Prev*. 2007;16:1954–1965.

197. National Cancer Institute: Fact Sheet- HPV and Cancer. http://www.cancer.gov/about-cancer/causes-prevention/risk/infectious-agents/hpv-fact-sheet. Accessed May 30, 2016.

198. CDC: Sexually Transmitted Diseases. Genital HPV infection—CDC fact sheet, 2014. http://www.cdc.gov/std/hpv/stdfact-hpv.htm. Accessed May 30, 2016.

199. Centers for Disease Control and Prevention (CDC) *Tracking the Hidden Epidemics 2000: Trends in STDs in the United States*. Hyattsville, MD: CDC; 2000. https://www.cdc.gov/std/trends2000/trends2000.pdf. Accessed July 31, 2016.

200. Centers for Disease Control and Prevention *National Center for Health Statistics: National Vital Statistics Report: Sexually Transmitted Infections*. Hyattsville, MD: CDC; 2009.

201. Markowitz LE, Dunne EF, Saraiya M, et al. Human papillomavirus vaccination: recommendations of the Advisory Committee on Immunization Practices (ACIP). *MMWR Morb Mortal Wkly Rep*. 2014;63(RR05):1–30.

202. HealthyPeople.gov. Healthy People 2020 Topics & Objectives. Immunization and Infectious Diseases. Objective IID–11.4. Increase the vaccination coverage level of 3 doses of human papillomavirus (HPV) vaccine for females by age 13 to 15 years. Objective IID–11.5. Increase the vaccination coverage level of 3 doses of human papillomavirus (HPV) vaccine for males by age 13 to 15 years. https://www.healthypeople.gov/2020/topics-objectives/topic/immunization-and-infectious-diseases/objectives. Accessed December 9, 2016.

203. Reagan-Steiner S, Yankey D, Jeyarajah J, et al. National, regional, state, and selected local area vaccination coverage among adolescents aged 13–17 years—United States, 2014. *MMWR Morb Mortal Wkly Rep*. 2015;64(29):784–792.

204. Baan YR, Grosse B, Lauby-Secretan F, et al. Carcinogenicity of radiofrequency electromagnetic fields. *Lancet Oncol*. 2011;12:624–626.

205. Baliatsas C, Van Kamp I, Hooiveld M, Yzermans J, Lebret E. Comparing non-specific physical symptoms in environmentally sensitive patients: prevalence, duration, functional status and illness behavior. *J Psychosom Res*. 2014;76:405–413.

206. National Safety Council (NSC) Environmental Health Center. Understanding radiation in our world. http://www.hpschapters.org/nochps/resources/radgdebk.pdf. Accessed July 31, 2016.

207. Gandini S, Autier P, Goniol M. Reviews of sun exposure and artificial light and melanoma. *Prog Biophys Mol Biol*. 2011;107:362–366.

208. Lazovich D. Indoor tanning and risk of melanoma: a case-control study in a highly exposed population. *Cancer Epidemiol Biomarkers Prev*. 2010;19(6):1557–1568.

209. Woo DK. Tanning beds, skin cancer, and vitamin D: an examination of the scientific evidence and public health implications. *Dermatol Ther*. 2010;23(1):61–71.

210. Schmutz J, Wheeler J, Grimwood J, et al. Quality assessment of the human genome sequence. *Nature*. 2004;429(6990):365–368.

211. Omenn GS. Genomics and prevention: a vision for the future. Medscape News and Perspective. http://www.medscape.com/viewarticle/501299. Accessed July 31, 2016.

212. Calzone K, Wattendorf D, Dunn BK. The application of genetics and genomics to cancer prevention. *Semin Oncol*. 2010;37:407–418.

213. Lindsey H. Environmental factors & cancer: research roundup. *Oncology Times*. 2005;27(4):8–10.

214. Joerger AC, Fersht AR. The tumor suppressor p53: from structures to drug discovery. *Cold Spring Harb Perspect Biol*. 2010;2(6):a000919.

215. Maslon MM, Hupp TR. Drug discovery and mutant p53. *Trends Cell Biol*. 2010;20(9):542–555.

216. Couzin J. Choices—and uncertainties—for women with BRCA mutations. *Science*. 2003;302:592.

217. Cancer Classification: National Cancer Institute–SEER. http://training.seer.cancer.gov/disease/categories/classification.html. Accessed July 31, 2016.

218. Ong MLH, Schofield JB. Assessment of lymph node involvement in colorectal cancer. *World J Gastrointest Surg*. 2016;8:179–192.

219. Kitagawa Y, Fujii H, Mukai M, et al. Intraoperative lymphatic mapping and sentinel lymph node sampling in esophageal and gastric cancer. *Surg Oncol Clin N Am*. 2002;11:293–304.

220. McGarvey CL. *Principles of Oncology for the Physical Therapist*. Long Island, NY: Stony Brook University (Course Presentation); 2003.

221. Lipton A. Bone continuum of cancer. *Am J Clin Oncol*. 2010;33(Suppl. 3):S1–S7.

222. Fagan A. Bone metastases in breast cancer. *Rehabil Oncol*. 2004;22:23–26.

223. Eatock AM, Scatzlein A, Kayes L. Tumour vasculature as a target for anticancer therapy. *Cancer Treat Rev*. 2000;26:191–204.

224. Springfield DS, Rosenberg A. Biopsy: complicated, risky (editorial). *J Bone Joint Surg.* 1996;78A:639–643.
225. Mankin HJ, Mankin CJ, Simon MA. The hazards of the biopsy revisited. *J Bone Joint Surg.* 1996;78A:656–663.
226. Abdu WA, Provencher M. Primary bone and metastatic tumors of the cervical spine. *Spine.* 1998;23:2767–2777.
227. Fischbein NJ. Recurrence of clival chordoma along the surgical pathway. *Am J Neuroradiol.* 2000;21:578–583.
228. Austin JP. Probable causes of recurrence in patients with chordoma and chondrosarcoma of the base of skull and cervical spine. *Int J Radiat Oncol Biol Phys.* 1993;25:439–444.
229. Bergh P. Prognostic factors in chordoma of the sacrum and mobile spine: a study of 39 patients. *Cancer.* 2000;88:2122–2134.
230. Cancer rehabilitation: Principles and practice. In Stubblefield M, O'Dell M, eds. New York: Demos Medical Publishing; 2009.
231. Slipman CW. Epidemiology of spine tumors presenting to musculoskeletal physiatrists. *Arch Phys Med Rehab.* 2003;84:492–495.
232. Melanoma: Statistics. http://www.cancer.net/cancer-types/melanoma/statistics. Accessed July 31, 2016.
233. American Cancer Society. How to spot skin cancer. http://www.cancer.org/cancer/news/features/how-to-spot-skin-cancer. Accessed August 5, 2016.
234. American Cancer Society. Melanoma skin cancer. http://www.cancer.org/cancer/skincancer-melanoma/detailedguide/melanoma-skin-cancer-key-statistics. Accessed July 31, 2016.
235. Chen K, Craig JC, Shumack S. Oral retinoids for the prevention of skin cancers in solid organ transplant recipients: a systematic review of randomized controlled trials. *Br J Dermatol.* 2005;152:518–523.
236. Thomas SS, Dunbar EM. Modern multidisciplinary management of brain metastases. *Curr Oncol Rep.* 2010;12(1):34–40.
237. Prasad D, Schiff D. Malignant spinal cord compression. *Lancet Oncol.* 2005;6:15–25.
238. Pigott KH, Baddeley H, Maher EJ. Pattern of disease in spinal cord compression on MRI scan and implications for treatment. *Clin Oncol (R Coll Radiol).* 1994;6:7–10.
239. Coleman RE. Management of bone metastases. *Oncologist.* 2000;5:463–470.
240. Schiff D. Spinal cord compression. *Neurol Clin.* 2003;21:67–86.
241. Ampil FL, Mills GM, Burton GV. A retrospective study of metastatic lung cancer compression of the cauda equina. *Chest.* 2001;120:1754–1755.
242. Orendacova J, Cizkova D, Kafka J, et al. Cauda equina syndrome. *Prog Neurobiol.* 2001;64:613–637.
243. Bagley CA, Gokaslan ZL. Cauda equina syndrome caused by primary and metastatic neoplasms. *Neurosurg Focus.* 2004;16(6):e3.
244. Small SA, Perron AD, Brady WJ. Orthopedic pitfalls: cauda equina syndrome. *Am J Emerg Med.* 2005;23:159–163.
245. McCarthy MJH, Aylott CEW, Grevitt MP, Hegarty J. Cauda equina syndrome. Factors affecting long-term functional and sphincteric outcome. *Spine.* 2007;32(2):207–216.
246. Hile ES. Persistent mobility disability after neurotoxic chemotherapy. *Phys Ther.* 2010;90(11):1649–1657.
247. Bataller A, Dalman J. Paraneoplastic disorders of the central nervous system: update on diagnosis and treatment. *Semin Neurol.* 2004;24:461–471.
248. Santacroce L. Paraneoplastic syndromes. Medscape. Updated Sept 30, 2015. http://emedicine.medscape.com/article/280744-overview. Accessed July 31, 2015.
249. Briani C. Spectrum of paraneoplastic disease associated with lymphoma. *Neurology.* 2011;76(8):705–710.
250. Maverakis E, Goodarzi H, Wehrli LN, Ono Y, Garcia MS. The etiology of paraneoplastic autoimmunity. *Clin Rev Allergy Immunol.* 2012;42(2):135–144.
251. Velez A, Howard MS. Diagnosis and treatment of cutaneous paraneoplastic disorders. *Dermatol Ther.* 2010;23(6):662–675.
252. Farrugia ME. Myasthenic syndromes. *J R Coll Physicians Edinb.* 2011;41(1):43–48.
253. Stummvoll GH, Aringer M, Machold KP, Smolen JS, Raderer M. Cancer polyarthritis resembling rheumatoid arthritis as a first sign of hidden neoplasms. *Scand J Rheumatol.* 2001;30:40–44.
254. Stummvoll GH, Graninger WB. Paraneoplastic rheumatism—musculoskeletal diseases as a first sign of hidden neoplasms. *Acta Med Austriaca.* 2002;29:36–40.
255. Henschke N, Maher CG, Refshauge KM. Screening for malignancy in low back pain patients: a systematic review. *Eur Spine J.* 2007;16(10):1673–1679.
256. Ross MD, Boissonnault WG. Red flags: to screen or not to screen? *J Orthop Sports Phys Ther.* 2010;40(11):682–684.
257. Cherny NI. The assessment of cancer pain. In: McMillan SC, Koltzenburg M, eds. *Wall and Melzack's Textbook of Pain.* 5 ed. Churchill Livingstone: Elsevier; 2006:1099–1125.
258. Montoya L. Managing hematologic toxicities in the oncologic patient. *J Infus Nurs.* 2007;30(3):168–172.
259. Stasi R, Abriani L, Beccaglia P, et al. Cancer-related fatigue: evolving concepts in evaluation and treatment. *Cancer.* 2003;98(9):1786–1801.
260. National Comprehensive Cancer Network (NCCN): Fatigue. https://www.nccn.org/patients/resources/life_with_cancer/managing_symptoms/fatigue.aspx. Accessed July 31, 2016.
261. Van Weert E. Cancer-related fatigue and rehabilitation. *Phys Ther.* 2010;90(10):1413–1425.
262. Blaney J. The cancer rehabilitation journey: barriers to and facilitators of exercise among patients with cancer-related fatigue. *Phys Ther.* 2010;90(8):1135–1147.
263. Schmitz KH, Courneya KS. American College of Sports Medicine roundtable on exercise guidelines for cancer survivors. *Med Sci Sports Exerc.* 2010;42(7):1409–1426.
264. Litterini AJ, Fieler VK. The change in fatigue, strength, and quality of life following a physical therapist prescribed exercise program for cancer survivors. *Rehabil Oncol.* 2008;26(3):11–17.
265. Lab Values Interpretation Resources. Acute Care Section, American Physical Therapy Association. http://c.ymcdn.com/sites/www.acutept.org/resource/resmgr/imported/labvalues.pdf. Accessed July 31, 2016.
266. Walsh K. Addressing psychosocial issues in cancer survivorship: past, present and future. *Future Oncol.* 2016;12(24):2823–2834. July epub ahead of print.
267. Jacobs AL. Adult cancer survivorship: evolution, research, and planning care. *CA Cancer J Clin.* 2009;59:391–410.
268. Miller KD, Triano LR. Medical issues in cancer survivors—a review. *Cancer J.* 2008;14(6):375–387.
269. Guerard EJ, Nightingale G, Bellizzi K, et al. Survivorship care for older adults with cancer: U13 conference report. *J Geriatr Oncol.* 2016;7(4):305–312.
270. Asher A. Cancer rehabilitation and survivorship: Cedars-Sinai Medical Center experience. *Oncol Nurse.* 2010;3(6):18–21. 1.
271. Shamley DR. Changes in shoulder muscle size and activity following treatment for breast cancer. *Breast Cancer Res Treat.* 2007;106(1):19–27.
272. Ahles TA. Candidate mechanisms for chemotherapy-induced cognitive changes. *Nat Rev Cancer.* 2007;7:192–201.
273. Ferguson RJ. Management of chemotherapy-related cognitive dysfunction. In: Feuerstein M, ed. *Handbook of Cancer Survivorship.* New York: Springer; 2006.
274. Kenney RJ, Cheney R, Stull MA, Kraybill W. Soft tissue sarcomas: current management and future directions. *Surg Clin North Am.* 2009;89(1):235–247.

275. Siegel HJ, Pressey JG. Current concepts on the surgical and medical management of osteosarcoma. *Expert Rev Anticancer Ther.* Aug 2008;8(8):1257–1269.

276. Roll L. Cancer in children and adolescents. In: Varricchio C, ed. *ACS: A Cancer Source Book for Nurses.* 8 ed. Boston: Jones and Bartlett; 2004:229–242.

277. American Cancer Society: Overview Osteosarcoma. http://www.cancer.org/acs/groups/cid/documents/webcontent/003069-pdf.pdf. Accessed July 31, 2016.

278. Maheshwari AV, Cheng EY. Ewing sarcoma family of tumors. *J Am Acad Orthop Surg.* 2010;18(2):94–107.

279. American Cancer Society – Ewing family of tumors. http://www.cancer.org/acs/groups/cid/documents/webcontent/003099-pdf.pdf. Accessed July 31, 2016.

280. Grubb MR, Currier BL, Pritchard DJ, Ebersold MJ. Primary Ewing sarcoma of the spine. *Spine.* 1994;19:309–313.

281. Lin PP, Moussallem CD, Deavers MT. Secondary chondrosarcoma. *J Am Acad Orthop Surg.* 2010;18(10):608–615.

282. Librodo G, Mehlman C, Gellman H. Osteoid Osteoma 2015. http://emedicine.medscape.com/article/1253443-overview. Accessed July 31, 2016.

283. Payne WT, Merrell G. Benign bone and soft tissue tumors of the hand. *J Hand Surg.* 2010;35(11):1901–1910.

284. Buckner JC, Brown PD, O'Neill BP, Meyer FB, Wetmore CJ, Uhm JH. Central nervous system tumors. *Mayo Clin Proc.* 2007;82(120):1271–1286.

285. Kasper D, Fauci A, Hauser S, Longo D, Jameson J, Loscalzo J. *Harrison's Principles of Internal Medicine.* 19 ed. New York: McGraw-Hill; 2015.

286. Volkow ND, Tomasi D, Wang G-H. Effects of cell phone radiofrequency signal exposure on brain glucose metabolism. *JAMA.* 2011;305(8):808–813.

287. Papadakis M, McPhee SJ, Rabow MW. *Current Medical Diagnosis and Treatment.* 53 ed. New York: McGraw Hill Medical; 2014.

288. Zaidi A, Vesole H. Multiple myeloma: an old disease with new hope for the future. *CA Cancer J Clin.* 2001;51:273–285.

289. Volker D. Other cancers: multiple myeloma. In: Varricchio C, ed. *ACS: Cancer Source Book for Nurses.* 8th ed. Boston: Jones and Bartlett; 2004:324–336.

290. Kennedy-Nasser AA, Hanley P, Bollard CM. Hodgkin disease and the role of the immune system. *Pediatr Hematol Oncol.* 2011;28(3):176–186.

291. Lim ST, Levine AM. Recent advances in acquired immunodeficiency syndrome (AIDS)-related lymphoma. *CA Cancer J Clin.* 2005;55:229–241.

292. Hardell L, Axelson O. Environmental and occupational aspects on the etiology of non-hodgkin lymphoma. *Oncol Res.* 1998;10:1–5.

293. Jones A. Lymphomas. In: Varricchio C, ed. *ACS: a Cancer Source Book for Nurses.* 8th ed. Boston: Jones and Bartlett; 2004:265–276.

294. Cesarman E. Pathology of lymphoma in HIV. *Curr Opin Oncol.* 2013;25(5):487–494.

295. Aboulafia AJ, Khan F, Pankowsky D, Aboulafia DM. AIDS-associated secondary lymphoma of bone: a case report with review of the literature. *Am J Orthop.* 1998;27:128–134.

296. Gapstur SM, Morrow M, Sellers TA. Hormone replacement therapy and risk of breast cancer with a favorable histology: results of the Iowa Women's Health Study. *JAMA.* 1999;281:2091–2097.

297. Rossouw JE, Anderson GL, Prentice RL, et al. Risks and benefits of estrogen plus progestin in healthy postmenopausal women: principal results from the Women's Health Initiative randomized controlled trial. *JAMA.* 2002;288:321–333.

298. Aubuchon M, Santoro N. Lessons learned from the WHI: HRT requires a cautious and individualized approach. *Geriatrics.* 2004;59:22–26.

299. Sweet's syndrome. Mayo Clinic. http://www.mayoclinic.org/diseases-conditions/sweets-syndrome/home/ovc-20165794. Accessed August 1, 2016.

300. Bourke JF, Keohane S, Long CC, et al. Sweet's syndrome and malignancy in the UK. *Br J Dermatol.* 1997;137:609–613.

301. Cohen PR, Kurzrock R. Sweet's syndrome revisited: a review of disease concepts. *Int J Dermatol.* 2003;42:761–778.

302. Paydas S. Sweet's syndrome: a revisit for hematologists and oncologists. *Crit Rev Oncol Hematol.* 2013;86(1):85–95.

CHAPTER

15

Screening the Head, Neck, and Back

In the United States, back pain is the fifth most common reason individuals seek medical care[1-3] and consumes 30 to 50 billion dollars on an annual basis. Half of all adults have reported low back pain (LBP) over 1 year and 20% have reported a complaint of frequent back pain.[4]

It has been suggested that 80% to 90% of individuals with back pain can be classified as mechanical LBP. Mechanical LBP means that the source of the pain is in the spine or its supporting structures.[5] Nonmechanical origins of LBP can be attributed to a neoplasm, infection, or inflammation in 1% of all cases with another 2% accounted for by visceral disorders (pelvic organs, gastrointestinal [GI] dysfunction, renal involvement, abdominal aneurysms).[6] Use of patient-reporting outcomes, such as the Optimal Screening for Prediction of Referral and Outcome-Review of Systems or OSPRO-ROS (Chapter 1), facilitates clinical decision-making by assisting in ruling in or out visceral systems that refer to the back or neck. Evidence suggests that 48% to 50% of therapists consider the use or patient-reporting outcomes potentially because clinicians are not familiar with the outcome measure, don't have the time to have the patient complete the form, or there is a lack of knowledge that the patient-reporting outcome exists.[7-9]

Most cases of back pain in adults are associated with age-related degenerative processes, physical loading, and muscular or ligamentous injuries. Many mechanical causes of back pain resolve within 1 to 4 weeks without serious problems. It has been estimated that fewer than 2% of individuals presenting with LBP present with significant neurologic involvement or other signs that require referral or imaging.[10] Up to 10% of individuals with LBP have no identifiable cause.[11]

Sacroiliac (SI) joint dysfunction can mimic LBP and discogenic disease with pain referred below the knee to the foot. Several studies have shown that SI joint dysfunction is the primary source of LBP in 18% to 30% of people with LBP.[11-16] It is important to remember that when conducting a physical examination the therapist must consider the possibility of a mechanical problem above or below the area of pain or symptom presentation. When there is involvement of a mechanical problem above or below the area of pain, the term *regional interdependence* is used. For example, many orthopedic causes of hip pain may be the referral of pain that comes from a proximal referral, such as from the lumbar spine. A neurodynamic screening is important especially for the consideration of lumbar involvement or entrapments that are influencing hip pain or symptoms

A smaller number of people will develop chronic pain without organic pathology or they may have an underlying serious medical condition. The therapist must be aware that many different diseases can appear as neck pain, back pain, or both at the same time (Table 15.1). For example, rheumatoid arthritis affects the cervical spine early in the course of the disease but may go unrecognized at first.[17-19] Neck pain may be a feature of any disorder or disease that occurs above the shoulder blades; it is a rare symptom of neoplasm or infection.[20]

In this chapter, general information is offered about spinal pain with a focus on clinical presentation, while being mindful of the risk factors and associated signs and symptoms typical of each visceral system capable of referring pain to the head, neck, and low back.

Additionally, LBP can be referred from abdominal or pelvic disease. Nonsteroidal antiinflammatory drug (NSAID) use is a typical cause of intraperitoneal or retroperitoneal bleeding causing LBP. People most often taking NSAIDs have a history of inflammatory conditions such as osteoarthritis.

Although the incidence of back pain from NSAIDs is fairly low (i.e., number of people taking NSAIDs who develop GI problems and referred pain), the prevalence (number seen in a physical therapist's practice) is much higher.[21-23] In other words, physical therapists are seeing a majority of people who have arthritis, are in pain, or have inflammatory conditions and are taking one or more prescription and/or over-the-counter (OTC) NSAIDs.[24]

TABLE 15.1	Viscerogenic Causes of Neck and Back Pain		
	Cervical	Thoracic/Scapular	Lumbar/Sacrum*
Cancer	Metastatic lesions (leukemia, Hodgkin's disease) Cervical bone tumors Cervical cord tumors Lung cancer; Pancoast's tumor Esophageal cancer Thyroid cancer	Mediastinal tumors Metastatic extension Pancreatic cancer Breast cancer Multiple myeloma	Primary bone tumors Neurogenic tumors (sacrum) Metastatic lesions Prostate cancer Testicular cancer Pancreatic cancer Colorectal cancer Multiple myeloma Lymphoma
Cardiovascular	Angina Myocardial infarction Aortic aneurysm Occipital migraine Cervical artery ischemia or dissection Arteritis	Angina Myocardial infarction Aortic aneurysm	Abdominal aortic aneurysm Endocarditis Myocarditis Peripheral vascular: • Postoperative bleeding from anterior spine surgery
Pulmonary	Lung cancer; Pancoast's tumor Tracheobronchial irritation Chronic bronchitis Pneumothorax Pleuritis involving the diaphragm	Respiratory or lung infection Empyema Chronic bronchitis Pleurisy Pneumothorax Pneumonia	
Renal/urologic		Acute pyelonephritis Kidney disease	Kidney disorders: • Acute pyelonephritis • Perinephritic abscess • Nephrolithiasis • Ureteral colic (kidney stones) • Urinary tract infection • Dialysis (first-use syndrome) • Renal tumors
Gastrointestinal	Esophagitis Esophageal cancer	Esophagitis (severe) Esophageal spasm Peptic ulcer Acute cholecystitis Biliary colic Pancreatic disease	Small intestine: • Obstruction (neoplasm) • Irritable bowel syndrome • Crohn's disease • Colon: • Diverticular disease • Pancreatic disease • Appendicitis
Gynecologic			Gynecologic disorders: • Cancer • Retroversion of the uterus • Uterine fibroids • Ovarian cysts • Endometriosis • Pelvic inflammatory disease (PID) • Incest/sexual assault • Rectocele, cystocele • Uterine prolapse • Normal pregnancy • Multiparity
Infection	Vertebral osteomyelitis Meningitis Lyme disease Retropharyngeal abscess; epidural abscess (poststeroid injection)	Vertebral osteomyelitis Herpes zoster Human immunodeficiency virus (HIV) Epidural abscess	Vertebral osteomyelitis Herpes zoster Spinal tuberculosis Candidiasis (yeast) Psoas abscess HIV
Other	Osteoporosis Fibromyalgia Psychogenic (nonorganic causes; see Chapter 3) Fracture Rheumatoid: • Rheumatoid arthritis and atlantoaxial subluxation • Psoriatic arthritis • Polymyalgia rheumatica • Ankylosing spondylitis Viral myalgia Cervical lymphadenitis Thyroid disease	Osteoporosis Fibromyalgia Psychogenic (nonorganic) Acromegaly Cushing's syndrome Fracture	Osteoporosis Fibromyalgia Psychogenic (nonorganic) Fracture Cushing's syndrome Type III hypersensitivity disorder (back/flank pain) Postregional anesthesia Ankylosing spondylitis

*Sacral sources of LBP are discussed separately in Chapter 16.

Screening for medical disease is an important part of the evaluation process that should be ongoing throughout all episodes of care as a reassessment process (see Fig. 1.4). The clues that a client provides about the quality of their pain, in addition to their age and the presence of systemic complaints or associated signs and symptoms, indicate the need to investigate further.

USING THE SCREENING MODEL TO EVALUATE THE HEAD, NECK, OR BACK

Past Medical History

A carefully taken, detailed medical history is the most important single element in the evaluation of a client who has musculoskeletal pain of unknown origin or cause. It is essential for the recognition of systemic disease or medical conditions that may be causing integumentary, muscle, nerve, or joint symptoms.

The history combined with the physical therapy examination provides essential clues in determining the need for referral to a physician or other appropriate health care provider. A history of cancer is most important, however long ago.[25] If a client has had a low backache for years, progressive serious disease is unlikely, though the therapist should not be misled by a chronic history of back pain because the client may be presenting with a new episode of serious back pain. Six weeks to 6 months of increasing backache, often in an older client, may be a signal of lumbar metastases, especially in a person with a history of cancer.[25]

Be alert for the history of diabetes mellitus, immunosuppression, rheumatologic disorders, tuberculosis, and any recent infection (Case Example 15.1). A history of fever and chills with or without previous infection anywhere in the body may indicate a low-grade infection.

Symptoms are likely to appear some time before striking physical signs of disease are evident and before laboratory tests are useful in detecting disordered physiology. Thus an accurate and sufficiently detailed history provides historical clues that can be significant in determining when the client should be referred to a physician or other appropriate health care provider.

The therapist must always ask about a history of motor vehicle accident, blunt impact, repetitive injury, sudden stress caused by lifting or pulling, or trauma of any kind. Even minor falls or lifting when osteoporosis is present can result in a severe fracture in older adults (Case Example 15.2). Anyone who cannot bear weight through the legs and hips should be considered for an immediate medical evaluation.[26]

Surgery of any kind can result in infection and abscess leading to hip, pelvic, abdominal, and/or LBP.[27] A recent history of spinal procedures (e.g., fusion, diskectomy, kyphoplasty, vertebroplasty) can be followed by back pain, motor impairment, and/or neurologic deficits when complicated by hematoma, infection, bone cement leakage, or subsidence (graft or instrumentation sinking into the bone).[28] Infection

---

CASE EXAMPLE 15.1
Bilateral Facial Pain

Background: A 79-year-old woman was in a rehabilitation facility following a stroke with resultant left hemiplegia. She told the therapist she was starting to have some new symptoms in her face. She could not smile on her "good" side and was having trouble closing her eyes, which was not a problem after her stroke.

Clinical Presentation: There were no apparent changes in hearing, sensation, or motor control of the right arm. The therapist conducted a new neurologic screening examination and found the following results:

Cranial Nerve VII: Client was unable to raise and lower either eyebrow or close the eyes tightly; there was bilateral facial drooping; as reported, the client was unable to smile with the right side of her face.

There was no change in sensory or motor findings from the initial evaluation post-cerebral vascular accident (post-CVA). However, deep tendon reflexes (DTR) were absent in both arms, leading the therapist to check DTR in the lower extremities, which were also absent. There were no other significant neurologic changes from the initial evaluation.

The therapist reviewed the Special Questions to Ask: Neck or Back (Pain Assessment and General Systemic) to look for any other screening questions and asked about a recent history of infection. The client reported a mild upper respiratory infection 2 weeks ago. There were no other obvious red-flag findings.

Result: The therapist reported the new episode of signs and symptoms. Red flags observed included bilateral symptoms, absent muscle stretch reflexes, and a recent history of infection. A medical evaluation was carried out, and a diagnosis of Guillain-Barré syndrome was made. The client continued to get worse with involvement of the respiratory muscles, foot drop, and numbness in the hands and feet.

A new episode of care was initiated to include physical therapy to strengthen facial musculature, prevent atrophy on the right side, and to prevent pneumonia from respiratory muscle involvement.

---

following spinal epidural injection is an infrequent but potentially serious complication.[29,30]

A few key questions to ask about the history might include:

 FOLLOW-UP QUESTIONS

- What do you think caused this pain?
- When did the pain (numbness, weakness, stiffness) start?
- Have you ever had this type of problem before?
- Have you ever had back surgery, seen a chiropractor (physical therapist or other health care professional), or had injection therapy for this problem?

Risk Factor Assessment

Understanding who is at risk and what the risk factors are for various illnesses, diseases, and conditions will alert the therapist early on as to the need for screening, education, and prevention as part of the plan of care. Educating clients about their risk factors is a key element in risk factor reduction.

CASE EXAMPLE 15.2

Minimal Trauma

Background: An inpatient acute care therapist was working with a 75-year-old woman who was 1-day status post (S/P) right total hip replacement (THR). The patient reported getting out of bed by herself early in the morning and falling against the night stand. She complained of low back pain (LBP) when the therapist arrived to help her sit up in bed and stand. The pain was in the left lumbar area without radiation.

Past Medical History: Past medical history included osteoporosis (treated with bisphosphonate medication, calcium, and vitamin D), breast cancer with mastectomy 30 years ago, and hypothyroidism treated with medication (Synthroid).

Clinical Presentation: No preoperative baseline information was available regarding the client's physical function, gait pattern, or range of motion (ROM) for the spine or hips. There was moderate tenderness to palpation and percussion of the sacrum on the left side. Mild tenderness was reported with percussion to the upper and lower lumbar spine. There were no apparent skin changes, bruising, warmth, or swelling.

The patient could ambulate slowly with a walker but reported pain in both hips with each step. She could only take small steps, moving approximately 2 to 4 inches forward with each step.

Lumbar ROM was very limited in flexion, side-bending, and extension. She was unable to straighten up to a fully upright standing position because of her low back/sacral pain.

Outcome: The therapist filed an incident report with the hospital unit clerk and spoke directly with the nursing supervisor requesting an orthopedic consult before continuing with the standard THR rehabilitation protocol.

The patient was diagnosed with a sacral insufficiency fracture on the left at S3. X-ray studies and magnetic resonance imaging (MRI) also revealed scoliosis of the lumbosacral spine, moderate degenerative arthritis, marked narrowing of the intervertebral disk spaces throughout the lumbar spine, and old compression fractures at T11 and T12. There was no evidence of bone lesions suggestive of breast cancer metastasis. Moderate foraminal stenosis was observed at the right L3 nerve root.

The client returned to physical therapy with an altered rehabilitation program consisting of weight-bearing exercises on the left (to stimulate osteoblastic bone formation), as tolerated, given the compromise on both sides. She had a minimally invasive hip procedure, so aquatic therapy was approved when no openings in the skin at the incision site were observed (1 week later).

Risk factors vary, depending on family history, previous personal history, and disease, illness, or condition present. For example, risk factors for heart disease will be different from risk factors for osteoporosis or vestibular/balance problems. In terms of back pain, risk factors, such as a history of cancer (positive likelihood ratio, 14.7), unexplained weight loss (positive likelihood ratio, 2.7), failure to improve after 1 month (positive likelihood ratio, 3.0), and age older than 50 years (positive likelihood ratio, 2.7) were each associated with a higher likelihood for cancer.[31] As a reminder of the interpretation of likelihood ratios, for a positive likelihood ratio, the higher the value, the more likely a client has a condition; for a negative likelihood ratio, the lower the value from 0, the less likely a client has a condition. Thus using the example above for a client with a history of cancer having a positive likelihood ratio of 14.7, this client is 14.7 times more likely to have cancer than a client that does not have back pain.

Always check medications for potential adverse side effects causing muscular, joint, neck, or back pain. Long-term use of corticosteroids can lead to vertebral compression fractures[25] (Case Example 15.3). Headache is a common side effect of many medications.

Keep in mind that physical and sexual abuse is a risk factor for central sensitization and chronic head, neck, and back pain for men, women, and children (see Appendix B-3 in the accompanying enhanced eBook version included with print purchase of this textbook).[32,33]

Age is a risk factor for many systemic, medical, and viscerogenic problems. The risk of certain diseases associated with back pain increases with advancing age (e.g., osteoporosis, aneurysm, myocardial infarction, cancer).[25] Under the age of 20 years or over the age of 50 years are both red-flag ages for serious spinal pathology. The highest likelihood of vertebral fracture occurs in females aged 75 years or older.[34]

As with all decision-making variables, a single risk factor may or may not be significant and must be viewed in context of the whole patient/client presentation. See Appendix A-2 in the accompanying enhanced eBook version included with print purchase of this textbook for a list of some possible health risk factors.

Routine screening for osteoporosis, hypertension, incontinence, cancer, vestibular or balance problems, and other potential problems can be a part of the physical therapist's practice. Therapists can advocate for disease prevention, wellness, and promotion of a healthy lifestyle by delivering health care services intended to prevent health problems or maintain health and by offering wellness screening as a part of primary prevention.

Clinical Presentation

During the examination the therapist will begin to get an idea of the client's overall clinical presentation. The client interview, systems review of the cardiopulmonary, musculoskeletal, neuromuscular, and integumentary systems, and assessment of pain patterns and pain types form the basis for the therapist's evaluation and eventual diagnosis.

Assessment of pain and symptoms is often a large part of the interview. In this final section of the text, pain and dysfunction associated with each anatomic part (e.g., back, chest, shoulder, pelvis, sacrum/SI, hip, and groin) are discussed and differentiated as systemic from musculoskeletal whenever possible.

Characteristics of pain such as onset, description, duration, pattern, and aggravating and relieving factors, and associated signs and symptoms are presented in Chapter 3 (see Table 3.2; see also Appendix C-7 in the accompanying enhanced eBook version included with print purchase of this textbook). Reviewing the comparison in Table 3.2 will assist

CASE EXAMPLE 15.3
Corticosteroid Use

Referral: A 73-year-old man was referred to a physical therapist by his family practitioner for evaluation of mid-to-low back pain that started when he stepped down from a curb. He was not experiencing radiating pain or sciatica and appeared to be in good general health. His medical history included bronchial asthma treated with oral corticosteroids and an abdominal hernia repaired surgically 10 years ago. There were no diagnostic imaging tests ordered.

Clinical Presentation: Vital signs were measured and appeared within normal limits for the client's age. There were no constitutional symptoms, no fever present, and no other associated signs or symptoms reported.

There was a marked decrease in thoracic and lumbar range of motion (ROM) from T10 to L1 and tenderness throughout this same area. No other objective findings were noted, despite a careful screening examination.

The client was treated conservatively over a 2-week period but without change in his painful symptoms and without improvement in spinal movement. A second therapist in the same clinic was consulted for a reevaluation without significant differences in findings. Several suggestions were made for alternative treatment techniques. After 1 more week without change in the client's symptoms, the client was reevaluated.

What is the next step in the screening process?

Using Table 15.1, the therapist can scan down the thoracic/scapular and lumbar columns for any screening clues. Prostate and testicular cancers are listed along with metastatic lesions. Given the client's age, questions should be asked about a past history of cancer and any associated urinary signs and symptoms.

Given his age, cardiovascular causes of back pain are also possible. Review past medical history, risk factors, and ask about signs and symptoms associated with angina, myocardial infarction, and aneurysm.

The therapist can continue to review Table 15.1 for potential pulmonary and gastrointestinal (GI) causes of this client's back pain and ask any further questions regarding possible risk factors and past history. Record all positive findings and conduct a final Review of Systems.

Use the Special Questions to Ask: Neck or Back at the end of this chapter to reassess the client's general health and clinical presentation. Not all questions must be asked; the therapist should use his or her judgment based on the known history for this client and current clinical findings.

Result: In this case the client's age, lack of improvement with a variety of treatment techniques, lack of diagnostic imaging studies to rule out fracture or infection, and a history of long-term corticosteroid use necessitated a return to the referring physician for further medical evaluation.

Long-term corticosteroid therapy and radiation therapy for cancer are risk factors for ischemic or avascular necrosis. Hip or back pain in the presence of these factors should be examined carefully.

Radiographic testing demonstrated ischemic vertebral collapse secondary to chronic corticosteroid administration. Diffuse osteopenia and a compression fracture of the tenth thoracic vertebral body were also mentioned in the medical report.

---

the therapist with recognition of a systemic versus musculoskeletal presentation of signs and symptoms.

Effect of Position

When seen early in the course of symptoms, neck or back pain of a systemic, medical, or viscerogenic origin is usually accompanied by full and painless range of motion (ROM) without limitations. When the pain has been present long enough to cause muscle guarding and splinting, then subsequent biomechanical changes occur.

Typically, systemic back pain or back pain associated with other medical conditions is not relieved by recumbency. Bone pain related to metastasis or multiple myeloma tends to be more continuous, progressive, and prominent when the client is recumbent.

Beware of the client with acute backache who is unable to lie still. Almost all clients with regional or nonspecific backache seek the most comfortable position (usually recumbency) and stay in that position to avoid pain or discomfort. In contrast, individuals with systemic backache tend to keep moving trying to find a comfortable position.

In particular, visceral diseases, such as pancreatic neoplasm, pancreatitis, and posterior penetrating ulcers, often have a systemic backache that causes the client to curl up, sleep in a chair, or pace the floor at night.

Back pain that is unrelieved by rest or a change in position, or pain that does not fit the expected mechanical or neuromusculoskeletal pattern, should raise a red flag. When the symptoms cannot be reproduced, aggravated, or altered in any way during the examination, additional questions to screen for medical disease are indicated.

Night Pain

Pain at night can signal a serious problem such as tumor, infection, or inflammation. Long-standing night pain unaltered by positional change suggests a space-occupying lesion such as a tumor.

Systemic back pain may get worse at night, especially when caused by vertebral osteomyelitis, septic diskitis, Cushing's disease, osteomalacia, primary and metastatic cancer, Paget's disease, ankylosing spondylitis, or tuberculosis of the spine (see Chapter 3 and Appendix B-25 in the accompanying enhanced eBook version included with print purchase of this textbook).

Associated Signs and Symptoms

After reviewing the client history and identifying pain types or pain patterns, the therapist must ask the client about the presence of additional signs and symptoms. Signs and symptoms associated with systemic disease or other medical conditions are often present but go unidentified, either because the client does not volunteer the information or the therapist does not seek to ask complete questions. To assess for associated signs and symptoms, the therapist can end the client interview with the following question:

The client with back pain and bloody diarrhea or the person with midthoracic or scapular pain in the presence of nausea and vomiting may not think the two symptoms are related. If the therapist only focuses on the chief complaint of back, neck, shoulder, or other musculoskeletal pain and does not ask about the presence of symptoms anywhere else, an important diagnostic clue may be overlooked.

Other possible associated symptoms may include fatigue, dyspnea, sweating after only minor exertion, and GI symptoms (see also Appendix A-2 on in the accompanying enhanced eBook version included with print purchase of this textbook for a more complete list of possible associated signs and symptoms).

If the therapist fails to ask about associated signs and symptoms, the Review of Systems offers one final step in the screening process that may bring to light important clues.

Review of Systems

Clusters of these associated signs and symptoms usually accompany the pathologic state of each organ system (see Box 4.19). As a part of the physical assessment, the therapist must conduct a Review of Systems. General questions about fevers, excessive weight gain or loss, and appetite loss should be followed by questions related to specific organ systems. Medications should be reviewed for possible adverse side effects. The OSPRO-ROS facilitates this process of identifying system involvement outside of musculoskeletal origin for the client with back pain.

Throughout the interview the therapist must remain alert to any yellow (caution) or red (warning) flags that may signal the need for further screening. Review of Systems is important even for clients who have been examined by a medical doctor. It has been reported that only 5% of physicians assess patients for "red flags."[35,36] In contrast, documentation of red flags by physical therapists (at least for patients with LBP) has been reported to be as high as 98%.[37]

During the Review of Systems a pattern of systemic, medical, or viscerogenic origin may be seen as the therapist combines information from the client history, risk factors present, associated signs and symptoms, and yellow or red-flag findings.

Yellow Flag Findings

Yellow flags are indicators that findings may be present requiring special attention, but not necessarily immediate action.[38]

One of the primary yellow flag findings that is important in clients with LBP, in terms of prognosis, is the presence of psychosocial risk factors (e.g., work, attitudes and beliefs, behaviors, affective presentation).[39–42] The presence of these yellow flags suggests a poor response to traditional intervention and the need to address the underlying psychosocial aspects of health and healing. A management approach using cognitive behavioral therapy and/or referral to a mental health professional may be warranted.[43,44] The Optimal Screening for Prediction of Referral and Outcome-Yellow Flags or OSPRO-YF is a useful tool to identify yellow flags in the client that facilitate referral of the client to appropriate care.

Work. In particular, belief that pain is harmful resulting in fear-avoidance behavior and belief that all pain must be gone before going back to work or normal, daily activities contribute to yellow (psychosocial) warning flags. Poor work history, unsupportive work environment, and belief that work is harmful all fall under the category of yellow work flags.[38]

Beliefs. People with chronic LBP who demonstrate yellow flag beliefs also have an increased risk for poor prognosis. This category includes catastrophizing, thinking the worst, a belief that pain is uncontrollable, poor compliance with exercise, low educational background, and the expectation of a quick fix for pain.

Behaviors. Beliefs extend into behaviors such as passive attitude toward rehabilitation, use of extended rest, reduced activity, increased intake of alcohol and other drugs to "manage" the pain, and avoidance or withdrawal from daily and/or social activities.

Affective. Depressed mood, irritability, and heightened awareness of bodily sensations along with anxiety represent affective psychosocial yellow flags (also prognostic of poor outcome for chronic LBP). Other affective yellow flags include feeling useless and not needed, disinterest in outside activities, and lack of family or personal support systems.

The assessment of psychosocial yellow flags should be part of any ongoing management of LBP at any time in the course of the problem. The New Zealand Guidelines[45] recommend the administration of a screening questionnaire at 2 to 4 weeks after the onset of pain (see Appendix C-4 in the accompanying enhanced eBook version included with print purchase of this textbook for a checklist of red/yellow flag indicators).

There is no evidence that this is the optimal time. This is early in the natural history of complaints of LBP, and other interventions may take this long to achieve their effects. In fact, over this time frame, practitioners may still be concerned about red-flag conditions, and their time with the client may still be consumed with ensuring compliance with home rehabilitation and analgesics.[42]

On the other hand, waiting until someone develops chronic pain (3 months) may be too late; the window of opportunity to prevent chronicity will have passed, by definition. Therefore in anyone with persisting pain, formal exploration of yellow flags should occur no later than 2 months after the onset of pain, and possibly by the end of the first month. A practical clinical approach would be to begin screening for yellow flag issues at the 1-month follow-up appointment.[46]

BOX 15.1   MOST COMMON RED FLAGS ASSOCIATED WITH BACK PAIN OF SYSTEMIC ORIGIN

- Age less than 20 years or over 50 years (malignancy)/ over 70 years (fracture)
- Previous history of cancer
- Constitutional symptoms (e.g., fever, chills, unexplained weight loss)
- Failure to improve with conservative care (usually over 4 to 6 weeks)
- Recent urinary tract infection, blood in urine (or stools), difficulty with urination
- History of injection drug use
- Immunocompromised condition (e.g., prolonged use of corticosteroids, transplant recipient, autoimmune diseases)
- Pain is not relieved by rest or recumbency
- Severe, constant nighttime pain
- Progressive neurologic deficit; saddle anesthesia; urinary or fecal incontinence
- Back pain accompanied by abdominal, pelvic, or hip pain
- History of falls or trauma (screen for fracture, osteoporosis, domestic violence, alcohol use)
- Significant morning stiffness with limitation in all spinal movements (ankylosing spondylitis or other inflammatory disorder)
- Skin rash (inflammatory disorder [e.g., Crohn's disease, ankylosing spondylitis])

❓ FOLLOW-UP QUESTIONS

- What do you understand is the cause of your back pain?
- What are you doing to cope with your symptoms?
- Do you expect to get back to work after treatment?
- (Alternate): Do you expect to fully return to work?

Red-Flag Signs and Symptoms

Watch for the most common red flags associated with back pain of a systemic origin or other medical condition (Box 15.1), but be aware that some recommended red flags have high false-positive rates when used in isolation.[47] Each condition (e.g., infection, malignancy, fracture) will likely have its own predictive risk factors. When multiple red flags are present, the probability of spinal fracture is higher. A systematic review by Downie et al. in the (medical) primary care setting reported that when three specific red flags were identified, there was a 90% probability (95% confidence interval 34%–99%) of spinal fracture (prolonged use of corticosteroids, age older than 70 years, and significant trauma).[48] Individuals with serious spinal pathology almost always have at least one red flag that may be missed when the clinician (physician or therapist) assumes that the client's symptoms are a result of mechanical-induced back pain (see also Appendix A-2 in the accompanying enhanced eBook version included with print purchase of this textbook).

Key findings are advancing age, significant recent weight loss, previous malignancy, and constant pain that is not relieved by positional change or rest and is present at night, disturbing the person's sleep. Poor response to conservative care, or poor success with comparable care, is an additional red flag in the diagnosis and management of musculoskeletal spine pain.[49] According to one source, cancer as a cause of LBP can be ruled out with 100% sensitivity when the affected individual is younger than 50 years old, has no prior history of cancer, no unexplained or unintended weight loss, and responds to conservative care.[6] A 2013 systematic review suggests that a red flag of a previous history of cancer increases the probability of malignancy to between 7% to 33%. Older age, failure to improve after 1 month of conservative care, and unexplained weight loss have post-test probabilities below 3%.[50]

According to the American College of Physicians guideline, three red flags have been identified to screen for vertebral fractures in clients presenting with acute LBP including age over 70 years, steroid use, and major trauma. In a 2013 systematic review, the authors suggest that prolonged steroid use and the appearance of a contusion or abrasion should be included when this guideline is revised. The presence of trauma in the history, along with neurological signs during the physical examination, such as weakness, sensory loss, reflex changes, bowel or bladder dysfunction increase the post-test probability to 43% for spinal fracture.[51]

Back pain in children is considered a red flag, especially in young children[52] and/or if it has been present for more than 6 weeks because of concern for infection or neoplasm.[53,54] Children are less likely to report associated signs and symptoms and must be interviewed carefully. Ask about any other joint involvement, swelling anywhere, change in ROM, and the presence of any constitutional and/or GI symptoms. A recent history of viral illness may be linked to myalgia and diskitis. Most common causes of back pain in children are listed in Table 15.2.

Red flags requiring medical evaluation or reevaluation include back pain or symptoms that are not improving as expected, steady pain irrespective of activity, symptoms that are increasing, or the development of new or progressive neurologic deficits such as weakness, sensory loss, change in reflexes, bowel or bladder dysfunction, or myelopathy.[55]

Indications for the use of plain films of the lumbar spine include any of the following features[56]:

- History of trauma
- History of cancer
- Older adults with minimal trauma
- Failure to respond to treatment

Use the Quick Screen Checklist (see Appendix A-1 in the accompanying enhanced eBook version included with print purchase of this textbook) to conduct a consistent and complete screening examination.

TABLE 15.2	Causes of Back Pain in Children			
Inflammatory Conditions	**Developmental Conditions**	**Trauma**	**Neoplastic Disease**	**Other**
Diskitis (most common before the age of 6 years) Vertebral osteomyelitis Spinal abscess Nonspinal infections (e.g., pancreatitis, pyelonephritis) Rheumatoid arthritis (cervical spine involved most often) Reactive Arthritis Psoriatic arthritis Ankylosing spondylitis (presents during adolescence) Inflammatory bowel disease	Spondylolysis Spondylolisthesis Scheuermann's syndromeScoliosis (especially left thoracic)	Muscle strain Vertebral stress or compression fracture Overuse syndrome Physical abuse	Leukemia Hodgkin's disease Non-Hodgkin's lymphoma Ewing's sarcoma (primary) Osteogenic sarcoma (osteosarcoma) [primary] Rhabdomyosarcoma (rare; skeletal metastasis)	Mechanical (hip and pelvic anomalies, upper cervical spine instability) Herniated disk Psychosomatic (conversion reaction) Benign tumors (osteoid osteoma) After lumbar puncture Juvenile osteoporosis

From Kliegman RM, editor: *Nelson essentials of pediatrics*, ed 5, Philadelphia, 2006, WB Saunders. Used with permission.

A few key screening questions might include:

 FOLLOW-UP QUESTIONS

- Have you had an injury or trauma to your head, face, neck, or back?
- Do you have (or have you recently had) a fever? Headache? Sore throat? Skin rash?
- Have you ever had cancer of any kind? Ever been treated with chemotherapy or radiation therapy?
- Are you taking any medications?
- Have you had any problems with your bowels or bladder?

For the Therapist[57]

- Is it possible/probable that there is a serious systemic disease or medical condition causing the pain?
- Is there neurologic compromise that might require surgical intervention?
- Is there social or psychologic distress that may amplify or prolong your pain?

LOCATION OF PAIN AND SYMPTOMS

There are many ways to examine and classify head, neck, and back pain. Pain can be divided into anatomic location of symptoms (where is it located?): cervical, thoracic, scapular, lumbar, and SI joint/sacral (as shown in Table15.1). For example, intrathoracic disease refers more often to the neck, mid-thoracic spine, shoulder, and upper trapezius areas. Visceral disease of the abdomen and/or pelvis is more likely to refer pain to the low back region. Later in this section, spine pain is presented by the source of symptoms (what is causing the problem?).

Whenever faced with the need to screen for medical disease the therapist can review Table 15.1. First, identify the location of the pain and then scan the list for possible causes. Given the client's history, risk factors, clinical presentation, and associated signs and symptoms, are there any conditions on this list that could be the possible cause of the client's symptoms? Is age or sex a factor? Is there a positive family or personal history?

Sometimes reviewing the possible causes of pain based on location gives the therapist a direction for the next step in the screening process. What other questions should be asked? Are there any tests that will help differentiate symptoms of one anatomical area from another? Are there any tests that will help identify symptoms that point to one system versus another?

Head

The therapist may evaluate pain and symptoms of the face, scalp, or skull. Headaches are a frequent complaint given by adults and children. Headaches account for 3% of emergency department visits annually and was the fourth or fifth leading reason for patients to visit the emergency department.[58] It may not be the primary reason for seeing a physical therapist but is often mentioned when asked if there are any other symptoms of any kind anywhere else in the body.

The brain itself does not feel pain because it has no pain receptors. Most often the headache is caused by an extracranial disorder and is considered "benign." Headache pain is related to pressure on other structures such as blood vessels, cranial nerves, sinuses, and the membrane surrounding the brain. Serious causes have been reported in 1% to 5% of the total cases, most often attributed to tumors and infections of the central nervous system (CNS).[59,60] In the past, headache was viewed as many disorders along a continuum. Better headache classifications have brought about the development of many discrete entities among these disorders.[61,62] The International Headache Society (HIS) published commonly used *International Classification of Headache Disorders* (third edition, revised) in 2018,[63] which divides headaches into three parts: primary headache, secondary headache, and cranial neuralgias.[64,65]

Primary headache includes migraine, tension-type headache, and cluster headache. Secondary headaches, of which there is a large number, are attributed to some other causative disorder specified in the diagnostic criteria attached to them.

The therapist often provides treatment for secondary headache called *cervicogenic headache* (CGH). This type of headache is defined as referred pain in any part of the head (e.g., musculoskeletal tissues innervated by these nerve roots) caused by spondylitic, fibrotic, or vascular compression or compromise of cervical nerves (C1-C4).[66] CGHs are frequently associated with postural strain or chronic tension, acute whiplash injury, intervertebral disk disease, or progressive facet joint arthritis (e.g., cervical spondylosis, cervical arthrosis) (Table 15.3).

Causes of Headaches

Headache can be a symptom of neurologic impairment, hormonal imbalance, neoplasm, a side effect of medication,[62] or other serious conditions (Box 15.2). Headache may be the only symptom of hypertension, cerebral venous thrombosis, or impending stroke.[67,68] Sudden, severe headache is a classic symptom of temporal vasculitis (arteritis), a condition that can lead to blindness if not recognized and treated promptly.

Recognizing associated signs and symptoms and performing vital sign assessment, especially blood pressure monitoring, are important screening tools for vascular-induced headaches (see Chapter 4 for information on monitoring blood pressure).

Stress and inadequate coping are risk factors for persistent headache. Headache can be part of anxiety, depression, panic disorder, and substance abuse.[69,70] Headaches have been linked with excessive caffeine consumption or withdrawal in children, adolescents, and adults.[71]

Therapists often encounter headaches as a complaint in clients with posttraumatic brain injury, postwhiplash injury, or postconcussion injury. A constellation of other symptoms is often present including dizziness, memory problems, difficulty concentrating, irritability, fatigue, sensitivity to noise, depression, anxiety, and problems with making judgments. Symptoms may resolve in the first 4 to 6 weeks following the injury but can persist for months to years causing permanent disability.[72,73]

Cancer. The greatest concern is always whether or not there is a brain tumor causing the headaches. Only a minority of individuals who have headaches have brain tumors. Risk factors include occupational exposure to gases and chemicals and a history of cranial radiation therapy for fungal infection of the scalp or other types of cancer.

A previous history of cancer, even long past history, is a red flag for insidious onset of head and occipital neck pain. Metastatic lesions of the upper cervical spine occur in less than 10% of all spinal metastases. Computed tomography

TABLE 15.3	Clinical Signs and Symptoms of Major Headache Types	
Migraine	Tension	Cervicogenic
Can be headache-free	Described as dull pressure	Pain starts in the occipital region and spreads anteriorly toward the frontal area
Migraines with headache are often described as throbbing or pulsating	Sensation of band or vise around the head; sometimes described as a painful, "tight" scalp	Usually bilateral
Often one-sided (unilateral); often around or behind one eye	Headache pain is bilateral or global (entire head)	Pain intensity fluctuates from mild to severe
Associated with nausea, vomiting	Muscular tenderness or soreness in soft tissues of the upper cervical spine	Often made worse by neck movements or sustained postures
Light and/or sound sensitivity (photophobia and phonophobia)	Not usually accompanied by associated signs and symptoms	Decreased neck range of motion
Common triggers:	May get worse with loud sounds or bright lights	Forward head posture
• Alcohol	Current diagnosis or history of anxiety, depression, or panic disorder	Trigger points or tender points in muscles
• Food		Cervical muscle weakness or dysfunction
• Hormonal changes		Can resemble migraines with throbbing pain, nausea, phonophobia, photophobia
• Hunger		History of trauma (e.g., whiplash), disk disease, or arthritis may be helpful
• Lack of sleep		
• Perfume		
• Stress		
• Medications		
• Environmental factors (e.g., pollutants, air pressure changes, temperature)		
May be preceded by prodromal symptoms:		
• Change in vision (aura): described as spots, balloons, lights, colors		
• Motor weakness		
• Dizziness		
• Paresthesia (numbness/tingling)		
• Confusion		
Facial pallor, cold hands and feet		
History of headaches in childhood; family history of migraines		

BOX 15.2 SYSTEMIC ORIGINS OF HEADACHE

Cancer
Primary neoplasm
Chemotherapy; brain radiation

Cardiovascular
Migraine
Ischemia (atherosclerosis; vertebrobasilar insufficiency; internal carotid artery dysfunction)
Cerebral vascular thrombosis
Arteriovenous malformation
Subarachnoid hemorrhage
Giant cell arteritis; vascular arteritis; temporal vasculitis
Hypertension
Febrile illnesses
Hypoxia
Systemic lupus erythematosus

Pulmonary
Obstructive sleep apnea
Hyperventilation (e.g., associated with anxiety or panic attacks)

Renal/Urologic
Kidney failure; renal insufficiency
Dialysis (first-use syndrome)

Gynecologic
Pregnancy
Dysmenorrhea

Neurologic
Postseizure
Disorder of cranium, cranial structures (e.g., nose, eyes, ears, teeth, neck)
Cranial neuralgia (e.g., trigeminal, Bell's palsy, occipital, herpes zoster, optic neuritis)
Brain abscess
Hydrocephalus

Other
History of physical or sexual abuse
Side effect of medication
Allergen/toxin (environmental or food)
Overuse of medication (analgesic rebound effect)
Psychogenic/psychiatric disorder
Substance abuse/withdrawal (drugs and/or alcohol)
Caffeine use/withdrawal
Candidiasis (yeast)
Trauma (e.g., cervicogenic headache, fracture, eating disorder with forced vomiting)
Infection (e.g., meningitis, sinusitis, syphilis, tuberculosis, sarcoidosis, herpes)
Postdural puncture
Scuba diving
Hantavirus
Paget's disease (when skull is affected)
Hypoglycemia
Fibromyalgia
Temporomandibular joint dysfunction

(CT) and magnetic resonance imaging (MRI) are routinely used for early detection of metastatic disease.[74]

The alert therapist may recognize the need for further imaging studies or medical evaluation. Persistent documentation of clinical findings and nonresponse to physical therapy intervention with repeated medical referral may be required.

Although primary head and neck cancers can cause headache, neck pain, facial pain, and/or numbness in the face, ear, mouth, and lips are more likely. Other signs and symptoms can include sore throat, dysphagia, a chronic ulcer that does not heal, a lump in the neck, and persistent or unexplained bleeding. Color changes in the mouth known as leukoplakia (white patches) or erythroplakia (red patches) may develop in the oral cavity as a premalignant sign.[75]

Cancer recurrence of the head and neck is common within the first 3 years after treatment; often these cancers are not diagnosed until an advanced stage, as a result of neglect on the part of the affected individual. Approximately 10% of patients with cancer develop metastases to the spine.[76,77] The most common site of spinal metastasis is the thoracic spine (50%–60%), followed by the lumbar spine (30%–35%), and the cervical spine (10%–15%).[78–81] Anyone with a history of head and neck cancer should be screened for cancer recurrence when seen by a therapist for any problem.

As always, prevention and early detection improve survival rates. Education is important because most of the risk factors (tobacco and alcohol use, betel nut, syphilis, nickel exposure, woodworking, sun exposure, dental neglect) are modifiable.

Tension-type or migraine headaches can occur with tumors. Rapidly growing tumors are more likely to be associated with headache and will eventually present with other signs and symptoms such as visual disturbances, seizures, or personality changes.[82,83] Headaches associated with brain tumors occur in up to half of all cases and are usually bioccipital or bifrontal, intermittent, and of increasing duration. Presence of tumor headache varies, depending on size, location, and type of tumor.[84] The headache is worse when awakening because of differences in CNS drainage in the supine and prone positions, but usually disappears soon after the person arises. It may be intensified or precipitated by any activity that increases intracranial pressure, such as straining during a bowel movement, stooping, lifting heavy objects, or coughing.

Often the pain can be relieved by taking aspirin, acetaminophen, or other moderate painkillers. Vomiting with or without nausea (unrelated to food) occurs in about 25% to 30% of people with brain tumors and often accompanies a headache when there is an increase in intracranial pressure. If the tumor invades the meninges, the headaches will be more severe.

Recognizing the need for medical referral for the client with complaints of headaches can be difficult. Past medical history can be complex in adults and screening clues are often confusing. Careful review of the clinical presentation is required. For example, although pain associated with the CGH can be constant (a red-flag symptom), the intensity often varies with activity and posture. Sustained posture consistently increases the intensity of painful symptoms.

Migraines. Approximately 15% of Americans experience migraines[85] and migraines were ranked as the sixth leading cause of years lost due to disability globally in 2013. Migraine headaches are often accompanied by nausea, vomiting, and visual disturbances, but the pain pattern is also often classic in description by the client. Age is a yellow (caution) flag because migraines generally begin in childhood to early adulthood. For those aged 45 to 64 years, the prevalence of migraine was 15.9% and this number decreased to 7.3% for those aged 65 to 74 years.[58] Migraines can first occur in an individual beyond the age of 50 years (especially in perimenopausal or menopausal women); advancing age makes other types of headaches more likely. Approximately 1 in 6 people and 1 in 5 women have reported severe headaches or migraines in the past 3 months. A family history is usually present, suggesting a genetic predisposition for migraine sufferers. In addition to the typical clinical presentation, normal examination results are likely.

Migraines can present with paralysis or weakness of one side of the body, mimicking a stroke. A medical examination is required to diagnose migraine, especially in cases of hemiplegic migraines. Medical evaluation and treatment for migraines, in general, is recommended.

There is a role for the physical therapist because the beneficial effects of exercise on migraine headaches have been documented.[86] More research needs to be done to determine the most effective intervention for treating migraine.

When present, associated signs and symptoms offer the best yellow or red flag warnings. For example, throbbing headache with unexplained diaphoresis and elevated blood pressure may signal a significant cardiovascular event. Daytime sleepiness, morning headache, and reports of snoring may point to obstructive sleep apnea. Headache-associated visual disturbances or facial numbness raises the suspicion of a neurologic origin of symptoms. Other red flags are listed in Box 15.3.

The therapist is advised to follow the same screening decision-making model introduced in Chapter 1 (see Box 1.7) and reviewed at the beginning of this chapter. Physical examination should include measurement of vital signs, a general assessment of cardiac and vascular signs, and a thorough head and neck examination. A screening neurologic examination should address mental status (including pain behavior), the cranial nerves, motor function, reflexes, sensory systems, coordination, and gait (see Chapter 4). Special Questions to Ask: Headache is listed at the end of

---

> ## BOX 15.3   RED-FLAG SIGNS AND SYMPTOMS ASSOCIATED WITH HEADACHE
>
> The therapist should watch for any of the following red flags (listed in descending order of importance) and report them to a medical doctor. A complete screening interview and examination can establish a baseline of information and aid in the medical referral decision-making process.
>
> - Headache that wakes the individual up or is present upon awakening (e.g., hypertension, tumor)
> - Headache accompanied by documented elevated blood pressure changes
> - Insidious or new onset of headache (less than 6 months)
> - New onset of headache with associated neurologic signs and symptoms (e.g., confusion, dizziness, gait or motor disturbances, fatigue, irritability or mood changes)
> - New onset of headache accompanied by constitutional symptoms (e.g., fever, chills, sweats) or stiff neck (infection, arteritis)
> - Episodes of "blacking out" during headache (seizures, hemorrhage, tumor)
> - Sudden severe headache accompanied by flu-like symptoms, aching muscles, jaw pain when eating, and visual disturbance (temporal arteritis)
> - No previous personal or family history of migraine headache

this chapter and in Appendix B-17 in the accompanying enhanced eBook version included with print purchase of this textbook.

Cervical Spine

Neck pain is the fourth leading cause of disability with a point prevalence in those aged 15 to 74 ranging from 5.9% to 38.7%.[87] Neck and shoulder pain and neck and upper back pain often occur together, making the differential diagnosis more difficult.

Traumatic and degenerative conditions of the cervical spine, such as whiplash syndrome and arthritis, are the major primary musculoskeletal causes of neck pain.[88] The therapist must always ask about a history of motor vehicle accident or trauma of any kind, including intimate partner violence.

Cervical or neck pain with or without radiating arm pain or symptoms may be caused by a local biomechanical dysfunction (e.g., shoulder impingement, disk degeneration, facet dysfunction) or a medical problem (e.g., infection, tumor, fracture). Referred pain presenting in these areas from a systemic source may occur from infectious disease, such as vertebral osteomyelitis, or from cancer, cardiac, pulmonary, or abdominal disorders (see Table 15.1).

Rheumatoid arthritis is often characterized by polyarthritic involvement of the peripheral joints, but the cervical spine is often affected early on (first 2 years) in the course of the disease. Deep aching pain in the occipital, retroorbital, or temporal areas may be present with pain referred to the face, ear, or subocciput from irritation of the C2 nerve root. Some clients may have atlantoaxial (AA) subluxation and report a sensation of the head falling forward during neck flexion or a clunking sensation during neck extension as the AA joint is reduced spontaneously. The most commonly involved nerve roots are C6 and C7, however, radiculopathy can occur at any cervical spine level.

Radicular symptoms accompanied by weakness, coordination impairment, gait disturbance, bowel or bladder retention or incontinence, and sexual dysfunction can occur whenever cervical myelopathy occurs, whether from a mechanical or medical cause. Cervical spondylotic myelopathy has been verified as a potential cause of LBP as well.[89] The combination of finger flexion, Hoffman's sign, and the Babinski test has a sensitivity of 91.7%, specificity of 87.5%, positive predictive value of 95.7% and a negative predictive value of 77.8% in detecting spinal cord compression.[90] An imaging study is usually needed to differentiate biomechanical from medical cause of radicular pain, especially when conservative care fails to bring about improvement.[91]

Torticollis of the sternocleidomastoid muscle may be a sign of underlying thyroid involvement. Anterior neck pain that is worse with swallowing and turning the head from side to side may be present with thyroiditis. Ask the client about associated signs and symptoms of endocrine disease (e.g., temperature intolerance; change in hair, nails, skin; joint or muscle pain; see Box 4.19) and a previous history of thyroid problems.[92]

Palpate the anterior spine and have the client swallow during palpation. Palpation of a soft tissue mass or lump should be noted. See guidelines for palpation in Chapter 4. Palpation of a firm, fixed, and immovable mass raises a red flag of suspicion for neoplasm. Visually inspect and palpate the trachea for lateral deviation to either side.[93]

Anterior disk bulge into the esophagus or pharynx and/or anterior osteophyte of the vertebral body may give the sensation of difficulty swallowing or feeling a lump in the throat when swallowing. Anxiety can also cause a sensation of difficulty swallowing with a lump in the throat. Conduct a cranial nerve assessment for cranial nerves V and VII (see chapter 5 for complete cranial nerve examination and explanation; see also Appendix B-21 in the accompanying enhanced eBook version included with print purchase of this textbook).

Vertebral artery syndrome caused by structural changes in the cervical spine is characterized by the client turning the whole body instead of turning the head and neck when attempting to look at something beyond his or her peripheral vision. Combined cervical motions, such as extension, rotation, and side-bending, cause dizziness, visual disturbance, and nystagmus. Rotational vertebral artery syndrome, or bow hunter syndrome, occurs when cervical spine rotation in certain clients compresses the vertebral artery at the atlantoaxial or lower levels of the cervical spine. The anatomy of the vertebral

CLINICAL SIGNS AND SYMPTOMS
Cervical Myelopathy

- Neck pain and/or shoulder pain, stiffness
- Wide-based clumsy, uncoordinated gait
- Loss of hand dexterity
- Paresthesia in one or both arms or hands
- Visible change in handwriting
- Difficulty manipulating buttons or handling coins
- Hyperreflexia
- Positive Babinski test
- Positive Hoffman's sign
- Lhermitte's sign (electric shock sensation down spine/arms with neck flexion/extension)
- Urinary retention followed by overflow incontinence (severe myelopathy)
- LBP[89]

artery is important to consider in this condition because the vertebral artery enters the transverse process of C6 and ascends through the transverse foramen of each cervical vertebrae up to C1 where the artery enters the foramen magnum. Clients that are older with more degenerative changes such as osteophytes are more prone to this condition, as well as those with hypertension, hyperlipidemia, diabetes, and a history of smoking or coronary artery disease. Most commonly, clients report dizziness, syncope, impaired vision, nystagmus, Horner's syndrome, and nausea with cervical spine rotation.[94–96]

Headache/neck pain may be the early presentation of underlying vascular pathology.[97] Decreased blood flow to the brain, referred to as cerebral ischemia, may be caused by vertebrobasilar insufficiency (VBI)/cervical arterial dysfunction,[97] secondary to atherosclerosis or some other arterial dysfunction. Arterial compression can also occur when decreased vertebral height, osteophyte formation, postural changes, and ligamentous changes reduce the foraminal space and encroach on the vertebral artery. Premanipulative screening tests for vertebral artery patency and other tests to "clear" the upper cervical spine before using upper cervical manipulative techniques (e.g., cervical rotation, alar and transverse ligament stress tests, tectorial membrane stress test) may help identify the underlying cause of neck pain. Consensus on the need to conduct these tests has not been reached because the validity of tests for VBI has not been established[98,99] and evidence suggests that high velocity thrusts do not affect the blood flow to the vertebral artery in healthy individuals.[100] More evidence is needed to confirm these findings.

Therapists are cautioned to screen clients before cervical spine manipulation to include taking the client's blood pressure, and to consider a premanipulative hold before manipulating a client, especially due to the prevalence of atherosclerosis in the United States. Caution is also advised with older adults, anyone with a history of hypertension, rheumatoid arthritis, or long-term use of corticosteroids. A careful history, blood pressure measurement, observation of vascular pain patterns, and conduction of a neurologic screening examination (possibly including cranial nerves) should be performed before upper cervical manipulation.

Thoracic Spine

As with the cervical spine and any musculoskeletal part of the body, the therapist must look for the cause of thoracic pain at the level above and below the area of pain and dysfunction. Possible musculoskeletal sources of thoracic pain include muscle strain, whiplash associated disorder,[101] vertebral or rib fracture, zygapophyseal joint arthropathy,[102] active trigger points, spinal stenosis, costotransverse and costovertebral joint dysfunction, ankylosing spondylitis, intervertebral disk herniation, intercostal neuralgia, diffuse idiopathic skeletal hyperostosis (DISH), and T4 syndrome.[103] Shoulder impingement and mechanical problems in the cervical spine can also refer pain to the thoracic spine.

Systemic origins of musculoskeletal pain in the thoracic spine (Table 15.4) are usually accompanied by constitutional symptoms and other associated symptoms. Often these additional symptoms develop after the initial onset of back pain and the client may not recognize their association, therefore failing to mention them.

The proximity of the thoracic spine to the chest and respiratory organs requires careful screening for pleuropulmonary symptoms in anyone with back pain of unknown cause or past medical history of cancer or pulmonary problems. Thoracic pain can also be referred from the kidney, biliary duct, esophagus, stomach, gallbladder, pancreas, and heart.

Thoracic aortic aneurysm, angina, and acute myocardial infarction (MI) are the most likely cardiac causes of thoracic back pain. Usually, there is a cardiac history and associated signs and symptoms such as a weak or thready pulse, extremely high or extremely low blood pressure, or unexplained perspiration and pallor.

Tumors occur most often in the thoracic spine because of its length, the proximity to the mediastinum, and direct metastatic extension from lymph nodes with lymphoma, breast, or lung cancer. The client may report symptoms typical of cancer. Tumor involvement in the thoracic spine may produce ischemic damage to the spinal cord or early cord compression because the ratio of canal diameter to cord size is small, resulting in rapid deterioration of neurologic status (Case Example 15.4).

Peptic ulcer can refer pain to the midthoracic spine between T6 and T10. The therapist should look for a history of NSAID use, ask about blood in the stools, and the effect of eating food on their pain and bowel function (see further discussion in Chapter 2).

Scapula

Most causes of scapular pain occur along the vertebral border and result from various primary musculoskeletal lesions. However, cardiac, pulmonary, renal, and GI disorders can cause scapular pain.

Specific questions to rule out potential systemic or medical origin of symptoms are listed in each chapter. For example, if the client reports any renal involvement, the therapist can use the questions at the end of Chapter 11 to screen further for urologic involvement. Appendix A in the accompanying enhanced eBook version included with print purchase of this textbook contains a series of screening questions based on the presence of specific factors (e.g., sex, joint pain, night pain, shortness of breath).

Lumbar Spine

LBP is the fifth most common reason individuals seek medical care with associated costs exceeding 200 billion dollars and up to 80% of adults experiencing acute LBP at some point in their lives.[1,104] In most cases, acute symptoms resolve within a few weeks to a few months. Individuals reporting persistent pain and activity limitation must be given a second screening examination.

As Table 15.1 shows, there is a wide range of potential systemic and medical causes of LBP. In one study, patients complaining of LBP in the emergency department were more likely to be males aged 20 to 39 years or females aged 65 to 94 years.[1] Older female adults with more comorbidities are at increased risk for LBP. Bone and joint diseases (inflammatory and noninflammatory), lung and heart diseases, and enteric diseases top the list of conditions contributing to LBP in older adults.[11,14,105]

Pain referred to the lumbar spine and low back region from the pelvic and abdominal viscera may come directly from the organ structures, but some experts suspect the referred pain pattern is produced by irritation of the posterior abdominal wall by pus, blood, or leaking enzymes. If that is the case, the pain is not referred but rather arises directly from the anterior aspect of the back.[38]

Sacrum/Sacroiliac

Sacral or SI pain in the absence of trauma and the presence of a negative spring test (posterior-anterior glide of sacrum between the innominates) must be evaluated more closely. The most common etiology of serious pathology in this anatomic region comes from the spondyloarthropathies (disease of the joints of the spine) such as ankylosing spondylitis, Reactive Arthritis, psoriatic arthritis, and arthritis associated with chronic inflammatory bowel (enteropathic) disease.

Spondyloarthropathy is characterized by pain occurring in the latter or second part of the night,[106] accompanied by prolonged stiffness that improves with activity. There is a limitation of motion in all directions and tenderness over the spine and SI joints

In addition to back pain, these rheumatic diseases usually include a constellation of associated signs and symptoms, such as fever, skin lesions, anorexia, and weight loss that alert the therapist to the presence of systemic disease or other medical conditions. Such symptoms present a red flag identifying clients who should be referred to a physician.

TABLE 15.4	Origin of Thoracic/Scapular Pain	
Systemic Origin	**Location**	**Neuromusculoskeletal**
CARDIAC Myocardial infarct Aortic aneurysm Angina	Midthoracic spine Thoracic spine; thoracolumbar spine Midthoracic spine; radiating down from shoulder (usually left side)	Trauma (including motor vehicle accident, domestic violence, assault) Muscle strain; overuse from repetitive motions Degenerative disk disease; disk calcification or other disk lesions Spinal stenosis Rib syndrome or zygapophyseal joint disorder (e.g., costovertebral [rib] dysfunction, slipping rib syndrome, twelfth rib syndrome, osteoarthritis, costovertebral or costotransverse joint hypomobility) Thoracic outlet syndrome Trigger points: trapezius (middle), multifidi, rotators, rectus abdominis, latissimus dorsi, rhomboids, infraspinatus, serratus posterior Vertebral or rib fracture or dislocation Bone or soft tissue ossification (e.g., spinal ligaments, bone spurs) Psychogenic (e.g., anxiety, depression, somatoform disorders) Scoliosis; spinal deformity; Scheuermann's disease Scapular dyskinesia
PULMONARY Basilar pneumonia Empyema Pleurisy Pneumothorax	Right upper back Scapula Scapula Ipsilateral scapula	
RENAL Acute pyelonephritis	Costovertebral angle (posterior)	
GASTROINTESTINAL Esophagitis Peptic ulcer: Stomach/duodenal Gallbladder disease Biliary colic Pancreatic carcinoma	Midback between scapulae Sixth through tenth thoracic vertebrae Midback between scapulae; right upper scapula or subscapular area Right upper back; midback between scapulae or subscapular areas Midthoracic or lumbar spine	
INFLAMMATORY/INFECTIOUS Rheumatoid arthritis Ankylosing spondylitis Osteomyelitis Pott's disease (tuberculosis of the spine) Spinal abscess or infection	Variable locations	
CANCER *Primary:* osteoid osteoma, spinal canal, spinal nerve roots *Metastases:* breast cancer, lung cancer, thyroid cancer, Hodgkin's disease, esophageal cancer, skin cancer	Variable locations	
OTHER Acromegaly Breast cancer Osteoporosis Paget's disease of bone Pregnancy Blood disorders (sickle cell disease)	Midthoracic or lumbar spine Midthoracic spine or upper back Variable locations Variable locations Variable locations Variable locations	

CASE EXAMPLE 15.4
Mid-Thoracic Back Pain

Background: A 55-year-old woman presents with sharp pain in the midback region around T5 to T6. The pain started after vacuuming her house last week. She has been taking Tylenol, but the pain is unrelieved. She reports being unable to find a comfortable position; the pain is keeping her awake at night.

History reveals a previous episode of pain in the same area 2 months ago. The pain started after she went grocery shopping and carried the heavy bags into her house. At that time, Tylenol quickly relieved her symptoms. The pain from the previous episode was described as "aching," not sharp like today.

Past Medical History: Past medical history includes breast cancer 15 years ago, surgical hysterectomy 10 years ago, and hypothyroidism. She does not remember what kind of breast cancer she had. She was treated with a lumpectomy and radiation. She has not had a mammogram or clinical breast examination in the past 5 years. She does not perform self-breast examination on a regular or consistent basis.

She takes Synthroid for her thyroid problem and does not take any other prescription medication. She takes a daily vitamin and 1200 mg of calcium but no other supplements. Tylenol is the only other over-the-counter (OTC) product she takes.

She does not smoke or drink, even socially. She does not use any other substances of any kind. She reports there are no other symptoms of any kind anywhere else in her body.

Clinical Presentation: Vital signs are normal. There are no visible or palpable lesions in the upper quadrant on either side. Axillary and supraclavicular lymph nodes are not enlarged or palpable. Submandibular lymph nodes are palpable but not tender or hard.

Neurologic screening examination is normal, including bowel and bladder function, although the client reports a sensation of intermittent "weakness" in her left arm. There is exquisite pain on palpation of the thoracic spine from T4 to T6. There was no apparent movement dysfunction observed.

How can you differentiate between a disk problem and bony metastases?

A differential diagnosis of this type is outside the scope of the physical therapist's practice and requires a medical evaluation. The physician's differential diagnosis may include mammography, x-ray studies, and computed tomography (CT) or magnetic resonance imaging (MRI) to assist in the diagnosis.

Severe back pain that is unrelieved by rest or change of position and is present at night in a woman with a past history of breast cancer requires immediate referral. Breast cancer has a predilection for axial skeletal bony metastases. Metastases can also occur hematogenously to the lungs (see Table 14.5). The therapist can perform a pulmonary system screening examination and ask about specific pulmonary signs and symptoms.

Reviewing Table 15.1 for possible viscerogenic causes of midthoracic back pain in a 55-year-old, the screening process can also include a brief cardiovascular examination and questions about gastrointestinal (GI) function. Baseline information of this type can be extremely helpful later when documenting change in status or condition.

Rather than providing physical therapy intervention and assessing the results, immediate medical evaluation is in the best interest of this client. If the medical tests come back negative or if there is a disk problem, then the appropriate physical therapy intervention can be prescribed.

Age, sex, and risk factors are important in assessing for systemic origin of symptoms associated with any of these inflammatory conditions. Clients with these diseases have a genetic predisposition to these arthropathies, which are triggered by environmental factors such as trauma and infection. Each of these clinical entities has been discussed in detail in Chapter 13.

Polymyalgia rheumatica and fibromyalgia syndrome are muscle syndromes associated with lumbosacral pain. Fibromyalgia syndrome refers to a syndrome of pain and stiffness that can occur in the low back and sacral areas with tender areas in multiple locations all over the body. Both of these disorders are also discussed in Chapter 13.

Anyone under the age of 45 years with low back, hip, buttock, and/or sacral pain lasting more than 3 months should be asked these four questions:

- Do you have morning back *stiffness* that lasts more than 30 minutes?
- Does the back pain wake you up during the second half of the night?
- Does the pain alternate from one buttock to the other (shift from side to side)?
- Does rest relieve the pain?

There is a 70% sensitivity and 81% specificity for inflammatory back pain if two of the four questions are positive.

Sensitivity drops to 33% if three of the four questions are answered as "yes," but the specificity increases to nearly 100%.[107]

SOURCES OF PAIN AND SYMPTOMS

Pain can be evaluated by the source of symptoms (what is causing the problem?). It could be visceral, neurogenic, vasculogenic, spondylogenic, or psychogenic in origin. Specific symptoms and characteristics of pain (frequency, intensity, duration, description) help identify sources of back pain (Table 15.5).[26,108]

The therapist must look at the history and risk factors, too. Any associated signs and symptoms that might reflect any one (or more) of these sources should be identified. Again, the therapist can use the tables in this chapter along with screening questions provided in Appendix A in the accompanying enhanced eBook version included with print purchase of this textbook to help guide the screening process.

Viscerogenic

Visceral pain may be confused with pain originating in the head, neck, and back. Physical therapists need to consider the referral of visceral pain to these areas and be vigilant in taking a thoughtful history and complete examination. It is

TABLE 15.5	Neck and Back Pain: Symptoms and Possible Causes
Symptom	**Possible Cause**
Night pain unrelieved by rest or change in position; made worse by recumbency; back pain, scoliosis, sensory and motor deficits in adolescents[108]	Tumor
Fever, chills, sweats	Infection
Unremitting, throbbing pain	Aortic aneurysm
Abdominal pain radiating to midback; symptoms associated with food; symptoms worse after taking NSAIDs	Pancreatitis, gastrointestinal disease, peptic ulcer
Morning stiffness that improves as day goes on	Inflammatory arthritis
Leg pain increased by walking and relieved by standing	Vascular claudication
Leg pain increased by walking, unaffected by standing but sometimes relieved by sitting or prolonged rest	Neurogenic claudication
"Stocking glove" numbness	Referred pain, nonorganic pain
Global pain	Nonorganic pain
Long-standing back pain aggravated by activity	Deconditioning
Pain increased by sitting	Discogenic disease
Sharp, narrow band of pain radiating below the knee	Herniated disk
Chronic spinal pain	Stress/psychosocial factors (unsatisfying job, fear-avoidance behavior, work or family issues, attitudes and beliefs)
Back pain dating to specific injury or trauma	Strain or sprain, fracture; failed back surgery
Back pain in athletic teenager[26]	Developmental, trauma, epiphysitis, juvenile discogenic disease, hyperlordosis, spondylosis, spondylolysis, or spondylolisthesis
Exquisite tenderness over spinous process	Tumor, fracture, infection
Back pain preceded or accompanied by skin rash	Inflammatory bowel disease

Modified from Nelson BW: A rational approach to the treatment of low back pain, *J Musculoskel Med* 10(5):75, 1993.
NSAIDs, Nonsteroidal antiinflammatory drugs.

an unusual presentation of systemic disease in the therapist's practice that will make it more difficult to recognize, therefore a systematic approach to consider the review of systems is paramount.

LBP is more likely to result from disease in the abdomen and pelvis than from intrathoracic disease, which usually refers pain to the neck, upper back, and shoulder. Disorders of the GI, pulmonary, urologic, and gynecologic systems can cause stimulation of sensory nerves supplied by the same segments of the spinal cord, resulting in referred back pain.[109] As discussed in Chapter 3, the CNS may not be able to distinguish which part of the body is responsible for the input into common neurons.

Back pain can be associated with distention or perforation of organs. Colicky pain is associated with spasm in a hollow viscus. Severe, tearing pain with sweating and dizziness may originate from an expanding abdominal aortic aneurysm (AAA). Burning pain may originate from a duodenal ulcer. Pain can occur from compression, ischemia, inflammation, or infection affecting any of the organs (Fig. 15.1).

Muscle spasm and tenderness along the vertebrae may be elicited in the presence of visceral impairment. For example, spasms on the right side at the ninth and tenth costal cartilages can be a symptom of gallbladder problems. The spleen can cause tenderness and spasm at the level of T9 through

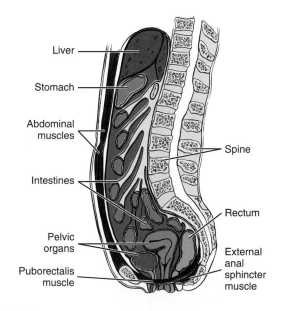

Fig. 15.1 Sagittal view of the abdominal and pelvic cavities to show the proximity of viscera to the spine. The abdominal muscles and muscles of the pelvic floor provide anterior and inferior support, respectively. Any dysfunction of the musculature can alter the relationship of the viscera; likewise anything that impacts the viscera can affect the dynamic tension and ultimately the function of the muscles. Pathology of the organs can refer pain through shared pathways or by direct distention as a result of compression from inflammation and tumor.

T11 on the left side. The kidneys are more likely to cause tenderness, spasm, and possible cutaneous pain or sensitivity at the level of the eleventh and twelfth ribs.

Most often, past medical history, clinical presentation, and associated signs and symptoms will alert the therapist to an underlying systemic origin of musculoskeletal symptoms. Any client older than 50 years of age with back pain, especially with insidious onset or unknown cause, must have their vital signs taken, including body temperature.

Careful questioning can elicit important information that the client withheld, thinking it was irrelevant to the problem, such as LBP alternating with abdominal pain at the same level, or back pain alternating with bouts of bloody diarrhea.

The therapist should look for clusters of signs and symptoms that may suggest an involvement of a particular system. The Review of Systems chart in Chapter 4 (see Box 4.19) can be very helpful in identifying visceral sources of symptoms, as well as the OSPRO-ROS.

Neurogenic

Neurogenic pain is not easily differentiated. Radicular pain results from irritation of axons of a spinal nerve or neurons in the dorsal root ganglion, whereas referred pain results from activation of nociceptive free nerve endings (nociceptors) in somatic or visceral tissue.

Neurologic signs are produced by a conduction block in motor or sensory nerves. This conduction block however does not cause pain. Thus even in a client with back pain and neurologic signs, whatever causes the neurologic signs is not causing the back pain by the same mechanism. Therefore, finding the cause of the neurologic signs does not always identify the cause of the back pain.[110] The therapist must look further.

Conditions such as radiculitis may cause both pain and neurologic signs, but in such a case the pain would occur in the lower limb, not in the back, upper extremity, or neck. If root inflammation also happens to involve the nerve root sleeve, neck or back pain might also arise. In such a case the individual will have three problems, each with a different mechanism: neurologic signs as a result of conduction block, radicular pain from nerve-root inflammation, and neck or back pain caused by inflammation of the dura.[110]

Identifying a mechanical cause of pain does not always rule out serious spinal pathology. For example, neurogenic pain can be caused by a metastatic lesion applying pressure or traction on any of the neural components. Positive neural dynamic tests do not reveal the underlying cause of the problem (e.g., tumor versus scar tissue restriction). The therapist must rely on history, clinical presentation, and the presence of any neurologic or other associated signs and symptoms to decide about the need for medical referral.

Sciatica alone or accompanying back pain is an important but unreliable symptom. Although 90% of cases of sciatica are caused by a herniated disk,[111] there are still the other 10%

the therapist must also be aware of in the screening process. For example, diabetic neuropathy can cause nerve root irritation. Prostatic metastases to the lumbar and pelvic regions or other neoplasms of the spine can create a clinical picture that is indistinguishable from sciatica of musculoskeletal origin (see Tables 17.1 and 17.6). This similarity may lead to long and serious delays in diagnosis. Such a situation may require persistence on the part of the therapist and client in requesting further medical follow-up.

Spinal stenosis caused by a narrowing of the vertebral (spinal) canal, lateral recess, or intervertebral foramina may produce neurogenic claudication (Fig. 15.2). The canal tends to be narrow at the lumbosacral junction, and the nerve roots in the cauda equina are tightly packed. Pressure on the cauda equina from a tumor, disk protrusion, spinal fracture or dislocation, infection, or inflammation can result in cauda equina syndrome, which is a neurologic medical emergency.[112,113] Cauda equina syndrome is defined as a constellation of symptoms that result from damage to the cauda equina, the portion of the nervous system below the conus medullaris (i.e., lumbar and sacral spinal nerves descending from the conus medullaris). The cauda equina is comprised of the lumbar nerves from L2 through L5, the sacral nerves and the coccygeal nerve. The incidence of cauda equina ranges from 1 in

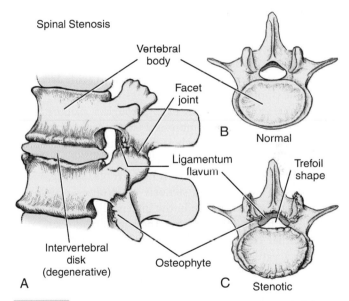

Spinal Stenosis

Fig. 15.2 *Spinal stenosis*. **A**, Aging causes a loss of disk height and compression of the vertebral body. The bone attempts to cushion itself by forming a lip or extra rim around the periphery of the endplates. This lipping can extend far enough to obstruct the opening to the vertebral canal. At the same time, the ligamentum flavum begins to hypertrophy or thicken and osteophytes (bone spurs) develop. Degenerative disease can cause the apophyseal (facet) joints to flatten out or become misshapen. Any or all of these variables can contribute to spinal stenosis. **B**, Normal, healthy vertebral body with a widely open vertebral canal. **C**, Stenotic spine from a variety of contributing factors. Many clients have all of these changes, but some do not. The presence of pathologic changes is not always accompanied by clinical symptoms.

33,000, making it a rare condition but one that physical therapists must be aware of to diagnose. Most clients with cauda equina are diagnosed in their 40 s with an increased likelihood of being female and obese. LBP is the most common clinical presentation but other symptoms include unilateral or bilateral sciatica, decreased perianal region sensation, fecal and bladder disruption, lower extremity weakness, and reduced sexual function.[114]

CLINICAL SIGNS AND SYMPTOMS
Cauda Equina Syndrome

- LBP
- Unilateral or bilateral sciatica
- Saddle anesthesia; perineal hypoesthesia
- Change in bowel and/or bladder function (e.g., difficulty initiating flow of urine, urine retention, urinary or fecal incontinence, constipation, decreased rectal tone and sensation)
- Sexual dysfunction:
  - Men: erectile dysfunction (inability to attain or sustain an erection)
  - Women: dyspareunia (painful intercourse)
- Lower extremity motor weakness and sensory deficits; gait disturbance
- Diminished or absent lower extremity deep tendon reflexes (DTR) (patellar, Achilles)

The medical diagnosis of cauda equina syndrome is not always straightforward. Decreased rectal tone may be delayed in individuals presenting with cauda equina syndrome. This is because sensory nerves are smaller and more sensitive than motor nerves; even so, some people present with decreased rectal tone (motor) without saddle anesthesia.[115]

The emerging nerve root exits through a shallow lateral recess and also may be compressed easily. Any combination of degenerative changes, such as disk protrusion, osteophyte formation, and ligamentous thickening reduces the space needed for the spinal cord and its nerve roots (see Fig. 15.2).

Confusion with spinal stenosis syndromes may occur when atheromatous change in the internal iliac artery results in ischemia to the sciatic nerve. The subsequent sciatic pain with vascular claudication-like symptoms may go unrecognized as a vascular problem. The therapist may be able to recognize the need for medical intervention by combining a careful subjective and objective examination with knowledge of vascular and neurogenic pain patterns (Table 15.6). This is especially true in the treatment of unusual cases of sciatica or back pain with leg pain.

The client with a neurogenic source of back pain may develop a characteristic pattern of symptoms, with back pain, discomfort in the buttock, thigh, or leg and numbness and paresthesia in the leg developing after the person walks a few hundred yards (neurogenic claudication). The person may be forced to stop walking and obtains relief after long periods of rest. The pattern of symptoms is similar to that of intermittent claudication associated with vascular insufficiency, the major

TABLE 15.6	Back Pain: Vascular or Neurogenic?
Vascular	**Neurogenic**
Throbbing	Burning
Diminished, absent pulses	No change in pulses
Trophic changes (skin color, texture, temperature)	No trophic changes; look for subtle strength deficits (e.g., partial foot drop, hip flexor or quadriceps weakness; calf muscle atrophy)
Pain present in all spinal positions	Pain increases with spinal extension, decreases with spinal flexion
Symptoms with standing: No	Symptoms with standing: Yes
Pain increases with activity; promptly relieved by rest or cessation of activity	Pain may respond to prolonged rest

differences being an immediate response to rest and position of the spine (see Fig. 15.4; see also Fig. 15.2).

The vertebral canal is wider when the spine is flexed, so relief from neurogenic pain may be obtained when the spine is flexed forward. Some individuals will bend over or squat as if to tie their shoelaces to assume a flexed spine position in public situations. Position of the spine (e.g., flexion, extension, side-bending, or rotation) does not affect symptoms of a cardiac origin.

Vasculogenic

Pain of a vascular origin may be mistaken for pain from a wide variety of musculoskeletal, neurologic, and arthritic disorders. Conversely, in a client with known vascular disease, a primary musculoskeletal disorder may go undiagnosed (e.g., discogenic disease, spinal cord tumor, peripheral neuritis, arthritis of the hip) because all symptoms are attributed to cardiovascular insufficiency.

Vasculogenic pain can originate from both the heart (viscera) and the blood vessels (soma), primarily as peripheral vascular disease. Back pain has been linked to atherosclerotic change in the posterior wall of the abdominal aorta in older adults.[116] The therapist can rely on special clues regarding vasculogenic-induced pain in the screening process (Box 15.4).

Vascular injury to the great vessels, which are in proximity to the vertebral column, can occur during lumbar disk surgery or can present as a complication postoperatively. In rare cases, severe bleeding can result in back pain and hypotension in the acute care phase. Late complications of back pain from pseudoaneurysm are rare (less than 0.05%) but can occur years after spine surgery (diskectomy).[117,118]

Once the history has been reviewed, the therapist assesses the pain pattern present during clinical examination, asks about associated signs and symptoms, and conducts a review of systems.

BOX 15.4 CLUES TO VASCULOGENIC PAIN

Pain of a vascular origin may be

- Described as "throbbing"
- Accompanied by leg pain that is relieved by standing still or rest
- Accompanied by leg pain that is described as "aching, cramping, or tired"
- Present in all spinal positions and increased by exertion
- Accompanied by a pulsing sensation in the abdomen or a palpable abdominal pulse
- Caused by a back injury (lifting) in someone with known heart disease or a past history of aneurysm
- Accompanied by pelvic pain, leg pain, or buttock pain
- Presented as arm pain when working with the arms overhead
- Accompanied by temperature changes in the extremities
- An early or late complication of lumbar surgery; ask about a history of previous spine surgery

Vascular back pain may be described as "throbbing" and almost always is increased with any activity that requires greater cardiac output and diminished or even relieved when the workload or activity is stopped. A "throbbing" headache may be a vascular headache from a variety of causes.

Women in the transitional menopause (perimenopause) state may experience vascular headaches from decreased estrogen levels.[119] Clients taking cardiac medication, such as glyceryl trinitrate (relaxes smooth muscle, especially the blood vessels), used to prevent angina, may also report episodes of throbbing headache. Vascular symptoms of this kind require medical evaluation.

Atherosclerosis and the resulting peripheral arterial disease are the underlying causes of most vascular back pain. Often the client history will reveal significant cardiovascular risk factors, such as smoking, hypertension, diabetes mellitus, advancing age, or elevated serum cholesterol (see Table 7.3 and discussion of peripheral vascular disease in Chapter 7).

Older age is an important red flag when assessing for pain of a vasculogenic origin. Most often, clients with back pain and any of the vascular clues previously listed are middle-aged or older. A personal or family history of heart disease is a second red flag. Continuous midthoracic pain can be a symptom of MI, especially in a postmenopausal woman with a positive family history of heart disease.

Older clients with long-term nonspecific LBP may have occluded lumbar/middle sacral arteries associated with disk degeneration. Back pain and neurogenic symptoms in the presence of a high serum low-density lipoprotein cholesterol level raise a red flag.[120]

Spondylogenic

Bone tenderness and pain during weight-bearing usually characterize spondylogenic back pain (or the symptoms produced by bone lesions). Associated signs and symptoms may include weight loss, fever, deformity, and night pain. There are numerous conditions capable of producing bone pain, but the most common pathologic disorders are fracture from any cause, osteomalacia, osteoporosis, Paget's disease, infection, inflammation, and metastatic bone disease (Case Example 15.5).[121–126]

The acute pain of a compression fracture superimposed by chronic discomfort, often in the absence of a history of trauma, may be the only presenting symptom. The client may recall a "snap" associated with mild pain, or there may have been no pain at all after the "snap." More intense pain may not develop for hours or until the next day.

Back pain over the thoracic or lumbar spine that is intensified by prolonged sitting, standing, and the Valsalva maneuver may resolve after 3 or 4 months as the fractures of the vertebral bodies heal. Clients who undergo kyphoplasty or vertebroplasty often have immediate pain relief.

The pain of untreated vertebral compression fractures may persist because of microfractures from the biomechanical effects of deformity. Other symptoms include pain during percussion over the fractured vertebral bodies, paraspinal muscle spasms, loss of height, and kyphoscoliosis.

When asking about the presence of any associated symptoms the therapist must keep in mind that older adults with vertebral compression fractures or kyphotic posture for any reason may report other pulmonary, digestive, and skeletal problems. These symptoms may not be indicative of back pain from a systemic or medical cause, but rather an organic dysfunction from a skeletal cause (i.e., somatovisceral response from the effect of a forward bent, kyphotic posture on the viscera).[127]

Sacral stress fractures should be considered in LBP of postmenopausal women with risk factors and athletes, particularly runners, volleyball players, and field hockey players (see further discussion on spondylogenic causes of sacral pain in Chapter 15).

Psychogenic

Psychogenic pain is observed in the client who has anxiety that amplifies or increases the person's perception of pain. Depression has been implicated in many painful conditions as the primary underlying problem. The prevalence of depression in physical therapy patients being treated for LBP has been reported to be as high as 26%.[128] There is a concern that depression may go unrecognized or inappropriately managed. Screening for depression can be done quickly and easily with the following two questions:

- During the past month, have you been bothered often by feeling down, depressed, or hopeless?
- During the past month, have you been bothered often by little interest or pleasure in doing things?

This two-question tool demonstrates a 96% sensitivity with a negative likelihood ratio (LR−) of 0.07, and a negative predictive value of 98%. Specificity was reported at 57% with a LR + of 2.2, and a positive predictive value of 33%.[129,130] A *yes* response to either or both of these questions warrants

CASE EXAMPLE 15.5

Osteoporosis

A 59-year-old man came to physical therapy for midthoracic back pain that seemed to come on gradually over the last few weeks and was starting to make his job as a janitor more difficult. There were no other symptoms to report: no neck, chest, or arm pain.

Past medical history was without incident. The client had never missed a day of work because of his illness, had never been hospitalized, and had no previous history of surgery. He has a 40-pack year history of smoking and "throws back a few beers" every night (six-pack daily for the last 15 years).

Clinical Presentation: Postural examination revealed a significant thoracic kyphosis with limited passive and active extension to neutral. Range of motion (ROM) in the lumbar spine was within normal limits. ROM in the hip and knee was also normal.

The client could take a deep breath without increasing his pain, but not without setting off a long spell of coughing. There was local tenderness palpable in the midthoracic paraspinal and rhomboid muscles without evidence of erythema, swelling, or other skin changes.

Neurologic screening examination was normal.

What are the red flags? Is a medical referral needed before initiating treatment?

Red flags include age and a significant history of tobacco and alcohol abuse. All three are risk factors for reduced bone mass and fracture. Osteopenia and osteoporosis are frequently overlooked in men and occur more often than previously appreciated.[121–125] Thirty percent of osteoporotic fractures occur in men.[126]

An x-ray would be a good idea in this case before beginning a program of back extension exercises or applying any manual therapy.

---

further evaluation.[128] (See additional questions in Appendices B-9 and B-10 on.)

Anxiety, depression, and panic disorder (see Chapter 3 for further discussion of anxiety, depression, and panic disorder) can lead to muscle tension, more anxiety, and then muscle spasm and guarding. Signs and symptoms of these conditions are listed in Tables 3.9 and 3.10. Other signs of psychogenic-induced back pain may be:

- Paraplegia with only stocking glove anesthesia
- Reflexes inconsistent with the presenting problem or other symptoms present
- Cogwheel motion of muscles for weakness
- Passive straight leg raise (SLR) in sitting versus the supine position (person is unable to complete SLR in supine but can easily perform an SLR in a sitting position)
- SLR supine with plantar flexion instead of dorsiflexion reproduces symptoms

The client may use words to describe painful symptoms characterized as "emotional." Recognizing these descriptors will help the therapist identify the possibility of an underlying psychologic or emotional etiology. An "exploding" or "vicious" headache, "agonizing" neck pain, or "punishing" backache are all red-flag descriptors of psychogenic origin (see Table 3.1).

The client who is unable to concentrate on anything except the symptoms and who reports that the symptoms interfere with every activity may need a psychologic/psychiatric referral. The therapist can screen for illness behavior as described in Chapter 3. Recognizing illness behavior helps the therapist clarify the physical assessment and alerts the therapist to the need for further psychologic assessment.[1]

Many studies have now shown a link between psychosocial distress and chronic neck or back pain.[131–136] Factors associated with chronic LBP may include job dissatisfaction, depression, fear-avoidance behavior, and compensation issues.[137,138] It may be necessary to conduct a social history to assess the client's recent life stressors and history of depression or drug or alcohol abuse.

The presence of psychosocial risk factors does not mean the pain is any less real nor does it reduce the need for symptom control. The therapist concentrates on pain management issues and improving function. Tools to screen for emotional overlay and fear-avoidance behavior are available in Chapter 3 of this text.

SCREENING FOR ONCOLOGIC CAUSES OF BACK PAIN

Cancer is a possible cause of referred pain. Tumors of the spine reportedly account for anywhere between 0.1% and 12% of back pain patients seen in a general medical practice.[139] Autopsy reports show up to 70% of adults who die of cancer have spinal metastases; up to 14% exhibit clinically symptomatic disease before death.[140]

Most reports place malignancy as a source of LBP in less than 1% of primary care patients.[141] Brain tumors (e.g., meningioma) in the motor cortex can present as LBP; abnormal symptom behavior and atypical responses to treatment may be observed and represent red flags for referral.[142] Head and neck pain from cancer is discussed earlier in this chapter (see the Causes of Headaches section).

Multiple myeloma is the most common primary malignancy involving the spine, often resulting in diffuse osteoporosis and pain with movement that is not relieved while the person is recumbent. Back pain with radicular symptoms can develop with spinal cord compression. There can be a long period of development (5 to 20 years) with a chronic presentation of LBP.

For most oncologic causes of back pain, the thoracic and lumbosacral areas are affected. As a general rule, thoracic pain must be screened for metastatic carcinoma. Pain and dysfunction in the lumbosacral area may be caused by direct spread of cancer from the abdomen or pelvic areas. When the lumbar spine is affected by metastasis, it is usually from a breast, lung, prostate, or kidney neoplasm. GI cancer, myelomas, and lymphomas can also spread to the spine via the paravertebral venous plexus. This thin-walled and valveless venous system probably accounts for the higher incidence of metastasis in the thoracic spine from breast carcinoma and in the lumbar region from prostatic carcinoma.

Past Medical History

Prompt identification of malignancy is important, starting with knowledge of previous cancers. A history of cancer anywhere in the body is a red-flag warning that careful screening is required. Always ask clients who deny a previous personal history of cancer about any previous chemotherapy or radiation therapy.

Early recognition and intervention does not always improve prognosis for survival from metastatic cancer, but it does reduce the risk of cord compression and paraplegia. It is important to remember that the history can be misleading. For example, almost 50% of clients with back pain from a malignancy have an identifiable (or attributable) antecedent injury or trauma[143] (Case Example 15.6).

It is unclear if this is a coincidence or merely reflective of weakness in the musculoskeletal system leading to loss of balance and strength and ultimately an injury. If the trauma results in significant injury (e.g., fracture), then the underlying cancer is usually identified quickly. But if soft tissue injury does not necessitate an x-ray or other imaging study, then the underlying oncologic cause may go undetected. The therapist may be the first to recognize the cluster of clinical signs and symptoms and/or red-flag findings to suggest a more serious underlying pathology.

Red Flags and Risk Factors

A combination of age (50 years or older), previous history of cancer, unexplained weight loss, and failure to improve after 1 month of conservative care has a reported sensitivity of 100%.[141] Of these four red flags, a previous history of cancer is the most informative with a pooled positive likelihood ratio of 23.7, compared with a positive likelihood ratio of 3 for age over 50 years, unexplained weight loss, and failure to improve after 1 month of conservative care.[136] Therefore, a previous history of cancer is the most important question to ask but if the client answers yes to this question and has an unexplained weight loss and a failure to improve after 1 month of conservative care, it is the therapist's responsibility to refer this patient to a physician because the sensitivity of these items is 100%.

Until now there has been an emphasis in this text on advancing age as a key red flag. Back pain at a young age (younger than 20 years old) has been considered a red flag in the previous editions of this text. As a general rule, persistent backache as a result of extraspinal causes is rare in children. As mentioned, mechanical back pain in children is possibly linked with heavy backpacks,[144,145] sports, and sedentary lifestyle. In 2020, Fabricant et al.[146] reported a prevalence of 33.7% of children and adolescents between the ages of 10 to 18 who reported back pain at some point during the year, with 13.8% seeking treatment. Fabricant et al. found that as adolescents aged, they were more likely to report back pain and that females were more likely than males to report back

---

CASE EXAMPLE 15.6

Multiple Myeloma Presenting as Back Pain

Background: A 41-year-old woman presented with low back pain (LBP) after a skiing accident 6 months ago. She continued skiing but reinjured her back a month later while loading bicycles onto a car.

She did not seek help at that time, thinking the pain would resolve with healing and time. She took acetaminophen and over-the-counter (OTC) nonsteroidal antiinflammatory drugs (NSAIDs) but did not think these helped with her symptoms.

She reports her stress level as "high" as a result of family problems. She reports her fatigue level to be "high" also because of caring for four preschool-aged children and a sick husband. She has lost 6 lbs in the last month trying to keep up with work and home activities. She currently reports her height and weight as 5 feet 4 inches tall and 108 lbs.

She reports her LBP is "always there," but it gets worse with activity or movement. There is no numbness or tingling, but the pain does radiate into the buttocks on both sides. When asked if there were any symptoms anywhere else in her body, she mentioned a mild discomfort in the lower thorax/chest that gets worse when she coughs or takes a deep breath.

She has seen her family physician and been told that the LBP is as a result of postrepetitive trauma and that she needs to give it time to heal. She was advised to avoid activities that could strain her back. She decided to see a physical therapist for exercises.

Past Medical History

- Benign breast cyst reported as negative 5 months ago
- Cesarean section delivery of all four children without complications

Clinical Presentation

- Posture: Standing and sitting postures appeared natural; normal lumbar lordosis
- Thin and pale but in no acute distress
- Vital signs: All normal
- Alert and oriented to time, place, and person

Neurologic Screen

Cranial nerves	Within normal limits (WNL)
Manual muscle testing (MMT)	WNL (5/5 all extremities)
Sensory examination	WNL (light touch, pinprick)
Deep tendon reflexes (DTR)	Brisk 3 +, equal in all four extremities
Straight leg raise (SLR)	Limited to 25 degrees, bilaterally because of back pain and apprehension
Romberg	WNL

Unable to test physiologic (accessory, joint play) motions of the spine because of a painful response

Unable to test for hip motion or overpressure of the sacroiliac (SI) joint because of pain

Positive tapping test (percussion over spinous processes) from L4 to S1

Walking pattern unremarkable; no antalgic gait

Able to walk in tandem and squat

Able to stand and walk on both heels and toes, bilaterally

Associated Signs and Symptoms

No report of fever, chills, night sweats, or night pain

No report of gastrointestinal (GI) or genitourinary (GU) dysfunction

Mild discomfort in the lower thorax/chest that gets worse when she coughs or takes a deep breath

What else do you need to know in the screening process?

Past history of infections of any kind? Cancer?

Recent or current medications besides OTC NSAIDs?

Tobacco use? Substance use (especially injection drugs with back pain)?

Did the physician examine your spine?

Were any x-rays or other imaging studies done?

Did you have a urinalysis or blood test done?

Recheck her vital signs on another day. Ask her to report any sweats, chills, or fever over the next 24 to 72 hours.

Any cough or shortness of breath? (Remember to ask about any functional limitations, not just ask if the client is having these symptoms.)

Any other respiratory signs and symptoms or red flags?

Take a more detailed birth/delivery history.

Type of birth control used (intrauterine contraceptive device?).

Date of last Pap smear and mammogram.

Has she had a hysterectomy (consider surgical menopause and osteoporosis)? Ask about STIs or the possibility of physical or sexual assault.

Any pelvic symptoms? Vaginal discharge? Unusual bleeding? Missed menses?

What other steps can you take in the screening process?

Turn to Table 15.1. As you look this over, does anything else come to mind given the client's age, sex, and history? Vertebral osteomyelitis is one possibility. Review the risk factors for this condition. Making a diagnosis of vertebral osteomyelitis would be outside the scope of a physical therapist's practice, but identifying risk factors and associated signs and symptoms aids the therapist in making a referral decision.

Review Clues to Screening Head, Neck, or Back Pain at the end of this chapter. After looking this list over, the therapist may be prompted to ask if there are any other painful or symptomatic joints anywhere else in the body.

The therapist can scan the Special Questions to Ask: Back to see if there have been any questions left out or that now seem appropriate to ask based on the information gathered so far. Review Special Questions for Women.

Given the information you have, would you treat or refer this client?

Even though the vital signs are unremarkable and the neurologic screen appears negative, there are plenty of red flags here.

Weight loss of 6 lbs even with emotional or psychologic stress in a thin person must be considered significant until proven otherwise.

Her age is borderline at 41 years, but there is an increased risk for diseases and illnesses with increasing age. Her pain appears to be constant but can be made worse with activity or movement. The fact that she injured her back 6 months ago but is still too acute to examine today is a red flag for possible orthopedic involvement that requires additional medical testing. This is not the expected clinical picture. The positive tapping test with percussion over the spine is another orthopedic red flag.

Radiating pain into the buttocks on both sides (bilateral) raises a red flag. It may be neurologic or from a disk problem. There is also the possibility of a vascular cause of bilateral buttock pain. The client is not as old as one might expect with vascular claudication, but at age 41 years it still must be considered. Palpate for an abdominal pulse (possible aneurysm). Check the width of the aortic pulse.

Pain during inspiration should prompt auscultation of respiratory sounds.

Screening for psychogenic or emotional overlay may be appropriate. If the therapist decides to treat the client as a part of the diagnostic process without the aid of imaging studies, caution is advised with any intervention. Obtaining the medical records is important, especially the physician's notes from the client's most recent visit.

Do not hesitate to contact the physician with your findings first and wait for agreement with your treatment plan. What the therapist observes during the examination may not be what the physician saw (e.g., acute presentation, positive tapping test, bilateral buttock pain).

If the client does not respond to physical therapy intervention, consider it the final red flag and refer immediately.

Result: The therapist made a judgment for immediate medical consultation by phone and by sending a faxed copy of the physical therapy evaluation. After conferring with the physician, a magnetic resonance imaging (MRI) was requested along with a complete blood cell count. The client had a compression fracture involving the central aspect of both the superior and inferior endplates of L5.

Blood cell counts were significantly decreased below normal (white blood cell [WBC], hemoglobin, hematocrit, and platelets). Erythrocyte sedimentation rate (ESR, or sed rate) and total protein levels were elevated.

Further diagnostic testing revealed a diagnosis of multiple myeloma. The diagnosis was confirmed by bone marrow biopsy, which showed infiltration of plasma cells. Further radiologic imaging revealed metastatic involvement of several ribs on both sides of the thoracic cage, right tibial head, and left ulna.

Physical therapy intervention was not appropriate in this case. A 41-year-old woman with LBP following repetitive injuries can be very deceiving. Multiple myeloma is unusual in people younger than 40 years of age and affects more men than women, and more African Americans than Caucasians.

Exposure to radiation, wood dust, or pesticides can contribute to the development of multiple myeloma. The therapist did not ask any questions about occupational or environmental exposures because there was nothing in the history or clinical presentation to suggest it.

Data from Dajoyag-Mejia MA, Cocchiarella A: Multiple myeloma presenting as low back pain. *J Musculoskel Med* 21(4):229–232, 2004.

pain.[146] Evidence suggests that this increasing trend of back pain is occurring on a global basis.[147]

It is important to consider that primary bone cancer occurs most often in adolescents and young adults. In considering this the authors of this text will continue to list that back pain in those younger than 20 years old should be a red flag. Bones of the appendicular skeleton (limbs) are affected more than the spine in this age group, but secondary metastases to the vertebrae can occur.

CLINICAL SIGNS AND SYMPTOMS

Oncologic Spine Pain

- Severe weakness without pain
- Weakness with full range
- Sciatica caused by metastases to the bones of the pelvis, lumbar spine, or femur
- Pain (nonmechanical) does not vary with activity or position (intense, constant); night pain
- Skin temperature differences from side to side
- Progressive neurologic deficits[148]
  - Sensory changes in myotome/dermatome pattern
  - Decreased motor function
  - Radiculopathy (rapid onset)
  - Myelopathy or cauda equina syndrome
- Positive percussive tap test to one or more spinous process
- Occipital headache, neck pain, palpable external mass in neck or upper torso
- Cervical pain or symptoms accompanied by urinary incontinence
- Look for signs and symptoms associated with other visceral systems (e.g., GI, genitourinary [GU], pulmonary, gynecologic)

Clinical Presentation

Back pain associated with cancer is usually constant, intense, and worse at night or with weight-bearing activities, although vague, diffuse back pain can be an early sign of non-Hodgkin's lymphoma and multiple myeloma. Pain with metastasis to the spine may become quite severe before any radiologic manifestations appear.[140]

Back pain associated with malignant retroperitoneal lymphadenopathy from lymphomas or testicular cancers is characterized as persistent, poorly localized LBP present at night, but relieved by forward flexion. Pain may be so excruciating while lying down that the person can sleep only if sitting in a chair hunched forward over a table.

Palpate the midline of the spinous processes for any abnormality or tenderness. Perform a tap test (percussion over the involved spinous process).[149] Reproduction of pain or exquisite tenderness over the spinous process(es) is a red-flag sign requiring further investigation and possible medical referral.

Neoplasm (whether primary or secondary) may interfere with the sympathetic nerves; if so, the foot on the affected side is warmer than the foot on the unaffected side. Paresis in the absence of nerve root pain suggests a tumor. Severe weakness without pain is very suggestive of spinal metastases. Gross muscle weakness with a full range of passive SLR and without

a history of recent acute sciatica at the upper two lumbar levels is also suggestive of spinal metastases.

A careful assessment of motor strength, sensory levels, proprioception, and reflexes is recommended. These findings can provide a baseline against which to compare future responses that might represent deterioration or undiagnosed lesions at other levels. Abnormal or new findings should be reported.[140]

A short period of increasing central backache in an older person is always a red-flag symptom, especially if there is a previous history of cancer. The pain spreads down both lower limbs in a distribution that does not correspond with any one nerve root level. Bilateral sciatica then develops, and the back pain becomes worse.

Radiographs do not show bone destruction from metastatic lesions until the lytic process has destroyed 30% to 50% of the bone. The therapist cannot assume metastatic lesions do not exist in the client with a past medical history of cancer now presenting with back pain and "normal" radiograph images.[150–152] In a 2020 systematic review, the combination of a history of cancer and/or the clinical suspicion of cancer resulted in a higher positive likelihood ratio (27.9; 17.5-44.6).[153,154]

Associated Signs and Symptoms

Clinical signs and symptoms accompanying back pain from an oncologic cause may be system related (e.g., GI, GU, gynecologic, spondylogenic), depending on where the primary neoplasm is located and the location of any metastases (Case Example 15.7).

The therapist must ask about the presence of constitutional symptoms, symptoms anywhere else in the body, and assess vital signs as a part of the screening process. Unexplained weight loss is a common feature in anyone with tumors of the spine. Review the red flags in Box 15.1 and conduct a Review of Systems to identify any clusters of signs and symptoms.

SCREENING FOR CARDIAC CAUSES OF NECK AND BACK PAIN

Vascular pain patterns originate from two main sources: cardiac (heart viscera) and peripheral vascular (blood vessels). The most common referred cardiac pain patterns seen in a physical therapy practice are angina, MI, and aneurysm.

Pain of a cardiac nature referred to the soma is based on multisegmental innervation. For example, the heart is innervated by the C3 through T4 spinal nerves. Pain of a cardiac source can affect any part of the soma (body) also innervated by these levels. This is why someone having a heart attack can experience jaw, neck, shoulder, arm, upper back, or chest pain. See Chapter 3 for an in-depth discussion of the origins of viscerogenic pain patterns affecting the musculoskeletal system for males and females.

On the other hand, pain and symptoms from a peripheral vascular problem are determined by the location of the underlying pathology (e.g., aortic aneurysm, arterial or venous obstruction). Peripheral vascular patterns will be reviewed later in this chapter.

CASE EXAMPLE 15.7

Skin Lesions

A 52-year-old woman presented in physical therapy with low back pain (LBP) radiating down the right leg to the knee. She had recently completed chemotherapy for acute myeloid leukemia and was referred to physical therapy by the oncology nurse. Bone marrow biopsy 1 month ago was negative for leukemic cells.

Clinical Presentation: The client presented with acute LBP described as "going across my low back area." She had a normal gait pattern but decreased lumbar motions in forward bending, right side-bending, and left rotation.

Her pain was relieved by forward bending. Pain was too intense to conduct accessory motion testing because the client was unable to lie down for more than 1 minute before having to sit up.

Neurologic screen revealed a positive straight leg raise (SLR) on the right, intact sensation, and decreased ankle reflex on the right (patellar tendon reflex was assessed as normal). Manual muscle strength testing was deferred as a result of the client's extreme agitation during testing. There were no reported changes in the bowel or bladder.

When asked if there were any other symptoms of any kind anywhere else in the body, the client raised her shirt and showed the therapist several nodules on her skin. They were not tender or oozing any discharge. The client reported she first noticed them about 1 week before her back pain started. She had not remembered to tell the nurse or her doctor about them.

Outcome: This is a good case to point out that even though the client has a known condition, such as cancer, and the referral comes from a health care professional, screening for medical disease as the cause of the pain or symptoms is still very important.

The therapist made phone contact with the referring nurse and reported findings from the evaluation. Of particular concern were the skin lesions and neurologic changes. The nurse was unaware of these changes. The therapist requested a medical evaluation before starting a physical therapy program.

The client was diagnosed with cancer metastasis to the spine and cauda equina syndrome. Cauda equina syndrome, caused by mechanical compression of the spinal nerve roots by tumor (or infection), requires immediate medical attention.

The client underwent urgent total spine irradiation, which did relieve her back pain. She declined further medical care (i.e., chemotherapy) and decided to continue with physical therapy to regain motion and strength.

CASE EXAMPLE 15.8

Back Pain and Dizziness after Colonoscopy

An 87-year-old woman visiting her daughter from out of town fell and suffered a compression fracture of L1. She reported having "heart problems" during a colonoscopy several weeks before this fall. She has had extreme back pain and is being given Vicodin (opioid analgesic for mild pain).

She is nauseated and attributes this to the pain medication. Blood pressure is 200/90 mm Hg with a pulse in the low 80s. There is no respiratory distress, no heart palpitations, and no fever. She reports taking many blood pressure and heart medications, and thyroid meds.

The family reports she has dizzy spells and is weak. She frequently loses her balance but does not fall. She is extremely tired and the family reports she sleeps much during the day.

She has been referred to physical therapy through a home health agency. Because she is from out of town, she does not have a primary care physician. The daughter took her to a local walk-in clinic. The nurse practitioner then referred her to home health. Physical therapy was prescribed for the dizziness and falling.

You suspect the symptoms of dizziness, drowsiness, and weakness may be drug-induced. What do you do in a case like this?

Conduct an evaluation and gather as much information as you can from the client and family members. Use the Quick Screen Checklist and complete a Review of Systems. Organize the information you obtain from the evaluation so that the need for any other screening questions can be identified.

Look up potential side effects of Vicodin and ask the client about the presence of any other symptoms of any kind. See if any of the reported signs and symptoms point to side effects of medication. Conduct a cardiovascular screening examination (see Chapter 4).

Do not hesitate to contact the local clinic/nurse practitioner and ask if the client's symptoms could be cardiac or drug-induced. Report the abnormal vital signs. There may be a change in drug dosage, suggested drug administration (with or without food, time of day), or change in prescribed drug that can alleviate symptoms while still controlling pain. Vital signs may return to normal with better pain control unless there is an underlying cardiovascular reason for her symptoms.

Assess muscle weakness, vestibular function, and balance. Look for modifiable risk factors. Offer as much intervention as possible, given the temporary visiting situation and short-term episode of care.

Document findings, problem list, and plan of care and communicate these results with the referring agency. Medical referral may be advised given the client's age, vital signs, history of heart disease, and use of multiple medications.

Angina

Angina may cause chest pain radiating to the anterior neck and jaw, sometimes appearing only as neck and/or jaw pain and misdiagnosed as temporomandibular joint (TMJ) dysfunction. Postmenopausal women are the most likely candidates for this type of presentation. If the jaw pain is steady, lasts a long time, or is worst when first waking up in the morning, it could be that the individual is grinding their teeth while sleeping. But jaw pain that comes and goes with physical activity or stress may be a symptom of angina.

Angina and/or myocardial infarction can appear as isolated midthoracic back pain in men or women (see Figs. 7.4 and 7.8). There is usually a lag time of 3 to 5 minutes between an increase in activity and onset of musculoskeletal symptoms caused by angina.

Myocardial Ischemia

Heart disease and MI, in particular, can be completely asymptomatic. Sudden death occurs without any warning in 50% of all MIs. Back pain from the heart (cardiac pain pattern) can be referred to the anterior neck and/or midthoracic spine in both men and women.

When pain does present, it may look like one of the patterns shown in Fig. 7.9. There are usually some associated signs and symptoms such as unexplained perspiration (diaphoresis), nausea, vomiting, pallor, dizziness, or extreme anxiety. Age and past medical history are important when screening for angina or MI as possible causes of musculoskeletal symptoms. Vital signs are key in clinical assessment (Case Example 15.8).

Abdominal Aortic Aneurysm

On occasion, an AAA can cause severe back pain (see Fig. 7.11 and additional discussion in Chapter 7). An aneurysm is an abnormal dilation in a weak or diseased arterial wall causing a sac-like protrusion. Prompt medical attention is imperative because rupture can result in death. Aneurysms can occur anywhere in any blood vessel, but the two most common places are the aorta and cerebral vascular system. AAA occurs most often in men aged 65 to 75 who have ever smoked in their life.[155] Authors define "ever smoker" as someone who has smoked 100 or more cigarettes. There is a dose-response relationship as greater smoking exposure is associated with an increased risk for AAA.

Risk Factors

The major risk factors for AAA include older age, male sex,[156] smoking, and having a first-degree relative with a AAA. The risk of developing an AAA is stronger with a female first-degree relative (odds ratio, 4.32) than with a male first-degree relative (odds ratio, 1.61).[157-162] Although the underlying cause is most often atherosclerosis, the therapist should be aware that aging athletes involved in weight lifting are at risk for tears in the arterial wall, resulting in an aneurysm.[163] There is often a history of intermittent claudication and decreased or absent peripheral pulses. Other risk factors include a history of vascular aneurysms, coronary artery disease, cerebrovascular disease, hypercholesterolemia, and hypertension.[164-166] Often the presence of these risk factors remains unknown until an aneurysm becomes symptomatic.[167] Factors that are associated with a reduced risk include African American race, Hispanic ethnicity, Asian ethnicity, and diabetes.[168-172]

Clinical Presentation

Pain presents as deep and boring in the midlumbar region. The pattern is usually described as sharp, intense, severe, or knife-like in the abdomen, chest, or anywhere in the back (including the sacrum). The location of the symptoms is determined by the location of the aneurysm (see Fig. 7.11).

Most aortic aneurysms (95%) occur just below the renal arteries. An objective examination may reveal a pulsing abdominal mass or abnormally widened aortic pulse width (see Fig. 4.55).

Obesity and abdominal ascites or distention make this examination more difficult. The therapist can also listen for bruits. Bruits are abnormal blowing or swishing sounds heard during auscultation of the arteries.

Bruits with both systolic and diastolic components suggest the turbulent blood flow of partial arterial occlusion. The client will be hypertensive if the renal artery is occluded as well. Peripheral pulses may be diminished or absent. Other historical clues of coronary disease or intermittent claudication of the lower extremities may be present.

Monitoring vital signs is important, especially among exercising older adults. Teaching proper breathing and abdominal support without using a Valsalva maneuver is important in any exercise program, but especially for those clients at increased risk for aortic aneurysm.

CLINICAL SIGNS AND SYMPTOMS

Impending Rupture or Actual Rupture of an Aortic Aneurysm

- Rapid onset of severe neck or back pain (buttock, hip, and/or flank pain possible)
- Pain may radiate to chest, between the scapulae, or to posterior thighs
- Pain is not relieved by a change in position
- Pain is described as "tearing" or "ripping"
- Other signs: cold, pulseless lower extremities, blood pressure differences between arms (more than 10 mm Hg diastolic)

The U.S. Preventive Services Task Force (USPSTF) updated its guidelines for medical screening for AAA in 2019.[173] The new guidelines recommend ultrasound screening for men ages 65 to 75 years who have ever smoked as a 1-time screening evaluation.[222] In 2015, a study investigating the use of the USPSTF guidelines indicates that AAA screening rates remain below 50% in primary care clinics.[174] The therapist should advise men in this age group who have ever smoked to discuss their risk for AAA with a medical doctor. Any male with these two risk factors, especially presenting with any of these signs or symptoms, must be referred immediately.

The cost-effectiveness of screening women for AAA is under investigation. The USPSTF recommends against routine screening for AAA with ultrasonography in women who have never smoked and have no family history of AAA. One trial reported a prevalence in women that was one-sixth of the prevalence in men (1.3% vs 7.6%), and most AAA-related deaths occurred in women 80 years or older (70% vs <50% in men). However when aneurysms occur in women, smaller AAAs have an increased risk of rupture, and rupture at an older age than in men.[175]

The orthopedic or acute care therapist must be aware that aortic damage (not an aneurysm but sometimes referred to as a *pseudoaneurysm*) can occur with any anterior spine surgery (e.g., spinal fusion, spinal fusion with cages). Blood vessels are moved out of the way and can be injured during surgery. If the client (usually a postoperative inpatient) has internal bleeding from this complication, there may be:

- Abdominal distention
- Change in blood pressure
- Change in stool
- Possible back and/or shoulder pain

In such cases, the client's recent history of anterior spinal surgery accompanied by any of these symptoms is enough to notify nursing or medical staff of concerns. Monitoring postoperative vital signs in these clients is essential.

SCREENING FOR PERIPHERAL VASCULAR CAUSES OF BACK PAIN

Most physical therapists are very familiar with the signs and symptoms of peripheral vascular disease (PVD) affecting the extremities, including both arterial and venous disease (see discussion in Chapter 7).

When assessing back pain for the possibility of a vascular cause, remember peripheral vascular disease can cause back pain. The location of the pain or symptoms is determined by the location of the pathology (Fig. 15.3).

With obstruction of the aortic bifurcation, the client may report back pain alone, back pain with any of the following features, or any of these signs and symptoms alone (Table 15.7):

- Bilateral buttock and/or leg pain or discomfort
- Weakness and fatigue of the lower extremities
- Atrophy of the leg muscles
- Absent lower extremity pulses
- Change in color and/or temperature of the feet and lower legs

Symptoms are often (but not always) bilateral because the obstruction occurs before the aorta divides (i.e., before it becomes the common iliac artery and supplies each leg separately). Frequently, someone with symptomatic atherosclerotic disease in one blood vessel has a similar pathology in other blood vessels. Over time there may be a progression of symptoms as the disease worsens and blood vessels become more and more clogged with plaque and debris.

With obstruction of the iliac artery, the client is more likely to present with pain in the low back, buttock, and/or leg of the affected side and/or numbness in the same area(s). Obstruction of the femoral artery can result in thigh and/or calf pain, again with distal pulses diminished or absent.

Ipsilateral calf/ankle pain or discomfort (intermittent claudication) occurs with obstruction of the popliteal artery and is a common first symptom of PVD.

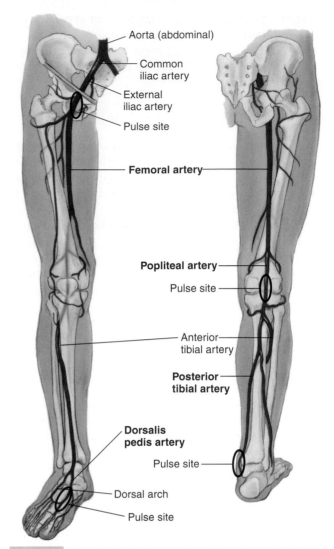

Fig. 15.3 **Arteries in the lower extremities.** As you look at this illustration, note the location of the arteries in the lower extremities starting with the aorta branching into the common iliac artery, which descends on both sides into the legs. Once the common iliac artery passes through the pelvis to the femur, it becomes the femoral artery and then the popliteal artery behind the knee before branching into the popliteal artery. The final split comes as the popliteal artery divides to form the anterior tibial artery down the front of the lower leg and the posterior tibial artery down the back of the lower leg. The anterior tibial artery also becomes the dorsalis pedis artery. Note the pulse points shown with bold, black ovals and remember that distal pulses disappear with aging and the presence of atherosclerosis causing peripheral vascular disease. (From Jarvis C: *Physical examination and health assessment*, ed 5, Philadelphia, 2008, WB Saunders.)

Adults over the age of 50 years presenting with back pain of unknown cause and mild-to-moderate elevation of blood pressure should be screened for the presence of PVD.

Back Pain: Vascular or Neurogenic?

The medical differential diagnosis is difficult to make between back pain of a vascular versus neurogenic origin. Frequently, vascular and neurogenic claudication occurs in the same age group (over 60 years of age and even more often, after the age of 70).

TABLE 15.7	Back and Leg Pain from Arterial Occlusive Disease

The location of discomfort, pain, or other symptoms is determined by the location of the pathology (arterial obstruction).

Site of Occlusion	Signs and Symptoms

Aortic bifurcation	• Sensory and motor deficits
	  • Muscle weakness and atrophy
	  • Numbness (loss of sensation)
	  • Paresthesia (burning, pricking)
	  • Paralysis
	• Intermittent claudication (pain or discomfort relieved by rest): bilateral buttock and/or leg, low back, gluteal, thigh, calf
	• Cold, pale legs with decreased or absent peripheral pulses

Iliac artery	• Intermittent claudication (pain or discomfort in the buttock, hip, thigh of the affected leg; can be unilateral or bilateral; relieved by rest) • Diminished or absent femoral or distal pulses • Impotence in males
Femoral and popliteal artery	• Intermittent claudication (pain or discomfort; calf and foot; may radiate) • Leg pallor and coolness • Dependent rubor • Blanching of feet with elevation • No palpable pulses in ankles and feet • Gangrene
Tibial and common peroneal artery	• Intermittent claudication (calf pain or discomfort; feet occasionally) • Pain at rest (severe disease); possibly relieved by dangling leg • Same skin and temperature changes in lower leg and foot as previously described • Pedal pulses absent; popliteal pulses may be present

(From Goodman CC, Fuller KS: *Pathology: implications for the physical therapist*, ed 3, Philadelphia, 2009, WB Saunders.)

Sometimes clients are referred to physical therapy to help make the differentiation (Case Example 15.9).

Vascular and neurogenic disease often coexists in the same person with an overlap of symptoms. There are several major differences to look for, but especially response to rest (i.e., activity pain), position of the spine, and the presence of any trophic (skin) changes (see Tables 15.6 and 16.5).

Vascular-induced back and/or leg pain or discomfort is alleviated by rest and usually within 1 to 3 minutes. Conversely, activity (usually walking) brings the symptoms on within 1 to 3 minutes, sometimes 3 to 5 minutes. Neurogenic-induced symptoms often occur immediately with the use of the affected body part and/or when adopting certain positions. The client may report the pain is relieved by prolonged rest or not at all.

What is the effect of changing the position of the spine on pain of a vascular nature? Are the vascular structures compromised in

any way by forward bending, side-bending, or backward bending (Fig. 15.4)? Are we asking the diseased heart or compromised blood vessels to supply more blood to this area?

It is not likely that movements of the spine will reproduce back pain of a vascular origin. What about back pain of a neurogenic cause? Forward bending opens the vertebral canal (vertebral foramen) giving the spinal cord (through L1) additional space. This is important in preventing painful symptoms when spinal stenosis is present as a cause of neurogenic claudication.

Unless there is a spinal neuroma, a true stenosis with spinal cord pressure does not occur in the lumbar region because the spinal cord ends at L1 in most people. Neural symptoms at L1 to L3 are rare and more likely indicate a spinal tumor rather than disk or facet pathology. Nerve pressure leading to radicular symptoms (e.g., pain, numbness, myotomal weakness) below L2 is not true stenosis of the vertebral canal, but rather intervertebral foraminal stenosis with encroachment of the peripheral nerve as it leaves the spinal canal through the neural foramina.

The position of comfort for someone with back pain associated with spinal stenosis is usually lumbar flexion. The client may lean forward and rest the hands on the thighs or lean the upper body against a table or cupboard.

The Bicycle Test

The Bicycle test of van Gelderen[176–178] is one way to assess the cause of back pain (Fig. 15.5). Although sensitivity, specificity, and LRs have not been established for this test, from clinical experience it is believed to offer clues to the source (neurogenic or vascular). It is not a definitive test by itself. The Bicycle test is based on two of the three variables listed earlier: (1) response to rest and (2) position of the spine. Trophic (skin) changes are assessed separately.

In theory, if someone has back/buttock pain of a vascular origin, what is the effect of pedaling a stationary bicycle? Increased demand for oxygen can result in back/buttock pain when the cardiac workload/oxygen need is greater than the ability of the affected coronary arteries to supply the necessary oxygen.

Normally, the response would be angina (chest pain or discomfort or whatever pattern the client typically experiences). In the case of referred pain patterns, the client may experience midthoracic or even lumbar pain. How soon do these symptoms appear? With musculoskeletal pain of cardiac origin, there is a 3- to 5-minute lag time before the onset of symptoms. Immediate reproduction of painful symptoms is more indicative of neuromusculoskeletal involvement.

After pedaling for 5 minutes and observing the client's response, ask him or her to lean forward and continue pedaling. What is the expected response if the back, buttock, or leg pain is vascular-induced? In other words, what is the response to a change in position when someone has back pain of a vascular origin?

Typically, there is no change because a change in position does not reproduce or alleviate vascular symptoms. The therapist can palpate pulses before and after the test to confirm the presence of vascular symptoms. What about neurogenic impairment? The client with neurogenic back pain may report

CASE EXAMPLE 15.9

Spinal Stenosis

Background: A 68-year-old woman with a long history of degenerative arthritis of the spine was referred to physical therapy for conservative treatment toward the goal of improving function despite her painful symptoms. She was a nonsmoker with no other significant previous medical history.

Her symptoms were diffuse bilateral lumbosacral back pain into the buttocks and thighs, which increased with walking or any activity and did not subside substantially with rest (except for prolonged rest and immobility).

Clinical Presentation: During the examination, this client moved slowly and with effort, complaining of the painful symptoms described. There was no tenderness of the sacroiliac (SI) joint or sciatic notch, but a subjective report of tenderness over L4-L5 and L5-S1. Tap test was negative; the client reported mild diffuse tenderness. There was no palpable step-off or dip of the spinous processes for spondylolisthesis and no paraspinal spasm, but a marked right lumbar scoliosis was noted. The client reported knowledge of scoliosis since she was a child.

A neurologic screening examination revealed normal straight leg raise (SLR) and normal sensation and reflexes in both lower extremities. Motor examination was unremarkable for an inactive 68-year-old woman. Dorsalis pedis and posterior tibialis pulses were palpable, but weak, bilaterally.

Despite physical therapy treatment and compliance on the part of the client with a home program, her symptoms persisted and progressively worsened.

What is the next step in the screening process?

Reevaluate the client's movement dysfunction and the selected intervention to date. Was the right treatment approach taken? Reassess red-flag findings (age, lack of improvement with intervention) and conduct a review of systems (if this has not already been done).

In this case the client's age, negative neurologic screening examination, and diminished lower extremity pulses suggested a second look for a vascular cause of symptoms.

Vital signs were assessed along with a peripheral vascular screening examination. The Bike test was administered, but the results were unclear with increased pain reported in both extension and flexion.

Result: She returned to her physician with a report of these findings. Further testing showed that in addition to degenerative arthritis of the lumbosacral spine, there was secondary stenosis and marked aortic calcification, indicating a vascular component to her symptoms.

Surgery was scheduled: an L4-L5 laminectomy with fusion, iliac crest bone graft, and decompression foraminotomies. Postoperatively, the client subjectively reported 80% improvement in her symptoms with an improvement in function, although she was still unable to return to work.

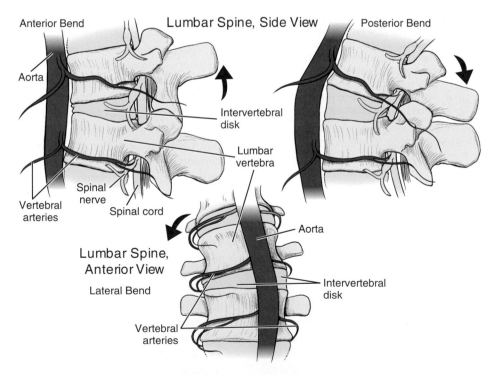

Fig. 15.4 Vascular supply is not compromised by position of the spine, so there is usually no change in back pain that is vascular-induced with change of position. Forward bend, extension, and side-bending do not aggravate or relieve symptoms. Rather, increased activity requiring increased blood supply to the musculature is more likely to reproduce symptoms; likewise, rest may relieve the symptoms. Watch for a lag time of 3 to 5 minutes after the start of activity or exercise before symptoms appear or increase as a sign of a possible vascular component.

a decrease in pain intensity or duration with forward flexion. Leaning forward (spinal flexion) can increase the diameter of the spinal canal, reducing pressure on the neural tissue.

When using the Bicycle test to look for neurogenic claudication, the client starts pedaling while leaning back slightly. This position puts the lumbar spine in a position of extension. If the pain is reproduced, the first part of the test is positive for a neurogenic source of symptoms. The client then leans forward while still pedaling. If the pain is less or goes away, the second part of the test is positive for neurogenic claudication. With neurogenic claudication, the pain returns when the individual sits upright again.

There is one major disadvantage to this test. Many clients in their sixth and seventh decades have both spinal stenosis and atherosclerosis contributing to painful back and/or leg symptoms. What if the client has back pain before even getting on the bicycle that is not relieved when bending forward? What diagnostic information does that provide?

The client could be experiencing neurogenic back pain that would normally feel better with flexion, but now while pedaling, vascular compromise occurs. In some cases, neurogenic pain lasts for hours or days, despite a change in position, because once the neurologic structures are irritated, pain signals can persist.

The Bicycle test has its greatest use when only one source of back pain is present: Either vascular or neurogenic and even then, chronic neurogenic pain may not be modulated by change in position. An alternate test to distinguish neurogenic claudication (pseudoclaudication) from vascular claudication is the Stoop test.[179] The individual being tested walks quickly until symptoms develop. Relief of symptoms in response to sitting or bending forward is a positive test for a neurogenic source of pain. Straightening up and/or extending the spine reproduces the symptoms.

The therapist must rely on results of the screening interview and examination, taking time to perform a Review of Systems to identify clients who may need further medical evaluation. In some cases, medical referral is not required. Identifying the underlying pathologic mechanism directs the therapist in choosing the most appropriate intervention.

In patients that are not able to tolerate the bicycle test or walking on a treadmill, an alternative test that will need validation is the pedal plantar flexion test. The pedal plantar flexion test consists of having the patient perform 50 sequential, symptom-limited calf raises. During the exercise, the ankle plantar flexors should continuously raise the heels maximally off the floor. Authors correlated this test with maximum exercise time and walking distance on a treadmill (R = 0.74).[180]

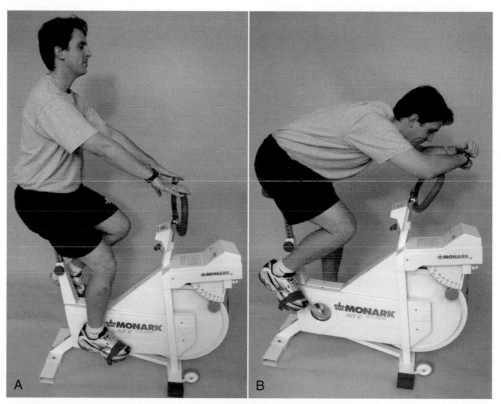

Fig. 15.5   Assessing the underlying cause of intermittent claudication: vascular or neurogenic? The effect of stooping over while pedaling on vascular claudication is negligible, whereas a change in spine position can aggravate or relieve claudication of a neurogenic origin. **A**, The client is seated on an exercise bicycle and asked to pedal against resistance without using the upper extremities, except for support. If pain into the buttock and posterior thigh occurs, followed by tingling in the affected lower extremity, the first part of the test is positive, but whether it is vascular or neurogenic remains undetermined. **B**, While pedaling, the client leans forward. If the pain subsides over a short time, the second part of the test is positive for neurogenic claudication but negative for vascular-induced symptoms. The test is confirmed for a neurogenic cause of symptoms when the client sits upright again and the pain returns. (From Magee DJ: *Orthopedic physical assessment*, ed 5, Philadelphia, 2008, WB Saunders.)

More research is required to find alternative tests for patients that can not tolerate different forms of exercise.

SCREENING FOR PULMONARY CAUSES OF NECK AND BACK PAIN

There are many potential pulmonary causes of back pain. The lungs occupy a large area of the upper trunk (see Fig. 8.1), with an equally large anterior and posterior thoracic area where pain can be referred. The most common conditions known to refer pulmonary pain in the somatic areas are pleuritis, pneumothorax, pulmonary embolus, cor pulmonale, and pleurisy.

Past Medical History

A recent history of one of these disorders in a client with neck, shoulder, chest, or back pain raises a red flag of suspicion. In keeping with the model for screening, the therapist should review the client's (1) past medical history, (2) risk factors, (3) clinical presentation, and (4) associated signs and symptoms (Box 15.5).

Clinical Presentation

Pulmonary pain patterns vary in their presentation based in part on the lobe(s) or segment(s) involved and on the underlying pathology. Several different pain patterns are presented in Chapter 8 (see Fig. 8.10).

Autosplinting is considered a valuable red flag of possible pulmonary involvement. Autosplinting occurs when the client prefers to lie on the involved side. Because pain of a pulmonary source is referred from the ipsilateral side, putting pressure on the involved lung field reduces respiratory movements and therefore reduces pain. It is uncommon for a person with a true musculoskeletal problem to find relief from symptoms by lying on the involved side.

The therapist should perform the following tests for clients with back pain who have a suspicious history or concomitant respiratory symptoms:

- Vital sign assessment
- Auscultation
- Assess the effect of reproducing respiratory movements on symptoms (e.g., does deep breathing, laughing, or coughing reproduce the painful symptoms?)
- ROM: Assess all active trunk movements (flexion, extension, side-bending, and rotation)
- Can pain or symptoms be reproduced with palpation (e.g., palpate the intercostals)?

Although reproducing pain, or increased pain, during respiratory movements is considered a hallmark sign of pulmonary involvement, symptoms of pleural, intercostal, muscular, costal, and dural origin all increase with coughing or deep inspiration.

Only pain of a cardiac origin is ruled out when symptoms increase in association with respiratory movements. For this reason, the therapist must always carefully correlate clinical

---

BOX 15.5 SCREENING FOR PULMONARY-INDUCED NECK OR BACK PAIN

History

Previous history of cancer (any kind, but especially lung, breast, bone, myeloma, lymphoma)

Previous history of recurrent upper respiratory infection (URI) or pneumonia

Recent scuba diving, accident, trauma, or overexertion (pneumothorax)

Risk Factors

Smoking

Trauma (e.g., rib fracture, vertebral compression fracture)

Prolonged immobility

Chronic immunosuppression (e.g., corticosteroids, cancer chemotherapy)

Malnutrition, dehydration

Chronic diseases: diabetes mellitus, chronic lung disease, renal disease, cancer

Upper respiratory infection or pneumonia

Pain Pattern

Sharp, localized

Aggravated by respiratory movements

Prefer to sit upright

Autosplinting decreases the pain

ROM does not reproduce symptoms (e.g., shoulder and/or trunk movements)

Associated Signs and Symptoms

Dyspnea

Persistent cough

Constitutional symptoms: fever, chills

Weak and rapid pulse with concomitant fall in blood pressure (e.g., pneumothorax)

---

presentation with client history and associated signs and symptoms when assessing for pulmonary disease.

Forceful coughing from an underlying pulmonary problem can cause an intercostal tear, which can be palpated. Even if some symptoms can be reproduced with palpation, the problem may still be pulmonary-induced, especially if the cause is repeated forceful coughing from a pulmonary etiology.

Pancoast's tumors of the lung may invade the roots of the brachial plexus causing entrapment as they enlarge, appearing as pain in the C8 to T1 region, possibly mimicking thoracic outlet syndrome. Faulty data collection leads to inaccurate findings or incorrect diagnosis and treatment, resulting in less than optimal outcomes.[181] Other signs may include atrophy of the muscles of the hand and/or Horner's syndrome with unilateral constricted pupil, ptosis, and loss of facial sweating.

Tracheobronchial irritation can cause pain to be referred to sites in the neck or anterior chest at the same levels as the points of irritation in the air passages (see Fig. 8.2). This irritation may be caused by inflammatory lesions, irritating foreign materials, or cancerous tumors.

Associated Signs and Symptoms

Assessing for associated signs and symptoms will usually bring to light important red flags to assist the therapist in recognizing an underlying pulmonary problem. Neck or back pain that is reproduced, increased with inspiratory movements, or accompanied by dyspnea, persistent cough, cyanosis, or hemoptysis must be evaluated carefully. Clients with respiratory origins of pain usually also show signs of general malaise or constitutional symptoms.

SCREENING FOR RENAL AND UROLOGIC CAUSES OF BACK PAIN

When considering the possibility of a renal or urologic cause of back pain, the therapist can use the same step-by-step approach of looking at the history, risk factors, clinical presentation, and associated signs and symptoms.

For example, in anyone with back pain reported in the T9 to L1 area, corresponding to pain patterns from the kidney or urinary tract (see Figs. 11.7 and 11.8), ask about a history of kidney stones, urinary tract infections (UTIs), and trauma (fall, blow, lift).

Origin of Pain Patterns

As discussed in Chapter 3, there can be at least three possible explanations for visceral pain patterns, including embryologic development, multisegmental innervation, and direct pressure on the diaphragm.

All three of these mechanisms are found in the urologic system. The *embryologic* origin of urologic pain patterns begins with the testicles and ovaries. These reproductive organs begin in utero where the kidneys are in the adult and then migrate during fetal development following the pathways of the ureters. A kidney stone down the pathway of the ureter causes pain in the flank radiating to the scrotum (male) or labia (female).

Evidence of the influence of *multisegmental innervation* is observed when skin pain over the kidneys is reported. Visceral and cutaneous sensory fibers enter the spinal cord close to each other and converge on the same neurons. When visceral pain fibers are stimulated, cutaneous fibers are stimulated, too. Thus visceral pain can be perceived as skin pain.

None of the components of the lower urinary tract comes in contact with the diaphragm, so the bladder and urethra are not likely to refer pain to the shoulder. Lower urinary tract impairment is more likely to refer pain to the low back, pelvic, or sacral areas. However, the upper urinary tract can impinge the diaphragm with resultant referred pain to the costovertebral area or shoulder.

Past Medical History

Kidney disorders such as acute pyelonephritis and perinephric abscess of the kidney may be confused with a back condition. Most renal and urologic conditions appear with a combination of systemic signs and symptoms accompanied by pelvic, flank, or LBP.

The client may have a history of recent trauma or a past medical history of UTIs to alert the clinician to a possible renal origin of symptoms.

Clinical Presentation

Risk factors associated with increased risk for pyelonephritis in healthy, nonpregnant women include frequent sexual activity, recent UTI, recent spermicide use, diabetes, and recent incontinence.[230] There may be a genetic component for increased susceptibility to these infections; a history of upper respiratory infection in female relatives is strongly and consistently associated with UTI recurrence and pyelonephritis.[231] *Acute pyelonephritis*, perinephric abscess, and other kidney conditions appear with aching pain at one or several costovertebral areas, posteriorly, just lateral to the muscles at T12 to L1, from acute distention of the capsule of the kidney.

The pain is usually dull and constant, with possible radiation to the pelvic crest or groin. The client may describe febrile chills, frequent urination, hematuria, and shoulder pain (if the diaphragm is irritated). Percussion to the flank areas reveals tenderness; the therapist can perform Murphy's percussion (punch) test (see Fig. 4.54). Although this test is commonly performed, its diagnostic value has never been validated. Results of at least one Finnish study[182] suggested that in acute renal colic, loin tenderness and hematuria (blood in the urine) are more significant signs than renal tenderness.[183] A diagnostic score incorporating independent variables, including results of urinalysis, presence of costovertebral angle tenderness and renal tenderness, duration of pain, and appetite level reached a sensitivity of 0.89 in detecting acute renal colic, with a specificity of 0.99 and an efficiency of 0.99.[182]

Nephrolithiasis (kidney stones) may appear as back pain radiating to the flank or the iliac crest (see Fig. 11.7) (Case Example 15.10). Clinical symptoms are the same for the various types of stones. The classic presentation of a kidney stone is acute "colicky" flank pain radiating to the groin or perineal areas (including the scrotum in males and labia in females) with hematuria. The pain is severe; most people are unable to find a comfortable position. Symptoms consistent with a UTI such as urinary urgency and frequency and dysuria are often present.

Kidney stones may occur in the presence of diseases associated with hypercalcemia (excess calcium in the blood) such as hyperparathyroidism, metastatic carcinoma, multiple myeloma, senile osteoporosis, specific renal tubular disease, hyperthyroidism, and Cushing's disease. Other conditions associated with calculus formation are infection, urinary

CASE EXAMPLE 15.10

Back and Flank Pain

Background and Description of Client: JH is a 57-year-old male with a history of mild mental retardation, seizure disorder, obesity, osteoarthritis, hypertension, and cervical disk disease (magnetic resonance imaging [MRI] reveals herniation at C7-T1 and spondylosis at C5-C6). He resides at a residential facility and is well known to physical therapy over the past 6 years because of five separate physical therapy examinations related to complaints of insidious onset of back pain.

These previous episodes of back pain resolved without physical therapy intervention. JH presented in physical therapy this time with complaints of low back and right hip pain that he and his primary physician attributed to a minor fall 2 months before the physical therapy examination. Physical therapy was not consulted during the initial period after the fall because x-rays were unremarkable and JH had not complained of any symptoms at that time.

When asked to point to the area of pain, JH indicated his right lower lumbar area and along the right hip and flank. He was unable to describe the pain as a result of some cognitive limitations, but he did report that it was unrelieved with rest and occurred intermittently.

JH works full-time in a sheltered workshop doing piecework. He reported that the pain kept him from performing his job fully, and he found that lifting boxes was particularly difficult because of the bending. He also reported that prolonged ambulation or exercise caused an increase in the flank pain. He was taking over-the-counter (OTC) ibuprofen for his pain; however, it was not effective.

JH is taking the following medications: Colace (for constipation), Allegra (for allergy), Tegretol (for seizures), Zoloft (for obsessive-compulsive disorder), Risperdal (for psychosis), BuSpar (for anxiety), and ibuprofen (as needed for pain).

Clinical Presentation: Vital signs were as follows: HR: 65 bpm; BP: 130/70 mm Hg; RR: 12; Temp: 99° F. These were not significantly different from JH's normal vital signs.

Gait analysis was significant for an antalgic gait, slight increase in base of support, decreased trunk and pelvic rotation, significant ankle pronation, and pes planus bilaterally (JH does not like to wear his orthotics). He is an independent ambulator on all surfaces without the use of an assistive device. He lives in a two-story home and is able to ascend and descend stairs independently without complaints of pain.

Posture while standing was significant for decreased lumbar lordosis, rounded shoulders, and forward head, left shoulder mildly depressed.

Strength testing revealed strength of 4 +/5 throughout the upper extremities, trunk, and left lower extremity. JH was very hesitant about resisted strength testing of his right lower extremity for fear of pain; therefore no formal data was obtained. JH did report pain upon mildly resisted right hip flexion, abduction, and adduction.

Passive range of motion (PROM) was all within functional limits. There was no apparent evidence of inflammation in the bilateral knees or hips. The physical therapist was unable to reproduce symptoms with palpation along the spine and bilateral hips and knees.

Right knee extension active ROM (AROM) while sitting revealed pain in the right flank. Right straight leg raise (SLR) test in the supine position also revealed similar pain in the right flank. Right side-bending produced right flank pain. Left side-bending produced no symptoms.

Neurologic examination revealed intact sensation to light touch along dermatomal pattern. Deep tendon reflexes (DTRs) were 1 + throughout.

Evaluation: JH's symptoms appeared inconsistent and dependent on the level of physical activity. It seemed counterintuitive that a minor fall 2 months before this examination could cause the current symptoms. The location of the pain also raised some concerns because JH had never before complained of flank pain.

The physical therapist did not have access to the prior x-rays taken at the time of the fall. Therefore the therapist requested further x-rays of JH's hip and spine from the orthopedic surgeon, serving as consultant to rule out a more serious orthopedic, systemic, or other medical issue. Physical therapy was deferred until the x-ray results were examined and reviewed by the orthopedic consultant and therapist.

Outcome and Discussion: Anteroposterior (AP) pelvis and frog view x-rays of hips were reviewed by the orthopedic consultant and the physical therapist, and it was concluded that the x-ray films were unremarkable. AP and lateral x-rays of JH's thoracolumbar spine (TLS) at first glance also appeared to be unremarkable, and the x-ray report agreed with our initial assessment.

However, upon closer inspection, there was a circular 2-cm suspicious area that appeared on film at the level and location of JH's right kidney. The orthopedic surgeon ordered further imaging to confirm a diagnosis of a kidney stone. An intravenous pyelogram (IVP) did confirm the diagnosis. After appropriate treatment for the kidney stone, JH reported that the pain on his right side had resolved.

JH was well known to the physical therapy department because of his previous examinations. JH was a challenging case because of previous "false alarms" and because he did not always accurately communicate his symptoms, as a result of his mild cognitive limits.

He also has comorbidities that warrant a more cautious approach in treating and assessing his complaints. These include hypertension, a seizure disorder, and the multitude of medications he takes.

It is up to the physical therapist to understand him and try to interpret his meanings as closely as he or she can. Fortunately in this case, JH's chief complaint of flank pain was different enough from his previous complaints and the films clearly showed a systemic cause of symptoms.

Instructor's Comments: Some additional screening questions/information that might help with a case like this:

1. Did he have any symptoms of genitourinary (GU) distress (pain during urination, blood in the urine, difficulty starting or continuing a flow of urine, nocturia, frequency, or changes in bladder function)?
2. Did he have a past medical history of kidney stones?
3. Was Murphy's percussion (punch) test positive?
4. Was there a report of any constitutional symptoms (night sweats, spiked temps, flu-like symptoms)?

From Yee J, DPT: Case report submitted as part of course requirements in fulfillment of DPT 910, New York, 2002, Stony Brook University. Used with permission.

stasis, dehydration, and excessive ingestion or absorption of calcium.

Ureteral colic, caused by passage of a kidney stone (calculus), appears as excruciating pain that radiates down the course of the ureter into the urethra or groin area. The pain is unrelieved by rest or change in position. These attacks are intermittent and may be accompanied by nausea, vomiting, sweating, and tachycardia. Localized abdominal muscle spasm may be present. The urine usually contains erythrocytes or is grossly bloody.

The pain from *Urinary tract infection* affecting the lower urinary tract is related directly to irritation of the bladder and urethra. The intensity of symptoms depends on the severity of the infection. Although LBP may be the client's chief complaint, further questioning usually elicits additional urologic symptoms. The therapist should ask about:

- Urinary frequency, urgency, dysuria (burning pain during urination), nocturia (frequency at night)
- Constitutional symptoms (fever, chills, nausea, vomiting)
- Blood in urine
- Testicular pain

Clients can be asymptomatic concerning urologic symptoms, making the physical therapy diagnosis more difficult. Risk factors for UTI include female gender (especially post menopausal and pregnant), frequency of vaginal penetration, history of previous UTI, spermicidal use, and diabetes treatment.

Screening Questions: Renal and Urologic System

It is important to ask questions about the presence of urologic symptoms (see Appendix B-5 in the accompanying enhanced eBook version included with print purchase of this textbook). Many people (therapists and clients alike) are uncomfortable discussing the details of bladder (or bowel) function. If presented professionally with a brief explanation, both parties can be put at ease. For example, the interview may go something like this:

"I am going to ask a few other questions. There are many possible causes of back pain and I want to make sure I do not leave anything out.

If I ask you anything you do not know, please pay attention over the next few days and see if you notice something. Do not hesitate to bring this information back to me. It could be very important."

To the therapist: The important thing to look for is CHANGE. Many people have problems with incontinence, nocturia, or frequency. If someone has always experienced a delay before starting a flow of urine, this may be normal for him or her.

Many women have nocturia after childbirth, but most men do not get up at night to empty their bladders until after the age of 65 years. They may not even be aware that this has changed for them. Often, it is the wife or partner who answers the question about getting up at night as "yes!" Likewise, if a man has always had a delay in starting a flow of urine, he may not be aware that the delay is now twice as long as before. Or he may not recognize that being unable to continue a flow of urine is not "normal" and in fact, requires medical evaluation.

Pseudorenal Pain

Sometimes clients appear to have classic symptoms of a kidney problem but without any associated signs and symptoms. Such a situation can occur with someone who has a mechanical derangement of the costovertebral or costotransverse joint or irritation of the costal nerve (radiculitis, T10-T12).

What does this look like in the clinic? How does the therapist make the differentiation? Use the same guidelines for decision-making in the screening process presented throughout this text (e.g., history, risk factors, associated signs and symptoms).

History

Trauma is often the underlying etiology. The client may or may not report assault. The individual may not remember any specific trauma or accident. Pseudorenal pain can occur when floating ribs become locked with the ribs above, but this is a rare cause of these symptoms. Radiculitis or mechanical derangement of the T10 to T12 costovertebral or costotransverse joint(s) is more likely.

Risk Factors

Unknown or none for this condition.

Clinical Presentation

Pain pattern is affected by change in position:

- Lying on that side increases pain (remember clients with renal pain prefer pressure on the involved side; musculoskeletal symptoms are often made worse by lying on the affected side).
- Prolonged sitting increases pain; slumped sitting especially increases pain; the therapist can have the client try this position and see what effect it has on symptoms.
- Symptoms are reproduced with movements of the spine (especially forward flexion and side-bending).
- Presence of costovertebral angle tenderness: The therapist may be able to reproduce pain with palpation; Murphy's percussion (punch) test is negative (see Fig. 4.54).

A positive Murphy's test for renal involvement elicits kidney pain or reproduces the referred back pain and must be reported to the physician. A negative response occurs when no discomfort or pain can be reproduced by local palpation at the costovertebral angle. The therapist must ask about the presence of signs and symptoms associated with renal disease.

One final note about pseudorenal back pain: Thoracic disk disease can mimic kidney disease and presents with flank, buttock, and/or leg pain. MRI is negative but may show only the lumbar spine.[184] If MRI is performed for only the lumbar region, lesions more cephalic may go undetected.

In the case of a possible thoracic disk mimicking renal involvement, the therapist can provide the physician with clinical findings and the reason for the referral. Look for a history of straining, lifting, accident, or other mechanical injuries to the thoracic spine.

The therapist must look carefully for evidence of neurologic involvement. Perform a screening neurologic assessment as outlined in Chapter 4. There may be a change in bladder function, which can be confusing; are these urologic-induced or disk-related? Report any suspicious symptoms.

Associated Signs and Symptoms

Usually, none when pseudorenal pain is present.

SCREENING FOR GASTROINTESTINAL CAUSES OF BACK PAIN

Back pain of a visceral origin may occur as a result of GI problems. Pain patterns associated with the GI system can present as sternal, shoulder, scapular, midback, low back, or hip pain and dysfunction. If the client had primary symptoms of GI impairment (abdominal pain, nausea, diarrhea, or constipation; see Fig. 9.18), he or she would see a medical doctor. Keep in mind the individual who has LBP with constipation could also be manifesting symptoms of pelvic floor muscle overactivity or spasm. In such cases, pelvic floor assessment should be a part of the screening examination. Consultation with a physical therapist skilled in this area should be considered if the primary care therapist is unable to perform this examination.

As it is, the referred pain patterns are quite convincing that the musculoskeletal region described is the problem. Referred pain patterns for the GI system are presented in Fig. 9.19 (anterior and posterior). These are the pain patterns the therapist is most likely to see.

Past Medical History and Risk Factors

Taking a closer look at past medical history, risk factors, and clinical presentation and asking about associated signs and symptoms may reveal important red flags and clues pointing to the GI system. The most significant and common history is one of long-term or chronic use of NSAIDs. Other significant

---

BOX 15.6　SIGNS AND SYMPTOMS OF GASTROINTESTINAL DYSFUNCTION

Anterior neck pain or back pain accompanied by any of the following is a red flag:

- Esophageal pain
- Epigastric pain with radiation to the back
- Dysphagia (difficulty swallowing)
- Odynophagia (pain with swallowing)
- Early satiety; symptoms associated with meals
- Bloody diarrhea
- Fecal incontinence
- Melena (dark, tarry, sticky stools caused by oxidized blood)
- Hemorrhage (blood in the toilet)

---

risk factors in the history include the long-term use of immunosuppressants, past history of cancer, history of Crohn's disease (also known as regional enteritis), or previous bowel obstruction.

Signs and Symptoms of Gastrointestinal Dysfunction

The most common signs and symptoms associated with the GI system are listed in Box 15.6 and discussed in greater detail in Chapter 8. Back pain (as well as hip, pelvic, sacral, and lower extremity pain) with any of these accompanying features should be considered a red flag for the possibility of GI impairment.

Anterior neck (esophageal) pain may occur, usually with a burning sensation ("heartburn") or other symptoms related to eating or swallowing (e.g., dysphagia, odynophagia). Esophageal varices associated with chronic alcoholism may appear as anterior neck pain but usually occur at the xiphoid process and are attributed to heartburn.

Anterior neck pain can also occur as a result of a discogenic lesion requiring a careful history and neurologic screening to document findings. Clients with eating disorders who repeatedly binge and then purge by vomiting may report anterior neck pain without realizing the correlation between eating behaviors and symptoms.

When assessing neck pain, the therapist should look for other associated signs and symptoms, such as sore throat; pain that is relieved with antacids, the upright position, fluids, or avoidance of eating; and pain that is aggravated by eating, bending, or recumbency.

Dysphagia or difficulty swallowing, *odynophagia* (painful swallowing), and *epigastric pain* are indicative of esophageal involvement. Certain types of drugs (e.g., antidepressants, antihypertensives, asthma medications) can make swallowing difficult, requiring a careful evaluation during the client interview.

Early satiety (the client takes one or two bites of food and is no longer hungry) is another red-flag symptom of the GI system (Case Example 15.11). In general, back pain made better, worse, or altered in any way by eating is a red-flag symptom. If the change in symptom(s) occurs immediately to within 30 minutes of eating, the upper GI tract or stomach/duodenum may be a possible cause. Change in symptoms 2 to 4 hours *after* eating is more indicative of the lower GI tract (intestines/colon).

Bloody diarrhea, new or sudden onset of fecal incontinence, and *melena* are three additional signs of lower GI involvement. It is important to ask the client about the presence of specific signs that may be too embarrassing to mention (or the client may not see the connection between back pain and bowel smears on the underwear). Asking someone with back pain about bowel function can be accomplished in a very professional manner. The therapist may tell the client:

"I am going to ask you a series of questions about your bowels. These are important questions to make sure we

have covered every possibility. If you do not know the answer to the question, pay attention over the next day or two to see how everything is working. If you notice anything unusual or different, please let me know when you come in next time."

 FOLLOW-UP QUESTIONS

- When was your last bowel movement? (Look for a change of any kind in the client's normal elimination pattern.) Additionally, failure to have a bowel movement over a much longer time than expected for that client may be a sign of impaction/obstruction/obstipation. Normal time for food to travel through the GI tract is 1 to 5 days.
- Are you having any diarrhea?
- Is there any blood in your stool?
- Have you ever been told you have hemorrhoids or do you know that you have hemorrhoids? Because blood in the stool might just be a chronic or reoccurring hemorrhoid
- Do you have large volume of stool leakage?

Again, when it comes to something like bowel smears on the underpants, it is important to distinguish between pathology and poor hygiene. The key to look for is change, such as the new appearance of a problem that was not present before the onset of back pain or other symptoms. With blood in the stools, a medical doctor must differentiate between internal versus external bleeding (i.e., hemorrhoid).

Melena is a dark, tarry stool caused by oxidation of blood in the GI tract (usually the upper GI tract, but it can be the lower GI tract). The most common causes of abdominal bleeding are chronic use of NSAIDs, leading to ulceration, Crohn's disease, or ulcerative colitis, and diverticulitis or diverticulosis. Anyone with a history of these problems presenting with new onset of back pain must be screened for medical disease.

Hemorrhage or visible blood in the toilet may be a sign of anal fissures, hemorrhoids, or colon cancer. The etiology must be determined by a medical doctor. Be aware that there is an increased incidence of rectal bleeding from anal fissures and local tissue damage associated with anal intercourse. This

CASE EXAMPLE 15.11

Early Satiety and Weight Loss

Background: A 78-year-old female was referred to physical therapy by her orthopedic surgeon 6 weeks status post (S/P) total knee replacement (TKR). Her active knee flexion was 70 degrees; passive knee flexion was only 86 degrees. There was a 15-degree extensor lag.

During the course of her rehabilitation program, her adult daughters took turns bringing her to the clinic. They all commented on how much weight she had lost, though the therapist thought she looked quite obese.

When asked about the weight loss, she replied, "Oh, I take a bite or two and then I am not very hungry." This symptom (early satiety with weight loss) had been present for the last 2 months (starting before the TKR).

She did not have any other signs or symptoms associated with the gastrointestinal (GI) system. There were no reported changes in bowel function or the appearance of her stools, no blood in the stools, no back or sacral pain, no night pain that was not directly related to her knee, and no other changes in her health.

Her social history included the recent death of a spouse. She had taken care of her husband at home for the last 3 years after he had a severe stroke. She knew she needed a knee replacement, but put it off because of her husband's poor health. Within 6 weeks of his death, she scheduled the needed operation.

Could her weight loss be a delayed grieving reaction? Emotional overlay? How can you tell?

The screening process often begins with the recognition and categorization of red flags. It is not within the scope of a physical therapist's practice to diagnose psychologic or emotional problems. Clearly, many of the clients and patients in our clinics have significant psychologic needs and emotional responses to their illnesses, injuries, or conditions.

Identifying a cluster of signs and symptoms suggestive of a psychologic or behavioral component may help determine the need for behavioral counseling or a psych consult. However, the therapist's plan of care may include the use of specific client

management skills based on observation of particular behavioral patterns.

What do you see in the history, clinical presentation, and associated signs and symptoms as they are presented here that raise a red flag?

- History: Age and positive social history for a recent personal loss
- Clinical presentation: Unremarkable; consistent with orthopedic diagnosis
- Associated signs and symptoms: Early satiety with weight loss

Viewing the whole client or patient and identifying the presence of emotional overlay to symptoms can be accomplished using the McGill Pain questionnaire, Waddell's nonorganic signs adapted for the knee, and listening to the client's response to her condition and the rehabilitation program (symptom magnification). These three assessment tools are discussed in Chapter 3.

There are really only two red flags here (age and early satiety with weight loss), but they are significant enough to warrant contact with her physician. The next question is: To whom do you send her? The referring orthopedist or her family doctor (if she has one)?

It may be best to communicate all findings with the referring physician or health care provider. The therapist can leave the door open by asking any one of the following questions:

- Do you want to see Mrs. So-and-So back in your office or shall I send her to her family physician?
- Do you want Mr. X/Mrs. Y to check with his/her family doctor or do you prefer to see him/her yourself?
- How do you want to handle this? or How do you want me to handle this?

Outcome: The orthopedic surgeon recommended referral to her primary care physician. Examination and diagnostic tests resulted in a diagnosis of esophageal cancer (early stage). The client was treated successfully for the cancer while completing her rehabilitation program.

occurs predominantly in the male homosexual or bisexual population, but can be seen in heterosexual partners who engage in anal intercourse. There are also increasing reports of adolescents engaging in oral and anal intercourse as a form of birth control.

It may be necessary to take a sexual history. The therapist should offer the client a clear explanation for any questions concerning sexual activity, sexual function, or sexual history. There is no way to know when someone will be offended or claim sexual harassment. It is in the therapist's best interest to maintain the most professional manner possible.

There should be no hint of sexual innuendo or humor injected into any of the therapist's conversations with clients at any time. The line of sexual impropriety lies where the complainant draws it and includes appearances of misbehavior. This perception differs broadly from client to client.[149]

You may need to include the following questions (see also Appendix B-32 in the accompanying enhanced eBook version included with print purchase of this textbook). Always explain the importance of taking a sexual history. For example, *"There are a few personal questions I will need to ask that may help sort out where your symptoms are coming from. Please answer these as best you can."*

 FOLLOW-UP QUESTIONS

- Are you sexually active?
  "Sexually active" does not necessarily mean engaging in sexual intercourse. Sexual touch is enough to transmit many STIs. The therapist may have to explain this to the client to clarify this question. Oral and anal intercourse are often not viewed as "sexual intercourse" and will result in the client answering the question with a "No" when, in fact, for screening purposes, the answer is "Yes."
- Have you had more than one sexual partner (one at a time or during the same time)?
- Have you ever been told you have an STI or STD such as herpes, chlamydia, gonorrhea, venereal disease, human immunodeficiency virus (HIV), or other disease?
- Is there any chance the bleeding you are having could be related to sexual activity?

For Women

- What form of birth control are you using? (Risk factor: intrauterine contraceptive device [IUCD])
- Is there any possibility you could be pregnant?
- Have you ever had an abortion?
  - *If* yes, follow up with careful (sensitive) questions about how many, when, where, and any immediate or delayed complications (physical or psychologic).

Back pain from any cause may impair sexual function. Many health care professionals do not address this issue; the therapist can offer much in the way of education, pain management, improved function, and proper positioning for work and recreation. Some publications are available to assist therapists in discussing sexual function and pain control for the client with back pain.[185,186]

Esophagus

Esophageal pain will occur at the level of the lesion and is usually accompanied by epigastric pain and heartburn. Severe esophagitis (see Fig. 9.15) may refer pain to the anterior cervical or more often, the midthoracic spine.

The pain pattern will most likely present in a band of pain starting anteriorly and spreading around the chest wall to the back. Rarely, pain will begin in the midback and radiate around to the front. Referred pain to the midthoracic spine occurs around T5-T6.

As with cervical pain of GI origin, there may be a history of alcoholism with esophageal varices, cirrhosis, or an underlying eating disorder. If liver impairment is an underlying factor, there may be signs such as asterixis (liver flap or flapping tremor), palmar erythema, spider angiomas, and carpal (tarsal) tunnel syndrome (see discussion in Chapter 10).

Keep in mind that this same type of midthoracic back pain can occur with thoracic disk disease. Look for a history of trauma and neurologic changes typically associated with disk degeneration (e.g., bowel and bladder changes, numbness and tingling or paresthesia in the upper extremities); these are not usually present with esophageal impairment. Lower thoracic disk herniation can cause groin pain, leg pain, or mimic kidney pain.

Stomach and Duodenum

Long-term use of NSAIDs is the most common cause of back pain referred from the stomach or duodenum. Ulceration and bleeding into the retroperitoneal area can cause pain in the back or shoulder. The primary and referred pain patterns for pain of a stomach or duodenal source are shown in Fig. 9.16.

The referred pain to the back is at the level of the lesion, usually between T6 and T10. For the client with midthoracic spine pain of unknown cause or which does not fit the expected musculoskeletal presentation, ask about associated signs and symptoms, such as:

- Blood in the stools
- Symptoms associated with meals
- Relief of pain after eating (immediately or 2 hours later)
- Increased symptoms with or during a bowel movement
- Decreased symptoms after a bowel movement

The pain of peptic ulcer (see Figs. 9.9 and 9.16) occasionally occurs only in the midthoracic back between T6 and T10, either at the midline or immediately to one side or the other of the spine. Posterior penetration of the retroperitoneum with blood loss and resultant referred thoracic pain is most often caused by long-term use of NSAIDs. The therapist should look for a correlation between symptoms and the timing of meals, as well as the presence of blood in the feces or relief of symptoms with antacids.

Small Intestine

Diseases of the small intestine (e.g., Crohn's disease, irritable bowel syndrome, obstruction from neoplasm) usually produce midabdominal pain around the umbilicus (see Fig. 9.3), but the pain may be referred to the back if the stimulus is sufficiently intense or if the individual's pain threshold is low (see Fig. 9.17) (Case Example 15.12).

For the client with LBP of unknown cause or suspicious presentation, ask if there is ever any abdominal pain present. Alternating abdominal/LBP at the same level is a red flag that requires medical referral. Because both symptoms do not always occur together, the client may not recognize the relationship or report the symptoms. The therapist must be sure and ask appropriate screening questions (Case Example 15.13).

Look for known history of Crohn's disease (regional enteritis), irritable bowel syndrome, bowel obstruction, or cancer. Low back, sacral, or hip pain may be a new symptom of an already established disease. The client may not be aware that 25% of people with GI disease have concomitant back or joint pain.

Enteric-induced arthritis can be accompanied by a skin rash that comes and goes. A flat red or purple rash or raised skin lesion(s) is possible, usually preceding the joint or back pain. The therapist must ask the client if he/she has had any skin rashes in the last few weeks.

The therapist may treat joint or back pain when there is an unknown or unrecognized enteric cause. Palliative intervention for musculoskeletal symptoms or apparent movement impairment can make a difference in the short-term, but does not affect the outcome.

Eventually, the GI symptoms will progress; symptoms that are unrelieved by physical therapy intervention are red flags. Medical treatment of the underlying disease is essential to correcting the musculoskeletal component.

SCREENING FOR LIVER AND BILIARY CAUSES OF BACK PAIN

The primary pain pattern for liver disease is located at the anatomic site over the liver. In primary liver pathology, palpation of the organ will reproduce the symptoms and the examiner can feel the liver distention. The normal, healthy liver is located up under the right side of the diaphragm and ribs. The gallbladder is tucked up under the liver (see also Fig. 10.2).

When a referred pain pattern occurs, there may be pain during palpation of the liver, but the primary complaint is of back pain. There is no report of anterior pain to alert the examiner to the need for liver palpation. In anyone with the referred pain patterns depicted and described in Fig. 10.11, liver palpation may be required as a part of the physical assessment (see Figs. 4.51 and 4.52). In addition to a painful and distended liver, the client may report:

- Pain/nausea 1 to 3 hours after eating (gallstones)
- Pain immediately after eating (gallbladder inflammation)
- Muscle guarding/tenderness and fever/chills in the right upper quadrant (posterior)

Other signs and symptoms associated with liver impairment are discussed in detail in Chapter 10 and include:

- Liver flap (asterixis)
- Nail bed changes (nail of Terry)
- Palmar erythema (liver palms)
- Spider angioma
- Ascites, jaundice

Crohn's Disease and Back Pain

A 23-year-old ballet dancer with "shin splints" comes to you from a sports medicine doctor. Besides anterior lower leg pain, she also reports low back pain (LBP) that seems to come and go with overuse. She has a history of Crohn's disease.

Can symptoms of anterior compartment syndrome be caused by Crohn's disease?

It is very unlikely. There are no reported cases to date. Crohn's disease is linked with low back, hip, and sometimes knee pain (knee pain is usually associated with hip pain and usually does not occur alone).

Anterior compartment syndrome is easily reproducible with tenderness during palpation of the anterior tibial region. The pain pattern and etiology is fairly typical and symptoms respond to treatment. If the soft tissues are acutely inflamed, surgical intervention may be required.

What questions can you ask to rule out a gastrointestinal (GI) cause for her back pain?

- Ask about the presence of GI signs and symptoms:
  Are you having any nausea, vomiting, diarrhea, or constipation?

Any change in your bowel movements? Any trouble wiping yourself clean after a bowel movement?
Any blood in the stools?

- Any other symptoms of any kind? (headache, sweats, fever)
- Is there abdominal pain and is it at the same level as the back pain?
- Does the abdominal and/or back pain change with food intake (assess from 30 minutes to 2 hours after eating)?
- Is there relief of back pain with passing gas or having a bowel movement?
- Is there a recent (chronic) history of antibiotic and/or nonsteroidal antiinflammatory drugs (NSAID) use?
- Has the client experienced any joint pain anywhere else in the body?
- Any skin rashes anywhere?

A "yes" answer to any of these questions is a significant red flag and must be evaluated in the context of the overall clinical presentation and findings from the Review of Systems.

CASE EXAMPLE 15.13

Abdominal and Back Pain at the Same Level

Background: A 68-year-old accountant came to physical therapy as a self-referral for low back pain (LBP). He reported slipping on a patch of ice as the mechanism of injury.

Symptoms were mild but distressing to this gentleman. He reported pain as "sore" and "aching" with any spinal twisting or side-bending to the right. The pain was present across the low back on both sides.

The client reported symptoms of stomach distress from time to time. He attributed this to his trips overseas, eating foods from Ireland, Scotland, Germany, and the Netherlands.

Lumbar range of motion (ROM) was fairly typical of a nearly 70-year-old man with most of his functional forward flexion from the hips and thoracic spine. True physiologic motion in the lumbar spine was negligible. Accessory spinal motions were also limited globally. Active rotation and sidebending were stiff and limited to both sides, but only painful to the right.

Neurologic screening examination was negative. The therapist did not ask about the presence of any other symptoms of any kind anywhere else in his body. No questions were asked about changes in the pattern of his bowel movements or appearance of his stools.

Given the examination results as tested, a conditioning exercise program seemed most appropriate. The client began a stationary bicycling program alternating with walking when the weather permitted. He reported gradual relief from his symptoms and return of motion and function to his previous levels.

Four months later this same client reported another injury while walking with subsequent back pain.

What are the red-flag findings? What is the next step in the screening process?

The client's age (over 50 years) is the first red flag. Back pain across both sides can be considered bilateral and therefore a red flag until further assessment is completed. The presence of back pain and abdominal pain or discomfort warrants some additional questions.

The therapist should conduct a more thorough pain assessment and ask about the location of the symptoms as well as the presence of any additional gastrointestinal (GI) symptoms. Back pain and abdominal pain at the same level is always a red flag.

Screening questions related to the back and GI dysfunction are available at the end of this chapter. Questions about changes in bowel function may reveal some important clues. A screening physical assessment of the abdomen including visual inspection, palpation, and auscultation, as described in Chapter 4, may be helpful. Vital sign assessment is always recommended.

Result: The key red flag in this case was alternating back and abdominal pain at the same level. The client did not see a connection between these two episodes of pain. When his back hurt, he did not have any abdominal pain and vice versa.

The client was advised to see his regular physician for an evaluation. He was diagnosed with advanced stage colon cancer and died 6 weeks later. Earlier detection may have made a difference in this case, but the cyclical nature of his presentation masked the true significance of his symptoms.

Gallbladder and biliary disease may also refer pain to the interscapular or right subscapular area. The therapist should be observant for any report of fever and chills, nausea and indigestion, changes in urine or stool, or signs of jaundice. The client may not associate GI symptoms with the scapular pain or discomfort. The therapist can use specific questions to rule out potential GI problems (see Special Questions to Ask in this chapter and greater detail in Chapter 9).

The Pancreas

Acute pancreatitis may appear as epigastric pain radiating to the midthoracic spine (see Fig. 9.19). Pain from the head of the pancreas is felt to the right of the spine, whereas pain from the body and tail is perceived to the left of the spine. More rarely, pain may be referred to the upper back and midscapular areas.

There may be a history of alcohol and tobacco use. Associated symptoms, which are usually GI related, may include diarrhea, anorexia, pain after a meal, and unexplained weight loss. The pain is relieved initially by heat, which decreases muscular tension, and may be relieved by leaning forward, sitting up, or lying motionless.

The therapist should remain alert for the client with LBP who reports benefit from a heating pad or other heat modalities who then suddenly gets worse and does not improve with physical therapy intervention.

SCREENING FOR GYNECOLOGIC CAUSES OF BACK PAIN

Gynecologic disorders can cause midpelvic or LBP and discomfort. Gynecologic-induced back pain occurs most often in women of childbearing age (commonly between the age of 20 and 45 years). How can the therapist recognize when a woman may be experiencing back pain from a gynecologic cause?

As always, the model for screening includes history, presence of any risk factors, clinical presentation, and associated signs and symptoms. Gynecologic involvement should be considered in females with back, pelvic, groin, hip, sacral or SI symptoms, especially with a history of insidious onset or previous history of reproductive cancer.

Whenever objective musculoskeletal findings are minimal, a history of gynecologic involvement, or associated signs and symptoms of gynecologic disorders, the therapist is encouraged to ask appropriate questions to determine the need for a gynecologic evaluation (Case Example 15.14).

The therapist should determine the stage of reproductive life cycle (see previous discussions of Life Cycles and Menopause in Chapter 2). If the client is an adolescent, has she begun her menstrual cycle (menses)? If a young to middle-aged adult, is she menstruating, or has she had a hysterectomy and experienced surgically-induced menopause?

CASE EXAMPLE 15.14

Human Movement Impairment

A 28-year-old woman in the twentieth week of her first pregnancy reported low back pain (LBP) of approximately 2 weeks' duration. She could not recall any injury or cause for her pain and attributed it to her pregnancy. She did report a 6-year history of back pain caused by exercise (military press); before this episode her back pain could be relieved by rest, heat, and massage therapy.

The current back pain was located bilaterally in the thoracolumbar paraspinal region and described as a "nagging ache." The client rated her pain as a 7 to 9 on the Numeric Rating Scale (NRS; see Fig. 3.6), worse in the afternoon and evening. Pain was aggravated by sitting more than 20 minutes and bending forward. She reported episodes of night pain that could be relieved by a change in position.

There were no other symptoms anywhere in her body; she was not taking any medications except for prenatal vitamins. She reported her pregnancy was "normal" with appropriate weight gain. There has been no spotting or vaginal bleeding during the pregnancy. Vital signs were within normal limits (WNL).

Is a medical screening examination needed?

The client's age is not a red flag at this time. Although she reports an insidious onset for her symptoms, the pain is not constant and can be relieved with a change in position. The pain wakes her up at night, but she is able to get back to sleep by getting up and walking or by changing position. Vital signs were normal and there were no constitutional symptoms.

At this point the evaluation can proceed as usual. The therapist should include a neurologic screening assessment as a part of the examination. Keep in mind that hormonal changes can unmask a preexisting, but asymptomatic, musculoskeletal condition, which is something the physical therapist can address. Movement testing further confirmed an extension syndrome with worse symptoms during trunk flexion and improved pain after repetitive trunk extension.

No further medical screening is required, unless additional red-flag symptoms develop. The client's improvement with physical therapy intervention confirmed the decision that medical referral was not necessary.

Data from Requejo SM, Barnes R, Kulig K, et al.: The use of a modified classification system in the treatment of low back pain during pregnancy: a case report, *J Orthop Sports Phys Ther* 32(7):318–326, 2002.

CASE EXAMPLE 15.15

Back Pain During Pregnancy

A 32-year-old Native American woman in the third trimester of her second pregnancy presented with acute onset of mid- to right-sided lumbar pain. She reported pain radiating around to the right side. An abdominal sonogram was negative and all laboratory values were within normal limits. The client declined any further imaging studies and requested a referral to physical therapy.

What will you need to do to make sure this client's problem is within the scope of a physical therapy practice?

Take a thorough history (including childbirth history) and evaluate pain pattern(s) carefully.

Screen for domestic abuse sometime during the evaluation or early treatment intervention.

Ask about the presence of any other symptoms, even if they seem unrelated to her pregnancy or back pain.

See if you can reproduce the symptoms by palpation or through position or movement; assess for trigger points.

Take all vital signs and ask about the presence of constitutional symptoms.

Assess for rectus abdominis diastasis (separation of the rectus abdominal muscles) as a possible contributing factor.

Outcome: During palpation of the ribs, the therapist noted an outward flaring of the lower ribs. There was pain and tenderness at the interchondral junctions, between the eighth and tenth ribs.

The history was significant for chronic cough from smoking. The woman reported feeling the child in a horizontal position pushing against the lower ribs.

Based on these findings, the therapist telephoned the physician and asked if there was any chance a rib fracture could be causing the painful symptoms. The client agreed to an x-ray and the radiograph showed a fracture of the right tenth rib.

Past Medical History

Gynecologic conditions causing back pain can include ovarian cysts, uterine fibroids, endometriosis, pelvic inflammatory disease, dysmenorrhea, or normal pregnancy, ectopic pregnancy, sexually transmitted disease (STD), or abortion (Case Example 15.15). Back pain can also occur with use of an Intra uterine contraceptive device (IUCD).

Usually there is a history of a chronic or long-standing gynecologic disorder and the association between back pain and gynecologic disorder has been established. Back pain has also been shown to be associated with a history of sexual assault, incest, and other childhood and adult trauma.

Having an understanding of the normal female reproductive anatomy (see Fig. 15.3) can help the therapist better appreciate musculoskeletal pain and dysfunction (see Fig. 15.4).

Taking a careful history and correlating symptoms with a woman's monthly cycle can help the therapist determine when to refer a client for a possible gynecologic cause of back, pelvic, or sacral pain/symptoms.

Pregnancy related LPB and pelvic girdle pain (PGP)

Back pain is common during pregnancy beginning most often during the second trimester between the fifth and seventh months of gestation; intensity varies throughout pregnancy.[187-190] Women who have had multiple pregnancies or births may have pelvic girdle pain (PGP) or LBP associated with poor abdominal muscle tone and ligamentous laxity. The most significant predictor of pregnancy related LBP is previous LBP (non pregnant, pregnant, and menstrual).[191] Risk factors for PGP include prior pregnancy, orthopedic dysfunctions, increased BMI, smoking, work dissatisfaction, and lack of belief in improvement. Studies repeated over time have not shown an increased risk of back pain in women who receive epidural anesthesia during delivery.[192,193]

PGP continues up to 11 years after delivery in 10% of women[191] and approximately one third of women have pregnancy related LBP 3 months after delivery.[194]

If the woman's history includes a recent birth or multiple previous births, she may not recognize the association with her current symptoms.[194]

Endometriosis

Endometriosis is an estrogen-dependent disorder defined by the presence of endometrial-like tissue outside of the uterus. Tissues form pockets called implants. Implants swell in response to the menstrual cyclic forming cysts that contain old blood called chocolate cysts. Inflammation appears to play a role, but it is unclear whether inflammation predisposes women to endometriosis or is the by-product of endometriosis. Implants often cause adhesions.

These implants can be deposited anywhere in the body. They are most commonly found coating the abdominal and pelvic viscera, however it is clear now that endometrial tissue migrates throughout the body. It has been recovered from bone, lungs, and even the brain.[195,196]

Pain can occur anywhere, but often the woman experiences back, pelvic, hip, and/or sacral pain that can be mistaken for a musculoskeletal, musculoligamentous, or neuromuscular impairment of the lumbar spine (Case Example 15.16).

The key to recognizing this condition is that it is cyclical, increasing during the second half of the menstrual cycle and decreasing after the first few days of menstrual flow. Any cyclical pain in menstruating women should be evaluated by a gynecologist. After menopause, pain can persist from scar tissue. There may be urinary tract and bowel involvement with associated symptoms ranging from urinary frequency, intermittent dysuria, and bloody stools to ureteral or bowel obstruction.

This condition is more common than previously thought. It is estimated that up to 50% of the female population who is infertile is affected by endometriosis.[195,197] Risk factors for endometrioses include early menarche, regular menstruation but 27-day or shorter cycles, and menstrual periods lasting 7 days or longer. There also appears to be a genetic link. A women with a maternal history of endometriosis is twice as likely to have the diagnosis herself. Endometriosis often co-exists with other health problems such as chronic fatigue syndrome, hypothyroidism, fibromyalgia, rheumatoid arthritis, multiple sclerosis, and systemic lupus erythematosus.[198-200] Endometriosis is a risk factor for ovarian and breast cancer.[195,201]

A cure has not been found at present, but for many women, it can be managed with medications and/or surgery. The therapist can help provide pain management strategies that can reduce sick leave and improve daily function. See Box 15.5 for more information on this condition.

CLINICAL SIGNS AND SYMPTOMS
Endometriosis

- Intermittent, cyclical, or constant pelvic and/or back pain (unilateral or bilateral)
- Pain during or after sexual intercourse
- Painful bowel movements or painful urination during menstrual period
- Small blood loss (spotting) before or between periods
- Heavy or irregular menstrual bleeding
- Bleeding anywhere else (nosebleeds, coughing up blood, blood in urine or stools)
- Fatigue
- History of ectopic pregnancy, miscarriage, infertility
- GI problems (abdominal bloating and cramping, nausea, diarrhea, constipation)

Ovarian Cysts and Uterine Fibroids

Ovarian cysts are often asymptomatic until they grow large enough to pull the ovary out of its normal position, sometimes cutting off the blood supply to the ovary and contributing to infertility. As the weight of the ovary causes a change in position, pressure is exerted against the uterus, bladder, intestines, or vagina, causing a variety of symptoms.

Lower abdominal or pelvic pain is most common, but back pain associated with ovarian cysts and uterine fibroids can occur, usually presenting in a cyclical pattern associated with the menstrual cycle similar to endometriosis. A physician must determine the underlying gynecologic cause of cyclical back, hip, pelvic, and sacral pain or symptoms.

In a screening context, we look for red-flag histories, clinical presentation, risk factors, and associated signs and symptoms. Risk factors for ovarian cysts include taking infertility medications, pregnancy, endometriosis, and severe pelvic infection. Risk factors for polycystic ovarian syndrome (PCOS) include obesity and genetic predisposition. Ovarian cysts present as a part of PCOS and place the woman at increased risk for insulin resistance and potentially at increased risk for cardiovascular disease as a result.[202-204] Other symptoms or conditions associated with PCOS include obstructive sleep apnea and daytime sleepiness and benign breast disease (formerly fibrocystic breast disease). There is a 2-fold increased risk for venous thrombosis embolism among women with PCOS who are taking combined oral contraceptives, and a 1.5-fold increased risk for women with PCOS who are not taking oral contraceptives. Several psychological symptoms have been reported, including depression, anxiety, and general decrease in quality of life.

If the Review of Systems points to a gynecologic source of pain/symptoms, further questions can be asked and a referral

CASE EXAMPLE 15.16

Endometriosis

Case Description: A 25-year-old female was referred for physical therapy with a diagnosis of nonspecific low back pain (LBP). She presented with the sudden onset of pain in the left lumbosacral region, left lower abdominal quadrant, and left buttock and anterior thigh which was constant and severe.

Medical examination ruled out a renal source of pain and diagnosed the client with a low back sprain. X-ray studies and magnetic resonance imaging (MRI) were negative and ruled out a spondylogenic, oncologic, or discogenic lesion. She was given an injection of Demerol, a prescription for nonsteroidal antiinflammatory drugs (NSAIDs) and antispasmodics, and a referral to physical therapy.

Past Medical History and Risk Factors: The client was a nonsmoker and consumed alcohol only on occasion. Personal family history was unremarkable; she reported that her mother had rheumatoid arthritis and hypothyroidism.

Clinical Presentation: The client was seen in physical therapy 3 weeks after the initial painful episode. She presented with a chief complaint of sharp, constant pain in the left lumbosacral region, which occasionally radiated into the left lower abdominal quadrant and into the left buttock and the anterior thigh as far distally as the knee.

The pain was worse when sitting or walking. She was only able to sleep 1 to 2 hours at a time because of the severity of the pain. There was no report of bowel or bladder changes. The hip and sacroiliac (SI) joint were ruled out as the sources of pain. A neurologic screening examination was negative.

Trunk motions were mildly restricted with increased pain during forward flexion. There was a positive left straight leg raise (SLR) test at 60 degrees. The client appeared to have a musculoskeletal-based movement impairment.

Physical examination determined the most significant clinical finding to be exquisite tenderness in the left lower abdominal quadrant. The client reported marked tenderness with palpation over the left lower abdominal quadrant, just proximal to the anterior superior iliac spine (ASIS). She also reported tenderness

with palpation directly over the left lumbar paraspinal region, just superior to the iliac crest.

Red Flags: The sudden onset, intensity, severity, and duration of the client's back pain raised a red flag. The left lower quadrant was the location of greatest tenderness and severe subjective pain, both experienced at rest and with activity. The client's sex and childbearing age raise yellow (caution) flags.

Should the therapist treat this client and reassess symptoms and clinical presentation in 2 weeks or refer immediately?

Once again, the decision to carry out a physical therapy plan of care with direct intervention versus making a medical referral is based on clinical judgment. Given the presentation of this case, either decision could be justified.

Because she was evaluated by a medical doctor who sent her to physical therapy, a telephone call would be more appropriate than suggesting the client go back to her doctor.

In this case the therapist made the decision not to treat the client given the fact that a delay in diagnosis with risk for increased morbidity and potential mortality is possible with LBP from serious pelvic pathology.

Outcomes: The therapist conferred with the referring orthopedic surgeon and a referral was made to a gynecologist. Further testing provided a diagnosis of endometriosis and ovarian cyst. The client underwent a laparoscopy; the diagnosis of endometriosis was confirmed.

Following medical and surgical intervention, the lower quadrant pain was abolished, and the LBP and leg pain significantly diminished in frequency and intensity, enabling the client to return to her normal activities.

Discussion: Given the prevalence of endometriosis, physical therapists are likely to encounter clients with this disorder in orthopedic physical therapy practice. Proper differential diagnosis is necessary to identify the risk factors and physical findings that would provide early diagnosis of endometriosis and avoid the morbidity associated with this and other pelvic disorders.

From Troyer MR: *Differential diagnosis of endometriosis in a patient with nonspecific low back pain.* Case report presented in partial fulfillment of DPT 910, Principles of Differential Diagnosis, Institute for Physical Therapy Education, Chester, PA, 2005, Widener University. Used with permission.

made if appropriate. LBP is a late finding for some women with ovarian cancer (see Chapter 16).

CLINICAL SIGNS AND SYMPTOMS

Ovarian Cysts

- Abdominal heaviness or pressure, pain, or bloating
- Discomfort during urination, bowel movement, or sexual intercourse
- Irregular menses, infertility
- Breat tenderness
- Urinary frequency or difficulty emptying the bladder
- Dysmenorrhea
- Dyspareunia
- Dull aching low back, buttock, pelvic, or groin pain
- Sudden, sharp pain with rupture or haemorrhage

Ectopic Pregnancy

An ectopic pregnancy is a live pregnancy that takes place outside of the uterus. As shown in Fig. 15.5, this may occur in a variety of places, such as the ovary, the tube (tubal pregnancy), outside lining of the uterus, or along the peritoneal cavity. None of these locations can sustain a viable ovum, and the woman will have a spontaneous abortion (miscarriage).

Risk factors include STDs, prior tubal surgery, and current use of an IUCD. Depending on the location of the ectopic pregnancy, symptoms can include back, hip, sacral, abdominal, pelvic, and/or shoulder pain. Shoulder pain is more likely to occur if there is retroperitoneal bleeding when rupture of the developing embryo and hemorrhage occurs with pressure on the diaphragm.

It is usually unilateral, on the same side as the bleeding, but can cause bilateral shoulder pain if the hemorrhage is significant enough to impinge both sides of the diaphragm. The pain is usually of sudden onset (when rupture and hemorrhage occur) with intense, constant pain. Situations of this type represent a medical emergency. Most likely the client did not come to the therapist for this problem but may develop emerging symptoms during treatment for some other orthopedic or neurologic problem.

Consider it a red flag when any woman of childbearing age who is sexually active has sudden, intense pain as described. Take her blood pressure and other vital signs while asking appropriate screening questions. Seek immediate medical assistance.

CLINICAL SIGNS AND SYMPTOMS
Ectopic Pregnancy

- Amenorrhea or irregular bleeding and spotting
- Diffuse, aching lower abdominal quadrant or LBP; can cause ipsilateral shoulder pain
- May progress to a sharper, intermittent type of pain

Intrauterine Contraceptive Device

The intrauterine contraceptive device (IUCD is the current medical term; known by most women as an IUD) has become popular once again, having gone out of favor in the 1970s when the copper T caused so many problems. Although this contraceptive device has been improved, there are still potential problems (Fig. 15.6). The body may recognize this as a foreign object and set up an immune response or try to wall it off. The IUCD can become embedded in the tissue of the uterus, causing inflammation, infection, and scarring.

For any woman with low back, pelvic, sacral, or hip pain who is in the reproductive age range, it may be necessary to ask about her method of birth control: Are you using an IUD for birth control?

Clinical Presentation

Normally occurring back pain that is associated with the menstrual cycle occurs most often at or around the point of ovulation (between day 10 and day 14 for most women) and again just before or during menstrual flow (between days 23 and 28 for most women). Day 1 is counted as the first day the woman experiences bleeding with her menstrual cycle.

Back pain associated with the menstrual cycle may be a regular feature for a woman, it may occur intermittently, or it may be new onset. The woman may be unaware of the link between the two until she charts her monthly cycle and correlates menstrual pain with her back pain.

A woman may have back pain accompanied by or alternating with sharp, bilateral, and cramping pain in the lower abdominal and/or pelvic quadrants. Menstrual pain can be referred to the rectum, lower sacrum, or coccyx. Tumors, masses, or even endometriosis may involve the sacral plexus or its branches, causing severe, burning pain.

After gathering information during the examination, the therapist performs a Review of Systems looking for clusters of

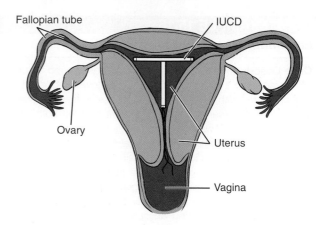

Fig. 15.6 Intrauterine contraceptive device (IUCD or IUD), a potential source of low back, pelvic, sacral, or even hip pain in any woman of reproductive age who is using this form of birth control.

signs and symptoms suggesting a gynecologic cause of LBP. If appropriate, the next step is to ask a few final screening questions.

CLINICAL SIGNS AND SYMPTOMS
Gynecologic Disorders

- Missed menses, irregular menses, history of menstrual disturbance, painful menstruation
- Tender breasts
- Nausea, vomiting
- Chronic constipation (with laxative and enema dependency)
- Pain on defecation
- Fever, night sweats, chills
- Low blood pressure (hemorrhaging with ectopic pregnancy)
- Vaginal discharge
- Abnormal vaginal bleeding
  - Late menstrual periods with persistent bleeding
  - Spotting before period or between periods
  - Irregular, longer, heavier menstrual periods, no specific pattern
  - Any postmenopausal bleeding
- Urinary problems (intermittent dysuria, frequency, urgency, hematuria)

SCREENING FOR MALE REPRODUCTIVE CAUSES OF BACK PAIN

Men can experience back pain (as well as hip, groin, SI, and sacral pain) caused by referred pain from the male reproductive system. See Chapter 11 for a complete discussion of prostate impairments (e.g., prostatitis, benign prostatic hypertrophy, chronic pelvic pain syndrome, prostate and testicular cancer).

Prostate cancer is the third most common cancer in males over the age of 60 years in the United States.[205] The mortality associated with prostate cancer has decreased by 51% since the initiation of widespread prostate-specific antigen (PSA) screening in the 1990s.[206]

Testicular cancer, though relatively rare, is the most common cancer in males ages 15 to 35 years and is on the rise.[207] Details of both conditions are discussed in Chapter 11. Benign prostatic hyperplasia (BPH) is one of the most common disorders of the aging male population affecting 50% of men over the age of 50 years.

Risk Factors

Risk factors for prostate dysfunction include advancing age, family history, ethnicity (greater risk for African American men), diet, and possibly exposure to chemicals. Not all disorders of this system occur with aging, so the therapist must remain alert for red-flag symptoms in males of any age.

Clinical Presentation

Back pain, changes in bladder function, and sexual dysfunction are the most common symptoms associated with male reproductive disorders. Any obstruction, growth, or inflammation of the prostate can directly affect the urethra, resulting in difficulty starting a flow of urine, continuing a flow of urine, frequency, and/or nocturia.

Prostate cancer is often asymptomatic and only diagnosed when the man seeks medical assistance because of symptoms of urinary obstruction or sciatica. Sciatic pain affects the low back, hip, and leg and is caused by metastasis to the bones of the pelvis, lumbar spine, or femur.

Associated symptoms may include melena, sudden moderate to high fever, chills, and changes in bowel or bladder function. Men who have reached the fifth decade of life or more are most commonly affected.

Testicular cancer presents most often as a painless swelling nodule in one gonad, noted incidentally by the client or his sexual partner. This is described as a lump or hardness of the testis, with occasional heaviness or a dull, aching sensation in the lower abdomen or scrotum. Acute pain is the presenting symptom in about 10% of affected men.

Involvement of the epididymis or spermatic cord may lead to pelvic or inguinal lymph node metastasis, although most tumors confined to the testis itself will spread primarily to the retroperitoneal lymph nodes. Subsequent cephalad drainage may be to the thoracic duct and supraclavicular nodes. Hematogenous spread to the lungs, bone, or liver may occur as a result of direct tumor invasion.

In about 10% of affected individuals, dissemination along these pathways results in thoracic, lumbar, supraclavicular, neck, or shoulder pain or mass as the first symptom. Other symptoms related to this pathway of dissemination may include respiratory symptoms or GI disturbance.

As discussed earlier, back pain caused by a neoplasm is typically progressive, is more pronounced at night, and may not have a clear association with activity level (as is more characteristic of mechanical back pain). The usual progression of symptoms in clients with cord compression is back pain followed by radicular pain, lower extremity weakness, sensory loss, and finally, loss of sphincter (bowel and bladder) control.

Associated Signs and Symptoms

Besides changes in urinary patterns, the therapist should ask about discharge from the penis, constitutional symptoms, and pain in any of the nearby soft tissue areas (groin, rectum, scrotum). Is there any blood in the urine (or change in color from yellow to orange or red)? Recurrent UTI is common in prostatitis but does not lead to prostate cancer.

Because the therapist is not going to treat back pain related to dysfunction of the male reproductive system, any red flags should be reported to the physician. A rectal examination may be needed. Access to the prostate is easiest through this type of examination. By pressing on the inflamed or infected prostate, the physician can reproduce painful symptoms as a part of the differential diagnosis (see Fig. 11.5).

Many men are reluctant to pursue diagnosis and treatment whenever the male reproductive system is involved. Early detection and treatment of these conditions can result in a good outcome. Screening questions for men are a good way to elicit red-flag history, risk factors, and signs or symptoms. The therapist must follow-up with the client and make sure contact is made with the appropriate health care professional.

CLINICAL SIGNS AND SYMPTOMS
Prostate Pathology

- May be asymptomatic early on
- Urinary dysfunction (hesitancy, frequency, urgency, nocturia, dysuria)
- Low back, inner thigh, or perineal pain or stiffness
- Suprapubic or pelvic pain
- Testicular or penis pain
- Sciatica (prostate cancer metastases)
- Bone pain, lymphedema of the groin, and/or lower extremities (prostate cancer metastases)
- Neurologic changes from spinal cord compression (prostate cancer metastases to the vertebrae)
- Sexual dysfunction (difficulty having an erection, painful ejaculation, cramping/discomfort after ejaculation)
- Constitutional symptoms with prostatitis
- Blood in urine or semen
- See full discussion in Chapter 11; see also Appendices B-24 and B-30

SCREENING FOR INFECTIOUS CAUSES OF BACK PAIN

Drug abuse, immune suppression, and human immunodeficiency virus (HIV) may predispose one to infection. Fever in anyone taking immunosuppressants is a red-flag symptom indicating a possible underlying infection. Many people with a spinal infection do not have a fever; they are more likely to have a red-flag history or risk factors.[1]

Vertebral Osteomyelitis

Vertebral osteomyelitis is a bone infection most often affecting the first and second lumbar vertebrae, causing LBP.[208] There are many causative factors. Osteomyelitis may occur in individuals with diabetes mellitus, injection drug users, alcoholics, clients taking corticosteroid drugs, clients with spinal cord injury and neurogenic bladder, and otherwise debilitated or immune-suppressed clients. Older children can be affected, although the most common peak is after the third decade of life.

Vertebral osteomyelitis is increasingly being reported as a complication of nosocomial bacteremia. Methicillin-resistant *Staphylococcus aureus* (MRSA) is the most common causative organism. Osteomyelitis also can occur after surgery, open fractures, penetrating wounds, skin breakdown and ulcers, and systemic infections. It may result from a hematogenous spread through arterial and venous routes secondary to surgically implanted hardware for internal fixation of the spine, pelvic inflammatory disease, or GU tract infection.

A physician should evaluate new onset of back pain in anyone who has been treated with vancomycin therapy for MRSA. Vancomycin therapy may give the appearance of being effective with resolution of fever and the return of white blood cell counts to normal ranges, but in fact is insufficient to prevent or reverse the progression of hematogenous MRSA vertebral osteomyelitis.[209,210]

In the adult, usually two adjacent vertebrae and their intervening disk are involved, and the vertebral body/bodies may undergo destruction and collapse. Abscess formation may result, with possible neurologic involvement. The abscess can advance anteriorly to produce an abscess that can extend to the psoas muscle producing hip pain.

The most consistent clinical finding is marked local tenderness over the spinous process of the involved vertebrae with "nonspecific backache." The classic history describes pain that has been increasing in severity over 1 to 3 weeks. Movement is painful and there is marked muscular guarding and spasm of the paravertebral muscles and the hamstrings. The involved vertebrae are usually exquisitely sensitive to percussion, and pain is more severe at night.

There may be no rise in temperature or abnormality in white blood cell count because generalized sepsis is not present, but an elevated erythrocyte sedimentation rate (ESR) is likely. A low-grade fever is most common in adults when body temperature changes do occur.

Children are more likely to present with acute, severe complaints including high fever, intense pain, and localized manifestations such as edema, erythema, and tenderness. Acute hematogenous osteomyelitis seen in children usually originates in the metaphysis of a long bone. Precipitating trauma is often present in the history, and well-localized, acute bone pain of 1 day to several days' duration is the primary symptom. The pain is most commonly severe enough to limit or restrict the use of the involved extremity, and fever and malaise consistent with sepsis are usual.

CLINICAL SIGNS AND SYMPTOMS
Vertebral Osteomyelitis

- Pain and local tenderness over the involved spinous process(es); possible swelling, redness, and warmth in the affected area
- Night pain
- Stiff back with difficulty bearing weight, moving, walking
- Paravertebral muscle guarding or spasm
- Positive SLR
- Hip pain if infection spreads to the psoas muscle
- May be constitutional symptoms (fever, malaise)
- Recent history of bacterial infection (e.g., pharyngitis, otitis media in children)

Disk Space Infection

Disk space infection is a form of subacute osteomyelitis involving the vertebral endplates and the disk in both children and adults. The lower thoracic and lumbar spines are the most common sites of infection.

Symptoms associated with postoperative disk space infection occur 2 to 8 weeks after diskectomy. Diskitis of an infectious type occurs following bacteremia secondary to UTI, with or without instrumentation (e.g., catheterization or cystoscopy). Low-grade viral or bacterial infection (e.g., gastroenteritis, upper respiratory infection, UTI) is most often implicated in young children with diskitis (4 years old and younger). Ask the parent, guardian, or caretaker of any young child with back pain if there has been a recent history of sore throat, cold, ear infection, or other upper respiratory illness.

Adults with disk space infection often complain of LBP localized around the disk area. The pain can range from mild to "excruciating" and sometimes is described as "knife-like." Such severe pain is accompanied by restricted movement and constant pain, present both day and night. The pain is usually made worse by activity, but unlike most other causes of back pain, it is *not* relieved by rest. If the condition becomes chronic, pain may radiate into the abdomen, pelvis, and lower extremities.

Children present with a history of increasingly severe localized back pain often accompanied by a limp or refusal to walk. There may be an increased lumbar lordosis. Pain may occur in the flank, abdomen, or hip. Symptoms may get worse with passive SLR testing or other hip motion. A neurologic screening examination is usually negative.

Physical examination may reveal localized tenderness over the involved disk space, paraspinal muscle spasm, and restricted lumbar motion. SLR may be positive and fever is common (Case Example 15.17).

CASE EXAMPLE 15.17

Septic Diskitis

Background: A 72-year-old man with leg myalgia and stabbing back pain of 2 weeks' duration was referred to physical therapy for evaluation by a rural nurse practitioner. When questioned about past medical history, the client reported a prostatectomy 22 years ago with no further problems. He was not aware of any other associated signs and symptoms but reported a recurring dermatitis that was being treated by his nurse practitioner. There were no skin lesions associated with the dermatitis present at the time of the physical therapist's evaluation.

Clinical Presentation: The examination revealed spasm of the thoracolumbosacral paraspinal muscles bilaterally. The client reported extreme sensitivity to palpation of the spinous processes at L3 and L4; tap test reproduced painful symptoms. Spinal accessory motions could not be tested because of the client's state of acute pain and immobility.

Hip flexion and extension reproduced the symptoms and produced additional radiating flank pain. A straight leg raise (SLR) caused severe back pain with each leg at 30 degrees on both sides. A neurologic examination was otherwise within normal limits. Vital signs were taken: blood pressure of 180/100 mm Hg; heart rate of 100 bpm; temperature of 101° F.

What are the red flags in this case?

- Age
- Recurring dermatitis
- Positive tap test
- Bilateral SLR
- Vital signs

Result: The therapist contacted the nurse practitioner by telephone to report the findings, especially the vital signs and results of the SLR. It was determined that the client needed a medical evaluation, and he was referred to a physician's center in the nearest available city. A summary of findings from the physical therapist was sent with the client along with a request for a copy of the physician's report.

The client returned to the physical therapist's clinic with a copy of the physician's report with the following diagnosis: *Clostridium perfringens* septic diskitis (made on the basis of blood culture). The prescribed treatment was intravenous antibiotic therapy for 6 weeks, progressive mobilization, and a spinal brace to be provided and fitted by the physical therapist. The client's back pain subsided gradually over the next 2 weeks and he followed-up at intervals until he was weaned from the brace and resumed normal activities.

Septic diskitis may occur following various invasive procedures, or it may be related to occult infections, urinary tract infections, septicemia, and dermatitis. Contact dermatitis was the most likely underlying cause in this case.

Bacterial Endocarditis

Bacterial endocarditis often initially presents with musculoskeletal symptoms, including arthralgia, arthritis, LBP, and myalgia. Half of these clients will have only musculoskeletal symptoms, without other signs of endocarditis.

The early onset of joint pain and myalgia is more likely if the client is older and has had a previously diagnosed heart murmur or prosthetic valve (risk factors). Other risk factors include injection drug use, previous cardiac surgery, recent dental work, and recent history of invasive diagnostic procedures (e.g., shunts, catheters).

Almost one-third of clients with bacterial endocarditis have LBP. In many persons, LBP is the principal musculoskeletal symptom reported. Back pain is accompanied by decreased ROM and spinal tenderness. Pain may affect only one side, and it may be limited to the paraspinal muscles.

Endocarditis-induced LBP may be very similar to the pain pattern associated with a herniated lumbar disk; it radiates to the leg and may be accentuated by raising the leg, coughing, or sneezing. The key difference is that neurologic deficits are usually absent in clients with bacterial endocarditis. The therapist can review history and risk factors and conduct a Review of Systems to help in the screening process.

PHYSICIAN REFERRAL

Most adults with an episode of acute back pain experience recovery within 1 to 4 weeks. As many as 90% of affected individuals resume normal activity levels during this time.[211,212]

All clients who have not regained usual activity after 4 weeks should be formally reassessed, including a review of the history and examination, looking for yellow (caution) or red (warning) flags, testing for any neurologic deficit, and conducting a Review of Systems to identify any evidence of systemic disease or other medical condition requiring referral.

Reassessment of movement dysfunction is critical at this stage to look for alternate impairments not previously observed or identified. The therapist must consider whether the underlying primary problem is spinal or nonspinal, mechanical or medical, and what specific structures are involved.

Review the concepts from the screening physical assessment in Chapter 4 to make sure the evaluation is complete. Inspection, palpation, and auscultation may reveal key findings previously missed. Assessment of fear-avoidance may be needed as discussed in Chapter 3. The therapist should not rely on his or her perception of patient's/client's fear-avoidance behaviors. Tools such as the Fear-Avoidance Beliefs Questionnaire (FABQ; see Table 3.7), Tampa Scale of Kinesophobia (TSK-11), and Pain Catastrophizing Scale (PSC) are available to identify fear-avoidance beliefs.[213]

Medical referral is made based on a comparison of baseline data with findings upon reassessment. Providing the physician with concise but comprehensive information about findings and concerns is a helpful part of the medical differential diagnostic process.

Guidelines for Immediate Medical Attention

Immediate medical referral is not always required when a client presents with any one of the red flags listed in Box 15.1.

When viewed as a whole, the history, risk factors, and any cluster of red-flag findings will guide the therapist in making a final intervention versus referral decision.

- Neck pain with evidence of VBI (e.g., reproduction of symptoms with vertebral artery testing such as vertigo, change in vision, headache, nausea) requires medical attention. VBI can develop into cerebral or brain stem ischemia, leading to severe morbidity or death.[214]
- Immediate medical attention is required when anyone with LBP presents with symptoms of cauda equina syndrome (e.g., saddle anesthesia, new onset of fecal incontinence, motor weakness of the legs, radiculopathy, unable to heel or toe walk, altered knee or ankle DTR). Acute mechanical compression of nerves in the lower extremities, bowel, and bladder as they pass through the caudal sac may be a surgical emergency.
- Massive midline rupture of a disk in the lower lumbar levels can lead to LBP, rapidly progressive bilateral motor weakness and sciatica, saddle anesthesia (buttock and medial and posterior thighs; the area that would come in contact with a saddle when sitting on a horse), and new onset of bowel and bladder incontinence or urinary retention.[215]
- Men between the ages of 65 and 75 years who ever smoked should undergo medical screening for AAA. Any male with these two risk factors, especially presenting with signs or symptoms of AAA, must be referred immediately.
- Sudden, intense back and/or shoulder pain in a sexually active woman of childbearing age may signal the end of an ectopic pregnancy. Sudden change in blood pressure, pallor, pain, and dizziness will alert the therapist to the need for immediate medical attention.
- Inability to bear weight, especially with fever and/or a history of cancer, diabetes mellitus, immunosuppression, or trauma (even if radiographs have already been obtained and declared "negative" [infection, fracture]).

Guidelines for Physician Referral

- Red flags requiring physician referral or reevaluation include back pain or symptoms that are not improving as expected, steady pain irrespective of activity, symptoms that are increasing, or the development of new or progressive neurologic deficits such as weakness, sensory loss, reflex changes, bowel or bladder dysfunction, or myelopathy.
- A positive Sharp-Purser test for AA subluxation in the client with rheumatoid arthritis (sensation of head falling forward during neck flexion and clunking during neck extension) must be evaluated by an orthopedic surgeon.[17]
- The ESR, serum calcium level, and alkaline phosphatase level are usually elevated if bone cancer is present.[216] Back pain in the presence of elevated alkaline phosphatase levels can also indicate hyperparathyroidism, osteomalacia, pregnancy, and/or rickets.
- Reproduction of pain or exquisite tenderness over the spinous process(es) is a red-flag sign requiring further investigation and possible medical referral.

Clues to Screening Head, Neck, or Back Pain

General

- Age younger than 20 years and older than 50 years with no history of a precipitating event
- Back pain in children is uncommon and constitutes a red-flag finding, especially back pain that lasts more than 6 weeks.
- Nocturnal back pain that is constant, intense, and unrelieved by change in position
- Pain that causes constant movement or makes the client curl up in the sitting position
- Back pain with constitutional symptoms: fatigue, nausea, vomiting, diarrhea, fever, sweats
- Back pain accompanied by unexplained weight loss
- Back pain accompanied by extreme weakness in the leg(s), numbness in the groin or rectum, or difficulty controlling bowel or bladder function (**cauda equina syndrome;** rare but requires immediate medical attention)
- Back pain that is insidious in onset and progression (remember to assess for unreported sexual assault or physical abuse)
- Back pain that is unrelieved by recumbency
- Back pain that does not vary with exertion or activity
- Back pain that is relieved by sitting up and leaning forward (**pancreas**)
- Back pain that is accompanied by multiple joint involvement (**GI, rheumatoid arthritis, fibromyalgia**) or by sustained morning stiffness (**spondyloarthropathy**)
- Severe, persistent back pain with full and painless movement of the spine
- Sudden, localized back pain that does not diminish in 10 days to 2 weeks in postmenopausal women or osteoporotic adults (**osteoporosis with compression fracture**)

Past Medical History

- Previous history of cancer, Crohn's disease, or bowel obstruction
- Long-term use of NSAIDs (**GI bleeding**), steroids, or immunosuppressants (**infectious cause**)
- Recent history or previous history of recurrent upper respiratory infection or pneumonia
- Recent history of surgery, especially back pain 2 to 8 weeks after diskectomy (**infection**)
- History of osteoporosis and/or previous vertebral compression fracture(s) (**fracture**)
- History of heart murmur or prosthetic valve in an older client who currently has LBP of unknown cause (**bacterial endocarditis**)
- History of intermittent claudication and heart disease in a man with deep midlumbar back pain; assess for pulsing abdominal mass (**AAA**)
- History of diseases associated with hypercalcemia such as hyperparathyroidism, multiple myeloma, senile osteoporosis, hyperthyroidism, Cushing's disease, or specific renal tubular disease not appearing with back pain radiating to the flank or iliac crest (**kidney stone**)

Oncologic

- Back pain with severe lower extremity weakness without pain, with full ROM and recent history of sciatica in the absence of a positive SLR

- Bilateral leg pain with motor and reflex impairments
- Bone tenderness over the spinous processes **(infection or neoplasm)**
- Temperature differences: involved side warmer when tumor interferes with sympathetic nerves
- Associated signs and symptoms: significant weight loss; night pain disturbing sleep; extreme fatigue; constitutional symptoms such as fever, sweats; other organ/system-dependent symptoms such as urinary changes (urologic), cough, and dyspnea (pulmonary); abdominal bloating or bloody diarrhea (GI)

Cardiovascular

- Back pain that is described as "throbbing"
- Back pain accompanied by leg pain that is relieved by standing still or resting
- Back pain that is present in all spinal positions and increased by exertion
- Back pain accompanied by a pulsating sensation or palpable abdominal pulse (possibly a palpable pulsating abdominal mass)
- Low back, pelvic, and/or leg pain with temperature changes from one leg to the other (involved side warmer: venous occlusion or tumor; involved side colder: arterial occlusion)
- Back injury that occurred during weight lifting in someone with known heart disease or past history of aneurysm

Pulmonary

- Associated signs and symptoms (dyspnea, persistent cough, fever and chills)
- Back pain aggravated by respiratory movements (deep breathing, laughing, coughing)
- Back pain relieved by breath holding or Valsalva maneuver
- Autosplinting by lying on the involved side or holding firm pillow against the chest/abdomen that decreases the pain
- Spinal/trunk movements (e.g., trunk rotation, trunk sidebending) do not reproduce symptoms (exception: an intercostal tear caused by forceful coughing from underlying diaphragmatic pleurisy can result in painful movement but is also reproduced by local palpation).
- Weak and rapid pulse accompanied by fall in blood pressure (pneumothorax)

Renal/Urologic

- Renal and urethral pain is felt throughout T9 to L1 dermatomes; pain is constant but may crescendo (kidney stones).
- Kidney pain of an inflammatory nature can be relieved by a change in position. However, renal colic (e.g., infection) remains unchanged by a change in position. But there are usually constitutional symptoms associated with either inflammation or infection to tip off the alert therapist.
- Back pain at the level of the kidneys can be caused by ovarian or testicular cancer
- Back pain and shoulder pain, either simultaneously or alternately, may be renal/urologic in origin
- Side-bending to the same side and pressure placed along the spine at that level is "more comfortable"; pain may

be reduced, but it is not eliminated when the kidney is involved. The client with kidney disease/disorder may prefer this position because it moves the kidney out away from the spine and away from any compressive forces causing painful symptoms.
- Associated signs and symptoms (blood in urine, fever, chills, increased urinary frequency, difficulty starting or continuing stream of urine, testicular pain in men, painful erection and/or ejaculation)
- Assess for costovertebral angle tenderness; pain is affected by change of position **(pseudorenal pain)**.
- History of traumatic fall, blow, lift **(musculoskeletal)**
- Persistent back (pelvic, groin, or testicular) pain in a male with history of chronic prostatitis that does not respond to medical treatment such as antibiotics suggests the need to assess (or reassess) for pelvic floor muscle impairment; watch for a history of improved symptoms without complete resolution with an orthopedic treatment approach

Gastrointestinal

- Back and abdominal pain at the same level (may occur simultaneously or alternately); check for GI history or associated signs and symptoms
- Back pain with abdominal pain at a lower level than the back pain; look for its source in the back
- Back pain associated with food or meals (increase or decrease in symptoms)
- Back pain accompanied by heartburn or relieved by antacids
- Associated signs and symptoms (dysphagia, odynophagia, melena, unexplained or unintended weight loss, especially if accompanied by early satiety, abdominal distention, tenderness over McBurney's point, positive iliopsoas or obturator sign, bloody diarrhea, nausea, vomiting)
- LBP accompanied by constipation may be a manifestation of pelvic floor muscle overactivity or spasm; this requires a pelvic floor screening examination.
- Sacral pain occurs when the rectum is stimulated, such as during a bowel movement or when passing gas, and relieved after each of these events.

Gynecologic

- History or current gynecologic disorder (e.g., ovarian cysts, uterine fibroids, endometriosis, pelvic inflammatory disease, sexual assault/incest, and IUCD)
- Associated signs and symptoms (missed or irregular menses, tender breasts, cyclic nausea and vomiting, chronic constipation, vaginal discharge, abnormal uterine bleeding or bleeding in a postmenopausal woman)
- Low back and/or pelvic pain developing soon after a missed menstrual cycle; blood pressure may be significantly low, and there may be concomitant shoulder pain when hemorrhaging occurs **(ectopic pregnancy)**
- Low back and/or pelvic pain occurring intermittently but with regularity in response to menstrual cycle (e.g., ovulation around days 10 to 14 and onset of menses around days 23 to 28) **(endometriosis)**

Nonorganic (Psychogenic) (see discussion in Chapter 3)

- Widespread, nonanatomic low back tenderness with over-reaction to superficial palpation
- Assess for nonorganic signs such as axial loading (downward pressure on the top of the head) or shoulder-hip rotation (client rotates shoulder and hips with feet planted); Waddell's nonorganic signs (see Table 3.12)
- Regional (whole leg) pain, numbness, weakness, sensory disturbances
- Chronic use of (or demand for) narcotics

Infectious

- Infection, such as osteomyelitis or inflammatory arthritis (e.g., ankylosing spondylitis, psoriatic or reactive arthritis), may present as back pain with intermittent reports of fever, chills, sweats, fatigue, and/or adenopathy. Watch for other associated signs and symptoms specific to each condition (e.g., urethritis, psoriasis, severe morning stiffness).

Pediatrics

- Children presenting with back pain are very different from adults with the same problem; children are less likely than adults to report symptoms when there is no organic cause for the complaint.[217]
- Eighty-five percent of children with back pain lasting more than 2 months have a diagnosable lesion.[218]
- Children with persistent reports of LBP must be evaluated and reevaluated until a diagnosis is reached; x-rays and laboratory values are needed.

REFERRED BACK PAIN PATTERNS (FIG. 15.7)

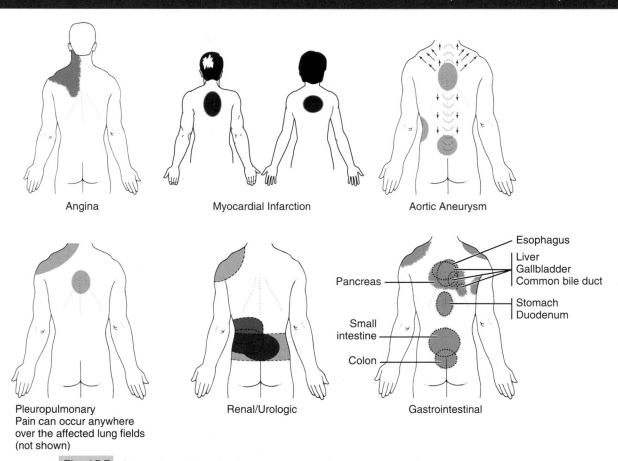

Angina

Myocardial Infarction

Aortic Aneurysm

Pleuropulmonary
Pain can occur anywhere
over the affected lung fields
(not shown)

Renal/Urologic

Gastrointestinal
Esophagus
Liver
Gallbladder
Common bile duct
Pancreas
Stomach
Duodenum
Small intestine
Colon

Fig. 15.7 Composite picture of referred back pain patterns. Not pictured: gynecologic pain patterns.

■ Key Points to Remember

1. Clients may inaccurately attribute symptoms to a particular incident or activity, or they may fail to recognize causative factors.
2. At presentation, any person with musculoskeletal pain of unknown cause and/or a past medical history of cancer should be screened for medical disease. Special Questions for Men and Women may be helpful in this screening process.
3. Consider visceral origin of back pain in the absence of muscular spasm, tenderness, and impaired movement.[149]

Continued

■ **Key Points to Remember—Cont'd**

4. Ask the client about nipple discharge or dimpling of the breast as these are red flags and require further medical evaluation.
5. Backache may be the earliest and only manifestation of visceral disease.[149]
6. Neck or back pain in the presence of normal ROM and strength is a yellow (caution)-flag symptom.
7. Persistent backache as a result of extraspinal pathology is rare in children but common in adults.[52,149]
8. Children, adolescents, and especially athletes reporting back pain of more than 3 weeks' duration may need medical referral, depending on the history and clinical presentation.[52,219]
9. Lumbar spasm may occur in the presence of severe pain from retroperitoneal diseases (e.g., renal tumors, abscesses, appendicitis, kidney stones, lymphoma).[149]
10. Back pain accompanied by recent history of infection (especially UTI) or in the presence of constitutional symptoms (e.g., fever, chills, nausea; see Box 1.3) must be screened more carefully.
11. Nonpainful paresthesia can be the result of neural compression but can also occur from ischemia (atherosclerosis, tumor, prodromal sign of a migraine headache); painful paresthesia is more likely indicative of an inflammatory or mechanical process.
12. When symptoms seem out of proportion to the injury, or if they persist beyond the expected time for the nature of the injury, medical referral may be indicated.
13. Pain that is unrelieved by rest or change in position or pain/symptoms that do not fit the expected mechanical

or neuromusculoskeletal pattern should serve as red-flag warnings.
14. When symptoms cannot be reproduced, aggravated, or altered in any way during the examination, additional questions to screen for medical disease are indicated.
15. Always rule out trigger points as a possible cause of musculoskeletal symptoms before referring the client elsewhere.
16. Postoperative infection of any kind may not appear with any clinical signs/symptoms for weeks or months.
17. Muscle weakness without pain, without history of sciatica, and without a positive SLR is suggestive of spinal metastases.
18. Sciatica may be the first symptom of prostate cancer metastasized to the bones of the pelvis, lumbar spine, or femur.
19. Back pain may be a symptom of depression.
20. Urinary incontinence concomitant with cervical spine pain requires a neurologic screening examination and possible medical referral.
21. Anterior neck pain, movement dysfunction, and torticollis of the sternocleidomastoid muscle may be a sign of underlying thyroid involvement.
22. The therapist may need to screen for illness behavior and the need for psychologic evaluation. Many clients with chronic back pain have both a physical problem and varying degrees of illness behavior. A single behavioral sign or symptom may be normal; multiple findings of several different kinds are much more significant.[59]
23. Remember to screen for fear-avoidance behaviors; this is considered a yellow flag pointing to psychosocial factors that can direct treatment.

CLIENT HISTORY AND INTERVIEW

SPECIAL QUESTIONS TO ASK: HEADACHE

See Appendix C-7 in the accompanying enhanced eBook version included with print purchase of this textbook for a complete pain assessment.

History

- Do other family members have similar headaches?
- What major life changes or stressors have you had in the last 6 months?
- Have you ever had a head injury? Cancer of any kind? A hysterectomy? High blood pressure? A stroke? Seizures?
- Have you been hit or kicked in the head, neck, or face? Pushed against a wall or other object? Pulled or thrown by the hair?
- For women of childbearing age: Is it possible you are pregnant?

Site

- Where do you feel the headache? Can you point to it with one finger (localized versus diffuse)? Does it move?

Onset

- Do you recall your first headache of this type?
- Was it caused by a fall or trauma? (Therapist may have to screen for trauma associated with domestic violence as a potential cause.)

Frequency

- How often do you have this type of headache?

Intensity

- On a scale from 0 (no pain) to 10 (worst pain), how would you rate your headache now? Worst it has been?
- Does the pain keep you from your daily activities? From exercise or recreation? From work?

Continued

CLIENT HISTORY AND INTERVIEW—Cont'd

Duration
- How long do your headaches last?

Description
- What do your headaches feel like? (The client may have more than one type of headache.)
- Alternate question: What words would you use to describe the pain?

Pattern
- Is there a pattern to your headaches (e.g., Weekly? Monthly? Morning to evening?)
- Do you wake up in the early morning hours with a headache? (**Occipital pain: hypertension**)
- For women who are perimenopausal or menopausal (natural or surgically induced): Are the headaches cyclical? (Monthly? Right before or right after the menstrual flow?)

Aggravating Factors
- What makes the headache worse?
- Are you aware of any triggers that can bring the headache on? (Alcohol, noise, lights, food, coughing or sneezing, fatigue or lack of sleep, stress, caffeine withdrawal; for women: menstrual cycle)
- Do you grind your teeth during the day or at night?
  - *If yes*, assessment of the cervical spine and temporomandibular joints is indicated. Referral to a dentist may be required.
- Are you taking any medications? (Headache can be a side effect of many different medications, but especially NSAIDs, muscle relaxants, antianxiety and antidepressant agents, and food and drugs containing nitrates, calcium, and beta-blockers.)

Relieving Factors
- Is there anything you can do to make the headache better?
  - *If yes*, how? (caffeine, medications, sleep, avoid certain foods, alcohol, cigarettes) (Ask follow-up questions about use of OTC or prescription drugs and/or herbs or pharmaceuticals.)
  - How does rest affect your symptoms?

Associated Symptoms
- Do you have any symptoms of any kind anywhere else in your head or body? (Follow-up with questions about any change in vision, dizziness, ringing in the ears, change in mood, nausea, vomiting, nasal congestion, nosebleeds, light or sound sensitivity, paresthesia such as numbness and tingling of the face or fingers, difficulty swallowing, hoarseness, fever, chills.)

For the Therapist
- Take the client's blood pressure and pulse and assess for cardiovascular risk factors.

- Auscultate for bruits in the temporal and carotid arteries (**temporal arteritis, carotid stenosis**).
- Headaches that cannot be linked to a neuromuscular or musculoskeletal cause (e.g., dysfunction of the cervical spine, thoracic spine, or temporomandibular joints; muscle tension, poor posture, nerve impingement) may need further medical referral and evaluation.

SPECIAL QUESTIONS TO ASK: NECK OR BACK

To the Therapist: If a more complete screening interview is required, see *Special Questions to Ask* at the end of each chapter for further questions related to the individual organ systems.

Pain Assessment (see also Appendix C-7 in the accompanying enhanced eBook version included with print purchase of this textbook)
- When did the pain or symptoms start?
- Did it (they) start gradually or suddenly? (**Vascular versus trauma problem**)
- Was there an illness or injury before the onset of pain?
- Have you noticed any changes in your symptoms since they first started to the present time?
- Is the pain aggravated or relieved by coughing or sneezing? (**Nerve root involvement, muscular**)
- Is the pain aggravated or relieved by activity?
- Are there any particular positions (sitting, lying, standing) that make your back pain feel better or worse?
- Does the pain go down the leg? *If so*, how far does it go?
- Have you noticed any muscular weakness?
- Have you been treated previously for back disorders?
- How has your general health been, both before the beginning of your back problem and today?
- How does rest affect the pain or symptoms?
- Do you feel worse in the morning or evening ... **OR** ... What difference do you notice in your symptoms from the morning when you first wake up until the evening when you go to bed?

General Systemic
Most of these questions may be asked of clients who have pain or symptoms anywhere in the musculoskeletal system.
- Have you ever been told that you have osteoporosis or brittle bones?
- Have you ever fractured your spine?
- Have you ever been diagnosed or treated for cancer in any part of your body?
  - *If no*, have you ever had chemotherapy or radiation therapy for anything? (**Rectal bleeding is a sign of radiation proctitis.**)
- Do you ever notice sweating, nausea, or chest pains when your current symptoms occur?

CLIENT HISTORY AND INTERVIEW—Cont'd

- What other symptoms have you had with this problem? Wait for an answer but consider offering, for example, have you had:
  - Numbness
  - Burning, tingling
  - Nausea, vomiting
  - Loss of appetite
  - Unexpected or significant weight gain or loss
  - Diarrhea, constipation, blood in your stool or urine
  - Difficulty in starting or continuing the flow of urine
  - Incontinence (inability to hold your urine, using a pad for urine leakage)
  - Hoarseness or difficulty in swallowing
  - Heart palpitations or fluttering
  - Difficulty in breathing while just sitting or resting or with mild effort (e.g., when walking from the car to the house)
  - Unexplained sweating or perspiration
  - Night sweats, fever, chills
  - Change in vision: blurred vision, black spots, double vision, temporary blindness
  - Fatigue, weakness, sudden paralysis of one side of your body, arm, or leg **(transient ischemic attack)**
  - Headache
  - Dizziness or fainting spells
- Have you had a recent cold, sore throat, upper respiratory infection, or the flu? Have you ever been diagnosed with HIV?

Cardiovascular

- Have you ever been told you have high blood pressure or heart trouble?
- Do you ever have chest pain or discomfort when your back hurts or just before your back starts hurting?
- Do you ever have swollen feet or ankles? *If yes*, are they swollen when you get up in the morning? **(Edema/congestive heart failure)**
- Do you ever get cramps in your legs if you walk for several blocks or in your arms if you work with your arms overhead? **(Intermittent claudication)**
- Do you ever have bouts of rapid heart action, irregular heartbeats, or palpitations of your heart?
- Have you ever felt a "heartbeat" in your abdomen when you lie down?
  - *If yes*, is this associated with LBP or left flank pain? **(Abdominal aneurysm)**
- Do you ever notice sweating, nausea, or chest pain when your current symptoms (e.g., head, neck, jaw, back pain) occur?

Pulmonary

- Are you able to take a deep breath?
- Do you ever have shortness of breath or breathlessness with your back pain?
  - How far can you walk before you feel breathless?
  - What symptoms stop your walking/activities (e.g., shortness of breath, heart pounding, chest tightness, or weak arms/legs)?

- Have you had any trouble with coughing lately?
  - *If yes*, have you strained your back from coughing?

Renal/Urologic

- Have you noticed any changes in the flow of urine since your back/groin pain started?
  - If *no*, it may be necessary to provide prompts or examples of what changes you are referring to (e.g., difficulty in starting or continuing the flow of urine, numbness or tingling in the groin or pelvis, increased frequency, getting up at night)
- Have you had burning with urination during the last 3 to 4 weeks? Fever and/or chills?
- Do you ever have blood in your urine or notice blood in the toilet going to the bathroom?
- Have you noticed any changes in color or blood in your urine?
- Do you have any problems with your kidneys or bladder? *If so*, describe.
- Have you ever had kidney or bladder stones? *If so*, how were these stones treated?
- Have you ever had an injury to your bladder or to your kidneys? *If so*, how was this treated?
- Have you had any infections of the bladder, and how were these infections treated?
  - Were they related to any specific circumstances (e.g., pregnancy, intercourse)?
- Have you had any kidney infections, and how were these treated?
  - Were they related to any specific circumstances (e.g., pregnancy, after bladder infections, a strep throat, or strep skin infections)?
- Do you ever have pain, discomfort, or a burning sensation when you urinate? **(Lower urinary tract irritation)**

Gastrointestinal

- Are you having any stomach or abdominal pain either at the same time as the back pain or at other times?
  - *If yes*, assess the location and the presence of any GI symptoms.
- Have you noticed any association between when you eat and when your symptoms increase or decrease?
  - Do you notice any change in your symptoms 1 to 3 hours after you eat?
  - Do you notice any pain beneath the breastbone (epigastric) or just beneath the shoulder blade (subscapular) 1 to 2 hours after eating?
- Do you have a feeling of fullness after only one or two bites of food? **(Early satiety)**
- Is your back pain relieved after having a bowel movement? **(GI obstruction)**
- Do you have rectal, low back, or SI pain when passing stool or having a bowel movement?
- Do you have any blood in your stools or change in the normal color of your bowel movements (e.g., black, red,

Continued

CLIENT HISTORY AND INTERVIEW—Cont'd

mahogany color, gray color)? (**Hemorrhoids, prostate problems, cancer**)

- Are you having any diarrhea, constipation, or other changes in your bowel function?
- Do you have frequent heartburn or take antacids to relieve heartburn or acid indigestion?
- Have you had any skin rashes or skin lesions in the last 6 weeks? (**Regional enteritis or Crohn's disease**)

To the therapist: It may be necessary to conduct a risk factor assessment for NSAID-induced back pain (see discussion in Chapter 9) or screen for eating disorders (see Appendix B-13, A in the accompanying enhanced eBook version included with print purchase of this textbook).

SPECIAL QUESTIONS TO ASK: SEXUAL HISTORY

There are a wide range of reasons why it may be necessary to ask questions about sexual function, birth control, and STDs. For example, joint pain can be caused by STIs. Low back, sacral, and pelvic pain can be caused by sexual trauma or sexual violence. Sciatica accompanied by unreported impotence can be caused by prostate cancer metastasized to the skeletal system.

Whenever taking a sexual history seems appropriate, remember to offer your clients a clear explanation for any questions asked concerning sexual activity, sexual function, or sexual history. The therapist may want to introduce the series of questions by saying, "When evaluating LBP sometimes it is necessary to ask some more personal questions. Please answer as accurately as you can."

The personal nature of some questions sometimes leads clients to feel embarrassed. It is important to assure them they will not be judged and that providing accurate information is crucial to providing good care. Investing in good history taking can lead to early detection and early treatment with less morbidity and better outcomes.[220]

Try to avoid medical terminology and jargon—a common pitfall among health care providers when they feel embarrassed. Listen to the words the clients use to describe sexual activities and practices and then use their preferred words when appropriate.

Men who have sex with men may identify as homosexual, bisexual, or heterosexual. No matter what label is used, these men are at increased risk for STDs, as well as psychologic and behavioral disorders, drug abuse, and eating disorders. Avoid terms such as "gay," "queer," and "straight" when talking about sexual practices or sexual identity.[221]

There is no way to know when someone will be offended or claim sexual harassment. It is in your own interest to behave in the most professional manner possible. There should be no hint of sexual innuendo or humor injected into any of your conversations with clients at any time. The line of sexual impropriety lies where the complainant draws it and includes appearances of misbehavior. This perception differs broadly from client to client.[149]

It is also true that clients sometimes behave inappropriately; there may be times when the therapist must remind clients of appropriate personal boundaries. At the same time, the therapist must be prepared to hear just about anything if and when it is necessary to ask questions about sexual history or sexual practices. Be aware of your facial expressions, body language, and verbal remarks in response to a client's answers.

What if a man or woman with pelvic or sacral pain tells you he or she has been the victim of repeated violent sexual acts? What if a client admits to being the victim of physical or emotional assault? The therapist must be prepared to respond in a professional and responsible way. Additional training in this area may be helpful. Many local organizations, such as Planned Parenthood, Lambda Alliance, and AIDS Council may offer helpful information and/or training.

The therapist may want to introduce the series of questions by saying, "*When evaluating low back pain sometimes it is necessary to ask some more personal questions. Please answer as accurately as you can.*"

- Are you sexually active?
  - Follow-up question: How does sexual activity affect your symptoms?

"Sexually active" does not necessarily mean engaging in sexual intercourse. Sexual touch is enough to transmit many STIs. You may have to explain this to your client to clarify this question. Oral and anal intercourse are often not viewed as "sexual intercourse" and will result in the client answering the question with a "No" when, in fact, for screening purposes, the answer is "Yes."

- Do you have pain with certain positions? (e.g., for the therapist: a position with the woman on top can be more difficult with **prolapsed uterus; the penis or other object touching an inflamed cervix also can cause pain**)
- Have you had more than one sexual partner? (**Increases risk of STDs**)
- Have you ever been told you have an STI or STD such as herpes, genital warts, Reactive Arthritis, syphilis, "the clap," chlamydia, gonorrhea, venereal, HIV, or other disease?
- Have you ever had sexual intercourse without wanting to? Alternate question: Have you ever been raped?
- Do you have any blood in your urine or your stools? Alternate question: Do you have any bleeding when you go to the bathroom?
  - *If yes*, do you have a history of hemorrhoids?
  - What do you think could be causing this?

SPECIAL QUESTIONS TO ASK: WOMEN EXPERIENCING BACK, HIP, PELVIC, GROIN, SACROILIAC, OR SACRAL PAIN

Not all of these questions will need to be asked. Use your professional judgment to decide what to ask based on what the female client has told you and what you have observed during the examination.

CLIENT HISTORY AND INTERVIEW—Cont'd

Past Medical History

Have you ever been told that you have:

- Ovarian cysts
- Fibroids or tumors
- Endometriosis
- Cystocele (sagging bladder)
- Rectocele (sagging rectum)
- Pelvic inflammatory disease (PID)?
- Have you had vaginal surgery or a hysterectomy? (**Vaginal surgery: incontinence**)
- Have you had a recent history of bladder or kidney infections? (**Referred back pain**)
- Have you ever been told you have "brittle bones" or osteoporosis?
- Have you ever had a compression fracture of your back?

Menstrual History

A menstrual history may be helpful when evaluating back or shoulder pain of unknown cause in a woman of reproductive age. Not all of these questions will need to be asked. Use your professional judgment to decide what to ask based on what the woman has told you and what you have observed during the examination.

- Is there any connection between your (back, hip, SI) pain/symptoms and your menstrual cycle (related to either ovulation, midcycle, or menses)?
- Since your back/SI (or other) pain/symptoms started, have you seen a gynecologist to rule out any gynecologic cause of this problem?
- Where were you in your menstrual cycle when your injury or illness occurred?
- Where are you in your menstrual cycle today (premenstrual/midmenstrual/postmenstrual)? (**Appropriate question for shoulder or back pain of unknown cause**)
- Please describe any other menstrual irregularity or problems not already discussed.

For the Young Female Adolescent/Athlete

- Have you ever had a menstrual period?
  - *If yes*, do you have a menstrual period every month? (Amenorrhea or irregular cycles can be a natural part of development but also the result of an eating disorder.)
- Have you ever gone 3 months without having a period?
- Do your periods change with your training regimen?
  - *If yes*, please describe.
- Are you taking birth control pills or using a patch or injection?
  - *If yes*, are you using them for birth control, to regulate your menstrual cycle, or both?
  - Assess risk factors and monitor blood pressure.
  - How long have you been taking birth control?
  - When was the last time you saw the doctor who prescribed birth control for you?

- Please describe any other menstrual irregularity or problems not already discussed.

Reproductive History

- Is there any possibility you could be pregnant?
- Was your last period normal for you?
- What form of birth control are you using? (If the client is using birth control pills, patches, or injections check her blood pressure.)
- Do you have an intrauterine coil or loop contraceptive device (IUD or IUCD)? (**PID and ectopic pregnancy can occur.**)
- **For the pregnant woman:** Are you under the care of a physician? Have you had any spotting or bleeding during your pregnancy?
- Have you recently had a baby? (**Birth trauma**)
  - *If yes*, did you have any significant medical problem during your pregnancy or delivery?
- Have you ever had a tubal or ectopic pregnancy? Is it possible that you may be pregnant now?
- How many pregnancies have you had?
- How many live births have you had?
- Have you ever had an abortion or miscarriage?
  - *If yes*, follow-up with careful (sensitive) questions about how many, when, where, and any immediate or delayed complications (physical or psychologic). (Weakness secondary to blood loss, infection, scarring; blood in **peritoneum irritating diaphragm causing lumbar and/or shoulder pain**); ask about the onset of symptoms in relation to the incident.
- Do you ever experience a "falling out" feeling or pelvic heaviness after standing for a long time? (**Uterine prolapse; pelvic floor muscle weakness; incontinence**)
- Do you ever leak urine when coughing, laughing, lifting, exercising, or sneezing? (**Stress incontinence**)

If yes to incontinence: Ask several additional questions to determine the frequency, the amount of protection needed (as measured by the number and type of pads used daily), and how much this problem interferes with daily activities and lifestyle. See also Appendix B-5 in the accompanying enhanced eBook version included with print purchase of this textbook.

- Do you have an unusual amount of vaginal discharge or vaginal discharge with an obvious odor? (**Referred back pain**) (Note to reader: This one and the previous bullet are conditions that might indicate the need for a referral to a specialized Pelvic PT assessment to determine impact on function and symptoms.)
  - *If yes*, do you know what is causing this discharge? Is there any connection between when the discharge started and when you first noticed your back/SI (or other) symptoms?
- For the postmenopausal woman: Are you taking hormone replacement therapy (HRT) or any natural hormone products?

Continued

CLIENT HISTORY AND INTERVIEW—Cont'd

SPECIAL QUESTIONS TO ASK: MEN EXPERIENCING BACK, HIP, PELVIC, GROIN, OR SACROILIAC PAIN

- Have you ever had prostate problems or been told you have prostate problems?
- Have you ever been told you have a hernia? Do you think you have one now?
  - *If yes*, follow-up with medical referral. Strangulation of the bowel can lead to serious complications. If the client has been evaluated by a physician and has declined treatment (usually surgery), encourage him to follow-up on this recommendation.
- Have you recently had kidney stones or bladder or kidney infections?
- Have you had any changes in urination recently?
- Do you ever have blood in your urine?
- Do you ever have pain, burning, or discomfort during urination?

- Do you urinate often, especially during the night?
- Can you easily start a flow of urine?
- Can you keep a steady stream without stopping and starting?
- When you are done urinating, does it feel like your bladder is empty or do you feel like you still have to go, but you cannot get any more out?
- Do you ever dribble or leak urine?
- Do you have trouble getting an erection?
- Do you have trouble keeping an erection?
- Do you have trouble ejaculating? (Therapists beware; this term may not be understood by all clients.)
- Any unusual discharge from your penis?

To the therapist: If the client is having difficulty with sexual function, it may be necessary to conduct a screening examination for bladder or prostate involvement. See Appendices B-5 and B-30 on.

CASE STUDY

Steps in the Screening Process

REFERRAL

A 47-year-old man with LBP of unknown cause has come to you for exercises. After gathering information from the client's history and conducting the interview, you ask him:

 FOLLOW-UP QUESTIONS

- Are there any other symptoms of any kind anywhere else in your body?

  The client tells you he does break out into an unexpected sweat from time to time but does not think he has a temperature when this happens. He has increased back pain when he passes gas or a bowel movement, but then the pain goes back to the "regular" pain level (reported as a 5 on a scale from 0 to 10). Other reported symptoms include:

- Heartburn and indigestion
- Abdominal bloating after meals
- Chronic bronchitis from smoking (3 packs/day)
- Alternating diarrhea and constipation

  Use the list of signs and symptoms in Box 4.19 to review this case.

  Do these symptoms fall into any one category?

  It appears that many of the symptoms may be GI in nature.

  What is the next step in the screening process?

  Because the client has mentioned unexplained sweating but no known fevers, take the time to measure all vital signs, especially body temperature. Turn to Special Questions to Ask at the end of Chapter 9 and scan the list of questions for any that might be appropriate for this client.

  For example, find out about the use of NSAIDs (prescription and OTC; be sure to include aspirin). Follow-up with:

 FOLLOW-UP QUESTIONS

- Have you ever been treated for an ulcer or internal bleeding while taking any of these pain relievers?
- Have you experienced any unexpected weight loss in the last few weeks?
- Have you traveled outside of the United States in the last year?
- What is the effect of eating or drinking on your abdominal pain? Back pain?
- Have the client pay attention to his symptoms over the next 24 to 48 hours:
  - Immediately after eating
  - Within 30 minutes of eating
  - 1 to 2 hours after eating
- Do you have a sense of urgency so that you have to find a bathroom for a bowel movement or diarrhea right away without waiting?

Ask any further questions that may be appropriate as listed in this chapter or from the more complete Special Questions to Ask section of Chapter 9 (see the subsection: Associated Signs and Symptoms: Change in bowel habits).

You will make your decision to refer this client to a physician depending on your findings from the clinical examination and the client's responses to these questions. Use the Quick Screen Checklist in Appendix A-1 in the accompanying enhanced eBook version included with print purchase of this textbook to see if you have left anything out that might be important.

This does not appear to be an emergency because the client is not in acute distress. An elevated temperature or other unusual vital signs might speed the referral process along.

PRACTICE QUESTIONS

1. The most common sites of referred pain from systemic diseases are:
   a. Neck and back
   b. Shoulder and back
   c. Chest and back
   d. None of the above

2. To screen for back pain caused by systemic disease:
   a. Perform special tests (e.g., Murphy's percussion, Bicycle test)
   b. Correlate client history with clinical presentation and ask about associated signs and symptoms
   c. Perform a Review of Systems
   d. All of the above

3. What are two ways of classifying back pain (as presented in the text)?

4. Which statement is the most accurate?
   a. Arterial disease is characterized by intermittent claudication, pain relieved by elevating the extremity, and history of smoking.
   b. Arterial disease is characterized by loss of hair on the lower extremities, throbbing pain in the calf muscles that goes away by using heat and elevation.
   c. Arterial disease is characterized by painful throbbing of the feet at night that goes away by dangling the feet over the bed.
   d. Arterial disease is characterized by loss of hair on the toes, intermittent claudication, and redness or warmth of the legs that is accompanied by a burning sensation.

5. Pain associated with pleuropulmonary disorders can radiate to:
   a. Anterior neck
   b. Upper trapezius muscle
   c. Ipsilateral shoulder
   d. Thoracic spine
   e. All of the above

6. Which of the following are clues to the possible involvement of the GI system?
   a. Abdominal pain alternating with TMJ pain within a 2-week period of time
   b. Abdominal pain at the same level as back pain occurring either simultaneously or alternately
   c. Shoulder pain alleviated by a bowel movement
   d. All of the above

7. Percussion of the costovertebral angle resulting in the reproduction of symptoms signifies:
   a. Radiculitis
   b. Pseudorenal pain
   c. Has no significance
   d. Medical referral is advised

8. A 53-year-old woman comes to physical therapy with a report of leg pain that begins in her buttocks and goes all the way down to her toes. If this pain is of a vascular origin she will most likely describe it as:
   a. Sore, hurting
   b. Hot or burning
   c. Shooting or stabbing
   d. Throbbing, "tired"

9. Twenty-five percent of the people with GI disease, such as Crohn's disease (regional enteritis), irritable bowel syndrome, or bowel obstruction, have concomitant back or joint pain.
   a. True
   b. False

10. Skin pain over T9 to T12 can occur with kidney disease as a result of multisegmental innervation. Visceral and cutaneous sensory fibers enter the spinal cord close to each other and converge on the same neurons. When visceral pain fibers are stimulated, cutaneous fibers are stimulated, too. Thus visceral pain can be perceived as skin pain.
    a. True
    b. False

11. Autosplinting is the preferred mechanism of pain relief for back pain caused by kidney stones.
    a. True
    b. False

12. Back pain from pancreatic disease occurs when the body of the pancreas is enlarged, inflamed, obstructed, or otherwise impinging on the diaphragm.
    a. True
    b. False

13. A 53-year-old postmenopausal woman with a history of breast cancer and mastectomy 5 years ago presents with a report of sharp pain in her midback. The pain started after she lifted her 2-year-old granddaughter 3 days ago. Tylenol seems to help, but the pain is keeping her awake at night. Once she wakes up, she cannot find a comfortable position to go back to sleep. What are the red flags? What will you do to screen for a medical cause of her symptoms?

REFERENCES

1. Waterman BR, Belmont PJ, Schoenfeld AJ. Low back pain in the United States: incidence and risk factors for presentation in the emergency setting. Spine. 2012;12:63–70.
2. Chou R, Chekelle P. Will this patient develop persistent disabling low back pain? JAMA. 2010;303:1295–1302.
3. Dickman RD, Zigler JE. Discogenic back pain. In: Spivak JM, Connolly PJ, eds. Orthopaedic knowledge update: spine 3, Rosemont, H; 2006319–329. N Am Spine Society.
4. Deyo RA, Von Korff M, Duhrkoop D. Opioids for low back pain. BMJ. 2015;350:g6380.
5. Maas ET, Juch JNS, Groeneweg JG, et al. Cost-effectiveness of minimal interventional procedures for chronic mechanical low back pain: design of four randomized controlled trials with an economic evaluation. BMC Musculoskeletal Disorders. 2012;13:260.
6. Jarvik J, Deyo R. Diagnostic evaluation of low back pain with emphasis on imaging. Ann Intern Med. 2002;137:586–597.
7. Jette DU, Halbert J, Iverson C, Miceli E, Shah P. Use of standardized outcome measures in physical therapist practice: perceptions and applications. Phys Ther. 2009;89(2):125–135.

8. Russek L, Wooden M, Ekedahl S, Bush A. Attitudes toward standardized data collection. Physical therapy. 1997;77(7):714–729.

9. Michener LA, Leggin BG. A review of self-report scales for the assessment of functional limitation and disability of the shoulder. J Hand Ther. 2001;14(2):68–76.

10. Spitzer WO. Quebec Task Force on Spinal Disorders: scientific approach to the assessment and management of activity-related spinal disorders: a monograph for clinicians. Spine. 1987;12(Suppl 1):51–59.

11. Sembrano JN, Polly DW. How often is low back pain not coming from the back? Spine. 2009;34:E27–E32.

12. Bernard Jr. TN, Kirkaldy-Willis WH. Recognizing specific characteristics of nonspecific low back pain. Clin Orthop. 1987;217:266–280.

13. Shaw JA. The role of the sacroiliac joint as a cause of low back pain and dysfunction et al.. In: Vleeming A, Mooney V, Snijders C, eds. The First Interdisciplinary World Congress on low back pain and its relation to the sacroiliac joint. Rotterdam, Netherlands: ECO; 1992:67–80.

14. Depalma MJ. What is the source of chronic low back pain and does age play a role? Pain Med. 2011;12(2):224–233.

15. Vora AJ. Functional anatomy and pathophysiology of axial low back pain: discs, posterior elements, sacroiliac joint, and associated pain generators. Phys Med Rehabil Clin N Am. 2010;21(4):679–709.

16. Vanelderen P. Sacroiliac joint pain. Pain Pract. 2010;10(5):470–478.

17. Kim DH, Hilibrand AS. Rheumatoid arthritis in the cervical spine. J Am Acad Orthop Surg. 2005;13(7):463–474.

18. Magarelli N. MR imaging of atlantoaxial joint in early rheumatoid arthritis. Radiol Med. 2010;115(7):1111–1120.

19. Krauss WE. Rheumatoid arthritis of the craniovertebral junction. Neurosurgery. 2010;66(Suppl 3):83–95.

20. Guzman J. A new conceptual model of neck pain. Spine. 2008;33(4S):S14–S23.

21. Boissonnault WG, Koopmeiners MB. Medical history profile: orthopaedic physical therapy outpatients. J Orthop Sports Phys Ther. 1994;20:2–10.

22. Boissonault WG. Prevalence of comorbid conditions, surgeries, and medication use in a physical therapy outpatient population: a multi-centered study. J Orthop Sports Phys Ther. 1999;29(506–519):520–525.

23. Boissonnault WG, Meek PD. Risk factors for antiinflammatory drug or aspirin induced gastrointestinal complications in individuals receiving outpatient physical therapy services. J Orthop Sports Phys Ther. 2002;32:510–517.

24. Biederman RE. Pharmacology in rehabilitation: nonsteroidal antiinflammatory agents. J Orthop Sports Phys Ther. 2005;35:356–367.

25. Downie A, et al. Red flags to screen for malignancy and fracture in patients with low back pain: systematic review. BMJ. 2013;347:f7095.

26. Daniels JM. Evaluation of low back pain in athletes. Sports Health. 2011;3(4):336–345.

27. Witkin LR. Abscess after a laparoscopic appendectomy presenting as low back pain in a professional athlete. Sports Health. 2011;3(1):41–45.

28. Cosar M. The major complications of transpedicular vertebroplasty. J Neurosurg: Spine. 2009;11(5):607–613.

29. Johnson BA. Epidurography and therapeutic epidural injections: technical considerations and experience with 5334 cases. Am J Neuroradiol. 1999;20:697–705.

30. Davenport TE. Subcutaneous abscess in a patient referred to physical therapy following spinal epidural injection for lumbar radiculopathy. J Orthop Sports Phys Ther. 2008;38(5):287.

31. Deyo RA, Diehl AK. Cancer as a cause of back pain: frequency, clinical presentation, and diagnostic strategies. J Gen Intern Med. 1988;3:230–238.

32. Hart-Johnson MS T, Green MD CR. The Impact of Sexual or Physical Abuse History on Pain-Related Outcomes Among Blacks and Whites with Chronic Pain: Gender Influence. Pain Medicine. 2012;13(3):229–242.

33. Chandan JS, Thomas T, Raza K, et al. Association between child maltreatment and central sensitivity syndromes: a systematic review protocol. BMJ Open. 2019;9(2):e025436 Published online February 3, 2019.33.

34. van den Bosch MAAJ. Evidence against the use of lumbar spine radiography for low back pain. Clin Radiol. 2004;59:69–76.

35. Bishop PB, Wing PC. Compliance with clinical practice guidelines in family physicians managing worker's compensation board patients with acute lower back pain. Spine J. 2003;3(6):442–450.

36. Bishop PB, Wing PC. Knowledge transfer in family physicians managing patients with acute low back pain: a prospective randomized control trial. Spine J. 2006;6(3):282–288.

37. Leerar PJ, Boissonnault W. Domholdt E et al. Documentation of red flags by physical therapists for patients with low back pain. J Man Manip Ther. 2007;15(1):42–49.

38. Bogduk N, McQuirk B. Medical management of acute and chronic low back pain: an evidence based approach. Amsterdam: Elsevier; 2002.

39. Burton AK. Psychosocial predictors of outcome in acute and subchronic low back trouble. Spine. 1995;20:722–728.

40. McCarthy CJ. The reliability of the clinical tests and questions recommended in International Guidelines for Low Back Pain. Spine. 2007;32(6):921–926.

41. Moore JE. Chronic low back pain and psychosocial issues. Phys Med Rehabil Clin N Am. 2010;21(4):801–815.

42. Kendall NAS, Linton SJ, Main CJ. Guide to assessing psychosocial yellow flags in acute low back pain: risk factors for long-term disability and work loss. Wellington, New Zealand: Accident Rehabilitation and Compensation Insurance Corporation of New Zealand and the National Health Committee; 1998.

43. Burns SA. A treatment-based classification approach to examination and intervention of lumbar disorders. Sports Health. 2011;3(4):363–372.

44. George SZ, Fritz JM, Childs JD. Investigation of elevated fear-avoidance beliefs for patients with low back pain: a secondary analysis involving patients enrolled in physical therapy clinical trials. J Orthop Sports Phys Ther. 2008;38(2):50–58.

45. Grimmer-Somers K, Prior M, Robertson J. Yellow flag scores in a compensable New Zealand cohort suffering acute low back pain. J Pain Res. Dec 2008;1(1):15–25.

46. Bogduk N. Evidence-based clinical guidelines for the management of acute low back pain: the national musculoskeletal medicine initiative. Australia: Australian Association of Musculoskeletal Medicine; 2002.

47. Henschke N. Prevalence of and screening for serious spinal pathology in patients presenting to primary care settings with acute low back pain. Arthritis Rheum. 2009;60(10):3072–3080.

48. Downie A, Williams CM, Henschke N, et al. Red flags to screen for malignancy and fracture in patients with low back pain. Br J Sports Med. 2014;48:1518.

49. Sizer PS, Brismee JM, Cook C. Medical screening for red flags in the diagnosis and management of musculoskeletal spine pain. Pain Pract. 2007;7(1):53–71.

50. Downie A, Williams CM, Henschke N, et al. Red flags to screen for malignancy and fracture in patients with low back pain: a systematic review. BMJ. 2013;347:f7095.

51. Gibson M, Zoltie N. Radiography for back pain presenting to accident and emergency departments. Arch Emerg Med. 1992;9:28–31.

52. Micheli LJ. Back pain in young athletes: significant differences from adults in causes and patterns. Arch Pediatr Adolesc Med. 1995;149(1):15–18.

53. Bhatia N. Diagnostic modalities for the evaluation of pediatric back pain: a prospective study. J Pediatr Orthop. 2008;28(2):230–233.

54. Nigrovic P.A.: Evaluation of the child with back pain. Available online at http://www.uptodate.com/index. Published January 25, 2010. Accessed July 15, 2011.

55. Henschke N. A systematic review identifies five "red flags" to screen for vertebral fracture in patients with low back pain. J Clin Epidemiol. 2008;61:110–118.

56. Deyo RA, Diehl AK. Lumbar spine films in primary care: current use and effects of selective ordering criteria. J Gen Intern Med. 1986;1:20–25.

57. Royal College of General Practitioners: Clinical guidelines of the management of acute low back pain, National Low Back Pain Clinical Guidelines, 1997.

58. Burch R, Rizzoli P, Loder E. The prevalence and impact of migraine and severe headache in the United States: figures and trends from government health studies. Headache. 2018;58(4):496–505. https://doi.org/10.1111/head.1328.

59. Waddell G, ed. The back pain revolution. ed 2 Edinburgh: Churchill Livingstone; 2004.

60. Leon-Diaz A, Gonzalez-Rabelino G, Alonso-Cervino M. Analysis of the etiologies of headaches in a pediatric emergency service. Rev Neurol. 2004;39(3):217–221. 1–15.

61. Olesen J, Steiner TJ. The international classification of headache disorders, ed 2 (ICHD-II). J Neurol Neurosurg Psychiatry. 2004;75(6):808–811.

62. Silberstein SD, Olesen J, Bousser MG, et al. The international classification of headache disorders, ed 2 (ICHD-II)—revision of criteria for 8.2 medication overuse headache. Cephalalgia. 2005;25(6):460–465.

63. Headache Classification Committee of the International Headache Society the international classification of headache disorders ed 3 (beta version). Cephalalgia. Jul 2013;33(9):629–808.

64. Headache Classification Committee of the International Headache Society classification and diagnostic criteria for headache disorders, cranial neuralgias, and facial pain. Cephalalgia. 1988;8(Suppl 7):1–96.

65. Headache Classification Committee of the International Headache Society classification and diagnostic criteria for headache disorders, cranial neuralgias and facial pain ed 2 (revised). Cephalalgia. 2004;25(12):460–465.

66. Petersen SM. Articular and muscular impairments in cervicogenic headache. J Orthop Sports Phys Ther. 2003;33(1):21–30.

67. Agostoni E. Headache in cerebral venous thrombosis. Neurol Sci. 2004;25(Suppl 3):S206–S210.

68. Agostoni E, Aliprandi A. Alterations in the cerebral venous circulation as a cause of headache. Neurol Sci. 2009;30(Suppl 1):S7–S10.

69. Jacobson SA, Folstein MF. Psychiatric perspectives on headache and facial pain. Otolaryngol Clin North Am. 2003;36(6):1187–1200.

70. Farmer K. Psychologic factors in childhood headaches. Semin Pediatr Neurol. 2010;17(2):93–99.

71. Hering-Hanit R, Gadoth N. Caffeine-induced headache in children and adolescents. Cephalalgia. 2003;23(5):332–335.

72. Ryan LM, Warden DL. Post concussion syndrome. Int Rev Psychiatry. 2003;15(4):310–316.

73. Seiffert TD, Evans RW. Posttraumatic headache: a review. Curr Pain Headache Rep. 2010;14(4):292–298.

74. Zwolak P, Kröber M. Acute neck pain caused by atlantoaxial instability secondary to pathologic fracture involving odontoid process and C2 vertebral body: treatment with radiofrequency thermoablation, cement augmentation and odontoid screw fixation. Arch Orthop Trauma Surg. Sep 2015;135(9):1211–1215.

75. O'Reilly MB. Nonresectable head and neck cancer. Rehab Oncology. 2004;22(2):14–16.

76. Greenlee RT, Murray T, Bolden S, et al. Cancer statistics, 2000. CA Cancer J Clin. 2000;50:7–33.

77. Landis SH, Murray T, Bolden S, et al. Cancer statistics, 1999. CA Cancer J Clin. 1999;49:8–31.

78. Bartanusz V, Porchet F. Current strategies in the management of spinal metastatic disease. Swiss Surg. 2003;9:55–62.

79. Heidecke V, Rainov NG, Burkert W. Results and outcome of neurosurgical treatment for extradural metastases in the cervical spine. Acta Neurochir (Wien). 2003;145:873–880. discussion 880–881.

80. Sciubba DM, Gokaslan ZL, Suk I, et al. Positive and negative prognostic variables for patients undergoing spine surgery for metastatic breast disease. Eur Spine J. 2007;16:1659–1667.

81. Moulding HD, Bilsky MH. Metastases to the craniovertebral junction. Neurosurgery. 2010;66:113–118.

82. Purdy RA, Kirby S. Headaches and brain tumors. Neurol Clin. 2004;22(1):39–53.

83. Kirby S. Headache and brain tumours. Cephalalgia. 2010;30(4):387–388.

84. Valentinis L. Headache attributed to intracranial tumours: a prospective cohort study. Cephalalgia. 2010;30(4):389–398.

85. Peters GL. Migraine overview and summary of current and emerging treatment options. Am J Manag Care. 2019;25(2):S23–S34.

86. Fernández-de-Las-Peñas C, Cuadrado ML. Physical therapy for headaches. Cephalalgia. 2016;36(12):1134–1142.

87. Popescu A, Lee H. Neck pain and lower back pain. Med Clin North Am. 2020;104(2):279–292.

88. Gorski JM, Schwartz LH. Shoulder impingement presenting as neck pain. J Bone Joint Surg. 2003;85A(4):635–638.

89. Lee L, Elliott R. Cervical spondylotic myelopathy in a patient presenting with low back pain. J Orthop Sports Phys Ther. 2008;38(12):798.

90. Tejus MN, Singh V, Ramesh A, et al. An evaluation of the finger flexion, Hoffman's and platar reflexes as markers of cervical spinal cord compression—a comparative clinical study. Clin Neurol Neurosurg. 2015;134:12–16.

91. Slipman CW, Issac Z, Patel R, et al. Chronic neck pain: the specific syndromes. J Musculoskel Med. 2003;20(1):24–33.

92. Koopmeiners M.B. Personal communication, 2003.

93. Boissonnault W.G. Personal communication, 2003.

94. Duan G, Xu J, Shi J, Cao Y. Advances in the Pathogenesis, Diagnosis and Treatment of Bow Hunter's Syndrome: A Comprehensive Review of the Literature. Interv Neurol. 2016;5(1-2):29–38.

95. Rastogi V, Rawls A, Moore O, et al. Rare Etiology of Bow Hunter's Syndrome and Systematic Review of Literature. J Vasc Interv Neurol. 2015;8(3):7–16.

96. Velat GJ, Reavey-Cantwell JF, Ulm AJ, Lewis SB. Intraoperative dynamic angiography to detect resolution of Bow Hunter's syndrome: Technical case report. Surg Neurol. 2006;66(4):420–423. discussion 423.

97. Rushton A, Rivett D, Carlesso L, et al. International framework for examination of the cervical region for potential of cervical arterial dysfunction prior to orthopaedic manual therapy intervention. Manual Therapy. 2014;19:222–228.

98. Kerry R, Taylor AJ. Cervical arterial dysfunction assessment and manual therapy. Man Ther. 2006;11:243–253.

99. Kerry R, Taylor AJ. Cervical arterial dysfunction: knowledge and reasoning for manual physical therapists. J Orthop Sports Phys Ther. 2009;39(5):378–387.

100. Earhardt JW, Windsor BA, Kerry R, et al. The immediate effect of atlanto-axial high velocity thrust techniques on blood flow in the vertebral artery: a randomized controlled trial. Manual Therapy. 2015;20:614–622.

101. Heneghan NR, Smith R, Tyros I, Falla D, Rushton A. PLoS One. 2018;23(13):e0194235.

102. Mooney V, Robertson J. The facet syndrome. Clin Orthop. 1976;115:149–156.

103. Fruth SJ. Differential diagnosis and treatment in a patient with posterior upper thoracic pain. *Phys Ther.* 2006;86(2):154–268.

104. Nicol AL, Adams MCB, Gordon DB, et al. AAAPT diagnostic criteria for acute low back pain with and without lower extremity pain. *Pain Med.* 2020;239 http://doi.org/10.1093.

105. Hartvigsen J, Christensen K, Frederiksen H. Back pain remains a common symptom in old age: a population-based study of 4,486 Danish twins aged 70–102. *Eur Spine J.* 2003;12(5):528–534.

106. Braun A, Gnann H, Saracbasi E, et al. Optimizing the identification of patients with axial spondyloarthritis in primary care—the case for a two-step strategy combining the most relevant clinical items with HLA B27. *Rheumatology.* 2013;52:1418–1424.

107. Braun J, Inman R. Clinical significance of inflammatory back pain for diagnosis and screening of patients with axial spondyloarthritis. *Ann Rheum Dis.* 2010;69(7):1264–1268.

108. Ozgen S. Lumbar disc herniation in adolescence. *Pediatr Neurosurg.* 2007;43:77–81.

109. O'Neill CW, Kurgansky ME, Derby R, et al. Disc stimulation and patterns of referred pain. *Spine.* 2002;27(24):2776–2781.

110. Bogduk N. On the definitions and physiology of back pain, referred pain, and radicular pain. *Pain.* 2009;147:17–19.

111. Koes BW. Diagnosis and treatment of sciatica. *BMJ.* 2007;334:1313–1317.

112. Crowell MS, Gill NW. Medical screening and evacuation: cauda equina syndrome in a combat zone. *J Orthop Sports Phys Ther.* 2009;39(7):541–549.

113. O'Laughlin SJ, Kokosinski E. Cauda equina syndrome in a pregnant woman referred to physical therapy for low back pain. *J Orthop Sports Phys Ther.* 2008;38(11):721.

114. Long B, Koyfman A, Gottlieb M. Evaluation and management of cauda equine syndrome in the emergency department. *Am J Emerg Med.* 2020;38(1):143–148.

115. McCarthy MJH. Cauda equina syndrome: factors affecting long-term functional and sphincteric outcome. *Spine.* 2007;32(2):207–216.

116. Kauppila LI. Atherosclerosis and disc degeneration/low-back pain—a systematic review. *Eur J Endovasc Surg.* 2009;37(6):661–670.

117. Bingol H, Cingoz F, Yilmaz AT, et al. Vascular complications related to lumbar disc surgery. *J Neurosurg: Spine.* 2004;100(3):249–253.

118. Lacombe M. Vascular complications of lumbar disk surgery. *Ann Chir.* 2006;131(10):583–589.

119. Delaruelle Z, Ivanova TA, Khan S, Negro A, Ornello R, Raffaelli B, Terrin A, Mitsikostas DD, Reuter U, Delaruelle Z, Ivanova TA, Khan S, et al. on behalf of the European **Headache** Federation School of Advanced Studies (EHF-SAS):. Male and female sex hormones in primary **headaches**. *J Headache Pain.* 2018;19(1):117 Published online November 29, 2018.

120. Kauppila LI, Mikkonen R, Mankinen P, et al. MR aortography and serum cholesterol levels in patients with long-term nonspecific lower back pain. *Spine.* 2004;29(19):2147–2152.

121. Seeman E. The dilemma of osteoporosis in men. *Am J Med.* 1995;98(2A):765S–788S.

122. Orwoll ES, Klein RF. Osteoporosis in men. *Endocr Rev.* 1995;16:87–116.

123. Kiebzak G, Beinart G, Perser K, et al. Undertreatment of osteoporosis in men with hip fracture. *Arch Intern Med.* 2002;162(19):2217–2222.

124. Ebeling PR. Osteoporosis in men. *N Engl J Med.* 2008;358(14):1474–1482.

125. Ebeling PR. Androgens and osteoporosis. *Curr Opin Endocrinol Diabetes Obes.* 2010;17(3):284–292.

126. Blain H. Osteoporosis in men: epidemiology, physiopathology, diagnosis, prevention, and treatment. *Rev Med Interne.* 2005;25(Suppl 5):S552–S559.

127. Silverman SL. The clinical consequences of vertebral compression fracture. *Bone.* 1992;13:S27–S31.

128. Badke MB, Boissonnault WG. Changes in disability following physical therapy intervention for patients with low back pain: dependence on symptom duration. *Arch Phys Med Rehab.* 2006;87(6):749–756.

129. Whooley MA. Case-finding instruments for depression. Two questions are as good as many. *J Gen Intern Med.* 1997;12:439–445.

130. Haggman S. Screening for symptoms of depression by physical therapists managing low back pain. *Phys Ther.* 2004;84:1157–1165.

131. Hoogendoorn WE, van Poppel MN, Bongers PM, et al. Systematic review of psychosocial factors at work and private life as risk factors for back pain. *Spine.* 2000;25:2114–2125.

132. Marras WS, Davis KG, Heaney CA, et al. The influence of psychosocial stress, gender, and personality on mechanical loading of the lumbar spine. *Spine.* 2000;25(23):3045–3054.

133. Thorbjornsson CO, Alfredsson L, Fredriksson K, et al. Physical and psychosocial factors related to low back pain during a 24-year period. *Occup Environ Med.* 1998;55(2):84–90.

134. McCarthy CJ. The reliability of the clinical tests and questions recommended in International Guidelines for Low Back Pain. *Spine.* 2007;32(6):921–926.

135. Ramond A. Psychosocial risk factors for chronic low back pain in primary care—a systematic review. *Fam Prac.* 2011;28(1):12–21.

136. van Tulder M. European guidelines for the management of acute nonspecific low back pain in primary care. European Commission, Geneva. *Eur Spine J.* 2006;15(Suppl 2):S169–S191.

137. Kendall NAS, Linton SJ, Main CJ. *Guide to assessing psychological yellow flags in acute low back pain: risk factors for long-term disability and work loss.* Wellington, New Zealand: Accident Rehabilitation and Compensation Insurance Corporation of New Zealand and the National Health Committee; 1997.

138. Borkan J, Van Tulder M, Reis S, et al. Advances in the field of low back pain in primary care: a report from the fourth international forum. *Spine.* 2002;27(5):E128–E132.

139. Slipman C. Epidemiology of spine tumors presenting to musculoskeletal physiatrists. *Arch Phys Med Rehabil.* 2003;84:492–495.

140. Rose PS, Buchowski JM. Metastatic disease in the thoracic and lumbar spine: evaluation and management. *J Am Acad Orthop Surg.* 2011;19(1):37–48.

141. Henschke N. Screening for malignancy in low back pain patients: a systematic review. *Eur Spine J.* 2007;16(10):1673–1679.

142. Briggs HK. The physical therapist's management of a patient with low back pain following an atypical response to treatment: a case report. *J Orthop Sports Phys Ther.* 2011;41(1):A16.

143. Mazanec DJ, Segal AM, Sinks PB. Identification of malignancy in patients with back pain: red flags. *Arthritis Rheum.* 1993;36(Suppl):S251–S258.

144. Skoffer B. Low back pain in 15- to 16-year-old children in relation to school furniture and carrying of the school bag. *Spine.* 2007;32(24):E713–E717.

145. Neuschwander TB. The effect of backpacks on the lumbar spine in children. *Spine.* 2009;35(1):83–88.

146. Fabricant PD, Heath MR, Schachne JM, et al. The epidemiology of back pain in American children and adolescents. *Spine.* 2020;45(16):1135–1142.

147. Calvo-Muñoz I, Gómez-Conesa A, Sánchez-Meca J. Prevalence of low back pain in children and adolescents: a meta-analysis. *BMC Pediatr.* 2013;13:14.

148. Patchell RA. Direct decompressive surgical resection in the treatment of spinal cord compression caused by metastatic cancer: a randomized trial. *Lancet.* 2005;366(9486):643–648.

149. Rex L. *Evaluation and treatment of somatovisceral dysfunction of the gastrointestinal system.* Edmonds WA: URSA Foundation; 2004.

150. Deyo RA, Diehl AK. Cancer as a cause of back pain: frequency, clinical presentation, and diagnostic strategies. *J Gen Intern Med.* 1988;3(3):230–238.

151. Wong DA, Fornasier VL, MacNab I. Spinal metastases: the obvious, the occult, and the imposters. *Spine.* 1990;15(1):1–4.

152. Ross MD, Bayer E. Cancer as a cause of low back pain in a patient seen in a direct access physical therapy setting. *J Orthop Sports Phys Ther.* 2005;35(10):651–658.

153. Galliker G, Scherer DE, Trippolini MA, et al. Low back pain in the emergency department: prevalence of serious spinal pathologies and diagnostic accuracy of red flags. *Am J Med.* 2020;133(1):60–72.

154. Reinus WR, Strome G, Zwemer Jr FL. Use of lumbosacral spine radiographs in a level II emergency department. *AJR. American journal of roentgenology.* 1998;170:443–447.

155. Owens DK. Screening for abdominal aortic aneurysm. US Preventive Services Task Force Recommendation Statement. *JAMA.* 2019;322(22):2211–2218.

156. Cosford PA, Leng GC. Screening for abdominal aortic aneurysm. *Cochrane Database Syst Rev.* 2007;18(2):CD002945.

157. Guirguis-Blake JM, Beil TL, Senger CA, Coppola EL. *Primary Care Screening for Abdominal Aortic Aneurysm: Updated Systematic Review for the US Preventive Services Task Force: Evidence Synthesis No. 184.* Rockville, MD: Agency for Healthcare Research and Quality; 2019. AHRQ publication 19-05253-EF-1.

158. Joergensen TM, Houlind K, Green A, Lindholt JS. Abdominal aortic diameter is increased in males with a family history of abdominal aortic aneurysms: results from the Danish VIVA-trial. *Eur J Vasc Endovasc Surg.* 2014;48(6):669–675. https://doi.org/10.1016/j.ejvs.2014.09.005.

159. Lindholt JS, Juul S, Fasting H, Henneberg EW. Screening for abdominal aortic aneurysms: single centre randomised controlled trial. *BMJ.* 2005;330(7494):750. https://doi.org/10.1136/bmj.38369.620162.82.

160. Kent KC, Zwolak RM, Egorova NN, et al. Analysis of risk factors for abdominal aortic aneurysm in a cohort of more than 3 million individuals. *J Vasc Surg.* 2010;52(3):539–548. https://doi.org/10.1016/j.jvs.2010.05.090.

161. Wilmink AB, Hubbard CS, Day NE, Quick CR. The incidence of small abdominal aortic aneurysms and the change in normal infrarenal aortic diameter: implications for screening. *Eur J Vasc Endovasc Surg.* 2001;21(2):165–170. https://doi.org/10.1053/ejvs.2000.1285.

162. Vardulaki KA, Walker NM, Day NE, et al. Quantifying the risks of hypertension, age, sex and smoking in patients with abdominal aortic aneurysm. *Br J Surg.* 2000;87(2):195–200. https://doi.org/10.1046/j.1365-2168.2000.01353.x.

163. Ahmadi H, Shirani S, Yazdanifard P. Aortic dissection type 1 in a weightlifter with hypertension: a case report. *Cases J.* 2008;1:99.

164. van Vlijmen-van Keulen CJ, Pals G, Rauwerda JA. Familial abdominal aortic aneurysm: a systematic review of a genetic background. *Eur J Vasc Endovasc Surg.* 2002;24(2):105–116. https://doi.org/10.1053/ejvs.2002.1692.

165. MacSweeney ST, O'MearaM Alexander C, et al. High prevalence of unsuspected abdominal aortic aneurysm in patients with confirmed symptomatic peripheral or cerebral arterial disease. *Br J Surg.* 1993;80(5):582–584. https://doi.org/10.1002/bjs.1800800510.

166. Lederle FA, Johnson GR, Wilson SE, et al. The Aneurysm Detection and Management (ADAM) Veterans Affairs Cooperative Study Investigators. Relationship of age, gender, race, and body size to infrarenal aortic diameter. *J Vasc Surg.* 1997;26(4):595–601. https://doi.org/10.1016/S0741-5214(97)70057-0.

167. Mechelli F, Preboski Z, Boissonnault W. Differential diagnosis of a patient referred to physical therapy with low back pain: abdominal aortic aneurysm. *J Orthop Sports Phys Ther.* 2008;38(9):551–557.

168. Lindholt JS, Juul S, Fasting H, Henneberg EW. Screening for abdominal aortic aneurysms: single centre randomised controlled trial. *BMJ.* 2005;330(7494):750. https://doi.org/10.1136/bmj.38369.620162.82.

169. De Rango P, Farchioni L, Fiorucci B, Lenti M. Diabetes and abdominal aortic aneurysms. *Eur JVasc Endovasc Surg.* 2014;47(3):243–261. https://doi.org/10.1016/j.ejvs.2013.12.007.

170. Lederle FA, Johnson GR, Wilson SE, et al. Aneurysm Detection and Management Veterans Affairs Cooperative Study Investigators. The aneurysm detection and management study screening program: validation cohort and final results. *Arch Intern Med.* 2000;160(10):1425–1430. https://doi.org/10.1001/archinte.160.10.1425.

171. akagi H, Umemoto T. ALICE (All-Literature Investigation of Cardiovascular Evidence) Group: Negative association of diabetes with rupture of abdominal aortic aneurysm. *Diab Vasc Dis Res.* 2016;13(5):341–347. https://doi.org/10.1177/1479164116651389.

172. Xiong J, Wu Z, Chen C, et al. Association between diabetes and prevalence and growth rate of abdominal aortic aneurysms: a meta-analysis. *Int J Cardiol.* 2016;221:484–495. https://doi.org/10.1016/j.ijcard.2016.07.016.

173. Owens DK. Screening for abdominal aortic aneurysm. US Preventive Services Task Force Recommendation Statement. *JAMA.* 2019;322(22):2211–2218.

174. Ruff AL, Teng K, Hu B, et al. Screening for abdominal aortic aneurysms in outpatient primary care clinics. *Am J Med.* 2015;128(3):283–288.

175. Guirguis-Blake JM, Beil TL, Senger CA, Coppola EL. *Primary Care Screening for Abdominal Aortic Aneurysm: Updated Systematic Review for the US Preventive Services Task Force: Evidence Synthesis No. 184.* Rockville, MD: Agency for Healthcare Research and Quality; 2019. AHRQ publication 19-05253-EF-1.

176. Dyck P, Doyle JB. "Bicycle test" of van Gelderen in diagnosis of intermittent cauda equina compression syndrome. *J Neurosurg.* 1977;46:667–670.

177. Huml EL, Davies RA, Kearns GA, et al. Common iliac artery occlusion presenting with back and leg pain: case report and differential diagnosis considerations for neurogenic/vascular claudication. *J Man Manip Ther.* 2018;26(5):249–253.

178. Tanishima S, Fukada S, Ishii H, et al. Comparison between walking test and treadmill test for intermittent claudication associated with lumbar spinal canal stenosis. *Eur Spine J.* 2015;24(2):327–332.

179. Dyck P. The stoop-test in lumbar entrapment radiculopathy. *Spine.* 1979;4:89–92.

180. Yamamoto K, Miyata T, Onozuka A, et al. Plantar flexion as an alternative to treadmill exercise for evaluating patients with intermittent claudication. *Eur J Vasc Endovasc Surg.* 2007;33:325–329.

181. Yung E. Screening for head, neck, and shoulder pathology in patients with upper extremity signs and symptoms. *J Hand Ther.* 2010;23(2):173–186.

182. Eskelinen M. Usefulness of history-taking, physical examination and diagnostic scoring in acute renal colic. *Eur Urol.* 1998;34(6):467–473.

183. Houppermans RP, Brueren MM. Physical diagnosis—pain elicited by percussion in the kidney area. *Ned Tijdschr Geneeskd.* 2001;145(5):208–210.

184. Herkowitz HN, ed. *The spine*. Philadelphia: WB Saunders; 1999.

185. Sex and back pain video. IMPACC, Inc. Dixfield, Maine. Available online at www.impaccusa.com. Accessed March 9, 2011.

186. Sex and back pain patient manual. IMPACC, Inc. Dixfield, ME. Available online at www.impaccusa.com. Accessed March 9, 2011.

187. Padua L, Caliandro P, Aprile I, et al. Back pain in pregnancy. *Eur Spine J*. 2005;14(2):151–154.

188. Borg-Stein J, Dugan SA, Gruber J. Musculoskeletal aspects of pregnancy. *Am J Phys Med Rehabil*. 2005;84(3):180–192.

189. Quaresma C. Back pain during pregnancy: a longitudinal study. *Acta Rheumatol Port*. 2010;35(3):346–351.

190. Han IH. Pregnancy and spinal problems. *Curr Opin Obstet Gynecol*. 2010;22(6):477–481.

191. Elden H, et al. Predictors and consequences of long-term pregnancy-related pelvic girdle pain: a longitudinal follow-up study. *BMC Musculoskeletal Disorders*. 2016;17:276.

192. Macarthur AJ. Is epidural anesthesia in labor associated with chronic low back pain? A prospective cohort study. *Anesth Analg*. 1997;85(5):1066–1070.

193. Leighton BL, Halpern SH. The effects of epidural analgesia on labor, maternal, and neonatal outcomes: a systematic review. *Am J Obstet Gynecol*. 2002;186(5 Suppl Nature):S69–S77.

194. Mogren IM. BMI, pain and hyper-mobility are determinants of long-term outcome for women with low back pain and pelvic pain during pregnancy. *Eur Spine J*. 2006;15(7):1093–1102.

195. Giudice LC, Kao LC. Endometriosis. *Lancet*. 2004;364(9447):1789–1799.

196. Sarma D. Cerebellar endometriosis. *Am Roentgen Ray Society*. 2004;182:1543–1546.

197. Carrell DT, Peterson CM, eds. *Reproductive endocrinology and infertility*. New York: Springer Science; 2010.

198. Sinaii N, Cleary SD, Ballweg ML, et al. High rates of autoimmune and endocrine disorders, fibromyalgia, chronic fatigue syndrome, and atopic diseases among women with endometriosis: a survey analysis. *Hum Reprod*. 2002;17(10):2715–2724.

199. Sundqvist J. Endometriosis and autoimmune disease. *Fertil Steril*. 2011;95(1):437–440.

200. Barrier BF. Immunology of endometriosis. *Clin Obstet Gynecol*. 2010;53(2):397–402.

201. Nissenblatt M. Endometriosis-associated ovarian carcinomas. *N Engl J Med*. 2011;364(5):482–485.

202. Svendsen PF, Nilas L. Norgaard Ket al.: Polycystic ovary syndrome. New pathophysiological discoveries. *Ugeskr Laeger*. 2005;167(34):3147–3151.

203. Dokras A, Bochner M, Hollinrake E, et al. Screening women with polycystic ovary syndrome for metabolic syndrome. *Obstet Gynecol*. 2005;106(1):131–137.

204. Wild RA. Assessment of cardiovascular risk and prevention of cardiovascular disease in women with the polycystic ovary syndrome: a consensus statement by the androgen excess and polycystic ovary syndrome society. *J Clin Endocrinol Metab*. 2010;95(5):2038–2049.

205. Siegel RL, Miller KD, Jemal A. Cancer statistics, 2016. *CA Cancer J Clin*. 2016;66:7–30.

206. Welch HG, Albertsen PC. Reconsidering prostate cancer mortality-the future of PSA screening. *N Engl J Med*. 2020;382(16):1557–1563.

207. Nigam M, Aschebrook-Kilfoy B, Shikanov S, et al. Increasing incidence of testicular cancer in the United States and Europe between 1992 and 2009. *World J Urol*. 2015;33:623–631.

208. Cornett CA, Vincent SA, Crow J, et al. Bacterial spine infections in adults: evaluation and management. *J Am Acad Orthop Surg*. 2016;24:11–18.

209. Gelfand MS, Cleveland KO. Vancomycin therapy and the progression of methicillin-resistant *Staphylococcus aureus* vertebral osteomyelitis. *South Med J*. 2004;97(6):593–597.

210. Van Hal SJ. Emergence of daptomycin resistance following vancomycin-unresponsive *Staphylococcus aureus* bacteraemia in a daptomycin-naive patient—a review of the literature. *Eur J Clin Microbiol Infect Dis*. 2011;30(5):603–610.

211. Patel RK, Everett CR. Low back pain: 20 clinical pearls. *J Musculoskel Med*. 2003;20(10):452–460.

212. Walton DM. Recovery from acute injury: clinical, methodological and philosophical considerations. *Disabil Rehabil*. 2010;32(10):864–874.

213. Calley D. Identifying patient fear-avoidance beliefs by physical therapists managing patients with low back pain. *J Orthop Sports Phys Ther*. 2010;40(12):774–783.

214. Asavasopon S, Jankoski J, Godges JJ. Clinical diagnosis of vertebrobasilar insufficiency: resident's case problem. *J Orthop Sports Phys Ther*. 2005;35(10):645–650.

215. Wiesel BB, Wiesel SW. Radiographic evaluation of low back pain: a cost-effective approach. *J Musculoskel Med*. 2004;21(10):528–538.

216. Mazanec DJ. Recognizing malignancy in patients with low back pain. *J Musculoskel Med*. 1996;13(1):24–31.

217. King H. Evaluating the child with back pain. *Pediatr Clin North Am*. 1986;33(6):1489–1493.

218. Behrman R, Kliegman RM, Arvin AM, eds. *Nelson's textbook of pediatrics*. ed 17 Philadelphia: WB Saunders; 2004.

219. McTimoney CA, Micheli LJ. Managing back pain in young athletes. *J Musculoskel Med*. 2004;21(2):63–69.

220. Goode B. *Personal communication*. Raleigh, NC: Centers for Disease Control and Prevention; 2006.

221. Knight D. Health care screening for men who have sex with men. *Amer Fam Phys*. 2004;69(9):2149–2156.

222. Fleming C, Whitlock EP, Biel TL, et al. Screening for abdominal aortic aneurysm: A best evidence systematic review for the United States preventive services task force. *Ann Intern Med*. 2005;142(3):203–211.

223. Lederle FA. Smokers' relative risk for aortic aneurysm compared with other smoking-related diseases: a systematic review. *J Vasc Surg*. 2003;38:329–334.

224. Dua MM, Dalman RL. Identifying aortic aneurysm risk factors in postmenopausal women. *Women's Health*. 2009;5(1):33–37.

225. Lederle FA. Abdominal aortic aneurysm events in the women's health initiative: cohort study. *BMJ*. 2008;337:1724–1734.

Screening the Sacrum, Sacroiliac, and Pelvis

Following the model for decision making in the screening process outlined in Chapter 1 (see Box 1.7), we now turn our attention to pain from medical conditions, illnesses, and diseases referred to the sacrum, sacroiliac (SI), and pelvic regions.

The basic premise is that physical therapists must be able to identify signs and symptoms of systemic origin or associated with medical conditions that can mimic neuromuscular or musculoskeletal (neuromusculoskeletal) impairment in these areas.

In the screening process, therapists will watch for yellow (caution) or red (warning) flags to direct them. Clinicians rely on special questions to ask men and women with significant risk factors, significant past medical history, suspicious clinical presentation, or associated signs and symptoms.

With a careful interview and the right screening questions, the therapist can identify clues suggestive of a problem outside the scope of a physical therapist's practice that may require medical referral. Specific tests to screen for an underlying infectious or inflammatory source of pelvic or abdominal pain are also presented with a suggested order of testing.

When dealing with painful symptoms of the sacral and pelvic areas, the therapist may need to ask questions about sexual history or sexual practices. The therapist must remain aware of facial expressions, body language, and verbal remarks in response to a client's answers.

The therapist must be prepared to respond professionally if a man or woman with pelvic or sacral pain reports that he or she has been the victim of repeated violent sexual acts, or if a client admits to physical or emotional assault. More about the client interview, the screening interview, and screening for assault and domestic (intimate partner) violence is included in Chapter 2 (see also Appendices B-3 and B-32 in the accompanying enhanced eBook version included with print purchase of this textbook).

THE SACRUM AND SACROILIAC JOINT

The main function of the SI joint is to transmit a load from the trunk to the extremities.[1] Load transfer from the trunk to the extremities can reach 300% of an individual's body weight during gait.[2] Evaluating the SI joint can be difficult in that no single physical examination finding can predict a disorder of the SI joint. Pain originating from the SI joint can mimic pain referred from lumbar disk herniation, spinal stenosis, facet joint impairment, or even a disorder of the hip.[3-5]

The most common clinical presentation of SI pain is associated with a memorable *physical event* that initiated the pain such as a misstep off a curb, a fall on the hip or buttocks, lifting of a heavy object in a twisted position, or childbirth (Case Example 16.1). A history of previous spine surgery is very common in clients with SI intraarticular pain.[3]

The most typical *medical conditions* that refer pain to the sacrum and SI joint include endocarditis, prostate cancer or other neoplasm,[6] gynecologic disorders, rheumatic diseases that target the SI area (e.g., spondyloarthropathies such as ankylosing spondylitis, reactive arthritis, or psoriatic arthritis), and Paget's disease (Table 16.1).[7]

Disorders of the large intestine and colon, such as ulcerative colitis, Crohn's disease (regional enteritis), carcinoma of the colon, and irritable bowel syndrome (IBS) can refer pain to the sacrum when an abscess develops or when the rectum is stimulated.[8] Likewise, primary SI problems can refer pain to the lower abdomen.[9]

A medical differential diagnosis may be needed to exclude a fracture, infection, or tumor. Insufficiency fractures of the sacrum can occur after pelvic radiotherapy for cancer[10] and in osteoporotic bone with minimal or unremembered trauma.[11] (See further discussion in this chapter on spondylogenic causes of sacral pain.)

Using the Screening Model to Evaluate Sacral/Sacroiliac Symptoms

The principles guiding evaluation of SI joint or sacral pain are consistent with the information presented throughout this text and is enhanced with tools such as the OSPRO-ROS (see Chapter 1). The connection of SI joint dysfunction was also presented in the chapter on back pain (see Chapter 15).

Each disorder listed in Table 16.1 typically has its unique *clinical presentation* with clues available in the *past medical history*. The presence of *associated signs and symptoms* is always a red flag. Most of these conditions have clear red-flag clues that come to light if the client is interviewed carefully with these conditions in mind during the history portion of the interview.

CASE EXAMPLE 16.1

Sacroiliac Pain Caused by Pelvic Floor Muscle Impairment

Background: A 33-year-old woman referred by her orthopedic surgeon presented with low back pain centered over the sacroiliac (SI) region. She described it as "sharp" and "knife-like." It comes and goes with no warning. Sometimes, it is so severe she cannot catch her breath and falls to her knees. After that, she cannot stand up straight for several hours and walks "hunched over."

The pain presented on both sides intermittently, but the primary pain pattern was localized in the left SI area. Heat seems to help for a short time, but nothing brings complete relief all the time.

She has a previous history of disk herniation with diskectomy and laminectomy and complete resolution of symptoms. No cause is known for this new onset of SI symptoms. No radiating symptoms are apparent, and recent magnetic resonance imaging (MRI) shows no sign of disk protrusion at this time. (She tried doing her previous program of McKenzie exercises, but no change in symptoms occurred.)

Clinical Presentation: Physical therapy examination reveals the following:

Antalgic gait secondary to pain. Trendelenburg sign: Negative. Slight left lumbar lateral shift; posture is otherwise within normal limits. Active lumbar motions are full, with a normal capsular end feel and no reproduction of symptoms. Repeated trunk and lumbar motions do not elicit painful symptoms.

Neurologic screen: Negative for abnormal reflexes, abnormal sensation, decreased strength, or altered neural tension. Hamstrings are tight bilaterally, but a straight leg raise does not increase symptoms. In fact, it is the only time in the assessment when the client reports a slight decrease in pain.

Examination of the SI area revealed an upslip on the left (anterior superior iliac spine [ASIS] and posterior superior iliac spine [PSIS] on the left are higher than ASIS and PSIS on the right, indicating an upward movement of the ilium on the sacrum on the high side; leg length discrepancy or muscle spasm from a disk lesion can also cause an upslip). Given her past history of diskogenic lesion, altered muscle activation may be the cause. This will have to be examined further.

Is a screening examination for systemic origin of symptoms warranted? Why, or why not?

Using our screening model, review the past medical history. Are there any red flags here? No, but the history is very incomplete. We know she had a previous diskogenic lesion treated operatively. Nothing of her personal or family history is included.

Even in a musculoskeletal assessment, we will want to know about pregnancy and birth histories; use of medications, over-the-counter drugs (OTC), and illicit drugs; smoking and drinking history or current use; levels of activity before the onset of symptoms; correlation of symptoms with menses or births; occupation and work-related activities; and history of cancer.

A general screening interview will ask about recent history of infection, the presence of joint pain or skin rash anywhere else, and the presence of any constitutional or other symptoms.

Next, review the clinical presentation. Are there any red flags here? Not really. There is no night pain. There is the fact that nothing seems to make it better or worse, but one red flag by itself usually is not highly significant. We will tuck that bit of information in the back of our minds as we continue the evaluation process.

Hamstring stretching brings some mild, temporary relief. This suggests a muscular component, but that has to be further evaluated. The SI upslip could be the cause of the symptoms, but this will not be determined until the alignment and cause of the upslip are corrected.

A trigger point assessment may be needed as well.

Step three involves a review of associated signs and symptoms. We do not know about constitutional symptoms, relationship of SI pain to menses, or the presence of any other symptoms associated with the viscera (e.g., gastrointestinal [GI], urologic). It is always recommended to take the client's temperature in the presence of pain of unknown cause.

What to Do: Several strategies are presented here. Intervention for the upslip may be the first step with reassessment of symptoms. If a lack of progress occurs, the therapist can go back and ask more specific questions, or the therapist can treat the upslip and continue to interview the client each day, obtaining additional pertinent information before making a final decision.

Result: When the client was directly questioned about painful intercourse, she did admit significant pain. The client finally described a sensation of "trying to deliver a baby through my rectum" during intercourse. The woman also reported symptoms of overactive bladder with urinary incontinence. She reported a complicated birth history with her first child, which was repeated with less severity during the births of her second and third children.

The therapist suggested she share the signs and symptoms with her gynecologist. An internal vaginal examination reproduced her symptoms exactly. The evaluating therapist was not trained in pelvic floor muscle assessment but knew enough to refer the woman for further assessment. In the end, it was discovered that the client had significant pelvic floor impairment with overactivity of the pelvic floor muscles and detrusor imbalance with urinary incontinence.

Looking back, it is likely that development of the discogenic lesion was linked to birth/delivery problems (or perhaps, vice versa; it is not known for sure). Closer examination revealed a loss of lumbar stabilization because of multifidus impairment. Muscle impairment at the time of the disk lesion and births probably contributed to the gradual development of pelvic floor impairment.

Changes were also noted in the abdominal muscles with a loss of cocontraction between the multifidus and the transversus abdominis. The pelvic floor muscles were in a contract-hold pattern, contributing to the painful symptoms described.

Heat relaxed the muscles, but only for a short time.

A program directed at restoring normal muscle tone and function in the lumbar spine, abdominal muscles, and pelvic floor muscles resulted in immediate reduction and eventual elimination of painful symptoms and return of comfortable coitus. Symptoms of urinary incontinence also were resolved.

Although the SI upslip could be corrected, the client could not maintain the correction. Because she was pain-free, she did not return to physical therapy for further evaluation of the underlying biomechanics around the SI upslip.

TABLE 16.1	Causes of Sacral and Sacroiliac Pain
Systemic	Neuromuscular/ Musculoskeletal[17]
INFECTIOUS/INFLAMMATORY	Idiopathic (unknown)
Spondyloarthropathy:	Trauma
• Ankylosing spondylitis	Myofascial or kinetic chain
• Reactive arthritis	imbalance
• Psoriatic arthritis	Enthesis (tendon insertion)/
• IBD (arthritis associated	ligamentous sprain
with IBD)	Degenerative joint disease
Vertebral osteomyelitis	Bone harvesting for grafts
Endocarditis	(may cause secondary
Tuberculosis (uncommon)	instability)
	Lumbar spine fusion or hip
SPONDYLOGENIC	arthrodesis
Fracture (traumatic, insufficiency,	Myofascial syndromes
pathologic), metabolic bone	(mimics SI joint pain)
disease	Pelvic floor muscle spasm/
• Osteoporosis (insufficiency	myalgia
fractures)	Diskogenic disease (mimics
• Paget's disease	SI joint pain)
• Osteodystrophy	Nerve root compression
• Osteoarthritis	(mimics SI joint pain)
Gynecologic	Zygapophyseal joint pain
Reproductive cancers	(mimics SI joint pain)
Uterine fibroids	
Ovarian cysts	
Endometriosis	
PID	
Incest/sexual assault	
Rectocele, cystocele	
Uterine prolapse	
Normal pregnancy; multiparity	
(more than one pregnancy)	
GASTROINTESTINAL	
Ulcerative colitis	
Colon cancer	
IBS	
Crohn's disease (regional enteritis)	
CANCER	
Primary tumors* (rare: giant	
cell, chondrosarcoma,	
chondroma, synovial	
villoadenomas, schwannoma,	
neurofibroma, ependymomas,	
ganglioneuromas)	
Metastatic lesions (history of	
cancer):	
• Prostate	
• Lung	
• Thyroid	
• Colorectal	
• Breast	
• Gastrointestinal	
• Multiple myeloma	
• Kidney	
OTHER	
Fibromyalgia	

IBD, Inflammatory bowel disease; *IBS*, irritable bowel syndrome; *PID*, pelvic inflammatory disease; *SI*, sacroiliac.
*Includes benign and malignant osseous and neurogenic tumors affecting the sacrum.

BOX 16.1 RED FLAGS ASSOCIATED WITH SACROILIAC/SACRAL PAIN OR SYMPTOMS

History

- Sacroiliac/sacral pain without a history of trauma or overuse (rule out assault, anal intercourse)
- Previous history of cancer
- Previous history of gastrointestinal (GI) disease (ulcerative colitis, Crohn's disease, irritable bowel syndrome)
- Previous history of infection (skin, genitourinary tract, heart, septic sacroiliitis)

Risk Factors

- Osteoporosis
- Sexually transmitted infection or other organ system infection
- Intravenous drug abuse
- Long-term use of antibiotics (colitis)

Clinical Presentation

- Insidious onset/unknown cause
- Lack of objective findings
- Anterior pelvic, suprapubic, or low abdominal pain at the same level as the sacrum

Associated Signs and Symptoms

- Pain relieved by passing gas or having a bowel movement
- Presence of GI, gynecologic, or urologic signs and symptoms
- Fever (septic sacroiliitis); other constitutional symptoms

Clinical Presentation

Insidious onset or unknown cause is always a red flag. Without a clear cause, the therapist looks for something else in the history or accompanying signs and symptoms. Even with a known or assigned cause, it is important to keep other possibilities in mind and to watch for red flags (Box 16.1). Sacral pain in the absence of a history of trauma or overuse is a clue to the presentation of systemic backache.

The amount and direction of pain radiation can offer helpful clues. Low back or sacral pain radiating around the flank suggests the renal or urologic system. In such cases, the therapist should ask questions about bladder or urologic function.

Low back or sacral pain radiating to the buttock or legs may be vascular. Questions about the effects of activity on symptoms and history of cardiovascular or peripheral vascular diseases (PVDs) are important. Sorting out pain of a vascular versus neurogenic cause is discussed in Chapter 15.

Most commonly, unless pain causes muscle spasm, splinting, and subsequent biomechanical changes, clients affected by systemic, medical, or viscerogenic causes of sacral or SI pain demonstrate a remarkable lack of objective findings to

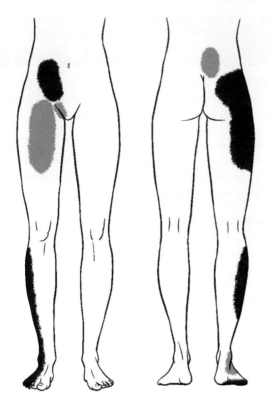

Fig. 16.1 Unilateral sacroiliac (SI) pain pattern. Pain coming from the SI joint is usually centered over the area of the posterior superior iliac spine (PSIS), with tenderness directly over the PSIS. Lower lumbar pain occurs in 72% of all cases; it rarely presents as upper lumbar pain above L5 (6%). It may radiate over the buttocks (94%), down the posterior–lateral thigh (50%), and even past the knee to the ankle (14%) and lateral foot (8%). Paresthesias in the leg are not a typical feature of SI joint pain. The affected individual may report abdominal (2%), groin or pubic (14%), or anterior thigh pain (10%). Anterior symptoms may occur alone or in combination with posterior symptoms. Occasionally, a client will report bilateral pain. (Data from Slipman CW, Jackson HB, Lipetz JS, et al.: Sacroiliac joint pain referral zones, *Arch Phys Med Rehab* 81:334–338, 2000.)

implicate the SI joint or sacrum as the causative factor for the presenting symptoms. Pain elicited by mobilizations to the sacrum with the client in a prone position suggests sacroiliitis (inflammation of the SI joint) or mechanical derangement.

Sacroiliac Joint Pain Pattern. Whether from a mechanical or a systemic origin, the patient usually experiences pain over the posterior SI joint and buttock, with or without lower extremity pain. Pain may be unilateral or bilateral (Fig. 16.1)[12] and can be referred to a wide referral zone, including the lumbar spine, abdomen, groin, thigh, foot, and ankle.[3,13]

Clients with SI joint pain rarely have pain at or above the level of the L5 spinous process, although it is possible. The presence of midline lumbar pain tends to exclude the SI joint as a potential pain generator.[13–15]

A wide range of SI joint–referred pain patterns occur because innervation is highly variable and complex, or because pain may be somatically referred, as discussed in Chapter 3. Adjacent structures, such as the piriformis muscle, sciatic nerve, posterior long SI ligament, and L5 nerve root,

may be affected by intrinsic joint disease and can become active nociceptors. Pain referral patterns also may be dependent on the distinct location of injury within the SI joint.[15,16]

SI pain can mimic diskogenic disease with radicular pain down the leg to the posterior calf or the foot.[13,17] People who report midline lumbar pain when they rise from a sitting position are likely to have diskogenic pain. Clients with unilateral pain below the level of the L5 spinous process and pain when they rise from sitting are likely to have a painful SI joint.[14,15]

Pain from SI joint syndrome may be aggravated by sitting or lying on the affected side. Pain gets worse with prolonged driving or riding in a car, weight-bearing on the affected side, the Valsalva maneuver, and trunk flexion with the legs straight.[16]

SI pain can also mimic the pain pattern of kidney disease with anterior thigh pain, but with SI impairment, no signs and symptoms (e.g., constitutional symptoms, bladder dysfunction) are associated, as would be the case with thigh pain referred from the renal system.

Screening for Infectious/Inflammatory Causes of Sacroiliac Pain

Joint infections spread hematogenously through the body and can affect the SI joint. Usually, the infection is unilateral and is caused by *Pseudomonas aeruginosa*, *Staphylococcus aureus*, *Cryptococcus* organisms, or *Mycobacterium tuberculosis*.

Risk factors for joint infection include trauma, endocarditis, intravenous drug use, and immunosuppression. Postoperative infection of any kind may not appear with any clinical signs or symptoms for weeks or months. Infections causing bacterial sacroiliitis as a complication of dilatation and curettage after incomplete abortions have been reported.[18]

Infection can cause distention of the anterior joint capsule, irritating the lumbosacral nerve roots.[19] Inflammation of the SI joint may result from metabolic, traumatic, or rheumatic causes. Sacroiliitis is present in all individuals with ankylosing spondylitis.[20]

Rheumatic Diseases as a Cause of Sacral or Sacroiliac Pain

The most common systemic causes of sacral pain are noninfected, inflammatory erosive rheumatic diseases that target the SI, including ankylosing spondylitis, Reiter's syndrome, psoriatic arthritis, and arthritis associated with inflammatory bowel disease (IBD) such as regional enteritis (Crohn's disease).

Reactive arthritis (see Chapter 13) occurs most often in young men with venereal disease. Reiter's syndrome often presents as a triad of symptoms, including arthritis, conjunctivitis, and urethritis. These three symptoms in the presence of sacral pain raise a red flag. The therapist must ask about pain in other joints, urologic symptoms, and a recent (or current) history of conjunctivitis (red, painful inflammation of the eye).

A positive sexual history or known diagnosis of venereal disease is helpful information. With sacral or SI pain, the therapist should always consider taking a sexual history (see Special Questions to Ask in Chapter 15 or Appendix B-32 in the accompanying enhanced eBook version included with print purchase of this textbook).

BOX 16.2 RISK FACTORS FOR SACRAL FRACTURES

- Osteoporosis (see also Box 12.3)
- Paget's disease
- Sex (female)
- Athletes, military personnel (overuse, overtraining, improper footwear or training surface)
- Athletic, pregnant, or postpartum women
- Pelvic radiation
- Lumbosacral fusion (early postoperative)
- Osteomyelitis
- Multiple myeloma
- Trauma (motor vehicle accident, fall, assault)
- Prolonged use of corticosteroids

Crohn's disease (see Chapter 9) may be accompanied by skin rash and joint pain. This enteric condition is well known for its arthritic component, which is present in up to 25% of all cases. The client may have had Crohn's disease for years and may not recognize the onset of these new symptoms as a part of that condition. Skin rash may precede joint pain by days or weeks. The hips, thighs, and legs are affected most often; the rash may be raised or flat, purple or red. Knowing the history and association between skin lesions and joint pain can help the therapist direct screening questions and make a reasonable decision about referral.

Screening for Spondylogenic Causes of Sacral/Sacroiliac Pain

Metabolic bone disease (MBD) such as osteoporosis, Paget's disease, and osteodystrophy can result in loss of bone mineral density and deformity or fracture of the sacrum. The therapist should review cases of sacral pain for the presence of risk factors for any of these MBDs (see the discussion on MBD in Chapter 12). Neoplasm and fracture are two other possible bony causes of sacral pain. Neoplasm is discussed separately in this chapter.

Metabolic Bone Disease

Mild-to-moderate MBD may occur with no visible signs. Advanced cases of MBD include constipation, anorexia, fractured bones, and deformity.

Osteoporosis. Osteoporosis can cause insufficiency fractures of the sacrum. The therapist must assess for risk factors (Box 16.2; see Box 11.3) in anyone with sacral pain, especially those in whom pain has an unknown cause, in postmenopausal women, older men (over 65), and anyone with a known history of osteoporosis or Paget's disease. See further discussion on osteoporosis in Chapter 12 and discussion on fractures at the end of this section.

Paget's Disease. Paget's disease as a cause of lumbar, sacral, SI, or pelvic pain occurs most commonly in men over 70 years of age (although it can occur earlier and in women). It is the second most common MBD after osteoporosis. The bones that are most frequently involved are the pelvis, femur, lumbar spine, and skull.[21]

Characterized by slowly progressive enlargement and deformity of multiple bones, it is associated with unexplained acceleration of bone deposition and resorption. The bones become weak, spongy, and deformed. Redness and warmth may be noted over involved areas, and the most common symptom is bone pain (see further discussion on Paget's disease in Chapter 12 and an excellent online article as referenced here).[22]

Fracture

Three types of fractures affect the sacrum: traumatic, insufficiency, and pathologic. Trauma resulting in fracture occurs most often with lateral compression injuries seen in motor vehicle accidents or vertical shear injuries resulting from a fall from a height onto the lower limbs. Less commonly, direct stress to the sacrum from a fall landing on the buttocks or athletic injury can cause traumatic sacral fracture.[23,24] Other risk factors for sacral fracture are listed in Box 16.2.

Trauma-related fatigue or stress fracture of the sacrum occurs most often in young active persons and older adults with osteoporosis. Fatigue or stress fractures can develop as a result of submaximal repetitive forces over time, such as those that occur from overuse or overtraining as seen in military personnel and athletes (e.g., runners, volleyball and field hockey players). Less often, pregnant or postpartum women experience sacral stress fractures, especially if they are participating in athletic training activities or running.[25-27] The most common stress fractures in runners occur in the tibia (16.2%), femur (6.6%), and pelvis (1.6%).[28]

Insufficiency fractures of the sacrum result from a normal stress acting on the bone with decreased density.[29] Reduced bone integrity is most often associated with postmenopausal or corticosteroid-induced osteoporosis and radiation therapy.[21] Insufficiency fractures occur insidiously or as a result of minor trauma, possibly even from weight-bearing transmitted through the spine.[30]

Pathologic fracture describes fractures that occur as a result of bone weakened by neoplasm or other disease conditions (e.g., osteomyelitis, giant cell tumor, chordoma, Ewing sarcoma, multiple myeloma). Insufficiency fractures are a subset of pathologic fractures confined to bones with structural alterations as a result of MBD.[23,31]

Clinical manifestations of sacral fractures can present with a wide range of signs and symptoms, many of which are present inconsistently and are considered nonspecific.[29,32] Bilateral or multiple stress fractures of the sacrum or pelvis have been reported.[33]

The client may report or demonstrate localized pain, tenderness with palpation, antalgic gait, and leg length discrepancy. With all sacral fractures, hip, low back, sacral, groin, or buttock, pain may occur, especially with multiple stress fractures of the pelvic and sacral bones. Symptoms may mimic other conditions such as disk disease, recurrence of a local tumor, or metastatic disease.[23]

Diagnostic imaging may be needed to make the final medical diagnosis. In two thirds of patients complaining of symptoms, radiographs are initially negative for a stress fracture and only half ever develop positive radiograph findings. The most common radiologic sign in initial stress fractures is a focal periosteal bone formation. Advanced imaging such as a bone scan or magnetic resonance imaging (MRI) should be used to confirm the diagnosis of a stress fracture.[34]

New onset of sacral or buttock pain 1 to 2 weeks after multilevel lumbosacral fusion with instrumentation should be evaluated for sacral insufficiency fractures, especially if the patient has a recent history of osteoporosis, prolonged sitting, and kyphosis.[35-37]

Screening for Gynecologic Causes of Sacral Pain

See later discussion on gynecologic causes of pelvic pain in this chapter.

Screening for Gastrointestinal Causes of Sacral/Sacroiliac Pain

The *primary* pain pattern for gastrointestinal (GI) disease involves the midabdominal region around the umbilicus. It is not common for the therapist to see clients with this chief complaint as they are more likely to see a doctor or go to the emergency department.

However, the therapist may be evaluating or treating a client for an orthopedic or neurologic problem who reports GI symptoms. When a client relates symptoms associated with the viscera or abdomen, the therapist must think in terms of screening questions to discern whether these symptoms require immediate medical assessment and intervention.

The therapist is more likely to see clients with *referred* low back or sacral pain from the small or large intestine as it presents in the low back or sacral area (see Figs. 9.17 and 9.18). Although these illustrations depict the pain in small, very round areas, actual pain patterns can vary quite a bit. The location will be approximately the same, but individual variation does occur.

The therapist must ask about the presence of abdominal pain or GI symptoms, occurring either simultaneously or alternating, but at the same anatomic level as back or sacral pain. See Case Example 15.13 to review the importance of looking for this particular red flag.

Sacral pain from a GI source may be reduced or relieved after the person passes gas or completes a bowel movement. It may be appropriate to ask a client the following:

❓ FOLLOW UP QUESTIONS

- Is your pain relieved by passing gas or having a bowel movement?
- The patient may have a history of GI disease and medication used to treat such a condition. Keep the following conditions or past histories in mind when asking questions of anyone with lumbar spine or sacral pain patterns:
- Ulcerative colitis
- Crohn's disease
- Irritable bowel syndrome
- Colon cancer
- Long-term use of antibiotics (colitis)

Screening for Tumors as a Cause of Sacral/Sacroiliac Pain

Primary sacral tumors include benign and malignant growths and account for less than 7% of all spinal tumors.[38,39] Benign neoplasms include osteochondroma, giant cell tumor, and osteoid osteoma. The more common primary malignant lesions directly affecting the sacrum include chordoma, chondrosarcoma, osteosarcoma, and myeloma.

MBD to the sacrum from primary breast, lung, colon, and prostate is far more common. Sacral insufficiency fractures after pelvic radiation for rectal, prostate, or reproductive cancers can occur, although these are rare.[8,40]

Although rare, sacral neoplasms are usually not diagnosed early in the disease course because of mild symptoms resembling low back, buttock, or leg pain (sciatica).[38,41,42] Sacral tumors are not easy to see on x-ray films and are easily overlooked because of the curvature of the sacrum, location deep within the pelvis, and frequent presence of overlying bowel gas. It is common for diagnostic delays to occur as the person is treated for a presumed lumbar pathology before the sacrum is finally identified as the source of pathology.[39,42] Referral to a physical therapist before a correct medical diagnosis is made is common because of the clinical presentation.

Giant cell tumor is a highly aggressive local tumor of the bone and accounts for 5% to 10% of all primary bone tumors.[43] The sacrum is the third most common site of involvement.[44] Clients present with localized pain in the low back and sacrum that may radiate to one or both legs. Swelling may be noted in the involved area. When asked about the presence of other symptoms anywhere else in the body, the client may report abdominal complaints and neurologic signs and symptoms (e.g., bowel and bladder or sexual dysfunction, numbness and weakness of the lower extremity).[4,43,45]

Colorectal or anorectal cancer as a cause of sacral pain is possible as the result of local invasion. Severe sacral pain in the presence of a previous history of uterine, abdominal, prostate, rectal, or anal cancer requires immediate medical referral.

Prostatic (males) *or reproductive cancers* in men and women can result in sacral pain. See further discussions on testicular cancer in Chapters 11 and 15, prostate cancer in Chapter 11, and gynecologic conditions in this chapter.

THE COCCYX

The coccyx or tailbone is a small triangular bone that articulates with the bottom of the sacrum at the sacrococcygeal joint. Injury or trauma to this area can cause coccygeal pain called *coccygodynia*.

Coccygodynia

Most cases of coccygodynia or coccydynia (pain in the region of the coccyx) seen by the physical therapist occur as a result of trauma, such as a fall directly on the tailbone, or events associated with childbirth.

Symptoms include localized pain in the tailbone that is usually aggravated by direct pressure such as that caused by sitting,

BOX 16.3   CAUSES OF COCCYGEAL PAIN

- Degenerative spondylolysis or spondylolisthesis
- Lumbar spinal stenosis
- Sacroiliac joint impairment
- Anal fissures
- Inflammatory cysts
- Prostatitis
- Thrombosed hemorrhoids
- Chordoma (neoplasm)
- Pilonidal cysts
- Trauma (fall, childbirth, anal intercourse)
- Nonunion fracture (sacrum, coccyx)
- Coccygeal disk injury (rare)
- Pelvic floor muscle and inferior gluteal trigger points

Data from Wood KB, Mehbod AA: Operative treatment for coccygodynia, *J Spinal Disord Tech* 17(6):511–515, 2004.

defecation, standing, or sexual intercourse.[46] Moving from sitting to standing may also reproduce or aggravate painful symptoms related to the gluteal fibers at the coccyx, and soft tissue mobilization is effective to improve this origin of pain.

In the case of *persistent* coccygodynia with a history of trauma, the therapist must keep in mind the possibility of rectal or bladder lesions (Box 16.3). When asked about the presence of other symptoms, clients with coccygodynia after a traumatic fall may also report bladder, bowel, or sexual symptoms. The therapist must ask whether bladder, bowel, or rectal symptoms were present before the fall. Because 50% of all clients with back or sacral pain from a malignancy have preceding trauma or injury, the apparent trauma (especially if the client reports associated symptoms that were present before the trauma) may be something more serious.

For possible clues to treating a client with coccygodynia, the therapist should review Box 16.3, keeping in mind the risk factors for each of these conditions. The therapist should also conduct a neurologic screening examination to identify any signs or symptoms of disk disease. Past history of any of the problems listed is a yellow (warning) flag. Blood in the toilet after a bowel movement may be a sign of anal fissures, hemorrhoids, or colorectal cancer and requires medical evaluation. Pain with intercourse is a symptom of overactive pelvic floor muscle (PFM) or spasm. It may also be related to medical conditions such as dryness, infection, or skin lesions.

THE PELVIS

Once again, the principles used in screening for systemic, medical, or viscerogenic causes of back, sacral, and SI pain also apply to pelvic pain. The history and associated signs and symptoms may vary somewhat according to the cause, but many of the causes are the same (e.g., cancer, GI, vascular, urogenital) (Table 16.2).

The most common primary causes of pelvic pain are musculoskeletal, neuromuscular, gynecologic, infectious, vascular, neoplastic, and GI (in descending order). For example, chronic pelvic pain is most commonly associated with endometriosis, adhesions, IBS, and interstitial cystitis. Infectious disease is the most common systemic cause of pelvic pain.[47,48]

The goal of screening is to identify individuals with infectious, vascular, or neoplastic causes of pelvic pain and to refer appropriately, simultaneously making sure that those individuals treated have a problem within the scope of our practice. Therapists must keep in mind that pelvic pain and symptoms can be referred to the pelvis from the hip, sacrum, SI area, or lumbar spine. At the same time, pelvic diseases can refer pain or symptoms to the abdomen, low back, buttocks, groin, and thigh. This means that anytime a client presents with pain or impairment in any of these areas, pelvic disease must be considered as a possible cause. At the same time, keep in mind that PFM spasm can be associated with disorders such as IBS or interstitial cystitis; such problems can be aided by the therapist who is skilled in management of PFM impairments.

The anterior pelvic wall is part of the musculature of the abdominal cavity. The lateral walls are covered by the iliopsoas and obturator muscles; inferiorly, the outlet is guarded by the PFMs of which the pubococcygeus, illiococcygeus, puborectalis, and coccygeus are the largest and are collectively known as the levator ani muscles.

These two anatomic regions are separated only by walls of muscle. Because the pelvic cavity is in direct communication with the abdominal cavity (see Fig. 15.1), any organ disease or systemic condition of the pelvic or abdominal cavity can cause primary pelvic pain or referred musculoskeletal pain, as is described in this section.

The therapist should keep in mind that pelvic pain, pelvic girdle pain (PGP), and low back pain often occur together or alternately. Whenever discussing pelvic pain, the therapist should ask about the presence of unreported low back pain (including PGP). PGP can occur separately or combined with low back pain and is defined as generally present between the posterior iliac crest (posterior superior iliac spine [PSIS]) and the gluteal fold in the vicinity of the SI joint.

Using the Screening Model to Evaluate the Pelvis

When our screening model is followed, the same steps are always taken. A personal or family history is obtained and risk factor assessment is performed. Once the history has been established, the pelvic pain pattern is reviewed. The therapist looks for red flags that may suggest systemic, medical, or viscerogenic causes. Additional questions may be needed to complete the screening process. These questions are presented for all causes of pelvic pain at the end of this chapter.

History Associated With Pelvic Pain

With so many possible causes of pelvic pain, many different factors in the past medical history can raise a red flag. Pelvic pain is a very complex problem. Many medical texts are written about just this one anatomic area.

This text does not attempt to explain or discuss all the possible causes of PFM or PGP. Rather, the intent is for the reader to learn how to screen for the possibility of systemic or viscerogenic sources of pelvic pain or symptoms. With a good understanding of what is important in the history and a list of possible follow-up questions, the therapist assesses each client, keeping in mind that medical referral may be needed.

Some of the more common red-flag histories associated with pelvic pain are listed in Box 16.4. With the use of

categories from the screening model, risk factors, clinical presentation, and associated signs and symptoms also are listed.

It is useful to separate pelvic floor dysfunction from PFM impairments. Pelvic floor dysfunction is related to organ problems such as urinary incontinence or retention, whereas PFM impairments are specific to the PFMs being overactive

TABLE 16.2	Causes of Pelvic Pain	
Systemic	**Neuromuscular/Musculoskeletal/Soft Tissue**

Systemic	Neuromuscular/Musculoskeletal/Soft Tissue

GYNECOLOGIC
Pregnancy (including ectopic, ruptured or unruptured)
Uterovaginal, urethral, and/or rectal prolapse (rare)
Vulvodynia
Dysmenorrhea
Endometriosis
Premenstrual tension syndrome
Uterine or cervical tumors, fibroids, adhesions, polyps, stenosis
Ovarian cysts, varicosities, torsion, ovulation; any ovarian anomaly
Intrauterine contraceptive device
Adnexal torsion (ovaries, fallopian tubes twisted) (rare)
 	
INFECTION/INFLAMMATION
Spontaneous, therapeutic, or incomplete abortion; postabortion syndrome
Septic arthritis; reactive arthritis
Ankylosing spondylitis
Ileal Crohn's disease
Acute or chronic appendicitis
Herpes zoster
Osteomyelitis
PID
Sexually transmitted infection
Postpartum infection
 	
VASCULAR DISORDERS
Arterial occlusion; ischemia
Abdominal angina
Abdominal aneurysm
Pelvic congestion
Varicosities or pelvic thrombophlebitis
Cancer
Reproductive
Urologic
 	
GASTROINTESTINAL DISORDERS
IBD
   • Crohn's disease
   • Ulcerative colitis
   • IBS
Diverticular disease
Constipation (common in older adults)
Neoplasm
Hernia
Bowel obstruction
 	
UROGENITAL
Chronic urinary tract infection
Detrusor-sphincter dyssynergia (bladder spasm)
Interstitial cystitis/painful bladder syndrome
Radiation cystitis
Acute pyelonephritis
Kidney stones (ureteric calculus, urolithiasis)
Chronic nonbacterial prostatitis, prostatodynia, prostate cancer
Chronic orchalgia
Urethral strictures
	Hip, sacroiliac joint, low back, sacral, or coccyx impairment*
	Muscle impairment (hamstrings, abdominals, rectus femoris, piriformis, adductor muscles, pelvic floor muscles, pelvic girdle, iliopsoas, quadratus lumborum)†
	Psoas abscess (abdominal or pelvic infectious process)
	Total hip arthroplasty (polyethylene wear debris)
	Stress reaction/fracture
	Vertebral compression fracture (lumbar spine)
	Spondylolysis
	Pubic strain/sprain/separation (pubis symphysis)
	Osteitis pubis
	Sexual, birth, or activity-related trauma or injury:
	Overactive PFM syndromes: Levator ani syndrome
	Tension myalgia
	Coccygodynia, vaginismus, anismus
	Neurologic disorders:
	Nerve entrapment (surgical scar in lower abdomen)
	Incomplete spinal cord lesion; neoplasia of spinal cord or sacral nerve
	Multiple sclerosis
	Pudendal neuralgia
	Shingles (herpes zoster)
	Diskogenic lesions (herniation)
	Complex regional pain syndrome
	Abdominal migraine
	Scoliosis
	Osteoporosis
	Somatization disorders
	Adhesions
	Abdominal wall myofascial pain, trigger points
	Postural alignment issues
	Hernia (obturator, sciatic, inguinal, femoral, umbilical)

TABLE 16.2	Causes of Pelvic Pain—cont'd	
Systemic	Neuromuscular/Musculoskeletal/Soft Tissue

OTHER

Psychogenic; somatization disorder; depression
Sleep disorder
Trauma/sexual assault; physical abuse
Surgery (abdominal/laparoscopic, tubal, pelvic)
Fibromyalgia
Autonomic nervous system impairment
Paget's disease
Lead or mercury toxicity
Substance abuse (cocaine)
Sickle cell anemia
Chronic visceral pain syndrome

IBD, Inflammatory bowel disease, *IBS*, irritable bowel syndrome; *PID*, pelvic inflammatory disease.
The combined medical and physical therapy differential diagnosis includes many origins of pathokinesiologic conditions, including joint laxity; subluxations or displacements; thoracolumbar hypermobility; bursitis; osteoarthritis; spondyloarthropathy; fracture; and postural, ligamentous, or osteoporosis/osteomalacia. (This list is not exhaustive.)
†As with joint impairment, the differential diagnosis of muscle pathokinesiologic conditions can include many origins (e.g., trigger points, tendinous avulsion, strain/sprain/tear, weakness, loss of flexibility, pelvic floor overactivity [pain and spasm] or underactivity [laxity, weakness, and leaking], diastasis recti).

BOX 16.4   RED FLAGS ASSOCIATED WITH PELVIC PAIN OR SYMPTOMS

History*
- History of reproductive, colon, or breast cancer
- History of dysmenorrhea, ovarian cysts, pelvic inflammatory disease, sexually transmitted disease
- Endometriosis
- Chronic bladder or urinary tract infections
- Irritable bowel syndrome
- Previous history of pelvic/bladder surgery, especially hysterectomy and mesh with pelvic organ prolapse
- Recent abortion or miscarriage
- History of assault, incest, trauma
- Chronic yeast/vaginal infection
- History of varicose veins in the lower extremities (risk factor for pelvic congestion syndrome)

Risk Factors
- Recent intrauterine contraceptive device (rejection) or long-term use, especially without medical follow-up (scar tissue)
- Transitional menopause (perimenopause), menopause (vaginitis, vaginal atrophy)
- Sexual activity without use of a condom (sexually transmitted disease [STD], pelvic inflammatory disease [PID])
- Multiple sexual partners (STD, PID)
- Pregnancy, childbirth, recent abortion, multiple abortions

Clinical Presentation
- Insidious onset; unknown cause
- Poorly localized, diffuse; client unable to point to one spot
- Aggravated by increased intraabdominal pressure (e.g., standing, walking, sexual intercourse, coughing, constipation, Valsalva maneuver)
- Pelvic pain is not affected by specific movements but gets worse toward the end of the day or after standing for a long time
- May be temporarily relieved by position change (e.g., getting off feet, resting or elevating the legs, putting the feet up)
- Pelvic pain is not reduced or eliminated by scar or soft tissue mobilization or by trigger point release of myofascial structures in the pelvic cavity
- Positive McBurney's, pinch an inch test, or iliopsoas/obturator sign (see Chapter 9)
- Presence of vulvar varicosities (seen most often in women with pelvic floor congestion syndrome and pregnancy)

Associated Signs and Symptoms
- Discharge from vagina or penis
- Urologic signs or symptoms
- Unreported abdominal pain
- Dyspareunia (painful or difficult intercourse)
- Constitutional symptoms
- Missed menses or unexplained/unexpected spotting (light staining of blood) (e.g., ectopic pregnancy), ask about shoulder pain
- Headache, fatigue, irritability

*Many of the histories listed are also *risk factors* for pelvic pain. Regarding pelvic girdle pain, according to the European Guidelines for the Diagnosis and Treatment of Pelvic Girdle Pain, red and yellow flags are the same for low back pain and pelvic girdle pain, with the possible exception of age (pelvic girdle pain affects younger individuals less than 30 years old and is less likely to be caused by malignancy).[38]

or underactive. Most conditions that affect the pelvic structures are found in women, but men may also experience PFM impairment and pain. Sexual assault, anal intercourse, prostate infection, prostate or colon cancer in advanced stages, bladder or kidney infection, and sexually transmitted disease (STD) are the most common causes for men. Prostate problems such as benign prostatic hyperplasia or prostatitis can cause lower abdominal, back, thigh, or pelvic pain. These conditions are discussed in Chapter 11.

Clinical Presentation

In the screening process, clinical presentation and especially pain patterns are very important. Mechanisms of viscerogenic pain (i.e., how these patterns develop) are discussed in Chapter 3.

Pelvic pain may be visceral pain, caused by stimulation of autonomic nerves (T11-S3); somatic pain, caused by stimulation of sensory nerve endings in the pudendal nerves (S2, S3); or peritoneal pain, caused by pressure from inflammation, infection, or obstruction of the lining of the pelvic cavity.

Peritoneal pain may be caused by disruption of the autonomic nerve supply of the visceral pelvic peritoneum, which covers the upper third of the bladder, the body of the uterus, and the upper third of the rectum and the rectosigmoid junction. It is not sensitive to touch but responds with pain on traction, distention, spasm, or ischemia of the viscus.

Peritoneal pain may also occur in relation to the parietal pelvic peritoneum, which covers the upper half of the lateral wall of the pelvis and the upper two thirds of the sacral hollow—all supplied by somatic nerves. These somatic nerves also supply corresponding segmental areas of the skin and muscles of the trunk and the anterior abdominal wall. Painful stimulation of the parietal pelvic peritoneum may cause referred segmental pain and spasm of the iliopsoas muscle and muscles of the anterior abdominal wall.

Abdominal pain can be classified as intraabdominal pain (related to the organs), abdominal wall pain (related to the abdominal muscle itself or its related connective tissue), or referred pain. Studies show abdominal wall tenderness is present in up to 28% of patients with abdominal pain.[49] Multiple case series have been published over the years on abdominal wall pain.[50,51] Carnett's test can be useful in distinguishing abdominal muscle pain and dysfunction from organ pain. The test has a sensitivity of 81% and a specificity of 88%.[52] It is performed with the patient in the hook-lying position while the therapist systematically palpates the abdominal wall. When a painful area is located, the therapist holds pressure on the tender spot while the patient engages the abdominal muscle with a straight leg raise or a head lift. The patient is asked to report the change in pain.

Increased pain in the palpated area with abdominal contraction is a positive Carnett's test and is indicative of abdominal muscle pathology. In this case, physical therapy treatments directed at the abdominal muscle are often effective in alleviating the pain. Injections have also been used with good success.[53] A decrease in pain reported by the patient during abdominal contraction is related to organ dysfunction

as the abdominal muscle has lifted the therapist's finger off of the painful structure below. In some cases the patient may feel the pain is unchanged. This may be related to abdominal muscle dysfunction and/or organ dysfunction. Therapists should work closely with physicians to ensure comprehensive treatment.[49-53]

Knowing the characteristics of pain patterns typical of each system is essential. When the client describes these patterns, the therapist can recognize them for what they are and to see how the clinical presentation differs from neuromuscular or musculoskeletal impairment and dysfunction.

Pelvic disease may cause primary pelvic pain and may also refer pain to the low back, thigh, groin, and rectum. Usually, pelvic disease appears as an acute illness with sudden onset of severe pain accompanied by nausea and vomiting, fever, and abdominal pain. Mild-to-moderate back or pelvic pain that becomes worse as the day progresses may be associated with a gynecologic disorder. The therapist is more likely to see the atypical presentation of systemically related central lumbar and sacral pain, which is easily mistaken for mechanical pain.

Associated Signs and Symptoms

When collecting pertinent personal and family history, conducting a risk factor assessment, and evaluating the client's pain pattern, the therapist should listen and look for any yellow or red flags. From there, the therapist should formulate any additional questions that may be appropriate based on data collected so far. Before leaving the screening task, the therapist should ask a few final questions. The first is about the presence of any associated signs and symptoms.

For example, perhaps the client has pelvic pain and unreported shoulder pain. The client may not think their previously unreported shoulder pain has any connection to the current pelvic pain. Furthermore, the female client may not recognize that the presence of vaginal discharge is linked in any way to her low back and pelvic pain. Discharge from the vagina or penis (yellow or green, with or without an odor) in the presence of low back, pelvic, or sacral pain may be a red flag.

To bring this information out and make any of these connections, the therapist must ask about the presence of any associated signs and symptoms. Ask the client the following:

❓ FOLLOW UP QUESTIONS

- Do you have any symptoms anywhere else in your body? Tell me even if you do not think they are related to your pelvic pain.

If the client says "No," then ask about the presence of urologic symptoms and constitutional symptoms, and look for a connection between the menstrual cycle and symptoms. If it appears that there may be a gynecologic basis for the client's symptoms, the therapist may want to ask some additional questions about missed menses, shoulder pain, and spotting or bleeding.

The therapist should assess for the presence of dysmenorrhea, defined as painful cramping during menstruation. Dysmenorrhea may be primary (of unknown cause) or secondary, as a result of a pelvic pathologic condition related to endometriosis, intrauterine tumors or polyps (myomas), uterine prolapse, pelvic inflammatory disease (PID), cervical stenosis, and adenomyosis (benign invasive growths of the endometrium into the muscular layers of the uterus).

Dysmenorrhea is characterized by spasmodic, cramp-like pain that comes and goes in waves and radiates over the lower abdomen and pelvis, thighs, and low back, sometimes accompanied by headache, irritability, mental depression, fatigue, and GI symptoms. Most women have some discomfort during menstruation. Clients with dysmenorrhea have significant pain that limits function.

Screening for Neuromuscular and Musculoskeletal Causes of Pelvic and Pelvic Floor Muscle and Pelvic Girdle Pain

Neurologic disorders (e.g., nerve entrapment, incomplete spinal cord lesion, multiple sclerosis, Parkinson's, stroke, pudendal neuralgia) can cause pelvic pain and dysfunction. Pudendal nerve entrapment is characterized by perineal pain while sitting on hard surfaces and pain relief when sitting on a toilet seat or standing; elimination of symptoms after a pudendal nerve block is diagnostic.

Muscles most likely to cause or refer pain to the pelvic area include the levator ani, abdominals, quadratus lumborum, and iliopsoas.[54-56] The therapist looks for a contributing history, such as a fall on the buttocks, pregnancy, or trauma. Avulsion of hamstrings from a sports injury may be reported. Trauma from physical or sexual assault may remain unreported and screening for assault is an important part of many evaluations (see Chapter 2).

PFM tension myalgia can present suprapubically, perineally, and/or in the low buttock/anal areas. Excessive PFM tension can be the origin or missing piece of nonresolving musculoskeletal pelvic pain.

When evaluating low back or pelvic pain, the therapist should assess for pelvic floor laxity or tension, psoas abscess, tender points, history of birth or sexual trauma, and the presence of any associated signs and symptoms.

Prevention and treatment of symptoms is an important issue for therapists who work in the area of women's health.[57,58] PFM tension myalgia may manifest as dyspareunia (pain during or after intercourse). Overactivity (pain and spasm; muscles contract when they should relax or do not relax completely)[59] of the PFM and pelvic floor tender points can contribute to superficial or deep dyspareunia. Deep thrust dyspareunia may also be related to organ disease, SI, or low back impairment. Dyspareunia symptoms that are reduced in alternate positions may indicate a musculoskeletal component, especially when other signs and symptoms characteristic of musculoskeletal impairment are also present.[60,61] It is very helpful to screen all pelvic and low back pain patients for dyspareunia.

Other symptoms that can indicate the need for a PFM examination include pain in the perineum especially while sitting, pain with ejaculation, painful defecation and constipation, and urinary urgency.

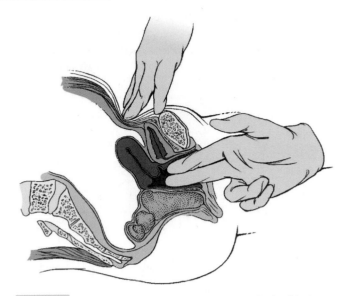

Fig. 16.2 Pelvic examination. With the woman in the lithotomy position (supine with hips and knees flexed and feet in stirrups), the examiner inserts one or two gloved fingers into the vaginal canal up to the point of the cervix or soft tissue obstruction. The examiner applies firm pressure in the lower abdomen above the bladder while the woman bears down slightly as if performing a Valsalva maneuver. The examiner evaluates the tone of the pelvic floor and the position of the uterus during this test. Integrity of the pelvic floor (e.g., muscle tone, laxity, trigger points) can also be tested.

For therapists trained in PFM examination, external and internal palpation of the pelvic floor musculature is helpful.[62,63] Examination also includes observation for varicosities and assessment of muscle tone (muscle overactivity [pain and spasm] or underactivity [laxity with weakness and leaking]) and the presence of tender points (Fig. 16.2).[54,64,65]

Many clients who experience low back, pelvic, SI, sacral, or groin pain have unrecognized pelvic floor impairment.[66] Fig. 16.3 gives a simple representation of how the puborectalis muscle acts as a sling around various structures of the pelvis. The condition and position of the pelvic sling are very important in the maintenance of normal pelvic floor health.

Fig. 15.1 provides a visual reminder that the muscles of the pelvic floor support the reproductive organs and the viscera in the peritoneum. Any impairment of these organs may cause impairment of the PFM and vice versa. PGP can occur separately or be combined with low back pain and is defined as generally present between the posterior iliac crest (PSIS) and the gluteal fold in the vicinity of the SI joint. Pain may radiate to the posterior thigh; endurance for standing, walking, and sitting is decreased.[67] PGP occurs most often during pregnancy and postpartum and may continue many years postpartum. Pain provocation tests for the symphysis pubis and SI joint (e.g., Patrick's/Faber's, modified Trendelenburg, Gaenslen's, shear, posterior pelvic pain provocation test [P4], gapping, and compression tests), palpation, and mobility testing help point to pelvic girdle impairment. The P4 test or thigh thrust is a SI dysfunction test which can be used for nonpregnant and pregnancy-related PGP.[52] Reliability and validity of the provocation tests mentioned here have been evaluated

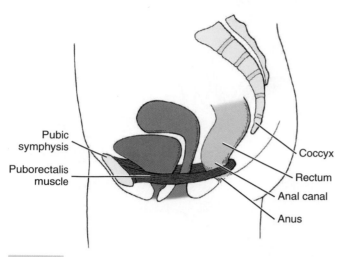

Pubic symphysis

Puborectalis muscle

Coccyx

Rectum

Anal canal

Anus

Fig. 16.3 Pelvic sling. Puborectalis muscle forms a U-shaped sling encircling the posterior aspect of the rectum and returns along the opposite side of the levator hiatus to the posterior surface of the pubis. This shows how the condition and position of the pelvic sling contribute to the function of the pelvic floor and the encircled viscera. Obesity, multiparity, and prolonged pushing during labor and delivery are just a few of life's events that can disrupt the integrity of the pelvic sling and the pelvic floor. (From Myers RS: *Saunders manual of physical therapy practice*, Philadelphia, 1995, WB Saunders.)

and reported; for details see the Vleeming and Olsen references.[67,68] Imaging tests, such as x-rays, computed tomography, and MRI help rule out problems such as fractures, ankylosing spondylitis, and reactive arthritis.[67] The therapist must be able to identify pain originating from the SI and pubic symphysis joints (PGP), avoiding the under-reporting or over-reporting of the condition to achieve an accurate diagnosis and subsequently an effective treatment.

Many women have both PFM tension myalgia and PGP, requiring each to be addressed externally and internally. These conditions have a significant effect on daily life for many women.[57,58,68]

It is always important to screen for PFM tension myalgia. In the absence of reported associated factors, the treatment strategy may be to address the PGP first; if it does not resolve, then a PFM examination may be needed to confirm pelvic floor impairment.

Anterior Pelvic Pain

Anterior pelvic pain occurs most often as a result of disorders of the hip joint, including inflammatory arthritis; upper lumbar vertebrae disk disease (rare at these segments); pregnancy with separation of the symphysis pubis; local injury to the insertion of the rectus abdominis, rectus femoris, or adductor muscle; femoral neuralgia; abdominal muscle tender points (Carnett's test); and psoas abscess.

Stress reactions of the pubis or ilium, sometimes called *stress fractures* (disruption of the bone at the tendon-bone interface without displacement from repetitive contraction), can occur during traumatic labor and delivery, but they are more common in osteomalacia and Paget's disease and produce anterior pelvic pain. Traumatic stress reactions may also occur in joggers, military personnel, and athletes.

Although the underlying pathology differs, symptoms are similar to separation of the symphysis pubis and pelvic ring disruption, and may include pain in the involved areas that is aggravated by active motion of the limb or deep pressure and weight-bearing during ambulation. Symptoms from pelvic instability, as a result of pelvic ring injury or disruption (whether from birth trauma in women of childbearing age or pelvic stress fracture in an older adult with osteoporosis), may be aggravated by a single leg stance.[69,70]

Femoral hernia, considered rare, accounting for less than 5% of all hernias, is typically seen in women (4:1 ratio to men) because of their wider hip bone structure and enlarged femoral ring. Femoral hernias are more common in multiparous women than in nonparous women.[71] Interestingly, 60% of femoral hernias occur on the right side, 30% on the left, and 10% bilaterally.[72] Typically, femoral hernias occur just below the inguinal ligament and the referred pain pattern may be located down the medial side of the thigh to the knee; inguinal hernias are likely to cause groin pain. Immediate surgical repair is indicated.

Posterior Pelvic Pain

Posterior pelvic pain originating in the lumbosacral, SI, coccygeal, and sacrococcygeal regions usually appears as localized in the lower lumbar spine, pelvic girdle, and over the sacrum, often radiating over the SI ligaments. Pain radiating from the SI joint can commonly be felt in both the buttock and the posterior thigh and is often aggravated by rotation of the lumbar spine on the pelvis. A proximal hamstring injury, including avulsion of the ischial epiphysis in the adolescent, may also cause posterior pelvic and buttock pain.

Coccygodynia and sacrococcygeal pain are more common in women and are often associated with a fall on the buttocks or traumatic childbirth. They manifest with the person having difficulty sitting on firm surfaces and having pain in the coccygeal region during defecation or straining.

PFM tension myalgia (aka levator ani syndrome) may produce symptoms of pain, pressure, and discomfort in the rectum, vagina, perirectal area, or low back. The levator ani refers to a group of muscles deep in the pelvic floor and includes the puborectal and coccygeous. Overactivity in the PFMs, levator ani syndrome, and tension myalgia all refer to overactivity (pain and spasm) and tenderness in the muscles of the pelvic floor. These conditions may occur in men and women and may be caused by chronic prostatitis that does not resolve with antibiotics (men), vaginal infections (women), bladder dysfunction (interstitial cystitis), bowel dysfunction (IBS), neurologic abnormalities in the lumbosacral spine, sexual assault or trauma, or anal fissures from anal intercourse. Pain or rectal pressure may occur during sexual intercourse, as may throbbing pain during bowel movement with accompanying constipation and impaired bowel and bladder function.

Screening for Gynecologic Causes of Pelvic Pain

Pregnancy, multiparity, and prolonged labor and delivery (especially combined with obesity) are risk factors for

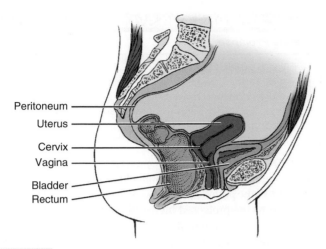

Fig. 16.4 Normal female reproductive anatomy (sagittal view). Locate the rectum, uterus, bladder, vagina, and cervix in this illustration. Note the size, shape, and orientation of each of these structures. The rectum turns away from the viewer in this sagittal section, giving it the appearance of ending with no connection to the intestines. Understanding the normal orientation of these structures will help when each of the diseases that can cause low back pain is considered.

gynecologic conditions that can alter the normal position of the bladder, uterus, and rectum in relation to one another (Fig. 16.4), resulting in pelvic organ prolapse such as rectocele, cystocele, and prolapsed uterus with concomitant pelvic floor pain and impairment.

Gynecologic causes of PFM pain are most often produced by inflammatory processes (including infection), neoplasia, or trauma. Also, PGP may be associated with pregnancy and endometriosis. Variations in the angle and position of the uterus occur from woman to woman and from day to day in the same woman (Fig. 16.5). Uterine position rarely causes pain.

Children younger than 14 years rarely experience pelvic pain of gynecologic origin. Infection is the most likely cause and is limited to the vulva and vagina. Theoretically, infection can ascend to involve the peritoneal cavity, causing iliopsoas abscess and pelvic, hip, or groin pain, but this rarely happens in this age group.

Ectopic Pregnancy

Pelvic pain associated with a normal pregnancy is similar to low back pain, as was discussed earlier in Chapter 15. About 1% of all pregnancies occur outside of the endometrium (ectopic), with most ectopic implantations occurring in the fallopian tube (Fig. 16.6). Risk factors include tubal ligation; STD; PID; infertility or infertility treatment; previous tubal, pelvic, or abdominal surgery; or the use of intrauterine contraceptive devices (IUCDs) such as rings, loops, coils, or T-shaped devices (see Fig. 15.6).

Symptoms of ectopic pregnancy most often include unexplained vaginal spotting, bursts of bleeding, and sudden lower abdominal and pelvic cramping shortly after the first missed menstrual period. At first, the pain may be a vague "twinge" or soreness on the affected side; later it can be sharp and severe.

CLINICAL SIGNS AND SYMPTOMS
Ectopic Pregnancy

- Unexplained vaginal bleeding (spotting), missed menses
- Sudden, unexplained lower abdominal and pelvic cramping (especially after first missed menstrual period); usually unilateral
- Pain may be mild, progressing to severe over a matter of hours to days
- Low back (unilateral or bilateral) or shoulder pain (unilateral)
- Hypotension (low blood pressure and pulse rate), shock (tubal rupture)

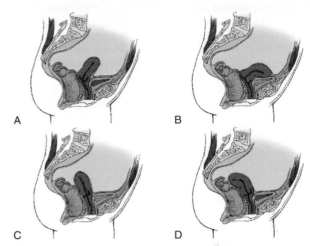

Fig. 16.5 Abnormal positions of the uterus. Variations in the angle and position of the uterus occur from woman to woman. Each illustration depicts a slightly different anatomic position of the uterus. **A**, Midline position. Usually, the uterus is above and parallel to the bladder. In the midline position, the uterus is more vertical. **B**, Anteflexed uterus. The uterus is in its proper position above the bladder, but the upper one third to one half of the body is flexed forward. **C**, Retroverted uterus. About 20% of American women have a tilted, or retroverted, uterus. The top of the uterus naturally slants toward the spine rather than toward the umbilicus. **D**, Retroflexed uterus. An extremely tilted uterus called *retroflexion* may even bend down toward the tailbone. A woman with a retroflexed uterus may be unable to use a tampon or a diaphragm. Back pain is more likely to occur with pregnancy and labor for the woman with a retroverted or retroflexed uterus.

Gradual hemorrhage causes pelvic (and sometimes low back or shoulder) pain and pressure, but rapid hemorrhage results in hypotension or shock. Tubal rupture is common and requires medical attention and diagnosis.

Prolapsed Conditions

Prolapse is the collapse, or downward displacement of structures such as the uterus, bladder, or rectum. This condition occasionally causes low back pain, often causes perineal pressure but rarely causes pain.

Uterovaginal prolapse may rarely cause low-grade and persistent pelvic pain. Prolapse may result from a combination of the effects of pregnancy and delivery, postmenopausal hormone changes, surgical cutting of pelvic ligaments (i.e., during hysterectomy), and poor PFM support. Obesity combined with chronic cough, constipation, and multiparity is a

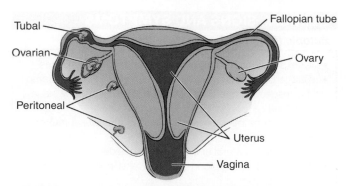

Fig. 16.6 Ectopic pregnancy. An ectopic pregnancy can occur when the egg is fertilized and implanted outside of the uterus. The ovum can be embedded inside the ovary (ovarian pregnancy), inside the fallopian tube (tubal pregnancy), or anywhere between the ovary and the uterus, including along the outside lining of the uterus (extrauterine) or inside the abdominal cavity along the peritoneum as shown. Rupture of the ovum and hemorrhage is the usual result. If this occurs early in the menstrual cycle, the woman may experience heavier bleeding than usual but remain unaware of the failed pregnancy.

common contributing factor to prolapse. All prolapse can be graded as first, second, or third degree.

Uterine Prolapse. Uterine prolapse occurs most often after childbirth (Fig. 16.7). Secondary prolapse may occur with prolonged pushing during labor and delivery, large intrapelvic tumors, or sacral nerve trauma, or it may follow pelvic or abdominal surgery.

The pain of prolapse is central, suprapubic, and dragging in the groin, and a sensation of a lump at the vaginal opening is noted. Pain is primarily as a result of stretching of the ligamentous support structures (uterosacral ligament attaches to the sacrum; loss of ligamentous integrity contributes to significant biomechanical changes) and secondarily to excoriation (scratch or abrasion) of the prolapsed cervical or vaginal tissue, which may occur.

Third-degree prolapse may be accompanied by low back pain with pelvic, sacral, or abdominal heaviness. Symptoms are relieved by rest and lying down and are often aggravated by prolonged standing, walking, coughing, or straining. Urinary incontinence may be associated with uterine prolapse.

Some women use a removable device called a *pessary* for a prolapsed uterus, bladder, or rectum. It is placed in the vagina to support the prolapsed structure. These devices may be considered temporary and should be used in conjunction with a program to rehabilitate the PFM impairment. Long-term use of such devices may be required when surgical repair is not possible or the woman is not a good surgical candidate.

Identifying the presence of uterine prolapse does not necessarily require medical referral. Conservative care provided by a specialized pelvic physical therapist can be very helpful for the woman and may be the first step in treatment. Client education about gravity-assisted positions for repositioning the uterus can be very helpful. For example, the supine position with a pillow or wedge support under the pelvis is a helpful rest position and can be used while the patient is doing PFM exercises. It is also a more comfortable position for sexual intercourse for some women.

CLINICAL SIGNS AND SYMPTOMS
Uterine Prolapse

- Bulge in vaginal opening
- Pelvic pressure, perineal heaviness, backache
- Symptoms relieved by lying down
- Symptoms made worse by prolonged standing, walking, coughing, or straining

Cystocele and Rectocele. Cystocele is the protrusion of the anterior vaginal wall against the wall of the vagina. Rectocele is a protrusion of the posterior vaginal wall into the vagina (Fig. 16.8).

Similar to the prolapsed uterus, these two pelvic floor disorders occur most often after pregnancy and childbirth but may also be associated with surgery and obesity (especially obesity combined with multiple pregnancies and births). These conditions are the result of PFM weakness or structural overstretching of the pelvic musculature or ligamentous structures. Patient history may include prolonged labor, bearing down before full dilation, instrument delivery (e.g., forceps, vacuum suction), chronic cough, or lifting of heavy objects.

Trauma to the pudendal or sacral nerves during birth and delivery is an additional risk factor. Decreased muscle tone as a result of aging, complications of pelvic surgery, or excessive straining during bowel movements may also result in prolapse. Pelvic tumors and neurologic conditions, such as spina bifida and diabetic neuropathy, which interrupt the innervation of pelvic muscles, can also increase the risk of prolapse.

CLINICAL SIGNS AND SYMPTOMS
Cystocele

- Urinary frequency and urgency
- In advanced stages, difficulty emptying the bladder
- Cystitis (bladder infection)
- Bulge or pressure sensation in the perineal area
- Urinary incontinence

Rectocele

- Perineal pressure and bulge
- Straining to defecate
- Feeling of incomplete rectal emptying
- Constipation

Endometriosis

Endometriosis (see Chapter 15) is a pathologic condition of retrograde menstruation. Tissue resembling the mucous membrane lining the uterus occurs outside the normal location in the uterus but within the pelvic cavity, including the ovaries, pelvic peritoneum, bowel, and diaphragm. It occurs most often during the reproductive years and in up to 50% of women with infertility.[73–75] Severity of pain is related more to the site than to the extent of disease.

Pelvic pain associated with endometriosis can be referred to the low back, rectum, and lower sacral or coccygeal region, starting each month several days up to a week before onset of menstruation and improving after cessation of menstrual flow. As the condition progresses, pain continues throughout the cycle, with exacerbation at menstruation and, finally, constant severity.

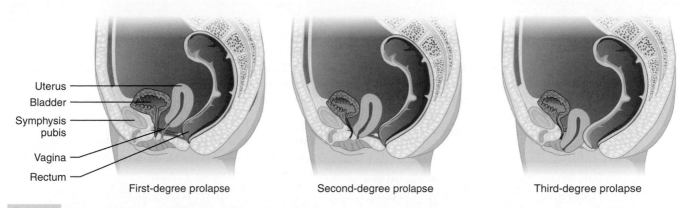

Fig. 16.7   Stages of uterine prolapse. Herniation of the uterus through the pelvic floor resulting in protrusion into the vagina. First-degree: the cervix remains in the vagina. Second-degree: the cervix appears at the perineum on straining. Third-degree: the entire uterus protrudes outside the body, and there is total inversion of the vagina. (From Goodman CC, Fuller KS: *Pathology: implications for the physical therapist*, ed 4, St Louis, 2013, Elsevier.)

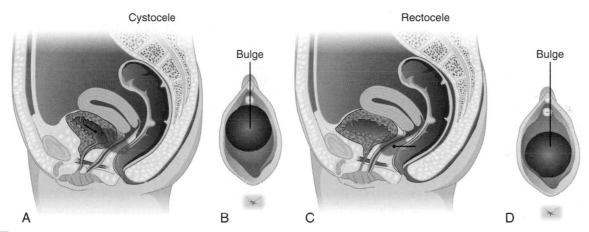

Fig. 16.8   **A**, Cystocele (sagittal view). Note the bulging of the anterior vaginal wall. The urinary bladder is displaced downward. **B**, Lithotomy view. The bladder pushes the anterior vaginal wall downward into the vagina. **C**, Rectocele (sagittal view). **D**, Note the bulging of the posterior vaginal wall associated with rectocele (lithotomy view). (From Goodman CC, Fuller KS: *Pathology: implications for the physical therapist*, ed 4, St Louis, 2013, Elsevier.)

Other symptoms may include rectal discomfort during bowel movements, diarrhea, constipation, recurrent miscarriage, and infertility. Box 16.5 has more information on this condition.

Chronic Pelvic Pain

Although a pathologic cause can be identified for most cases of chronic pelvic pain, a small percentage remains for which no physical cause can be determined. Women with chronic pelvic pain are usually 25 to 40 years of age and have at least one child. The symptoms are of at least 2 years' duration (and often many more), with acute exacerbation from time to time.

Pain associated with chronic pelvic pain is vague and poorly localized, although it is usually confined to the lower abdomen and pelvis, radiating to the groin and upper and inner thighs. Other symptoms include dyspareunia, menstrual changes, low back pain, urinary and bowel changes, fatigue, and obvious anxiety and depression.

Screening for Infectious Causes of Pelvic Girdle Pain

Infection is the most common cause of systemically induced pelvic pain. Infection or inflammation within the pelvis from acute appendicitis, diverticulitis, Crohn's disease, osteomyelitis, septic arthritis of the SI joint, urologic disorders, sexually transmitted infection (STI; e.g., *Chlamydia trachomatis*), and salpingitis (inflammation of the fallopian tube) can produce visceral and somatic pelvic pain because of the involvement of the parietal peritoneum.

Secondary pelvic infection may follow surgery, septic abortion, pregnancy, or recent birth as a result of the entry of endogenous bacteria into the damaged pelvic tissues. PID and STI are the most common causes of infection in women.

All of these disorders have similar signs and symptoms during the acute phase. The client may not have any pain but will report low back or pelvic "discomfort," or there may be a report of acute, sharp, severe aching on both sides of the

---

BOX 16.5   RESOURCES

Endometriosis*

- Endometriosis Zone, a service of The Universe of Women's Health—a commercial organization directed by a board of obstetricians and gynecologists. Information is directed at medical professionals, the medical industry, and women. The Endometriosis Zone is found at both of the following websites:
  http://www.endozone.org
  http://www.endometriosiszone.org
- Endometriosis Research Center (ERC) was started as a lobbying organization. The goal of the ERC is to bring science and support together through education. http://www.endocenter.org or call (800) 239-7280.
- The International Endometriosis Association (IEA) was established by Mary Lou Ballweg, RN, PhD, as an advocacy organization for endometriosis; offers online support for women diagnosed with endometriosis. http://www.endometriosisassn.org
- The National Library of Medicine offers an interactive tutorial about endometriosis in both English and Spanish online at
  http://www.nlm.nih.gov/medlineplus/tutorials/endometriosis

Pelvic Inflammatory Disease (PID)

- The National Women's Health Information Center (NWHIC) offers information on all aspects of women's health, including PID; (1-800-994-9662) or online at http://www.4woman.gov/
- Centers for Disease Control and Prevention (CDC) provides a PID fact sheet online at http://www.cdc.gov/std/PID/STDFact-PID.htm

- Mount Auburn Obstetrics & Gynecologic Associates, Cincinnati, OH, a group of obstetric and gynecologic (OBGYN) professionals offers online education about endometriosis and other OBGYN topics online at http://www.mtauburnobgyn.com/pid.html

Pelvic Pain

- Fall M, Baranowski AP, Elneil S: *Guidelines on chronic pelvic pain*, Arnhem, The Netherlands, 2008, European Association of Urology (EAU).
- Vleeming A: European guidelines for the diagnosis and treatment of pelvic girdle pain, *Eur Spine J* 17(6):794–819, 2008.
- The American College of Obstetricians and Gynecologists (ACOG) offers information, education, and publications related to a wide variety of women's health issues online at
  http://www.acog.org/
  The ACOG has recently issued a new practice bulletin on chronic pelvic pain in women. The guidelines were published as ACOG Practice Bulletin No. 51. Chronic Pelvic Pain, *Obstet Gynecol* 103(3):589–605, 2004. To read more about these guidelines, go to the following website: http://www.medscape.com/viewarticle/471545
- The International Pelvic Pain Society is a professional organization with the goal to enhance and improve the treatment of diseases that cause pelvic pain in men and women. Education for health care professionals is a major focus of this organization, which can be reached online at http://www.pelvicpain.org/

*Data from Deevey S: Endometriosis: Internet resources. *Med Ref Serv Q* 24(1):67–77, Spring 2005.

---

pelvis. Accompanying groin discomfort may radiate to the inner aspects of the thigh.

Keep in mind that in the older adult, the first sign of any infection might not be an elevated temperature, but rather, confusion, increased confusion, or some other change in mental status.

Right-sided abdominal or pelvic inflammatory pain is often associated with appendicitis, whereas left-sided pain is more likely associated with diverticulitis, constipation, or obstipation (left sigmoid impaction). Left-sided appendicitis is possible and not that uncommon.[76] Bilateral pain may indicate infection. The pain may be aggravated by increased abdominal pressure (e.g., coughing, walking). Knowing these pain patterns helps the therapist quickly decide what questions to ask and which associated signs and symptoms to look for. The therapist should test for iliopsoas or obturator abscesses (see Chapter 9).

Other red-flag symptoms may be reported in response to specific questions about disturbances in urination, odorous vaginal discharge, tachycardia, dyspareunia (painful or difficult intercourse), or constitutional symptoms such as fever, general malaise, and nausea and vomiting.

Pelvic Inflammatory Disease

PID consists of a variety of conditions (i.e., it is not a single entity), including endometritis, salpingitis, tubo-ovarian abscess, and pelvic peritonitis. Any inflammatory condition that affects the female reproductive organs (uterus, fallopian tubes, ovaries, cervix) may come under the diagnostic label of PID.[77]

PID is a bacterial infection of the female reproductive organs and is often associated with an STI/STD. Infection can be introduced through the skin, vagina, or GI tract. It can be an acute, one-time episode or may be chronic with multiple recurrences.

It is estimated that two thirds of all cases are caused by STIs such as chlamydia and gonorrhea.[78] Chlamydia is a bacterial STI that is acquired through vaginal, oral, or anal intercourse. It is often asymptomatic but can present with vaginal bleeding and discharge and burning during urination. Pelvic pain does not occur until chlamydia leads to PID. When detected and treated early, chlamydia is relatively easy to cure.

A direct relationship has been observed between early age of first sexual intercourse, the number of sexual partners a woman has, a recent new partner (within previous 3 months), and a history of STD (in the client or her partner) or risk of STD (especially human papillomavirus [HPV], a risk factor for cervical cancer).[79–81] PID may occur if chlamydia is not treated; even if it is treated, damage to the pelvic cavity cannot be reversed. The more partners a woman has, the greater the risk of PID.[77]

Other risk factors include interruption of the cervical barrier through pregnancy termination, insertion of an intra-uterine device within the past 6 weeks, in vitro fertilization/intrauterine insemination, or any other instrumentation of the uterus.[77]

PID associated with scarring in the pelvic organs, including the ovaries, fallopian tubes, bowel, and bladder, may cause chronic pain. Women can be left infertile because of damage and scarring to the fallopian tubes. After a single episode of PID, a woman's risk of ectopic pregnancy increases sevenfold compared with the risk for women who have no history of PID.[82,83]

CLINICAL SIGNS AND SYMPTOMS

Pelvic Inflammatory Disease

- Often asymptomatic
- Abnormal vaginal discharge or bleeding
- Burning during urination (dysuria)
- Moderate (dull aching) to severe lower abdominal and/or pelvic pain; back pain is possible
- Painful intercourse (dyspareunia)
- Painful menstruation
- Constitutional symptoms (fever, chills, nausea, vomiting)

STIs such as chlamydia and syphilis are on the rise among America's sexually active young adult population (ages 18 to 25 years).[84] In fact, chlamydia was the most commonly reported infectious disease in the United States in 2004. According to the Centers for Disease Control and Prevention annual report, the highest rates of chlamydia occur in sexually active women aged 15 to 19 years. Syphilis predominates in men who engage in risky sexual behavior (e.g., unprotected vaginal, anal, oral sex) with men or with men and women.[83,85–88]

It does not happen often, but there may be times when the therapist must ask about the possibility of an STI. Sexually active women with vague symptoms are the most likely group to be interviewed about STIs/STDs. See specific screening questions in Chapter 15 and Appendix B-32 in the accompanying enhanced eBook version included with print purchase of this textbook.

Any of the red flags listed in Box 16.4 in the presence of pelvic pain raises the suspicion of a medical problem. Medical referral must be made as quickly as possible. Early medical intervention can prevent the spread of infection and septicemia, and can preserve fertility. See Box 16.5 for resources that can provide more information on this and other conditions.

Screening for Vascular Causes of Pelvic Girdle Pain

Vascular problems that affect the pelvic cavity and pelvic floor musculature have two primary causes. The first is the general condition of PVD; the second is a specific example of PVD called *pelvic congestion syndrome* (PCS) from ovarian and/or vulvar varicosities (abnormal enlargement of veins). Other conditions, such as abdominal angina and abdominal aneurysm, are less common vascular causes of pelvic pain; these conditions are discussed in greater detail in Chapter 7.

Peripheral Vascular Disease

The iliac arteries may become gradually occluded by atherosclerosis or may be obstructed by an embolus. The resultant ischemia produces pain in the affected limb but may also give rise to pelvic pain. Whether the occlusion is thrombotic or embolic, the client may report pain in the pelvis, affected limb, and possibly the buttocks.

The pain is characteristically aggravated by exercise (claudication). Typically, symptoms develop 5 or 10 minutes after the client has started the activity. This lag time is characteristic of a vascular pain pattern associated with atherosclerosis or blood vessel occlusion.

Musculoskeletal causes of pelvic pain are also made worse by activity and exercise, especially weight-bearing exercise, but the timing is not as predictable as it is with pain from vascular causes. Musculoskeletal conditions may cause pain immediately (e.g., with muscle strain or trigger points) or, more likely, after prolonged activity or exercise. With vascular occlusion, the affected limb becomes colder and paler. In sudden occlusion, diminished sensation to pinprick may be observed during the examination. Femoral and distal arteries should be palpated for pulsation.

Thrombosis of the large iliac veins may occur spontaneously after injury to the lower limb and pelvis, or it may appear after pelvic surgical procedures. An estimated 30% of clients have asymptomatic deep vein thrombosis after major surgery. Thrombosis that occludes the iliac vein produces an enlarged, warm, and painful leg; occasionally, discomfort in the pelvis is noted.

Anyone with PVD can demonstrate the same kind of symptoms in the pelvic floor structures. The most likely age group to be affected by vascular disease is adults over 60 years of age, especially women who are postmenopausal.

Watch for a history of heart disease with a clinical presentation of pelvic, buttock, and leg pain that is aggravated by activity or exercise (claudication). Look for changes in skin and temperature on the affected side (arterial occlusion or venous thrombosis), especially in the presence of known heart disease or recent pelvic surgery (see Box 4.13; Case Example 16.2).

Pelvic Congestion Syndrome

Varicose veins of the ovaries (varicosities) cause the blood in the veins to flow downward rather than up toward the heart. They are a manifestation of PVD and a potential cause of chronic pelvic pain. The condition has been called PCS or ovarian varicocele. PCS is manifested as intermittent or constant pain of at least 3 to 6 months' duration, localized in the abdomen or pelvis. It is not limited to any period of the menstrual cycle or intercourse, and is not associated with

CASE EXAMPLE 16.2

Pelvic and Buttock Pain

A 34-year-old man with leukemia had a routine bone marrow biopsy near the left posterior superior iliac crest. No problems were noted at the time of biopsy, but 2 days later, the man came into physical therapy complaining of pelvic girdle pain.

He said his platelet count was 50,000/uL and international normalized ratio (INR), a measure of clotting time, was "normal." Laboratory values were recorded on the day of the biopsy.

The only clinical findings were a positive Faber's (Patrick's) test on the left and tenderness to palpation over the left sciatic notch, about 1 inch below the biopsy site. No abnormal neurologic signs were observed.

What are the red flags in this scenario?

Use the screening model to find the red flags and decide what to do.

History: Current history of cancer; recent history of biopsy

Clinical Presentation: Reduced platelet count (normal is >100,000 uL); new onset of painful symptoms within 48 hours of biopsy; tenderness to palpation in left buttock

Associated Signs and Symptoms: None. Client had no other signs and symptoms.

The therapist has to make a clinical judgment in a case like this. The platelet level is low, putting the client at risk for poor clotting and spontaneous bleeding, but the INR suggests that the body can initiate the coagulation cascade.

Given the timing between the biopsy and the symptoms, it is likely that the procedure caused an intramuscular hematoma. The diagnosis can be made with a computed tomography (CT) scan. The location of biopsy needle entry indicates that the gluteus medius was punctured. No major blood vessel is located in this area, so the problem is rare.

Pain after bone marrow biopsy is usually mild to moderate and gradually gets better. The use of ice, massage, and later, moist heat is safe when properly applied. Worsening buttock pain over the next 24 to 48 hours would necessitate a medical referral.

It is always a good idea to contact the primary care physician and report your findings and intended intervention. This gives the doctor the option to follow-up with the client immediately if he or she thinks it is warranted.

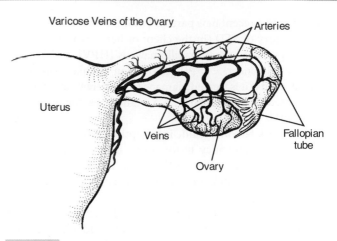

Fig. 16.9 Ovarian varicosities associated with pelvic congestion syndrome are the cause of chronic pelvic pain for women. This form of venous insufficiency is often accompanied by prominent varicose veins elsewhere in the lower quadrant (buttocks, thighs, calves). Men may have similar varicosities of the scrotum (not shown).

symptoms include pelvic pain that worsens toward the end of the day or after standing for a long time, pain after intercourse, sensation of heaviness in the pelvis, and prominent varicose veins elsewhere on the body, especially the buttocks and thighs.[90,93–95]

CLINICAL SIGNS AND SYMPTOMS

Pelvic Congestion Syndrome (Ovarian Varicosities)

- Lower abdominal/pelvic pain (intermittent or continuous, described as "dull aching" but can be sharp and severe)
- Tenderness during deep palpation of the ovarian point (located on the imaginary line drawn from the anterior superior iliac spine (ASIS) to the umbilicus where the upper one third meets the lower two thirds)[96]
- Unilateral or bilateral
- Pain that worsens with prolonged standing or at the end of the day
- Pain that is worse before or during menses
- Pain or "aching" that occurs after intercourse (dyspareunia)
- Presence of varicose veins in the buttocks, thighs, or lower extremities
- Low backache is a common feature, made worse by standing
- Other associated signs and symptoms (these vary; see text in the next section)

Other associated symptoms may vary and include vaginal discharge, headache, emotional distress, GI distress, constipation, and urinary frequency and urgency. An undetermined number of women also have endometriosis, but the relationship is unknown.[97,98] Varicosities may be large enough to compress the ureter, leading to these urologic symptoms. Fatigue (loss of energy) and insomnia are common in women who experience headache with PCS (Case Example 16.3).

Screening for Cancer as a Cause of Pelvic Pain

The female pelvis is a depository for malignant tissue after incomplete removal of a primary carcinoma within the pelvis,

pregnancy. PCS typically affects women of reproductive age who have had at least one child. PCS prevalence ranges from 2.1% to 24% in women aged 18 to 50 years.[89]

The specific impairment associated with PCS is an incompetent and dilated ovarian vein with retrograde blood flow (Fig. 16.9). Ovarian venous reflux and stasis produce venous dilatation, congestion, and pelvic pain. Imaging studies have verified that very few venous valves are found in the blood vessels of the pelvic area.[90–93]

Any compromise of the valves (or blood vessels) in the area can lead to this condition. It can also occur as the result of kidney removal or donation because the ovarian vein is cut when the kidney is removed. Varicosity of the gonadal venous plexus can occur in men and is more readily diagnosed by the presentation of observable varicosities of the scrotum.

Symptoms of ovarian varicosities reflect the vascular incompetence associated with venous insufficiency. These

CASE EXAMPLE 16.3

Pelvic Congestion Syndrome

If a woman presents with chronic pelvic girdle pain, how would you assess for a vascular problem? Or ovarian varicosities as a possible cause? Remember, we are not trying to make a medical diagnosis, but rather to look for clues to suggest when medical referral is required. Use the overall clues in our screening model.

What kind of *past medical history* and *risk factors* would you expect to see? With a vascular cause of pelvic girdle pain, a history of heart disease is often reported in a postmenopausal woman. With ovarian varicosities, multiparity is usually present (i.e., a woman who has had several full-term pregnancies and deliveries).

What would you expect to see in the *clinical presentation?* With a vascular cause of pelvic girdle pain, the client often reports pelvic, buttock, and leg pain or "discomfort" that is aggravated by activity or exercise. With varicosities, the client usually has a generalized dull ache in the lower abdominal/low back area that is worse after standing, after intercourse, or just at the end of the day.

When you ask the client what other symptoms are present, she may not have any other symptoms, but if she does, look for a cluster of vascular signs and symptoms. These can be found in Box 4.19.

With ovarian varicocele, visually observe for varicose veins in the legs. These are a prominent feature in the clinical presentation of most women with ovarian varicosities. Ask about the presence of associated signs and symptoms such as vaginal discharge, headache, gastrointestinal (GI) distress, insomnia, and urologic symptoms.

---

for recurrence of cancer after surgical resection or radiotherapy of a pelvic neoplasm, or metastatic deposits from a primary lesion elsewhere in the abdominal cavity.

Metastatic spread can occur from any primary tumor in the abdominal or pelvic cavity (see Fig. 14.2). For example, colon cancer can metastasize to the pelvic cavity by direct extension through the bowel wall to the musculoskeletal walls of the pelvic cavity or surrounding organs. This may produce fistulas into the small intestine, bladder, or vagina. Advanced rectal tumors can become "fixed" to the sacral hollow. Deep pain within the pelvis may indicate spread of neoplasm into the sacral nerve plexuses.

Cancer recurrence can also occur after radiotherapy or surgery to the abdominal or pelvic cavity. This happens most often when incomplete removal of the primary carcinoma has occurred.

Using the Screening Model for Cancer

In the case of cancer as a cause of pelvic pain, a *past history* of cancer is usually present, most commonly, cancer within the pelvic or abdominal cavity (e.g., GI, renal, reproductive). A history of cancer with recent surgical removal of tumor tissue followed by back, hip, sacral, pelvic, or PGP within the next 6 months is a major red flag. Even if it appears to be a clear

neuromuscular or musculoskeletal problem, referral is warranted for medical evaluation.

A common *clinical presentation* of pelvic or abdominal cancer referred to the soma is one of back, sacral, or pelvic pain described as one or more of the following: deep aching, colicky, constant with crescendo waves of pain that come and go, or diffuse pain. Usually, the client cannot point to it with one finger (i.e., pain does not localize).

The therapist must remember to ask whether the client is having any symptoms of any kind anywhere else in the body. This is vitally important! Signs and symptoms associated with pelvic pain can range from constitutional symptoms to symptoms more common with the GI, genitourinary, or reproductive system.

The therapist must ask about blood in the urine or stools. Once the physical therapy examination has been completed, including the history, risk factor assessment, pain patterns, and any associated signs and symptoms, it is time to step back and conduct a Review of Systems (see Chapters 1 and 4).

The *Review of Systems* is a part of the evaluation described in the *Guide's* Elements of Patient/Client Management that leads to optimal outcomes (see Fig. 1.4). It is a part of the dynamic process in which the therapist makes clinical judgments based on data gathered during the examination.

In the screening process, the therapist reviews the following:

- Do any red flags in the history or clinical presentation suggest a systemic origin of symptoms?
- Are any red flags associated signs and symptoms?
- What additional screening tests or questions are needed (if any)?
- Is referral to another health care provider needed, or is the therapist clear to proceed with a planned intervention (Case Example 16.4)?

Keep in mind the Clues to Screening the Pelvis, which are listed at the end of this chapter. If hip or groin pain is an accompanying feature with pelvic pain, review Clues to Screening Lower Quadrant Pain (see Chapter 17); likewise for anyone with pelvic and back pain see Clues to Screening Head, Neck, or Back Pain (see Chapter 15).

The therapist can use the Special Questions to Ask at the end of Chapter 15. It may not be necessary to ask all these questions. The therapist can use the overall clues gathered from the *history, risk factor assessment, clinical presentation*, and *associated signs and symptoms*, and review the list of special questions to see whether there is anything appropriate to ask the individual client.

Gynecologic Cancers

Cancers of the female genital tract account for about 12% of all new cancers diagnosed in women. Although gynecologic cancers are the fourth leading cause of death from cancer in women in the United States, most of these cancers are highly curable when detected early. The most common cancers of the female genital tract are uterine endometrial cancer, ovarian cancer, and cervical cancer.[99]

Endometrial (Uterine) Cancer. Cancer of the uterine endometrium, or lining of the uterus, is the most common gynecologic cancer, usually occurring in postmenopausal

CASE EXAMPLE 16.4

Peripheral Neuropathy of the Pelvic Floor

A 57-year-old woman presented with an unusual triad of symptoms. She reported numbness and tingling of the feet, urinary incontinence, and migrating arthralgias and myalgias of the lower body (e.g., low back or hip, sometimes hip adductor spasm or aching, a "heavy" sensation in the pelvic region).

Past Medical History: Significant previous medical history included a hysterectomy 10 years ago for uncontrolled bleeding, and oophorectomy 2 years ago followed by pelvic radiation for ovarian cancer.

She is a nonsmoker and a nondrinker and is in apparent good health after cancer treatment. She is not taking any medications or using any drugs or supplements. All follow-up checks have detected no signs of cancer recurrence. She is active in a women's cancer support group and exercises four or five times a week.

She has kept a journal of activities, foods, and symptoms but cannot find a pattern to explain any of her symptoms. Urinary incontinence is present continually with constant dripping and leaking. It is not made worse by exercise, the sound or feel of running water, putting the key in the door, or other triggers of urge or stress incontinence.

Bowel function is reportedly "normal." The client is a widow and is not currently sexually active.

Where do you go from here? What are the red flags? What questions do you ask? What tests do you perform? Is medical referral needed?

Red Flags
- Age
- Previous history of cancer
- Bilateral symptoms (numbness and tingling in both feet)

Screening Questions
Menstrual history, including pregnancies, miscarriages or abortions, births; current menstrual status (perimenopausal, postmenopausal, hormone replacement therapy)

Any symptoms or other problems anywhere else in the body?

Screening Tests
Can you reproduce any of the muscle or joint pain?

Neurologic Screen: Besides the usual manual muscle testing, deep tendon reflexes, and sensation, the therapist should test for lower extremity proprioception and assess feet more closely to identify the level of peripheral nerve impairment.

- Ask about the presence of other neurologic symptoms such as headache, muscle weakness, confusion, depression, irritability, blurred vision, balance/coordination problems, change in memory status, and sleepiness.
- Some of these are more likely when the central nervous system is impaired; for now, it looks as though we are looking at a problem in the peripheral nervous system, but paraneoplastic syndrome or metastases to the central nervous system can occur.

Assess for signs of skin or soft tissues, including the presence of lymphedema

Palpate the lymph nodes

Assess vital signs

Medical Referral
Immediate medical referral is warranted if the patient has not been evaluated recently. It is impossible to tell whether her symptoms are radiation-induced or are signs of cancer recurrence. A phone conversation between the therapist and the oncologist may be all that is needed. Information gathered during the interview and examination should be summarized for the physician.

Result: The client had peripheral neuropathies that affected the bladder, pelvic floor muscles, and feet because the same nerves innervate these two areas. Physical therapy intervention remained appropriate, and cancer recurrence was ruled out.

Radiation therapy is well known to cause significant delayed, chronic effects on connective tissue and the nervous system. Fibrosis of connective tissue can result in impairment of the soft tissues, such as pelvic adhesions, with subsequent functional limitations.

The incidence of plexopathy after radiation therapy has been reduced significantly with improved treatment, but it still occurs in a small number of cases. Younger women seem more vulnerable to radiation-induced peripheral neuropathy.

---

women between the ages of 50 and 70 years. Its occurrence is associated with obesity, endometrial hyperplasia, prolonged unopposed estrogen therapy (hormone replacement therapy without progesterone), and more recently, tamoxifen used in the treatment of breast cancer.[100,101]

Clinical Signs and Symptoms. Seventy-five percent of all cases of endometrial cancer occur in postmenopausal women. The most common symptom is abnormal vaginal bleeding or discharge at presentation. However, 25% of these cancers occur in premenopausal women, and 5% occur in women younger than 40 years.

In a physical therapy practice, the most common presenting complaint is pelvic pain without abnormal vaginal bleeding. Abdominal pain, weight loss, and fatigue may occur but remain unreported. Unexpected or unexplained vaginal bleeding in a woman taking tamoxifen (chemoprevention for breast cancer) is a red-flag sign. Tamoxifen as a risk factor for endometrial carcinoma has come under question.[102]

CLINICAL SIGNS AND SYMPTOMS

Endometrial (Uterine) Cancer

- Unexpected or unexplained vaginal bleeding or vaginal discharge after menopause (extremely significant sign)
- Persistent irregular or heavy bleeding between menstrual periods, especially in obese women
- Watery pink, white, brown, or bloody discharge from the vagina
- Abdominal or pelvic pain (more advanced disease)
- Weight loss, fatigue

Ovarian Cancer. Ovarian cancer is the second most common reproductive cancer in women and the leading cause of death from gynecologic malignancies, accounting for more than half of all gynecologic cancer deaths in the Western world.[99] It affects women of all races and ethnic groups.

Risk Factors. Risk increases with advancing age, and the incidence of ovarian cancer peaks between the ages of 40 and 70 years. Other factors that may influence the development of ovarian cancer include the following:

- Nulliparity (never being pregnant), giving birth to fewer than two children, giving birth for the first time when over the age of 35 years
- Personal or family history of breast, endometrial, or colorectal cancer
- Family history of ovarian cancer (mother, sister, daughter; especially at a young age); carrying the *BRCA1* or *BRCA2* gene mutation
- Infertility
- Early menarche, late menopause, prolonged postmenopausal hormone (estrogen) therapy (long-term, additive exposure to estrogen)
- Obesity (body mass index of 30 or more)
- Exposure to cosmetic talc or asbestos (conflicting evidence)[103–107]

Identification of the *BRCA1* or *BRCA2* genetic mutation and subsequent evidence for a family of genes that may play a role in the breast–ovarian syndrome and familial ovarian cancer offer the possibility of identifying women truly at risk for this disease.[108,109]

No reliable screening test can detect ovarian cancer in its early, most curable stages. Two diagnostic tests are used, but both lack sensitivity and specificity. The CA-125 blood test (carcinoembryonic antigen, a biologic marker) shows elevation in about half of women with early-stage disease and about 80% of those with advanced disease. Transvaginal ultrasonography helps determine whether an existing ovarian growth is benign or cancerous. Because early-stage symptoms are nonspecific, most women do not seek medical attention until the disease is advanced.

The ovaries begin to develop in utero, where the kidneys are located in the fully developed human, and then migrate along the pathways of the ureters. Following the viscero-somatic referral patterns discussed in Chapter 3, ovarian cancer can cause back pain at the level of the kidneys. Murphy's percussion test (see Chapter 10) would be negative; other symptoms of ovarian cancer might be present but remain unreported if the woman does not recognize their significance.

An ovarian symptom index for advanced ovarian cancer has also been developed.[113]

Rarely, reproductive carcinomas, including ovarian carcinoma, will present first with a paraneoplastic syndrome such as polyarthritis syndrome, carpal tunnel syndrome, myopathy, plantar fasciitis, or palmar fasciitis (swelling, digital stiffness or contractures, palmar erythema). The condition may be misdiagnosed as chronic regional pain syndrome (formerly reflex sympathetic dystrophy), Dupuytren's contracture, or a rheumatologic disorder.[114,115]

Hand and upper extremity manifestations often appear before the tumor is clinically evident. Treatment of the symptoms will have little effect on these conditions. Only successful treatment of the underlying neoplasm will affect symptoms favorably.[114]

The therapist should consider it a red flag whenever someone does not improve with physical therapy intervention. Failure to respond or worsening of symptoms requires a second screening examination. Progression of disease is often accompanied by a cluster of new signs and symptoms.

Extraovarian Primary Peritoneal Carcinoma. Extraovarian primary peritoneal carcinoma (EOPPC) is abdominal cancer (peritoneal carcinomatosis) without ovarian involvement. It arises in the peritoneum and mimics the symptoms, microscopic appearance, and pattern of spread of endothelial ovarian cancer with no identifiable disease of the ovaries.[116]

EOPPC develops only in women and accounts for most extraovarian causes of symptoms with a presumed but inaccurate diagnosis of ovarian cancer.[117] EOPPC has been reported after bilateral oophorectomy performed for benign disease or prophylaxis.[118] The occurrence of EOPPC with the same histology as neoplasms arising within the ovary may be explained by the common origin of the peritoneum and the ovaries from the coelomic epithelium.[119]

Cervical Cancer. Cancer of the cervix is the third most common gynecologic malignancy in the United States. It is the most common cause of death from gynecologic cancer in the world. Since the widespread introduction of the Papanicolaou (Pap) smear as a standard screening tool, the diagnosis of cervical cancer at the invasive stage has decreased significantly. In 2012 the American Society for Colposcopy and Cervical Pathology and the American Society for Clinical Pathology

CLINICAL SIGNS AND SYMPTOMS

Ovarian or Primary Peritoneal Cancer

Retrospective studies indicate that more than 70% of women with ovarian cancer have symptoms for 3 months or longer before diagnosis.[110] Over two thirds of women have late-stage cancer with metastatic disease at the time of diagnosis. Early symptoms are often vague, nonspecific, and easily overlooked.

In one study, when the symptoms listed next were present for less than 1 year and occurred more than 12 days per month, there was a cancer symptom index with a sensitivity of 56.7% for early-stage disease and 79.5% for advanced-stage disease. Specificity was 90% for women older than 50 years of age and 86.7% for women younger than 50 years of age.[111] Even early-stage ovarian cancer can produce these signs and symptoms:[112]

- Persistent vague GI complaints
- Pelvic/abdominal discomfort, bloating, increase in abdominal or waist size (ascites)
- Indigestion, belching
- Early satiety
- Mild anorexia in a woman 40 years of age or older
- Vaginal bleeding
- Change in bowel or bladder habits, especially constipation, urinary frequency, or severe urinary urgency
- Pelvic discomfort or pressure; back pain
- Ascites, pain, and pelvic mass (advanced disease)

issued a joint guideline for cervical cancer screening based on the evidence. Based on these guidelines, it is recommended that women aged 21 to 39 years should receive cervical screening every 3 years. Even so, nearly half of all women diagnosed with cervical cancer are diagnosed at a late stage, with locally or regionally advanced disease and a poor prognosis.[99]

At the same time that rates of invasive cervical carcinoma have been on the decline, the highly curable preinvasive carcinoma in situ (CIS) has increased. CIS is more common in women 30 to 40 years of age, and invasive carcinoma is more frequent in women over age 40 years.

Risk Factors. Risk factors associated with the development of cervical cancer are many, and varied, and include the following:
- Early age at first sexual intercourse
- Early age at first pregnancy
- Tobacco use, including exposure to passive smoke[120]
- Low socioeconomic status (lack of screening)
- History of any STD, especially HPV and human immuno-deficiency virus (HIV)
- History of multiple sex partners
- History of childhood sexual abuse
- Intimate partner abuse
- Women whose mothers used the drug diethylstilbestrol (DES) during pregnancy

Research into the health effects of intimate partner abuse points to a higher risk of STD and prevention of women from seeking health care; both contribute to an increased risk of cervical cancer.[121] Women with a history of childhood sexual abuse may avoid regular gynecologic care because being examined triggers painful memories. A history of childhood sexual abuse also increases a woman's risk of exposure to STIs that may contribute to the development of cervical cancer.[121]

The American Cancer Society (ACS) has issued updated recommendations for the early detection of cervical cancer.[122,123] The ACS advises all women to start cervical cancer screening starting at the age of 21 years. Pap smears should be done regularly, usually every 3 years. After a total hysterectomy (including removal of the cervix) or after age 70 years, the Pap smear is discontinued.[124] Women with certain risk factors for cervical cancer (e.g., HIV infection, long-term steroid use, immunocompromised status, DES exposure before birth) should be advised to have an annual Pap smear.[122,124]

Clinical Signs and Symptoms. Early cervical cancer has no symptoms. Clinical symptoms related to advanced disease include painful intercourse; postcoital, coital, or intermenstrual bleeding; and a watery, foul-smelling vaginal discharge.

Disease usually spreads by local extension and through the lymphatics to the retroperitoneal lymph nodes (see Table 14.4). Metastases to the central nervous system can occur hematogenously late in the course of the disease and are generally rare. Clinical presentation of brain metastases depends on the site of the metastasized lesion; hemiparesis and headache are the most commonly reported signs and symptoms.[125]

CLINICAL SIGNS AND SYMPTOMS
Cervical Cancer

- May be asymptomatic (early stages)
- Painful intercourse or pain after intercourse
- Unexplained or unexpected bleeding
- Watery, foul-smelling vaginal discharge
- Hemiparesis, headache (cancer recurrence with brain metastases)

Screening for Gastrointestinal Causes of Pelvic Pain

GI conditions can cause pelvic pain. The most common causes of pelvic pain referred from the GI system are the following:
- Acute appendicitis
- IBD, Crohn's disease or regional enteritis, ulcerative colitis
- Diverticulitis
- IBS

The small bowel, sigmoid, and rectum can be affected by gynecologic disease; abdominal, low back, and/or pelvic pain may result from pressure or displacement of these organs. Swelling, reaction to an adjacent infection, or reaction to the spilling of blood, menstrual fluid, or infected material into the abdominal cavity can cause pressure or displacement.

Bowel function is usually altered, but sometimes, the client experiences periods of normal bowel function alternating with intermittent bowel symptoms, and the client does not see a pattern or relationship until asked about current (or recent) changes in bowel function.

For all of these conditions, the symptoms as seen or reported in a physical therapy practice are usually the same. The client may present with one or more of the following:
- GI symptoms (see Box 4.19)
- Symptoms aggravated by increased abdominal pressure (coughing, straining, lifting, bending)
- Iliopsoas abscess (see Figs. 9.4 and 9.8; a positive test is indicative of an inflammatory/infectious process)
- Positive McBurney's point (see Figs. 9.10 and 9.11; appendicitis)
- Rebound tenderness or Blumberg's sign (see Fig. 9.13; appendicitis or peritonitis)

Appendicitis can cause peritoneal inflammation with psoas abscess, resulting in referred pain to the low back, hip, pelvis, or groin area (Case Example 16.5). The position of the vermiform appendix in the abdominal cavity is variable (see Fig. 9.11). Negative tests for appendicitis that use McBurney's point may occur when the appendix is located somewhere other than at the end of the cecum. See Fig. 9.13 for an alternate test (Blumberg's sign). Clinical signs and symptoms of appendicitis are listed in Chapter 9.

Blumberg's sign, a test for rebound tenderness, is usually positive in the presence of peritonitis, appendicitis, PID, or any other infection or inflammation associated with abdominal or pelvic conditions. Acute appendicitis is rare in older adults, but half of all those who die of a ruptured appendix are over the age of 65 years.[126]

The test for rebound tenderness can be very painful for the client. The therapist is advised to do this test last. Some clinicians prefer to start with this test (the only screening test used for abdominal or pelvic inflammation or infection) and to make a medical referral immediately when it is positive.

This is a matter of professional preference based on experience and clinical judgment. In our experience, the iliopsoas and obturator tests are useful tools. If back pain (rather than abdominal quadrant pain) is the response, the therapist is alerted to the need to assess these muscles further and to consider their role in low back pain.

If the iliopsoas test is negative for lower quadrant pain, the therapist can palpate the integrity of the iliopsoas muscle and assess for trigger points (See Fig. 9.7). If the tests are negative (i.e., they do not cause abdominal pain), then the therapist can palpate McBurney's point for the appendix. If McBurney's is negative but an infectious cause of symptoms is suspected, the test for rebound tenderness can be conducted last.

Clients with symptoms of possible inflammatory or infectious origin usually have a history of the conditions mentioned earlier (e.g., appendicitis, IBD or IBS, other GI disease). PID is another common cause of pelvic pain that can cause psoas abscess and a subsequent positive iliopsoas or obturator test. In this case, it is most likely a young woman with multiple sexual partners who has a known or unknown case of untreated chlamydia.

Crohn's disease, chronic inflammation of all layers of the bowel wall (see Chapter 9), may affect the terminal ileum and cecum or the rectum and sigmoid colon in the pelvis. In addition to pelvic and low back pain, systemic manifestations of Crohn's disease may include intermittent fever with sweats, malaise, anemia, arthralgia, and bowel symptoms.

Diverticular disease of the colon (diverticulosis), an acquired condition most common in the fifth to seventh decades, appears with intermittent symptoms. Moderate-to-severe pain in the left lower abdomen and the left side of the pelvis may be accompanied by a feeling of bowel distention and bowel symptoms such as hard stools, alternating diarrhea and constipation, mucus in the stools, and rectal bleeding.

IBS produces persistent, colicky lower abdominal and pelvic pain associated with anorexia, belching, abdominal distention, and bowel changes. Symptoms are produced by excessive colonic motility and spasm of the bowel (spastic colon).

See Chapter 9 for additional details about the referred pain patterns and most common associated signs and symptoms for each of these diseases.

Screening for Urogenital Causes of Pelvic Pain

Infection of the bladder or kidney, kidney stones, renal failure (chronic kidney disease), spasm of the urethral smooth muscle, interstitial cystitis, and tumors in any of the urogenital organs can refer pain to the lower lumbar and pelvic regions, mimicking musculoskeletal impairment. Pelvic floor tension myalgia can develop in response to these conditions and create pelvic pain. The primary pain pattern may radiate around the flanks to the lower abdominal region, the genitalia, and the anterior/medial thighs (see Figs. 11.7–11.10).

Usually, the most common diseases of this system appear as obvious medical problems. In the physical therapy setting, past medical history, risk factors, and associated signs and symptoms provide important red-flag clues. The therapist needs to ask the client about the presence of painful urination or changes in urination and constitutional symptoms such as fever, chills, sweats, and nausea or vomiting.

Deep, aching pelvic pain that is worse if weight-bearing or is accompanied by sciatica or numbness and tingling in the groin or lower extremity may be associated with cancer recurrence or cancer metastases.

Screening for Other Conditions as a Cause of Pelvic Girdle Pain

Psychogenic pain is often ill-defined, and its anatomic distribution depends more on the person's concepts than on clinical disease processes. Pelvic pain may coevolve with psychologic impairments.[127]

Such pain does not usually radiate; commonly, the client has multiple unrelated symptoms, and fluctuations in the course of symptoms are determined more by crises in the person's psychosocial life than by physical changes. (See also Screening for Emotional and Psychologic Overlay in Chapter 3.) Central sensitization can easily occur with conditions of pelvic pain, especially if the diagnosis takes several months or even years. During that time, the patient may fear the worst as the medical community is slowly working through the diagnosis. Stress and worry contribute to the formation of central sensitization. Physical therapists can offer suggestions to decrease the effects of a sensitive nervous system, even as the physician is treating the organ dysfunction.

A history of sexual abuse in childhood or adulthood (men and women) may contribute to chronic pelvic pain or symptoms of a vague and diffuse nature.[128] In some cases, the link between abuse and pelvic pain may be psychologic or neurologic, or may result from biophysical changes that heighten a person's physical sensitivity to pain. Taking a history of sexual abuse may be warranted.[128,129]

Occasionally, a woman has been told there is no organic cause for her distressing pelvic pain. Chronic vascular pelvic congestion, enhanced by physical or emotional stress, may be the underlying problem. The therapist may be instrumental in assessing for this condition and providing some additional clues to the medical community that can lead to a medical diagnosis.

Surgery, in particular hysterectomy, is associated with varying amounts of pain from problems such as nerve damage, scar formation, or hematoma formation with infection, which can cause backache and pelvic pain. Lower abdominal discomfort, vaginal discharge, and fatigue may accompany pelvic pain or discomfort months after gynecologic surgery.

Other types of abdominal, pelvic, or tubal surgery, such as laparotomy, tubal ligation, or laminectomy, can also be followed by pelvic pain, usually associated with low back pain.

CASE EXAMPLE 16.5

Appendicitis

Background: A 23-year-old woman who was training for a marathon developed groin and pelvic girdle pain—first just on the right side, but then on both sides. She reported that the symptoms came on gradually over 2 weeks. She could not point to a particular spot as the source of the pain, but rather indicated a generalized lower abdominal, pelvic, and inner thigh area.

She denied ever being sexually active and had never been diagnosed with a sexually transmitted disease (STD). She was on a rigorous training schedule for the marathon, did not appear anorexic, and seemed in overall good health.

No signs of swelling, inflammation, or temperature change were noted in the area. Running made the pain worse, rest made it better.

Range of motion of the hip and back was full and painless. A neurologic screening examination was normal. Resisted hip abduction was "uncomfortable" but did not exactly reproduce the symptoms.

What are the red flags here? What do you ask about or do next?

Not very many red flags are present: The bilateral presentation and overall size and location of the symptoms are the first two to be considered. Aggravating and relieving factors seem consistent with a musculoskeletal problem, but objective findings to support impairment of the movement system are significantly lacking.

What do you ask about or do next?

Take the client's vital signs, including body temperature, blood pressure, respiratory rate, and heart rate. If you are pressed for time, at least take the body temperature and blood pressure.

Perform one or more of the tests for abdominal or pelvic infection/inflammation. You can go right to the rebound (Blumberg's) test, or you can assess the soft tissues one at a time as discussed in the text. If this is negative, consider trigger points as a possible source of painful symptoms.

Ask the client about constitutional symptoms or other symptoms anywhere else in the body.

Your next step or steps in interviewing or assessing the client will depend on the results of your evaluation so far. Once you have compiled the clinical presentation, step back and conduct a Review of Systems. If a cluster of signs and symptoms is associated with a particular visceral system, look over the Special Questions to Ask at the end of the chapter that address that system.

Check the Special Questions for Men and Women (Appendices A-24 and B-37). Have you left out or missed any special questions that might be appropriate to this case?

Results: The client had normal vital signs but reported "night and day sweats" from time to time. The iliopsoas and obturator tests caused some general discomfort but were considered negative.

McBurney's point was positive, eliciting extreme pain. Blumberg's test for rebound was not performed. The client was referred to the emergency department immediately because she did not have a primary care physician.

It turned out that this client had peritonitis from a ruptured appendix. The doctors think she was in such good shape with a high pain threshold that she presented with minimal symptoms (and survived). Her white blood count was almost 100,000/mm³ when laboratory work was finally ordered.

The use of "candy cane" stirrups that wrap around the foot, ankle, and calf and place the hip in extreme hip abduction may contribute to hip labral tears and subsequent hip and/or pelvic pain. There is evidence that these stirrups are linked with lumbosacral nerve plexus injuries and transient postoperative neuropathy.[130] The association between the stirrups and labral tears is based on clinical observation and anecdotal data. Research is needed to verify this relationship. During the client interview, the therapist must include questions about recent surgical procedures.

PHYSICIAN REFERRAL

Guidelines for Immediate Medical Attention

- Immediate medical attention is required anytime the therapist identifies signs and symptoms that point to fracture, infection, or neoplasm. For example, a positive rebound test for appendicitis or peritonitis requires immediate medical referral. Likewise, severe sacral pain in the presence of a previous history of uterine, abdominal, prostate, rectal, or anal cancer requires immediate medical referral.

- Suspicion of any infection (e.g., STD, PID) requires immediate medical referral. Early medical intervention can prevent the spread of infection and septicemia and preserve fertility.

- A sexually active female with shoulder or back pain of unknown cause may need to be screened for ectopic pregnancy. Onset of symptoms after a missed menstrual cycle or in association with unexplained or unexpected vaginal bleeding requires immediate medical attention. Hemorrhage from ectopic pregnancy can be a life-threatening condition.

Guidelines for Physician Referral

- Any vaginal bleeding more than 12 months after menstruation stops should be evaluated by a physician.

- Blood in the toilet after a bowel movement may be a sign of anal fissures or hemorrhoids but can also signal colorectal cancer. A medical differential diagnosis is needed to make the distinction. History of an unrepaired hernia or suspected undiagnosed hernia requires medical referral. Lateral wall pelvic pain referred down the anteromedial side of the thigh to the knee can occur with femoral hernias; inguinal hernias are more likely to cause groin pain.

- A history of cancer with recent surgical removal of tumor tissue followed by back, hip, sacral, or pelvic pain within 6 months of surgery is a red flag for possible cancer recurrence. Even in the presence of apparent movement system impairment, referral for medical evaluation is warranted.
- All adolescent females and adult women who are sexually active or over the age of 21 years should be asked when their last Pap smear was done and what the results were. The therapist can play an important part in client education and disease prevention by teaching women about the importance of a Pap smear every 3 years and encouraging them to schedule one, if appropriate.
- Women with conditions such as endometriosis, PCS, STI, and PID can be helped with medical treatment. Medical referral is advised anytime a therapist identifies signs and symptoms that suggest any of these conditions.
- Failure to respond to physical therapy intervention is usually followed by reevaluation that includes a second screening and a Review of Systems. Any red flags or cluster of suspicious signs and symptoms must be reported. Depending on the therapist's findings, medical evaluation may be the next step.

Clues to Screening the Sacrum/Sacroiliac

Past Medical History

- Previous history of Crohn's disease; presence of skin rash with new onset of sacral, hip, or leg pain
- Previous history of other GI disease
- Previous history of rheumatic disease
- Previous history of conjunctivitis or venereal disease (reactive arthritis)
- History of heart disease or PVD; the therapist should ask about the effect of activity on symptoms
- Remember to consider unreported assaults or anal intercourse (partnered rape, teens, homosexual men with men). Please note that many of today's teens are resorting to anal intercourse and oral sex to prevent pregnancy. These forms of sexual contact do not prevent STD. Also, they can result in sacral pain and other lesions (e.g., rectal fissures) caused by trauma.

Clinical Presentation

- Constant (usually intense) pain; pain with a "catch" or "click" (sacral fracture)
- Sacral pain occurs when the rectum is stimulated (pain occurs when passing gas or having a bowel movement).
- Pain relief occurs after passing gas or having a bowel movement.
- Sacral or SI pain in the absence of a (remembered) history of trauma or overuse
- Assess for trigger points, a common musculoskeletal (not systemic) cause of sacral pain. If trigger point therapy relieves, reduces, or eliminates the pain, further screening may not be necessary.
- Lack of objective findings; special tests (e.g., Patrick's test, Gaenslen's maneuver, Yeoman's test, central posterior–anterior overpressure or spring test on the sacrum) are negative. Soft tissue and contractile tissue can usually be provoked during a physical examination by palpation, resistance, overpressure, compression, distraction, or motion.
- Look for other PFM spasm.

Associated Signs and Symptoms

- Presence of urologic or GI symptoms along with sacral pain (the therapist must ask to find out)

Clues to Screening the Pelvis

Frequently, pelvic and low back pain occur together or alternately. Whenever pelvic pain is listed, the reader should consider this as pelvic pain with or without PGP, low back, or sacral pain.

Past Medical History/Risk Factors

- History of dysmenorrhea, ovarian cysts, inflammatory disease, STD, fibromyalgia, sexual assault/incest/trauma, chronic yeast/vaginal infection, chronic bladder or urinary tract infection, chronic IBS
- History of abdominal, pelvic, or bladder surgery
- History of pelvic or abdominal radiation
- Recent therapeutic or spontaneous abortion
- Recent IUCD in the presence of PID or women with a history of PID
- History of previous gynecologic, colon, or breast cancer
- History of prolonged labor, use of forceps or vacuum extraction, and/or multiple births
- Obesity, chronic cough

Clinical Presentation

- Pelvic pain that is described as "achy" or "comes and goes in waves" and is poorly localized (person cannot point to one spot)
- Pelvic pain that is aggravated by walking, sexual intercourse, coughing, or straining
- Pain that is not affected by position changes or specific movements, especially when accompanied by night pain unrelieved by change in position
- Pelvic pain that is not reduced or eliminated by scar tissue mobilization, soft tissue mobilization, or release of trigger points of the myofascial structures in the pelvic cavity

Associated Signs and Symptoms

- Pelvic pain in the presence of yellow, odorous vaginal discharge
- Positive McBurney's or iliopsoas/obturator tests (see Chapter 9)
- Pelvic pain with constitutional symptoms, especially nausea and vomiting, GI symptoms (possible enteropathic origin)
- Presence of painful urination; urinary incontinence, urgency, or frequency; nocturia; blood in the urine; or other urologic changes

Gynecologic

- Pelvic pain that is relieved by rest, placing a pillow or support under the hips and buttocks in the supine position, or "getting off your feet"
- Pelvic pain that is correlated with menses or sexual intercourse
- Pelvic pain that occurs after the first menstrual cycle is missed, especially if the woman is using an IUCD or has had a tubal ligation (see text for other risk factors), with shoulder pain also present (ruptured ectopic pregnancy); assess for low blood pressure
- Presence of unexplained or unexpected vaginal bleeding, especially after menopause
- Presence of pregnancy

Vascular

- History of heart disease with a clinical presentation of pelvic, buttock, and leg pain that is aggravated by activity or exercise (claudication)
- Pelvic pain accompanied by buttock and leg pain with a change in skin and temperature on the affected side (arterial occlusion or venous thrombosis), especially in the presence of known heart disease or recent pelvic surgery
- Pain that worsens toward the end of the day, accompanied by pain after intercourse and in the presence of varicose veins elsewhere in the body (ovarian varicosities)

■ Key Points to Remember

Many of the Key Points to Remember in Chapter 15 also apply to the sacrum and SI joints. These will not be repeated here.

Sacrum/Sacroiliac Joint

1. Sacral pain, in the absence of a history of trauma or overuse that is not reproduced with anterior–posterior overpressure (spring test) on the sacrum, is a red-flag presentation that indicates a possible systemic cause of symptoms.
2. Pain above the L5 spinous process is not likely from the sacrum or SI joint.
3. Midline lumbar pain, especially if present when rising from sitting, more often comes from a diskogenic source; clients with unilateral pain below L5 when rising from sitting are more likely to have a painful SI joint.
4. Insufficiency fractures of the spine are not uncommon with individuals who have osteoporosis or who are taking corticosteroids; apparent insidious onset or minor trauma is common.
5. The most common cause of noninfected, inflammatory sacral/SI pain is ankylosing spondylitis; other causes may include reactive arthritis, psoriatic arthritis, and arthritis associated with IBD.
6. Infection can seed itself into the joints, including the SI joint. Watch for a history of recent dental surgery (endocarditis), intravenous drug use, trauma (including surgery), and chronic immunosuppression.

7. Anyone with joint pain of unknown cause should be asked about a recent history of skin rash (delayed allergic reaction, Crohn's disease).
8. Referred pain from PFM spasm is often felt at the sacrum and SI region.

Pelvis

1. Pelvic and low back pain often occur together; either may be accompanied by unreported abdominal pain, discomfort, or other symptoms. The therapist must ask about the presence of any unreported pain or symptoms.
2. Yellow or green discharge from the vagina or penis (with or without an odor) in the presence of low back, pelvic, or sacral pain may be a red flag. The therapist must ask additional questions to determine the need for medical evaluation.
3. The first sign of pelvic infection in the older adult might not be an elevated temperature, but rather, confusion, increased confusion, or some other change in mental status.
4. Bilateral anterior pelvic pain may be a symptom of inflammation; the therapist can test for iliopsoas or obturator abscess, appendicitis, or peritonitis (see discussion in Chapter 9).
5. PGP that is aggravated by exercise and starts 5 or more minutes after exercise begins may be vascularly induced.
6. A history of sexual abuse at any time in the person's past may contribute to chronic pelvic pain or nonspecific symptoms. Taking a history of sexual abuse may be needed.

CLIENT HISTORY AND INTERVIEW

SPECIAL QUESTIONS TO ASK: SACRUM, SACROILIAC, AND PELVIS

See Special Questions to Ask: Neck or Back, and Special Questions to Ask Men/Women Experiencing Back, Hip, Pelvic, Groin, SI, or Sacral Pain in Chapter 15.

Not all the special questions listed in Chapter 15 will have to be asked. Use your professional judgment to decide what to ask based on what the client has told you and what you have observed during the examination.

Sacral/Sacroiliac Pain

- Have you ever been diagnosed with ulcerative colitis, Crohn's disease, IBS, or colon cancer?
- Are you taking any antibiotics? (Long-term use of antibiotics can result in colitis.)
- Have you ever been diagnosed or treated for cancer of any kind? **(Metastases to the bone, especially common with breast, lung, or prostate cancer, but also with pelvic or abdominal cancer)**
- Do you have any abdominal pain or GI symptoms? (Assess for lower abdominal or suprapubic pain at the same level as the sacral pain; if the client denies GI symptoms, follow-up with a quick list: Any nausea? Vomiting? Diarrhea? Change in stool color or shape? Ever have blood in the toilet?)
- If sacral pain occurs when the rectum is stimulated:
  - Is your pain relieved by passing gas or by having a bowel movement?
- Sacral or SI pain without a history of trauma or overuse

Remember to consider unreported assault, anal intercourse (partnered rape; adolescents may use anal intercourse to prevent pregnancy, homosexual men with men). Please note that many of today's teens are resorting to anal intercourse and oral sex to prevent pregnancy.

These forms of sexual contact do not prevent STD. Also, they can result in sacral pain and other lesions (e.g., rectal fissures) resulting from trauma.

Pelvic Pain

- Have you ever been diagnosed or treated for cancer of any kind?
- Have you had recent abdominal or pelvic surgery (including hysterectomy, bladder reconstruction, prostatectomy)?
- Have you ever been told that you have (or do you have) varicose veins? **(Pelvic congestion syndrome)**
- Do you ever have blood in the toilet?

For women with low back, sacral, or pelvic pain: See Special Questions to Ask: Women Experiencing Back, Hip, Pelvic, Groin, SI, or Sacral Pain in Chapter 15.

For anyone with low back, sacral, or pelvic pain of unknown cause: It may be necessary to conduct a sexual history as a part of the screening process (see Chapter 15 or Appendix B-32 in the accompanying enhanced eBook version included with print purchase of this textbook).

For men with sciatica, pelvic, sacral, or low back pain: See Special Questions to Ask: Men Experiencing Back, Hip, Pelvic, Groin, or SI Pain (Chapter 15 or Appendix B-24 in the accompanying enhanced eBook version included with print purchase of this textbook).

PRACTICE QUESTIONS

1. Pelvic pain that is made worse after 5 to 10 minutes of physical activity or exertion but goes away with rest or cessation of the activity describes:
   a. A constitutional symptom
   b. An infectious process
   c. A symptom of osteoporosis
   d. A vascular pattern of ischemia
2. Pain that is relieved by placing a pillow or support under the hips and buttocks describes:
   a. A constitutional symptom
   b. An infectious process
   c. A response to vascular congestion
   d. A trigger point pattern
3. A positive Blumberg's sign indicates:
   a. Pelvic infection
   b. Ovarian varicosities
   c. Arthritis associated with IBD
   d. Sacral neoplasm

4. A 33-year-old pharmaceutical sales representative reports pain over the midsacrum radiating to the right PSIS. Overpressure on the sacrum does not reproduce symptoms. This signifies:
   a. The presence of a neoplasm
   b. A red flag for sacral insufficiency fracture
   c. A lack of objective findings
   d. Coccygodynia
5. A 67-year-old man was seen by a physical therapist for low back pain rated 7 out of 10 on the visual analog scale. He was evaluated and a diagnosis was made by the physical therapist. The client attained immediate relief of symptoms, but after 3 weeks of therapy, the symptoms returned. What is the next step from a screening perspective?
   a. The client can be discharged. Maximum benefit from physical therapy has been achieved.
   b. The client should be screened for systemic disease, even if you have already included screening during the initial evaluation.
   c. The client should be sent back to the physician for further medical follow-up.
   d. The client should receive an additional modality to help break the pain–spasm cycle.

PRACTICE QUESTIONS—cont'd

6. McBurney's point for appendicitis is located:
   a. Approximately one third the distance from the ASIS toward the umbilicus, usually on the left side.
   b. Approximately one half the distance from the ASIS toward the umbilicus, usually on the left side.
   c. Approximately one third the distance from the ASIS toward the umbilicus, usually on the right side.
   d. Approximately one half the distance from the ASIS toward the umbilicus, usually on the right side.
   e. Impossible to tell because the appendix can be located anywhere in the abdomen

7. Which one of the following is a yellow (caution) flag?
   a. Sacral pain occurs when the examiner performs a sacral spring test (posterior-anterior glide of the sacrum).
   b. Sacral pain is relieved when the client passes gas or has a bowel movement.
   c. Sacral pain occurs following a history of overuse.
   d. Sacral pain is reduced or relieved by release of trigger points.

8. Cancer as a cause of sacral or pelvic pain is usually characterized by:
   a. A previous history of reproductive cancer
   b. Constant pain
   c. Blood in the urine or stools
   d. Constitutional symptoms
   e. All of the above

9. Reproduced or increased abdominal or pelvic pain when the iliopsoas muscle test is performed suggests:
   a. An iliopsoas trigger point
   b. Inflammation or abscess of the muscle from an inflamed appendix or peritoneum
   c. An abdominal aortic aneurysm
   d. The presence of a neoplasm

10. A 75-year-old woman with a known history of osteoporosis has pain over the sacrum radiating to the right PSIS and right buttock. How do you rule out an insufficiency fracture?
    a. Perform Blumberg's test.
    b. Conduct a sacral spring test (posterior–anterior overpressure of the sacrum).
    c. Perform Murphy's percussion test.
    d. Diagnostic imaging is the only way to know for sure.

11. What is the importance of the pelvic floor musculature to the abdominal and pelvic viscera?

CASE STUDY

STEPS IN THE SCREENING PROCESS

When a client presents with pelvic pain, how do you get started with the screening process?

First, review the possible causes of pelvic pain (see Table 16.2).
- Was there anything in the history or presentation to suggest one of the categories in this table?
- From looking at the table, do additional questions come to mind?
- Review Special Questions to Ask: Sacrum, SI, or Pelvis presented in this chapter. Are any of these questions appropriate or needed?
- Did you ask about associated signs and symptoms?
- Remember to ask the client the following:
  - Is there anything else about your general health that concerns you?
  - What other symptoms are you having that may or may not be connected to your current problem?

Next, review Clues to Screening the Pelvis. Is there anything here to raise your suspicion of a systemic disorder?
- If necessary, conduct a general health screening examination:
  - Have you had any recent infections or illnesses?
  - Have you had any fevers, sweats, or chills?
  - Any unusual discharge from the vagina or penis?
  - Any unusual skin rashes or muscle/joint pain?
  - Any unusual fatigue, irritability, or difficulty sleeping?
- Is there anything to suggest a pelvic organ disease or dysfunction or pelvic floor muscle dysfunction as the source of symptoms? Look for the following:
  - Pain that comes and goes and changes location
  - Pain that is not predictably reproducible (Note to reader: more likely to be systemic pain than for this to be the case for pelvic floor muscle dysfunction)
  - Pain made worse by hip flexion or straight leg raise (muscle impairment associated with disk pathology)
  - Rectal pain
  - Discomfort in the pelvis or vagina that is worse during intercourse or penetration
  - Pain or discomfort (better or worse) before, during, or after menstrual cycle (more likely to be a uterus condition)
- Mentally conduct a Review of Systems
  - Did the past medical history, age, medications, or associated signs and symptoms point to anything?
  - Use your Review of Systems table (see Box 4.19) to look for possible clusters of symptoms, or to remind you what to look for
  - If you identify a specific system in question, ask additional questions for that system:
  - For example, if a significant past medical history or current signs and symptoms of GI involvement are reported, review the Special Questions to Ask in Chapter 9. Would any questions listed be appropriate to ask, given your client's clinical presentation? Or, if you suspected a renal/urologic cause of symptoms, look at the questions posed in Chapter 11.

Sometimes, the initial screening process does not raise any suspicious history or red-flag symptoms. As discussed in Chapter 1, screening can take place anywhere in the Guide's patient/client management model (see Box 1.5).

CASE STUDY—cont'd

The therapist may begin to carry out the intervention without seeing any red flags that suggest a systemic disorder and may then find that the client does not improve with physical therapy. This in itself is a red flag.

If someone is not improving with physical therapy intervention, the therapist should review the findings (i.e., what you are doing and why you are doing it) and evaluate the need to repeat some steps in the screening process. Because systemic disease progresses over time, new signs and symptoms may have developed since the time of the first interview and client history taking.

The therapist may want to have someone else review the case. Often, this can provide some clarity and add insight to the evaluation process. Asking a few screening questions may bring to light some new information to be included in the ongoing evaluation. Now may be the time to repeat (or perform for the first time) specific and appropriate screening tests and measures.

REFERENCES

1. Casaroli G, Bassani T, Brayda-Bruno M, Luca A, Galbusera F. What do we know about the biomechanics of the sacroiliac joint and of sacropelvic fixation? A literature review. *Med Eng Phys.* 2020;76:1–12.
2. Phillips ATM, Pankaj P, Howie CR, Usmani AS, Simpson AHRW. Finite element modelling of the pelvis: inclusion of muscular and ligamentous boundary conditions. *Med Eng Phys.* 2007;29:739–748.
3. Buchowski JC, Kebaish KM, Sinkov V, Cohen DB, Sieber AN, Kostuik JP. Functional and radiographic outcome of sacroiliac arthrodesis for the disorders of the sacroiliac joint. *Spine J.* 2005;5(5):520–528.
4. Vora AJ. Functional anatomy and pathophysiology of axial low back pain: discs, posterior elements, sacroiliac joint, and associated pain generators. *Phys Med Rehabil Clin N Am.* 2010;21(4):679–709.
5. Vanelderen P. Sacroiliac joint pain. *Pain Pract.* 2010;10(5):470–478.
6. Martin C, McCarthy EF. Giant cell tumor of the sacrum and spine: series of 23 cases and a review of the literature. *Iowa Orthop.* 2010;30:69–75.
7. Haanpaa M, Paavonen J. Transient urinary retention and chronic neuropathic pain associated with genital herpes simplex virus infection. *Acta Obstet Gynecol Scand.* 2004;83(10):946–949.
8. Smith C, Kavar B. Extensive spinal epidural abscess as a complication of Crohn disease. *J Clin Neurosci.* 2010;17(1):144–166.
9. Norman GF. Sacroiliac disease and its relationship to lower abdominal pain. *Am J Surg.* 1968;116:54–56.
10. Igdem S. Insufficiency fractures after pelvic radiotherapy in patients with prostate cancer. *Int J Radiat Oncol Biol Phys.* 2010;77(3):818–823.
11. Blake SP, Connors AM. Sacral insufficiency fracture. *Br J Radiol.* 2004;77(922):891–896.
12. Fortin J, Aprill CN, Dwyer A, West S, Pier J. Sacroiliac joint: pain referral maps upon applying a new injection/arthrography technique. I. Asymptomatic volunteers. *Spine.* 1994;19(13):1475–1482.
13. Palsson TS, Graven-Nielsen T. Experimental pelvic pain facilitates pain provocation tests and causes regional hyperalgesia. *Pain.* 2012;153:2233–2240.
14. Young S, Aprill C, Laslett M. Correlation of clinical examination characteristics with three sources of low back pain. *Spine J.* 2003;3(6):460–465.
15. Depalma MJ. Does location of low back pain predict its source? *PM R.* 2011;3(1):3–39.
16. Slipman CW, Patel RK, Whyte WS. Diagnosing and managing sacroiliac pain. *J Musculoskel Med.* 2001;18(6):325–332.
17. Cheng DS. Sacral insufficiency fracture: a masquerader of diskogenic low back pain. *PM R.* 2010;2(2):162–164.
18. Yansouni CP. Bacterial sacroiliitis and gluteal abscess after dilation and curettage for incomplete abortion. *Obstet Gynecol.* 2009;114(2 Pt 2):440–443.
19. Dreyfuss P, Dreyer SJ, Cole A, Mayo K. Sacroiliac joint pain. *J Am Acad Orthop Surg.* Jul/Aug 2004;13(4):255–265.
20. Schumacher Jr. HR, Klippel JH, Koopman WJ, eds. *Primer on the Rheumatic Diseases.* 12th ed. Atlanta: Arthritis Foundation; 2001.
21. Zaas AK, Marrie TJ. The physical therapist's leg pain: Paget's disease. *Am J Med.* 2015;2(128):130–132.
22. Betancourt-Albrecht M, Roman F, Marcelli M. Grand rounds in endocrinology, diabetes, and metabolism from Baylor College of Medicine: a man with pain in his bones. *Medscape Diabetes Endocrinol.* 2003;5(1). http://www.medscape.com/viewarticle/445158. Accessed March 10, 2011.
23. White JH, Hague C, Nicolaou S, Gee R, Marchinkow LO, Munk PL. Imaging of sacral fractures. *Clin Radiol.* 2003;58:914–921.
24. Southam JD. Sacral stress fracture in a professional hockey player. *Orthopedics.* 2010;33(11):846.
25. Lin JT, Lane JM. Sacral stress fractures. *J Womens Health (Larchmt).* 2003;12(9):879–888.
26. Beltran LS, Bencardino JT. Lower back pain after recently giving birth: postpartum sacral stress fractures. *Skeletal Radiol.* 2011;40(4):481–482.
27. Rodrigues LM. Sacral stress fracture in a runner. *Clinics (Sao Paulo).* 2009;64(11):1127–1129.
28. Kahanov L, Eberman LE, Games KE, Wasik M. Diagnosis, treatment, and rehabilitation of stress fractures in the lower extremity in runners. *Open Access J Sports Med.* 2015;6:87–95.
29. Yoder K, Bartsokas J, Averell K, McBride E, Long C, Cook C. Risk factors associated with sacral stress fractures: a systematic review. *J Man Manip Ther.* 2015;23(2):84–92.
30. Leroux JL, Denat B, Thomas E, Blotman F, Bonnel F. Sacral insufficiency fractures presenting as acute low-back-pain-biomechanical aspects. *Spine.* 1993;18(16):2502–2506.
31. Andresen R, Ludtke CW, Radmer S, Kamusella P, Schober HC. Radiofrequency sacroplasty for the treatment of osteoporotic insufficiency fractures. *Eur Spine J.* Apr 2015;24(4):759–763.
32. Boissonnault WG, Thein-Nissenbaum JM. Differential diagnosis of a sacral stress fracture. *J Orthop Sports Phys Ther.* 2002;12(32):613–621.
33. Ahovuo JA, Kiuru MJ, Visuri T. Fatigue stress fractures of the sacrum: diagnosis with MR imaging. *Eur Radiol.* 2004;14(3):500–505.
34. Wilder RP, Sethi S. Overuse injuries: tendinopathies, stress fractures, compartment syndrome, and shin splints. *Clin Sports Med.* 2004;23:55–81.
35. Khan MH, Smith PN, Kang JD. Sacral insufficiency fractures following multilevel instrumented spinal fusion. *Spine.* 2005;30(16):E484–E488.
36. Klineberg E. Sacral insufficiency fractures caudal to instrumented posterior lumbosacral arthrodesis. *Spine.* 2008;33(16):1806–1811.

37. Vavken P. Sacral fractures after multi-segmental lumbosacral fusion: a series of four cases and systematic review of literature. *Eur Spine J.* 2008(Suppl 2):S285–S290.

38. Bederman SS, Shah KN, Hassan JM, Hoang BH, Kiester PD, Bhatia NN. Surgical techniques for spinopelvic reconstruction following total sacrectomy: a systematic review. *Eur Spine J.* 2014;23:305–319.

39. Manaster BJ, Graham T. Imaging of sacral tumors. *Neurosurg Focus.* 2003;15(2):E2.

40. Parikh VA, Edlund JW. Sacral insufficiency fractures—rare complication of pelvic radiation for rectal carcinoma. *Dis Colon Rectum.* 1998;41(2):254–257.

41. Zileli M, Hoscoskun C, Brastiano P, Sabah D. Surgical treatment of primary sacral tumors: complications with sacrectomy. *Neurosurg Focus.* 2003;15(5):E9.

42. Scuibba DM. Diagnosis and management of sacral tumors. *J Neurosurg Spine.* 2009;10(3):244–256.

43. Randall RL. Giant cell tumor of the sacrum. *Neurosurg Focus.* 2003;15(2):E13.

44. Thangaraj R, Grimer RJ, Carter SR, Stirling AJ, Spilsbury J, Spooner D. Giant cell tumour of the sacrum: a suggested algorithm for treatment. *Eur Spine J.* 2010;19:1189–1194.

45. Payer M. Neurological manifestation of sacral tumors. *Neurosurg Focus.* Aug, 2003;15(2):E1.

46. Elkhashab Y, Ng A. A review of current treatment options for coccygodynia. *Curr Pain Headache Rep.* 2018;22:28.

47. Howard FM, El-Minawi AM, Sanchez RA. Conscious pain mapping by laparoscopy in women with chronic pelvic pain. *Obstet Gynecol.* 2000;96(6):934–939.

48. Howard FM. Chronic pelvic pain. *Obstet Gynecol.* 2003; 101(3):594–611.

49. Gray DWR, Seabrook G, Dixon JM, Collins J. Is abdominal wall tenderness a useful sign in the diagnosis of non-specific abdominal pain? *An R Coll Surg Engl.* 1988;70:233–234.

50. Msonda HT, Laczek JT. Medical evacuation for unrecognized abdominal wall pain: a case series. *Mil Med.* 2015; 180(5):e605–e607.

51. Thomson WH, Dawes RF, Carter SS. Abdominal wall tenderness: a useful sign in chronic abdominal pain. *Br J Surg.* 1991;78(2):223–225.

52. Matsunaga S, Eguchi Y. Importance of a physical examination for efficient differential diagnosis of abdominal pain: diagnostic usefulness of Carnett's test in psychogenic abdominal pain. *Intern Med.* 2011;50:177–178.

53. Mishriki YY. Reminder of important clinical lesson abdominal wall pain in obese women: frequently missed and easily treated. *BMJ Case Rep.* 2009 Published online 2009 Feb 27.

54. Simons DG, Travell JG. *Travell & Simons' Myofascial Pain and Dysfunction: the Trigger Point Manual.* vol. 2. Baltimore: Williams & Wilkins; 1993.

55. Bassaly R. Myofascial pain and pelvic floor dysfunction in patients with interstitial cystitis. *Int Urogynecol J Pelvic Floor Dysfunc.* 2011;22(4):413–418.

56. Anderson RU. Painful myofascial trigger points and pain sites in men with chronic prostatitis/chronic pelvic pain syndrome. *J Urol.* 2009;182(6):2753–2758.

57. Vollestad NK, Stuge B. Prognostic factors for recovery from postpartum pelvic girdle pain. *Eur Spine J.* 2009;18(5):718–726.

58. Stuge B, Hilde G, Vollestad N. Physical therapy for pregnancy-related low back and pelvic pain: a systematic review. *Acta Obstet Gynecol Scand.* 2003;82(11):983–990.

59. Messelink B. Standardization of terminology of pelvic floor muscle function and dysfunction: report from the pelvic floor clinical assessment group of the International Continence Society. *Neurourol Urodyn.* 2005;24:374–380.

60. Baker PK. Musculoskeletal problems. In: Steege JF, Metzger DA, Levy BS, eds. *Chronic Pelvic Pain: An Integrated Approach.* Philadelphia: WB Saunders; 1998:215–240.

61. Steege JF, Zolnoun DA. Evaluation and treatment of dyspareunia. *Obstet Gynecol.* 2009;113(5):1124–1136.

62. Bø K, Sherburn M. Evaluation of female pelvic-floor muscle function and strength. *Phys Ther.* Mar 2005;85(3):269–282.

63. Riesco ML. Perineal muscle strength during pregnancy and postpartum: the correlation between perineometry and digital vaginal palpation. *Rev Lat Am Enfermagem.* 2010; 18(6):1138–1144.

64. Headley B. *When Movement Hurts: A Self-help Manual for Treating Trigger Points.* Minneapolis, MN: Orthopedic Physical Therapy Products; 1997.

65. Kostopoulos D, Rizopoulos K. *The Manual of Trigger Point and Myofascial Therapy.* Thorofare, NJ: Slack, Inc; 2001.

66. Arab AM. Correlation of digital palpation and transabdominal ultrasound for assessment of pelvic floor muscle contraction. *J Man Manip Ther.* 2009;17(3):e75–e79.

67. Vleeming A. European guidelines for the diagnosis and treatment of pelvic girdle pain. *Eur Spine J.* 2008;17(6):794–819.

68. Olsen MF. Self-administered screening test for pregnancy-related pain. *Europ Spine J.* 2009;18(8).

69. MacAvoy MC. Stability of open-book pelvic fractures using a new biomechanical model of single-limb stance. *J Orthop Trauma.* 1997;11:590–593.

70. Siegel J. Single-leg-stance radiographs in the diagnosis of pelvic instability. *J Bone Joint Surg.* 2008;90(1):2119–2125.

71. Pillay Y. Laparoscopic repair of an incarcerated femoral hernia. *Int J Surg Case Rep.* 2015;17:85–88.

72. Mahajan A, Luther A. Incarcerated femoral hernia in male: a rare case report. *Int Surg J.* 2014;1:25–26.

73. Giudice LC. Status of current research on endometriosis. *J Reprod Med.* 1998;43(3 Suppl):252–262.

74. Giudice LC, Kao LC. Endometriosis. *Lancet.* 2004;364(9447): 1789–1799.

75. Carrell DT, Peterson CM, eds. *Reproductive Endocrinology and Infertility.* New York: Springer Science; 2010.

76. Akbulut S. Left-sided appendicitis: review of 95 published cases and a case report. *World J Gastroenterol.* 2010; 16(44):5598–5602.

77. Ross J. European Guideline for the Management of Pelvic Inflammatory Disease. http://www.iusti.org/regions/europe/PID_v5.pdf, 2008. Accessed March 10, 2011.

78. Soper DE. Pelvic inflammatory disease. *Obstet Gynecol.* 2010;116(2 Pt 1):419–428.

79. Kahn JA, Kaplowitz RA, Goodman E, Emans SJ. The association between impulsiveness and sexual risk behaviors in adolescent and young adult women. *J Adolesc Health.* 2002;30(4):229–232.

80. Kahn JA, Rosenthal SL, Succop PA, Ho GYF, Burk RD. Mediators of the association between age of first sexual intercourse and subsequent papillomavirus infection. *Pediatrics.* 2002;109(1):E5.

81. Shikary T. Epidemiology and risk factors for human papillomavirus infection in a diverse sample of low-income young women. *J Clin Virol.* 2009;46(2):107–111.

82. Centers for Disease Control and Prevention (CDC) *Policy Guidelines for Prevention and Management of Pelvic Inflammatory Disease (PID).* Washington, DC: U.S. Department of Health and Human Services; 1991. http://www.cdc.gov/mmwr/preview/mmwrhtml/00031002.htm. Accessed March 10, 2011.

83. Centers for Disease Control and Prevention. *Sexually Transmitted Disease Surveillance: 2009.* Washington, DC: U.S. Department of Health and Human Services; 2011. http://www.cdc.gov/std/stats09/default.htm. Accessed March 14, 2011.

84. Newman L, Rowley J, Vander Hoorn S, et al. Global estimates of the prevalence and incidence of four curable sexually transmitted infections in 2012 based on systematic review and global reporting. *PLoS One.* Dec 2015;10(12):e0143303.

85. Anderton JP, Valdiserri RO. Combating syphilis and HIV among users of internet chat rooms. *J Health Commun.* Oct/Nov 2005;10(7):665–771.

86. Douglas Jr. JM, Peterman TA, Fenton KA. Syphilis among men who have sex with men: challenges to syphilis elimination in the United States. *Sex Transm Dis.* 2005;32(10 Suppl):S80–S83.

87. Centers for Disease Control and Prevention (CDC). Syphilis Profiles 2009. Updated February 28, 2011. http://www.cdc.gov/std/syphilis/. Accessed March 14, 2011.

88. Centers for Disease Control and Prevention (CDC). Syphilis & MSM (men who have sex with men)—CDC fact sheet. Updated April 28, 2010. http://www.cdc.gov/std/syphilis/STDFact-MSM-Syphilis.htm. Accessed March 14, 2011.

89. Borghi C, Dell'Atti L. Pelvic congestion syndrome: the current state of the literature. *Arch Gyn Obst.* 2016;293:291–301.

90. Tarazov PG, Prozorovskij KV, Ryzhkov VK. Pelvic pain syndrome caused by ovarian varices. *Acta Radiol.* 1997;38(6):1023–1025.

91. El-Minawi AM. Pelvic varicosities and pelvic congestion syndrome. In: Howard FM, Perry P, Carter JE, El-Minawi AM, eds. *Pelvic Pain Diagnosis and Management.* Philadelphia: Lippincott Williams & Wilkins; 2000:171–183.

92. Hobbs JT. Varicose veins arising from the pelvis due to ovarian vein incompetence. *Int J Clin Pract.* Oct 2005;59(10):1195–1203.

93. Freedman J. Pelvic congestion syndrome: the role of interventional radiology in the treatment of chronic pelvic pain. *Postgrad Med.* 2010;86(1022):704–710.

94. Gasparini D, Geatti O, Orsolon PG, et al. Female "varicocele. *Clin Nucl Med.* 1998;23(7):420–422.

95. Tu FF. Pelvic congestion syndrome-associated pelvic pain: a systematic review of diagnosis and management. *Obstet Gynecol Surv.* 2010;65(5):332–340.

96. Hantes J. History and physical of the chronic pelvic pain patient. VISION: The International Pelvic Pain. *Society.* 2004;9(1):1–4.

97. Hartung O, Grisoli D, Boufi M, et al. Endovascular stenting in the treatment of pelvic vein congestion caused by nutcracker syndrome: lessons learned from the first five cases. *J Vasc Surg.* 2005;42(2):275–280.

98. Singh MK. Chronic pelvic pain. Emedicine Specialties. Updated Sep 13, 2010. http://emedicine.medscape.com/article/258334-overview Accessed March 14, 2011.

99. Jemal A, Seigel R, Xu J, Ward E. Cancer statistics, 2010. *CA Cancer J Clin.* 2010;60(5):277–300.

100. Ferguson SE, Soslow RA, Amsterdam A, Barakat RR. Comparison of uterine malignancies that develop during and following tamoxifen therapy. *Gynecol Oncol.* 2006;101(2):322–326.

101. Carter J, Pather S. An overview of uterine cancer and its management. *Expert Rev Anticancer Ther.* 2006;6(1):33–42.

102. Creasman WT. Endometrial carcinoma. Emedicine Specialties, 2010. http://emedicine.medscape.com/article/254083-overview. Accessed March 14, 2011.

103. Huncharek M, Geschwind JF, Kupelnick B. Perineal application of cosmetic talc and risk of invasive epithelial ovarian cancer: a meta-analysis of 11,933 subjects from sixteen observational studies. *Anticancer Res.* 2003;23(2C):1955–1960.

104. Langseth H, Kjaerheim K. Ovarian cancer and occupational exposure among pulp and paper employees in Norway. *Scand J Work Environ Health.* 2004;30(5):356–361.

105. Mills PK, Riordan DG, Cress RD, Young HA. Perineal talc exposure and epithelial ovarian cancer risk in the Central Valley of California. *Int J Cancer.* 2004;112(3):458–464.

106. Wu AH. Markers of inflammation and risk of ovarian cancer in Los Angeles County. *Int J Cancer.* 2009;124(6):1409–1415.

107. Muscat JE, Huncharek MS. Perineal talc use and ovarian cancer: a critical review. *Eur J Cancer Prev.* 2008;17(2):139–146.

108. Study questions ovary removal during hysterectomy. Harvard Health Publications. Originally published March 2014. http://www.health.harvard.edu/newsletter_article/Study_questions_ovary_removal_during_hysterectomy. Accessed January 13, 2016.

109. Daly MB. Genetic/familial high risk assessment: breast and ovarian. *J Natl Comp Canc Netw.* 2010;8(5):562–594.

110. Goff BA, Mandel LS, Melancon CH, Muntz HG. Frequency of symptoms of ovarian cancer in women presenting to primary care clinics. *JAMA.* 2004;291(22):2705–2712.

111. Goff BA. Development of an ovarian cancer symptom index: possibilities for earlier detection. *Cancer.* 2007;109(2):221–227.

112. Liu S. Patterns of symptoms in women after gynecologic surgery. *Oncol Nurs Forum.* 2010;37(2):156.

113. Jensen SE. A new index of priority symptoms in advanced ovarian cancer. *Gynecol Oncol.* 2011;120(2):214–219.

114. Martorell EA, Murray PM, Peterson JJ, Menke DM, Calamia KT. Palmar fasciitis and arthritis syndrome associated with metastatic ovarian carcinoma: a report of four cases. *J Hand Surg.* 2004;29(4):654–660.

115. Krishna K. Palmar fasciitis with polyarthritis syndrome in a patient with breast cancer. *Clin Rheumatol.* 2011;30(4):569–572. https://doi.org/10.1007/s10067-010-1592-2. . Epub 2010 Oct 16.

116. Ozat M. Extraovarian conditions mimicking ovarian cancer. *Arch Gynecol Obstet.* 2011 Sep;284(3):713–719. https://doi.org/10.1007/s00404-010-1705-9. . Epub 2010 Oct 15.

117. Roffers SD, Wu XC, Johnson CH, Correa CN. Incidence of extra-ovarian primary cancers in the United States, 1992–1997. *Cancer.* 2003;97(10 Suppl):2643–2647.

118. Eltabbakh GH, Piver MS. Extraovarian primary peritoneal carcinoma. *Oncology (Williston Park).* June 1998;12(6):813–819.

119. Kunz J, Rondez R. Correlation between serous ovarian tumors and extra-ovarian peritoneal tumors of the same histology. *Schweiz Rundsch Med Prax.* 1998;87(6):191–198.

120. Trimble CL, Genkinger JM, Burke AE, et al. Active and passive cigarette smoking and the risk of cervical neoplasia. *Obstet Gynecol.* 2005;105(1):174–181.

121. Coker AL. Violence against women raises risk of cervical cancer. *J Womens Health (Larchmt).* 2009;18(8):1179–1185.

122. Saslow D, Runowicz CD, Solomon D, et al. American Cancer Society guideline for the early detection of cervical neoplasia and cancer. *CA Cancer J Clin.* 2002;52(6):342–362.

123. Schiffman M, Solomon D. Screening and prevention methods for cervical cancer. *JAMA.* 2009;302(16):1809–1810.

124. American Cancer Society (ACS): ACS cancer detection guidelines. Atlanta, Georgia. http://www.cancer.org/Healthy/FindCancerEarly/CancerScreeningGuidelines/american-cancer-society-guidelines-for-the-early-detection-of-cancer. Accessed March 10, 2011.

125. Amita M, Sudeep G, Rekha W, Yogesh K, Hemant T. Brain metastasis from cervical carcinoma – case report. *Med Gen Med.* 2005;7(1):26 http://www.medscape.com/viewarticle/496603_3. Accessed March 15, 2011.

126. Storm-Dickerson TL, Horattas MC. What have we learned over the past 20 years about appendicitis in the elderly? *Am J Surg.* 2003;185(3):198–201.

127. Mathias SD, Kuppermann M, Liberman RF, Lipschutz RC, Steege JF. Chronic pelvic pain: prevalence, health-related quality of life, and economic correlates. *Obstet Gynecol.* 1996;87(3):321–327.

128. Paras ML. Sexual abuse and lifetime diagnosis of somatic disorders: a systematic review and meta-analysis. *JAMA.* 2009;302(5):550–561.

129. Hilden M, Schei B, Swahnberg K, et al. A history of sexual abuse and health: a Nordic multicentre study. *BJOG.* 2004;111(10):1121–1127.

130. Bohrer JC. Pelvic nerve injury following gynecologic surgery: a prospective cohort study. *Am J Obstet Gynecol.* 2009;201(531):E1–E7.

CHAPTER 17

Screening the Lower Quadrant: Buttock, Hip, Groin, Thigh, and Leg

The causes of lower quadrant pain or dysfunction vary widely; presentation of symptoms is equally wide-ranging. Vascular conditions (e.g., arterial insufficiency, abdominal aneurysm), infectious or inflammatory conditions, gastrointestinal (GI) disease, and gynecologic and male reproductive systems may cause symptoms in the lower quadrant and lower extremity,[1] including the pelvis, buttock, hip, groin, thigh, and knee. Some overlap may occur, but unique differences exist.

Cancer may present as primary hip, groin, or leg pain or symptoms. Primary cancer can metastasize to the low back, pelvis, and sacrum, thus referring pain to the hip and groin. Primary cancer may also metastasize to the hip, causing hip or groin pain and related symptoms.

Pain may be referred from other locations such as the scrotum, kidneys, abdominal wall, abdomen, peritoneum, or retroperitoneal region. Lower quadrant pain may be referred through conditions that affect nearby anatomic structures, such as the spine, spinal nerve roots, or peripheral nerves, and overlying soft tissue structures (e.g., hernia, bursitis, fasciitis).[2]

One of the keys to accurate and quick screening is knowledge of the types of conditions, illnesses, and systemic disorders that can refer pain to the lower quadrant, especially the hip and groin. Much of the information related to screening of the back (see Chapter 15), sacrum, sacroiliac (SI), and pelvis (see Chapter 16) also applies to the hip and groin.

USING THE SCREENING MODEL TO EVALUATE THE LOWER QUADRANT

When screening is called for, the therapist looks at the client's personal and family history, clinical presentation, and associated signs and symptoms. Knowledge of problems that can affect the lower quadrant, along with the likely history, pain patterns, and associated signs and symptoms, should guide the therapist concerning the steps they should follow during screening.

In outpatient settings, the OSPRO-ROS can be used to gather information on the potential for systemic conditions. During the screening process, a series of special questions and special tests may help to identify systemic conditions. Recognition of red-flag signs and symptoms of systemic or viscerogenic problems can direct the client toward the

necessary medical attention early in the disease process. In many cases, early detection and treatment may result in improved outcomes.

Past Medical History

Some of the more common histories associated with lower extremity, hip, or groin pain of a visceral nature are listed in Box 17.1. A previous history of cancer, such as prostate cancer (men), reproductive cancer (women), or breast cancer, is a red flag as these cancers may be associated with metastases to the hip.

Past history of joint replacement (especially hip arthroplasty) combined with recent infection of any kind and new onset of hip, groin, or knee pain is suspicious. Postoperatively, orthopedic pins may migrate, referring pain from the hip to the back, tibia, or ankle. Loose components, improper implant size, muscular imbalance, and infection that occur any time after joint arthroplasty may cause lower quadrant pain or symptoms (Case Example 17.1).

There have been reports of hip, groin, and/or pelvic pain and/or mass associated with wear debris from hip arthroplasty. Polyethylene wear debris can also cause deep vein thrombosis, lower extremity edema, ureteral or bladder compression, or sciatic neuropathy.[3]

Risk Factors

Each condition, illness, or disease that can cause referred pain to the buttock, hip, thigh, groin, or lower extremity has its unique risk factors. Many of the items listed as past medical history are risk factors. For example, femoral artery catheterization used to monitor ongoing hemodynamic status (arterial line; status post burn injuries, and/or individuals in the intensive care unit [ICU]) or used for individuals with poor upper extremity intravenous access can cause retroperitoneal hematoma formation or septic arthritis and subsequent hip pain. Complications from femoral artery catheterization are rare (0.81%) and most likely to occur in older adults.[4]

Most known risk factors for systemically induced problems have been discussed in the individual chapters on each specific condition. For example, arterial insufficiency as a cause of low back, hip, buttock, or leg pain is presented as a part of the discussion of peripheral vascular disease (PVD)

BOX 17.1 RED-FLAG HISTORIES ASSOCIATED WITH THE LOWER EXTREMITY

- Previous history of cancer
- Previous history of renal or urologic disease such as kidney stones and urinary tract infections (UTIs)
- Trauma/assault (fall, blow, lifting)
- Femoral artery catheterization
- History of an infectious or inflammatory condition
  - Crohn's disease (regional enteritis) or ulcerative colitis
  - Diverticulitis
  - Pelvic inflammatory disease (PID)
  - Reactive Arthritis
  - Appendicitis
- History of gynecologic condition(s):
  - Recent pregnancy, childbirth, or abortion
  - Multiple births (multiparity)
  - Other gynecologic condition
- History of alcoholism (e.g., hip osteonecrosis)
- Long-term use of immunosuppressants (e.g., Crohn's disease, sarcoidosis, cancer treatment, organ transplant, autoimmune disorders)
- History of heart disease (e.g., arterial insufficiency, peripheral vascular disease)
- Receiving anticoagulation therapy (risk factor for hemarthrosis)
- History of acquired immunodeficiency syndrome (AIDS)-related tuberculosis
- History of hematologic disease such as sickle cell anemia or hemophilia

in Chapter 7 and again in Chapter 15 because it relates to low back pain. Likewise, known risk factors for bone cancer or metastases as a cause of hip, groin, or lower extremity pain are presented in Chapter 14.

Many conditions with overlap symptoms (e.g., back and hip pain, pelvic and groin pain) are presented throughout this third text section (Systemic Origins of Neuromusculoskeletal Pain and Dysfunction) as a part of the discussion of back pain (see Chapter 15) or pelvic pain (see Chapter 16).

Awareness of risk factors for various problems can help alert the therapist early to the need for medical intervention, as well as to the need for direct education and prevention efforts. Many risk factors for disease are modifiable. Exercise often plays a key role in prevention and treatment of pathologic conditions. Recognizing red flags in the history and clinical presentation and knowing when to refer versus when to treat are topics of focus in this chapter.

Clinical Presentation

If no neuromuscular or musculoskeletal cause of the client's symptoms can be identified, then the therapist must consider the following:

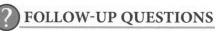

? FOLLOW-UP QUESTIONS

- Are red flags suggestive of a viscerogenic cause of pain or symptoms? (See Box 15.1; the lack of diagnostic testing or imaging studies may be an additional red flag.[5])
- What kind of pain patterns do we expect to see with each of the viscerogenic causes?
- Are any associated signs and symptoms suggestive of a particular organ system?

Hip and Buttock

The physical therapist is well acquainted with hip or buttock pain (Table 17.1) that occurs as a result of regional neuromuscular or musculoskeletal disorders. The therapist must be aware that disorders affecting the organs within the pelvic and abdominal cavities can also refer pain to the hip region, mimicking a primary musculoskeletal lesion. A careful history and physical examination usually differentiate these entities from true hip disease.[6]

Pain Pattern. True hip pain, whether from a neuromusculoskeletal or systemic cause (Table 17.2), is usually felt posteriorly deep within the buttock or anteriorly in the groin, sometimes with radiating pain down the anterior thigh. Pain perceived on the outer (lateral) side or posterior aspect of the hip is usually not caused by an intraarticular problem but more likely results from a trigger point, bursitis, knee, SI, or back problem.

With true hip joint disease, pain will occur with active or passive motion of the hip joint; this pain increases with weight-bearing.[7] Often, an antalgic gait pattern is observed as the individual leans away from the affected hip and shortens the swing phase to avoid weight-bearing.

When the underlying problem is related to soft tissue (e.g., abductor weakness) rather than to the joint as the source of symptoms, the client may lean toward the affected side to compensate for the downward rotation of the pelvis.[8] With soft tissue involvement of the bursa or tendons (e.g., gluteus medius, gluteus minimus), pain may radiate from the buttock, greater trochanter, and/or lateral thigh down the leg to the level of insertion of the iliotibial tract on the proximal tibia.[9–11]

Pain with medial rotation and decreased hip medial range of motion is associated with hip osteoarthritis.[12] Cyriax's "Sign of the Buttock" (Box 17.2) can help differentiate between hip and lumbar spine disease.[13–15] The presence of any of these signs may be an indication of osteomyelitis, neoplasm (upper femur, ilium), fracture (sacrum), abscess, or other infection.[14]

Neuromusculoskeletal Presentation. Identifying the hip as the source of a client's symptoms may be difficult because pain originating in the hip may not localize to the hip but rather may present as low back, buttock, groin, SI, anterior thigh, or even knee or ankle pain (Fig. 17.1).

On the other hand, regional pain from the low back, SI, sacrum, or knee can be referred to the hip. SI pain that localizes to the base of the spine may be accompanied by radicular pain extending across the buttock and down the leg. It can

CASE EXAMPLE 17.1

Screening After Total Hip Replacement

A 74-year-old retired homemaker had a total hip replacement (THR) 2 days ago. She remains an inpatient with complications related to congestive heart failure. She has a previous medical history of gallbladder removal 20 years ago, total hysterectomy 30 years ago, and surgically induced menopause with subsequent onset of hypertension.

Her medications include intravenous furosemide (Lasix), digoxin, and potassium replacement.

During the initial physical therapy intervention, the client reported muscle cramping and headache but was able to complete the entire exercise protocol. Blood pressure was 100/76 mm Hg (measured in the right arm while lying in bed). Systolic measurement dropped to 90 mm Hg when the client moved from supine to standing. Pulse rate was 56 bpm with a pattern of irregular beats. Pulse rate did not change with postural change. Platelet count was 98,000 cells/mm³ when it was measured yesterday.

How would you screen a client with this history and current comorbidities?

Neuromusculoskeletal	Systemic
Assess orthopedic complications such as signs of infection, increased skin temperature, localized swelling, pain.	Monitor all vital signs.
Observe patient's adherence to hip precautions; note surgical technique and approach used, type of implant, and location of incision.	Monitor platelet levels, international normalized ratio: if low, observe for bruising, joint bleeds, deep venous thrombosis; follow precautions and exercise guidelines.[133]
Be aware that orthostatic hypotension can cause dizziness, loss of balance, falls—a very dangerous situation with a recent THR. This can be compounded by osteoporosis, if present as a result of surgical menopause.	Watch for signs and symptoms of cardiovascular/pulmonary impairments such as: • Fatigue and muscle weakness • Tachycardia • Fluid migration from the legs to the lungs during the supine position • Dyspnea, orthopnea,* spasmodic cough (check sputum) • Peripheral edema; check jugular distention (see Fig. 4.44) • Check nail beds for signs of decreased perfusion

*Ask if the patient must use pillows and sit up or have the head of the bed elevated; often described as "1-pillow orthopnea" or "2-pillow orthopnea."

Neuromusculoskeletal	Systemic
	Observe for side effects of medications or drug interactions: • Diuresis from Lasix (loop diuretic) can result in potassium depletion and lead to increased sensitivity of myocardium to digoxin (digitalis); monitor serum electrolytes, and observe for signs/symptoms of potassium imbalance; observe for urinary frequency and headache. • Common adverse effects of Lasix include dehydration, muscle cramping, fatigue, weakness, headache, paresthesia, nausea, confusion, orthostatic hypotension, blurred vision, rash • Digoxin: headache, drowsiness, other central nervous system disturbance, bradycardia, arrhythmia, gastrointestinal upset, blurred vision, halos

What signs and symptoms should be reported to the medical staff?

Nurses will be closely monitoring the patient's signs and symptoms. Read the medical record to stay up with what everyone else knows or has observed about the patient. Read the physician's notes to see whether medical intervention has been ordered.

Report anything observed but not already recorded in the chart such as muscle cramping, headache, irregular heartbeat with bradycardia, low pulse, and orthostatic hypotension.

Bradycardia is one of the first signs of digitalis toxicity. In some hospitals, a pulse less than 60 bpm in an adult would indicate that the next dose of digoxin should be withheld and the physician contacted. The protocol may be different from institution to institution.

The therapist is advised to report the following:
• Irregular heartbeat with bradycardia (a possible sign of digoxin/ digitalis toxicity)
• Muscle cramping (possible adverse effect of Lasix) and headache (possible adverse effect of digoxin)
• Charting of vital signs; her blood pressure was not too unusual and pulse rate did not change with position change (probably because of medications), so she does not have medically defined orthostatic hypotension.
• Monitor vital signs throughout intervention; record the time it takes for vital signs to return to normal after exercise or treatment for your documentation of measurable outcomes.

---

also cross the lateral hip area. Additionally, SI joint dysfunction can cause groin pain and, with referred pain to the hip, may be accompanied by an ipsilateral decrease in hip joint internal rotation of 15 degrees or more, thereby confusing the clinical picture even further.[16,17]

Overlying soft tissue structure disorders such as femoral hernia, bursitis, or fasciitis; muscle impairments such as weakness, loss of flexibility, spasms, strain, or tears; and peripheral nerve injury or entrapment, including meralgia paresthetica, can also cause localized hip (and/or groin) pain.

TABLE 17.1	Causes of Buttock Pain
Systemic/Medical Conditions	**Neuromusculoskeletal**
Sciatica from tumor, infection, endometriosis (see Table 17.6)	Sciatica (nerve compression from surrounding soft tissues; piriformis syndrome; see Table 17.6)
Sacroiliitis (pyogenic infection, reactive arthritis, spondyloarthritis)	Posterior facet joint dysfunction
Neoplasm (primary or regional metastases via lymph nodes)	Hip joint disease
Osteoid osteoma of the upper femur	Disk disease (thoracic or lumbar)
Osteomyelitis of the upper femur	SI joint dysfunction
Fracture (sacrum, ilium, pubic ramus)	Bursitis (psoas, gluteal, ischial, trochanteric)
Septic arthritis (hip, SI)	Hamstring strain
Abscess from aseptic necrosis, Crohn's disease, or other retroperitoneal infection; anorectal abscess	Myofascial syndromes
	Spondylolisthesis
Sacral neuralgia from genital herpes	Direct trauma
Ischemia (e.g., claudication from PVD, peripheral arterial aneurysm)	

PVD, Peripheral vascular disease; *SI*, sacroiliac.

Hip pain referred from the upper lumbar vertebrae can radiate into the anterior aspect of the thigh, whereas hip pain from the lower lumbar vertebrae and sacrum is usually felt in the gluteal region, with radiation down the back or outer aspect of the thigh (Fig. 17.2).

The client with pain caused by component instability following total hip arthroplasty may report hip or groin pain with activity, pain at rest, or both. Clinically, a history of "start up" pain may indicate a loose component. After 5 or 10 steps, the groin pain subsides. Pain may increase again after a moderate amount of walking. Groin or thigh pain is most common with micromotion at the bone–prosthesis interface or other loose component, periosteal irritation, or an undersized femoral stem.[18-20]

The client reports a dull aching pain in the thigh with no history of systemic illness or recent trauma. Often, the pain is localized to the site of the prosthetic stem tip. The client points to a specific spot along the anterolateral thigh. Pain with initiation of activity that resolves with continued activity should raise suspicion of a loose prosthesis. Persistent pain that is not relieved with rest and continues through the night suggests infection, requiring medical referral.[18,21]

Systemic Presentation. A *noncapsular* pattern of restricted hip motion (e.g., limited hip extension, adduction, lateral rotation) may be a sign of pathology other than a joint problem associated with osteoarthritis, potentially a serious underlying disease (Case Example 17.2). The pattern

TABLE 17.2	Causes of Hip Pain
Systemic/Medical Conditions	**Neuromusculoskeletal†**
Cancer	Lumbar spine (especially spondylosis, stenosis, disk), SI joint, sacral, or knee pathology
• Metastasis	
• Bone tumor*	
Osteoid osteoma	Osteoarthritis
Chondrosarcoma	Synovitis
Giant cell tumor	Femoral, inguinal, or sports hernia/athletic pubalgia
Ewing's sarcoma	
Vascular	FAI
• Arterial insufficiency	Bursitis (trochanteric, iliopectineal, iliopsoas, ischial)
• Abdominal aortic aneurysm	
• Avascular necrosis	Fasciitis, myofascial pain
Urogenital	Muscle impairment (weakness, loss of flexibility, abnormal tone/strain/tear/ avulsion); snapping hip syndrome
• Kidney (renal) impairment; kidney stones	
• Testicular cancer	
Infectious/inflammatory conditions	
• Abdominal or peritoneal inflammation (psoas abscess; see Box 17.3)	Tendinopathy (tendinitis, tendinosis)
• Ankylosing spondylitis	Piriformis syndrome
• Appendicitis	Stress reaction/fracture
• Ischial rectal abscess*	Occult fracture of the femoral neck
• Crohn's disease; ulcerative colitis	Peripheral nerve injury or entrapment; meralgia paresthetica
• Diverticulitis	
• Osteomyelitis (upper femur)*	Total hip arthroplasty
• PID	• Infection
• Reactive arthritis	• Implant loosening
• Inflammatory arthritis (RA, SLE, seronegative arthropathy, gout)	• Intraoperative blood vessel injury
• Septic hip or SI arthritis*	• Bone loss; subsidence
• Septic hip bursitis*	Acetabular labral or cartilage lesion
• Tuberculosis	
Metabolic disease	Developmental hip dysplasia; hip dislocation
• Osteomalacia, osteoporosis	
• Gaucher's disease	Legg-Calvé-Perthes disease
• Paget's disease	
• Ochronosis	SCFE
• Hemochromatosis	Osteitis pubis (pubic pain radiates to anterior hip)
• Diabetes mellitus (associated with neuropathy)	
Other	
• Sickle cell crisis	
• Hemophilia	
• Ectopic pregnancy	
• Femoral artery catheterization	

FAI, Femoroacetabular impingement; *PID*, pelvic inflammatory disease; *RA*, rheumatoid arthritis; *SCFE*, slipped capital femoral epiphysis; *SI*, sacroiliac; *SLE*, systemic lupus erythematosus.
*Most common causes of the "Sign of the Buttock."
†This is not an exhaustive, all-inclusive list, but rather, it includes the most commonly encountered adult neuromuscular or musculoskeletal causes of hip pain.

BOX 17.2   SIGN OF THE BUTTOCK

James Cyriax, M.D., was the first to write about the "Sign of the Buttock," which is actually made up of seven signs that indicate serious disease posterior to the axis of flexion and extension of the hip. These signs of neural tension deficit suggest severe central nervous system compromise, requiring medical referral. When positive, this test may help the therapist to identify serious extracapsular hip or pelvic disease.

- Primary sign of the buttock: passive hip flexion more limited and more painful than the straight leg raise
- Limited (and painful) passive straight leg raise
- Trunk flexion limited to the same extent as hip flexion
- Painful weakness of hip extension
- Noncapsular pattern of restriction (hip); the capsular pattern is marked limitation of hip medial rotation first, then hip flexion with some limitation of abduction and little or no limitation of adduction and lateral rotation.
- Swelling (and tenderness) in the buttocks region
- Empty end feel with hip flexion

Data from Cyriax J: *Textbook of orthopaedic medicine. Diagnosis of soft tissue lesions,* ed 8, Philadelphia, 1983, WB Saunders.

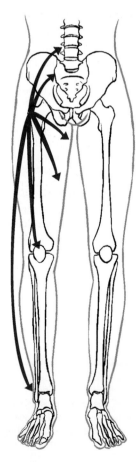

Fig. 17.1   Pain referred *from* the hip *to* other structures and anatomic locations. Pain from a pathologic condition of the hip can be referred to the low back, sacroiliac or sacral area, groin, anterior thigh, knee, or ankle.

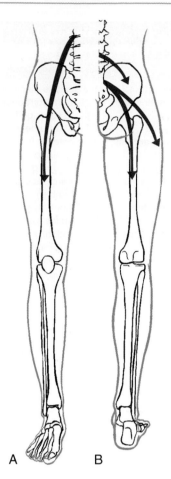

A   B

Fig. 17.2   Pain referred *to* the hip *from* other structures and anatomic locations. **A,** Hip pain referred from the upper lumbar vertebrae can radiate into the anterior aspect of the thigh. **B,** Hip pain from the lower lumbar vertebrae and sacrum is usually felt in the gluteal region, with radiation down the back or outer aspect of the thigh.

of movement restriction most common with a *capsular* pattern for the hip is limitation of hip medial rotation, flexion, abduction, and, sometimes, slight limitation of hip extension. Empty end feel can be an indicator of potentially serious disease such as infection or neoplasm. Empty end feel is described as limiting pain before the end range of motion is reached, but with no resistance perceived by the examiner.[14]

Whenever assessing hip joint pain for a systemic or viscerogenic cause, the therapist should look at hip rotation in the neutral position and perform the log-rolling test. With the client in the supine position, the examiner supports the client's heels in the examiner's hands and passively rolls the feet in and out. Decreased range of motion (usually accompanied by pain) is positive for an intraarticular source of symptoms. If normal hip rotation is present in this position but the motion reproduces hip pain, then an extraarticular cause should be considered.

Log-rolling of the hip back and forth, though not sensitive, is generally considered to be the most specific examination maneuver for intraarticular hip pathology because it rotates the femoral head back and forth in the acetabulum and capsule, not stressing any of the surrounding extraarticular

CASE EXAMPLE 17.2

Noncapsular Hip Pattern

A 46-year-old male long-distance runner developed sudden onset of right hip pain. He was given a diagnosis of trochanteric bursitis (greater trochanteric pain syndrome [GTPS]) by an orthopedic physician and was referred to physical therapy.

Objective Findings

(–) For tenderness on palpation over the greater trochanter

(–) Trigger points (TrPs) of the hip and low back region

(+) Noncapsular pattern of restriction of the hip (capsular pattern in the hip is flexion, abduction, and medial rotation); client was limited in extension and lateral rotation

(+) Heel strike test

The major criteria for a medical diagnosis of trochanteric bursitis (GTPS) consist of marked tenderness to deep palpation of the greater trochanter and relief of pain after peritrochanteric injection with a local anesthetic and corticosteroid.

The absence of greater trochanter tenderness and the presence of a noncapsular pattern of restriction of the hip were not consistent with the given diagnosis. Local injection was not administered. If an injection had been given, trochanteric bursitis/GTPS may have been eliminated from the list of possible diagnoses.

Objective findings are not consistent with trochanteric bursitis/GTPS. What do you do now?

More tests, of course, and more questions! Is there any history of cancer or prostate problems? Take his vital signs. Can he squat? Clear the hip. Conduct a Review of Systems to look for a pattern in the past medical history, clinical presentation, and any associated signs and symptoms.

Look for a pattern of symptoms that suggests a particular visceral system. Hip pain can be caused by gastrointestinal (GI), vascular, infectious, or cancerous causes. Ask a few screening questions directed at each of these systems. For example:

GI: Are you having any nausea? Vomiting? Abdominal pain? Change in bowel function? Blood in the stool? Test for psoas abscess.

Vascular: Any throbbing pain? Presence of varicose veins? Trophic changes? History of heart disease?

Infectious: Any history of inflammatory bowel conditions such as Crohn's disease, ulcerative colitis, or diverticulitis? Ever have appendicitis? Any recent skin rashes on the legs?

Cancerous: Previous history of cancer? Bone pain at night? Night sweats? Palpate the lymph nodes in the inguinal and popliteal regions.

Result: Red flags included:

- Age
- Past history of prostate cancer at the age of 44 years
- Positive heel strike test
- Noncapsular hip pattern
- Inconsistent symptoms with diagnosis

The results of the physical therapy examination warranted further medical evaluation, and the client was returned to the physician with a recommendation for imaging studies. Magnetic resonance imaging (MRI) results indicated a nondisplaced, complete fracture of the femoral neck from prostate cancer that had metastasized to the bone.

Data from Jones DL, Erhard RE: Differential diagnosis with serious pathology: a case report. Phys Ther 76:S89–S90, 1996.

structures.[22] The test does not identify the specific disease present but identifies the source of the symptoms as intraarticular.

Keep in mind that if normal rotations are present but painful, the problem may still be musculoskeletal in origin (e.g., SI, early sign of arthritic changes in the hip joint). Full motion is also possible in the early stages of avascular necrosis and sickle cell anemia. The log-rolling test should be combined with Patrick's or Faber's (flexion, abduction, and external rotation) test, long-axis distraction, compressive hip loading, and the scour (quadrant) test to determine whether the hip is a possible source of symptoms.

The presence of GI symptoms (e.g., nausea, vomiting, diarrhea, constipation, abdominal bloating or cramping) or urologic symptoms (e.g., urinary frequency, nocturia, dysuria, or flank pain) along with hip pain is cause to take a closer look. Palpable reproduction of painful symptoms is generally considered extraarticular.[23]

Negative radiographs of the hip may not rule out bone lesions. When intervention by the physical therapist does not yield relief of symptoms (or only temporary relief), further imaging studies or referral back to the physician may be needed. A careful review of risk factors and clinical presentation will guide this decision.[24,25]

Groin

The physical therapist may see a client with an isolated groin problem, especially in the sports or military populations (Case Example 17.3), but more often, the individual has low back, pelvic, hip, knee, or SI problems with a secondary complaint of groin pain. Possible systemic and/or visceral causes of groin pain are wide-ranging, appearing as an isolated symptom or in combination with pelvic, hip, low back, or thigh pain (Table 17.3 and Case Example 17.4).

Palpating the groin area is usually necessary in making a differential diagnosis. The therapist should explain the examination procedure and obtain the client's permission. A third person in the exam room can be offered but is not mandatory.

During examination of the groin, the physical therapist may palpate enlarged lymph nodes, or the client may indicate these nodes to the examiner. Painless, progressive enlargements of lymph nodes or lymph nodes that are aberrant or suspicious for any reason, especially if present in more than one area or the presence of a past medical history of cancer, are an indication of the need for medical referral.

Changes in lymph nodes without a previous history of cancer continue to represent a yellow or red flag. Tender, movable inguinal lymph nodes may be a sign of food intolerance or allergies or an indication that the body is fighting off an infectious process. The therapist should use his or her best clinical judgment in deciding what to do, but should always err on the side of caution. When doubt arises, one should contact the physician and communicate any concerns, observations, or questions.

Neuromusculoskeletal Presentation. Neuromuscular or musculoskeletal causes of groin pain should also be considered (Case Example 17.5).[26,27] Keep in mind that intraarticular pathology of the hip can manifest as groin pain owing

CASE EXAMPLE 17.3

Groin Pain in a 13-Year-Old Skateboarder

Referral: A 13-year-old boy presented with a 2-week history of left groin pain. He reported a skateboarding accident as the cause of the symptoms. He was coming down a flight of stairs, hit the last step by mistake, and caught his foot on the stair railing. His leg was forced into wide abduction and external rotation. No pop or snap was perceived (heard or felt) at the time of injury.

The client continued skateboarding but experienced increasing pain 2 hours later. At that time, he could "hardly walk" and has had trouble walking without limping ever since. He tried getting back to skateboarding but was stopped by sharp pain in the groin. No other symptoms were reported (no saddle anesthesia, no numbness and tingling, no bladder changes, no constitutional symptoms).

Clinical Presentation: An antalgic gait was observed as the boy avoided putting full weight through the hip during the stance phase. Trendelenburg gait or the Trendelenburg test was not positive. He could not do a squat test because of pain. He could not put enough weight on the left leg to try heel walking or toe walking.

Generalized pain occurred along the inner thigh and was described as "tenderness." The child cannot internally rotate the hip past midline. Abduction was limited to 30 degrees with painful empty end feel. During active hip flexion, the hip automatically flexes, abducts, and externally rotates. Pain increases with active-assisted or passive hip flexion when one is trying to keep the hip in neutral alignment.

Associated Signs and Symptoms: When asked about symptoms of any kind anywhere else in his body, the boy replied, "No." When offered a list of possible symptoms, these were all negative. He did admit to being slightly constipated because of the pain. Vital signs were all within normal limits.

Is referral indicated in the absence of any signs or symptoms of viscerogenic or systemic disease?

Some red flags are identified here, even though they do not point to a viscerogenic or systemic origin. Trauma, young age, and failure to complete a squat screening test for orthopedic clearance of the hip, knee, and ankle all suggest the need for medical referral before physical therapy intervention is initiated.

Turn to Table 17.3. As you look at the left column of Systemic Causes, what clinical presentation and signs and symptoms might be expected with each of these conditions? Does the current clinical presentation fit any of these?

Now look at the musculoskeletal causes of groin pain (right column, Table 17.3). Are past medical history, risk factors, or clinical presentation consistent for any of these problems? For example, pain in the hip or groin area in anyone who is not skeletally mature raises the suspicion of an orthopedic injury. Abduction and external rotation forces on the hip can produce a slipped capital femoral epiphysis (SCFE).

This is the case here, which required imaging studies for diagnosis. Anteroposterior x-ray films were negative, but a lateral view showed slippage to confirm SCFE.

Data from Learch T, Resnick D: Groin pain in a 13-year-old skateboarder. *J Musculoskel Med* 20:513–515, 2003.

TABLE 17.3	Causes of Groin Pain
Systemic/Medical Conditions	**Neuromusculoskeletal**
Cancer	Musculotendinous strain (adductors, hamstrings, iliopsoas, abdominals, tensor fascia lata, gluteus medius)[41]
• Spinal cord tumor	
• Osteoid osteoma	
• Hodgkin's disease/lymphoma	
• Leukemia	Internal oblique avulsion
• Testicular	Nerve compression or entrapment (ilioinguinal, obturator nerves)
• Prostate	
• Soft tissue mass	Stress reaction, stress fracture, avulsion fracture, or complete bone fracture (femoral neck, pubic ramus)
Osteoporosis	
Fluid in peritoneal cavity	
• Ascites (cirrhosis)	
• Congestive heart failure	Bursitis (iliopectineal)
• Cancer	Pubalgia*
• Hyperaldosteronism	Osteitis pubis
Hemophilia	Apophysitis (young athletes)
• GI bleeding	
Abdominal aortic aneurysm, peripheral arterial aneurysm	Trauma (physical, sexual, birth)
Gynecologic conditions	Sports, inguinal or femoral hernia
• Cancer (uterine/ovarian masses)	Hip joint impairment
• Uterine fibroids	• Subluxation, dislocation, dysplasia
• Ovarian cyst	• Avascular necrosis (osteonecrosis)
• Endometriosis (causing pubalgia)	• Total hip arthroplasty (loosening, infection, bone loss, subsidence)
• Ectopic pregnancy (not common)	
• Sexually transmitted infection	• SCFE
• PID	• Legg-Calvé-Perthes disease
Infection, usually intraabdominal or intraperitoneal infection (see Box 17.3)	• Labral tear with or without femoroacetabular impingement
Urologic	• Arthritis, arthrosis
• Prostate impairment (prostatitis, BPH, prostate cancer)	SI joint impairment
• Epididymitis; testicular torsion	Lumbar spine impairment (spinal stenosis, disk disease)
• Urethritis/urinary tract infection	Myofascial dysfunction
• Upper urinary tract problems affecting the kidneys or ureters (inflammation, infection, obstruction)	Thoracic disk disease (lower thoracic spine)
• Hydrocele/varicocele	
GI	
• Diverticulitis	
• Inflammatory bowel disease	
Seronegative spondyloarthropathy	

BPH, Benign prostatic hyperplasia; *GI*, gastrointestinal; *PID*, pelvic inflammatory disease; *SCFE*, slipped capital femoral epiphysis; *SI*, sacroiliac.

*Pubalgia is a description of painful symptoms of the groin that can be caused by a wide range of muscular, tendinous, osseous, and even visceral structures. This condition may be labeled osteitis pubis when there is articular involvement such as arthritis, articular instability, or other articular lesions involving the pubic symphysis.[41]

CASE EXAMPLE 17.4

Soft Tissue Sarcoma

A 38-year-old female patient was referred to physical therapy by a primary care clinic physician assistant with a diagnosis of "groin strain." The client denied any injury or trauma. Little to no pain was reported, but a feeling of "fullness" in the left proximal thigh was described. She was unable to cross her legs when sitting because of this fullness. No other constitutional or associated symptoms were noted.

When asked, "How long have you had this?" the client thought it had been present for the past 3 months. When asked, "Has it changed since you first noticed it?" she stated that she thought it was getting larger.

Examination: There was an obvious area of edema or tissue mass identified in the proximal medial left thigh. No tenderness, bruising, erythema, or skin temperature changes were reported. The area in question had a boggy feel during palpation. Lower extremity range of motion and manual muscle testing were within normal limits.

Screening and Differential Diagnosis: Look at Table 17.3. As you review the possible systemic and musculoskeletal causes of groin pain, what additional questions and tests or measures must be asked/carried out to complete your screening examination?

On the Systemic Side

- Spinal cord tumors—No temperature changes, dermatomal changes, or associated bowel and bladder changes; no further testing required at this time
- Hodgkin's disease/lymphoma/leukemia—Ask about previous history of cancer, family history of cancer; palpate lymph nodes (quick screen of lymph nodes above and below the groin and careful examination of inguinal lymph nodes)
- Urinary tract involvement—No history of recent fever, chills, difficulty urinating, or urinary tract infection; no blood in the urine; no further questions at this time
- Ascites—No apparent abdominal ascites, no history of alcoholism; check for asterixis, liver palms (palmar erythema); ask about symptoms of carpal tunnel syndrome, look for spider angiomas during inspection, and observe nail beds for any changes (nails of Terry)
- Hemophilia—It is a long shot, but ask about personal/family history
- Abdominal aortic aneurysm (AAA)—Ask about bounding pulse sensation in the abdomen; palpate aortic pulse width (see Fig. 4.54); ask about the presence of chest or back pain at any time, especially with exertion
- Gynecologic—Ask about a history of pelvic pain, pelvic inflammatory disease, or sexually transmitted infection

- Appendicitis—Perform McBurney's test, Blumberg's sign, and iliopsoas and obturator tests (see Chapter 8 for descriptions)

On the Musculoskeletal Side

- Muscle strain—As already tested, no loss of motion or strength; no pain with resisted movement; no history of trauma or overuse. Red flag: clinical presentation is not consistent with the medical diagnosis
- Internal oblique avulsion/stress reaction or fracture—As previously stated
- Pubalgia—As previously stated; no painful symptoms reported, no pain during palpation
- Sexual assault/domestic violence—Even though the client denies trauma, consider a screening interview for nonaccidental trauma (see Chapter 2 or Appendix B-3 on); absence of erythema, skin bruising, or other skin changes makes this type of trauma unlikely
- Total hip arthropathy—Negative history
- Avascular necrosis—Not likely, given the clinical presentation; ask about a history of long-term use of immunosuppressants (corticosteroids for Crohn's disease, sarcoidosis, autoimmune disorders)
- Trigger points (TrPs)—Atypical presentation for a trigger point; check for latent TrPs of the adductors, iliopsoas, vastus medialis, and sartorius

Special Questions to Ask: Take a final look at *Special Questions to Ask* in this chapter. Have you missed anything? Left anything out?

Result: Based on lack of objective findings and red flags of mass increasing in size and clinical presentation inconsistent with medical diagnosis, the therapist consulted with an orthopedic surgeon in the same health care facility. The orthopedic surgeon ordered radiographs, which were normal, and advised a short period of observation before ordering magnetic resonance imaging (MRI).

After 3 weeks, no changes were observed, and MRI was ordered. MRI showed a soft tissue tumor, later diagnosed by biopsy as a stage IIIB high-grade soft tissue sarcoma.

The client underwent multiple surgical procedures, including removal of the medial compartment musculature and limb salvage with an eventual hemiarthroplasty. Physical therapy included gait training, regaining safe hip active range of motion, an aquatic rehabilitation program, use of an underwater treadmill, and both open and closed kinetic chain strengthening.

Adapted from Baxter RE: Identification of neoplasm mimicking musculoskeletal pathology: A case report involving groin symptoms. Poster presented at Combined Sections Meeting, 2004, New Orleans, LA. Used with permission.

to the innervation of the hip capsule. Extraarticular hip conditions radiate to the lateral or posterior aspects of the hip.[28]

Groin pain is a common complaint in sports that involve kicking and rapid change of direction (e.g., soccer, hockey). The most common musculoskeletal cause of groin pain is strain of the adductor muscles, most often involving the adductor longus. The history includes a specific trauma, repetitive motion, or injury, which occurs primarily at the junction of the muscle fibers and the extended tendon of

origin. Acutely, this injury causes unilateral or bilateral pain during or after activity, with local palpation of the adductor longus origin, and during passive stretching or active contraction; eccentric activation may be even more painful.[29,30] Acute injury may be followed in several days by ecchymosis.

Chronic groin or inguinal pain in the active athletic, sports, or military groups is often referred to as *athletic pubalgia*. Athletic pubalgia is sometimes used interchangeably to describe a *sports* or *athletic hernia*, which is a tear in the

CASE EXAMPLE 17.5

Groin Pain—Musculoskeletal Cause

A 44-year-old male patient came to physical therapy with a 7-year history of right groin pain. X-ray films, a bone scan, and an arthrogram of the hip were all negative. At the time of initial examination, the client was taking morphine for pain that was described as constant, severe, and sharp and that was rated 8 out of 10 on the Numeric Rating Scale (NRS; see Chapter 3). Sitting and driving made the symptoms worse, and he was unable to work as a mechanic because prolonged squatting was required. Lying supine relieved the pain.

Physical examination revealed extreme hip medial rotation associated with active hip flexion, abduction, and knee extension; each of these movements reproduced his symptoms. Passive range of motion of the right hip was painful and was limited to 95 degrees of flexion and 0 degrees of lateral rotation.

Visual inspection during movement and palpation of the greater trochanter indicated that the proximal femur had medially rotated and moved anteriorly during hip flexion. Through application of a posteroinferior glide over the proximal femur during hip flexion, groin pain was decreased and motion increased. The client was able to moderate his symptoms by avoiding hip medial rotation during hip and knee movements.

Consider: Are any red flags present? Is further screening indicated to rule out systemic origin of symptoms? *If yes*, what questions or tests might you consider carrying out?

Red Flags: Age (over 40 years); constant, intense pain

Further Screening Required: The length of time that symptoms have been present without accompanying signs and symptoms of a urologic or gastrointestinal (GI) nature (7 years) is not typical of systemic origin of musculoskeletal symptoms.

The fact that no aggravating and relieving factors are known further rules out a viscerogenic cause of pain. It would be appropriate to ask the *Special Questions for Men* at the end of Chapter 15 (see also Appendix B-24 on).

It is always a good idea to ask one final question: *Are any other symptoms of any kind anywhere else in your body?* Special tests might include the heel strike test (fracture), translational rotation tests for stress reaction (fracture), iliopsoas and obturator tests (abscess; see Chapter 9), and trigger point assessment.

Result: The client was treated for femoral anterior glide with medial rotation (movement impairment diagnosis).[26] Training to teach the client to modify hip medial rotation during sustained postures and functional activities was a key component of the intervention. Exercises were given to strengthen the right iliopsoas muscle, hip lateral rotator muscles, and posterior gluteus medius muscle.

The client was pain-free and off pain medications 2 months later after six treatment sessions. He was able to return to full-time work.

Comment: Knowledge of red-flag signs and symptoms, risk factors for various systemic conditions and illnesses, associated signs and symptoms of viscerogenic pain, and typical clinical presentations for neuromuscular and musculoskeletal problems can guide the therapist in quickly sizing up a situation and deciding whether or not further screening is warranted.

In this case, the therapist can see that only a few screening questions are in order. The application of any additional special tests depends on the client's answers to screening questions. The client's immediate response to intervention is another way to verify a correct physical therapy diagnosis. Failure to progress with intervention is a red flag that indicates the need for reevaluation.

Data from Bloom NJ, Sahrmann SA: Groin pain caused by movement system impairments: A case report. Poster presented at the American Physical Therapy Association Combined Sections Meeting, 2004, New Orleans, LA. Used with permission.

---

muscles of the inner thigh, lower abdomen, and/or the fascia.[31] The term *sports hernia* may be a bit misleading because experts in this area do not consider this condition the same as a true inguinal or femoral hernia.[32]

Symptoms associated with athletic pubalgia are often described as deep groin or lower abdominal pain with exertion (usually unilateral). There may be a localized sharp burning sensation in the lower abdomen and/or inguinal region. Symptoms are relieved with rest but aggravated by activity, especially sport-related activities that involve cutting and pivoting, as well as lateral motions that involve rapid acceleration and deceleration, such as ice hockey, soccer, and rugby.[33] As the condition progresses, symptoms may radiate to the adductor region, testes (male), and labia (female).[34,35]

Labral tears of the acetabulum can also cause groin pain. There may be a history of trauma, but acetabular labral tears can occur without trauma. The clinical presentation can vary and include night pain, activity-related pain, positive Trendelenburg sign, and positive impingement sign (pain reproduced with hip flexion, adduction, and internal rotation: specificity 95.4%, sensitivity 14.8%). In contrast to this, as recent as 2015, several studies have found a high prevalence of labral pathology in the asymptomatic population.[36,37]

Femoroacetabular impingement presents as groin pain in young adults. Onset is gradual and progressive with intermittent groin pain after prolonged walking, prolonged sitting, or athletic activities that stress the hip. The most reliable hip tests to determine whether a client has femoroacetabular impingement from most reliable to least reliable was the log-roll test (0.99), the FABER test (0.84), hip internal rotation causing pain (0.84), and the anterior impingement test[38] (internal hip rotation and adduction while the hip is flexed, 0.76). Referral for a medical orthopedic examination and imaging studies may be warranted.[39]

Another common problem in the young athlete or long-distance runner is osteitis pubis. Repetitive stress of the adductor group can cause inflammation at the musculotendinous attachment on the pubic bone, contributing to sclerosis and bony changes.[40]

Osteitis pubis with inflammation and sclerosis of the pubic symphysis can cause both acute and chronic groin pain. Individuals affected most often include competitive sports athletes involved in running, leaping, and landing with force, repetitive kicking motions, or training on concrete, uneven, or other hard surfaces. Osteitis pubis can also occur as a result of leg length differences, faulty foot and body mechanics, or muscular imbalances and during pregnancy. Tenderness during palpation of the pubic symphysis helps identify this condition.[33] Onset of midline pain that radiates to the groin is typical. Pain is reproduced by palpation of the pubis (anterior), passive hip abduction, and resisted hip adduction. Articular lesions involving the pubis symphysis can also lead to pubalgia.[41]

Insertional injuries of the upper attachment of the rectus abdominis muscle over the anteroinferior pubis (just lateral to the pubic symphysis) can lead to tendinopathy presenting as pubalgia. Without magnetic resonance imaging (MRI), insertional abdominis pathology cannot be differentiated from adductor pathology as the abdominis pubic attachment and the thigh adductor tendon blend to form one unit.[41]

Chronic, unresolved groin pain in the athletic population also has been linked with altered neuromotor control.[42] The therapist may need to evaluate groin pain from a motor control point of view. See further discussion of stress reaction/fractures in the section on Trauma as a Cause of Hip, Groin, or Lower Quadrant Pain in this chapter.

Older adults are more likely to experience hip, buttock, or groin pain associated with arthritis, lumbar stenosis, insufficiency fractures, or hip arthroplasty. Arthritis is characterized by radiating pain to the knee, but not below, with decreased hip range of motion. Gait disturbances may be seen as arthritis progresses.[19] Insufficiency fracture of the pubic rami can also cause hip/groin pain, resulting in a reluctance to bear weight on the affected side along with an antalgic gait.[43]

Hip and groin pain secondary to lumbar stenosis can manifest as low back pain that radiates to the lower extremities. The pain begins and gets worse with ambulation. Standing and walking may also increase symptoms when the lumbar spine assumes a more lordotic position and the ligamentum flavum folds in on itself, pinching the foramina closed. The client who has stenosis bends forward or sits to avoid painful symptoms. Clients who have a total hip arthroplasty for hip pain may have continued groin and buttock pain, secondary to sciatica or lumbar spinal stenosis.[19]

Systemic Presentation. The clinical presentation of groin pain from a systemic source does not vary from musculoskeletally induced groin pain. Once again, the key is to look at the client's age (e.g., atherosclerotically induced vascular problems in the older adult), past medical history (e.g., previous history of cancer, liver disease, hemophilia), and sex (e.g., ectopic pregnancy, prostate or testicular problems).

In addition, asking about the presence of other symptoms and conducting a Review of Systems may help the therapist identify any one of the systemic causes listed in Table 17.3.

Thigh

Once again, the importance of conducting a thorough physical examination to rule out systemic or viscerogenic disease as the source of thigh pain cannot be emphasized enough; a client history and lower quadrant screening examination should be performed (see Box 4.16).

Anterior thigh pain is more common (Table 17.4), but posterior thigh pain may occur, with ruptured abdominal aortic aneurysm (AAA). Local anterior or posterior thigh pain of systemic origin generally occurs as a deep aching generated by soft tissue irritation or bone involvement. Radicular pain is usually a sharp, stabbing pain that projects in dermatomal distributions caused by compression of the dorsal nerve roots.

Neuromusculoskeletal Presentation. The lower lumbar vertebrae and sacrum can refer pain to the gluteal and hip region, with pain radiating down the posterior or posterolateral thigh. Pain down the lateral aspect of the thigh to the knee may also be caused by inflammation of the tensor fascia lata with iliotibial band syndrome.[7] A similar pattern has been reported in association with irritability, injury, or disease of the thoracolumbar transitional segments,[44,45] and at least one case of synovial cell sarcoma presenting as iliotibial band syndrome has been reported.[46]

Anterior thigh pain is commonly disk related, resulting from L3-L4 disk herniation and occurring most often in older

TABLE 17.4	Causes of Thigh Pain	
Systemic/Medical Conditions	**Neuromusculoskeletal**
Retroperitoneal or intraabdominal tumor or abscess (see Box 17.3)	Musculotendinous strains (e.g., adductor, abductor, quadriceps)
Kidney stones (nephrolithiasis, ureteral or renal colic)	Iliopectineal bursitis (anterior and medial thigh pain); trochanteric bursitis/greater trochanteric pain syndrome (lateral thigh)
Peripheral neuropathy (bilateral, symmetric) • Diabetes mellitus • Neoplasm • Chronic alcohol use	Peripheral neuropathy (unilateral, asymmetric) Contusions (collisions with balls, hockey pucks, the ground, other athletes) Nerve compression (e.g., meralgia paresthetica from compression of the LFCN, sciatic nerve, obturator nerve)
Thrombosis (femoral artery, great saphenous vein)	Myositis ossificans (injury with contusion and hematoma formation)
Bone tumor (primary or metastases)	Femoral shaft or subtrochanteric stress reaction or fracture; insufficiency fracture/stress reaction Hip disease (osteoarthritis, labral tear)
Bone fracture associated with long-term bisphosphonates (rare; under investigation)*	Total hip arthroplasty (loose component, polyethylene wear debris, undersized/oversized femoral stem, periosteal irritation) SI joint dysfunction Upper lumbar spine dysfunction; spondylolisthesis, herniated disk, previous surgery Myofascial dysfunction Inguinal hernia

LFCN, Lateral femoral cutaneous nerve; *SI*, sacroiliac.
*Reports of thigh pain and weakness in affected thigh for weeks to months before a low-energy fracture occurs. See Update: thigh bone fractures in women taking bisphosphonate drugs, *Harvard Women's Health Watch* 17(7):6–7, 2010; and Abrahamsen B: Subtrochanteric and diaphyseal femur fractures in patients treated with alendronate: a register-based national cohort study, *J Bone Miner Res* 24(6):1095–1102, 2009.

clients with a previous history of lumbar spine surgery. The clinical presentation varies among affected individuals, but thigh pain alone is most common (Case Example 17.6).

Use of the extreme lateral interbody fusion technique has been linked with thigh weakness and/or numbness postoperatively as a possible consequence of trauma to the psoas muscle or femoral nerve during the approach. Symptoms are temporary and appear to resolve with soft tissue healing following surgery.[47]

Back and thigh pain, a positive reverse straight leg raise (SLR) test, and a decreased knee reflex are described more often in clients with disk herniation at the L3-L4 level than in clients with disk herniation at L4-L5 and L5-S1 levels.[48,49] A positive reverse SLR is defined as pain traveling down the

ipsilateral leg when the person is prone and the leg is extended at the hip and the knee. A positive test is caused by tension on the femoral nerve and its roots.[50]

Objective neurologic findings, such as hyperreflexia or hyporeflexia, decreased sensation to light touch or pinprick, and decreased motor strength, can occur with soft tissue problems such as bursitis. However, clients with true nerve root irritation experience pain extending into the lower leg and foot. Clients with bursitis exhibit a positive "jump" sign when pressure is applied over the greater trochanter; no jump sign is seen with nerve root irritation.[9]

A common neuromuscular cause of anterior or anterolateral thigh pain is lateral femoral cutaneous nerve (LFCN) neuralgia. Entrapment or compression of the LFCN causes pain or dysesthesia, or both, in the anterolateral thigh—a condition called *meralgia paresthetica (MP)*. Compression of the LFCN may occur at the level of the L2 and L3 roots through upper lumbar disk herniation or tumor in the second lumbar vertebra. MP most commonly occurs in males 30 to 40 years old and has recently been classified as either idiopathic or iatrogenic. Idiopathic causes are mechanical causes that compress the LFCN related to the following factors: BMI > 30, pregnancy, tight garments, military armor, seat belts, direct trauma, scoliosis, iliacus hematoma, and leg length changes. Metabolic factors that are considered idiopathic include diabetes mellitus, alcoholism, and lead poisoning. Iatrogenic causes include postsurgical complications after hip joint replacement and spinal surgery.[51] For example, LFCN neuropathy may occur after spine surgery to repair nerve damage that occurred during harvesting of the iliac bone graft or that resulted from pressure on the pelvis from prone positioning or with use of the Relton-Hall frame.[52]

Other causes of injury to the LFCN include positioning during hip arthroplasty.[53] For clients with hip arthroplasty, implant loosening, fracture, or subsidence (sinking into the bone) can cause thigh pain as the first symptom of instability.[21] Both passive and active range of motion should be evaluated to assess implant stability. Radiograph imaging is needed to look at component position, bone–prosthesis interface, and signs of fracture or infection.[18]

Systemic Presentation. The pain pattern for anterior thigh pain produced by systemic causes is often the same as that presented for pain resulting from neuromusculoskeletal causes. The therapist must rely on clues from the history and the presence of associated signs and symptoms to help guide the decision-making process.

For example, obstruction, infection, inflammation, or compression of the ureters may cause a pattern of low back and flank pain that radiates anteriorly to the ipsilateral lower abdomen and upper thigh. The client usually has a past history of similar problems or additional urologic symptoms such as pain with urination, urinary frequency, low-grade fever, sweats, or blood in the urine. Murphy's percussion test (see Fig. 4.54) may be positive when the kidney is involved.

The same pain pattern can occur with lower thoracic disk herniation. However, instead of urologic signs and symptoms, the therapist should look for a history of back pain and

---

CASE EXAMPLE 17.6
Total Knee Arthroplasty

A 78-year-old woman went to the emergency department over a weekend for knee pain. She reported a knee joint replacement 6 months ago because of arthritis. Radiograph examination showed that the knee implant was intact with no complications (i.e., no infection, fracture, or loose components). She was advised to contact her orthopedic surgeon the following Monday for a follow-up visit. The woman decided instead to see the physical therapist who was involved with her postoperative rehabilitation.

The physical therapist's interview and examination revealed the following information: no pain was perceived or reported anywhere except in the knee; the pain pattern was constant (always present), but was made worse by weight-bearing activities; the knee was not warm, red, or swollen; no other associated or constitutional signs and symptoms were present; and vital signs were within normal limits for her age range.

Range of motion was better than at the time of previous discharge, but painful symptoms were elicited with a gross manual muscle screening examination. After a test of muscle strength, the woman was experiencing intense pain and was unable to put any weight on the painful leg.

The physical therapist insisted that the woman contact her physician immediately and arranged by phone for an emergency appointment that same day.

Result: Orthopedic examination and pelvic and hip films showed a hip fracture that required immediate total hip replacement the same day. The knee can be a site for referred pain from other areas of the musculoskeletal system, especially when symptoms are monoarticular. Systemic origin (or medical conditions causing) symptoms are more likely when multiple joints are involved or migrating arthralgias are present.

No history or accompanying signs and symptoms suggested a systemic origin of knee pain, but the pain during weight-bearing made worse after muscle testing was a red-flag symptom for bone involvement. Hip fractures or other hip disease can masquerade as knee pain.

Prompt diagnosis of hip fracture is important in preventing complications. This therapist chose the conservative approach with medical referral rather than proceeding with physical therapy intervention. Sometimes, the "treat-and-see" approach to symptom assessment works well, but if any red flags are identified, a physician referral is advised.

trauma and the presence of neurologic signs and symptoms accompanying discogenic lesions.

Retroperitoneal or intraabdominal tumor or abscess may also cause anterior thigh pain. A history of reproductive or abdominal cancer or the presence of any condition listed in Box 17.3 is a red flag.

Thigh pain has been reported as a prodromal symptom of unilateral low-energy subtrochanteric and femoral shaft (diaphyseal) stress reactions and fractures in a small number of people on long-term bisphosphonate therapy.[54]

Knee and Lower Leg

Pain in the lower leg is most often caused by injury, inflammation, tumor (malignant or benign), altered peripheral circulation, deep venous thrombosis (DVT), or neurologic impairment (Table 17.5). Assessment of limb pain follows the series of pain-related questions presented in Fig. 3.6. The therapist can use the information in Boxes 4.13 and 4.15 to conduct a screening examination.

Neuromusculoskeletal Presentation. In addition to screening for medical problems, the therapist must remember to clear the joint above and below the area of symptoms or dysfunction. True knee pain or symptoms are often described as mechanical (local pain and tenderness with locking or giving way of the lower leg) or loading (poorly localized pain with weight-bearing).

There are many musculoskeletal or neuromuscular conditions well known to the therapist as a potential cause of generalized knee pain, including muscle spasm, strain, or tear; patellofemoral pain syndrome; tendinitis; ligamentous disruption, meniscal tear, or osteochondral lesion; stress fracture[55]; and nerve entrapment.[56,57]

Degenerative joint disease of the hip[58] or other hip pathology can masquerade as knee pain in adults.[59] Neurologic problems, including spinal stenosis, complex regional pain syndrome (type 1), neurogenic claudication, and lumbar radiculopathy are common disorders that can produce knee pain. Isolated knee pain involving SI dysfunction has also been reported.[60]

Pain and impaired function from a variety of intraarticular or extraarticular etiologies can also develop following a total knee arthroplasty.[61] Client history and clinical examination will help establish the diagnosis. Assessment of trigger points (TrPs) is also essential as pain referral to the knee from TrPs in the lower quadrant is well recognized but sometimes forgotten.[62,63]

Many therapists over the years have shared stories of clients treated for knee pain with a total knee replacement only to discover later (when the knee pain was unchanged) that the problem was extraarticular (i.e., coming from the back or hip). On the flip side, it is not as likely but is still possible that hip pain can be caused by knee disease. Individual case reports of hip fracture presenting as isolated knee pain have been published[64] (Case Example 17.7).

Systemic Presentation. Systemic or pathologic conditions presenting as *generalized knee pain* can include fractures, Baker's cyst, tumors (benign or malignant), arthritis,

---

BOX 17.3 CAUSES OF PSOAS ABSCESS

- Diverticulitis
- Crohn's disease
- Appendicitis
- Pelvic inflammatory disease (PID)
- Diabetes mellitus
- Any other source of infection, including dental[112]
  - Renal infection
  - Infective spondylitis (vertebra)
  - Osteomyelitis
  - Sacroiliac (SI) joint infection

---

infection, and/or DVT.[56] Other types of cancer can also cause knee pain such as lymphoma, leukemia, and myeloma. Watch for unusual bleeding, easy bruising, unintentional weight loss, fatigue, fever, worsening pain (duration and intensity), sweats, dyspnea, and lymphadenopathy.[55]

A history of trauma accompanied by persistent or worsening symptoms despite restricted loading of the area are typical with bone or soft tissue tumors. *Night pain, localized swelling or warmth, locking,* and *palpable mass* with any of the other symptoms listed raise the suspicion of bone or soft tissue tumor.[65]

Burning and pain in the legs and feet at night are common in older adults; this is also a potential side effect of some chemotherapy drugs. The exact mechanism is often unknown; many factors should be considered, including allergic response to the fabric in clothing and socks, poorly fitted shoes, long-term alcohol use, adverse effects of medication, diabetes mellitus, pernicious anemia, and restless legs syndrome.

Leg cramps, especially those occurring in the lower leg and calf, are common in the adult population.[66,67] Older adults, athletes, and pregnant women are at increased risk.[68] The history and physical examination are key elements in identifying the cause. The most common causes of leg cramps include dehydration, arterial occlusion from PVD, neurogenic claudication from lumbar spinal stenosis,[68] neuropathy, medication, metabolic disturbance, nutritional (vitamin, calcium) deficiency, and anterior compartment syndrome from trauma, hemophilia, sickle cell anemia, burn, cast, snakebite, or revascular perfusion injury.

Athletes often experience leg cramps preceded by muscle fatigue or twitching. Fractures and ligament tears can mimic a cramp. Cramping associated with severe dehydration may be a precursor to heat stroke.[69]

Heel pain is often a symptom of plantar fasciitis, heel spurs, nerve compression (e.g., tarsal tunnel syndrome), or stress fractures. Heel pain can also be a symptom of systemic conditions such as rheumatoid arthritis (RA), seronegative arthritides, primary bone tumors or metastatic disease, gout, sarcoidosis, Paget's disease of the bone, inflammatory bowel disease, osteomyelitis, infectious diseases, sickle cell disease, and hyperparathyroidism.[70]

The resolution of heel pain of a musculoskeletal origin is variable and can take weeks to months. Knowing when to

TABLE 17.5	Symptoms and Differentiation of Leg Pain			
	Vascular Claudication	Neurogenic Claudication	Peripheral Neuropathy	Restless Legs Syndrome
Description	Pain* is usually bilateral No burning or dysesthesia	Pain is usually bilateral but may be unilateral Burning and dysesthesia in the back, buttocks, and/or legs	Pain, aching, and numbness of feet (and hands) Motor, sensory, and autonomic changes: burning, prickling, or tingling may be present; extreme sensitivity to touch (or numbness); weakness, falling (foot drop), muscle atrophy; infection, ulcers, gangrene	Crawling, creeping sensation in legs; involuntary Involuntary contractions of calf muscles, occurring especially at night Pain† can be mild to severe, lasting seconds, minutes, or hours Sleep disturbance, paresthesia
Associated signs and symptoms	Decreased or absent pulses Change in color and skin of the feet Normal DTRs; may be absent in people older than 60 Sciatica possible (ischemia)	Normal pulses Good skin nutrition Depressed or absent ankle jerks Positive SLR Sciatica Positive "shopping cart" sign (leaning forward on supportive surface; unable to straighten up because of painful symptoms)	Pulses may be affected, depending on underlying pathologic condition (e.g., diabetes) DTRs diminished or absent May have positive SLR May have sciatica	
Location	Usually calf first but may occur in the buttock, hip, thigh, or foot	Low back, buttock, thighs, calves, feet	Feet and hands in stocking-glove pattern	Feet, calves, legs
Aggravating factors	Pain is consistent in all spinal positions; brought on by physical exertion (e.g., walking, positive van Gelderen bicycle test); increased by climbing stairs or walking uphill (increased metabolic demand)	Increased in spinal extension Increased with walking; increased by walking downhill (increased lumbar lordosis); less painful when walking uphill	Depends on underlying cause (e.g., uncontrolled glucose levels with diabetes; progressive alcoholism)	Caffeine, pregnancy, iron deficiency
Relieving factors	Relieved promptly by standing still, sitting down, or resting (1–5 minutes)	Pain decreased by sitting, lying down, bending forward, or flexion exercises (may persist for hours)	Relieved by pain medication and relaxation techniques; treatment of underlying cause	Eliminate caffeine; increase iron intake, movement, walking, moderate exercise; medication; stretching; maintain hydration; heat or cold
Ages affected	40–60 +	40–60 +	Varies, depending on underlying cause	Variable
Cause	Atherosclerosis in peripheral arteries	Neoplasm or abscess Disk protrusion Osteophyte formation Ligamentous thickening	More than 100 causes: diabetes; medication; accident; nerve compression; metal toxicity; nutritional deficiency; diseases such as RA, SLE, AIDS; cancer, hypothyroidism, alcoholism	Cause unknown; may be a sleep disorder, arterial disorder, or dysautonomic disorder of the autonomic nervous system; may occur with dehydration or as a side effect of many medications

AIDS, Acquired immunodeficiency syndrome; *DTRs*, Deep tendon reflexes; *RA*, rheumatoid arthritis; *SLE*, systemic lupus erythematosus; *SLR*, straight leg raise.

*"Pain" associated with vascular claudication may also be described as an "aching," "cramping," or "tired" feeling.

†"Pain" associated with restless legs syndrome may not be painful but may be described as a "frantic," "unbearable," or "compelling" need to move the legs.

CASE EXAMPLE 17.7
Insufficiency Fracture

A 50-year-old Caucasian woman was referred to physical therapy with a 4-year history of rheumatoid arthritis (RA). She had been taking prednisone (5 mg to 30 mg per day) and sulfasalazine (1 g twice a day).

She has a history of hypertension, smokes a pack of cigarettes a day, and drinks a six-pack of beer every night. She lives alone and no longer works outside the home. She admits to very poor nutrition and does not take a multivitamin or calcium.

Clinical Presentation: Symmetric arthritis with tenderness and swelling of bilateral metacarpophalangeal (MCP) joints, proximal interphalangeal (PIP) joints, wrists, elbows, and metatarsophalangeal (MTP) joints.

The patient reported "hip pain," which started unexpectedly 2 weeks ago in the right groin area. The pain went down her right leg to the knee but did not cross the knee. Any type of movement made it hurt more, especially when walking.

Hip range of motion was limited because of pain; formal range of motion (active, passive, accessory motions) and strength testing were not possible.

What are the red flags in this case?
- Age
- Insidious onset with no known or reported trauma
- Cigarette smoking
- Alcohol use
- Poor diet
- Corticosteroid therapy

Result: The client exhibited multiple risk factors for osteoporosis. Further questioning revealed that surgical menopause took place 10 years ago; this is another risk factor.

The patient was unable to stand on the right leg unsupported. She could not squat because of her arthritic symptoms. Heel strike test was negative. Patrick's (Faber's) test could not be performed because of the acuteness of her symptoms.

The patient was referred to her rheumatologist with a request for a hip x-ray before any further physical therapy was provided. The therapist pointed out the risk factors present for osteoporosis and briefly summarized the client's current clinical presentation.

The client was given a diagnosis of insufficiency fracture of the right inferior and superior pubic rami. An insufficiency fracture differs from a stress fracture in that it occurs when a normal amount of stress is placed on abnormal bone. A stress fracture occurs when an unusual amount of stress is placed on normal bone.

Conservative treatment with physical therapy, pain medication, and treatment of the underlying osteoporosis was recommended. Weight-bearing as tolerated, a general conditioning program, and an osteoporosis exercise program were prescribed by the physical therapist. Client education about managing active RA and synovitis was also included.

Data from Kimpel DL: Hip pain in a 50-year-old woman with RA, *J Musculoskel Med* 16:651–652, 1999.

request additional diagnostic assessment is not always clear. The therapist must keep each potential systemic cause in mind when looking for clues in the client's profile that might point to any one of these conditions.

For example, RA is more common between the third and fifth decades, affecting women two to two and half times more often than men. Ankylosing spondylitis usually affects the spine and SI joints first. Heel pain as a secondary symptom would be suspicious. Men are affected with ankylosing spondylitis more often than women.

A history of inflammatory bowel disease (e.g., Crohn's disease or ulcerative colitis) or cancer with new onset of ankle and/or heel pain must be evaluated medically. The calcaneus is the most common site of metastasis to the foot.[71] Subdiaphragmatic disease (especially genitourinary [GU] or colorectal neoplasm) tends to metastasize to the feet,[72] but cases of supradiaphragmatic disease, such as breast cancer metastasizing to the heel, have been reported.[73] X-ray studies and blood tests will be needed to look for an inflammatory, infectious, or metastatic cause of heel pain.[70]

No matter what area of the lower quadrant is affected, asking about the presence of other signs and symptoms, utilization of the OSPRO-ROS and questioning the patient for a complete Review of Systems, and identifying red-flag signs and symptoms will help the therapist in the clinical decision-making process. The therapist can use the red flags (see Appendix A-2 on 784.e3) to guide screening questions. Always ask every client the following:

 FOLLOW-UP QUESTION

- Are there any other symptoms of any kind anywhere else in your body?

If the client says, "No," the therapist may want to ask some general screening questions, including questions about constitutional symptoms.

Failure to improve with physical therapy intervention may be a part of the medical differential diagnosis and should be reported within a reasonable length of time, given the particular circumstances of each client.

TRAUMA AS A CAUSE OF HIP, GROIN, OR LOWER QUADRANT PAIN

Trauma, including an accident, injury, physical or sexual assault, or birth trauma, can be the underlying cause of buttock, hip, groin, or lower extremity pain.

Birth Trauma

Birth trauma is one possible cause of pelvic girdle pain and includes pelvic, hip, or groin pain, with pain radiating down the leg in some cases. Multiple births, prolonged labor and delivery, forceps/vacuum delivery, and postepidural complications are just a few of the more common birth-related causes of hip, groin, and lower extremity pain. Gynecologic conditions are discussed more completely in Chapter 16.

Stress Reaction or Fracture

An undiagnosed stress reaction or stress fracture is a possible cause of hip, thigh, groin, knee, shin, heel, or foot pain. A stress reaction or fracture is a microscopic disruption, or break, in a bone that is not displaced; it is not seen initially on radiograph images. Exercise-induced groin, tibial, or heel pain are the most common stress fractures.

There are two types of stress fractures. *Insufficiency* fractures are breaks in abnormal bone under normal force. *Fatigue* fractures are breaks in normal bone that has been put under extreme force. Fatigue fractures are usually caused by new, strenuous, very repetitive activities such as marching, jumping, or distance running. The most common stress fractures in runners occur in the tibia (16.2%), femur (6.6%), and pelvis (1.6%).[74]

Fatigue fractures are more likely to occur in distance runners, sprinters,[75] military recruits, or other high-intensity athletes, affecting the pubic ramus, calcaneus, femoral neck, and anterior tibia most often.[76,77] Older adults are more likely to present with insufficiency hip fractures. Depending on the age of the client, the therapist should look for a history of high-energy trauma, prolonged activity, or abrupt increase in training intensity. Traction from attached muscles such as the adductor magnus on the inferior pubic ramus is a contributing factor to pubic ramus stress fractures.

Other risk factors include changes in running surface, use of inadequately cushioned footwear, and the presence of the female athlete triad of disordered eating, osteoporosis, amenorrhea, and menopause.[78-80] Anything that can lead to poor bone density should be considered a risk factor for insufficiency stress fractures including radiation and/or chemotherapy,[81] prolonged use of corticosteroids, renal failure, metabolic disorders affecting bone, Paget's disease, and coxa vara.[82,83] A smaller cross-sectional diameter of the long bones of the leg in male distance runners is a unique risk factor for tibial stress fractures.[84]

Femoral shaft stress fractures are rare in the general population but are common among distance runners and military recruits involved in repetitive loading activities such as running and marching. Pain presentation is not always predictable.[82] Vague anterior thigh pain that radiates to the hip or knee with activity or exercise is the most common clinical presentation. The affected individual usually has full but painful active hip motion.[85] The fulcrum test for the femur (Fig. 17.3) has high clinical correlation with femoral shaft stress injury.[86,87]

Likewise, heel pain from calcaneal fractures can occur in the athlete following significant increases in athletic activities or after a plantar fascia rupture. Posterior and plantar heel pain and swelling are often misdiagnosed as plantar fasciitis. A medial-lateral squeeze test may help identify the need for further imaging studies, especially when radiographs have been read as "normal."[88]

Osteopenia or osteoporosis, especially in the postmenopausal woman or older adult with arthritis, can result in injury and fracture or fracture and injury (Case Example 17.8). The client has a small mishap, perhaps losing her footing on a slippery surface or tripping over an object. As she tries to "catch herself," a torsional force occurs through the hip, causing a fracture and then a fall. This is a case of fracture then fall, rather than the other way around. Often, but not always, the client is unable to get up because of pain and instability of the fracture site.[89]

Pain on weight-bearing is a red-flag symptom for stress reaction or fracture in any individual. In the case of bone pain (deep pain, pain on weight-bearing), the therapist can perform a heel strike test. This is done by applying a percussive force with the heel of the examiner's hand through the heel of the client's foot in a non–weight-bearing (supine) position. Reproduction of painful symptoms with axial loading is positive and highly suggestive of a bone fracture or stress reaction.[90]

Therefore, if a stress reaction or fracture is suspected, it makes sense for the therapist to consider if a non–weight-bearing test such as the heel strike test and fulcrum test is negative to a weight-bearing test. The therapist can ask a physically capable client to first perform a full squat to clear the hip, knee, and ankle, followed by a hop on the uninvolved side. These tests are used to screen for pubic ramus or hip stress fracture

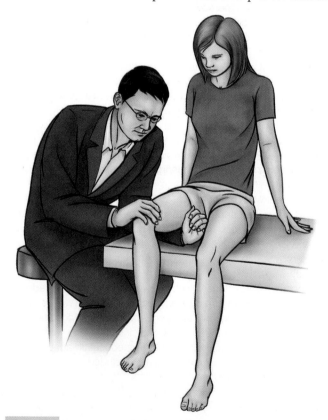

Fig. 17.3 Fulcrum test for femoral shaft stress reaction or fracture. With the client in a sitting position, the examiner places his or her forearm under the client's thigh and applies downward pressure over the anterior aspect of the distal femur. A positive test is characterized by reproduction of thigh pain often described as "sharp," with considerable apprehension on the part of the client.[86]

CASE EXAMPLE 17.8
Low Back Pain with Sciatica

A 52-year-old man with low back pain and sciatica on the left side has been referred to you by his family physician. He underwent diskectomy and laminectomy on two separate occasions about 5 to 7 years ago. No imaging studies have been done since that time.

What follow-up questions would you ask to screen for systemic disease?

1. The first question should always be, "Did you see your doctor?" (Of course, communication with the physician is the key here in understanding the physician's intended goal with physical therapy and his or her thinking about the underlying cause of the sciatica.)

2. Assess for the presence of constitutional symptoms. For example, after paraphrasing what the client has told you, ask, "Are you having any other symptoms of any kind in your body that you have not mentioned?" *If no*, ask more specifically about the presence of associated signs and symptoms; name constitutional symptoms one by one.

3. Follow-up with *Special Questions for Men* (see Appendix B-24 on). Include questions about past history of prostate health problems, cancer of any kind, and current bladder function.

4. Take a look at Table 17.6. By reviewing the possible systemic/extraspinal causes of sciatica, we can decide what additional questions might be appropriate for this man.

Vascular ischemia of the sciatic nerve can occur at any age as a result of biomechanical obstruction. It can also result from peripheral vascular disease. Check for skin changes associated with ischemia of the lower extremities. Ask about the presence of known heart disease or atherosclerosis.

Intrapelvic aneurysm: Palpate aortic pulse width and listen for femoral bruits.

Neoplasm (primary or metastatic): Consider this more strongly if the client has a previous history of cancer, especially cancer that might metastasize to the spine. Chapter 14 notes the three primary sites of cancer most likely to metastasize to the bone are lung, breast, and prostate. Other cancers that metastasize to the bone include thyroid, kidney, melanoma (skin), and lymphoma. A previous history of any of these cancers is a red-flag finding.

Primary bone cancer is not as likely in a middle-aged male as in a younger age group. Cancer metastasized to the bone is more likely and is most often characterized by pain during weight-bearing that is deep and does not respond to treatment modalities.

Diabetes mellitus (diabetic neuropathy): Ask about a personal history of diabetes mellitus. If the client has diabetes mellitus, assess further for associated neuropathy. If not, assess for symptoms of possible new-onset, but as of yet, undiagnosed diabetes mellitus.

Pregnancy: Not a consideration in this case.

Infection: Ask about a recent history of infection (most likely bacterial endocarditis, urinary tract infection, or sexually transmitted infection, but any infection can seed itself to the joints or soft tissues). Ask about any other signs or symptoms of infection (e.g., flu-like symptoms, such as fever and chills or skin rash, in the last few weeks).

Remember from Chapter 3 to ask the following:

? FOLLOW-UP QUESTIONS

- Are you having any pain anywhere else in your body?
- Are you having symptoms of any other kind that may or may not be related to your main problem?
- Have you recently (last 6 weeks) had any of the following:
  - Fracture
  - Bite (human, animal)
  - Antibiotics or other prescription medication
  - Infection [you may have to prompt with a specific infection such as strep throat, mononucleosis, urinary tract, upper respiratory (cold or flu), gastrointestinal (GI), hepatitis, sexually transmitted disease]

Total hip arthroplasty: Has the client had a recent (cemented) total hip replacement (e.g., cement extrusion, infection, implant fracture, loose component)?

Result: The client had testicular cancer that had already metastasized to the pelvis and femur. By asking additional questions, the physical therapist found out that the client was having swelling and hardness of the scrotum on the same side as the sciatica. He was unable to maintain an erection or to ejaculate. The physician was unaware of these symptoms because the client did not mention them during the medical examination.

Testicular carcinoma is relatively rare, especially in a man in his 50s. It is most common in the 15- to 39-year-old male group. Metastasis usually occurs via the lymphatics, with the possibility of an abdominal mass, psoas invasion, lymphadenopathy, and back pain. Palpation revealed a dominant mass (hard and painless) in the ipsilateral groin area.

Sending a client back to the referring physician in a case like this may require tact and diplomacy. In this case the therapist made telephone contact to express concerns about the reported sexual dysfunction and palpable groin lymphadenopathy.

By alerting the physician to these additional symptoms, further medical evaluation was scheduled, and the diagnosis was made quickly.

(reaction). Palpation over the injured bone may reproduce the painful symptoms, but when the stressed bone lies deep within the tissue, the therapist may be able to reproduce the pain by stressing the bone with translational (resisted active adduction) or rotational force (resisted active adduction combined with hip external rotation). Swelling is not usually evident early in the course of a stress reaction or fracture, but it does develop if the person continues athletic activity.

Look for the following clues suggestive of hip, groin, or thigh pain caused by a stress reaction or stress fracture.

Radiographs may not show the fracture, especially during its early stages.[41] The therapist should also keep in mind that some fractures of the intertrochanteric region do not show up on a standard anteroposterior or lateral radiograph image. An oblique view may be needed. If a radiograph image has been ruled negative for hip fracture but the client cannot put

CLINICAL SIGNS AND SYMPTOMS
Stress Reaction/Stress Fracture

- Pain described as aching or deep aching in hip and/or groin area; may radiate to the knee
- Pain increases with activity and improves with rest
- Muscle weakness (reduced grade during manual muscle testing; involved muscles vary depending on location of the fracture)
- Compensatory gluteus medius gait
- Pain localizing to a specific area of bone (localized tenderness)
- Positive Patrick's or Faber's test
- Pain reproduced by weight-bearing, heel strike, or hopping test; positive medial-lateral squeeze test (calcaneal stress test)
- Pain reproduced by translational/rotational stress (exquisite pain in response to active resistance to hip adduction/hip adduction combined with external rotation)
- Thigh pain reproduced by the fulcrum test (femoral shaft fracture)
- Possible local swelling
- Increased tone of hip adductor muscles; limited hip abduction
- Night pain (femoral neck stress fracture)

weight on that side and a heel strike test is positive, communication with the physician may be warranted.

Assault

The client may not report assault as the underlying cause, or he or she may not remember any specific trauma or accident. It may be necessary to take a sexual history (see Appendix B-32 on 784.e37) that includes specific questions about sexual activity (e.g., incest, partner assault or rape) or the presence of a sexually transmitted infection. Appropriate screening questions for assault or domestic violence are included in Chapter 2; see also Appendix B-3 on page xx.

SCREENING FOR SYSTEMIC CAUSES OF SCIATICA

Sciatica, described as pain radiating down the leg below the knee along the distribution of the sciatic nerve, is usually related to mechanical pressure or inflammation of lumbosacral nerve roots (Fig. 17.4). *Sciatica* is the term commonly used to describe pain in a sciatic distribution without overt signs of radiculopathy.

Radiculopathy denotes objective signs of nerve (or nerve root) irritation or dysfunction, usually resulting from involvement of the spine. Symptoms of radiculopathy may include weakness, numbness, or reflex changes. Sciatic *neuropathy* suggests damage to the peripheral nerve beyond the effects of compression, often resulting from a lesion outside the spine that affects the sciatic nerve (e.g., ischemia, inflammation, infection, direct trauma to the nerve, compression by neoplasm or piriformis muscle).

The terms *radiculopathy, sciatica,* and *neuropathy* are often used interchangeably, although there is a pathologic difference.[91] Electrodiagnostic studies, including nerve conduction studies, electromyography, and somatosensory evoked potential studies, are used to make the differentiation.

Sciatica has many neuromuscular causes, both diskogenic and nondiskogenic; systemic or extraspinal conditions can produce or mimic sciatica (Table 17.6). Risk factors for a mechanical cause of sciatica include previous trauma to the low back, taller height, tobacco use, pregnancy, obesity, overweight, and work- and occupational-related posture or movement.[92,93]

Risk Factors

Risk factors for systemic or extraspinal causes vary with each condition (Table 17.7). For example, clients with arterial insufficiency are more likely to be heavy smokers and to have a history of atherosclerosis. Increasing age, past history of

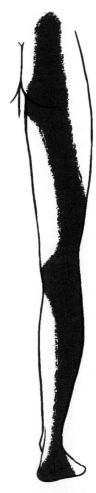

Fig. 17.4 Sciatica pain pattern. Perceived or reported pain associated with compression, stretch, injury, entrapment, or scarring of the sciatic nerve depends on the location of the lesion to the nerve root. The sciatic nerve is innervated by L4, L5, S1, S2, and sometimes S3 with several divisions (e.g., common fibular [peroneal] nerve, sural nerve, tibial nerve).

TABLE 17.6	Causes of Sciatica			

	NEUROMUSCULAR CAUSES			SYSTEMIC/ EXTRASPINAL CAUSES*
Disorder	Symptoms	Physical Signs		Disorders
DISCOGENIC				
Disk herniation	Low back pain with radiculopathy and paravertebral muscle spasm; Valsalva maneuver and sciatic stretch reproduce symptoms	Restricted spinal movement; restricted spinal segment; positive Lasègue's sign or restricted SLR		Vascular • Ischemia of sciatic nerve • PVD • Intrapelvic aneurysm (internal iliac artery) Neoplasm (primary or metastatic)
Lateral entrapment syndrome (spinal stenosis)	Buttock and leg pain with radiculopathy; pain often relieved by sitting, aggravated by extension of the spine	Similar to disk herniation		Diabetes mellitus (diabetic neuropathy Pregnancy; vaginal delivery Endometriosis Infection
NONDISCOGENIC				• Bacterial endocarditis
Sacroiliitis	Low back and buttock pain	Tender SI joint; positive lateral compression test; positive Patrick's test		• Wound contamination[97,98] • Herpes zoster (shingles)
Piriformis syndrome	Low back and buttock pain with referred pain down the leg to the ankle or midfoot	Pain and weakness during resisted abduction/external rotation of the thigh		• Psoas muscle abscess (see Box 17.3) • Reactive arthritis Total hip arthroplasty DVT (blood clot)
Iliolumbar syndrome	Pain in iliolumbar ligament area (posterior iliac crest); referred leg pain	Tender iliac crest and increased pain with lateral or side-bending		
Trochanteric bursitis	Buttock and lateral thigh pain; worse at night and with activity	Tender greater trochanter; rule out associated leg-length discrepancy; positive "jump sign" when pressure is applied over the greater trochanter		
GTPS	Mimics lumbar nerve root compression	Low back, buttock, or lateral thigh pain; may radiate down the leg to the iliotibial tract insertion on the proximal tibia; inability to sleep on the involved side[9]		
Ischiogluteal bursitis	Buttock and posterior thigh pain; worse with sitting	Tender ischial tuberosity; positive SLR and Patrick's tests; rule out associated leg-length discrepancy		
Posterior facet syndrome	Low back pain	Lateral bending in spinal extension increases pain; side-bending and rotation to the opposite side are restricted at the involved level		
Fibromyalgia	Back pain, difficulty sleeping, anxiety, depression	Multiple tender points (see Fig. 13.4)		

DVT, Deep venous thrombosis; *GTPS*, greater trochanteric pain syndrome; *PVD*, peripheral vascular disease; *SI*, sacroiliac; *SLR*, straight leg raise.
*Clinical symptoms of systemic/extraspinal sciatica can be very similar to those of sciatica associated with disk protrusion.
Data from Namey TC, An HC: Sorting out the causes of sciatica. *Mod Med* 52:132, 1984.

cancer, and comorbidities, such as diabetes mellitus, endometriosis, or intraperitoneal inflammatory disease (e.g., diverticulitis, Crohn's disease, pelvic inflammatory disease [PID]), are risk factors associated with sciatic-like symptoms (Case Example 17.9).

Total hip arthroplasty is a common cause of sciatica because of the proximity of the nerve to the hip joint. Possible mechanisms for nerve injury include stretching, direct trauma from retractors, infarction, hemorrhage, hip dislocation, and compression.[94] Sciatica referred to as sciatic nerve "burn" has been reported as a complication of hip arthroplasty caused by cement extrusion. The incidence of this complication has decreased with its increased recognition and the use of cementless implants,[21] but even small amounts of cement can cause heat production or direct irritation of the sciatic nerve.[95]

Propionibacterium acnes, a cause of spinal infection, has been linked to sciatica.[96] Bacterial wound contamination

TABLE 17.7	Risk Factors for Sciatica
Musculoskeletal or Neuromuscular Factors	**Systemic/Medical Factors**
Previous low back injury or trauma; direct fall on buttock(s); gunshot wound	Tobacco use
Total hip arthroplasty	History of diabetes mellitus
Pregnancy	Atherosclerosis
Work- or occupation-related posture or movement	Previous history of cancer (metastases)
Fibromyalgia	Presence of intraabdominal or peritoneal inflammatory disease (abscess):
Leg length discrepancy	• Crohn's disease
Congenital hip dysplasia; hip dislocation	• Pelvic inflammatory disease (PID)
Degenerative disk disease	• Diverticulitis
Piriformis syndrome	Endometriosis of the sciatic nerve
Spinal stenosis	Radiation therapy (delayed effects; rare)
Hypermobility syndromes such as Ehlers-Danlos syndrome	Recent spinal surgery, especially with instrumentation

CLINICAL SIGNS AND SYMPTOMS
Sciatica/Sciatic Radiculopathy

Symptoms are variable and may include the following:
- Pain along the sciatic nerve anywhere from the spine to the foot (see Fig. 17.4)
- Numbness or tingling in the groin, rectum, leg, calf, foot, or toes
- Diminished or absent deep tendon reflexes
- Weakness in the L4, L5, S1, S2 (and sometimes S3) myotomes (distal motor deficits more prominent than proximal)
- Diminished or absent deep tendon reflexes (especially of the ankle)
- Ache in the calf

Sciatic Neuropathy
- Symptoms of sciatica as just described
- Dysesthetic* pain described as constant burning or sharp, jabbing pain
- Foot drop (tibialis anterior weakness) with gait disturbance
- Flail lower leg (severe motor neuropathy)

*Dysesthesia is the distortion of any sense, especially touch; it is an unpleasant sensation produced by normal stimuli.

during spinal surgery has been traced to this pathogen on the patient's skin. Minor trauma to the disk with a breach of the mechanical integrity of the disk may also allow access by low-virulent microorganisms, thereby initiating or stimulating a chronic inflammatory response. These microorganisms may not only cause prosthetic hip infection but may also be associated with the inflammation seen in sciatica; they may even be a primary cause of sciatica.[97,98]

Endometriosis at the sciatic notch and pelvic endometriosis affecting the lumbosacral plexus or proximal sciatic nerve can present as sciatica/buttock pain that extends down the posterior aspect of the thigh and calf to the ankle. The pain is cyclic and corresponds with the menstrual cycle.[99,100]

Anyone with pain radiating from the back down the leg as far as the ankle has a greater chance that disk herniation is the cause of low back pain. This is true with or without neurologic findings. Unremitting, severe pain and increasing neurologic deficit are red-flag findings. Sciatica caused by extraspinal bone and soft tissue tumors is rare but may occur when a mass is present in the pelvis, sacrum, thigh, popliteal fossa, and calf.[101,102]

The therapist can conduct an examination to look for signs and symptoms associated with systemically induced sciatica. Box 4.13 offers guidelines on conducting an assessment for PVD. Box 4.16 provides a checklist for the therapist to use when examining the extremities. These tools can help the therapist define the clinical presentation more accurately.

The passive SLR test and other neurodynamic tests are widely used but do not identify the underlying cause of sciatica. For example, a positive SLR test does not differentiate between diskogenic disease and neoplasm.

Without a combination of imaging and laboratory studies, the clinical picture of sciatica is difficult to distinguish from that of conditions such as neoplasm and infection. Erythrocyte sedimentation rate (ESR or sed rate) is the rate at which red

blood cells settle out of unclotted blood plasma within 1 hour. A high ESR is an indication of infection or inflammation (see top table, Inside Front Cover). Elevated ESR and abnormal imaging are effective tools to use in screening for occult neoplasm and other systemic disease.[103]

Imaging studies are an essential part of the medical diagnosis, but even with these diagnostic tests, errors in conducting and interpreting imaging studies may occur. Symptoms can also result from involvement outside of the area captured by computed tomography or MRI.

SCREENING FOR ONCOLOGIC CAUSES OF LOWER QUADRANT PAIN

Many clients with orthopedic or neurologic problems have a previous history of cancer. The therapist must recognize signs and symptoms of cancer recurrence and those associated with cancer treatment such as radiation therapy or chemotherapy. The effects of these may be delayed by as long as 10 to 20 years or more (see Table 14.8; Case Example 17.10).

Cancer Recurrence

The therapist is far more likely to encounter clinical manifestations of metastases from cancer recurrence than from primary cancer. Breast cancer often affects the shoulder, thoracic vertebrae, and hip first, before other areas. Recurrence of colon (colorectal) cancer is possible with referred pain to the hip and/or groin area.

Beware of any client with a past history of colorectal cancer and recent (past 6 months) treatment by surgical removal. Reseeding the abdominal cavity is possible. Every effort is made to shrink the tumor with radiation or chemotherapy

Evaluating a Client for Cancer Recurrence

Referral: A 54-year-old man is self-referred to physical therapy on the recommendation of his trainer who is a friend of yours. He is experiencing leg weakness (greater on the right), with occasional pain radiating into the groin area on both sides.

He reports a twisting back injury 5 years ago when he was shoveling snow. At that time, he saw a physical therapist but did not get any better until he started working out at the fitness center.

Leg weakness has been present for about 2 weeks. Last weekend, he went to the emergency department because his leg was numb and he could not lift his ankle. He was told to rest. The leg was better the next day.

Past Medical History: Renal calculi, surgery for parathyroid and thyroid cancer 10 years ago, pneumonia 20 years ago. Currently seeing a counselor for emotional problems.

Objective Findings:
Neurologic Screen
- Alert; oriented to time, place, person
- Pupils equal and equally reactive to light; eye movements in all directions without difficulty
- No tremor, upper extremity weakness, or changes in deep tendon reflexes (DTRs)
- Straight leg raise (SLR) was mobile and pain free to 90 degrees bilaterally
- Iliopsoas, gluteal, hamstring manual muscle testing (MMT) = 3/5 on the right side. MMT within normal limits on the left side
- Tibialis anterior, plantar evertors and flexors: MMT = 2/5 (right); 3+ to 4 on the left
- No ankle clonus, no Babinski's, no changes in DTRs of lower extremities (LEs)
- Increased muscle tone in both LEs

No pain was reported with any movements performed during the examination.

Name three red-flag symptoms in this case:
Age is the first red flag: A man over 40 years of age (and especially over 50 years of age) with a previous history of cancer (second red flag) and new onset of painless neurologic deficit (third red flag) is significant.

Now that we have identified three red flags, what is next? Does this signify an automatic referral to the physician? We do not think so: the need for physician referral may depend on the specific red flags that are present. For example, in the case just presented, the three red flags are pretty significant. Take a closer look, and

gather as much information as possible. In this case it appears likely that an immediate referral is warranted.

Can we tell whether this is a recurrence of his previous cancer now metastasized or the presence of prostate cancer? No, but we can ask some additional questions to look for clusters of associated signs and symptoms that might point to prostate involvement. First, ask about bladder function, urination, and finally, sexual function. Remember, you may have to explain the need to ask a few personal questions.

- Have you ever had prostate problems or been told you have prostate problems?
- Have you had any changes in urination recently?
- Can you easily start a flow of urine?
- Can you keep a steady stream without stopping and starting?
- When you are finished urinating, does it feel as though your bladder is empty? Or, do you feel like you still have to go, but you cannot get any more out?
- Do you ever dribble urine?
- Do you have trouble getting an erection?
- Do you have trouble keeping an erection?
- Do you have trouble ejaculating?

Because the patient is seeing a counselor for emotional problems, you may wish to screen him for emotional overlay. You can use the three tools discussed in Chapter 3 (Symptom Magnification, McGill's Pain Questionnaire, Waddell's nonorganic tests).

After you have completed your examination, step back and put all the pieces together. Is there a cluster of signs and symptoms that point to any particular system? The answer to this question may lead you to ask some additional questions or to confirm the need for medical attention.

Special Note: Palpating the groin area is usually necessary when performing a thorough evaluation. This can be a sensitive issue. In today's litigious culture, you may want to have a third person in the examination area with you. You will certainly want to explain everything you are doing and obtain the client's permission.

For men, give the client time to make any necessary "adjustments" before beginning palpation. If the client has an erection during palpation, do not make any joking or unprofessional comments. This may seem self-evident but we have observed a wide range of responses when supervising others that supports the need to provide specific guidelines as stated here.

---

before attempts are made to remove the tumor. Even a small number of tumor cells left behind or introduced into a nearby (new) area can result in cancer recurrence.

Hodgkin's Disease

Hodgkin's disease arises in the lymph glands, most commonly on a single side of the neck or groin, but lymph nodes also enlarge in response to infection throughout the body. Lymph nodes in the groin area can become enlarged specifically as a result of sexually transmitted disease.

The presence of painless, hard lymph nodes that are also similarly present at other sites (e.g., popliteal space) is always

a red-flag symptom. As always, the therapist must question the client further regarding the onset of symptoms and the presence of any associated symptoms, such as fever, weight loss, bleeding, and skin lesions. The client must seek a medical diagnosis to be certain of the cause of enlarged lymph nodes.

Spinal Cord Tumors

Spinal cord tumors (primary or metastasized) present as dull, aching discomfort or sharp pain in the thoracolumbar area in a belt-like distribution, with pain extending to the groin or legs. Depending on the location of the lesion, symptoms may be unilateral or bilateral with or without radicular symptoms.

CASE EXAMPLE 17.10

Ischial Bursitis

Case Report courtesy of Jason Taitch, DDS, Spokane, WA, 2005.

Referral: A 30-year-old dentist was referred to physical therapy by an orthopedic surgeon for ischial bursitis, sometimes referred to as "Weaver's bottom." He reported left buttock pain and "soreness" that was intermittent and work related. As a dentist, he was often leaning to the left, putting pressure on the left ischium.

Background: Magnetic resonance imaging (MRI) showed local inflammation on the ischial tuberosity to confirm the medical diagnosis. He was given a steroid injection and was placed on an antiinflammatory (Celebrex) before he went to physical therapy.

The client reported a mild loss of hip motion, especially of hip flexion, but no other symptoms of any kind. The pain did not radiate down the leg. No significant past medical history and no history of tobacco use were reported; only an occasional beer in social situations was described. The client described himself as being "in good shape" and working out at the local gym four to five times per week.

Intervention/Follow-Up: Physical therapy intervention included deep friction massage, iontophoresis, and stretching. The client modified his dentist's chair with padding to take pressure off the buttock. Symptoms did not improve after 10 treatment sessions over the next 6 to 8 weeks; in fact, the pain became worse and was now described as "burning."

The client went back to the orthopedic surgeon for a follow-up visit. A second MRI was done with a diagnosis of "benign inflammatory mass." He was given a second steroid injection and was sent back to physical therapy. He was seen at a different clinic location by a second physical therapist.

The physical therapist palpated a lump over the ischial tuberosity, described as "swelling"; this was the only new physical finding since his previous visits with the first physical therapist.

Treatment concentrated deep friction massage in that area. The therapist thought the lump was getting better, but it did not resolve. The client reported increased painful symptoms, including pain at work and night. No position was comfortable; even lying down without pressure on the buttocks was painful. He modified every seat he used, including the one in his car.

Result: The orthopedic surgeon did a bursectomy and the pathology report came back with a diagnosis of epithelioid sarcoma. The diagnosis was made 2½ years after the initial painful symptoms. A second surgery was required because the first excision did not have clear margins.

It is often easier to see the red flags in hindsight. As this case is presented here with the outcome, what are the red flags?

Red Flags
- No improvement with physical therapy
- Progression of symptoms (pain went from "sore" to "burning," and intermittent to constant)
- Young age

Clinical signs of all types of bursitis are similar and include local tenderness, warmth, and erythema. The latter two signs may not be obvious when the inflamed bursa is located deep beneath soft tissues or muscles, as in this case.[108]

The presence of a "lump" or swelling as presented in this case caused a delay in medical referral and diagnosis because MRI findings were consistent with a diagnosis of an inflammatory mass. In this case symptoms progressed and did not fit the typical pattern for bursitis (e.g., pain at night, no position comfortable).

Other Tests

When a client is sent back a second time, the therapist's reevaluation is essential for documenting any changes from the original baseline and discharge findings. Reevaluation should include the following:
- Recheck levels above and below for possible involvement, including lumbar spine, sacroiliac joint, hip, and knee; perform range of motion and special tests, and conduct a neurologic screening examination (see Chapter 4).
- Test for the sign of the buttock to look for serious disease posterior to the axis of flexion and extension of the hip (see Box 17.2). A positive sign may be an indication of abscess, fracture, neoplasm, septic bursitis, or osteomyelitis.[15]

A noncapsular pattern is typical with bursitis and by itself is not a red flag. A capsular pattern with a diagnosis of bursitis would be more suspicious. Limited straight leg raise with no further hip flexion after bending the knee is a typical positive buttock sign seen with ischial bursitis. The absence of this sign would raise clinical suspicion that the diagnosis of bursitis was not accurate.[15]

With an ischial bursitis, expect to see equal leg length, negative Trendelenburg test, and normal sensation, reflexes, and joint play movements.[109] Anything outside of these parameters should be considered a yellow (caution) flag.
- Assess for myofascial dysfunction that may cause buttock pain, especially quadratus lumborum, gluteus maximus, and hamstrings, but also gluteus medius and piriformis.
- Reassess for the presence of constitutional symptoms or any associated signs and symptoms of any kind anywhere in the body.

The therapist should look for and ask about associated signs and symptoms (e.g., constitutional symptoms, bleeding or discharge, lymphadenopathy).

Symptoms of thoracic disk herniation can mimic spinal cord tumor. In isolated cases, thoracic disk extrusion has been reported to cause groin pain and lower extremity weakness that becomes progressively worse over time. A tumor is suspected if the client has painless neurologic deficit, night pain, or pain that increases when supine.

Testing the cremasteric reflex may help the therapist identify neurologic impairment in any male with suspicious back, pelvic, groin (including testicular), or anterior thigh pain. The cremasteric reflex is elicited by stroking the thigh downward with a cotton-tipped applicator (or handle of the reflex hammer). A normal response in males is upward movement of the testicle (scrotum) on the same side. The absence of a cremasteric reflex is an indication of disruption at the T12-L1 level.

Additionally, groin pain associated with spinal cord tumor is disproportionate to that normally expected with disk disease. No change in symptoms occurs after successful surgery for herniated disk. Age is an important factor: teenagers with symptoms of disk herniation should be examined closely for tumor.[104,105]

Spinal metastases to the femur or lower pelvis may appear as hip pain. Except for myeloma and rare lymphoma, metastasis to the synovium is unusual. Therefore, joint motion is not compromised by these bone lesions. Although any tumor of the bone may appear at the hip, some benign and malignant neoplasms have a propensity to occur at this location.

Bone Tumors

Osteoid osteoma, a small, benign but painful tumor, is relatively common, with 20% of lesions occurring in the proximal femur and 10% in the pelvis. Males are more commonly affected with a reported range of 67% to 80% of males being under the age of 25 years.[106,107] The client complains of chronic dull hip, thigh, or knee pain that is worse at night and is alleviated by activity and aspirin and nonsteroidal antiinflammatory drugs (NSAIDs). Usually, an antalgic gait is present, along with point tenderness over the lesion with restriction of hip motion.

Many varieties of benign and malignant tumors may appear differently, depending on the age of the client and the site and duration of the lesion (Case Example 17.11).[108,109] Malignant lesions compressing the LFCN can cause symptoms of MP, delaying diagnosis of the underlying neoplasm. Other bone tumors that cause hip pain, such as chondroblastoma, chondrosarcoma, giant cell tumor, and Ewing's sarcoma, are discussed in greater detail in Chapter 14.

CLINICAL SIGNS AND SYMPTOMS

Buttock, Hip, Groin, or Lower Extremity Pain Associated with Cancer

- Bone pain, especially during weight-bearing; positive heel strike test
- Antalgic gait
- Local tenderness
- Night pain (constant, intense; unrelieved by change in position)
- Pain relieved disproportionately by aspirin
- Fever, weight loss, bleeding, skin lesions
- Vaginal/penile discharge
- Painless, progressive enlargement of inguinal and/or popliteal lymph nodes

---

SCREENING FOR UROLOGIC CAUSES OF BUTTOCK, HIP, GROIN, OR THIGH PAIN

Ureteral pain usually begins posteriorly in the costovertebral angle but may radiate anteriorly to the upper thigh and groin (Fig. 17.6), or it may be felt just in the groin and genital area. These pain patterns represent the pathway that genitals take as they migrate during fetal development from their original position, where the kidneys are located in the adult, down the pathways of the ureters to their final location. Pain is referred to a site where the organ was located during fetal development. A kidney stone down the pathway of the ureters causes pain in the flank that radiates to the scrotum (male) or labia (female).

The lower thoracic and upper lumbar vertebrae and the SI joint can refer pain to the groin and anterior thigh in the same pain pattern as occurs with renal disease. Irritation of the T10-L1 sensory nerve roots (genitofemoral and ilioinguinal nerves) from any cause, especially from diskogenic disease, may cause labial (women), testicular (men), or buttock pain.[110] The therapist can evaluate these conditions by conducting a neurologic screening examination and using the screening model.

Referred symptoms from ureteral colic can be distinguished from musculoskeletal hip pain by the history, the presence of urologic symptoms, and the pattern of pain. Is there any history of urinary tract impairment? Is there a recent history of other infection? Are any signs and symptoms noted that are associated with the renal system?

Active tender points along the upper rim of the pubis and the lateral half of the inguinal ligament may lie in the lower internal oblique muscle and possibly in the lower rectus abdominis. These tender points can cause increased irritability and spasm of the detrusor and urinary sphincter muscles, producing urinary frequency, retention of urine, and groin pain.[65]

The therapist can perform Murphy's percussion test to rule out kidney involvement (see Chapter 11; see also Fig. 4.54). A positive Murphy's percussion test (pain is reproduced with percussive vibration of the kidney) points to the possibility of kidney infection or inflammation. When this test is positive, ask about a recent history of fever, chills, unexplained perspiration ("sweats"), or other constitutional symptoms.

SCREENING FOR REPRODUCTIVE CAUSES OF GROIN PAIN

Men can experience groin pain caused by disease of the male reproductive system such as prostate cancer, testicular cancer, benign prostatic hyperplasia, or prostatitis. Isolated groin pain is not as common as groin pain that is accompanied by low back, buttock, or pelvic pain. Risk factors, clinical presentation, and associated signs and symptoms for these conditions are discussed in Chapter 15.

SCREENING FOR INFECTIOUS AND INFLAMMATORY CAUSES OF LOWER QUADRANT PAIN

Anyone with joint pain of unknown cause who presents with current or recent (i.e., within the past 6 weeks) skin rash or recent history of infection (e.g., hepatitis, mononucleosis, urinary tract infection, upper respiratory infection, sexually transmitted infection, streptococcus, dental infection)[111,112] must be referred to a health care clinic or medical doctor for further evaluation.

Conditions affecting the entire peritoneal cavity such as PID or appendicitis may cause hip or groin pain in the young, healthy adult. Widespread inflammation or infection may be well tolerated by athletes, sometimes for up to several weeks (Case Example 17.12).

CASE EXAMPLE 17.11

Dancer with Appendicitis

A 21-year-old dance major was referred to the physical therapy clinic by the sports medicine clinic on campus with a medical diagnosis of "strained abdominal muscle."

She described her symptoms as pain with hip flexion when shifting the gears in her car. Some dance moves involving hip flexion also reproduced the pain, but this was not consistent. The pain was described as "deep," "aching," and "sometimes sharp, sometimes dull."

Past medical history was significant for Crohn's disease, but the client was having no gastrointestinal (GI) symptoms at this time. During the examination, no evidence of abdominal myofascial dysfunction was found. The pain was not reproduced with superficial palpation of the abdominal muscles on the day of the initial examination.

Intervention with stretching exercises did not change the clinical picture during the first week.

Result: The client was a no-show for her Monday afternoon appointment, and the physical therapy clinic receptionist received a phone call from the campus clinic with information that the client had been hospitalized over the weekend with acute appendicitis and peritonitis.

The surgeon's report noted massive peritonitis of several weeks' duration. The client had a burst appendix that was fairly asymptomatic until peritonitis developed with subsequent symptoms. Her white blood cell count was in excess of 100,000 cells/mm^3 at the time of hospitalization.

In retrospect, the client did relate some "sweats" occurring off and on during the last 2 weeks and possibly a low-grade fever.

What additional screening could have been conducted with this client?

1. Ask the client whether she is having any symptoms of any kind anywhere in her body. If she answers "No," be prepared to offer some suggestions such as:
   - Any headaches? Fatigue?
   - Any change in vision?
   - Any fevers or sweats, day or night?
   - Any blood in your urine or stools?
   - Burning with urination?
   - Any tingling or numbness in the groin area?
   - Any trouble sleeping at night?
2. Even though she has denied having any GI symptoms associated with her Crohn's disease, it is important to follow-up with questions to confirm this:
   - Any nausea? Vomiting?
   - Diarrhea or constipation?
   - Any change in your pattern of bowel movements?
   - Any blood in your stools? Change in color of your bowel movements?
   - Any foods or smells you cannot tolerate?
   - Any change in your symptoms when you eat or do not eat?
   - Unexpected weight gain or loss?
   - Is your pain any better or worse during or after a bowel movement?
3. As a part of the past medical history, it is important with hip pain of unknown cause to know whether the client has had any recent infections, sexually transmitted diseases, use of antibiotics or other medications, or skin rashes.
4. In a woman of reproductive years, it may be important to take a gynecologic history:
   - Have you been examined by a gynecologist since this problem started?
   - Is there any chance you could be pregnant?
   - Are you using an intrauterine contraceptive device (IUD or IUCD)?
   - Have you had an abortion or miscarriage in the last 6 weeks?
   - Are you having any unusual vaginal discharge?
5. Check vital signs. The presence of a fever (even low grade) is a red flag when the cause of symptoms is unknown. With a burst appendix, she may have had altered pulse and blood pressure that could alert the therapist of a systemic cause of symptoms.
6. Test for McBurney's point (Fig. 8.9), rebound tenderness using the pinch-an-inch test (Fig. 8.11), and the obturator or iliopsoas sign (Figs. 8.5 to 8.7). Check for Murphy's percussion (Fig. 4.54; kidney involvement).

Clinical Presentation

The clinical presentation can be deceptive in young people. The fever is not dramatic and may come and go. The athlete may dismiss excessive or unusual perspiration ("sweats") as part of a good workout. Loss of appetite associated with systemic disease is often welcomed by teenagers and young adults and is not recognized as a sign of physiologic distress.

With an infectious or inflammatory process, laboratory tests may reveal an elevated ESR. Questions about the presence of any other symptoms may reveal constitutional symptoms such as elevated nocturnal temperature, sweats, and chills, suggestive of an inflammatory process (Case Example 17.12).

Psoas Abscess

Any infectious or inflammatory process affecting the abdominal or pelvic region can lead to psoas abscess and irritation of the psoas muscle. For example, lesions outside the ureter, such as infection, abscess, or tumor, or abdominal or peritoneal inflammation, may cause pain with movement of the adjacent iliopsoas muscle that presents as hip or groin pain. (See discussion of Psoas Abscess in Chapter 11.)

PID is another common cause of pelvic, groin, or hip pain that can cause psoas abscess and a subsequent positive iliopsoas or obturator test. In this case, it is most likely a young woman with multiple sexual partners who has a known or unknown case of untreated *Chlamydia*.

The psoas muscle is not separated from the abdominal or pelvic cavity. Figure 9.4 shows how most of the viscera, including the kidneys, sigmoid colon, jejunum, appendix, pancreas, abdominal aorta, and ureter, lie adjacent to the psoas muscle. Therefore, any infectious or inflammatory process (see Box 17.3) can seed itself to the psoas muscle by direct extension, resulting in a psoas abscess—a localized collection of pus.

CASE EXAMPLE 17.12
Limp After Total Hip Arthroplasty

A 70-year-old man was referred to physical therapy by his doctor 1 year after a right total hip replacement (THR) for osteoarthritis. The client reports that he is in good general health without pain. His primary problem is a persistent limp, despite completion of a THR rehabilitation protocol.

How can you tell whether this is an infectious versus biomechanical problem?

First of all, laboratory tests, such as erythrocyte sedimentation rate (ESR or "sed" rate) and C-reactive protein level, can be done to screen for infection. The therapist can request this information from the medical record.

The absence of pain usually rules out infection or implant loosening. A radiograph image may be needed to rule out implant loosening. Again, check the record to see whether this was a part of the medical diagnostic workup.

Besides infection, a limp after THR may have many possible causes. Loosening of the prosthesis, neurologic dysfunction, altered joint biomechanics, and muscle weakness or dysfunction (e.g., hip abductors) are a few potential causes. As always, in an orthopedic examination, check the joints above (low back, sacrum, sacroiliac) and below (knee) the level of impairment. In the case of joint replacement, evaluate the contralateral hip as well.

Test for abdominal muscle weakness. This can be confirmed with manual muscle testing or a Trendelenburg test. An anterolateral approach to THR is more likely to cause partial or complete abductor muscle disruption than is a posterior approach.

With either approach, the superior gluteal nerve can be damaged by stretching or by cutting one of its branches. The therapist may be able to get some clues to this by looking at the incision site. Disruption of the nerve is more likely when the gluteus medius is split more than 5 cm proximal to the tip of the greater trochanter. If nerve damage has occurred, the client may not regain full strength. Electromyography (EMG) testing may be needed to document muscle denervation.

Physical therapy may be a diagnostic step for the physician. If muscle strengthening does not recondition the remaining intact muscle, a revision operation to repair the muscle may be needed. It may be helpful to communicate with the physician to see what his or her thinking is on this client.

Data from Farrell CM, Berry DJ: Persistent limping after primary total hip replacement. *J Musculoskel Med* 19:484–486, 2002.

Hip pain associated with such an abscess may involve the medial aspect of the thigh and femoral triangle areas (Fig. 17.5). Soft tissue abscess may cause pain and tenderness to palpation without movement. Once the abscess has formed, muscular spasm may be provoked, producing hip flexion and even contracture. The leg may also be pulled into internal rotation. Pain that increases with passive and active motion can occur when infected tissue is irritated. Pain elicited by stretching the psoas muscle through extension of the hip, called the *positive psoas sign*, may be present.

A positive response for any of these tests is indicative of an infectious or inflammatory process. Direct back, pelvic, or hip pain that results from these palpations is more likely to have a musculoskeletal cause. Besides the iliopsoas and obturator

CLINICAL SIGNS AND SYMPTOMS
Psoas Abscess

- Pain that is usually confined to the psoas fascia but that may extend to the buttock, hip, groin, upper thigh, or knee
- Pain located in the anterior hip in the area of the medial thigh or femoral triangle, often accompanied by or alternating with abdominal pain
- Psoas spasm causing functional hip flexion contracture
- Leg pulled into internal rotation
- Positive psoas sign (i.e., pain elicited by stretching the psoas muscle by extending the hip)
- Fever up and down (hectic fever pattern)
- Sweats
- Loss of appetite or other GI symptoms
- Palpable mass in the inguinal area (present with distal extension of the abscess)
- Positive iliopsoas or obturator test (see Figs. 9.6–9.8)
- Antalgic gait

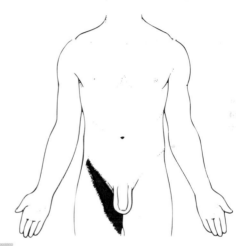

Fig. 17.5 Femoral triangle: Referred pain pattern from psoas abscess. Hip pain associated with such an abscess may involve the medial aspect of the thigh and femoral triangle areas. The femoral triangle is the name given to the anterior aspect of the thigh formed as different muscles and ligaments cross each other, producing an inverted triangular shape.

tests, another test for rebound tenderness used more often is the *pinch-an-inch* test (see Fig. 9.12). It may be appropriate to conduct these tests with a variety of clinical presentations involving the pelvic area, sacrum, hip, or groin.

Psoas abscess must be differentiated from tender points of the psoas muscle, causing the psoas minor syndrome, which is easily mistaken for appendicitis. Hemorrhage within the psoas muscle, either spontaneous or associated with anticoagulation therapy for hemophilia, can cause a painful compression syndrome of the femoral nerve. Endometrioses can also mimic psoas abscess and should be included in the differential diagnosis process.[113]

Systemic causes of hip pain from a psoas abscess are usually associated with loss of appetite or other GI symptoms, fever, and sweats. Symptoms from an iliopsoas trigger point are aggravated by weight-bearing activities and are relieved by recumbency or rest. Relief is greater when the hip is flexed.[63]

SCREENING FOR GASTROINTESTINAL CAUSES OF LOWER QUADRANT PAIN

The relationship of the gut to the joint is well known but poorly understood. Inflammatory bowel disease, ankylosing spondylitis, celiac disease, postdysenteric reactive arthritis, bowel bypass syndrome, and antibiotic-associated colitis all share the fact that some "interface" exists between the bowel and the hip articular surface. The clinical expression of immune-mediated joint disease may result from an immunologic response to an antigen that crosses the gut mucosa with an autoimmune response against self.[114-121]

For the client with hip pain of unknown cause or suspicious presentation, ask whether any back pain or abdominal pain is ever present. Alternating abdominal pain with low back pain at the same level, or alternating abdominal pain with hip pain is a red flag that requires medical referral.

The therapist may treat a client with joint or back pain with an underlying enteric cause before realizing the underlying problem. Palliative intervention can make a difference in the short term but does not affect the outcome. Symptoms that are unrelieved by physical therapy intervention are always a red flag. Symptoms that improve after physical therapy but then get worse again are also a red flag, revealing the need for further screening.

In the case of enterically induced joint pain, the client will get worse without medical intervention. Without early identification and referral, the client will eventually return to his or her gastroenterologist or primary care physician. Medical treatment for the underlying disease is essential in affecting the musculoskeletal component. Physical therapy intervention does not alter or improve the underlying enteric disease. It is better for the client if the therapist recognizes as soon as possible the need for medical intervention.

Crohn's Disease

In anyone with hip or groin pain of unknown cause, look for a history of PID, Crohn's disease (regional enteritis), ulcerative colitis, irritable bowel syndrome, diverticulitis, or bowel obstruction.

New onset of low back, sacral, buttock, or hip pain may be merely a new symptom of an already established enteric (GI) disease. About 25% of those with inflammatory enteric disease (particularly Crohn's disease) have concomitant back or joint pain that are symptoms of spondyloarthritis/spondyloarthropathy. Symptoms of Crohn's disease include diarrhea, fever, fatigue, abdominal pain and cramping, blood in the stool, mouth sores, reduced appetite, and weight loss.

A skin rash that comes and goes can accompany enterically induced arthritis. A flat rash or raised skin lesion of the lower extremities is possible; it usually precedes joint or back pain. Be sure to ask the client whether he or she has had skin rashes of any kind over the past few weeks.

Several tests can be done to assess for hip pain resulting from psoas abscess caused by abdominal or intraperitoneal infection or inflammation. These were discussed in the previous section.

A positive response for each of these tests is NOT a reproduction of the client's hip or groin pain, but rather, lower quadrant abdominal pain on the same side of the test. This is a symptom of an infectious or inflammatory process. Hip or back pain in response to these tests is more likely musculoskeletal in origin such as a trigger point of the iliopsoas or muscular tightness.

Reactive Arthritis

In the case of reactive arthritis, joint symptoms occur 1 to 4 weeks after an infection, usually GI or GU.[121] The joint is not septic (infected), but rather, it is aseptic (without infection). Affected joints often occur at a site that is remote from the primary infection. Prosthetic joints are not immune to this type of infection and may become infected years after the joint is implanted.

Whether the infection occurs in the natural joint or the prosthetic implant, the client is unable to bear weight on the joint. An acute arthritic presentation may occur, and the client often has a fever (commonly of low grade in older adults or in anyone who is immunosuppressed). Screening questions for clients with joint pain are listed in Box 3.5 and Appendix B-18 on page xx. These questions may be helpful for the client with joint pain of unknown cause or with an unusual presentation/history that does not fit the expected pattern for injury, overuse, or aging.

SCREENING FOR VASCULAR CAUSES OF LOWER QUADRANT PAIN

Vascular pain is often throbbing in nature and exacerbated by activity. With atherosclerosis, a lag time of 5 to 10 minutes occurs between when the body asks for increased oxygenated blood and when symptoms occur because of arterial occlusion. The client is older, often with a personal or family history of heart disease. Other risk factors include hyperlipidemia, tobacco use, and diabetes.

Peripheral Vascular Disease

PVD, also known as peripheral arterial disease or arterial insufficiency, in which the arteries are occluded by atherosclerosis, can cause unilateral or bilateral low back, hip, buttock, groin, or leg pain, along with intermittent claudication and trophic changes of the affected lower extremities.

Intermittent claudication of vascular origin may begin in the calf and gradually make its way up the lower extremity. The client may report the pain or discomfort as "burning," "cramping," or "sharp." Pain or other symptoms begin several minutes after the start of physical activity and resolve almost immediately with rest. As discussed in Chapter 15, the site of symptoms is determined by the location of the pathology (see Fig. 15.3) (Case Example 17.13).

PVD is a rare cause of lower quadrant pain in anyone under the age of 65 years, but leg pain in recreational athletes caused by isolated areas of arterial stenosis has been reported.[122]

The therapist must include assessment of vital signs and must look for trophic skin changes so often present with chronic

CASE EXAMPLE 17.13

Intermittent Claudication with Sciatica

Referral: A 41-year-old woman who was referred by her primary care physician with a medical diagnosis of sciatica reported bilateral lower extremity weakness with pain in the left buttock and left sacroiliac (SI) area. She also noted that she had numbness in her left leg after walking more than half a block.

She said both her legs felt like they were going to "collapse" after she walked a short distance and that her left would go "hot and cold" during walking. She also experienced cramping in her right calf muscle after walking more than half a block.

Symptoms are made worse by walking and better after resting or by standing still. Symptoms have been present for the last 2 months and came on suddenly without trauma or injury of any kind. No night pain was reported.

No medical tests or imaging studies have been done at this time.

Past Medical History: Significant positive for family history of heart disease (both sides of the family); smoking history: 1 pack of cigarettes/day for the past 26 years.

Clinical Presentation

Neurologic Screening Examination: Negative/within normal limits (WNL)

Neural Tissue Mobility: Tests were all negative; tissue tension WNL

Complete Lumbar Spine Examination: Unremarkable; ruled out as a source of client's symptoms

Diminished dorsalis pedis pulse on the left side

Bike Test (reviewed in Chapter 15; this test can be used to stress the integrity of the vascular supply to the lower extremities): Cycling in a position of lumbar forward flexion reproduced leg weakness and eliminated dorsalis pedis pulse on the left; no change was noted on the right.

Associated Signs and Symptoms

None.

What are the red flags in this case?

- Lower extremity (LE) weakness without pain accompanied by "giving out" sensation
- Symptoms brought on by specific activity, relieved by rest or standing still
- Significant family history of heart disease
- No known cause; onset of symptoms without trauma or injury
- Temperature changes in LEs
- Positive smoking history

Result: Given the severity of her family history of heart disease (sudden death at a young age was very common), she was sent back to the doctor immediately. The therapist briefly outlined the red flags and asked the physician to reevaluate for a possible vascular cause of symptoms.

Medical testing revealed a high-grade circumferential stenosis (narrowing) of the distal aorta at the bifurcation. The client underwent surgery for placement of a stent in the occluded artery. After the operation, the client reported complete relief from all symptoms, including buttock and SI pain.

Data from Gray JC: Diagnosis of intermittent vascular claudication in a patient with a diagnosis of sciatica: case report. *Phys Ther* 79:582–590, 1999.

arterial insufficiency. Pulse oximetry may be helpful when thrombosis is not clinically obvious; for example, pulses can be present in both feet with oxygen saturation (SaO_2) levels at 90% or less.[123] When assessing for PVD as a possible cause of back, buttock, hip, groin, or leg pain, look for other signs of PVD. See further discussion of this topic in Chapters 4, 7, and 15.

DVT as a cause of lower leg pain may present as loss of knee or ankle motion, swelling of the knee, calf, or ankle, with calf tenderness and erythema. There can be increased local skin temperature, local edema, and decreased distal pulses in the lower extremity.[51] Further discussion and information on assessment of DVT are presented in Chapters 4 and 7.

Abdominal Aortic Aneurysm

AAA may be asymptomatic; discovery occurs during physical or x-ray examination of the abdomen or lower spine for some other reason. The most common symptom is awareness of a pulsating mass in the abdomen, with or without pain, followed by abdominal and back pain. Groin pain and flank pain may occur because of increasing pressure on other structures. (For more detailed information, see Chapter 7.)

Be aware of the client's age. The client with an AAA can be of any age because this may be a congenital condition, but usually, he or she is over the age of 50 years and is more likely 65 years or older. The condition remains asymptomatic until the wall of the aorta grows large enough to rupture. If that happens, blood in the abdomen causes searing pain accompanied by a sudden drop in blood pressure. Other symptoms of impending rupture or actual rupture of the aortic aneurysm include the following:

- Rapid onset of severe groin pain (usually accompanied by abdominal or back pain)
- Radiation of pain to the abdomen or posterior thighs
- Pain not relieved by change in position
- Pain described as "tearing" or "ripping"
- Other signs such as cold, pulseless lower extremities

An increasingly prevalent risk factor in the aging adult population is initiation of a weight-lifting program without prior medical evaluation or approval. The presence of atherosclerosis, elevated blood pressure, or an unknown aneurysm during weight training can precipitate rupture.

The therapist can palpate the aortic pulse to identify a widening pulse width, which is suggestive of an aneurysm (see Fig. 4.55). Place one hand or one finger on either side of the aorta as shown. Press firmly deep into the upper abdomen just to the left of midline. The therapist should feel aortic pulsations. These pulsations are easier to appreciate in a thin person and are more difficult to feel in someone with a thick abdominal wall or a large anteroposterior diameter of the abdomen.

Obesity and abdominal ascites or distention make this more difficult. For therapists who are trained in auscultation, listen for bruits. Bruits are abnormal blowing or swishing sounds heard during auscultation of the arteries. Bruits with both systolic and diastolic components suggest the turbulent blood flow of partial arterial occlusion. If the renal artery is occluded as well, the client will be hypertensive.

Avascular Osteonecrosis

Avascular osteonecrosis (also known as *osteonecrosis* or *septic necrosis*) can occur without known cause but is often associated with trauma (e.g., hip dislocation or fracture) and various other nontraumatic risk factors.[124] Chronic use and abuse of alcohol is a common risk factor for this condition and screening for alcohol or drug use and abuse is discussed in Chapter 2 (see also Appendices B-1 and B-2 on 784.e5 and 784.e6).

Osteonecrosis is also associated with many other conditions such as systemic lupus erythematosus, pancreatitis, kidney disease, blood disorders (e.g., sickle cell disease, coagulopathies, leukemia), diabetes mellitus, Cushing's disease, and gout. Long-term use of corticosteroids, immunosuppressants, or use of medications for human immunodeficiency virus, acquired immunodeficiency syndrome, or any condition that causes immune deficiency, can also result in osteonecrosis.[124] Other individuals who are taking immunosuppressants include organ transplant recipients, clients with cancer, and those with RA or another chronic autoimmune disease.[125]

The femoral head is the most common site of this disorder. Bones with limited blood supply are at enhanced risk for this condition. Hip dislocation or fracture of the neck of the femur may compromise the already precarious vascular supply to the head of the femur. Ischemia leads to poor repair processes and delayed healing. Necrosis and deformation of the bone occur next.

The client may be asymptomatic during the early stages of osteonecrosis. Hip pain is the first symptom. At first, it may be mild, lasting for weeks. As the condition progresses, symptoms become more severe, with pain during weight-bearing, antalgic gait, and limited motion (especially internal rotation, flexion, and abduction). The client may report a distinct click in the hip when moving from the sitting position and increased stiffness in the hip as time goes by.

CLINICAL SIGNS AND SYMPTOMS

Osteonecrosis

- May be asymptomatic at first
- Hip pain (mild at first, progressively worse over time)
- Groin or anteromedial thigh pain possible
- Pain worse during weight-bearing
- Antalgic gait with a gluteus minimus limp
- Limited hip range of motion (internal rotation, flexion, abduction)
- Tenderness to palpation over the hip joint
- Hip joint stiffness
- Hip dislocation

SCREENING FOR OTHER CAUSES OF LOWER QUADRANT PAIN

Osteoporosis

Osteoporosis may result in hip fracture and accompany hip pain, especially in postmenopausal women who are not taking hormone replacement. Osteoporosis accompanying the postmenopausal period—when combined with circulatory

impairment, postural hypotension, or some medications—may increase a person's risk of falling and incurring hip fracture.

Transient osteoporosis of the hip can occur during third-trimester pregnancy or immediately postpartum, although the incidence is fairly low.[126] The prevalence of transient osteoporosis is rare but is slightly higher in males than in females and has been documented in nonpregnant women, children, and adolescents.[127] Symptoms include spontaneous acute and progressive hip pain. In some cases, pain is referred to the lateral thigh and severe enough to result in an antalgic gait (limp). There is usually minimal night discomfort. Hip range of motion is usually spared, though the individual may report pain at the end of internal rotation. Often, the pain subsides in 6 to 8 weeks; this corresponds with resolution of bone edema. During pregnancy, the pain develops shortly before or during the last trimester and is aggravated by weight-bearing. There is a classic left-sided predominance seen in pregnant women that is not present in nonpregnant individuals. The pain subsides, and radiographic appearance returns to normal within several months after delivery.[128,129]

The natural history in nonpregnant individuals is for spontaneous regression and recovery within 6 to 9 months with no permanent problems. Radiographs are often normal at presentation but later show progressive osteoporosis of the femoral head (and sometimes the femoral neck and acetabulum).[128]

Any evaluation procedures that produce significant shear through the femoral head of a pregnant woman must be performed by the physical therapist with extreme caution. The transient osteoporosis of pregnancy is not limited to the hip, and vertebral compression may also occur.

Extrapulmonary Tuberculosis

Tubercular disease of the hip or spine is rare in developed countries, but it may occur as an opportunistic disease associated with AIDS that causes hip or back pain. Usually, the diagnosis of AIDS and tuberculosis is known, which alerts the therapist about the underlying systemic cause.

With hip involvement, the client usually appears with a chronic limp and describes pain in the hip that persists at rest. Approximately 60% of affected individuals do not have constitutional symptoms, although the tuberculin skin test is usually positive, and radiographs are similar to those for septic arthritis.

Sickle Cell Anemia and Hemophilia

Sickle cell anemia resulting in avascular necrosis (death of cells caused by lack of blood supply) of the hip and hemarthrosis (blood in the joint) associated with *hemophilia* are two of the most common hematologic diseases that cause pain in the hip, groin, knee, or leg.

Hemophilia may involve GI bleeding accompanied by low abdominal, hip, or groin pain caused by bleeding into the wall of the large intestine or the iliopsoas muscle. This retroperitoneal hemorrhage produces a muscle spasm of the iliopsoas muscle. The subsequent bleeding–spasm cycle produces increased hip pain and hip flexion spasm or contracture. Other symptoms may include melena, hematemesis, and fever.

CLINICAL SIGNS AND SYMPTOMS
Hip Hemarthrosis

- Pain in the groin and thigh
- Fullness in the hip joint, both anterior in the groin and over the greater trochanter
- Limited motion in hip flexion, abduction, and external rotation (allows most room for the blood in the joint capsule)

Liver (Hepatic) Disease

Some hepatic conditions can influence musculoskeletal conditions. One example of this is in tarsal tunnel syndrome. *Tarsal tunnel syndrome* characterized by pain around the ankle that extends to the plantar surfaces of the toes possibly made worse by walking may be the result of tibial nerve compression from any space-occupying lesion. Causes of compression include a history of trauma (nonunion or displaced fracture), varicosities, lipomas, ganglion cysts, or tumors.[130]

Additional symptoms can include burning pain and numbness on the plantar surface of the foot. Similar symptoms misinterpreted as tarsal tunnel syndrome can occur with neuropathy associated with diabetes mellitus and/or alcoholism. Tinel's sign (reproduction of characteristic pain or tingling with tapping or compression of the tibial nerve) may be positive but does not differentiate between a musculoskeletal cause and systemic origin of symptoms.[131]

Ascites is an abnormal accumulation of serous (edematous) fluid in the peritoneal cavity; this fluid contains large quantities of protein and electrolytes as the result of portal backup and loss of proteins (see Fig. 9.8). This condition is associated with liver disease and alcoholism. For the physical therapist, the distended abdomen, abdominal hernias, and lumbar lordosis observed in clients with ascites may present musculoskeletal symptoms such as groin or low back pain.

The presence of ascites, as it is linked with groin pain, would be physically evident. If abdominal distention is present, then the therapist should ask about a past medical history of liver impairment, chronic alcohol use, and the presence of carpal or tarsal tunnel syndrome associated with liver impairment. The therapist can carry out the four screening tests for liver impairment discussed in Chapter 10, including the following:

- Liver flap (asterixis; see Fig. 10.8)
- Palmar erythema (liver palms; see Fig. 10.6)
- Scan for angioma(s) (upper body and abdomen; see Fig. 10.5)
- Assess nail beds for change in color (nail beds of Terry; see Fig. 10.7)
- Ask about the presence of tarsal tunnel (and carpal tunnel) symptoms

PHYSICIAN REFERRAL

Guidelines for Immediate Medical Attention

- Painless, progressive enlargement of lymph nodes, or lymph nodes that are suspicious for any reason and that persist or that involve more than one area (groin and popliteal areas); immediate medical referral is required for a client with a past medical history of cancer

- Hip or groin pain alternating or occurring simultaneously with abdominal pain at the same level (**aneurysm, colorectal cancer**)
- Hip or leg pain during weight-bearing with positive tests for stress reaction or fracture

Guidelines for Physician Referral

- Hip, thigh, or buttock pain in a client with a total hip arthroplasty that is brought on by activity but resolves with continued activity (**loose prosthesis**), or who has persistent pain that is unrelieved by rest (**implant infection**)
- Sciatica accompanied by extreme motor weakness, numbness in the groin or rectum, or difficulty controlling bowel or bladder function
- One or more of Cyriax's Signs of the Buttock (see Box 17.2)
- New onset of joint pain in a client with a known history of Crohn's disease, requiring careful screening and possible referral based on examination results

Clues to Screening Lower Quadrant Pain

- See also Clues to Screening Head, Neck, or Back Pain; general concepts from the back also apply to the hip and the groin (see especially the discussion on Cardiovascular Assessment in Chapter 4)
- Client does not respond to physical therapy intervention or becomes worse, especially in the presence of a past medical history of cancer or an unknown cause of symptoms

Past Medical History

- History of AIDS-related tuberculosis, sickle cell anemia, or hemophilia
- History of endometriosis in women (**extrapelvic endometriosis**)
- Hip or groin pain in a client who has a long-term history of use of NSAIDs or corticosteroids (**avascular necrosis**)
- History of alcohol abuse or injection drug abuse
- Femoral artery catheterization (**septic hip arthritis, retroperitoneal hematoma formation**)

Clinical Presentation

- Symptoms are unchanged by rest, movement, or change in position
- Limited passive hip range of motion with empty end feel, especially in someone with a previous history of cancer, insidious onset, or an unknown cause of painful symptoms
- Palpable soft tissue mass in the anterior hip or groin (**psoas abscess, hernia**)
- Presence of rebound tenderness, positive McBurney's, iliopsoas, or obturator test (see Chapter 9)
- Abnormal cremasteric response in male with groin or anterior thigh pain
- Hip pain in a young adult that is worse at night and is alleviated by activity and aspirin (**osteoid osteoma**)
- Sciatica in the presence of night pain and an atypical pattern of restricted hip range of motion[132]

- No change in symptoms of sciatica with trigger point release, neural gliding techniques, soft tissue stretching, or postural changes
- Painless neurologic deficit (**spinal cord tumor**)
- Insidious onset of groin or anterior thigh pain with a recent history of increased activity (e.g., runners who increase their mileage)
- Symptoms are cyclical and related to menstrual cycle (**endometriosis**)

Associated Signs and Symptoms

- Hip or groin pain accompanied by or alternating with signs and symptoms associated with the GI, urologic/ renal, hematologic, or cardiovascular system, or with constitutional symptoms, especially fever and night sweats
- Groin pain in the presence of fever, sweats, weight loss, bleeding, skin lesions, or vaginal/penile discharge; night pain
- Hip or groin pain, with any clues suggestive of cancer (see Chapter 14), especially anyone with a previous history of cancer and men between the ages of 18 and 24 years who experience hip or groin pain of unknown cause (**testicular cancer**)
- Buttock, hip, thigh, or groin pain accompanied by fever, weight loss, bleeding or other vaginal/penile discharge, skin lesions, or other discharge

REFERRED LOWER QUADRANT PAIN PATTERNS (FIG. 17.6)

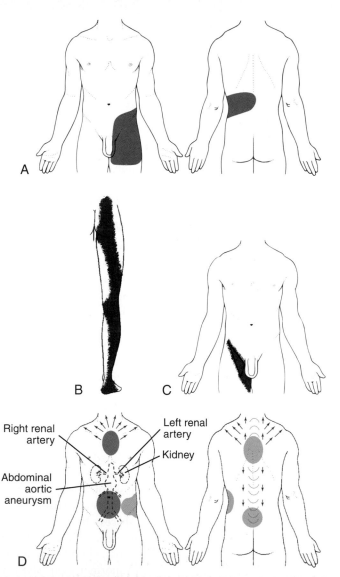

Fig. 17.6 Overview: Composite figure. **A,** Ureteral pain may begin posteriorly in the costovertebral angle, radiating anteriorly to the ipsilateral lower abdomen, upper thigh, or groin area. Isolated anterior thigh pain is possible, but uncommon. **B,** Pain pattern associated with sciatica from any cause. **C,** Pain pattern associated with psoas abscess from any cause. **D,** Abdominal aortic aneurysm can cause low back pain that radiates into the buttock unilaterally or bilaterally (not shown), depending on the underlying location and size of the aneurysm.

■ Key Points to Remember

1. See also Key Points to Remember in Chapter 15.

2. Identifying the hip as the source of a client's symptoms may be difficult, in that pain originating in the hip may not localize to the hip, but rather may present as low back, buttock, groin, SI, anterior thigh, or even knee or ankle pain.

3. Hip pain can be referred from other locations such as the scrotum, kidneys, abdominal wall, abdomen, peritoneum, or retroperitoneal region.

4. In addition to screening for medical problems, the therapist must remember to clear the joint above and below the area of symptoms or dysfunction.

5. True hip pain from any cause is usually felt in the groin or deep buttock, sometimes with pain radiating down the anterior thigh. Pain perceived on the outer (lateral) side of the hip is usually not caused by an intraarticular problem, but likely results from a tender point or from bursitis, SI, or back problems.

6. Hip pain referred from the upper lumbar vertebrae can radiate into the anterior aspect of the thigh, whereas hip pain from the lower lumbar vertebrae and sacrum is usually felt in the gluteal region, with radiation down the back or outer aspect of the thigh.

7. Systemic, medical, or viscerogenic causes of lower quadrant pain or symptoms mimic a neuromuscular or musculoskeletal cause, but usually, a red-flag history, risk factors, or associated signs and symptoms are identified during the screening process; this facilitates identification of the underlying problem.

8. Cancer recurrence most likely to metastasize to the hip includes breast, bone, and prostate.

9. Change in lymph node size with or without a previous history of cancer are a yellow or red flag.

10. Normal but painful log-rolling hip test present when the client is tested in the supine position with the hips in neutral extension (zero degrees of hip flexion) may be a yellow warning flag.

11. Cyriax's "Sign of the Buttock" can help differentiate between hip and lumbar spine disease.

12. Anyone with lower quadrant pain and a history of hip or knee arthroplasty must be evaluated for component problems (e.g., infection, subsidence, looseness), regardless of the client's perceived cause of the problem. Watch for pain during initiation of activity that improves with continued activity (loose prosthesis); also watch for signs of infection (recent history of infection anywhere else in the body, fever, chills, sweats, pain that is not relieved with rest, night pain, pain during weight-bearing).

13. A noncapsular pattern of restricted hip motion (e.g., limited hip extension, adduction, lateral rotation) may be a sign of serious underlying disease.

14. Anyone with pain radiating from the back down the leg as far as the ankle has a greater chance for disk herniation to be the cause of low back pain; this is true with or without neurologic findings.

15. The SLR and other neurodynamic tests are widely used but do not identify the underlying cause of sciatica. A positive SLR test does not differentiate between diskogenic disease and neoplasm; imaging studies may be needed.

16. Tests for the presence of hip pain caused by psoas abscess are advised whenever an infectious or inflammatory process is suspected based on past medical history, clinical presentation, and associated signs and symptoms.

17. New onset of low back, buttock, sacral, or hip pain in a client with a previous history of Crohn's disease, especially in the presence of a recent history of skin rash, requires screening for GI signs and symptoms.

18. Long-term use of corticosteroids or immunosuppressants or any condition that causes immune deficiency may also result in hip pain from osteonecrosis. As the condition progresses, symptoms become more severe with pain during weight-bearing, antalgic gait, and limited motion.

CLIENT HISTORY AND INTERVIEW

SPECIAL QUESTIONS TO ASK: LOWER QUADRANT

It is not necessary to ask every client every question listed. Sometimes, we ask some general screening questions because of something the client has told us. At other times, we screen because of something we saw in the clinical presentation. We may need to ask some specific questions based on gender. Finally, sometimes, the Review of Systems has pinpointed a particular system (e.g., GI, GU, vascular, pulmonary, gynecologic), and we go right to the end of the chapter dealing with that system and look for any screening questions that may be pertinent to the client.

The more often the therapist conducts screening interviews, the faster the process will get, and the easier it will become to remember which questions make the most sense to ask. The beginner may ask more questions than are needed, but with practice and experience, the screening process will smooth out. Generally, it takes about 3 to 5 minutes to

CLIENT HISTORY AND INTERVIEW—*cont'd*

conduct a screening interview and another 5 minutes to carry out any special tests.

As hip pain may be caused by referred pain from disorders of the low back, abdomen, and reproductive and urologic structures, special questions should include consideration of the following:

- Special Questions to Ask: Women Experiencing Back, Hip, Pelvic, Groin, or Sacroiliac Pain (see Appendix B-37 on 784.e43)
- Special Questions to Ask: Men Experiencing Back, Hip, Pelvic, Groin, or Sacroiliac Pain (see Appendix B-24 on 784.e29)
- Special questions for clients (see Chapter 15: Special Questions to Ask: Neck or Back):
- General systemic questions
- Pain assessment
- GI questions
- Urologic questions
- For anyone with lower quadrant pain of unknown cause:
  It may be necessary to conduct a sexual history as a part of the screening process (see Chapter 15 or Appendix B-32 on).
- A quick screening interview and additional questions may include the following:

PAIN ASSESSMENT

See Appendix C-7 on for a complete pain assessment.
- Have you had a recent injury?
  - *If yes*, tell me what happened.

- Did you hear any popping, snapping, or cracking when the injury occurred?
- How is the pain affected by putting weight on it?
- Does your leg "give out" on you (or feel like it is going to give out)?
- Does your pain feel better, the same, or worse after walking on it for a while? (**With joint arthroplasty, pain may improve after walking in the presence of loose components.**)

PAST MEDICAL HISTORY

- Have you ever been told (or have you known) that you have a sexually transmitted infection or disease?
- Have you been treated with cortisone, prednisone, other corticosteroids, or any other drug of that type?
- Do you have a known history of Crohn's disease, diverticulitis, or PID?
- Have you ever had cancer of any kind?
  If no, have you ever been treated with chemotherapy or radiation therapy?
- Have you ever had a bone tumor?

ASSOCIATED SIGNS AND SYMPTOMS

- Do you have any other symptoms anywhere else in your body?
- Any fatigue? Fever? Chills? Swollen joints?

CASE STUDY

STEPS IN THE SCREENING PROCESS

A 34-year-old woman was referred to physical therapy for pelvic pain from a nonrelaxing puborectalis muscle. She reported bilateral groin pain that was superficial and affected the skin area. She also said the area feels "warm." The pain was worse when sitting, better when standing, and had lasted longer than a month. The physician ruled out shingles and sent her to physical therapy for further evaluation.

WHAT ARE SOME STEPS YOU CAN TAKE TO START THE SCREENING PROCESS?

Have the client complete a past medical history form, and review it for any clues that might help direct the screening process. Ask the usual questions about bowel and bladder function, especially about constipation or pain with a bowel movement (see Appendices B-5 and B-6 on page 784.e9 and 784.e10).

Superficial skin changes are usually a sudomotor response; messages arrive via the spinal cord, but the system has no way

to know the specific source of the problem (i.e., viscerogenic versus somatic), so it sends out a "distress" signal that something is wrong at the S2-S3 level. The therapist must consider what could be involved.

Using Table 17.3 as a guide, the therapist can assess the likelihood of each condition listed based on age, sex, past medical history, and associated signs and symptoms. Screening tests may be conducted, as appropriate. For example, a neurologic screening examination may help identify discogenic disease or a possible spinal cord tumor.

The client is young to have developed an AAA from atherosclerosis, but a congenital aneurysm may be present. Palpating the abdomen and the aortic pulse and listening with a stethoscope for femoral bruits may be helpful.

A stress fracture would likely have a suspicious history such as prolonged activity requiring axial loading or trauma of some kind. It may be necessary to ask about physical or sexual assault. Conduct screening tests such as heel strike, rotational/translational stress test of the pubis, hop on one leg, and full squat. Assess for TrPs.

CASE STUDY—cont'd

Ureteral problems are usually accompanied by bladder changes (e.g., dysuria, hematuria, frequency) and constitutional symptoms such as fever, sweats, or chills. Take vital signs.

Gynecologic causes of low back, pelvic, groin, hip, or SI pain are usually accompanied by a significant history of gynecologic conditions or a traumatic or multiple birth/delivery history. Some additional questions along these lines may be needed if the past medical history form is not sufficient. Sexually transmitted infection or ectopic pregnancy is possible, although rare causes of groin pain may occur in sexually active women.

Appendicitis or another infectious process can cause a wide range of symptoms outside of the typical or expected right lower abdominal quadrant pain, including isolated groin pain or combined hip and groin pain. McBurney's test (see Fig. 9.10) or Blumberg's sign for rebound tenderness (see Figs. 9.12 and 9.13) can help the therapist to recognize when medical referral is required.

PRACTICE QUESTIONS

1. The screening model used to help identify viscerogenic or systemic origins of hip, groin, and lower extremity pain and symptoms is made up of:
   a. Past medical history, risk factors, clinical presentation, and associated signs and symptoms
   b. Risk factors, risk reduction, and primary prevention
   c. Enteric disease, systemic disease, and neuromusculoskeletal dysfunction
   d. Physical therapy diagnosis, Review of Systems, and physician referral referral
2. When would you use the iliopsoas, obturator, or Blumberg's test?
3. Hip and groin pain can be referred from:
   a. Low back
   b. Abdomen
   c. Retroperitoneum
   d. All of the above
4. Screening for cancer may be necessary in anyone with hip pain who:
   a. Is younger than 20 years of age or older than 50 years
   b. Has a past medical history of diabetes mellitus
   c. Reports fever and chills
   d. Has a total hip arthroplasty (THA)
5. Pain during weight-bearing may be a sign of hip fracture, even when radiographs are negative. Follow-up clinical tests may include:
   a. McBurney's, Blumberg's, Murphy's test
   b. Squat test, hop test, translational/rotational tests
   c. Psoas and obturator tests
   d. Patrick's or Faber's test
6. Abscess of the hip flexor muscles from intraabdominal infection or inflammation can cause hip and/or groin pain.

Clinical tests to differentiate the cause of hip pain resulting from psoas abscess include:
   a. McBurney's, Blumberg's, or Murphy's test
   b. Squat test, hop test, translational/rotational tests
   c. Iliopsoas and obturator tests
   d. Patrick's or Faber's test
7. Anyone with hip pain of unknown cause must be asked about:
   a. Previous history of cancer or Crohn's disease
   b. Recent infection
   c. Presence of skin rash
   d. All of the above
8. Vascular diseases that may cause referred hip pain include:
   a. Coronary artery disease
   b. Intermittent claudication
   c. Aortic aneurysm
   d. All of the above
9. True hip pain is characterized by:
   a. Testicular (male) or labial (female) pain
   b. Groin or deep buttock pain with active or passive range of motion
   c. Positive McBurney's test
   d. All of the above
10. Hip pain associated with primary or metastasized cancer is characterized by:
    a. Bone pain during weight-bearing; may not be able to stand on that leg
    b. Night pain that is relieved by aspirin
    c. Positive heel strike test with palpable local tenderness
    d. All of the above

REFERENCES

1. Hammond NA. Left lower-quadrant pain: guidelines from the American College of Radiology appropriateness criteria. *Am Fam Phys.* 2010;82(7):766–770.
2. Lachiewicz PF. Abductor tendon tears of the hip: evaluation and management. *J Am Acad Orthop Surg.* 2011;19(7):385–391.
3. Lachiewicz PF. Thigh mass resulting from polyethylene wear of a revision total hip arthroplasty. *Clin Orthop Relat Res.* 2007;455:274–276.
4. Smilowitz NR, Kirtane AJ, Guiry M, et al. Practices and complications of vascular closure devices and manual compression in patients undergoing elective transfemoral coronary procedures. *Am J Cardiol.* Jul 2012;15(2):177–782.
5. Browder DA, Erhard RE. Decision making for a painful hip: a case requiring referral. *J Orthop Sports Phys Ther.* 2005;35:738–744.
6. Lesher JM. Hip joint pain referral patterns: a descriptive study. *Pain Med.* 2008;9:22–25.
7. Kimpel DL. Hip pain in a 50-year-old woman with RA. *J Musculoskel Med.* 1999;16:651–652.
8. Bertot AJ, Jarmain SJ, Cosgarea AJ. Hip pain in active adults: 20 clinical pearls. *J Musculoskel Med.* 2003;20:35–55.
9. Tortolani PJ, Carbone JJ, Quartararo LG. Greater trochanteric pain syndrome in patients referred to orthopedic spine specialists. *Spine J.* 2002;2:251–254.
10. Strauss EJ. Greater trochanteric pain syndrome. *Sports Med Arthroscop.* 2010;18(2):113–119.
11. Williams BS, Cohen SP. Greater trochanteric pain syndrome: a review of anatomy, diagnosis, and treatment. *Anesth Analg.* 2009;108(5):1662–1670.
12. Lyle MA, Manes S, McGuinness M, Ziaei S, Iversen MD. Relationship of physical examination findings and self-reported symptom severity and physical function in patients with degenerative lumbar conditions. *Phys Ther.* 2005;85:120–133.
13. Greenwood MJ, Erhard RE, Jones DL. Differential diagnosis of the hip vs. lumbar spine: five case reports. *J Orthop Sports Phys Ther.* 1998;27:308–315.
14. Cyriax J. *Textbook of Orthopaedic Medicine.* 8 ed. London: Bailliere Tindall; 1982.
15. VanWye WR. Patient screening by a physical therapist for non-musculoskeletal hip pain. *Phys Ther.* 2009;89(3):248–256.
16. Cibulka MT, Sinacore DR, Cromer GS, Delitto A. Unilateral hip rotation range of motion asymmetry in patients with sacroiliac joint regional. *Spine.* 1998;23:1009–1015.
17. Cibulka MT. Symmetrical and asymmetrical hip rotation and its relationship to hip rotator muscle strength. *Clin Biomech.* 2010;25(1):56–62.
18. Brown TE, Larson B, Shen F, Moskal JT. Thigh pain after cementless total hip arthroplasty: evaluation and management. *J Am Acad Orthop Surg.* 2002;10:385–392.
19. Fogel GR, Esses SI. Hip spine syndrome: management of coexisting radiculopathy and arthritis of the lower extremity. *Spine J.* 2003;3:238–241.
20. Kim YH, Oh SH, Kim JS, Koo K-H. Contemporary total hip arthroplasty with and without cement in patients with osteonecrosis of the femoral head. *J Bone Joint Surg.* 2003;85:675–681.
21. Khanuja HS. Cementless femoral fixation in total hip arthroplasty. *J Bone Joint Surg.* 2011;93(5):500–507.
22. Byrd JWT. Investigation of the symptomatic hip: Physical examination. In: Byrd JWT, ed. *Operative Hip Arthroscopy.* 2 ed New York: Springer; 2005:36–50.
23. Kelly BT. Hip arthroscopy: current indications, treatment options, and management issues. *Am J Sports Med.* 2003;31:1020–1037.
24. Hair LC, Deyle G. Eosinophilic granuloma in a patient with hip pain. *J Orthop Sports Phys Ther.* 2011;41(2):119.
25. Heick JD, Bustillo KL, Farris JW. Recognition of signs and symptoms of a type 1 chondrosarcoma: a case report. *Physiother Theory Pract.* 2014;30(1):49–55.
26. Sahrmann SA. *Diagnosis and Treatment of Movement Impairment Syndromes.* 1 ed. St. Louis: Mosby; 2002.
27. Sahrmann S. *Movement System Impairment Syndromes of the Extremities, Cervical, and Thoracic Spines.* 1 ed. St. Louis: Mosby; 2010.
28. Grumet RC. Lateral hip pain in an athletic population: differential diagnosis and treatment options. *Sports Health.* 2010;2(3):191–196.
29. Schilders E. Adductor-related groin pain in recreational athletes. *J Bone Joint Surg.* 2009;91A(10):2455–2460.
30. Kluin J. Endoscopic evaluation and treatment of groin pain in the athlete. *Am J Sports Med.* 2004;32(4):944–949.
31. Swan KG, Wolcott M. The athletic hernia: a systematic review. *Clin Ortho Relat Res.* 2006;455:78–87.
32. Larson CM. Athletic pubalgia: current concepts and evolving management. *Orthop Today.* 2011;31(2):46–52.
33. Ross JR, Stone RM, Larson CM. Core muscle injury/sports hernia/athletic pubalgia, and femoroacetabular impingement. *Sports Med Arthrosc Rev.* 2015;23:213–220.
34. Van Veen RN. Successful endoscopic treatment of chronic groin pain in athletes. *Surg Endosc.* 2007;21:189–193.
35. Kachingwe AF, Grech S. Proposed algorithm for the management of athletes with athletic pubalgia (sports hernia): a case series. *J Orthop Sports Phys Ther.* 2008;38(12):768–781.
36. Lee AJJ, Armour P, Thind D, Coates MH, Kang ACL. The prevalence of acetabular labral tears and associated pathology in a young asymptomatic population. *Bone Joint J.* 2015;97-B:623–627.
37. Mayes S, Ferris AR, Smith P, Garnham A, Cook J. Similar prevalence of acetabular labral tear in professional ballet dancers and sporting participants. *Clin J Sport Med.* 2015;26(4):307–313.
38. Ratzlaff C, Simatovic J, Wong H, et al. Reliability of hip examination test for femoroacetabular impingement. *Arthritis Care Res.* 2013;65(10):1690–1696.
39. Parvizi J. Femoroacetabular impingement. *J Am Acad Ortho Surg.* 2007;15(69):561–570.
40. Mcintyre J. Groin pain in athletes. *Curr Sports Med Report.* 2006;5(6):293–299.
41. Zajick D, Zoga A, Omar I, Meyers WC. Spectrum of MRI findings in clinical athletic pubalgia. *Sem Musculoskel Radiol.* 2008;12(1):3–12.
42. Cowan SM, Schache P, Brukner KL, et al. Onset of transversus abdominis in long-standing groin pain. *Med Sci Sports Exerc.* 2004;36:2040–2045.
43. Mabry LM. Insufficiency fracture of the pubic rami. *J Orthop Sports Phys Ther.* 2010;40(10):666.
44. Maigne J-Y. Upper thoracic dorsal rami: anatomic study of their medial cutaneous branches. *Surg Radiol Anat.* 1991;13:109–112.
45. Giles LGF, Singer KP. *The Clinical Anatomy and Management of Thoracic Spine Pain.* 1 ed. Oxford: Butterworth-Heinemann; 2000.
46. Mesiha M. Synovial sarcoma presenting as iliotibial band friction syndrome: case report. *J Knee Surg.* 2009;22(4):376–378.
47. Youssef JA. Minimally invasive surgery: lateral approach interbody fusion. *Spine.* 2010;35(26S):S302–S311.
48. Tamir E, Anekshtein Y, Melamed E, Halperin N, Mirovsky Y. Clinical presentation and anatomic position of L3-L4 disc herniation. *J Spinal Disord Tech.* 2004;17:467–469.
49. Reverse straight leg raise test. http://courses.washington.edu/hubio553/glossary/reverse.html. Accessed March 16, 2011.
50. Foster MR. Herniated nucleus pulposus. eMedicine Specialties. Updated Jan 8, 2010. http://emedicine.medscape.com/article/1263961-overview. Accessed March 16, 2011.

51. Cheatham SW, Kolber MJ, Salamh PA. Meralgia paresthetica: a review of the literature. *Int J Sport Phys Ther*. 2013;8(6):883–893.

52. Cho KT. Prone position-related meralgia paresthetica after lumbar spinal surgery: a case report and review of the literature. *J Korean Neurosurg Soc*. 2008;44(6):392–395.

53. Weier CA. Meralgia paresthetica of the contralateral leg after total hip arthroplasty. *Orthopedics*. 2010;16:265–268.

54. Capeci CM, Tejwani NC. Bilateral low-energy simultaneous or sequential femoral fractures in patients on long-term alendronate therapy. *J Bone Joint Surg*. 2009;91A(11):2556–2561.

55. Rosenthal MD. Diagnosis of medial knee pain: atypical stress fracture about the knee joint. *J Orthop Sports Phys Ther*. 2006;36(7):526–534.

56. Constantinou M. Differential diagnosis of a soft tissue mass in the calf. *J Orthop Sports Phys Ther*. 2005;35:88–94.

57. Fink ML, Stoneman PD. Deep vein thrombosis in an athletic military cadet. *J Orthop Sports Phys Ther*. 2006;36(9):686–697.

58. Poppert E, Kulig K. Hip degenerative joint disease in a patient with medial knee pain. *J Orthop Sports Phys Ther*. 2011;41(1):33.

59. Emms NW. Hip pathology can masquerade as knee pain in adults. *Age Ageing*. 2002;31:67–69.

60. Vaughn DW. Isolated knee pain: a case report highlighting regional interdependence. *J Orthop Sports Phys Ther*. 2008;38(10):616–623.

61. Brown EC. The painful total knee arthroplasty: diagnosis and management. *Orthopedics*. 2006;29(2):129–138.

62. Cummings M. Referred knee pain treated with electroacupuncture to iliopsoas. *Acupunct Med*. 2003;21:32–35.

63. Travell JG, Simons DG. *Myofascial Pain and Dysfunction: The Lower Extremities*. Vol. 2. Baltimore: Williams and Wilkins; 1992.

64. Guss DA. Hip fracture presenting as isolated knee pain. *Ann Emerg Med*. 1997;29:418–420.

65. Muscolo DL. Tumors about the knee misdiagnosed as athletic injuries. *J Bone Joint Surg Am*. 2003;85A:1209–1214.

66. Abdulla AJ. Leg cramps in the elderly: prevalence, drug, and disease associations. *Int J Clin Pract*. 1999;53:494–496.

67. Butler JV. Nocturnal leg cramps in older people. *Postgrad Med J*. 2002;78:596–598.

68. Matsumoto M. Nocturnal leg cramps. *Spine*. 2009; 34(5):E189–E194.

69. Steele MK. Relieving cramps in high school athletes. *J Musculoskel Med*. 2003;20:210.

70. Lui E. Systemic causes of heel pain. *Clin Podiatr Med Surg*. 2010;27:431–441.

71. Maheshwari AV. Metastatic skeletal disease of the foot: case reports and literature review. *Foot Ankle Int*. 2008;29:699–710.

72. Berlin SJ. Tumors of the heel. *Clin Podiatr Med Surg*. 1990;7:307–321.

73. Groves MJ. Metastatic breast cancer presenting as heel pain. *J Am Podiatr Med Assoc*. 1998;88:400–405.

74. Kahanov L, Eberman LE, Games KE, Wasik M. Diagnosis, treatment, and rehabilitation of stress fractures in the lower extremity in runners. *Open Access J Sports Med*. 2015;6:87–95.

75. Krause DA, Newcomer KL. Femoral neck stress fracture in a male runner. *J Orthop Sports Phys Ther*. 2008;38(8):517.

76. Thelen MD. Identification of a high-risk anterior tibial stress fracture. *J Orthop Sports Phys Ther*. 2010;40(12):833.

77. Duquette TL, Watson DJ. Femoral neck stress fracture in a military trainee. *J Orthop Sports Phys Ther*. 2010;40(12):834.

78. Brukner P, Bennell KM, Matheson G. *Stress Fractures*. Australia: Blackwell Publishing; 1999.

79. Seidenberg PH, Childress MA. Managing hip pain in athletes. *J Musculoskel Med*. 2005;22:246–254.

80. Kelly AK, Hame SL. Managing stress fractures in athletes. *J Musculoskel Med*. 2010;27(12):480–486.

81. Cho CH. Sacral fractures and sacroplasty. *Neuroimaging Clin N Am*. 2010;20(2):179–186.

82. Gurney B, Boissonnault WG, Andrews R. Differential diagnosis of a femoral neck/head stress fracture. *J Orthop Sports Phys Ther*. 2006;36(2):80–88.

83. Carpintero P. Stress fractures of the femoral neck and coxa vara. *Arch Orthop Trauma Surg*. 2003;123(6):273–277.

84. Tommasini SM. Relationship between bone morphology and bone quality in male tibias: implications for stress fracture risk. *J Bone Min Res*. 2005;20(8):1372–1380.

85. Weishaar MD, McMillian DJ, Moore JH. Identification and management of 2 femoral shaft stress injuries. *J Orthop Sports Phys Ther*. 2005;35:665–673.

86. Johnson AW, Weiss Jr. CB, Wheeler DL. Stress fractures of the femoral shaft in athletes—more common than expected: a new clinical test. *Am J Sports Med*. 1994;22:248–256.

87. Ivkovic A, Bojanic I, Pecina M. Stress fractures of the femoral shaft in athletes: a new treatment algorithm. *Br J Sports Med*. 2006;40:518–520.

88. Hunt KJ, Anderson RB. Heel pain in the athlete. *Sports Health*. 2009;1(5):427–434.

89. Blain H, Rolland Y, Beauchet O, et al. Usefulness of bone density measurement in fallers. *J Bone Spine*. 2014;81:403–408.

90. Ozburn MS, Nichols JW. Pubic ramus and adductor insertion stress fractures in female basic trainees. *Milit Med*. 1981;146.332–334.

91. Valat JP. Sciatica. *Best Pract Res Clin Rheum*. 2010;24(2):241–252.

92. Jewell DV, Riddle DL. Interventions that increase or decrease the likelihood of a meaningful improvement in physical health in patients with sciatica. *Phys Ther*. 2005;85(11):1139–1150.

93. Shiri R, Lallukka T, Karppinen J, Viikari-Juntura E. Obesity as a risk factor for sciatica: a meta-analysis. *Am J Epidemiol*. 2014;179(8):929–937.

94. Yuen EC, So YT. Sciatic neuropathy. *Neurol Clin*. 1999;17:617–631.

95. Martin WN, Dixon JH, Sandhu H. The incidence of cement extrusion from the acetabulum in total hip arthroplasty. *J Arthroplasty*. 2003;18:338–341.

96. Carricajo A. Propionibacterium acnes contamination in lumbar disc surgery. *J Hosp Infect*. 2007;66(3):275–277.

97. Stirling A, Worthington T, Rafiq M, Lambert PA, Elliott TS. Association between sciatica and. *Propionibacterium acnes*. *Lancet*. 2001;357:2024–2025.

98. McLorinn GC, Glenn JV, McMullan MG, Patrick S. *Propionibacterium acnes* wound contamination at the time of spinal surgery. *Clin Orthop Relat Res*. 2005;437:67–73.

99. Hulbert A, Deyle GD. Differential diagnosis and conservative treatment for piriformis syndrome: a review of the literature. *Curr Orthop Pract*. 2009;20(3):313–319.

100. Floyd 2nd JR. Cyclic sciatica from extrapelvic endometriosis affecting the sciatic nerve. *J Neurosurg Spine*. 2011;14(2):281–289.

101. Bickels J, Kahanvitz N, Rubert CK, et al. Extraspinal bone and soft-tissue tumors as a cause of sciatica: clinical diagnosis and recommendations: analysis of 32 cases. *Spine*. 1999;24:1611.

102. Chin KR, Kim JM. A rare anterior sacral osteochondroma presenting as sciatica in an adult: a case report and review of the literature. *Spine J*. 2010;10(5):e1–e4.

103. Deyo RA, Diehl AK. Cancer as a cause of back pain: Frequency, clinical presentation, and diagnostic strategies. *J Gen Intern Med*. 1988;3:230–238.

104. Guyer RD, Collier RR, Ohnmeiss DD, et al. Extraosseous spinal lesions mimicking disc disease. *Spine*. 1988;13:328–331.

105. Bose B. Thoracic extruded disc mimicking spinal cord tumor. *Spine J*. 2003;3:82–86.

106. Jordan RW, Koc T, Chapman AWP, Taylor HP. Osteoid osteoma of the foot and ankle—a systematic review. *Foot Ankle Surg*. 2015;21:228–234.

107. Ilyas I, Younge DA. Medical management of osteoid osteoma. *Can J Surg.* 2002;45:435–437.
108. Arromdee E, Matteson EL. Bursitis: Common condition, uncommon challenge. *J Musculoskel Med.* 2001;18:213–224.
109. Magee DJ. *Orthopedic Physical Assessment.* 5 ed Philadelphia: WB Saunders; 2008.
110. Doubleday KL, Kulig K, Landel R. Treatment of testicular pain using conservative management of the thoracolumbar spine: a case report. *Arch Phys Med Rehabil.* 2003;84:1903–1905.
111. Keulers BJ, Roumen RH, Keulers MJ, Vandermeeren L, Bekke JPH. Bilateral groin pain from a rotten molar. *Lancet.* 2005;366:94.
112. Todkar M. Case report: psoas abscess—unusual etiology of groin pain. *Medscape Gen Med.* Jul 2005 http://www.medscape.com/viewarticle/507610_print. Accessed Online March 12, 2011.
113. Bhat SN, Mohanty SP, Kustagi P. Endometriosis presenting like a psoas abscess. *Saudi Med J.* 2007;28(6):952–954.
114. Inman RD. Arthritis and enteritis—an interface of protean manifestations. *J Rheumatol.* 1987;14:406–410.
115. Inman RD. Antigens, the gastrointestinal tract, and arthritis. *Rheum Dis Clin North Am.* 1991;17:309–321.
116. Gran JT, Husby G. Joint manifestations in gastrointestinal diseases. 1. Pathophysiological aspects, ulcerative colitis and Crohn's disease. *Dig Dis.* 1992;10:274–294.
117. Gran JT, Husby G. Joint manifestations in gastrointestinal diseases. 2. Whipple's disease, enteric infections, intestinal bypass operations, gluten-sensitive enteropathy, pseudomembranous colitis and collagenous colitis. *Dig Dis.* 1992;10:295–312.
118. Keating RM, Vyas AS. Reactive arthritis following *Clostridium difficile* colitis. *West J Med.* 1995;162:61–63.
119. Tu J. Bowel bypass syndrome/bowel-associated dermatosis arthritis syndrome post laparoscopic gastric bypass surgery. *Australas J Dermatol.* 2011;52(1):e5–e7.
120. Brakenhoff LK. The joint-gut axis in inflammatory bowel disease. *J Crohns Colitis.* 2010;4(3):257–268.
121. Prati C. Reactive arthritis due to Clostridium difficile. *Joint Bone Spine.* 2010;77(2):190–192.
122. Lundgren JM, Davis BA. End artery stenosis of the popliteal artery mimicking gastrocnemius strain. *Arch Phys Med Rehabil.* 2004;85:1548–1551.
123. Brau SA, Delamarter RB, Schiffman ML, Williams LA, Watkins RG. Vascular injury during anterior lumbar surgery. *Spine J.* 2004;4:409–441.
124. Babis GC. Osteonecrosis of the femoral head. *Orthopedics.* 2011;34(1):39–48.
125. Norton R. Hip pain in young adults: making a difficult diagnosis. *J Musculoskel Med.* 2006;23(12):857–872.
126. Hadji P, Boekhoff J, Hahn M, Hellmeyer L, Hars O, Kyvernitakis I. Pregnancy-associated transient osteoporosis of the hip: results of a case-control study. *Arch Osteoporos.* 2017;12(1):11 https://doi.org/10.1007/s11657-017-0310-y. Epub 2017 Jan 21. PMID: 28110481.
127. Asadipooya K, Graves L, Greene LW. Transient osteoporosis of the hip: review of the literature. *Osteoporos Int.* 2017;28(6):1805–1816. https://doi.org/10.1007/s00198-017-3952-0. . Epub 2017 Mar 17. PMID: 28314897 Review.
128. Holzer I. Transient osteoporosis of the hip: long-term outcomes in men and nonpregnant women. *Curr Orthop Pract.* 2009;20(2):161–163.
129. Boissonnault WB, Boissonnault JS. Transient osteoporosis of the hip associated with pregnancy. *J Orthop Sports Phys Ther.* 2001;31:359–367.
130. Kline AJ. Current concepts in managing chronic ankle pain. *J Musculoskel Med.* 2007;24(11):477–484.
131. Bilstrom E. Injection of the carpal and tarsal tunnels. *J Musculoskel Med.* 2007;24(11):472–474.
132. Ross MD, Bayer E. Cancer as a cause of low back pain in a patient seen in a direct access physical therapy setting. *J Orthop Sports Phys Ther.* 2005;35:651–658.
133. Goodman CC, Snyder TEK. Laboratory Tests and Values. In: Goodman CC, Fuller K, eds. *Pathology: Implications for the Physical Therapist.* 4 ed. Philadelphia: WB Saunders; 2015.

Screening the Chest, Breasts, and Ribs

Clients do not present in an outpatient physical therapy clinic with chest or breast pain as the primary symptom very often. It is more common for those patients to report to an emergency or urgent care clinic. The therapist is more likely to see the client with an orthopedic or neurologic impairment who experiences chest or breast pain during exercise or interventions by the therapist.

In other situations, the client reports chest or breast pain as an additional symptom during the screening interview. The pain may occur along with (or alternating with) the presenting symptoms of jaw, neck, upper back, shoulder, breast, or arm pain. When chest pain is the primary complaint, it is often an atypical pain pattern (possibly in a young athlete) that has misled the client and/or the physician.[1]

On the other hand, it is also possible for clients to have primary chest pain from a human movement system impairment, particularly spinal referred pain.[2] Symptoms persist or recur, often with months in between when the client is free of any symptoms. Countless medical tests are performed and repeated with referral to numerous specialists before a physical therapist is consulted (see Case Example 1.7).

Finally, so many of today's aging adults with movement system impairments have multiple medical comorbidities that the therapists must be able to identify signs and symptoms of systemic disease that can mimic neuromuscular or musculoskeletal dysfunction. Systemic or viscerogenic pain or symptoms that can be referred to the chest or breast include the cardiovascular, pulmonary, and upper gastrointestinal (GI) systems, as well as other causes such as cancer, anxiety, steroid use, and cocaine use (Table 18.1).[3] Various neuromusculoskeletal (NMS) conditions, such as thoracic outlet syndrome (TOS), costochondritis, tender points, and cervical spine disorders, can also affect the chest and breast.[4]

When faced with chest pain, the therapist must know how to assess the situation quickly and decide if referral is required and whether medical attention is needed immediately. As experts in understanding and assessing the human movement system, we are the most capable health care professional when it comes to differentiating an NMS condition from a systemic origin of symptoms.

The therapist must especially know how and what to look for to screen for cancer, cancer recurrence, and/or the delayed effects of cancer treatment. Cancer can present as primary chest pain with or without accompanying neck, shoulder, and/or upper back pain/symptoms. Basic principles of cancer screening are presented in Chapter 14; specific clues related to the chest, breast, and ribs will be discussed in this chapter. Breast cancer is always a consideration with upper quadrant pain or dysfunction.

USING THE SCREENING MODEL TO EVALUATE THE CHEST, BREASTS, OR RIBS

There are many causes of chest pain, both cardiac and noncardiac in origin (see Table 18.1). Two conditions may be present at the same time, each contributing to chest pain. For example, someone with cervicodorsal arthritis could also experience reflux esophagitis or coronary disease. Either or both of these conditions can contribute to chest pain.

Chest pain can be evaluated in one of two ways: cardiac versus noncardiac, or systemic versus NMS. Physicians and nurses assess chest pain from the first paradigm: cardiac versus noncardiac. The therapist must understand the basis for this screening method and also view each problem as potentially systemic versus NMS. Throughout the screening process, it is important to remember we are not medical cardiac specialists; we are just screening for systemic disease masquerading as NMS symptoms or dysfunction.

Paying attention to past medical history (PMH), recognizing unusual clinical presentation for a neuromuscular or musculoskeletal condition, and keeping in mind the clues to differentiating chest pain will help the therapist evaluate difficult cases.

Additionally, the woman with chest, breast, axillary, or shoulder pain of unknown origin at presentation must be questioned regarding breast self-examination. Any recently discovered lumps or nodules must be examined by a physician. The client may need to be educated regarding breast self-examination, and the physical therapist can provide this valuable information.[5,6] Breast self-examination techniques are commonly available in written form for the physical therapist or the client who is unfamiliar with these methods (see Appendix D-6 in the accompanying enhanced eBook version included with print purchase of this textbook).

TABLE 18.1	Causes of Chest Pain
Systemic/Medical Conditions	**Neuromusculoskeletal**

Systemic/Medical Conditions	Neuromusculoskeletal
Cancer • Mediastinal tumors Cardiac • Myocardial ischemia (unstable angina) • Myocardial infarct • Cardiomyopathy • Myocarditis • Pericarditis • Dissecting aortic aneurysm • Aortic aneurysm • Aortic stenosis or regurgitation • Mitral valve prolapse* • Tachycardia Pleuropulmonary • Asthma/COPD • Pulmonary embolism • Pneumothorax • Pulmonary hypertension* • Cor pulmonale • Pneumonia with pleurisy or pleuritis • Mediastinitis Epigastric/upper GI • Esophagitis* • Esophageal spasm* • Reflux or other motility disorder • Hiatal hernia • Upper GI ulcer • Cholecystitis • Pancreatitis Breast (see Table 18.2) Hematologic • Anemia • Polycythemia • Sickle cell crisis Other • Rheumatic disease (sternoclavicular joint) • Infection (sepsis): sternoclavicular joint (injection drug use) • Anxiety, panic attack* • Vertebroplasty (possible pulmonary embolism) • Cocaine use • Anabolic steroids • Collagen vascular disorder with pleuritis or pericarditis • Fibromyalgia • Hyperthyroidism • Dialysis (first-use syndrome) • Type III hypersensitivity reaction • Herpes zoster (shingles) • Psychogenic	Tietze's syndrome Costochondritis, sternochondritis Sternoclavicular joint strain Hypersensitive xiphoid, xiphodynia Slipping rib syndrome TrPs (see Table 18.4) Myalgia Cervical spine disorder, arthritis Neurologic • Nerve root compression • Intercostal neuritis • Dorsal nerve root irritation • TOS • Thoracic disk disease Postoperative pain Breast • Mastodynia • TrPs • Trauma (including motor vehicle accident, assault) • Rib fracture, costochondral • Dislocation, chest contusion

COPD, Chronic obstructive pulmonary disease; *GI*, gastrointestinal; *TOS*, thoracic outlet syndrome; *TrPs*, trigger points.
*Relieved by nitroglycerin because it relaxes smooth muscle.

Past Medical History

Although the PMH is important, it cannot be relied upon to confirm or rule out medical causes of chest pain. PMH does alert the therapist to an increased risk of systemic conditions that can masquerade as NMS disorders. Like risk factors, PMH varies according to each system affected, or condition present, and is reviewed individually in each section of this chapter.

Risk Factors

Any suspicious findings should be checked by a physician, especially in the case of the client with identified risk factors for cancer or heart disease. Identifying red-flag risk factors, the PMH, and correlation of this information with objective findings are important steps in the screening process.

Risk for cardiac-caused symptoms increases with advancing age, tobacco use, menopause (women), family history of hypertension or premature coronary artery disease (CAD), and high cholesterol. Risk factors associated with noncardiac conditions vary with each condition (e.g., infectious, rheumatologic, pulmonary, or other systemic causes).

Clinical Presentation

When the clinical presentation suggests further screening is needed, the therapist can follow the guide to pain assessment (see Chapter 3) and physical assessment for the upper quadrant as presented in Table 4.13. Assess vital signs and watch for trends in heart rate and blood pressure. Keep in mind that tachycardia may be a compensatory response to reduced cardiac output and bradycardia may be an indication of myocardial ischemia or (unreported) trauma.

The client's general appearance, along with vital sign assessment, will offer some idea of the severity of the condition. Watch for uneven pulses from side to side, diminished or absent pulses, elevated blood pressure, or extreme hypotension. Auscultation for breath or lung sounds and chest percussion may provide additional cardiovascular or pulmonary clues to aid in decision-making.

Check to see if the pain can be reproduced or made worse by palpation or with pressure on the chest; and, of course, ask about associated symptoms such as nausea and shortness of breath. The key features that point to spinal referred pain are chest pain reproduced during movement (especially with resistive movement), tenderness and tightness of musculoskeletal structures at a spinal level supplying the painful area, and an absence or lack of symptoms suggestive of a nonmusculoskeletal cause.[2]

Chest Pain Patterns

From the previous discussion in Chapter 3, there are at least three possible mechanisms for referred pain patterns to the soma from the viscera (embryologic development, multisegmental innervations, or direct pressure on the diaphragm).

Pain in the chest may be derived from the chest wall (dermatomes T1-T12), the pleura, the trachea and main airways, the mediastinum (including the heart and esophagus), and the abdominal viscera. From an embryologic point of view, the lungs are derived from the same tissue as the gut, so problems can occur in both areas (lung or gut), causing chest pain and other related symptoms.

Certain chest pain patterns are more likely to point to a medical rather than musculoskeletal cause. For example, pain that is positional or reproduced by palpation is not as suspicious as pain that radiates to one or both shoulders or arms, or that is precipitated by exertion. Physicians agree that the chest pain history by itself is not enough to rule out cardiac or some other systemic origin of symptoms. In most cases, some diagnostic testing is needed.[7]

Chest pain associated with increased activity is a red flag for possible cardiovascular involvement. In such cases, the onset of pain is not immediate but rather occurs 5 to 10 minutes after activity begins. This is referred to as the "lag time" and is a screening clue used by the physical therapist to assess when chest pain may be caused by musculoskeletal dysfunction (immediate chest pain occurs with movement of the arms and/or trunk) or by possible vascular compromise (chest pain occurs 5 to 10 minutes after activity begins).

Parietal pain may appear as unilateral chest pain (rather than midline only) because at any given point the parietal peritoneum obtains innervation from only one side of the nervous system. It is usually not reproduced by palpation. Thoracic disk disease can also present as unilateral chest pain, requiring careful screening.[8,9]

The four types of pain discussed in Chapter 3 (cutaneous, deep somatic or parietal, visceral, and referred) also apply to the chest. *Parietal (somatic) chest pain* is the most common systemic chest discomfort encountered in physical therapy practice. Parietal pain refers to pain generating from the wall of any cavity, such as the chest or pelvic cavity (see Fig. 7.5). Although the visceral pleura is insensitive to pain, the parietal pleura is well supplied with pain nerve endings. It is usually associated with an infectious disease, but is also seen in pneumothorax, rib fracture, pulmonary embolism with infarction, and other systemic conditions.

Pain fibers, originating in the parietal pleura, are conveyed through the chest wall as fine twigs of the intercostal nerves. Irritation of these nerve fibers results in pain in the chest wall that is usually described as knife-like and is sharply localized close to the chest wall, occurring cutaneously (in the skin).

Pain from the thoracic viscera and true chest wall pain are both felt in the chest wall, but *visceral pain* is referred to the area supplied by the upper four thoracic nerve roots. Report of pain in the lower chest usually indicates local disease, but upper chest pain may be caused by disease located deeper in the chest.

There are few nerve endings (if any) in the visceral pleurae (linings of the various organs), such as the heart or lungs. The exception to this statement is in the area of the pericardium (sac enclosed around the entire heart), which is adjacent to the diaphragm (see Fig. 7.5). Extensive disease may develop within the body cavities without the occurrence of pain until the process extends to the parietal pleura. Neuritis (constant irritation of nerve endings) in the parietal pleura then produces the pain described in this section.

Pleural pain may be aggravated by any respiratory movement involving the diaphragm, such as sighing, deep breathing, coughing, sneezing, laughing, or from hiccups. It may be referred along the costal margins or into the upper abdominal quadrants. Palpation usually does not reproduce pleural pain; change in position does not relieve or exacerbate the pain. In some cases of pleurisy, the individual can point to the painful spot, but deep breathing (not palpation) reproduces it.

Associated Signs and Symptoms

If the client has an underlying infectious or inflammatory process causing chest or breast pain or symptoms, there may be a change in vital signs and/or constitutional symptoms such as chills, night sweats, fever, upper respiratory symptoms, or GI distress.

Signs and symptoms associated with noncardiac causes of chest pain vary according to the underlying system involved. For example, cough, sputum production, and a recent history of upper respiratory infection (URI) may point to a pleuropulmonary origin of chest or breast pain. Anyone with persistent coughing or asthma can experience chest pain related to the strain of the chest wall muscles.

Chest or breast pain associated with GI disease is often food-related in the presence of a history of peptic ulcer, gastroesophageal reflux disease (GERD), or gallbladder problems. Blood in the stool or vomitus, combined with a history of chronic nonsteroidal antiinflammatory drug (NSAID) use, may point to a GI problem.

Many of the conditions affecting the breast are not accompanied by other systemic signs and symptoms. Risk factors, PMH, and clinical presentation provide the major clues in differentiating between a viscerogenic, systemic, or cancerous origin of chest and/or breast pain or symptoms.

SCREENING FOR ONCOLOGIC CAUSES OF CHEST OR RIB PAIN

Cancer can present as primary chest, neck, shoulder, and/or upper back pain and symptoms. A previous history of cancer of any kind is a major red flag (Case Example 18.1). Primary cancer affecting the chest with referred pain to the breast is not as common as cancer metastasized to the pulmonary system with subsequent pulmonary and chest/breast symptoms.

Clinical Presentation

The most common symptoms associated with metastasis to the pulmonary system are pleural pain, dyspnea, and persistent cough. As with any visceral system, symptoms may not occur until the neoplasm is quite large or invasive because the lining surrounding the lungs has no pain perception. Symptoms first appear when the tumor is large enough to

CASE EXAMPLE 18.1

Rib Metastases Associated with Ovarian Cancer

Referral: A 53-year-old university professor came to the physical therapy clinic with complaints of severe left shoulder pain radiating across her chest and down her arm. She rated the pain a 10 on the numeric rating scale (NRS; see explanation in Chapter 3).

Past Medical History (PMH): She had a significant personal and social history, including ovarian cancer 10 years ago, death of a parent last year, filing for personal bankruptcy this year, and a divorce after 30 years of marriage.

Clinical Presentation (First Visit): During the screening examination for vital signs, the client's blood pressure was 220/125 mm Hg. Pulse was 88 bpm. Pulse oximeter measured 98%. Oral temperature: 98.0° F. She denied any previous history of cardiovascular problems or current feelings of stress.

Intervention: She was referred for medical attention immediately based on her blood pressure readings but returned a week later with a medical diagnosis of "rib bruise." Electrocardiography (ECG) and heart catheterization ruled out a cardiac cause of symptoms. She was put on Prilosec for gastroesophageal reflux disease (GERD) and an antiinflammatory for her rib pain.

Clinical Presentation (Second Visit): The therapist was able to reproduce the symptoms just described with moderate palpation of the eighth rib on the left side and side-bending motion to the left side. The client described the symptoms as constant, sharp, burning, and intense. She had pain at night if she slept too long on either side.

Sidelying on the involved side and slump sitting did not reproduce the symptoms. There was no obvious mechanical cause for the painful symptoms (e.g., intercostal tear, costovertebral dysfunction, neuritis from nerve entrapment).

The therapist considered the possibility of a somato-visceral reflex response (e.g., a biomechanical dysfunction of the 10th rib can cause gallbladder changes), but there were no accompanying associated signs and symptoms and the 10th rib was not painful.

Result: The therapist decided to contact the referring physician to discuss the client's clinical presentation before initiating treatment, especially given the constancy and intensity of the pain in the presence of a PMH of cancer.

The physician directed the therapist to have the client return for further testing. A bone scan revealed metastases to the ribs and thoracic spine. Physical therapy intervention was not appropriate at this time.

press on other nearby structures or against the chest wall. The presence of any skin changes, lesions, or masses should be documented using the information presented in Fig. 4.6. Skeletal pain from metastases to the bone, or primary cancers such as multiple myeloma affecting the sternum, can present much like costochondritis.

Skin Changes

Ask the client about any recent or current skin changes. Metastatic carcinoma can present with a cellulitic appearance on the anterior chest wall as a result of carcinoma of the lung

(see Fig. 4.26). The skin lesion may be flat or raised and any color from brown to red or purple.

Liver impairment from cancer or any liver disease can also cause other skin changes, such as an angioma over the chest wall. An angioma is a benign tumor with blood (or lymph, as in lymphangioma) vessels. Spider angioma (also called spider nevus) is a form of telangiectasis, a permanently dilated group of superficial capillaries (or venules; see Fig. 10.5).

In the presence of skin lesions, ask about a recent history of infection of any kind, use of prescription drugs within the last 6 weeks, and previous history of cancer of any kind. Look for lymph node changes. Report all of these findings to the physician.

Palpable Mass

Occasionally, the therapist may palpate a painless sternal or chest wall mass when evaluating the head and neck region. Most mediastinal tumors are the result of a metastatic focus from a distant primary tumor and remain asymptomatic unless they compress mediastinal structures or invade the chest wall.

The primary tumor is usually a lymphoma (Hodgkin's lymphoma in a young adult or non-Hodgkin's lymphoma in a child or older adult; see Fig. 4.29), multiple myeloma (primarily observed in people over 60 years of age), or carcinoma of the breast, kidney, or thyroid.

When involvement of the chest wall and nerve roots results in pain, the pattern is more diffuse, with radiation of pain to the affected nerve roots (Case Example 18.2). Irritation of an intercostal nerve from rib metastasis produces burning pain that is unilateral and segmental in distribution. Sensory loss or hyperesthesia over the affected dermatomes may be noted.

SCREENING FOR CARDIOVASCULAR CAUSES OF CHEST, BREAST, OR RIB PAIN

Cardiac-related chest pain may arise secondary to angina, myocardial infarction (MI), pericarditis, endocarditis, mitral valve prolapse, or aortic aneurysm. Despite diagnostic advances, acute coronary syndromes and MIs are missed in 2% to 10% of patients[7]; emergency room physicians predict which client has an acute coronary syndrome better than by chance. There is no single element of chest pain history powerful enough to predict who is or who is not having a coronary-related incident; attempts made to construct clinical decision rules to determine this are currently not successful.[10] Medical referral is advised whenever there is any doubt and medical diagnostic testing is almost always required.[7]

Cardiac-related chest pain can also occur when there is normal coronary circulation, as in the case of clients with pernicious anemia. Affected clients may have chest pain or angina during physical exertion because of the lack of nutrition to the myocardium.

Risk Factors

Sex and age are nonmodifiable risk factors for chest pain caused by heart disease. The rate of CAD is rising among

CASE EXAMPLE 18.2

Lymphoma Masquerading as Nerve Entrapment

Referral: A 72-year-old woman was referred to physical therapy for a postural exercise program and home traction by her neurologist with a diagnosis of "nerve entrapment." She was experiencing symptoms of left shoulder pain with numbness and tingling in the ulnar nerve distribution. She had a moderate forward head posture with slumped shoulders and loss of height from known osteoporosis.

Past Medical History (PMH): The woman's PMH was significant for right breast cancer treated with a radical mastectomy and chemotherapy 20 years ago. She had a second cancer (uterine) 10 years ago that was considered separate from her previous breast cancer.

Clinical Presentation: The physical therapy examination was consistent with the physician's diagnosis of nerve entrapment in a classic presentation. There were significant postural components to account for the development of symptoms. However, the therapist palpated several large masses in the axillary and supraclavicular fossa on both the right and left sides. There was no local warmth, redness, or tenderness associated with these lesions. The therapist requested permission to palpate the client's groin and popliteal spaces for any other suspicious lymph nodes. The rest of the examination findings were within normal limits.

Associated Signs and Symptoms: Further questioning about the presence of associated signs and symptoms revealed a significant disturbance in sleep pattern over the last 6 months with unrelenting shoulder and neck pain. There were no other reported constitutional symptoms, skin changes, or noted lumps anywhere. Vital signs were unremarkable at the time of the physical therapy evaluation.

Result: Returning this client to her referring physician was a difficult decision to make given that the therapist did not have the benefit of the medical records or results of neurologic examination and testing. With the significant PMH for cancer, the woman's age, presence of progressive night pain, and palpable masses, no other reasonable choice remained. When asked if the physician had seen or felt the masses, the client responded with a definite "no."

There are several ways to approach handling a situation like this one, depending on the physical therapist's relationship with the physician. In this case, the therapist had never communicated with this physician before. It is possible that the physician was aware of the masses, knew from medical testing that there was extensive cancer, and chose to treat the client palliatively.

Because there was no indication of such, the therapist notified the physician's staff of the decision to return the client to the physician. A brief (one-page) written report summarizing the findings was given to the client to hand-carry to the physician's office.

Further medical testing was performed, and a medical diagnosis of lymphoma was made.

cancer, but in truth, they are 10 times more likely to die of cardiovascular disease. Whereas 1 in 30 women's deaths is from breast cancer, 1 in 2.5 deaths is from heart disease.[12] The annual cardiovascular disease mortality rate has remained greater for women than for men since 1984.[13]

Women do not seem to do as well as men after taking medication to dissolve blood clots or after undergoing heart-related medical procedures. In 2020, a systematic review noted that the class of medications prescribed differed in men and women.[14] Women were more likely to be prescribed diuretics but not aspirin, statins or angiotensin-converting enzyme inhibitors. Men were more likely to receive these medications but less likely to be prescribed diuretics. Of the women who survive a heart attack, 46% will be disabled by heart failure within 6 years.[15] African-American women have a 70% higher death rate from CAD than Caucasian women.[12] When screening individuals who have chest pain, keep in mind that older men and women, menopausal women, and African-American women are at greatest risk for cardiovascular causes.

A common treatment for CAD after heart attack is angioplasty with insertion of a stent. A stent is a wire mesh tube that props open narrowed coronary arteries. Sometimes, the stent malfunctions or gets scarred over. Cardiologists have realized that such treatments, although effective at alleviating chest pain, do not reduce the risk of heart attacks for most people with stable angina.

When the client presents with chest pain, he or she often does not think it can be from the heart because there is a stent in place, but this may not be true. Anyone with a history of stent insertion presenting with chest pain should be assessed carefully. The physical therapist in doubt needs to take vital signs and ask about associated signs and symptoms. Evaluate the effect of exercise on symptoms. For example, does the chest, neck, shoulder, or jaw pain start 3 to 5 minutes after exercise or activity? What is the effect on pain in the upper body when the individual is using just the lower extremities, such as walking on a treadmill or up a flight of stairs?

Other risk factors for CAD are listed in Table 7.3. Efforts are being made to determine evidence-based risk factors for low-versus high-risk chest pain of unknown origin. Predictive values for ischemia resulting in MI or death include two or more episodes of chest pain typical of a heart attack in an adult aged 55 years or older who has a family history of heart disease and/or a personal history of diabetes.[16]

Clinical Presentation

There are some well-known pain patterns specific to the heart and cardiac system. Sudden death can be the first sign of heart disease. In fact, according to the American Heart Association, 63% of women who died suddenly of cardiovascular disease had no previous symptoms. Sudden[14] death is the first symptom for half of all men who have a heart attack. Cardiac arrest strikes immediately and without warning.

middle-aged women[11] and falling among men. Men develop CAD at a younger age than women, but women make up for it after menopause. Many women know about the risk of breast

CLINICAL SIGNS AND SYMPTOMS
Cardiac Arrest

- Sudden loss of responsiveness; no response to gentle shaking
- No normal breathing; client does not take a normal breath when you check for several seconds
- No signs of circulation; no movement or coughing

Cardiac Pain Patterns

Cardiac disease is the leading cause of death in the United States,[17] but 1.5% of clients presenting to a primary care clinic with chest pain will have unstable angina or an acute MI. In primary care clinics, the clinical impression is shaped by the presenting symptoms, physical examination, and initial echocardiogram (ECG), combined with the client's risk of acute coronary syndrome.[18,19] Doctors and nurses often use "the three Ps" when screening for chest pain during the physical examination to determine whether the chest pain is cardiac. The presence of any or all of these Ps suggests that the client's pain or symptoms are *not* caused by an MI:

- **P**leuritic pain (exacerbation by deep breathing is more likely pulmonary)
- Pain during **p**alpation (musculoskeletal cause)
- Pain with changes in **p**osition (musculoskeletal cause)

Cardiac pain patterns may differ for men and women. For many men, the most common report is a feeling of pressure or discomfort under the sternum (substernal), in the midchest region, or across the entire upper chest. It can feel like uncomfortable pressure, squeezing, fullness, or pain.

Pain may occur just in the jaw, upper neck, midback, or down the arm without chest pain or discomfort. Pain may also radiate from the chest to the neck, jaw, midback, or down the arm(s). Pain down the arm(s) affects the left arm most often in the pattern of the ulnar nerve distribution. Radiating pain down both arms is also possible and may indicate an MI.

For women, symptoms can be more subtle or atypical (Box 18.1). Chest pain or discomfort is less common in women, but is still a key feature for some. They often have prodromal symptoms (e.g., pain in the chest, pain in the shoulder or back, radiating pain or numbness in the arms, dyspnea, and fatigue) 12 months prior and up to 1 month before having a heart attack (see Table 7.4).[20-22] African-American women younger than 50 years are more likely to report frequent and intense prodromal symptoms.[23]

Fatigue, nausea, and lower abdominal pain may signal a heart attack. Many women pass these off as the flu or food poisoning. Other symptoms for women include a feeling of intense anxiety, isolated right biceps pain, or midthoracic pain. Heartburn; sudden shortness of breath or the inability to talk, move, or breathe; shoulder or arm pain; or ankle swelling or rapid weight gain are also common symptoms associated with MI.

Chest Pain Associated with Angina

The therapist should keep in mind that coronary disease may go unnoticed because the client has no anginal or infarct pain

BOX 18.1 SIGNS AND SYMPTOMS OF MYOCARDIAL ISCHEMIA IN WOMEN

- Heart pain in women does not always follow classic patterns.
- Many women do experience classic chest discomfort.
- In older women, change in mental status or confusion may be common.
- Dyspnea (at rest or with exertion)
- Weakness and lethargy (unusual fatigue; fatigue that interferes with ability to perform activities of daily living)
- Indigestion or heartburn; mistakenly diagnosed or assumed to have gastroesophageal reflux disease (GERD)
- Lower abdominal pain
- Anxiety or depression
- Sleep disturbance (woman awakens with any of the symptoms listed here)
- Sensation similar to inhaling cold air; unable to talk or breathe
- Isolated midthoracic back pain
- Symptoms may be relieved by antacids (sometimes antacids work better than nitroglycerin).

associated with ischemia. This situation occurs when collateral circulation is established to counteract the obstruction of the blood flow to the heart muscle. Anastomoses (connecting channels) between the branches of the right and left coronary arteries eliminate the person's perception of pain until challenged by physical exertion or exercise in the physical therapy setting.

Chest pain caused by angina is often confused with heartburn or indigestion, hiatal hernia, esophageal spasm, or gallbladder disease, but the pain of these other conditions is not described as sharp or knife-like. The client often says the pain feels like "gas," "heartburn," or "indigestion." Referred pain from a trigger point (TrP) in the external oblique abdominal muscle can cause a sensation of heartburn in the anterior chest wall (see Fig. 18.7).

Episodes of stable angina usually develop slowly and last 2 to 5 minutes. Discomfort may radiate to the neck, shoulders, or back (Case Example 18.3). Shortness of breath is common. Symptoms of angina may be similar to the pattern associated with a heart attack. One primary difference is duration. Angina lasts a limited time (a few minutes up to half an hour) and can be relieved by rest or nitroglycerin. When screening for angina, a lack of objective musculoskeletal findings is always a red flag:

- Active range of motion, such as trunk rotation, side-bending, or shoulder motions, does not reproduce symptoms.
- Resisted motion does not reproduce symptoms (horizontal shoulder abduction/adduction).
- Heat and stretching do not reduce or eliminate symptoms.

CASE EXAMPLE 18.3
Adhesive Capsulitis

Referral: A 56-year-old man returned to the same physical therapist with his third recurrence of left shoulder adhesive capsulitis of unknown cause.

Past Medical History (PMH): There was no reported injury, trauma, or repetitive motion as a precipitating factor in this case. The client was a car salesman with a fairly sedentary job. He reported a PMH of prostatitis, peptic ulcers, and a broken collarbone as a teenager. He reported being a "social" drinker at work-related functions but did not smoke or use tobacco products. He was taking ibuprofen for his shoulder but no other over-the-counter or prescription medications or supplements.

The two previous episodes of shoulder problems resolved with physical therapy intervention. The client had a home program to follow to maintain range of motion and normal movement. At the time of his most recent discharge 6 months ago, he had attained 80% of motion available on the uninvolved side with some continued restricted glenohumeral movement and altered scapulohumeral rhythm. The client reported that he did not continue with his exercise routine at home and "that's why I got worse again."

Clinical Presentation

Shoulder flexion and abduction	Left: 105/100 degrees	Right: 170/165 degrees
Shoulder medial (internal) rotation	0–70 degrees	0–90 degrees
Shoulder lateral (external) rotation	0–45 degrees	0–80 degrees

Accessory motions: Reduced inferior and anterior glide on the left; within normal limits on the right. The client reports pain during glenohumeral flexion, abduction, and medial and lateral rotations.

Clinical impressions: Decreased physiologic motion with capsular pattern of restriction and compensatory movements of the shoulder girdle; humeral superior glide syndrome.

Associated Signs and Symptoms: When asked if there were any symptoms of any kind anywhere else in the body, the client reported "chest tightness" whenever he tried to use his arm for more than a few minutes. Previously, he was used to "working through the pain," but he cannot seem to do that anymore.

He also reported "a few bouts of nausea and sweating" when his shoulder started aching. He denied any shortness of breath or constitutional symptoms such as fever or sweats. There were no other gastrointestinal-related symptoms.

What are the red flags in this case? How would you screen further?

- Age over 50 years

- Nausea and sweating concomitant with shoulder pain; chest tightness
- Insidious onset
- Recurring pattern of symptoms

Screening can begin with something as simple as vital sign assessment. The therapist can consult Box 4.19 for a list of other associated signs and symptoms and look for a cluster or pattern associated with a particular system.

Given his age, sedentary lifestyle, and particular clinical presentation, a cardiovascular screening examination seems most appropriate. The therapist can also consult the Special Questions to Ask box at the end of Chapter 7 for any additional pertinent questions based on the client's response to questions and the examination results. A short (3- to 5-minute) bike test also can be used to assess the effect of lower extremity exertion on the client's symptoms.

Result: The client's blood pressure was alarmingly high at 185/120 mm Hg. Although this is an isolated (one time) reading, he was under no apparent stress, and he revealed that he had a history of elevated blood pressure in the past. The bike test was administered while his heart rate and blood pressure were being monitored. Symptoms of chest and/or shoulder pain were not reproduced by the test, but the therapist was unwilling to stress the client without a medical evaluation first.

Referral was made to his primary care physician with a phone call, fax, and report of the therapist's findings and concerns. Although there is a known viscero-somatic effect between heart and chest and heart and shoulder, there is no reported direct cause and effect link between heart disease and adhesive capsulitis. Comorbid factors, such as diabetes mellitus or heart disease, have been shown to affect pain levels and function.[24]

Likewise, adhesive capsulitis is known to occur in some people following immobility associated with intensive care, coronary artery bypass graft, or pacemaker complications/revisions.

The physician considered this an emergency and admitted the client to the cardiology unit for immediate workup. The electrocardiogram results were abnormal during the exercise stress test. Further testing confirmed the need for a triple bypass procedure. Following the operation and phase 1 cardiac rehab in the cardiac rehab unit, the client returned to the original outpatient physical therapist for his phase 2 cardiac rehab program. Shoulder symptoms were gone, and range of motion was unimproved but regained rapidly as the rehab program progressed.

The therapist shared this information with the cardiologist, who agreed that there may have been a connection between the chest/shoulder symptoms before surgery, although he could not say for sure.

The therapist should also watch for unstable angina in a client with known angina. Unlike stable angina, rest or nitroglycerin do not relieve symptoms associated with MI, unless administered intravenously. Without intervention, symptoms of MI may continue without stopping. A sudden change in the client's typical anginal pain pattern suggests unstable angina.

Pain that occurs without exertion, lasts longer than 10 minutes, or is not relieved by rest or nitroglycerin signals a higher risk for a heart attack. Clients complaining of pain radiating down both upper extremities, an S3 sound, or unusual hypotension need to be medically cleared by a physician.[25] Immediate medical referral is required under these circumstances.

SCREENING FOR PLEUROPULMONARY CAUSES OF CHEST, BREAST, OR RIB PAIN

Pulmonary chest pain usually results from obstruction, restriction, dilation, or distention of the large airways or large pulmonary arterial walls. Specific diagnoses include pulmonary artery hypertension, pulmonary embolism, mediastinal emphysema, asthma, pleurisy, pneumonia, and pneumothorax. Pleuropulmonary disorders are discussed in detail in Chapter 8.

Past Medical History

A previous history of cancer of any kind, recent history of pulmonary infection, or recent accident or hospitalization may be significant. Look for other risk factors, such as age, smoking, prolonged immobility, immune system suppression (e.g., cancer chemotherapy, corticosteroids), and eating disorders (or malnutrition from some other cause).

Mechanical alterations related to the overload of respiratory muscles with chronic asthma can lead to chest pain from musculoskeletal dysfunction and alterations in muscle length and posture.[26]

Clinical Presentation

Pulmonary pain patterns differ slightly depending on the underlying pathology and the location of the disease. For example, tracheobronchial pain is referred to the anterior neck or chest at the same levels as the points of irritation in the air passages. Chest pain that tends to be sharply localized or that worsens with coughing, deep breathing, or with other respiratory movement or motion of the chest wall and that is relieved by maneuvers that limit the expansion of a particular part of the chest (e.g., autosplinting) is likely to be pleuritic in origin.

Symptoms that increase with deep breathing and activity or the presence of a productive cough with bloody or rust-colored sputum are red flags. The therapist should ask about a new onset of wheezing at any time or difficulty breathing at night. Be careful when asking clients about changes in breathing patterns. It is not uncommon for the client to deny any shortness of breath.

Often, the reason for this is because the client has stopped doing anything that will bring on the symptoms. It may be necessary to ask what activities he or she can no longer do that were possible 6 weeks or 6 months ago. Symptoms that are relieved by sitting up are indicative of pulmonary impairment and must be evaluated more carefully.

SCREENING FOR GASTROINTESTINAL CAUSES OF CHEST, BREAST, OR RIB PAIN

GI causes of upper thorax pain are a result of epigastric or upper GI conditions. GERD ("heartburn" or esophagitis) accounts for a significant number of cases of noncardiac chest pain, in the young as well as older adults.[3,27–29] Stomach acid or gastric juices from the stomach enter the esophagus, irritating the protective lining of the lower esophagus. Whether the client is experiencing GERD or some other cause of chest pain, there is usually a telltale history or associated signs and symptoms to red flag the case.

Past Medical History

Watch for a history of alcoholism, cirrhosis, esophageal varices, and esophageal cancer or peptic ulcers. Any risk factors associated with these conditions are also red flags, such as long-term use of NSAIDs as a cause of peptic ulcers or chronic alcohol use associated with cirrhosis of the liver.

Clinical Presentation

The GI system has a broad range of referred pain patterns based on embryologic development and multisegmental innervations, as discussed in Chapter 3. Upper GI and pancreatic problems are more likely than lower GI disease to cause chest pain. Chest pain referred from the upper GI tract can radiate from the chest posteriorly to the upper back or interscapular or subscapular regions from T10 to L2 (Fig. 18.1).

Esophagus

Esophageal dysfunction will present with symptoms such as anterior neck and/or anterior chest pain, pain during swallowing (odynophagia), or difficulty swallowing (dysphagia) at the level of the lesion. Symptoms occur anywhere a lesion is present along the length of the esophagus. Early satiety, often with weight loss, is a common symptom associated with esophageal carcinoma.

Lesions of the upper esophagus may cause pain in the (anterior) neck, whereas lesions of the lower esophagus are more likely to be characterized by pain originating from the xiphoid process, radiating around the thorax to the middle of the back.

Chest pain with or without accompanying or alternating midthoracic back pain from an esophageal or other upper GI problem is usually red flagged by a suspicious history or

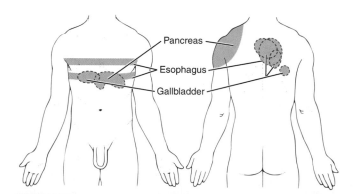

Fig. 18.1 Chest pain caused by gastrointestinal (GI) disease with referred pain to the shoulder and back. Upper GI problems can refer pain to the anterior chest with radiating pain to the thoracic spine at the same level. Look for accompanying GI symptoms and a red-flag history.

cluster of associated signs and symptoms. The pain pattern associated with thoracic disk disease can be the same as for esophageal pathology. In the case of disk disease, there may be bowel and/or bladder changes and sometimes numbness and tingling in the upper extremities. The therapist should ask about a traumatic injury to the upper back region and conduct a neurologic screening examination to assess for this possibility as a cause of the symptoms.

Epigastric Pain

Epigastric pain is typically characterized by substernal or upper abdominal (just below the xiphoid process) discomfort (see Fig. 18.1). This may occur with radiation posteriorly to the back, secondary to long-standing duodenal ulcers. Gastric duodenal peptic ulcer may occasionally cause pain in the lower chest rather than in the upper abdomen. Antacid and food often immediately relieve pain caused by an ulcer. Ulcer pain is not produced by effort and lasts longer than angina pectoris. The therapist will not be able to provoke or eliminate the client's symptoms. Likewise, physical therapy intervention will not have any long-lasting effects unless the symptoms were caused by TrPs.

Pain in the lower substernal area may arise as a result of reflux esophagitis (regurgitation of gastroduodenal secretions), a condition known as *gastroesophageal reflux disease*, or GERD. It may be gripping, squeezing, or burning, described as "heartburn" or "indigestion." Like that of angina pectoris, the discomfort of reflux esophagitis may be precipitated by recumbency or by meals; however, unlike angina, it is not precipitated by exercise and is relieved by antacids.

Hepatic and Pancreatic Systems

Epigastric pain or discomfort may occur in association with disorders of the liver, gallbladder, common bile duct, and pancreas, with referral of pain to the interscapular, subscapular, or middle/low back regions. This type of pain pattern can be mistaken for angina pectoris or MI (e.g., hypotension occurring with pancreatitis produces a reduction in coronary blood flow with the production of angina pectoris).

Hepatic disorders may cause chest pain with radiation of pain to the shoulders and back. Cholecystitis (gallbladder inflammation) appears as discrete attacks of epigastric or right upper quadrant pain, usually associated with nausea, vomiting, and fever and chills. Dark urine and jaundice indicate that a stone has obstructed the common duct.

The pain has an abrupt onset, is either steady or intermittent, and is associated with tenderness to palpation in the right upper quadrant. The pain may be referred to the back and right scapular areas. A gallbladder problem can result in a sore 10th rib tip (right side anteriorly) as described in Chapter 10 (also please see Case Example 18.4). Rarely, pain in the left upper quadrant and anterior chest can occur.

Acute pancreatitis causes pain in the upper part of the abdomen that radiates to the back (usually anywhere from T10 to L2) and may spread out over the lower chest. Fever and abdominal tenderness may develop.

CASE EXAMPLE 18.4
Chest Pain During Pregnancy

Referral: A 33-year-old woman in her twenty-ninth week of gestation with her first pregnancy was referred to a physical therapist by her gynecologist. Her abdominal sonogram and laboratory tests were normal. A chest x-ray was read as negative.

Past Medical History (PMH): None. The client had the usual childhood illnesses but had never broken any bones and denied use of tobacco, alcohol, or substances of any kind. There was no recent history of an infection, cold, virus, cough, trauma or accident, change in gastrointestinal (GI) function, and no history of cancer.

Clinical Presentation: Although there were no signs and symptoms associated with the respiratory system, the client's symptoms were reproduced when she was asked to take a deep breath. Palpation of the upper chest, thorax, and ribs revealed pain during palpation of the right tenth rib (anterior).

Thinking about the role of the gallbladder causing tenth rib pain, the therapist asked further questions about PMH and current GI symptoms. The client had no red-flag symptoms or history in this regard.

Knowing that transient osteoporosis can be associated with pregnancy,[30–35] the therapist gave the client the Osteoporosis Screening Evaluation (see Appendix C-6 in the accompanying enhanced eBook version included with print purchase of this textbook). The client replied "yes" to three questions (Caucasian or Asian, mother diagnosed with osteoporosis, physically inactive), suggesting the possibility of rib fracture.[31,33]

Result: The therapist initiated a telephone consultation with the physician to review her findings. Although the original x-ray film was read as negative, the physician ordered a different view (rib series) and identified a fracture of the tenth rib.

The physician explained that the mechanical forces of the enlarging uterus on the ribs pull the lower ribs into a more horizontal position. Any downward stress from above (e.g., forceful cough or pull from the external oblique muscles) or upward force from the serratus anterior and latissimus dorsi muscles can increase the bending stress on the lower ribs.[31]

An aquatics therapy program was initiated and continued throughout the remaining weeks of this client's pregnancy.

CLINICAL SIGNS AND SYMPTOMS
Gastrointestinal Disorders

- Chest pain (may radiate to back)
- Nausea
- Vomiting
- Blood in stools
- Pain during swallowing or associated with meals
- Jaundice
- Heartburn or indigestion
- Dark urine

SCREENING FOR BREAST CONDITIONS THAT CAUSE CHEST OR BREAST PAIN

Occasionally, a client may present with breast pain as the primary complaint, but most often the description is of shoulder,

CASE EXAMPLE 18.5

Breast Pain and Trigger Points

Referral: A 67-year-old woman came to physical therapy after seeing her primary care physician with a report of decreased functional left shoulder motion. She was unable to reach the top shelf of her kitchen cabinets or closets. She felt that at 5 feet 7 inches this is something she should be able to do.

Past Medical History (PMH): During the PMH portion of the interview, she mentioned that she had had a stroke 10 years ago. Her referring physician was unaware of this information. She had recently moved here to be closer to her daughter, and no medical records have been transferred. There was no other significant history.

At the end of the interview, when asked, "Is there anything else you think I should know about your health or current situation that we have not discussed?" she replied, "Well, actually the reason I really went to see the doctor was for pain in my left breast."

She had not reported this information to the physician.

Clinical Presentation: Examination revealed mild loss of strength in the left upper extremity accompanied by mild sensory and proprioceptive losses. Palpation of the shoulder and pectoral muscles produced breast pain. The client had been aware of this pain, but she had attributed it to a separate medical problem. She was reluctant to report her breast pain to her physician. Objectively, there were positive trigger points (TrPs) of the left pectoral muscles and loss of accessory motions of the left shoulder (see Fig. 18.7).

- Active TrP of the left pectoralis major with pain centered in the left breast
- Decreased left shoulder accessory motions (caudal glide, posterior glide and lateral traction); no shoulder pain or discomfort reported
- Range of motion limited by 20% compared with the right shoulder in flexion, external rotation, and abduction
- Mild strength deficit
- Mild sensory and proprioceptive loss
- Vital signs:

Blood pressure (sitting, left arm)	142/108 mm Hg
Heart rate	72 bpm
Pulse oximeter	98%
Oral temperature	98.0° F

Intervention: Physical therapy treatment to eliminate TrPs and restore shoulder motion resolved the breast pain during the first week.

Should you make a medical referral for this client? If so, on what basis?

Despite this woman's positive response to physical therapy treatment, given her age, significant PMH for cerebrovascular injury (reportedly unknown to the referring physician), current blood pressure (although an isolated measurement), report of breast pain (also unreported to her physician), and the residual paresis, medical referral was still indicated.

At the first follow-up visit, a letter was sent with the client that briefly summarized the initial objective findings, her progress to date, and the current concerns. She returned for an additional week of physical therapy to complete the home program for her shoulder. A medical evaluation ruled out breast disease, but medical treatment (medication) was indicated to address cardiovascular issues.

---

arm, neck, or upper back pain. When asked if any symptoms occur elsewhere in the body, the client may mention breast pain (Case Example 18.5).

During examination of the upper quadrant, the therapist may observe suspicious or aberrant changes in the integument, breast, or surrounding soft tissues. The client may report discharge from the nipple. Discharge from both nipples is more likely to be from a benign condition; discharge from one nipple can be a sign of a precancerous or malignant condition.

Asking the client about PMH, risk factors, and the presence of other signs and symptoms is the next step (see Box 4.15). Knowing possible causes of breast pain can help guide the therapist during the screening interview (Table 18.2).

Past Medical History

A PMH of breast cancer, heart disease, recent birth, recent URI, overuse, or trauma (including assault) may be significant for the client presenting with breast pain or symptoms. Any component of heart disease, such as hypertension, angina, MI, and/or any heart procedure such as angioplasty, stent, or coronary artery bypass, is considered a red flag.

TABLE 18.2	Causes of Breast Pain
Systemic/Medical Conditions	**Neuromusculoskeletal**
Infection	Pectoral myalgia or other
• Mastitis (lactating women)	conditions affecting the
• Abscess	pectoralis muscles
Paget's disease	TrPs
Tumor, cyst, calcific change	Mastodynia (mammary
Inflammatory carcinoma of the	neuralgia)
breast	Breast implants,
Acute fat necrosis (after trauma)	augmentation,
Lymph disease	reduction
PMS, menstrual or hormonal	Scar tissue
influence (including early	Trauma or injury (e.g.,
pregnancy)	assault, breast biopsy,
Shingles (herpes zoster)	or surgery)
Pleuritis	Cervical radiculopathy
GERD	TOS
Other:	Costochondritis
• Medication (e.g., some	Connective tissue
hormone, cardiovascular,	disorders
psychiatric drugs)	Heavy, pendulous breasts
• Anxiety	

GERD, Gastroesophageal reflux disease; *PMS*, premenstrual syndrome; *TOS*, thoracic outlet syndrome; *TrPs*, trigger points.

Any woman experiencing chest or breast pain should be asked about a personal history of previous breast surgeries, including mastectomy, breast reconstruction, or breast implantation or augmentation. A PMH of breast cancer is a red flag even if the client has completed all treatment and has been cancer-free for 5 years or more.

On the contrary, a PMH of breast cancer in a client who presents with musculoskeletal symptoms with or without a history of trauma does not always mean cancer metastasis. A complete evaluation with advanced imaging may be needed to uncover the true underlying etiology as in the reported case of fibular pain in a patient with a history of breast cancer that turned out to be an incomplete nondisplaced distal fibular stress fracture with no evidence of tumor or mass (Case Example 18.6).[36]

Breast cancer and cysts develop more frequently in individuals who have a family history of breast disease. A previous history of cancer is always cause to question the client further regarding the onset and pattern of current symptoms. This is especially true when a woman with a previous history of breast cancer or cancer of the reproductive system appears with shoulder, chest, hip, or sacroiliac pain of unknown cause.

If a client denies a PMH of cancer, the therapist should still ask whether that person has ever received chemotherapy or radiation therapy. It is surprising how often the answer to the question about a PMH of cancer is "no" but the answer to the question about prior cancer treatment is "yes."

Clinical Presentation

For the most part, breast pain (mastalgia), tenderness, and swelling are the result of monthly hormone fluctuations. Cyclical pain may become worse during perimenopause when hormone levels change erratically. These same symptoms may continue after menopause, especially in women who use hormone replacement therapy. Noncyclical breast pain is not linked to menstruation or hormonal fluctuations. It is unpredictable and may be constant or intermittent, affecting one or both breasts in a small area or the entire breast.

The typical referral pattern for breast pain is around the chest into the axilla, to the back at the level of the breast, and occasionally into the neck and posterior aspect of the shoulder girdle (Fig. 18.2). The pain may continue along the medial aspect of the ipsilateral arm to the fourth and fifth digits, mimicking pain of the ulnar nerve distribution.

Jarring or movement of the breasts and movement of the arms may aggravate this pain pattern. Pain in the upper inner arm may arise from outer quadrant breast tumors, but pain in the local chest wall may point to any pathologic condition of the breast.

Nipple discharge in women is common, especially in pregnant or lactating women, and does not always signal a serious underlying condition. It may occur as a result of some medications (e.g., estrogen-based drugs, tricyclic antidepressants, and benzodiazepines).

The fluid may be thin to thick in consistency and in various colors (e.g., milky white, green, yellow, brown, or bloody). Any unusual nipple discharge should be evaluated by a medical doctor. Injury, hormonal imbalance, underactive thyroid, infection or abscess, or a tumor are just a few possible causes of nipple discharge.

CLINICAL SIGNS AND SYMPTOMS
Breast Pathology

- Family history of breast disease
- Palpable breast nodule(s) or lump(s) and previous history of chronic mastitis
- May be painless
- Breast pain with possible radiation to the inner aspect of the arm(s)
- Skin surface over a tumor may be red, warm, edematous, firm, and painful
- Firm, painful site under the skin surface
- Skin dimpling over the lesion with attachment of the mass to surrounding tissue, preventing normal mobilization of skin, fascia, and muscle
- Unusual nipple discharge or bleeding from the nipple(s)
- Pain aggravated by jarring or movement of the breasts
- Pain that is not aggravated by resistance to isometric movement of the upper extremities

Causes of Breast Pain

There is a wide range of possible causes of breast pain, including systemic or viscerogenic, and NMS etiologies (see Table 18.2). Not all conditions are life-threatening or even require medical attention.

Although it is more typical in women, both men and women can have chest, back, scapular, and shoulder pain

CASE EXAMPLE 18.6
Fibular Pain with History of Breast Cancer

In a published case report, physical therapists evaluated a 46-year-old woman with left ankle pain who also had a past medical history (PMH) of breast cancer. The client gave a month-old history of an ankle sprain while running; symptoms were made worse by running and there were no advanced imaging studies to rule out cancer metastases.

Standard radiographs of the ankle were read as normal by the radiologist, but the therapist was suspicious of an observed irregularity in the distal fibula. Local tenderness was palpated just above the distal tip of the fibula.

A bone scan was ordered to differentiate between an old injury and new pathology. There was increased metabolic activity around the area in question. A follow-up magnetic resonance imaging (MRI) showed an incomplete, nondisplaced stress fracture of the distal fibula. No metastatic lesions were present.

This is a case where bone fracture could not be ruled out with a standard x-ray. Age over 40 years, PMH of breast cancer, and new onset of unresolving bone pain led to a differential diagnosis that confirmed a true musculoskeletal problem.

From Ryder M, Deyle GD. Differential diagnosis of fibular pain in a patient with a history of breast cancer. J Orthop Sports Phys Ther 2009;39(3):230.

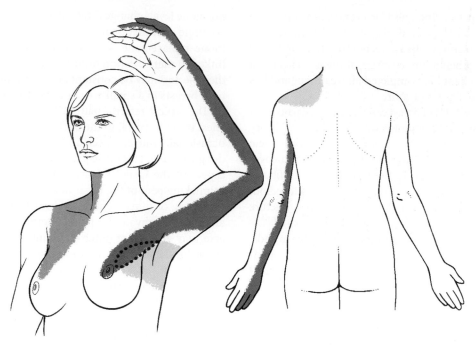

Fig. 18.2   Pain arising from the breast (mastalgia) can be referred to the axilla along the medial aspect of the arm. The referral pattern can also extend to the supraclavicular level and the neck. Breast pain may be diffuse around the thorax through the intercostal nerves. Pain may be referred to the back and the posterior shoulder. Ask the client about the presence of lumps, nipple discharge, distended veins, or puckered or red skin (or any other skin changes).

referred by a pathologic condition of the breast. Only those conditions most likely to be seen in a physical therapist's practice are included in this discussion.

Mastodynia

Mastodynia (irritation of the upper dorsal intercostal nerve) that causes chest pain is almost always associated with ovulatory cycles, especially premenstrually. The association between symptoms and menses may be discovered during the physical therapist's interview when the client responds to Special Questions to Ask: Breast (see end of this chapter or Appendix B-7 in the accompanying enhanced eBook version included with print purchase of this textbook). The presentation is usually unilateral breast or chest pain and occurs initially at the premenstrual period, and later, more persistently throughout the menstrual cycle.

Mastitis

Mastitis is an inflammatory condition associated with lactation (breastfeeding). Mammary duct obstruction causes the duct to become clogged. The breast becomes red, swollen, and painful. The involved breast area is often warm or even hot. Constitutional symptoms such as fever, chills, and flu-like symptoms are common. Acute mastitis can occur in males (e.g., nipple chafing from jogging) and the presentation is the same as for females.

Risk factors include previous history of mastitis; cracked, bleeding, painful nipples; and stress or fatigue. Bacteria can enter the breast through cracks in the nipple during trauma or nursing. Subsequent infection may lead to abscess formation.

Obstructive and infectious mastitis are considered to be two conditions on a continuum. Mastitis is often treated symptomatically, but the client should be encouraged to let her doctor know about any breast-related signs and symptoms present. Antibiotics may be needed in the case of a developing infection.

Benign Tumors and Cysts

A benign tumor and cyst were once lumped together and called "fibrocystic breast disease." With additional research over the years, scientists have come to realize that a single label is not adequate for the variety of benign conditions possible, including fibroadenoma, cyst, and calcification that can occur in the breast.

An unchanged lump of long duration (years) is more likely to be benign. Many lumps are hormonally induced cysts and resolve within two or three menstrual cycles. Cyclical breast cysts are less common after menopause.

Other conditions can include intraductal papilloma (wartlike growth inside the breast), fat necrosis (fat breaks down and clumps together), and mammary duct ectasia (ducts near the nipple become thin-walled and accumulate secretions). Some of these breast changes are a variation of the norm, and others are pathologic but nonmalignant. A medical diagnosis is needed to differentiate between these changes.

Paget's Disease

Paget's disease of the breast is a rare form of ductal carcinoma arising in the ducts near the nipple. The woman experiences itching, redness, and flaking of the nipple with occasional

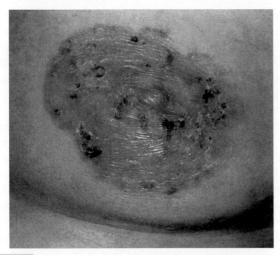

Fig. 18.3   Paget's disease of the breast is a rare form of breast cancer affecting the nipple. It is characterized by a red (sometimes scaly) rash on the breast that often surrounds the nipple and areola, as seen in this photograph. Other presentations are possible, such as a red pimple or sore on the nipple that does not heal. Symptoms are unilateral and the breast may be sore, itch, or burn. Diagnosis is often delayed because the symptoms seem harmless or the condition is misdiagnosed as dermatitis. (From Callen JP, Jorizzo J, Greer KE, et al. Dermatological Signs of Internal Disease. Philadelphia: Saunders; 1988.)

TABLE 18.3	Factors Associated With Breast Cancer
Sex	Women > men
Race	White
Age	Advancing age, >60 years; younger age at menarche, at first live birth, and diagnosis is associated with inflammatory breast cancer[40]
	Peak incidence: 45–70 years
	Mean and median age:
	60–61 years (women)
	60–66 years (men)
Genetic	BRCA-1/BRCA-2 gene mutation
Family history	First-degree relative with breast cancer
	Premenopausal
	Bilateral
	Mother, daughter, or sister
Previous medical history	Previous personal history of cancer
	Breast
	Uterine
	Ovarian
	Colon
	Number of previous breast biopsies (positive or negative)
Exposure to estrogen	Age at menarche < 12 years
	Age at menopause > 55 years
	Nulliparous (never pregnant)
	First live birth after the age of 35 years
	Environmental estrogens (esters)

For a more detailed guide to risk factors for breast cancer, see the American Cancer Society's document, *What are the risk factors for breast cancer?*
Available online at http://www.cancer.org/docroot/CRI/content/CRI_2_4_2x_what_are_the_risk_factors_for_breast_cancer 5.asp.

bleeding (Fig. 18.3). Paget's disease of the breast is not related to Paget's disease of the bone, except that the same physician (Dr. James Paget, a contemporary of Florence Nightingale, 1877) named both conditions after himself.

Breast Cancer

The breast is the most common *site* of cancer in women, the second most common cause of death from cancer, and a leading cause of premature mortality from cancer in women measured by average and total years of life lost.[37] The American Cancer Society (ACS) estimates there was 281,550 cases of invasive breast cancer diagnosed in US women and 43,600 deaths in 2021.[38] Male breast cancer is possible but rare, accounting for 1% of all new cases of breast cancer.

Although the frequency of breast cancer in men is strikingly less than that in women, the disease in both sexes is remarkably similar in epidemiology, natural history, and response to treatment. Men with breast cancer are 5 to 10 years older than women at the time of diagnosis, with mean or median ages between 60 and 66 years. This apparent difference may occur because symptoms in men are ignored for a longer period and the disease is diagnosed at a more advanced state.

Risk Factors. Despite the discovery of a breast cancer gene (BRCA-1 and BRCA-2), researchers estimate that only 5% to 10% of breast cancers are a result of inherited genetic susceptibility. Normally, BRCA-1 and BRCA-2 help prevent cancer by making proteins that keep cells from growing abnormally. Inheriting either mutated gene from a parent does increase the risk of breast cancer.[39] A much larger proportion of cases are attributed to other factors, such as advancing age, race, smoking, obesity, physical inactivity, excess alcohol intake, exposure to ionizing radiation, and exposure to estrogens (Table 18.3).[41]

Women who received multiple fluoroscopies for tuberculosis or radiation treatment for mastitis during their adolescent or childbearing years are at increased risk for breast cancer as a result of exposure to ionizing radiation. In the past, irradiation was used for a variety of other medical conditions, including gynecomastia, thymic enlargement, eczema of the chest, chest burns, pulmonary tuberculosis, mediastinal lymphoma, and other cancers. Most of these clients are in their 70s now and at risk for cancer because of advancing age as well.

As a general principle, the risk of breast cancer is linked to a woman's total lifelong exposure to estrogen. The increased incidence of estrogen-responsive tumors (tumors that are rich in estrogen receptors proliferate when exposed to estrogen) has been postulated to occur as a result of a variety of factors, such as prenatal and lifelong exposure to synthetic chemicals and environmental toxins, earlier age of menarche (first menstruation), improved nutrition in the United States, delayed and decreased childbearing, and longer average lifespan.

Women at higher than average risk of breast cancer include women with significant family history,[42] women with a prior diagnosis of benign proliferative breast disease,[43] and women with significant mammographic breast density.[44]

Risk factors for men are similar to those for women, but at least half of all cases do not have an identifiable risk factor. Risk factors for men include heredity, obesity, infertility, late onset of puberty, frequent chest x-ray examinations, history of testicular disorders (e.g., infection, injury, or undescended testes), and increasing age. Men who have several female relatives with breast cancer and those in families who have the BRCA-2 mutation have a greater risk potential.[45]

The presence of any of these factors may become evident during the interview with the client and should alert the physical therapist to the potential for NMS complaints from a systemic origin that would require a medical referral. There are several easy-to-use screening tools available. In addition to screening for current risk, clients should be given this information for future use (Box 18.2).

Clinical Presentation. Breast cancer may be asymptomatic in the early stages. The discovery of a breast lump with or without pain or tenderness is significant and must be investigated. Physical signs associated with advanced breast cancer have been summarized using the acronym BREAST: **B**reast mass, **R**etraction, **E**dema, **A**xillary mass, **S**caly nipple, and **T**ender breast.[46] Less common symptoms are breast pain; nipple discharge; nipple erosion, enlargement, itching, or redness; and generalized hardness, enlargement, or shrinking of the breast. Watery, serous, or bloody discharge from the nipple is an occasional early sign but is more often associated with benign disease.

Breast cancer usually consists of a nontender, firm, or hard lump with poorly delineated margins that is caused by local infiltration. Breast cancer in women has a predilection for the outer upper quadrant of the breast and the areola (nipple) area (Fig. 18.4) involving the breast tissue overlying the pectoral muscle. During palpation, breast tissue lumps move easily over the pectoral muscle compared with a lump within the muscle tissue itself. Later signs of malignancy include fixation of the tumor to the skin or underlying muscle fascia.

Male breast cancer begins as a painless induration, retraction of the nipple, and an attached mass progressing to include lymphadenopathy and skin and chest wall lesions. A tumor of any size in male breast tissue is associated with skin fixation and ulceration and deep pectoral fixation more often than a tumor of similar size in female breast tissue is because of the small size of male breasts.

BOX 18.2 RESOURCES FOR ASSESSING AND LOWERING BREAST CANCER RISK

Breastcancer.org
- www.breastcancer.org

Breastcancer.org is a nonprofit organization with a website dedicated to providing current and accurate information on every aspect of cancer. A professional advisory board that consists of more than 60 practicing medical professionals around the world review all information available on the website.

National Cancer Institute
- http://bcra.nci.nih.gov/brc/

The National Cancer Institute (NCI) offers a Breast Cancer Risk Assessment, which is an interactive tool to measure the risk of invasive breast cancer. This tool was designed to assist health care professionals in guiding individual clients to estimate the risk of invasive breast cancer. It is only part of a woman's options for assessing risk and screening for breast cancer. More information is available by calling the Cancer Information Service (CIS) at 1-800-4-CANCER.

Breast Cancer Risk Calculator
- http://www.halls.md/breast/risk.htm

This calculator uses the Gail model but with some added risk modifier questions. The author of the website (Steven B. Halls, MD) notes that the methods on the website have been gathered from peer-reviewed journals but have not been peer reviewed. Results provided are estimates.

Oncolink
- http://www.oncolink.com/

Abramson Cancer Center of the University of Pennsylvania offers a comprehensive website with information about various types of cancers, risk factors, cancer treatment, and cancer resources. Click on Cancer Types>Breast Cancer.

Susan G. Komen for the Cure
- www.komen.org

This is a website devoted to detecting and understanding breast cancer. This website provides the consumer with interactive tools and videos in many different languages to teach women (and men) how to examine their own breasts, what their individual risk factors are, and tips on making healthy lifestyle choices for cancer prevention. Regarding the controversy over self-breast examination, Susan G. Komen for the Cure says: Women should be aware of how their breasts normally look and feel. Knowing what is normal for you may enable you to note changes in your breast in the time between your yearly mammogram and/or clinical breast examination. Breast self-examination (BSE) is a tool that may help you become familiar with the way your breasts normally look and feel. Women who practice BSE should also be sure to get mammograms and clinical breast examinations at the appropriate age. BSE should not be substituted for these screening tests.

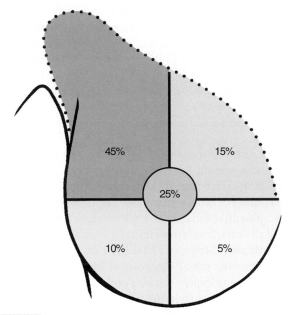

Fig. 18.4   Most breast cancer presents in the upper outer quadrant of the breast (45%) or around the nipple (25%). Metastases occur via the lymphatic system at the axillary lymph nodes to the bones (shoulder, hip, ribs, vertebrae) or central nervous system (brain, spinal cord). Breast cancer can also metastasize hematogenously to the lungs, pleural cavity, and liver.

CLINICAL SIGNS AND SYMPTOMS

Breast Cancer

- Nontender (painless), firm, or hard lump
- Unusual discharge from nipple
- Skin or nipple retraction dimpling; erosion, retraction, itching of nipple
- Redness or skin rash over the breast or nipple
- Generalized hardness, enlargement, shrinking, or distortion of the breast or nipple
- Unusual prominence of veins over the breast
- Enlarged rubbery lymph nodes
- Axillary mass
- Swelling of arm
- Bone or back pain
- Weight loss

Clinical Breast Examination. Breast cancer mortality is reduced when women are screened by both clinical breast examination (CBE) and mammography. CBE alone detects 4.6% to 5.7% of diagnosed breast cancers that screening mammography does not capture.[47-49] Studies show that the sensitivity of CBE is 80.3% (test's ability to determine a true positive) and specificity is 76% (test's ability to determine a true negative).[50] However, the rate of false-positive tests may be higher when CBE is performed without mammography.[51] In the United Kingdom, the standard of care is a triple assessment approach, i.e., the combination of CBE with imaging and tissue sampling. CBE helps to determine whether tissue sampling is needed if a palpable abnormality is identified.

A previous edition of this text (*Differential Diagnosis in Physical Therapy*, edition 3) specifically stated, "breast examination is not within the scope of a physical therapist's practice." This practice is changing. As the number of cancer survivors increases in the United States, physical therapists treating women who are postmastectomy and clients of both sexes with lymphedema are on the rise.

With direct and unrestricted access of consumers to physical therapists in many states, advanced skills have become necessary. For some clients, performing a CBE is an appropriate assessment tool in the screening process.[52] The ACS and National Cancer Institute (NCI) support the provision of cancer screening procedures by qualified health specialists. With additional training, physical therapists can qualify.[52,53]

Therapists who are trained to perform CBEs must make sure this examination is allowed according to the state practice act. In some states, it is allowed by exclusion, meaning it is not mentioned and therefore included. Discussion of the role of the physical therapist in primary care and cancer screening as it relates to integrating CBE into an upper quarter examination is available.[52] A form for recording findings from the CBE is provided in Fig. 4.48 and in Appendix C-10 in the accompanying enhanced eBook version included with print purchase of this textbook.

The physical therapist does not diagnose any kind of cancer, including breast cancer; only the pathologist can make a cancer diagnosis. The therapist can identify aberrant soft tissue and refer the client for further evaluation. Early detection and intervention can reduce morbidity and mortality.

For the therapist who is not trained in CBE, the client should be questioned about the presence of any changes in the breast tissue (e.g., lumps, distended veins, skin rash, open sores or lesions, or other skin changes) and the nipple (e.g., rash or other skin changes, discharge, distortion). Visual inspection is also possible and may be very important postmastectomy (Fig. 18.5). Ask the client if he or she has noticed any changes in the scar. Continue by asking:

? FOLLOW-UP QUESTION

- Would you have any objections if I looked at (or examined) the scar tissue?

If the client declines or refuses, the therapist should follow up with counsel to perform self-inspection, emphasizing the need for continued CBEs and the importance of reporting any changes to the physician immediately.

Therapists have an important role in primary prevention and client education. The ACS offers recommendations for breast cancer screening. The therapist can encourage women (and men) to follow these guidelines (Box 18.3).

Lymph Node Assessment. Palpation of the underlying soft tissues (chest wall, axilla) and lymph nodes in the supraclavicular and axillary regions should be a part of the screening examination in any client with chest pain (see Chapter 4 for description of lymph node palpation). Any report of palpable breast nodules, lumps, or changes in the appearance of the breast requires medical follow-up, especially when there is a personal or family history of breast disease.[54]

"Normal" lymph nodes are not palpable or visible, but not all palpable or visible lymph nodes are a sign of cancer.

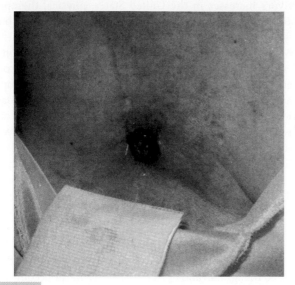

Fig. 18.5 This photo shows the chest of a woman who has had a right radical mastectomy. There is a metastatic nodule in the mastectomy scar as a result of local cancer recurrence. Breast cancer can occur (recur) if a mastectomy has been done. A closer look at the lesion suggests that the skin changes have been present for quite some time. Even in this black and white photo, the change in skin coloration is obvious in a large patch around the nodule. Any time a woman with a PMH of cancer develops neck, back, upper trapezius or shoulder pain, or other symptoms, examining the site of the original cancer removal is a good idea. (From Callen JP, Jorizzo J, Greer KE, et al. Dermatological Signs of Internal Disease. Philadelphia: Saunders; 1988.)

Infections, viruses, bacteria, allergies, and food intolerances can cause changes in the lymph nodes. Lymph nodes that are hard, immovable, irregular, and nontender raise the suspicion of cancer, especially in the presence of a previous history of cancer. The skin surface over a tumor may be red, warm, edematous, firm, and painful. There may be skin dimpling over the lesion, with attachment of the mass to surrounding tissues preventing normal mobilization of the skin, fascia, and muscle.

In the past, therapists were taught that any change in the lymph nodes present for more than 1 month in more than one region was a red flag. This has changed with the increased understanding of cancer metastases via the lymphatic system and the potential for cancer recurrence. A physician must evaluate all suspicious lymph nodes.

Metastases. Metastases have been known to occur up to 25 years after the initial diagnosis of breast cancer. On the other hand, breast cancer can be a rapidly progressing, terminal disease. Approximately 40% of clients with stage II tumors experience relapse.

Knowledge of the usual metastatic patterns of breast cancer and the common complications can aid in early recognition and effective treatment. Because bone is the most frequent site of metastasis from breast cancer in men and women, a PMH of breast cancer is a major red flag in anyone presenting with new onset or persistent findings of NMS pain or dysfunction.

All distant visceral sites are potential sites for metastasis. Other primary sites of involvement are lymph nodes, remaining breast tissue, lung, brain, central nervous system (CNS), and liver. Women with metastases to the liver or CNS have a poorer prognosis.

BOX 18.3 SUMMARY OF GUIDELINES FOR BREAST CANCER SCREENING

From Practice Bulletin no. 122; breast cancer screening. *Obstet Gynecol* 118(Pt. 1):372–382, 2011 and Smith RA: Cancer screening in the United States, 2010: A review of current American Cancer Society guidelines and issues in cancer screening, *CA Cancer J Clin* 60(2):99–119, 2010. Available online at www.cancer.org.

The debate is not over about these revised recommendations. Some experts advise using these guidelines as a starting point for discussion but should not be used to justify delaying or avoiding screening. Recognizing that the majority of cancers that would be missed by postponing mammography would not be immediately life-threatening, many physicians advise women to make an individual decision about screening based on these guidelines and their own risk factors and to do so in consultation with their primary care physician.

From the American College of Obstetricians and Gynecologists (ACOG), the American Cancer Society, and the National Comprehensive Cancer Network:
- Routine (annual) screening mammography is still recommended for women beginning at the age of 40 years and continuing for as long as a woman is in good health;

however, evidence is lacking in determining guidelines for screening mammography after the age of 74 years.
- Mammography may begin before the age of 40 years based on individual risk factors and personal preferences. Women younger than 40 years should become aware of the benefits and harms of routine mammograms when making this decision.
- Clinical breast examination (CBE) about every 3 years for women in their 20s and 30s and every year for women 40 years of age and over is recommended.
- Women should know how their breasts normally look and feel and report any breast change promptly to their health care provider. Breast self-examination (BSE) is an option for women starting in their 20s.
- Insufficient evidence makes it impossible to develop guidelines at this time regarding the effectiveness of digital mammography or breast magnetic resonance imaging (MRI) instead of film mammography. Some women (because of a family history, genetic tendency, or other risk factors) may be encouraged by their physicians to be screened with MRI in addition to mammography.

Spinal cord compression, usually from extradural metastases, may appear as back pain, leg weakness, and bowel/bladder symptoms. Rarely, an axillary mass, swelling of the arm, or bone pain from metastases may be the first symptom. Back or bone pain, jaundice, or weight loss may be the result of systemic metastases, but these symptoms are rarely seen during initial presentation.

Medical referral is advised before initiating treatment for anyone with a PMH of cancer presenting with symptoms of unknown cause, especially without an identifiable movement system impairment.

A medical evaluation is still needed in light of new findings, even if the client has been rechecked by a medical oncologist recently. It is better to err on the side of caution. Failure to recognize the need for medical referral can result in possible severe and irreversible consequences of any delay in diagnosis and therapy.[55]

CLINICAL SIGNS AND SYMPTOMS
Metastasized Breast Cancer

- Palpable mass in supraclavicular, chest, or axillary regions
- Unilateral upper extremity numbness and tingling
- Back, hip, or shoulder pain
- Pain during weight-bearing
- Leg weakness or paresis
- Bowel/bladder symptoms
- Jaundice

SCREENING FOR OTHER CONDITIONS AS A CAUSE OF CHEST, BREAST, OR RIB PAIN

Breast Implants

Scar tissue or fibrosis from a previous breast surgery, such as reconstruction following mastectomy for breast cancer or augmentation or reduction mammoplasty for cosmetic reasons, is an important history to consider when assessing chest, breast, neck, or shoulder symptoms. Likewise, the client should be asked about a history of radiation to the chest, breast, or thorax.

Women who have silicone or saline implants for reconstruction following mastectomy for breast cancer are more likely to have complications, including late complications[56] (e.g., pain, capsular contracture, rupture, rippling, infection, hematoma, seroma), than those who receive implants for cosmetic reasons only.[57,58] The rate of fibrosis and capsular contracture is significantly higher for irradiated breasts than for nonirradiated breasts.[59,60]

Studies show that ruptures are rare (0.4%) in women who have breast implants after mastectomy; thick, tight scarring, implant malposition, and infection are more common.[61,62]

Other complications of breast implantation may include gel bleed, implant leaking, calcification around the implant, chronic breast pain, prolonged wound healing, and formation of granulation tissue.

Anxiety

A state of anxiety, or in its extreme form, a panic attack, can cause chest or breast pain typical of a heart attack. The client experiences shortness of breath, perspiration, and pallor. It is the most common noncardiac cause of chest pain, accounting for half of all emergency department admissions each year for chest or breast pain (just ahead of chest pain caused by cocaine use). It is important to consider anxiety as a potential noncardiac cause of chest pain. In one study, 67.5% of adolescents aged 11 to 18 years had a normal cardiac examination (electrocardiogram [ECG]), blood tests, history and examination, and echo with anxiety determined to be the cause of their chest pain.[63]

Risk Factors

The first panic attack often follows a period of extreme stress, sometimes associated with being the victim of a crime or the loss of a job, partner, or close family member. The presence of another mental health disorder, such as depression or substance abuse (drugs or alcohol), increases the risk of developing panic disorder. There may be a familial component, but it is not clear if this is hereditary or environmental (learned behavior).[64,65]

Drugs such as over-the-counter (OTC) decongestants and cold remedies can trigger panic attacks. Excessive use of caffeine and stimulants, such as amphetamines and cocaine combined with a lack of sleep, can also trigger an attack. Menopause, quitting smoking, or caffeine withdrawal can also bring on new onset of panic attacks in someone who has never experienced this problem before. See Chapter 3 for further discussion.

Clinical Presentation

There are several types of chest or breast discomfort caused by anxiety. The pain may be sharp, intermittent, or stabbing and located in the region of the left breast. The area of pain is usually no larger than the tip of the finger but may be as large as the client's hand. It is often associated with a local area of hyperesthesia of the chest wall. The client can point to it with one finger. It is not reproduced with palpation or activity. It is not changed or altered by a change in position.

Anxiety-related pain may be located precordially (region over the heart and lower part of the thorax) or retrosternally (behind the sternum). It may be of variable duration, lasting no longer than a second or for hours or days. This type of pain is unrelated to effort or exercise. Distinguishing this sensation from myocardial ischemia requires medical evaluation.

Discomfort in the upper portion of the chest, neck, and left arm, again unrelated to effort, may occur. There may be a sense of persistent weakness and unpleasant awareness of the heartbeat. In the past, radiation of chest discomfort to the neck or left arm was considered to be diagnostic of atherosclerotic coronary heart disease. More recently, stress testing and coronary arteriography have shown that chest discomfort of this type can occur in clients with normal coronary arteriograms.

Some individuals with anxiety-related chest pain may have a choking sensation in the throat caused by hysteria. There may be associated hyperventilation. Palpitation, claustrophobia, and the occurrence of symptoms in crowded places are common.

Hyperventilation occurs in persons with and without heart disease and may be misleading. Such clients have numbness and tingling of the hands and lips and feel as if they are going to "pass out." For a more detailed explanation of anxiety and its accompanying symptoms (e.g., hyperventilation), see Chapter 3.

CLINICAL SIGNS AND SYMPTOMS

Chest Pain Caused by Anxiety

- Dull, aching discomfort in the substernal region and in the anterior chest
- Sinus tachycardia
- Fatigue
- Fear of closed-in places
- Diaphoresis
- Dyspnea
- Dizziness
- Choking sensation
- Hyperventilation: numbness and tingling of hands and lips

Cocaine

Cocaine (also methamphetamine, known as *crank*, and phencyclidine [PCP]) is a stimulant that has profound effects on all organ systems of the body, especially cardiotoxic effects, including cocaine-dilated cardiomyopathy, angina, and left ventricular dysfunction. Injection or inhalation can precipitate MI, cardiac arrhythmias, and even sudden cardiac death.[66–69]

Chronic use of cocaine or any of its derivatives is the leading cause of stroke in young people today. The incidence of stroke associated with substance use and abuse is increasing. Use of these stimulants also affects anyone with a congenital cerebral aneurysm and can lead to rupture.

The physiologic stress of cocaine use on the heart accounts for an increasing number of heart transplants. Acute effects of cocaine include increased heart rate, blood pressure, and vasomotor tone.[68,70] Cocaine remains the most common illicit drug–related cause of severe chest pain bringing the person to the emergency department.[66,69] In fact, chest pain is the most common cocaine-related medical complaint.

Many people with chest pain have used cocaine within the last week but deny its use. The use of these substances is not uncommon in middle-aged and older adults of all socioeconomic backgrounds. The therapist should not neglect to ask clients about their use of substances because of preconceived ideas that only teenagers and young adults use drugs. Careful questioning (see Chapter 2; see also Appendix B-36 in the accompanying enhanced eBook version included with print purchase of this textbook) may assist the physical therapist in identifying a possible correlation between chest pain and cocaine use.

Always end this portion of the interview by asking:

? FOLLOW-UP QUESTION

- Are there any drugs or substances you take that you have not mentioned?

Anabolic-Androgenic Steroids

Anabolic steroids are synthetic derivatives of testosterone used to enhance athletic performance or cosmetically shape the body. Used in supraphysiologic doses (more than the body produces naturally), these drugs have a potent effect on the musculoskeletal system, including the heart, potentially altering cardiac cellular and physiologic function.[71,72] Effects persist long after their use has been discontinued.[73]

The use of self-administered anabolic-androgenic steroids (AASs) is illegal but continues to increase dramatically among both athletes and nonathletes.[72] It is used among preteens who do not compete in sports for cosmetic reasons. The goal is to advance to a more mature body build and enhance their looks. AASs do have medical uses and were added to the list of prescribed controlled substances in 1990 under the control of the Drug Enforcement Administration.

Despite stricter control of the manufacture and distribution of AASs, illegal supplies come from unlicensed sources all over the world. When dispensed without a regulating agency, the purity and processing of chemicals are unknown. The quality of black market supplies is a major concern. There is no guarantee that the products obtained are correctly labeled. Contents and dosage may be inaccurate. Some athletes are using injectable anabolic steroids intended for veterinary use only. There is a trend for self-administration of higher doses and for combining AASs with other potentially harmful drugs.[74]

Clinical Presentation

Any young adult with chest pain of unknown cause, possibly accompanied by dyspnea and elevated blood pressure and without clinical evidence of NMS involvement, may have a history of anabolic steroid use. Consider anabolic steroid use as a possibility in men and women presenting with chest pain in their early 20s who have used this type of steroid since the age of 11 or 12 years.

In the pediatric population, there is a risk of decreased or delayed bone growth. Tendon and muscle strains are common and take longer than normal to heal. *Injuries that take longer than the expected physiologic time to heal* are an important red flag. Delayed healing occurs because the soft tissues are working under the added strain of extra body mass.

The alert therapist may recognize the associated signs and symptoms accompanying chronic use of these steroids. A personality change is the most dramatic sign of steroid use. The user may become more aggressive or experience mood swings (hypomanic or manic symptoms) and psychologic delusions (e.g., believe he or she is indestructible; sometimes referred to as "steroid psychosis"). "Roid rages," characterized by sudden outbursts of uncontrolled emotion, may be observed. Severe depression leading to suicide can occur with AAS withdrawal.[72]

CLINICAL SIGNS AND SYMPTOMS
Anabolic Steroid Use

- Chest pain
- Elevated blood pressure
- Ventricular tachycardia
- Weight gain (10 to 15 lbs in 2 to 3 weeks)
- Peripheral edema
- Acne on the face, upper back, chest
- Altered body composition with marked development of the upper torso
- Stretch marks around the back, upper arms, and chest
- Needle marks in large muscle groups (e.g., buttocks, thighs, deltoids)
- Development of male pattern baldness
- Gynecomastia (breast tissue development in males); breast tissue atrophy in females
- Frequent hematoma or bruising
- Change in personality, called "steroid psychosis" (rapid mood swings, sudden increased aggressive or even violent tendencies)
- Females: secondary male characteristics (deeper voice, breast atrophy, abnormal facial and body hair); menstrual irregularity
- Jaundice (chronic use)

The therapist who suspects a client may be using anabolic steroids should report findings to the physician or coach if one is involved. The therapist can begin by asking about the use of nutritional supplements or performance-enhancing agents. In the well-muscled male athlete, observe for common side effects of AAS such as acne, gynecomastia, and cutaneous striae in the deltopectoral region. Women who use AAS may exhibit muscular hypertrophy; male pattern baldness; excess hair growth on the face, breasts, and arms; and breast tissue atrophy.[71] Asking about the presence of common side effects of AAS and testing for elevated blood pressure may provide an opportunity to ask if the client is using these chemicals.

SCREENING FOR MUSCULOSKELETAL CAUSES OF CHEST, BREAST, OR RIB PAIN

It is estimated that half of all chest pain is noncardiac and 20% to 25% of noncardiac chest pain has a musculoskeletal basis.[75] Musculoskeletal causes of chest (wall) pain must be differentiated from pain of cardiac, pulmonary, epigastric, and breast origin (see Table 18.1) before physical therapy treatment begins. Careful history taking to identify red-flag conditions differentiates those who require further investigation.

Movement system impairment is most often characterized by pain during a specific posture, motion, or physical activity. Reproducing the pain by movement or palpation often directs the therapist in understanding the underlying problem.

Chest pain can occur as a result of cervical spine disorders because nerves originating as high as C3 and C4 can extend as far down as the nipple line. Pectoral, suprascapular, dorsal scapular, and long thoracic nerves originate in the lower cervical spine, and impingement of these nerves can cause chest pain.

Musculoskeletal disorders such as myalgia associated with muscle exertion, myofascial TrPs, costochondritis, osteomyelitis, or xiphoiditis can produce pain in the chest and arms. Compared with angina pectoris, the pain associated with these conditions may last for seconds or hours, and prompt relief does not occur with the ingestion of nitroglycerin.

Tietze's syndrome, costochondritis, a hypersensitive xiphoid, and the slipping rib syndrome must be differentiated from problems involving the thoracic viscera, particularly those of the heart, great vessels, mediastinum, and from illness originating in the head, neck, or abdomen.[76]

Rib pain (with or without neck, back, or chest pain or symptoms) must be evaluated for a systemic versus musculoskeletal origin (Box 18.4). The same screening model used for all conditions can be applied.

Costochondritis

Costochondritis, also known as *anterior chest wall syndrome, costosternal syndrome,* and *parasternal chondrodynia* (pain in a cartilage), is used interchangeably with Tietze's syndrome, although these two conditions are not the same. Costochondritis is more common than Tietze's syndrome.

Although both disorders are characterized by inflammation of one or more costal cartilages (costochondral joints where the ribs join the sternum), costochondritis refers to pain in the costochondral articulations without swelling. This disorder can occur at almost any age but is observed most often in people older than 40 years of age. It tends to affect the second, third, fourth, and fifth costochondral joints; women are affected in 70% of all cases (Fig. 18.6).[77] Other risk factors include trauma (e.g., driver striking steering wheel with chest during a motor vehicle accident, upper chest surgery, helmet tackle in sports, or other sports injury to the chest)[78] or repetitive motion (e.g., grocery-store clerk lifting and scanning items, competitive swimming).[79]

Costochondritis is characterized by a sharp pain along the front edges of the sternum, especially on the left side with possible radiation to the arms, back, or shoulders, often misinterpreted as a heart attack.

BOX 18.4   CAUSES OF RIB PAIN

Systemic/Medical Conditions
- Gallbladder disease (tenth rib)
- Shingles (herpes zoster)
- Pleurisy
- Osteoporosis
- Cancer (metastasized to the bone)

Musculoskeletal
- Trauma (e.g., bruise, fracture)
- Slipping rib syndrome
- Tietze's syndrome or costochondritis
- Trigger points (TrPs)
- Thoracic outlet syndrome (TOS)

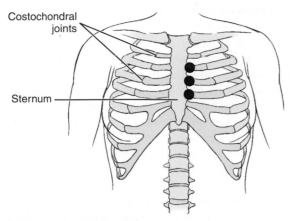

Fig. 18.6 Costochondritis is an inflammation of any of the costochondral joints (also called *costal cartilages*) where the rib joins the sternum. Sharp, stabbing, or aching pain can occur on either side of the sternum, but tends to affect the left more often, sometimes even radiating down the left arm or up to the upper back. Many people mistake the symptoms for a heart attack. In most cases, symptoms occur at a single site involving the second or third costochondral joint, although any of the joints can be affected as shown.

It is estimated that almost half of all people who present to a primary care clinic with chest pain have costochondritis.[77] The pain may radiate widely (to the arms, back, shoulders), stimulating intrathoracic or intraabdominal disease. It differs from MI because during a heart attack, the initial pain is usually in the center of the chest, under the sternum, not along the edges.

Costochondritis can be similar to muscular pain and (unlike cardiac-related pain) is elicited by palpatory pressure over the costochondral junctions. Occasionally, the affected individual will report a burning sensation in the breast(s) associated with this condition. Absence of associated signs and symptoms such as dyspnea, nausea, vomiting, and diaphoresis helps differentiate this condition from cardiac- or pulmonary-related chest pain.

Costochondritis may follow trauma or may be associated with systemic rheumatic disease. It can come and go (especially in conjunction with activities involving the upper extremities or rest) or persist for months. Inflammation of upper costal cartilages may cause chest pain, whereas inflammation of lower costal cartilages is more likely to cause abdominal or low back discomfort. In some cases, costochondritis is associated with an URI, but may be a result of the stress of coughing rather than the body's response to the virus.

Tietze's Syndrome

Tietze's syndrome (inflammation of a rib and its cartilage; costal chondritis) may be one possible cause of anterior chest wall pain, manifested by painful swelling of one or more costochondral articulations.

In most cases, the cause of Tietze's syndrome is unknown. Other causes of sternal swelling may include an infectious process in the immunocompromised person resulting from

tuberculosis, aspergillosis, brucellosis, staphylococcal infection, or pseudomonal disease producing sternal osteomyelitis. Onset is usually before 40 years of age, with a predilection for the second and third decades which differs from costochondritis.[77] However, it can occur in children.

Approximately 80% of clients have only single sites of involvement, most commonly the second or third costal cartilage (costochondral joint). Anterior chest pain may begin suddenly or gradually and may be associated with increased blood pressure, increased heart rate, and pain radiating down the left arm. Pain is aggravated by sneezing, coughing, deep inspirations, twisting motions of the trunk, horizontal shoulder abduction and adduction, or the "crowing rooster" movement of the upper extremities.[77]

These symptoms may seem similar to those of a heart attack, but the raised blood pressure, reproduction of painful symptoms with palpation or pressure, and aggravating factors differentiate Tietze's syndrome from MI (Case Example 18.7). In rare cases, the individual has been diagnosed with Tietze's syndrome only to find out later the precipitating cause was cancer (e.g., lymphoma, squamous cell carcinoma of the mediastinum).[80,81] Tietze's syndrome can also be confused with tender points of the pectoralis major or internal intercostalis as it is associated with the cartilage of the second or third ribs in 70% of the patients.[82]

CLINICAL SIGNS AND SYMPTOMS
Tietze's Syndrome or Costochondritis

- Sudden or gradual onset of upper anterior chest pain
- Pain/tenderness of costochondral joint(s)
- Bulbous swelling of the involved costal cartilage (Tietze's syndrome)
- Mild-to-severe chest pain that may radiate to the left shoulder and arm
- Pain aggravated by deep breathing, sneezing, coughing, inspiration, bending, recumbency, or exertion (e.g., push-ups, lifting grocery items)

Hypersensitive Xiphoid

The hypersensitive xiphoid (xiphodynia) is tender to palpation, and local pressure may cause nausea and vomiting. This syndrome is manifested as epigastric pain, nausea, and vomiting.

Slipping Rib Syndrome

The slipping, or painful, rib syndrome (sometimes also referred to as the *clicking rib syndrome*) can present as chest pain and occurs most often when there is hypermobility of the lower ribs.[76] In this condition, inadequacy or rupture of the interchondral fibrous attachments of the anterior ribs allows the costal cartilage tips to sublux, impinging on the intercostal nerves. This condition can occur alone or can be associated with a broader phenomenon such as myofascial pain syndrome.[83]

CASE EXAMPLE 18.7
Tietze's Syndrome

Referral: A 53-year-old woman was referred by her physician with a diagnosis of left anterior chest pain. The woman is employed at a sawmill and performs tasks that require repetitive shoulder flexion and extension when using a hydraulic apparatus on a sliding track. Lifting (including overhead lifting) is required occasionally, but is limited to items less than 20 lbs.

Past Medical History (PMH): Her PMH was significant for a hysterectomy 10 years ago with prolonged bleeding. She has been a 4- to 5-pack/day smoker for 30 years but has cut down to 1 pack/day for the last 2 months.

Clinical Presentation

Pain Pattern: The woman described the onset of her pain as sudden, crushing chest pain radiating down the left arm, occurring for the first time 6 weeks ago. She was transported to the emergency department, but tests were negative for cardiac incident. Blood pressure at the time of the emergency admittance was 195/110 mm Hg. She was released from the hospital with a diagnosis of "stress-induced chest pain."

The client experienced the same type of episode of chest pain 10 days ago but described radiating pain around the chest and under the armpit to the upper back. Today, her symptoms include extreme tenderness and pain in the left chest with deep pain described as penetrating straight through her chest to her back. There is no numbness or tingling and no pain down the arm but a residual soreness in the left arm.

The client believes that her symptoms may be "stress-induced" but expresses some doubts about this because her symptoms persist and no known cause has been found. She relates that because of divorce proceedings and child custody hearings, she is under extreme stress at this time.

Examination: The neurologic screen was negative. The deep tendon reflexes were within normal limits; strength testing was limited by pain but with a strong initial response elicited; and no change in sensation, two-point discrimination, or proprioception was observed.

There was exquisite pain during palpation of the left pectoral muscle with tenderness and swelling noted at the second, third, and fourth costochondral joints. Painful and radiating symptoms were reproduced with resisted shoulder horizontal adduction. Active shoulder range of motion was full, but with a positive painful arc on the left. There was also painful reproduction of the radiating symptoms down the arm with palpation of the left supraspinatus and biceps tendons.

The painful chest/arm/upper back symptoms were not altered by respiratory movement (deep breathing or coughing), but the client was unable to lie down without extreme pain.

Result: The physical therapy assessment was suggestive of Tietze's syndrome secondary to repetitive motion and exacerbated by emotional stress with concomitant shoulder dysfunction. Physical therapy intervention resulted in initial rapid improvement of symptoms with full return to work 6 weeks later.

It should be noted that although the physical therapist's assessment recognized emotional stress as a factor in the client's symptoms, it may not be in the client's best interest to include this information in the documentation. Although the medical community is increasingly aware of the research surrounding the mind-body connection, worker's compensation and other third-party payers may use this information to deny payment.

Rib syndrome can occur at any age, including during childhood,[84] but most commonly occurs during the middle-aged years. Repetitive trunk motion in individuals participating in running sports can cause rib syndrome manifesting as severe, sharp pain.[77] The physical therapist is usually able to readily identify a rib syndrome as the cause of chest pain after a careful musculoskeletal examination. In some cases, persistent upper abdominal and/or low thoracic pain occurs, leaving physicians, chiropractors, and therapists puzzled.[85,86] A sonogram may be needed to make the diagnosis. Pain is made worse by slump sitting or side-bending to the affected side. Reduction or elimination of symptoms following rib mobilization helps confirm the differential diagnosis.

Gallbladder impairment can also cause tenderness or soreness of the tip of the 10th rib on the right side. The affected individual may or may not have gallbladder symptoms. Because visceral and cutaneous fibers enter the spinal cord at the same level for the ribs and gallbladder, the nervous system may respond to the afferent input with sudomotor changes such as pruritus (itching of the skin) or a sore rib instead of gallbladder symptoms.

The clinical presentation appears as a biomechanical problem, such as a rib dysfunction, instead of nausea and food intolerances normally associated with gallbladder dysfunction. Symptoms will not be alleviated by physical therapy intervention, eventually sending the client back to his or her physician.

Trigger Points

The most common musculoskeletal cause of chest pain is TrPs, sometimes referred to as *myofascial TrPs*. TrPs (hypersensitive spots in the skeletal musculature or fascia) involving a variety of muscles (Table 18.4) may produce precordial pain (Fig. 18.7). Abdominal muscles have multiple referred pain patterns that may reach up into the chest or midback and produce heartburn or deep epigastric pain that mimics cardiac pain.

TABLE 18.4	Trigger Point Pain Guide
Location	Potential Muscles Involved
Front of chest pain	Pectoralis major
	Pectoralis minor
	Scaleni
	Sternocleidomastoid (sternal)
	Sternalis
	Iliocostalis cervicis
	Subclavius
	External abdominal oblique
Side of chest pain	Serratus anterior
	Latissimus dorsi
Upper abdominal/lower chest pain	Rectus abdominis
	Abdominal obliques
	Transversus abdominis

Modified from Travell JG, Simons DG. Myofascial Pain and Dysfunction: The Trigger Point Manual. Baltimore: Williams & Wilkins; 1983:574.

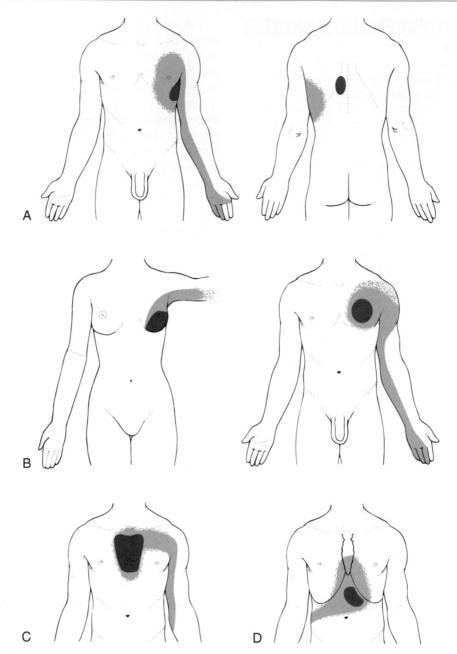

Fig. 18.7   (A) Referred pain pattern from the left serratus anterior muscle. (B) Left pectoralis major muscle: referred pain pattern in a woman and a man. (C) Referred pain pattern from the left sternalis muscle. (D) Referred pain from the external oblique abdominal muscle can cause "heartburn" in the anterior chest wall. Marathon runners may report chest pain mimicking a heart attack from this trigger point (TrP).

In addition to mimicking pain of a cardiac nature, TrPs can occur in response to cardiac disorders. A viscero-somatic response can occur when biochemical changes associated with visceral disease affect somatic structures innervated by the same spinal nerves (see Chapter 3). In such cases, the individual has a PMH of visceral disease. TrPs accompanied by symptoms such as vertigo, headache, change in vision, nausea, and syncope are yellow-flag warnings of autonomic involvement not usually present with TrPs strictly from a somatic origin.

Chest pain that persists long after an acute MI may be as a result of myofascial TrPs. In acute MI, pain is commonly referred from the heart to the midregion of the pectoralis major and minor muscles (see discussion of viscero-somatic sources of pain in Chapter 3). The injury to the heart muscle initiates a viscero-somatic process that activates TrPs in the pectoral muscles.[87]

After recovery from the infarction, these self-perpetuating TrPs tend to persist in the chest wall. As with all myofascial syndromes, inactivation of the TrPs eliminates the client's symptoms of chest pain. If the client's symptoms are eliminated with TrP release, medical referral may not be required. However, communication with the physician is essential; the therapist is advised to document all findings and report them to the client's primary care physician.

Past Medical History

There may be a history of URI with repeated forceful coughing. There is often a history of immobility (e.g., cast immobilization after fracture or injury). The therapist should also ask about muscle strain from lifting weights overhead, from push-ups, and from prolonged, vigorous activity that requires forceful abdominal breathing, such as severe coughing, running a marathon, or repetitive bending and lifting.

Clinical Presentation

TrPs are reproduced with palpation or resisted motions. During the examination, the physical therapist should palpate for tender points and taut bands of muscle tissue, squeeze the involved muscle, observe for increased pain with palpation, test for increased pain with resisted motion, and correlate symptoms with respiratory movements.

Chest pain from serratus anterior TrPs may occur at rest in severe cases. Clients with this myofascial syndrome may report that they are "short of breath" or that they are in pain when they take a deep breath. *Serratus anterior* TrPs on the left side of the chest can contribute to the pain associated with MI. This pain is rarely aggravated by the usual tests for range of motion at the shoulder but may result from a strong effort to protract the scapula. Palpation reveals tender points that increase symptoms, and there is usually a palpable taut band present within the involved muscles.

One of the most extensive patterns of pain from irritable TrPs is the complex pattern from the *anterior scalene* muscle. This may produce ipsilateral sternal pain, anterior chest wall pain, breast pain, or pain along the vertebral border of the scapula, shoulder, and arm, radiating to the thumb and index finger.

Breast pain may be differentiated from the aching pain arising from the scalene or pectoral muscles by a history of upper extremity overuse usually associated with myalgia. Resistance to isometric movement of the upper extremities reproduces the symptoms of a myalgia but does not usually aggravate pain associated with the breast tissue. Additionally, palpation of the underlying muscle reproduces the painful symptoms.

When active TrPs occur in the left *pectoralis major* muscle, the referred pain (anterior chest to the precordium and down the inner aspect of the arm) is easily confused with that of coronary insufficiency. Pacemakers placed superficially can cause pectoral TrPs. In the case of pacemaker-induced TrPs, the physical therapist can teach the client TrP self-treatment to carry out at home.

Myalgia

Myalgia, or muscular pain, can cause chest pain separate from TrP pain but with a similar etiologic basis of prolonged or repeated movement. As mentioned earlier, the physical therapy interview must include questions about recent URI with repeated forceful coughing and recent activities of a repetitive nature that could cause sore muscles (e.g., painting or washing walls; calisthenics, including push-ups; or lifting heavy objects or weights).

Three tests must be used to confirm or rule out muscle as the source of symptoms: (1) palpation, (2) stretch, and (3) contraction. If the muscle is not sore or tender during palpation, stretch, or contraction, the source of the problem most likely lies somewhere else.

With true myalgia, squeezing the muscle belly will reproduce painful chest symptoms. The discomfort of myalgia is almost always described as aching and may range from mild to intense. Diaphragmatic irritation may be referred to the ipsilateral neck and shoulder, lower thorax, lumbar region, or upper abdomen as muscular aching pain. Myalgia in the respiratory muscles is well localized, reproducible by palpation, and exacerbated by movement of the chest wall.

Rib Fractures

Periosteal (bone) pain associated with fractured ribs can cause sharp, localized pain at the level of the fracture with an increase in symptoms associated with trunk motions and respiratory movements, such as deep inspiration, laughing, sneezing, or coughing. The pain may be accompanied by a grating sensation during breathing. This localized pain pattern differs from bone pain associated with chronic disease affecting bone marrow and endosteum, which may result in poorly localized pain of varying degrees of severity.

Occult (hidden) rib fractures may occur, especially in a client with a chronic cough or someone who has had an explosive sneeze. Fractures may occur as a result of trauma (e.g., motor vehicle accident, assault), but painful symptoms may not be perceived at first if other injuries are more significant.

A history of long-term steroid use in the presence of rib pain of unknown cause should raise a red flag. For those clients who have a history of long-term steroid use or osteoporosis, spinal manipulation to the thorax is a contraindication. Also, clients over the age of 65 who fracture a rib, have an increased risk of pneumonia by 27% for each rib that is fractured.[88] Rib fractures must be confirmed by radiographs as a useful first step in imaging. If the physician has a high suspicion of a rib fracture, a computed tomography scan may be obtained.[88] Rib pain without fracture may indicate bone tumor or disease affecting bone, such as multiple myeloma.

Cervical Spine Disorders

Cervicodorsal arthritis may produce chest pain that is seldom similar to that of angina pectoris. It is usually sharp and piercing but may be described as a deep, boring, dull discomfort. There is usually unilateral or bilateral chest pain with flexion or hyperextension of the upper spine or neck. The chest pain may radiate to the shoulder girdle and down the arms and is not related to exertion or exercise. Rest may not alleviate the symptoms, and prolonged recumbency makes the pain worse.

Diskogenic disease can also cause referred pain to the chest, but there is usually evidence of disk involvement observed with diagnostic imaging and the presence of neurologic symptoms (Case Example 18.8).

CASE EXAMPLE 18.8

Pediatric Occupational Therapist with Chest Pain

Referral: A 42-year-old woman presented with primary chest pain of unknown cause. She is employed as an independent pediatric occupational therapist. She has been seen by numerous medical doctors who have ruled out cardiac, pulmonary, esophageal, upper gastrointestinal (GI), and breast pathology as underlying etiologies.

Because her symptoms continue to persist, she was sent to physical therapy for an evaluation.

She reports symptoms of chest pain/discomfort across the upper chest rated as a 5 or 6 and sometimes as an 8 on a scale of 0 to 10. The pain does not radiate down her arms or up her neck. She cannot bring the symptoms on or make them go away. She cannot point to the pain, but reports it as being more diffuse than localized.

Past Medical History (PMH): She denies any shortness of breath, but admits to being "out of shape" and has not been able to exercise because of a failed bladder neck suspension surgery 2 years ago. She reports fatigue, but states that this is not unusual for her with her busy work schedule and home responsibilities.

She has not had any recent infection, no history of cancer or heart disease, and her mammogram and clinical breast examination are up to date and normal. She does not smoke or drink, but by her own admission has a "poor diet" as a result of time pressure, stress, and fatigue.

How do we proceed in the screening process with a client like this?

First review Table 18.1. According to the client, the doctors have ruled out most of the systemic causes in the left column. We know that medical specialization and progression of disease can account for missed cases of somatic symptoms of a viscerogenic or systemic origin.

In the case of medical specialization, the doctors can be looking so carefully for a problem within their specialty area that they miss the obvious somewhere else. Progression of disease means that if enough time passes and the disease process goes unchecked, eventually the client will present with additional signs and symptoms to clear up the diagnostic mystery.

In the case of disease progression, it is possible that what the physician observed in his or her office is not the same as what you see weeks to months later. By carefully interviewing the client, you may be able to bring to light any new changes and report these to the physician.

Systemic Causes

Anemia: She has complained of fatigue, a hallmark finding in anemia. You may think the doctors would have already found any evidence of anemia, but symptoms may not be recognized until hemoglobin concentration is reduced to half of the normal. Because this is a Caucasian woman, we can skip looking at sickle cell anemia at this time.

As we look at the general information about anemia in Chapter 6, we are reminded to ask the following questions:

- Have you experienced any unusual or prolonged bleeding from any part of your body?
- Have you noticed any blood in your urine or stools? Have you noticed any change in the color of your stools (dark, tarry, sticky stools may signal melena from blood loss in the GI tract)?

- Have you been taking any over-the-counter or prescribed antiinflammatory drugs (NSAIDs and peptic ulcer with GI bleeding)?
- Have you ever been told you have rheumatoid arthritis, lupus, HIV/AIDS, or anemia?

You notice from the text that there can be nail bed changes. Quickly inspect the nail beds, palms, and skin. Remember, observation of the hands should be done at the level of the client's heart, and the hands should be warm if possible.

Be sure to assess ALL vital signs. This includes pulse, respirations, oxygen saturation, skin temperature, core body temperature, and blood pressure. For a review of vital signs as a red flag, see Vital Signs in Chapter 4.

Cancer: Palpate lymph nodes for generalized lymphadenopathy.

As we look at the items listed under "Other" in Table 18.1, are there any conditions here that might apply to this woman? What additional questions will you want to ask this client?

Rheumatic Diseases: First under "Other" is "Rheumatic diseases." Ask if the client has ever been diagnosed with arthritis of any kind or had any arthritic-like symptoms anywhere in her body. When you conduct your examination, keep in mind that RA is a systemic condition that can cause chest pain. Osteoarthritis of the cervical spine can also cause chest pain, so we will make a note to look at that more closely later.

Fibromyalgia: While you are asking about arthritis, go ahead and ask about fibromyalgia also in this list. You may want to ask about the presence of symptoms commonly associated with fibromyalgia.

Pain patterns typical of fibromyalgia can be found in Chapter 13. You can find a list of clinical signs and symptoms of fibromyalgia in that section.

Anxiety, Cocaine, or Steroid Use: Finally, from the list in the left column of Table 18.1, we have anxiety and cocaine or anabolic steroid use. We have already discussed anxiety as a potential cause of chest pain, but cocaine and steroid use are also covered in this chapter.

Additional signs and symptoms present with anxiety, anxiety as a factor in pain assessment, and screening for anxiety are discussed in Chapter 3. Table 3.9 lists the physical, behavioral, cognitive, and psychologic symptoms of anxiety. You may just want to take a look at this list and ask your client if she experiences any of these symptoms regularly.

Anabolic steroid use is not likely in this client, but cocaine use may be an issue. Do not neglect to ask about the use of any recreational drugs of any kind, including cocaine, crack, PCP, marijuana, hash, and so forth.

Neuromusculoskeletal (NMS) Causes: Now use the NMS causes of chest pain listed in the right column as a springboard for your examination. Perform appropriate orthopedic and other clinical tests and measures to identify any of the conditions listed.

Most of these conditions are associated with painful symptoms that can be reproduced if you know what movements to suggest and/or where and when to palpate. In the case of rib fractures or breast pain from trauma, do not forget to screen for domestic violence or assault as covered in Chapter 2.

Use Table 18.4 to identify trigger points (TrPs) in muscles that can cause chest pain. Sometimes, failure to respond to physical

Continued

therapy intervention is considered a red flag for systemic origin of somatic symptoms.

Beware when your client fails to respond to TrP therapy. This may not be a red flag suggesting screening for systemic or other causes of muscle pain. Muscle recovery from TrPs is not always so simple.

According to Headley, muscles with active TrPs fatigue faster and recover more slowly. They show more abnormal neural circuit dysfunction. The pain and spasm of TrPs may not be relieved until the aberrant circuits are corrected.[89]

Results: After completing the evaluation with appropriate questions, tests and measures, a Review of Systems pointed to the cervical spine as the most likely source of this client's symptoms. The jaw and shoulder joint were cleared, although there were signs of shoulder movement dysfunction from a possible impingement syndrome.

She had limited cervical spine range of motion with obvious limitations in passive intervertebral movements (joint play or accessory motions) at the C4-C5 level. There were no neurologic findings except for global neck muscle weakness, which was consistent with a chronic pain pattern. There were latent TrPs of the pectoralis major and minor, but eliminating these did not change the primary chest pain pattern.

A trial course of manual therapy improved the client's symptoms temporarily. The client was discharged with a home program to maintain neck range of motion and gradually increase neck musculature strength. Symptoms returned intermittently over the next 6 weeks.

After relaying these findings to the client's primary care physician, radiographs of the cervical spine were ordered. Interestingly, despite the thousands of dollars spent on repeated diagnostic workup for this client, a simple x-ray had never been taken.

Results showed significant spurring and lipping throughout the cervical spine from early osteoarthritic changes of unknown cause. Cervical spine fusion was recommended and performed for instability in the midcervical region.

The client's chest pain was eliminated and did not return even up to 2 years after the cervical spine fusion. The physical therapist's contribution in pinpointing the location of referred symptoms brought this case to a successful conclusion and closure.

SCREENING FOR NEUROMUSCULAR OR NEUROLOGIC CAUSES OF CHEST, BREAST, OR RIB PAIN

Several possible neurologic disorders can cause chest and/or breast pain, including nerve root impingement or inflammation, herpes zoster (shingles), thoracic disk disease, postoperative neuralgia, and TOS (see Table 18.1).

Neurologic disorders such as intercostal neuritis and dorsal nerve root radiculitis or a neurovascular disorder such as TOS also can cause chest pain. The two most commonly recognized noncardiac causes of chest pain seen in the physical therapy clinic are herpes zoster (shingles) and TOS.

Intercostal Neuritis

Intercostal neuritis, such as herpes zoster or shingles produced by a viral infection of a dorsal nerve root, can cause neuritic chest wall pain, which can be differentiated from coronary pain.

Risk Factors

Shingles may occur or recur at any age, but there has been a recent increase in the number of cases in two distinct age groups: college-aged young adults and older adults (over 70 years). Health care experts suggest that stress is the key factor in the first group, and immune system failure is the key factor in the second group.

Anyone who is immunocompromised as a result of advancing age, underlying malignancy, organ transplantation, or acquired immunodeficiency syndrome (AIDS) is at risk for shingles. There is an increased incidence of herpes zoster in clients with lymphoma, tuberculosis, and leukemia, but it can be triggered by trauma or injection drugs or can occur with no known cause.

Anyone in good health who had the chickenpox as a child is not at great risk for shingles. The risk of developing shingles increases for anyone who is immunocompromised for any reason or who has never had chickenpox.

Herpes zoster is a communicable disease and requires some type of isolation. Anyone in contact with the client before the outbreak of the skin lesions has already been exposed. Specific precautions depend on whether the disease is localized or disseminated and the condition of the client. Persons susceptible to chickenpox should avoid contact with the affected client and stay out of the client's room.

Clinical Presentation

Herpes zoster is characterized by raised fluid-filled clusters of grouped vesicles that appear unilaterally along cranial or spinal nerve dermatomes 3 to 5 days after transmission of the virus (see Figs. 4.23 and 4.24). The affected individual experiences 1 to 2 days of pain, itching, and hyperesthesia before the outbreak of skin lesions.

The skin changes are referred to as "shingles" and are easily recognizable as they follow a dermatome anywhere on the body. The lesions do not cross the body midline as they follow nerve pathways, although nerves of both sides may be involved. The skin eruptions evolve into crusts on the skin and clear in about 2 weeks unless the period between the pain and the eruption is longer than 2 days. Postherpetic neuralgia, with its burning and paroxysmal stabbing pain, may persist for long periods.

Neuritic pain occurs unrelated to effort and lasts longer (weeks, months, or years) than angina. The pain may be constant or intermittent and can vary from light burning to a deep visceral sensation. It may be associated with chills, fever, headache, and malaise. Symptoms are confined to the somatic distribution of the involved spinal nerve(s).

CLINICAL SIGNS AND SYMPTOMS
Herpes Zoster (Shingles)

- Fever, chills
- Headache and malaise
- 1 to 2 days of pain, itching, and hyperesthesia before skin lesions develop
- Skin eruptions (vesicles) that appear along dermatomes 4 or 5 days after the other symptoms

---

Dorsal Nerve Root Irritation

Dorsal nerve root irritation of the thoracic spine is another neuritic condition that can refer pain to the chest wall. This condition can be caused by infectious processes (e.g., radiculitis or inflammation of the spinal nerve root dural sheath; shingles can also fit in this category). However, the pain is more likely to be the result of mechanical irritation caused by spinal disease or deformity (e.g., bone spurs secondary to osteoarthritis or the presence of cervical ribs placing pressure on the brachial plexus).

The pain of dorsal nerve root irritation can appear as lateral or anterior chest wall pain with referral to one or both arms through the brachial plexus. Although it mimics the pain pattern of coronary heart disease, such pain is more superficial than cardiac pain. Like cardiac pain, dorsal nerve root irritation can be aggravated by exertion of only the upper extremities. However, unlike cardiac pain, exertion of the lower extremities has no exacerbating effect. It is usually accompanied by other neurologic signs such as muscle atrophy and numbness or tingling.

CLINICAL SIGNS AND SYMPTOMS
Dorsal Nerve Root Irritation

- Lateral or anterior chest wall pain
- History of back pain
- Pain that is aggravated by exertion of only the upper body
- May be accompanied by neurologic signs:
  - Numbness
  - Tingling
- Muscle atrophy

Thoracic Outlet Syndrome

TOS refers to compression of the neural and/or vascular structures that leave or pass over the superior rim of the thoracic cage (see Fig. 18.10). Various names have been given to this condition according to the presumed site of major neurovascular compression: first thoracic rib, cervical rib, scalenus anticus, costoclavicular, and hyperabduction syndromes.

Past Medical History

History of associated back pain may be the only significant PMH. The presence of anatomic anomalies, such as an extra rib or unusual sternoclavicular and/or acromioclavicular angle, may be the only known history linked to the development of TOS.

Risk Factors

Symptoms may be related to occupational activities (e.g., carrying heavy loads, working with arms overhead), poor posture, sleeping with arms elevated over the head, or acute injuries such as cervical flexion/extension (whiplash). Athletes such as swimmers, volleyball players, tennis players, and baseball pitchers are also at increased risk for compression of the neurovascular structures. Most people become symptomatic in the third or fourth decade, and women (especially during pregnancy) are affected three times more often than are men.

Clinical Presentation

Chest/breast pain can occur (and may be the only symptom of TOS) as a result of cervical spine disorders, an underlying etiology in TOS. This is because spinal nerves originating as high as C3-C4 can extend down as low as the nipple line.

The compressive forces associated with this problem usually affect the upper extremities in the ulnar nerve distribution but can result in episodic chest pain mimicking coronary heart disease. Neurogenic pain associated with TOS may be described as stabbing, cutting, burning, or electric. The pain is often unrelated to effort and lasts hours to days.[90] Pectoralis minor syndrome has been identified as one cause of recurrent neurogenic TOS contributing to an estimated 75% or more of all cases.[91] Pectoralis minor syndrome occurs when the bracial plexus is compressed inferior to the clavicle under the pectoralis minor, whereas TOS refers to compression to the brachial plexus or vessels above the clavicle.[92]

There may be radiating pain to the neck, shoulder, scapula, or axilla, but usually the superficial nature of the pain and associated changes in sensation and neurologic findings point to chest pain with an underlying neurologic cause (Table 18.5). Paresthesias (burning, pricking sensation) and hypoesthesia (abnormal decrease in sensitivity to stimulation) are common. Anesthesia and motor weakness are reported in about 10% of all cases.

When a vascular compressive component is involved, there may be more diffuse pain in the limb, with associated fatigue and weakness. With more severe arterial compromise, the client may describe coolness, pallor, cyanosis, or symptoms of Raynaud's phenomenon. Although vascular in origin, these symptoms are differentiated from CAD by the local or regional presentation, affecting only a single extremity or only the upper extremities.

Palpation of the supraclavicular space may elicit tenderness or may define a prominence indicative of a cervical rib. The effect on the pulse of the Halstead maneuvers (Fig. 18.8), the hyperabduction or Wright test (Fig. 18.9), and the costoclavicular test

TABLE 18.5	Assessing Symptoms of Thoracic Outlet Syndrome*
Component	Symptoms
Vascular component	3-minute elevated test
	Swelling (arm/hand)
	Discoloration of hand
	Costoclavicular test
	Hyperabduction test
	Upper extremity claudication
	Difference in blood pressure
	Change in skin temperature
	Cold intolerance
Neural	**Upper plexus**
	Point tenderness of C5-C6
	Pressure over lateral neck elicits pain and/or numbness
	Pain with head turned and/or tilted to opposite side
	Weak biceps
	Weak triceps
	Weak wrist
	Hypoesthesia in radial nerve distribution
	3-minute abduction stress test
	Lower plexus
	Pressure above clavicle elicits pain
	Ulnar nerve tenderness when palpated under axilla or along inner arm
	Tinel's sign for ulnar nerve in axilla
	Hypoesthesia in ulnar nerve distribution
	Serratus anterior weakness
	Weak hand grip

*Although no specific testing for thoracic outlet syndrome has proven valid in detecting upper extremity pain of a neurogenic origin, the use of these special tests may help identify patterns of positive objective findings to help characterize it.

(exaggerated military attention posture) should be compared in both arms. Authors have suggested that the Adson's and Roos test should be discontinued to differentiate TOS.[93]

Despite the widespread use of these tests, the reliability remains unknown. Specificity reported ranges from 18% to 87%, but sensitivity has been documented at 94%.[94] During assessment for vascular origin of symptoms, a change in pulse rate or rhythm is a positive test; however, because more than 50% of normal, asymptomatic individuals have pulse rate changes, it is better to reproduce the client's symptoms as a true indicator of TOS.[94,95]

Other clinical tests are described in orthopedic assessment texts.[94,96] With the use of special tests, patterns of positive objective findings may help characterize TOS as vascular, neural, or a combination of both (neurovascular).

Response to nerve blocks has not proved to be a predictable or reliable diagnostic or treatment approach to neurogenic TOS.[97] Although no specific testing for thoracic outlet has proven valid in detecting upper extremity pain of a neurogenic origin, Table 18.5 may help guide the therapist in assessing for this condition.

Knowing what the tests are for can help guide intervention. For example, Fig. 18.10 gives a visual representation of the effect of the hyperabduction test. A positive hyperabduction test may point to the need to restore normal function and movement of the pectoralis minor muscle.

Likewise, if there is a neural component, assess for location (upper versus lower plexus). Reproduction of pain or paresthesia with light pressure on the scalene, supraclavicular area, and pectoralis minor points to TOS rather than a cervical radiculopathy or more distal entrapment, but several pathologic conditions can be present at the same time.[98]

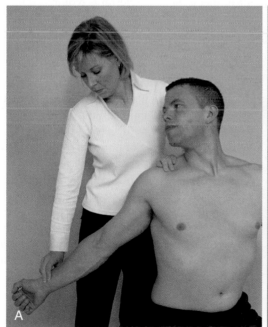 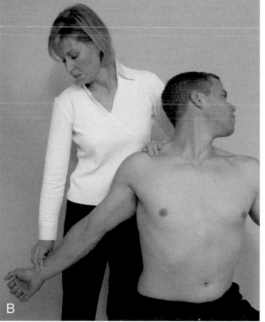

Fig. 18.8 Halstead maneuver. Baseline radial pulse is obtained before the client hyperextends and rotates his head to the opposite side. The examiner applies a downward, traction force on the involved side. Once again, the test is considered positive for a vascular component of a TOS when there is a change in pulse rate or rhythm. (From Magee D. Orthopedic Physical Assessment. 5 ed. Philadelphia: Saunders; 2008.)

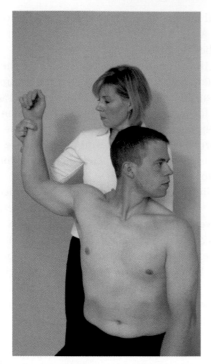

Fig. 18.9 Modified Wright test, also known as the Allen test or maneuver. The hyperabduction test can help screen for vascular compromise in thoracic outlet syndrome (TOS). Start with the client's arm resting at his or her side. Take the client's resting radial pulse for a full minute. Make note of any irregular or skipped beats. Raise the client's arm as shown with the client's face turned away, and recheck the pulse. This test is used to detect compression in the costoclavicular space. A diminished or thready pulse or an absence of a pulse is a positive sign for (vascular) TOS. In the standard test, the examiner waits up to 3 minutes before palpating to give time for an accurate assessment. In our experience, clients with a positive hyperabduction test almost always demonstrate an early change in symptoms, skin color, and skin temperature. Having the client take a breath and hold it may have an additional effect. Tests for other aspects of neurologic or vascular compromise are available.[93,94] (From Magee D. Orthopedic Physical Assessment. 5 ed. Philadelphia: Saunders; 2008.)

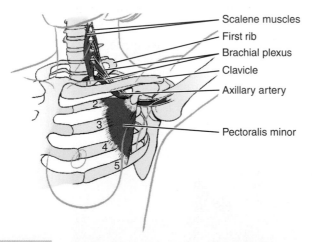

Scalene muscles
First rib
Brachial plexus
Clavicle
Axillary artery
Pectoralis minor

Fig. 18.10 The neurovascular bundle associated with thoracic outlet syndrome (TOS) can become compressed by nearby soft tissue structures such as the pectoralis minor. This illustration shows why the hyperabduction test can alter the client's pulse or reproduce symptoms. Effecting a change in the pectoralis minor may result in a change in the client's symptoms and can be measured by a return of the normal pulse rate and rhythm in the hyperabducted position.

TOS should be considered when persistent chest pain occurs in the presence of a normal coronary angiogram and normal esophageal function tests. Other conditions in the differential diagnosis include cervical degenerative disk disease or abnormality of the lung or chest wall.[99]

CLINICAL SIGNS AND SYMPTOMS
Thoracic Outlet Syndrome

Vascular
- Swelling, sometimes described as "puffiness," of the supra-clavicular fossa, axilla, arm, and/or hand
- Cyanotic (blue or white) appearance of the hand; especially notable when the arm is elevated over head; sometimes referred to as the white hand sign
- Coldness or blanching of the hand during exercise
- Subjective report of "heaviness" in arm or hand
- Chest, neck, and/or arm pain described as "throbbing" or deep aching
- Upper extremity fatigue and weakness
- Difference in blood pressure from side to side (more than 10 mm Hg difference in diastolic)

Neurologic
- Numbness and/or tingling, usually ulnar nerve distribution
- Atrophy of the hand; difficulty with fine motor skills
- Pain in the upper extremity (proximal to distal); described as stabbing, cutting, burning, or electric
- Numbness and tingling down the inner aspect of the arm (ulnar nerve distribution)

A vascular component to TOS may present with significant differences in blood pressure from side to side (a change of 10 mm Hg or more in diastolic is most likely). This does not mean that a medical referral is required immediately. Assess client age, PMH, and presence of comorbidities (e.g., known hypertension), and ask about any associated signs and symptoms that might point to heart disease as a cause of the underlying symptoms.

Physical therapy intervention can bring about a change in the soft tissue structures, putting pressure on the blood vessels in this area. Blood pressure can be used as an outcome measure to document the effectiveness of the intervention. If blood pressure does not normalize and equalize from side to side, then medical referral may be required.

If there is a cluster of cardiac symptoms, especially in the presence of a significant history of hypertension or heart disease, medical referral may be required before initiating treatment. If the Review of Systems does not provide cause for concern, documentation and communication with the physician are still important when initiating a plan of care.

Postoperative Pain

Postoperative chest pain following cardiac transplantation or other open heart procedures usually occurs as a result of the sternal incision and musculoskeletal manipulation during surgery. Coronary insufficiency does not appear as chest pain because of cardiac denervation.

PHYSICIAN REFERRAL

Never dismiss chest pain as insignificant. Chest pain that falls into any of the categories in Table 7.5 requires medical evaluation. This table offers some helpful clues in matching client's clinical presentation with the need for medical referral.

It may be impossible for a physician to differentiate anxiety from myocardial ischemia without further testing; such a differentiation is outside the scope of a physical therapist's practice. The therapist must confine himself or herself to a screening process before conducting a differential diagnosis of movement system impairments.

The therapist is not making the differential diagnosis between angina, MI, mitral valve prolapse, or pericarditis. The therapist is screening for systemic or viscerogenic causes of chest, breast, shoulder or arm, jaw, neck, or upper back symptoms.

Knowing the chest and breast pain patterns and associated signs and symptoms of conditions that masquerade as NMS dysfunction will help the therapist recognize a condition requiring medical attention. Likewise, quickly recognizing red-flag signs and symptoms is important in providing early medical referral and intervention, preferably with improved outcomes for the client.

Guidelines for Immediate Medical Attention

- Sudden onset of acute chest pain with sudden dyspnea could be a life-threatening condition (e.g., pulmonary embolism, MI, ruptured abdominal aneurysm), especially in the presence of red-flag risk factors, PMH, and vital signs.
- A sudden change in the client's typical anginal pain pattern suggests unstable angina. For the client with known angina, pain that occurs without exertion, lasts longer than 10 minutes, or is not relieved by rest or nitroglycerin signals a higher risk for a heart attack.
- The woman with chest, breast, axillary, or shoulder pain of unknown origin at presentation must be questioned regarding breast self-examinations. Any recently discovered breast lumps or nodules or lymph node changes must be examined by a physician.

Guidelines for Physician Referral See (See Figure 18.11)

- No change is noted in uneven blood pressure from one arm to the other after intervention for a vascular TOS component.
- The therapist who suspects a client may be using anabolic steroids should report findings to the physician or coach if one is involved.
- Symptoms are unrelieved or unchanged by physical therapy intervention.
- Medical referral is advised before initiating treatment for anyone with a PMH of cancer presenting with symptoms of unknown cause, especially without an identifiable movement system impairment.

Clues to Screening Chest, Breast, or Rib Pain

Past Medical History

- History of repetitive motion; overuse; prolonged activity (e.g., marathon); long-term use of steroids, assault, or other trauma
- History of flu, trauma, URI, shingles (**herpes zoster**), recurrent pneumonia, chronic bronchitis, or emphysema
- History of breast cancer or any other cancer; history of chemotherapy or radiation therapy
- History of heart disease, hypertension, previous MI, heart transplantation, bypass surgery, or any other procedure affecting the chest/thorax (including breast reconstruction, implantation, or reduction)
- Prolonged use of cocaine or anabolic steroids
- Nocturnal pain, pain without precise movement aggravation, or pain that fails to respond to treatment
- Weight loss in the presence of immobility when weight gain would otherwise be expected
- Recent childbirth and/or lactation (breastfeeding) (**Pectoral myalgia, mastitis**)

Risk Factors (see also Table 7.3)

- Age
- Tobacco use
- Obesity
- Sedentary lifestyle, prolonged immobilization

Clinical Presentation

- Range of motion (e.g., trunk rotation of side-bending, shoulder motions) does not reproduce symptoms (exception: intercostal tear caused by forceful coughing associated with diaphragmatic pleurisy)
- There is a lack of musculoskeletal objective findings; squeezing the underlying pectoral muscles does not reproduce symptoms; resisted motion (e.g., horizontal shoulder abduction or adduction) does not reproduce symptoms; heat and stretching do not reduce or eliminate the symptoms; pain or symptoms are not altered or eliminated with TrP therapy or other physical therapy intervention
- Chest pain relieved by antacid (**reflux esophagitis**), rest from exertion or taking nitroglycerin (**angina**), recumbency (**mitral valve prolapse**), squatting (**hypertrophic cardiomyopathy**), passing gas (**gas entrapment syndrome**)
- Presence of painless sternal or chest wall mass or painless, hard lymph nodes
- Unusual vital signs; change in breathing

Cardiovascular

- Timing of symptoms to physical or sexual activity (immediate, 5 to 10 minutes after engaging in activity, after activity ends). (**Lag time is associated with angina; symptoms occurring immediately or after an activity may be a sign of TOS, asthma, myalgia, or TrP**)
- Assess the effect of exertion; reproduction of chest, shoulder, or neck symptoms with exertion of only the lower extremities may be cardiovascular

- Chest, neck, or shoulder pain that is aggravated by physical exertion, exposure to temperature changes, strong emotional reactions, or a large meal (**coronary artery disease**)
- Atypical chest pain associated with dyspnea, arrhythmia, and light-headedness or syncope
- Other signs and symptoms such as pallor, unexplained profuse perspiration, inability to talk, nausea, vomiting, sense of impending doom, or extreme anxiety
- Symptoms can be precipitated by working with arms overhead; the client becomes weak or short of breath 3 to 5 minutes after raising the arms above the heart

Pleuropulmonary (see also Clues to Screening in Chapter 8)

- Autosplinting (lying on the involved side) quiets chest wall movements and reduces or eliminates chest or rib pain; symptoms are worse with recumbency (supine position)
- Pain is not reproduced by palpation
- Assess for the three *ps*: pleural pain, palpation, position (*p*leuritic pain exacerbated by respiratory movements, pain during *p*alpation associated with musculoskeletal condition, pain with change in neck, trunk, or shoulder *p*osition, indicating musculoskeletal origin)
- Musculoskeletal: symptoms do not increase with pulmonary movements (unless there is an intercostal tear or rib dysfunction associated with forceful coughing from a concomitant pulmonary problem) but can be reproduced with palpation
- Pleuropulmonary: symptoms increase with pulmonary movements and cannot be reproduced with palpation (unless there is an intercostal tear or rib dysfunction associated with forceful coughing)
- Increased symptoms occur with recumbency (abdominal contents push up against diaphragm and in turn push against the parietal pleura)
- Increased chest pain with exercise or increased movement can also be a sign of asthma; ask about a personal or family history of asthma or allergies
- Presence of associated signs and symptoms such as persistent cough, dyspnea (rest or exertional), or constitutional symptoms
- Chest pain with sudden drop in blood pressure or symptoms such as dizziness, dyspnea, vomiting, or unexplained sweating while standing or ambulating for the first time after surgery, an invasive medical procedure, assault, or accident involving the chest or thorax (**Pneumothorax**)

Gastrointestinal (Upper GI/Epigastric; see also Clues to Screening in Chapter 9)

- Effect of food on symptoms (better or worse); presence of GI symptoms, simultaneously or alternately with somatic symptoms
- Pain during swallowing
- Symptoms are relieved by antacids, food, passing gas, or assuming the upright position.
- Supine position aggravates symptoms (**upper GI problem**); symptoms are relieved by assuming an upright position.

- Symptoms radiate from the chest posteriorly to the upper back, interscapular, subscapular, or T10 to L2 areas
- Symptoms are not reproduced or aggravated by effort or exertion
- Presence of associated signs and symptoms such as nausea, vomiting, dark urine, jaundice, flatulence, indigestion, abdominal fullness or bloating, blood in stool, pain during swallowing

Breast (alone or in combination with chest, neck, or shoulder symptoms)

- Appearance (or report) of a lump, nodule, discharge, skin puckering, or distended veins
- Jarring or movement of the breast tissue increases or reproduces the pain
- Pain is palpable within the breast tissue
- Assess for TrPs (sternalis, serratus anterior, pectoralis major; see Fig. 18.7); breast pain in the absence of TrPs or failure to respond to TrP therapy must be investigated further
- Resisted isometric shoulder, horizontal adduction or abduction does *not* reproduce breast pain
- Breast pain is reproduced by exertion of the lower extremities (**Cardiac**)
- Association between painful symptoms and menstrual cycle (**Ovulation or menses**)
- Presence of aberrant or suspicious axillary or supraclavicular lymph nodes (e.g., large, firm, hard, or fixed)
- Skin dimpling especially with adherence of underlying tissue; ask about or visually inspect for:
  - Lump or nodule
  - Red, warm, edematous, firm, and painful area over or under skin
  - Change in size, shape, or color of either breast or surrounding area
  - Unusual rash or other skin changes (e.g., puckering, dimpling, peau d'orange)
  - Distended veins
  - Unusual sensation in nipple or breast
  - Unusual nipple ulceration or discharge

Anxiety (see Table 3.9)

- Pain pattern:
  - Sharp, stabbing pain: left breast region
  - Dull aching: substernal
  - Discomfort: upper chest, neck, left arm
  - Fingertip size; does not radiate
  - Unable to palpate locally
  - Lasts seconds to hours to days
- Not aggravated by respiratory or other (shoulder, arm, back) movements
- Unchanged by rest or change in position
- Unrelated to effort or exertion
- Associated signs and symptoms:
  - Local hyperesthesia of chest wall
  - Choking sensation (hysteria/panic)
  - Claustrophobia
  - Sense of persistent weakness
  - Unpleasant awareness of heartbeat

- Hyperventilation (can also occur with heart attack; watch for sighing respiration and numbness/tingling of face and fingertips)

Neuromusculoskeletal

- Symptoms described using words typical of NMS origin (e.g., aching, burning, hot, scalding, searing, cutting, electric shock)
- Pain is superficial compared with pain of a cardiac or pleuropulmonary origin
- Symptoms are confined to somatic or spinal nerve root distribution
- History of associated back pain
- Positive hyperabduction test or other tests for TOS
- Presence of TrPs; elimination of TrPs reduces or eliminates symptoms (see Table 18.4 and Fig. 18.7)
- Symptoms are elicited easily by palpation (e.g., squeezing the pectoral muscle belly, palpating the chest wall, intercostal space, or costochondral junction)

- Symptoms are reproduced by resisted horizontal shoulder abduction, adduction, or other shoulder movement
- Symptoms are relieved by heat and stretching
- Soft tissues (tendon and muscle) take longer than the expected time to heal (**Anabolic steroids**)
- Costochondritis or Tietze's syndrome may be accompanied by an increase in blood pressure but is usually palpable and aggravated by trunk movements
- Presence of neurologic involvement (e.g., numbness, tingling, muscle atrophy); consider age and history of trauma or injury (**Degenerative disk disease**)
- Pain referred along peripheral nerve pathway (**Dorsal nerve root irritation**)
- Pain is unrelated to effort and lasts hours or weeks to months
- Associated signs and symptoms: numbness and tingling, muscle atrophy (**Neurologic**); rash, fever, chills, headache, malaise (**Constitutional symptoms; neuritis or shingles**)

REFERRED CHEST, BREAST, RIB PAIN PATTERNS

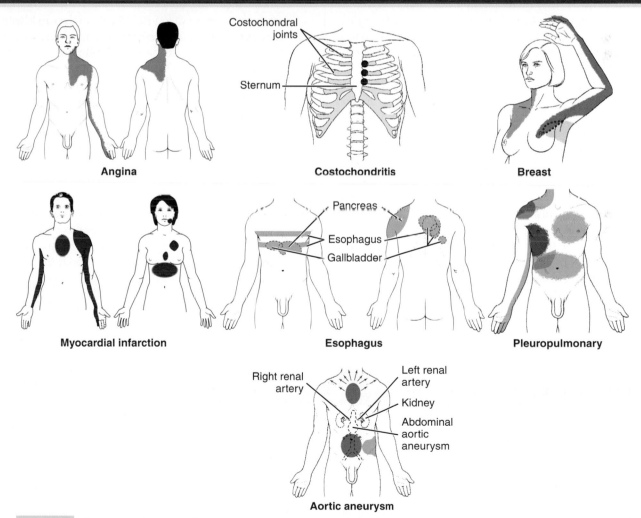

Fig. 18.11 Composite picture of referred chest, breast, and rib pain patterns. Not shown: TrP patterns (see Fig. 18.7).

■ Key Points to Remember

1. When faced with chest pain, the therapist must know how to assess the situation quickly and decide if medical referral is required and whether medical attention is needed immediately. Therapists must be able to differentiate NMS from a systemic origin of symptoms.
2. Although the PMH is important, it cannot be relied upon to confirm or rule out medical causes of chest pain. PMH does alert the therapist to an increased risk of systemic conditions that can masquerade as NMS disorders.
3. Likewise, chest pain history by itself is not enough to rule out cardiac or other systemic origin of symptoms; in most cases, some diagnostic testing is needed. The physical therapist can offer valuable information from the screening process to aid in the medical differential diagnosis.
4. Chest pain associated with increased activity is a red flag for possible cardiovascular involvement. The physical therapist can assess when chest pain may be caused by musculoskeletal dysfunction (immediate chest pain occurs with use) or by possible vascular compromise (chest pain occurs 5 to 10 minutes after activity begins).
5. Anyone with a history of stent insertion presenting with chest pain should be screened carefully. The stent can get scarred over and/or malfunction. Stents are effective at alleviating chest pain but do not reduce the risk of heart attack for most people with stable angina.
6. Cardiac pain patterns may differ for men and women; the therapist should be familiar with known pain patterns for both genders.
7. TrPs can cause chest, breast, or rib pain, even mimicking cardiac pain patterns; a viscero-somatic response can also occur following an MI, causing persisting symptoms of myocardial ischemia (angina); releasing the TrP relieves the symptoms.
8. The therapist must especially know how and what to look for to screen for cancer, cancer recurrence, and/or the delayed effects of cancer treatment. Cancer can present as primary chest pain with or without accompanying neck, shoulder, and/or upper back pain/symptoms.
9. When a woman with a PMH of cancer develops neck, back, upper trapezius or shoulder pain, or other symptoms, examining the site of the original cancer removal is a good idea.
10. The ACS and the NCI support breast cancer screening by qualified health care specialists. With adequate training, the physical therapist can incorporate CBE as a screening tool in the upper quarter examination for appropriate clients (e.g., individuals with neck, shoulder, upper back, chest, and/or breast signs or symptoms of unknown cause or insidious onset).[6]
11. A physical therapist conducting a CBE could miss a lump (false negative), but this will most certainly happen if the therapist does not conduct a CBE at all to assess skin integrity and surrounding soft tissues of the breast or axilla.[6]
12. The physical therapist does not diagnose any kind of cancer, including breast cancer; only the pathologist can make a cancer diagnosis. The therapist can identify aberrant soft tissue and refer the client for further evaluation. Early detection and intervention can reduce morbidity and mortality.
13. Thoracic disk disease can also present as unilateral chest pain and requires careful screening.
14. Chest pain of unknown cause in the adolescent or young adult athlete may be the result of anabolic steroid use. Watch for injuries that take longer than expected to heal, a personality change, and any of the physical signs listed in the text.
15. A history of long-term steroid use in the presence of rib pain of unknown cause raises a red flag for rib fracture.
16. Many people with chest pain have used cocaine within the last week but deny its use; the therapist should not neglect asking clients of all ages about their use of substances.

CLIENT HISTORY AND INTERVIEW

SPECIAL QUESTIONS TO ASK: CHEST/THORAX

Musculoskeletal

- Have you strained a muscle from (repeated, forceful) coughing?
- Have you ever injured your chest?
- Does it hurt to touch your chest or to take a deep breath (e.g., coughing, sneezing, sighing, or laughing)? (**Myalgia, fractured rib, costochondritis, myofascial TrP**)

- Do you have frequent attacks of heartburn, or do you take antacids to relieve heartburn or acid indigestion? (**Noncardiac cause of chest pain, abdominal muscle TrP, GI disorder**)
- Does chest movement or body/arm position make the pain better or worse?

Neurologic

- Do you have any trouble taking a deep breath? (Weak chest muscles secondary to polymyositis, dermatomyositis, myasthenia gravis)
- Does your chest pain ever travel into your armpit, arm, neck, or wing bone (scapula)? (TOS, TrPs)
  - *If yes*, do you ever feel burning, prickling, numbness, or any other unusual sensation in any of these areas?

Pulmonary

- Have you ever been treated for a lung problem?
  - *If yes*, describe what this problem was, when it occurred, and how it was treated.
- Do you think your chest or thoracic (upper back) pain is caused by a lung problem?
- Have you ever had trouble with breathing?
- Are you having difficulty with breathing now?
- Do you ever have shortness of breath, breathlessness, or difficulty catching your breath?
  - *If yes*, does this happen when you rest, lie flat, walk on level ground, walk up stairs, or when you are under stress or tension?
  - How long does it last?
  - What do you do to get your breathing back to normal?
- How far can you walk before you feel breathless?
- What symptom stops your walking (e.g., shortness of breath, heart pounding, or weak legs)?
- Do you have any breathing aids (e.g., oxygen, nebulizer, humidifier, or ventilation devices)?
- Do you have a cough? (Note whether the person smokes, for how long, and how much.) Do you have a smoker's hack?
  - *If yes* to having a cough, distinguish it from a smoker's cough. Ask when it started.
  - Does coughing increase or bring on your symptoms?
  - Do you cough anything up? *If yes*, please describe the color, amount, and frequency.
  - Are you taking anything for this cough? *If yes*, does it seem to help?
  - Do you have periods when you cannot seem to stop coughing?
  - Do you ever cough up blood?
  - *If yes*, what color is it? (Bright red: fresh; brown or black: older)
  - *If yes*, has this been treated?
- Have you ever had a blood clot in your lungs?
  - *If yes*, when and how was it treated?
- Have you had a chest x-ray film taken during the last 5 years?
  - *If yes*, when and where did it occur? What were the results?
- Do you work around asbestos, coal, dust, chemicals, or fumes? *If yes*, describe.

- Do you wear a mask at work? *If yes*, approximately how much of the time do you wear a mask?
- If the person is a farmer, ask what kind of farming (because some agricultural products may cause respiratory irritation).
- Have you ever had tuberculosis or a positive skin test for tuberculosis?
  - *If yes*, when did it occur and how was it treated? What is your current status?
- When was your last test for tuberculosis? Was the result normal?

Cardiac

- Has a physician ever told you that you have heart trouble?
- Have you recently (or ever) had a heart attack? *If yes*, when? Describe.
  - *If yes*, to either question: Do you think your current symptoms are related to your heart problems?
- Do you have angina (pectoris)?
  - *If yes*, describe the symptoms, and tell me when it occurs.
  - *If no*, pursue further with the following questions.
- Do you ever have discomfort or tightness in your chest? **(Angina)**
- Have you ever had a crushing sensation in your chest with or without pain down your left arm?
- Do you have pain in your jaw, either alone or in combination with chest pain?
- If you climb a few flights of stairs fairly rapidly, do you have tightness or pressing pain in your chest?
- Do you get pressure, pain, or tightness in the chest if you walk in the cold wind or face a cold blast of air?
- Have you ever had pain, pressure, or a squeezing feeling in the chest that occurred during exercise, walking, or any other physical or sexual activity?
- Do you ever have bouts of rapid heart action, irregular heartbeats, or palpitations of your heart?
  - *If yes*, did this occur after a visit to the dentist? **(Endocarditis)**
- Have you noticed any skin rash or dots under the skin on your chest in the last 3 weeks? **(Rheumatic fever, endocarditis)**
- Have you noticed any other symptoms (e.g., shortness of breath, sudden and unexplained perspiration, nausea, vomiting, dizziness or fainting)?
- Have you used cocaine, crack, or any other recreational drug in the last 6 weeks?
- Does your pain wake you up at night? (Therapist: distinguish between awakening *from* pain and awakening *with* pain; awakening from pain is more likely with **cardiac ischemia**, whereas awakening with pain is characteristic of sleep disturbance and more common with **psychogenic or stress-induced** chest pain; this information will help in

CLIENT HISTORY AND INTERVIEW—cont'd

deciding whether referral is needed immediately or at the next follow-up appointment)

Epigastric

- Have you ever been told that you have an ulcer?
- Does the pain under your breast bone radiate (travel) around to your back, or do you ever have back pain at the same time that your chest hurts?
- Have you ever had heartburn or acid indigestion?
  - *If yes*, how is this pain different?
  - *If no*, have you noticed any association between when you eat and when this pain starts?

Special Questions to Ask: Breast

- Have you ever had any breast surgery (implants, lumpectomy, mastectomy, reconstructive surgery, or augmentation)?
  - *If yes*, has there been any change in the incision line, nipple, or breast tissue?
  - May I look at the incision during my examination?
- Do you have a history of cystic or lumpy breasts?
  - *If yes*, do the lumps come and go or change with your periods?
- Is there a family history of breast disease?
  - *If yes*, ask about type of disease, age of onset, treatment, and outcome.
- Have you ever had a mammogram or ultrasound?
  - *If yes*, when was your last test? What were the results?
- Have you ever had a lump or cyst drained or biopsied?
  - *If yes*, what was the diagnosis?
- Have you ever been treated for cancer of any kind? *If yes*, when? What?
- Have you examined yourself for any lumps or nodules and found any thickening or lump in the breast or armpit area?
  - *If yes*, has your physician examined/treated this?
  - *If no*, do you examine your breasts? (Follow-up questions regarding last breast examination by self or other health care professional)
- Do you have any discharge from your breasts or nipples?
  - *If yes*, do you know what is causing this discharge? Have you received medical treatment for this problem?
- Are you nursing or breastfeeding an infant (lactating)?
  - *If yes*, are your nipples sore or cracked?
  - Is your breast painful or hot? Are there any areas of redness?
  - Have you had a fever? (**Mastitis**)
- Have you noticed any other changes in your breast(s)? For example, are there any noticeable bulging or distended veins, puckering, swelling, tenderness, rash, or any other skin changes?
- Do you have any pain in your breasts?
  - *If yes*, does the pain come and go with your period? (**Hormone-related**)
  - Does squeezing the breast tissue cause the pain?

- Does using your arms in any way cause the pain?
- Have you been involved in any activities of a repetitive nature that could cause sore muscles (e.g., painting, washing walls, push-ups or other calisthenics, heavy lifting or pushing, overhead movements, prolonged running, or fast walking)?
- Have you recently been coughing excessively? (**Pectoral myalgia**)
- Have you ever had angina (chest pain) or a heart attack? (**Residual TrPs**)
- Have you been in a fight or hit, punched, or pushed against any object that injured your chest or breast? (**Assault**)

Special Questions to Ask: Lymph Nodes

Use the lymph node assessment form (Fig. 4.48) to record and report baseline findings.
- General screening question: Have you examined yourself for any lumps or nodules and found any thickening or lump?
  - *If yes*, has your physician examined/treated this?

If any suspicious or aberrant lymph nodes are observed during palpation, ask the following questions.
- Have you recently had any skin rashes anywhere on your face or body?
- Have you recently had a cold, URI, the flu, or other illness? (**Enlarged lymph nodes**)
- Have you ever had:
  - Cancer of any kind?

If no, have you ever been treated with radiation or chemotherapy for any reason?
- Breast implants
- Mastectomy or prostatectomy
- Mononucleosis
- Chronic fatigue syndrome
- Allergic rhinitis
- Food intolerance, food allergy, or celiac sprue
- Recent dental work
- Infection of any kind
- Recent cut, insect bite, or infection in the hand or arm
- A sexually transmitted disease of any kind
- Sores or lesions of any kind anywhere on the body (including genitals)

Special Questions to Ask: Soft Tissue Lumps or Skin Lesions

- How long have you had this?
- Has it changed in the last 6 weeks to 6 months?
- Has your doctor seen it?
- Does it itch, hurt, feel sore, or burn?
- Does anyone else in your household have anything like this?
- Have you taken any new medication (prescribed or over-the-counter) in the last 6 weeks?
- Have you traveled somewhere new in the last month?

CLIENT HISTORY AND INTERVIEW—cont'd

- Have you been exposed to anything in the last month that could cause this? (consider exposure from occupational, environmental, and hobby interests)
- Do you have any other skin changes anywhere else on your body?

- Have you had a fever or sweats in the last 2 weeks?
- Are you having any trouble breathing or swallowing?
- Have you had any other symptoms of any kind anywhere else in your body?

CASE STUDY

STEPS IN THE SCREENING PROCESS

If a client comes to you with chest pain, breast pain, or rib pain (either alone or in combination with neck, back, or shoulder pain), start by looking at Tables 18.1 and 18.2 and Box 18.4. As you look down these lists, does your client have any red-flag histories, unusual clinical presentation, or associated signs and symptoms to point to any particular category? Just by looking at these lists, you may be prompted to ask some additional questions that have not been asked yet.

COULD IT BE CANCER?

The therapist does not determine whether or not a client has cancer; only the pathologist can make this determination. The therapist's assessment determines whether the client has a true neuromuscular or musculoskeletal problem that is within the scope of our practice.

However, knowing red flags for the possibility of cancer helps the therapist know what questions to ask and what red flags to look for. Early detection often means reduced morbidity and mortality for many people. Watch for the following:

- Previous history of cancer (any kind, but especially breast or lung cancer).
- Be sure to assess for TrPs. Reassess after TrP therapy (e.g., Were the symptoms alleviated? Did the movement pattern change?).
- Conduct a neurologic screening examination.
- Look for skin changes or other trophic changes, and ask about recent rashes or lesions (see Box 4.11).

COULD IT BE VASCULAR?

- Consider the client's age, menopausal status (women), PMH, and the presence of any cardiac risk factors. Do any of these components suggest the need to screen further for a vascular cause?
- Are there any reported associated signs and symptoms (e.g., unexplained perspiration without physical activity, nausea, pallor, unexplained fatigue, palpitations; see Box 4.19)?

- Is there a significant difference in blood pressure from one arm to the other? Have you checked? Do the symptoms suggest the need to conduct this assessment?
- Have you assessed for the three Ps? (*p*leuritic pain, *p*alpation, *p*osition)

COULD IT BE PULMONARY?

- Consider the age of the client and any recent history of pneumonia or other URIs. Again, consider the three Ps.
- Have you observed or heard any reports from the client to suggest changes in the breathing pattern? Are there other pulmonary symptoms present (e.g., dry or productive cough, symptoms aggravated by respiratory movement)?
- Are the symptoms made better by sitting up, worse by lying down, or better in sidelying on the affected side (autosplinting)? *If yes*, further screening may be warranted.

COULD IT BE UPPER GI?

- Follow the same line of thinking in terms of mentally reviewing the client's PMH (e.g., chronic NSAID use, GERD, gallbladder, or liver problems) and the presence of any GI signs or symptoms. Is there anything here to suggest a potential GI cause of the current symptoms? *If yes*, then review the Special Questions to Ask box for any further screening questions.
- Have you asked the client about the effect of eating or drinking on their symptoms? It is a quick and simple screening question to help identify any GI component.
- Be sure and assess for TrPs as a potential cause of what might appear to be GI-induced symptoms.

COULD IT BE BREAST PATHOLOGY?

- Consider red-flag histories, risk factors, and the pain pattern for men and women when considering breast tissue as a possible cause of upper quadrant pain.
- Is there any cyclical aspect to the symptoms linked to menstruation or hormonal fluctuations?
- Ask if jarring or squeezing the breast reproduces the pain.

CASE STUDY—cont'd

- Ask if there have been any obvious changes in the breast tissue or nipple.
- Have you palpated the axillary or supraclavicular lymph nodes? This is a quick and easy screening test that can easily be incorporated into your examination.

COULD IT BE TRAUMA OR OTHER CAUSES?

- Remember to consider trauma (including assault) as a possible cause of symptoms.
- Is there any reason to suspect drug use (e.g., cocaine, anabolic steroids)?

Should you consider screening for emotional overlay or psychogenic source of symptoms (see Chapter 3; see Appendix B-31 in the accompanying enhanced eBook version included with print purchase of this textbook

- Consider anemia as a possible cause; without a laboratory test, this is impossible to know for certain. In the screening process, the therapist can ask some questions to help formulate a referral decision. For example, has the client complained of fatigue, a hallmark finding in anemia? Some additional questions may include the following:
  - Have you experienced any unusual or prolonged bleeding from any part of your body?

- Have you noticed any blood in your urine or stools? Have you noticed any change in the color of your stools? (Dark, tarry, sticky stools may signal melena from blood loss in the GI tract.)
- Have you been taking any OTC or prescribed antiinflammatory drugs (NSAIDs and peptic ulcer with GI bleeding)?

Have you ever been told you have rheumatoid arthritis (RA), lupus, human immunodeficiency virus/acquired immunodeficiency syndrome (HIV/AIDS), or anemia?

RA is a systemic condition that can cause chest pain; osteoarthritis of the cervical spine, fibromyalgia, and anxiety can also cause chest pain. When completing the Review of Systems, look for a cluster of associated signs and symptoms that might suggest any of these conditions.

Do not forget to consider screening for anabolic steroid use, cocaine or other substance use, and domestic violence or assault.

Finally, review the clues to differentiating chest, breast, or rib pain, and then scan the Special Questions to Ask: Chest/Thorax or Special Questions to Ask: Breast in this chapter (depending on the chief complaint and presenting symptoms). Have you left anything out?

PRACTICE QUESTIONS

1. Chest pain can be caused by TrPs of the:
   a. Sternocleidomastoid.
   b. Rectus abdominis.
   c. Upper trapezius.
   d. Iliocostalis thoracis.
2. During examination of a 42-year-old woman's right axilla, you palpate a lump. Which characteristics most suggest the lump may be malignant?
   a. Soft, mobile, tender.
   b. Hard, immovable, nontender.
3. A client complains of throbbing pain at the base of the anterior neck that radiates into the chest and interscapular areas and increases with exertion. What should you do first?
   a. Monitor vital signs and palpate pulses.
   b. Call the physician or 911 immediately.
   c. Continue with the examination; find out what relieves the pain.
   d. Ask about PMH and associated signs and symptoms.
4. A 55-year-old grocery store manager reports becoming extremely weak and breathless whenever stocking groceries on overhead shelves. What is the possible significance of this complaint?
   a. TOS.
   b. Myocardial ischemia.

   c. TrP.
   d. All of the above.
5. Chest pain of a pleuritic nature can be distinguished by:
   a. Increases with autosplinting (lying on the involved side).
   b. Reproduced with palpation.
   c. Exacerbated by deep breathing.
   d. All of the above.
6. A 66-year-old woman has come to you with a report of anterior neck pain radiating down the left arm. Her PMH is significant for chronic diabetes mellitus (insulin dependent), coronary artery disease, and peripheral vascular disease. About 6 weeks ago, she had an angioplasty with stent placement. Which test will help you differentiate a musculoskeletal cause from a cardiac cause of neck and arm pain?
   a. Stair climbing or stationary bike test.
   b. Using arms overhead for 3 to 5 minutes.
   c. TrP assessment.
   d. All of the above.
7. You are evaluating a 30-year-old woman with left chest pain that starts just below the clavicle and extends down to the nipple line. The majority of test results point to TOS. Her blood pressure is 120/78 mm Hg on the right (sitting) and 125/100 on the left (sitting). She is in apparent good health with no history of surgeries

PRACTICE QUESTIONS—cont'd

or significant health problems. What plan of action would you recommend?

a. Refer her to a physician before initiating treatment.

b. Carry out a plan of care, and reassess after three sessions or 1 week, whichever comes first.

c. Document your findings, and contact the physician by phone or by fax while initiating treatment.

d. Eliminate TrPs and then reassess symptoms.

8. A 60-year-old woman with a history of left breast cancer (10 years postmastectomy) presents with pain in her midback. The pain is described as "sharp" and radiates around her chest to the sternum. She gets some relief from her pain by lying down. Her vital signs are normal, and there are no palpable or aberrant lymph nodes. She denies any change in breast tissue on the right or the scar and soft tissue on the left. You do not have adequate training to perform a CBE, but the client agrees to visual inspection, which reveals nothing unusual. All other findings are within normal limits; you are unable to provoke or aggravate her symptoms. Neurologic screening examination is within normal limits. The client denies any history of trauma. What plan of action would you recommend?

a. Refer her to a physician before initiating treatment.

b. Carry out a plan of care and reassess after three sessions or 1 week, whichever comes first.

c. Document your findings, and contact the physician by phone or by fax while initiating treatment.

d. Eliminate TrPs and then reassess symptoms.

9. You are working with a client in his home who had a total hip replacement 2 weeks ago. He describes chest pain with increased activity. Knowing what could cause this symptom will help guide you in asking appropriate screening questions. Can this be a symptom of:

a. Asthma.

b. Angina.

c. Pleuritis or pleurisy.

d. All of the above.

10. Cardiac pain in women does not always follow classic patterns. Watch for this group of symptoms in women at risk:

a. Indigestion, food poisoning, jaw pain.

b. Nausea, tinnitus, night sweats.

c. Confusion, left biceps pain, dyspnea.

d. Unusual fatigue, shortness of breath, weakness, or sleep disturbance.

REFERENCES

1. Sik EC. Atypical chest pain in athletes. *Curr Sports Med Rep.* 2009;8(2):52–58.
2. Harding G, Yelland M. Back, chest, and abdominal pain—is it spinal referred pain? *Aust Fam Phys.* 2007;36(6):422–429.
3. Lenfant C. Chest pain of cardiac and noncardiac origin. *Metabolism.* 2010;59(Suppl 1):S41–S46.
4. Bono CM. An evidence-based clinical guideline for the diagnosis and treatment of cervical radiculopathy from degenerative disorders. *Spine J.* 2011;11(1):64–72.
5. Lovelace-Chandler V, Bassar M, Dow D, et al. The role of physical therapists assisting women in skill development in performing breast self-examination. New Orleans: Poster presentation. Combined Sections Meeting; February 2005.
6. Goodman CC, McGarvey CL. The role of the physical therapist in primary care and cancer screening: integrating clinical breast examination (CBE) in the upper quarter examination. *Rehabil Oncol.* 2003;21(2):4–11.
7. Swap C, Nagurney JT. Value and limitations of chest pain history in the evaluation of patients with suspected acute coronary symptoms. *JAMA.* 2005;294(20):2623–2629.
8. Bruckner FE, Greco A, Leung AW. Benign thoracic pain syndrome: role of magnetic resonance imaging in the detection and localization of thoracic disc disease. *J R Soc Med.* 1989;82:81–83.
9. Baranto A. Acute chest pain in a top soccer player due to thoracic disc herniation. *Spine.* 2009;34(10):E359–E362.
10. Lee CP, Hoffmann U, Bamberg F, et al. Emergency physician estimates of the probability of acute coronary syndrome in a cohort of patients enrolled in a study of coronary computed tomographic angiography. *CJEM.* 2012;14(3):147–156.
11. Towfighi A, Zheng L, Ovbiagele B. Sex-specific trends in midlife coronary heart disease risk and prevalence. *Arch Intern Med.* 2009;169(19):1762–1766.
12. American Heart Association: Heart News. http://www.americanheart.org. Accessed March 17, 2011.
13. Mehta LS, Beckie TM, DeVon HA, et al. Acute myocardial infarction in women. a scientific statement from the American Heart Association. *Circulation.* 2016;133:916–947.
14. Zhao M, Woodward M, Vaartjes I, et al. Sex differences in cardiovascular medication prescription in primary care: a systematic review and meta-analysis. *J Am Heart Assoc.* 2020;9(11):e014742.
15. Heart and stroke statistics: American Heart Association 2011. http://www.heart.org/HEARTORG/General/Heart-and-Stroke-Association-Statistics_UCM_319064_SubHomePage.jsp#. Accessed March 17, 2011.
16. Sanchis J. Identification of very low risk chest pain using clinical data in the emergency department. *Int J Cardiol.* 2011;150(3):260–263.
17. Hsiao CJ, Cherry DK, Beatty PC, Rechtsteiner A. National ambulatory medical care survey: 2007 summary. *Natl Health Stat Report.* 2010;27:1–32.
18. Kontos MC, Diercks DB, Kirk JD. Emergency department and office-based evaluation of patients with chest pain. *Mayo Clin Proc.* 2010;85(3):284–299.
19. Cooper A, Timmis A, Skinner J, Guideline Development Group Assessment of recent onset chest pain or discomfort of suspected cardiac origin: summary of NICE guidance. *BMJ.* 2010;340:c1118.
20. Marrugat J, Sala J, Masiá R, et al. Mortality differences between men and women following first myocardial infarction. *JAMA.* 1998;280:1405–1409.

21. McSweeney JC. Women's early warning symptoms of acute myocardial infarction. *Circulation*. 2003;108(21):2619–2623.

22. Lovlien M. Early warning signs of an acute myocardial infarction and their influence on symptoms during the acute phase, with comparisons by gender. *Gend Med*. 2009;6(3):444–453.

23. McSweeney JC. Cluster analysis of women's prodromal and acute myocardial infarction symptoms by race and other characteristics. *J Cardiovasc Nurs*. 2010;25(4):311–312.

24. Wolf JM, Green A. Influence of comorbidity on self-assessment instrument scores of patients with idiopathic adhesive capsulitis. *J Bone Joint Surg*. 2002;84A(7):1167–1173.

25. McConaghy JR, Oza RS. Outpatient diagnosis of acute chest pain in adults. *Am Fam Physician*. 2013;87(3):177–182.

26. Lunardi AC. Musculoskeletal dysfunction and pain in adults with asthma. *J Asthma*. 2011;48(1):105–110.

27. Rathod NR. Extra-oesophageal presentation of gastro-oesophageal reflux disease. *J Indian Med Assoc*. 2010;108(1):18–22.

28. Chait MM. Gastroesophageal reflux disease: important considerations for the older patients. *World J Gastrointest Endosc*. 2010;2(12):388–396.

29. Seo TH. Clinical distinct features of noncardiac chest pain in young patients. *J Neurogastroenterol Motil*. 2010;16(2):166–171.

30. Smith R, Athanasou NA, Ostlere SJ, Vipond SE. Pregnancy-associated osteoporosis. *QJM*. 1995;88:865–878.

31. Baitner AC, Bernstein AD, Jazrawi AJ. Spontaneous rib fracture during pregnancy: a case report and review of the literature. *Bull Hosp Jt Dis*. 2000;59(3):163–165.

32. Boissonnault WG, Boissonnault JS. Transient osteoporosis of the hip associated with pregnancy. *J Orthop Sports Phys Ther*. 2001;31(7):359–367.

33. Michalakis K. Pregnancy- and lactation-associated osteoporosis: a narrative mini review. *Endocr Regul*. 2011;45(1):43–47.

34. Kovacs CS. Calcium and bone metabolism during pregnancy and lactation. *J Mammary Gland Biol Neoplasia*. 2005;10(2):105–118.

35. Debnah UK, Kishore R, Black RJ. Isolated acetabular osteoporosis in TOH in pregnancy: a case report. *South Med J*. 2005;98(11):1146–1148.

36. Ryder M, Deyle GD. Differential diagnosis of fibular pain in a patient with a history of breast cancer. *J Orthop Sports Phys Ther*. 2009;39(3):230.

37. Howlander N, Noone A, Krapcho M, et al. *SEER Cancer Statistics Review, 1975–2012*. Bethesda, MD: National Cancer Institute; 2015.

38. https://www.cancer.org/cancer/breast-cancer/about/how-common-is-breast-cancer.html.

39. American Cancer Society (ACS): What are the risk factors for breast cancer? http://www.cancer.org/cancer/breastcancer/detailedguide/breast-cancer-risk-factors. Accessed January 17, 2017.

40. Robertson FM. Inflammatory breast cancer. The disease, the biology, the treatment. *CA Cancer J Clin*. 2010;60(6):351–375.

41. Travis RC. Gene-environment interactions in 7610 women with breast cancer: prospective evidence from the Million women study. *Lancet*. 2010;375(9732):2143–2151.

42. Holm J, Humphreys K, Li J, et al. Risk factors and tumor characteristics of interval cancers by mammographic density. *J Clin Oncol*. 2015;33(9):1030–1037.

43. Hartmann LC, Degnim AC, Santen RJ, Dupont WD, Ghosh K. Atypical hyperplasia of the breast: risk assessment and management options. *Engl J Med*. 2015;372(1):78–89.

44. Boyd NF, Guo H, Martin LJ, et al. Mammographic density and the risk and detection of breast cancer. *Engl J Med*. 2007;356(3):227–236.

45. Mitri ZI, Jackson M, Garby C, et al. BRCAPRO 6.0 Model Validation in male patients presenting for BRCA testing. *Oncologist*. 2015;20(6):593–597. https://doi.org/10.1634/theoncologist.2014-0425. Epub 2015 May 6.

46. Coleman EA, Heard JK. Clinical breast examination: an illustrated educational review and update. *Clin Excell Nurse Pract*. 2001;5:197–204.

47. Bancej C, Decker K, Chiarelli A, Harrison M, Turner D, Brisson J. Contribution of clinical breast examination to mammography screening in the early detection of breast cancer. *J Med Screen*. 2003;10(1):16–21.

48. Bobo J, Lee N. Factors associated with accurate cancer detection during a clinical breast examination. *Ann Epidemiol*. 2000;10(7):463.

49. Oestreicher N, White E, Lehman CD, Mandelson MT, Porter PL, Taplin SH. Predictors of sensitivity of clinical breast examination (CBE). *Breast Cancer Res Treat*. 2002;76(1):73–81.

50. Tasoulis MK, Zacharioudakis KE, Dimopoulos NG, Hadjiminas DJ. Diagnostic accuracy of tactile imaging in selecting patients with palpable breast abnormalities: a prospective comparative study. *Breast Cancer Res Treat*. 2014;147:589–598.

51. Chiarelli AM. The contribution of clinical breast examination to the accuracy of breast screening. *J Natl Cancer Inst*. 2009;101(18):1236–1243.

52. Goodman CC, McGarvey CL. An introductory course to breast cancer and clinical breast examination for the physical therapist is available. (Charlie McGarvey, PT, MS and Catherine Goodman, MBA, PT present the course in various sites around the U.S. and upon request.).

53. A certified training program is also available through *MammaCare* Specialist. The program is offered to health care professionals at training centers in the United States. The course teaches proficient breast examination skills. For more information, contact: http://www.mammacare.com/index.php.

54. Schwartz GF. Proceedings of the international consensus conference on breast cancer risk, genetics, and risk management. *Breast J*. 2009;15(1):4–16.

55. Rubin RN. Woman with sharp back pain. *Consultant*. 1999;39(11):3065–3066.

56. Hall-Findlay EJ. Breast implant complication review: double capsules and late seromas. *Plast Reconstr Surg*. 2011;127(1):56–66.

57. Gabriel SE, Woods JE, O'Fallon WM, Beard CM, Kurland LT, Melton 3rd LJ. Complications leading to surgery after breast implantation. *Engl J Med*. 1997;336(10):718–719.

58. Codner MA. A 15-year experience with primary breast augmentation. *Plast Reconstr Surg*. 2011;127(3):1300–1310.

59. Benediktsson K, Perback L. Capsular contracture around saline-filled and textured subcutaneously-placed implants in irradiated and non-irradiated breast cancer patients: five years of monitoring of a prospective trial. *J Plast Reconstr Aesthet Surg*. 2006;59(1):27–34.

60. Lipa JE. Pathogenesis of radiation-induced capsular contracture in tissue expander and implant breast reconstruction. *Plast Reconstr Surg*. 2010;125(2):437–445.

61. Henriksen TF, Fryzek JP, Holmich LR, et al. Reconstructive breast implantation after mastectomy for breast cancer: clinical outcomes in a nationwide prospective cohort study. *Arch Surg*. 2005;140(12):1152–1159.

62. Scuderi N. Multicenter study on breast reconstruction outcome using Becker implants. *Aesthetic Plast Surg*. 2011;35(1):66–72.

63. Khairandish Z, Jamali L, Haghbin S. Role of anxiety and depression in adolescents with chest pain referred to a cardiology clinic. *Cardiol Young*. 2016;16:1–6.

64. National Institute of Mental Health: Health Information—Anxiety Disorders. http://www.nimh.nih.gov/. Updated 3/16/11. Accessed March 18, 2011.

65. Rubio M. *Psychopathology risk and protective factors research program*. National Institute of Mental Health (NIMH); 2009. http://www.nimh.nih.gov/about/organization/datr/adult-psycho-pathology-and-psychosocial-intervention-research-branch/

psychopathology-risk-and-protective-factors-research-program.shtml. Accessed March 18, 2011.

66. Velasquez EM, Anand RC, Newman WP, Richard SS, Glancy DL. Cardiovascular complications associated with cocaine use. *J La State Med Soc.* 2004;156(6):302–310.

67. Bamberg F. Presence and extent of coronary artery disease by cardiac computed tomography and risk for acute coronary syndrome in cocaine users among patients with chest pain. *Am J Cardiol.* 2009;103(5):620–625.

68. Milroy CM, Parai JL. The histopathology of drugs of abuse. *Histopathology.* 2011;59(4):579–593. 2011 Oct. https://doi.org/10.1111/j.1365-2559.2010.03728.x. Epub 2011 Jan 25.

69. Schwartz BG. Cardiovascular effects of cocaine. *Circulation.* 2010;122(24):2558–2569.

70. Pletcher MJ, Kiefe CI, Sidney S, Carr JJ, Lewis CE, Hulley SB. Cocaine and coronary calcification in young adults: the coronary artery risk development in young adults (CARDIA) study. *Am Heart J.* 2005;150(5):921–926.

71. van Amsterdam J. Adverse health effects of anabolic-androgenic steroids. *Regul Toxicol Pharmacol.* 2010;57(1):117–123.

72. Kanayama G. Illicit anabolic-androgenic steroid use. *Horm Behav.* 2010;58(1):111–121.

73. Sullivan ML, Martinez CM, Gennis P, Gallagher EJ. The cardiac toxicity of anabolic steroids. *Prog Cardiovasc Dis.* 1998;41(1);1–15.

74. Sanchez-Orio M. Anabolic-androgenic steroids and liver injury. *Liver Int.* 2008;28(2):278–282.

75. Eslick GD. Classification, natural history, epidemiology and risk factors of noncardiac chest pain. *Dis Mon.* 2008;54(9):593–603.

76. Stochkendahl MJ. Chest pain in focal musculoskeletal disorders. *Med Clin North Am.* 2010;94(2):259–273.

77. Ayloo A, Cvengros T, Marella S. Evaluation and treatment of musculoskeletal chest pain. *Prim Care.* 2013;40(4):863–887.

78. Peterson LL, Cavanaugh DG. Two years of debilitating pain in a football spearing victim: slipping rib syndrome. *Med Sci Sports Exerc.* 2003;35(10):1634–1637.

79. Cubos J. Chronic costochondritis in an adolescent competitive swimmer: a case report. *J Can Chiropr Assoc.* 2010;54(4):271–275.

80. Thongngarm T, Lemos LB, Lawhon N, Harisdangkul V. Malignant tumor with chest pain mimicking Tietze's syndrome. *Clin Rheumatol.* 2001;20(4):276–278.

81. Fioravanti A, Tofi C, Volterrani L, Marcolongo R. Malignant lymphoma presenting as Tietze's syndrome. *Arthritis Rheum.* 2003;49(5):737.

82. Rosenberg M, Conermann T. *Tietze Syndrome. 2020 Oct 21. StatPearls [Internet].* Treasure Island (FL): StatPearls Publishing; 2020. PMID: 33232033.

83. Hughes KH. Painful rib syndrome: a variant of myofascial pain syndrome. *AAOHN.* 1998;46(3):115–120.

84. Saltzman DA, Schmitz ML, Smith SD, Wagner CW, Jackson RJ, Harp S. The slipping rib syndrome in children. *Paediatr Anaesth.* 2001;11(6):740–743.

85. Meuwly JY, Wicky S, Schnyder P, Lepori D. Slipping rib syndromes: a place for sonography in the diagnosis of a frequently overlooked cause of abdominal or low thoracic pain. *J Ultrasound Med.* 2002;21(3):339–343.

86. Udermann BE, Cavanaugh DG, Gibson MH, Doberstein ST, Mayer JM, Murray SR. Slipping rib syndrome in a collegiate swimmer: a case report. *J Athl Train.* 2005;40(2):120–122.

87. Simons DG, Travell JG, Simons LS. *Travell & Simons' Myofascial Pain And Dysfunction: The Trigger Point Manual. Volume 1: Upper half of body.* 2 ed. Baltimore: Williams & Wilkins; 1999.

88. Baiu I, Spain D. Rib Fractures. *JAMA.* 2019;321(18):1836 https://doi.org/10.1001/jama.2019.2313. PMID: 31087024.

89. Headley BJ. *When Movement Hurts: A Self-help Manual for Treating Trigger Points.* Minneapolis: Orthopedic Physical Therapy Products; 1997.

90. Christo PJ, McGreevy K. Updated perspectives on neurogenic thoracic outlet syndrome. *Curr Pain Headache Rep.* 2011;15(1):14–21.

91. Sanders RJ. The forgotten pectoralis minor syndrome: 100 operations for pectoralis minor syndrome alone or accompanied by neurogenic thoracic outlet syndrome. *Ann Vasc Surg.* 2010;24:701–708.

92. Sanders RJ, Annest SJ. Pectoralis minor syndrome: subclavicular brachial plexus compression. *Diagnostics (Basel).* 2017;7(3):46 https://doi.org/10.3390/diagnostics7030046. PMID: 28788065.

93. Hixson KM, Horris HB, McLeod TCV, Bacon CEW. The diagnostic accuracy of clinical diagnostic tests for thoracic outlet syndrome. *J Sport Rehabil.* 2017;26(5):459–465. https://doi.org/10.1123/jsr.2016-0051. Epub 2016 Aug 24. PMID: 27632823.

94. Dutton M. *Orthopaedic Examination, Evaluation, and Intervention.* 2 ed. New York: McGraw-Hill; 2008.

95. Selke FW, Kelly TR. Thoracic outlet syndrome. *Am J Surg.* 1988;156:54–57.

96. Magee D. *Orthopedic Physical Assessment.* 5 ed. Philadelphia: Saunders; 2008.

97. Sanders RJ. Recurrent neurogenic thoracic outlet syndrome stressing the importance of pectoralis minor syndrome. *Vasc Endovascular Surg.* 2011;45(1):33–38.

98. Yung E. Screening for head, neck, and shoulder pathology in patients with upper extremity signs and symptoms. *J Hand Ther.* 2010;23(2):173–186.

99. Braun RM. Thoracic outlet syndrome: a primer on objective methods of diagnosis. *J Hand Surg.* 2010;35A(9):1539–1541.

CHAPTER 19

Screening the Shoulder and Upper Extremity

The therapist is well aware that many primary neuromuscular and musculoskeletal conditions in the neck, cervical spine, axilla, thorax, thoracic spine, and chest wall can refer pain to the shoulder and arm. For this reason, the physical therapist's examination usually includes assessment above and below the involved joint for referred musculoskeletal pain (Case Example 19.1).

In this chapter, systemic and viscerogenic causes of shoulder and arm pain are explored as well as each system that can refer pain or symptoms to the shoulder. This will include vascular, pulmonary, renal, gastrointestinal (GI), and gynecologic causes of shoulder and upper extremity pain and dysfunction. Primary or metastatic cancer as an underlying cause of shoulder pain also is included. The therapist must know how and what to look for to screen for cancer.

Systemic diseases and medical conditions affecting the neck, breast, and any organs in the chest or abdomen can present clinically as shoulder pain (Table 19.1).[1] Peptic ulcers, heart disease, ectopic pregnancy, and myocardial ischemia are only a few examples of systemic diseases that can cause shoulder pain and movement dysfunction. Each disorder listed can present clinically as a shoulder problem before ever demonstrating systemic signs and symptoms.

USING THE SCREENING MODEL TO EVALUATE SHOULDER AND UPPER EXTREMITY

Past Medical History

As you look over the various potential systemic causes of shoulder symptomatology listed in Table 19.1, think about the most common risk factors and red-flag histories you might see with each of these conditions. For example, a history of any kind of cancer is always a red flag. Breast and lung cancer are the two most common types of cancer to metastasize to the shoulder.[2,3]

Heart disease can cause shoulder pain, but it usually occurs in an age-specific population.[4,5] Anyone over 50 years old, postmenopausal women, and anyone with a positive first-generation family history is at increased risk for symptomatic heart disease. Younger individuals may be more likely to demonstrate atypical symptoms such as shoulder pain without chest pain.[6]

Alternately, although atherosclerosis has been demonstrated in the blood vessels of children, teens, and young adults, they are rarely symptomatic unless some other heart anomaly is present.[7,8]

Hypertension, diabetes mellitus, and hyperlipidemia are other red-flag histories associated with cardiac-related shoulder pain. Of course, a history of angina,[9] heart attack, angiography, stent or pacemaker placement, coronary artery bypass graft (CABG), or other cardiac procedure is also a yellow (caution) flag to alert the therapist of the potential need for further screening. Use of screening tools like the OSPRO-YF is suggested to inform the therapist regarding potential yellow flags for the patient with an upper extremity impairment.

Knowledge of risk factors associated with pathologic conditions, illnesses, and diseases helps the therapist navigate the screening process. For example, pulmonary tuberculosis (TB) is a possible cause of shoulder pain.[10–12] Who is most likely to develop TB? Risk factors include:
- Health care workers
- Homeless population
- Prison inmates
- Immunocompromised individuals (e.g., transplant recipients, long-term users of immunosuppressants, anyone treated for long-term rheumatoid arthritis [RA], anyone treated with chemotherapy for cancer)
- Older adults (over 65 years of age)
- Immigrants from areas where TB is endemic
- Injection drug users
- Malnourished individuals (e.g., eating disorders, alcoholism, drug users, cachexia)

In a case like TB, there will usually be other associated signs and symptoms such as fever, sweats, and cough. When completing a screening examination for a client with shoulder pain of unknown origin or an unusual clinical presentation, the therapist should look at vital signs, auscultate the client, and see what effect increased respiratory movements have on shoulder symptoms (Case Example 19.2).

Clinical Presentation

Differential diagnosis of shoulder pain is sometimes especially difficult because any pain that is felt in the shoulder often affects the joint as though the pain were originating in

CASE EXAMPLE 19.1

Evaluation of a Professional Golfer

Referral: A 38-year-old male professional golfer presented to physical therapy with a diagnosis of left shoulder impingement syndrome, with partial thickness tears of the supraspinatus tendon.

Before the physical therapy intervention, x-ray films were reported as negative for fracture or tumor. Magnetic resonance imaging (MRI) was reported as positive for bursitis and supraspinatus tendinitis with some partial tears. The shoulder specialist also provided the client with one corticosteroid injection, which gave him some relief of shoulder pain.

Past Medical History: Past medical history and Review of Systems were negative for any systemic issues. He was not taking any medication at the time of evaluation.

Clinical Presentation: Functional deficits were reported as pain with the take-away phase of the golf swing and with the adduction motion of the shoulder in follow-through. He also reported a loss of distance associated with his drive by 20 to 30 yards. He had trouble sleeping and reported pain would wake him up if his head was turned into left rotation. He also had pain when turning his head to the left (e.g., when driving a car).

Upper Quarter Screen
Shoulder Range of Motion (ROM)

Active ROM:

Left		Right
160 degrees	Flexion (flex)	170 degrees
165 degrees	Abduction (abd)	170 degrees
50 degrees	Internal rotation (IR)	55 degrees
55 degrees	External rotation (ER)	85 degrees

Passive ROM:

Left		Right
170 degrees	Flex	175 degrees
170 degrees	Abd	175 degrees
55 degrees	IR	60 degrees
60 degrees	ER	75 degrees

Isometric muscle testing of rotator cuff

Abd	Painful/strong
Abd with IR	Painful/strong
IR	Painless/strong
ER	Painless/strong

Special tests

Hawkins/Kennedy (+)

Neer (+)

Speed (+)

ER lag test (–)

IR lag test (–)

Cervical ROM

Flexion 40 degrees	
Extension (ext) 20 degrees	Report of left scapular pain
Left side bend 20 degrees	Report of left scapular pain
Right side bend 25 degrees	No report of pain
Left rotation 45 degrees	Report of left scapular pain
Right rotation 70 degrees	No report of pain
Quadrant position	Right and left: Reproduced left posterior scapular pain with radicular pain to the thumb and second finger area

Deep Tendon Reflexes (DTRs)

Left	DTRs	Right
2+	Biceps	2+
0	Triceps	2+
2+	Brachioradialis	2+

Strength

Left		Right
5/5	Shoulder flex	5/5
4/5	Shoulder abd	5/5
5/5	Elbow flex	5/5
2/5	Elbow ext	5/5
3/5	Wrist ext	5/5
5/5	Wrist flex	5/5
5/5	Thumb ext	5/5
5/5	Finger abd	5/5

He did have intact sensation to light touch and proprioceptive sense. Strength testing during use of the Cybex weight-lifting machines showed he was able to do 10 triceps extensions on the right with four plates, but on the left he was only able to do one repetition with one plate.

Result: With the data obtained in the examination, the conclusion was made that he did have an impingement syndrome as described by Neer, with involvement of the bursa and rotator cuff tendons.[81] Cyriax muscle testing revealed some musculotendon involvement with the strong/painful tests.[70]

The cervical findings required consultation with the referring physician. A provisional medical diagnosis was made of cervical radiculopathy with a C5-C6 herniated disk. The client was referred to a neurosurgeon for evaluation. An MRI confirmed the diagnosis and the client underwent an anterior cervical fusion with diskectomy.

Summary: This case example helps highlight the importance of a complete examination process, even if a physician specialist refers a client for physical therapy services. The therapist must "clear" or examine the joints above and below the region thought to be the cause of the dysfunction. The major reason for the symptoms or a secondary diagnosis may be missed if the screening step is left out because of a lack of time or assuming someone else checked out the entire client.

Voshell S: Case report presented in fulfillment of DPT 910, Institute for Physical Therapy Education, Widener University, Chester, PA, 2005. Used with permission.

TABLE 19.1	Systemic and Medical Conditions as Causes of Shoulder and Upper Extremity Symptoms		
	Neck	Chest/Trunk/Back	Abdomen
Cancer	Metastasis (leukemia, Hodgkin's lymphoma) Cervical cord tumor Bone tumor	Metastasis to nodes in axilla or mediastinum Metastasis to lungs from: Bone Breast Kidney Colorectal Pancreas Uterus Bone metastasis to thoracic spine: Breast Lung Thyroid Breast cancer Lung cancer	Pancreatic cancer Spinal metastases Kidney Testicle Prostate
Cardiovascular/ vascular	TOS	Angina/MI Acute coronary syndrome ICU s/p CABG Pacemaker (complications) Bacterial endocarditis Pericarditis Thoracic aortic aneurysm Empyema and lung abscess Collagen vascular disease	Dissecting aortic aneurysm
Pulmonary	Pulmonary tuberculosis	Pulmonary embolism Pulmonary tuberculosis Spontaneous pneumothorax Pancoast's tumor Pneumonia	
Renal/urologic			Kidney stones Obstruction, inflammation, or infection of upper urinary tract
Gastrointestinal/ hepatic		Hiatal hernia	Peptic/duodenal ulcer (perforated) Ruptured spleen Liver disease Gallbladder disease Pancreatic disease
Infection		Septic arthritis Necrotizing fasciitis Mononucleosis Osteomyelitis/transverse myelitis Syphilis/gonorrhea Herpes zoster (shingles) Pneumonia Cellulitis (skin anywhere on neck, chest, arm, hand)	Subphrenic abscess
Gynecologic			Ectopic pregnancy (rupture) Endometriosis [cyst(s)]
Other	Cervical central cord lesion Trauma: Cervical fracture or ligamentous instability; whiplash	Mastodynia (breast) Diabetes mellitus (adhesive capsulitis) Sickle cell disease Hemophilia	Diaphragmatic hernia Anterior spinal surgery (postoperative hemorrhage)

ICU s/p CABG, Intensive care unit status post coronary artery bypass graft; *MI*, myocardial infarction; *TOS*, thoracic outlet syndrome.

the joint.[5] Shoulder pain with any of the components listed in this chapter should be approached as a manifestation of systemic visceral illness, even if shoulder movements exacerbate the pain or if there are objective findings at the shoulder.

Many visceral diseases present as unilateral shoulder pain (Table 19.2). Esophageal, pericardial (or other myocardial diseases), aortic dissection, and diaphragmatic irritation from thoracic or abdominal diseases (e.g., upper GI, renal, hepatic/biliary) can all appear as unilateral pain.

Adhesive capsulitis, a condition in which both active and passive glenohumeral motions are restricted, can be associated with diabetes mellitus, hyperthyroidism,[13,14] ischemic heart disease, infection, and lung diseases (TB, emphysema, chronic bronchitis, Pancoast's tumors) (Case Example 19.3).[11,12,15–17]

CASE EXAMPLE 19.2

Homeless Man with Tuberculosis

Referral: A 36-year-old man was referred to physical therapy as an inpatient for a short-term hospitalization. He was a homeless man brought to the hospital by the police and admitted with an extensive medical problem list including:

- Malnutrition
- Alcoholism
- Depression
- Hepatitis A
- Broken wrist
- Shoulder pain
- Dehydration

There was no past medical history of cancer. The client was a smoker when he could get cigarettes. He would like to support a 1-pack/day habit.

Medical service requested an evaluation of the client's shoulder pain. X-ray films were not taken because the man had full active range of motion (ROM), no history of trauma, and no insurance to cover additional testing.

Clinical Presentation: The therapist was unable to reproduce the shoulder pain with palpation, position, or provocation testing. There was no sign of rotator cuff dysfunction, adhesive capsulitis, tendinitis, or TrPs in the upper quadrant. There was a noticeable stiffening of the neck with very limited cervical ROM in all planes and directions.

Vital signs were unremarkable, but the client was perspiring heavily, despite being in threadbare clothing and at rest. He reported getting the "sweats" every day around this same time.

The therapist asked the client to take a deep breath and cough. He went into a paroxysm of coughing, which he said caused his shoulder to start aching. The cough was productive, but the client swallowed the sputum. Auscultation of lung sounds revealed rales (crackles) in the right upper lung lobe. Supraclavicular lymph nodes were palpable, tender, and moveable on both sides.

The therapist contacted the charge nurse and reported the following concerns:

- Constitutional symptoms of sweats and fatigue (although fatigue could be caused by his extreme malnutrition)
- Pulmonary impairment with reproduction of symptoms with respiratory movement
- Suspicious (aberrant) lymph nodes (bilateral)

Cervical spine involvement with no apparent cause or recognizable musculoskeletal pattern

Result: Consulting with the physician on-call resulted in a medical evaluation and x-ray. Client was diagnosed with pulmonary tuberculosis (TB), which was confirmed by a skin test. Shoulder and neck pain and dysfunction were attributed to a pulmonary source and not considered appropriate for physical therapy intervention.

The client was sent to a halfway house where he could receive adequate nutrition and medical services to treat his TB.

TABLE 19.2 | Location of Shoulder Pain

Systemic Origin	Right Shoulder Location	Systemic Origin	Left Shoulder Location

Peptic ulcer	Lateral border, right scapula	Internal bleeding:
		  Spleen (trauma, rupture)
		  Postoperative laparoscopy
			Left shoulder (Kehr's sign)

Myocardial ischemia	Right shoulder, down arm	Myocardial ischemia	Left pectoral/left shoulder
		Thoracic aortic aneurysm	Left shoulder (or between shoulder blades)
Hepatic/biliary:		Pancreas	Left shoulder
Acute cholecystitis	Right shoulder; between scapulae; right subscapular area		
Gallbladder	Right upper trapezius, right shoulder	Infectious mononucleosis (hepatomegaly, splenomegaly)	Left shoulder/left upper trapezius
Liver disease (hepatitis, cirrhosis, metastatic tumor, abscess)	Right shoulder, right subscapular		

Pulmonary:
  Pleurisy
  Pneumothorax
  Pancoast's tumor
  Pneumonia
	Ipsilateral shoulder; upper trapezius	Pulmonary: Pleurisy
		  Pneumothorax
		  Pancoast's tumor
		  Pneumonia
			Ipsilateral shoulder; upper trapezius

Kidney	Ipsilateral shoulder	Kidney	Ipsilateral shoulder

Gynecologic:
  Endometriosis
	Reported in right shoulder[77]; possible in either shoulder, depending on location of cyst(s)	Gynecologic:
		  Ectopic pregnancy
			Ipsilateral shoulder

CASE EXAMPLE 19.3

Cardiac Cause of Shoulder Pain

A 65-year-old retired railroad engineer has come to you with a left "frozen shoulder." During the subjective examination, he tells you he is taking two cardiac medications.

What questions would you ask that might help you relate these two problems or rule out a cardiac condition as a possible cause? (shoulder/cardiac)

Try to organize your thoughts using these categories:
- Onset/history of shoulder involvement
- Medical testing
- Clinical presentation
- Past medical history

Physical Therapy Screening Interview

Onset/History
- What do you think is the cause of your shoulder problem?
- When did it occur, or how long have you had this problem (sudden or gradual onset)?
- Can you recall any specific incident when you injured your shoulder, for example, by falling, being hit by someone or something, automobile accident?
- Did you ever have a snapping or popping sensation just before your shoulder started to hurt? **(Ligamentous or cartilaginous lesion)**
- Did you injure your neck in any way before your shoulder developed these problems?
- Have you had a recent heart attack? Have you had nausea, fatigue, sweating, chest pain, or pressure? Any pain in your neck, jaw, left shoulder, or down your left arm?
- Has your left hand ever been stiff or swollen? **(CRPS after myocardial infarction [MI])**
- Do you think your shoulder pain is related to your heart problems?
- Shortly before you first noticed difficulty with your shoulder, were you involved in any kind of activity that would require repetitive movement, such as painting, gardening, playing tennis or golf?

Medical Testing
- Have you had any recent x-rays taken of the shoulder or your neck?
- Have you received medical or physical therapy treatment for shoulder problems before?
  - If yes, where, when, why, who, and what (see Chapter 2 for specific questions)?
- Have you had any (extensive) medical testing during the past year?

Clinical Presentation

Pain/Symptoms
Follow the usual line of questioning regarding the pattern, frequency, intensity, and duration outlined in Fig. 3.6 to establish necessary information regarding pain.
- Is your shoulder painful?
  - If yes, how long has the shoulder been painful?
  Aggravating/Relieving Activities
- How does rest affect your shoulder symptoms? **(True muscular lesions are relieved with prolonged rest [i.e., more**

than 1 hour], **whereas angina is usually relieved more immediately by cessation of activity or rest [i.e., usually within 2 to 5 minutes, up to 15 minutes].)**
- Does your shoulder pain occur during exercise (e.g., walking, climbing stairs, mowing the lawn or any other physical or sexual activity? **(Evaluate the difference between total body exertion causing shoulder symptoms versus movement of the upper extremities only reproducing symptoms. Total body exertion causing shoulder pain may be secondary to angina or MI, whereas movement of just the upper extremities causing shoulder pain is indicative of a primary musculoskeletal lesion.)**

Past Medical History
- Have you had any surgery during the past year?
- How has your general health been? (**Shoulder pain is a frequent site of referred pain from other internal medical problems;** see Fig. 19.2.)
- Did you have rheumatic fever when you were a child?
- What is your typical pattern of chest pain or angina?
- Has this pattern changed in any way since your shoulder started to hurt? For example, does the chest pain last longer, come on with less exertion, and/or feel more intense?
- What medications are you taking?
- Do your heart medications relieve your shoulder symptoms, even briefly?
  - If yes, how long after you take the medication do you notice a difference?
  - Does this occur every time that you take your medication?

Evaluating subacute/acute/chronic musculoskeletal lesion versus systemic pain pattern (see Chapter 3 for specific meaning to the client's answers to these questions):
- Can you lie on that side?
- Does the shoulder pain awaken you at night?
  - If yes, is this because you have rolled onto that side?
- Do you notice any chest pain, night sweats, fever, or heart palpitations when you wake up at night?
- Have you ever noticed these symptoms (e.g., chest pain, heart palpitations) with your shoulder pain during the day?
- Do these symptoms wake you up separately from your shoulder pain, or does your shoulder pain wake you up and you have these additional symptoms? **(As always, when asking questions about sleep pattern, the person may be unsure of the answers. In such cases, the physical therapist is advised to ask the client to pay attention to what happens related to sleep during the next few days up to 1 week and report back with more information.)**

Other Clinical Tests: In addition to an orthopedic screening examination, the therapist should review potential side effects and interactions of cardiac medications, take vital signs, and auscultate (including femoral bruits) and palpate for the aortic pulse (see Fig. 4.54).

Shoulder pain (unilateral or bilateral) progressing to adhesive capsulitis can occur 6 to 9 months after CABG. Similarly, anyone immobile in the intensive care unit (ICU) or coronary care unit (CCU) can experience loss of shoulder motion resulting in adhesive capsulitis (Case Example 19.4). Clients with pacemakers who have complications and revisions that result in prolonged shoulder immobilization can also develop complex regional pain syndrome (CRPS) and/or adhesive capsulitis.[18]

The Shoulder Is Unique

It has been stressed throughout this text that the basic clues and approaches to screening are similar, if not the same, from system to system and anatomic part to anatomic part.

So, for example, much of what was said about screening the neck and back (Chapter 15) applied to the sacrum, sacroiliac (SI), and pelvis (Chapter 16); buttock, hip, and groin (Chapter 17); and chest, breast, and rib (Chapter 18). Presenting the shoulder last in this text is by design.

It is not uncommon for the older adult to attribute "overdoing" it to the appearance of physical pain or neuromusculoskeletal (NMS) dysfunction. Any adult over the age of 65 years presenting with shoulder pain and/or dysfunction must be screened for systemic or viscerogenic origin of symptoms, even when there is a known (or attributed) cause or injury.

In Chapter 2, it was stressed that clients who present with no known cause or insidious onset must be screened along with anyone who has a known or assumed cause of symptoms. Whether the client presents with an unknown etiology of injury or impairment, or with an assigned cause, always ask yourself these questions:

❓ FOLLOW-UP QUESTIONS

- Is it insidious?
- Is it caused by such and such (whatever the client told you)?

CASE EXAMPLE 19.4

Pleural Effusion with Fibrosis, Late Complication of Coronary Artery Bypass Graft

Referral: A 53-year-old man was referred to physical therapy by his primary care physician for left shoulder pain.

Past Medical History: The client had a recent (6 months ago) history of cardiac bypass surgery (also known as coronary artery bypass graft [CABG]) and had completed phase 1 and phase 2 cardiac rehabilitation programs. He was continuing to follow an exercise program (phase 3 cardiac rehabilitation) prescribed for him at the time of his physical therapy referral.

Clinical Presentation: The client looked in good health and demonstrated good posture and alignment. Shoulder range of motion (ROM) was equal and symmetric bilaterally, but the client reported pain when the left arm was raised over 90 degrees of flexion or abduction. His position of preference was left sidelying. The pain could be reduced in this position from a rated level of 6 to a 2 on a scale of 0 (no pain) to 10 (worst pain).

Scapulohumeral motion on the left was altered when compared with the right. Medial and lateral rotations were within normal limits (WNL) with the upper arm against the chest. Lateral rotation reproduced painful symptoms when performed with the shoulder in 90 degrees of abduction. Physiologic motions were fully present in all directions on the left but seemed "sluggish" compared with the right. Neurologic screen was negative.

Vital signs:

Blood pressure:	122/68 mm Hg
Resting pulse:	60 bpm
Body temperature:	98.6° F

Cardiopulmonary screening examination:
Diminished basilar (lower lobes) breath sounds on the left compared with the right
Decreased chest wall excursion on the left; increased shoulder pain with deep inspiration
Dyspnea was not observed at rest

When asked if there were any symptoms of any kind anywhere else in the body, the client reported ongoing but intermittent chest pain and shortness of breath for the last 3 months. The client had not reported these "new" symptoms to the physician.

What are the red flags (if any)? Is an immediate medical referral indicated?
Red Flags:
- Age over 40 years
- Previous (recent) history of cardiac surgery
- Unequal basilar breath sounds
- Unreported symptoms of chest pain and dyspnea
- Autosplinting (lying on the affected side diminishes lung movement, reducing shoulder pain)

Medical Consultation: Shoulder problems are not uncommon following CABG, but the number and type of red flags present caught the therapist's attention. The client was not in any apparent physiologic distress and vital signs were WNL (although he was taking antihypertensive medication). Because he was referred by his primary care physician, the therapist made telephone contact with the physician's office and faxed a summary of findings immediately.

A program of physical therapy intervention was determined, but the therapist insisted on speaking with the physician before proceeding with the program. The physician approved the therapist's treatment plan but requested immediate follow-up with the client who was seen the next day.

Result: The client was diagnosed with pleural effusion causing pleural fibrosis, a rare long-term complication of cardiac bypass surgery. The physician noted that the left lower lobe was adhered to the chest wall.

Pleural effusion is a common complication of cardiac surgery and is associated with other postoperative complications. It occurs more often in women and individuals with associated cardiac or vascular comorbidities and medications used to treat those conditions.[82-86]

The client was treated medically but also continued in physical therapy to restore full and normal motion of the shoulder complex. The physician also asked the therapist to review the client's cardiac rehab program and modify it accordingly because of the pulmonary complications.

The client may wrongly attribute the onset of symptoms to an activity. The alert therapist may recognize a true causative factor.

Shoulder Pain Patterns

In Chapter 3, we presented three possible mechanisms for referred pain patterns from the viscera to the soma (embryologic development, multisegmental innervations, and direct pressure on the diaphragm). Multisegmental innervations (see Fig. 3.3) and direct pressure on the diaphragm (see Fig. 3.4 and 3.5) are two key mechanisms for referred shoulder pain.

Multisegmental Innervations. As the shoulder is innervated by the same spinal nerves that innervate the diaphragm (C3 to C5), any messages to the spinal cord from the diaphragm can result in referred shoulder pain. The nervous system can only tell what nerves delivered the message. It does not have any way to tell if the message sent along via spinal nerves C3 to C5 came from the shoulder or the diaphragm. So it takes a guess and sends a message back to one or the other.

This means that any organ in contact with the diaphragm that gets obstructed, inflamed, or infected can refer pain to the shoulder by putting pressure on the diaphragm, stimulating afferent nerve signals, and telling the nervous system that there is a problem.

Diaphragmatic Irritation. Irritation of the peritoneal (outside) or pleural (inside) surface of the central diaphragm refers sharp pain to the ipsilateral upper trapezius, neck, and/or supraclavicular fossa (Fig. 19.1). Shoulder pain from diaphragmatic irritation usually does not cause anterior shoulder pain. Pain is confined to the suprascapular, upper trapezius, and posterior portions of the shoulder.

If the irritation crosses the midline of the diaphragm, then it is possible to have bilateral shoulder pain. This does not happen very often and is most common with cardiac ischemia or pulmonary pathology affecting the lower lobes of the lungs on both sides. Irritation of the peripheral portion of the diaphragm is more likely to refer pain to the costal margins and lumbar region on the same side.

As you review Fig. 3.4, note how the heart, spleen, kidneys, pancreas (both the body and the tail), and the lungs can put pressure on the diaphragm. This illustration is key to remembering which shoulder can be involved based on organ pathology. For example, the spleen is on the left side of the body, so pain from spleen rupture or injury is referred to the left shoulder (called *Kehr's sign*) (Case Example 19.5).[19]

Either shoulder can be involved with renal colic or distention of the renal cap from any kidney disorder, but it is usually an ipsilateral referred pain pattern depending on which kidney is impaired (see Fig. 11.7; again, via pressure on the diaphragm). Bilateral shoulder pain from renal disease would only occur if and when both kidneys are compromised at the same time.

Look for history of a recent surgery as a part of the past medical history and the presence of accompanying urologic symptoms.

The body of the pancreas lies along the midline of the diaphragm. When the body of the pancreas is enlarged, inflamed, obstructed, or otherwise impinging on the diaphragm, back pain is a possible referred pain pattern. Pain felt in the left shoulder may result from activation of pain fibers in the left diaphragm by an adjacent inflammatory process in the tail of the pancreas.

Postlaparoscopic shoulder pain (PLSP) frequently occurs after various laparoscopic surgical procedures. During the procedure, air is introduced into the peritoneum to expand the area and move the abdominal contents out of the way. The mechanism of PLSP is commonly assumed to be overstretching of the diaphragmatic muscle fibers as a result of the pressure of a pneumoperitoneum (residual carbon dioxide [CO_2] gas after surgery).[20] Pressure from distention causes phrenic nerve–mediated referred pain to the shoulder.[21] Recent evidence suggests that risk factors for PLSP include patients receiving laparoscopic surgery who are below 50 years of age and are in surgery for over 3 hours.[22]

Keep in mind that shoulder pain also can occur from diaphragmatic dysfunction. For anyone with shoulder pain of an unknown origin, or which does not improve with intervention, palpate the diaphragm and assess its excursion and timing during respiration. Reproduction of shoulder symptoms with direct palpation of the diaphragm and the presence of altered diaphragmatic movement with breathing offer clues to the possibility of diaphragmatic (muscular) involvement.

Shoulder pain can be referred from the neck, back, chest, abdomen, and elbow (Fig. 19.2; see also Shoulder and Upper Extremity Pain Patterns later in the chapter). During orthopedic assessment, the therapist always checks "above and below" the impaired level for a possible source of referred pain. With this guideline in mind, we know to look for potential musculoskeletal or neuromuscular causes from the cervical and thoracic spine[23] and elbow.

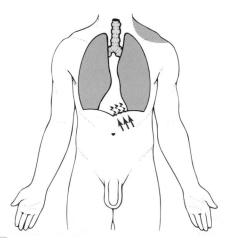

Fig. 19.1 Irritation of the peritoneal (outside) or pleural (inside) surface of the *central* area of the diaphragm can refer sharp pain to the upper trapezius muscle, neck, and supraclavicular fossa. The pain pattern is ipsilateral to the area of irritation. Irritation to the *peripheral* portion of the diaphragm can refer sharp pain to the ipsilateral costal margins and lumbar region (not shown).

CASE EXAMPLE 19.5

Rugby Injury: Kehr's Sign

Referral: A 27-year-old male accountant who has an office in the same complex with a physical therapy practice stopped by early Monday morning complaining of left shoulder pain.

When asked about repetitive motion or recent trauma or injury, he reported playing in a rugby tournament over the weekend. "I got banged up quite a few times, but I had so much beer in me, I did not feel a thing."

Clinical Presentation: Pain was described as a deep, sharp aching over the upper trapezius and shoulder area on the left side. There were no visual bruises or signs of bleeding in the upper left quadrant.

Vital signs:

Pulse:	89 bpm
Respirations:	12 per minute
Blood pressure:	90/48 mm Hg (recorded sitting, left arm)
Temperature:	97° F (reported as the client's "normal" morning temperature)
Pain:	Rated as a 5 on a scale of 0–10

Range of motion (ROM) was full in all planes and movements. No particular movement increased or decreased the pain. Gross manual muscle test of the upper extremities was normal (5/5 for flexion, abduction, extension, rotations).

Neurologic screen was negative. All special shoulder tests (e.g., impingement, anterior and posterior instability, quadrant position) were unremarkable.

What are the red flags here? What are your next questions, steps, or screening tests?

Red Flags
- Hypotension
- Left shoulder pain within 24 hours of possible trauma or injury
- Unable to alter, provoke, or palpate painful symptoms
- Clinical presentation is not consistent with expected picture for a shoulder problem; lack of objective findings.

What are your next questions, steps, or screening tests?
Repeat blood pressure measurements, bilaterally. Perform percussive tests for the spleen (see Fig. 4.53).

Depending on the results of these clinical tests, referral might be needed immediately. In this case the percussive test for an enlarged spleen was inconclusive, but there was an observable and palpable "fullness" in the left flank compared with the right.

Result: This client was told:

"Mr. Smith, your examination does not look like what I would expect from a typical shoulder injury. Because I cannot find any way to make your pain better or worse and I cannot palpate or feel any areas of tenderness, there may be some other cause for your symptoms.

Given your history of playing rugby over the weekend, you may have some internal injuries. I am not comfortable treating you until a medical doctor examines you first. Bleeding from the spleen can cause left shoulder pain. When I tapped over the area of your spleen, it did not sound quite like I expected it to, and it seems like there is some fullness along your left side that I am not seeing or feeling on the right.

I do not want to alarm you, but it may be best to go over to the emergency department of the hospital and see what they have to say. You can also call your primary care doctor and ask if you can be seen right away. You can do that right from our clinic phone."

Final Result: This accountant had clients already scheduled starting in 10 minutes. He did not feel he had the time to go check this out until his lunch hour. About 45 minutes later an ambulance was called to the building. Mr. Smith had collapsed and his coworkers called 9-1-1.

He was rushed to the hospital and diagnosed with a torn and bleeding spleen, which the doctor called a "slow leak." It eventually ruptured, leaving him unconscious from blood loss.

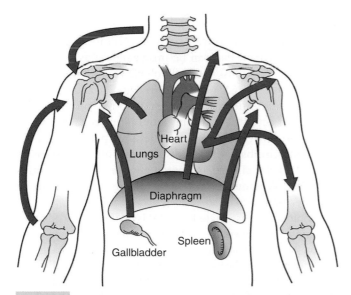

Fig. 19.2   Musculoskeletal and systemic structures referring pain to the shoulder.

Associated Signs and Symptoms

One of the most basic clues in screening for a viscerogenic or systemic cause of shoulder pain is to look for shoulder pain accompanied by any of the following features:
- Pleuritic component
- Exacerbation by recumbency
- Recent history of laparoscopic procedure (risk factor)[19,22,24,25,]
- Coincident diaphoresis (cardiac)
- Associated GI signs and symptoms
- Exacerbation by exertion unrelated to shoulder movement (cardiac)
- Associated urologic signs and symptoms

Shoulder pain with any of these features present should be approached as a manifestation of systemic visceral illness. This is true even if the pain is exacerbated by shoulder movement or if there are objective findings at the shoulder.[26]

Using the past medical history and assessing for the presence of associated signs and symptoms will alert the therapist to any red flags suggesting a systemic origin of shoulder symptoms. For example, a ruptured ectopic pregnancy with abdominal hemorrhage can produce left shoulder pain (with or without chest pain) in a woman of childbearing age.[27-30] The woman is sexually active, and there is usually a history of missed menses or recent unexplained/unexpected bleeding.

The client may not recognize the connection between painful urination and shoulder pain or the link between gallbladder removal by laparoscopy and subsequent shoulder pain. It is the therapist's responsibility to assess musculoskeletal symptoms, making a diagnosis that includes ruling out the possibility of systemic disease.

Review of Systems

In ruling out systemic disease, we must rely on the Review of Systems. Associated signs and symptoms of a systemic disease present with a cluster of signs and symptoms and the therapist must recognize this cluster. The patient will be unaware of the association between shoulder pain and particular organ-dependent signs and symptoms. Based on the results of this review, we formulate our final screening questions, tests, and measures. Always remember to end each client interview with the following (or similar) question:

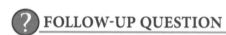

? FOLLOW-UP QUESTION

- Do you have any symptoms of any kind anywhere else in your body that we have not talked about yet?

SCREENING FOR PULMONARY CAUSES OF SHOULDER PAIN

Extensive disease may occur in the periphery of the lung without pain until the process extends to the parietal pleura. Pleural irritation then results in sharp, localized pain that is aggravated by any respiratory movement.

Clients usually note that the pain is alleviated by lying on the affected side, which diminishes the movement of that side of the chest (called "autosplinting"), whereas shoulder pain of musculoskeletal origin is usually aggravated by lying on the symptomatic shoulder.

Shoulder symptoms made worse by recumbence are a yellow flag for pulmonary involvement. Lying down increases the venous return from the lower extremities. A compromised cardiopulmonary system may not be able to accommodate the increase in fluid volume. Referred shoulder pain from the taxed and overworked pulmonary system may result.

At the same time, recumbency or the supine position causes a slight shift of the abdominal contents in the cephalic direction. This shift may put pressure on the diaphragm, which in turn presses up against the lower lung lobes. The combination of increased venous return and diaphragmatic pressure may be enough to reproduce the musculoskeletal symptoms.

Pneumonia in the older adult may appear as shoulder pain when the affected lung presses on the diaphragm; usually there are accompanying pulmonary symptoms, but in older adults, confusion (or increased confusion) may be the only other associated sign.

The therapist should look for the presence of a pleuritic component such as a persistent or productive cough and/or chest pain. Look for tachypnea, dyspnea, wheezing, hyperventilation, or other noticeable changes. Chest auscultation is a valuable tool when screening for pulmonary involvement.

SCREENING FOR CARDIOVASCULAR CAUSES OF SHOULDER PAIN

Pain of cardiac and diaphragmatic origin is often experienced in the shoulder because the heart and diaphragm are supplied by the C5 to C6 spinal segment, and the visceral pain is referred to the corresponding somatic area (see Fig. 3.3).

Exacerbation of the shoulder symptoms from a cardiac cause occurs when the client increases activity that does not necessarily involve the arm or shoulder. Although it is known that using the upper extremities increases systolic blood pressure,[31] physical activity such as walking up stairs or riding a stationary bicycle can bring on cardiac-induced shoulder pain.

In cases like this, the therapist should ask about the presence of nausea, unexplained sweating, jaw pain or toothache, back pain, or chest discomfort or pressure. For the client with known heart disease, ask about the effect of taking nitroglycerin (men) or antacids/acid-relieving drugs (women) on their shoulder symptoms.

Vital signs and physical examination, including chest auscultation, are important screening tools. See Chapter 4 for details.

Angina or Myocardial Infarction

Angina and/or myocardial infarction (MI) can appear as arm and shoulder pain that can be misdiagnosed as arthritis or some other musculoskeletal pathologic condition (see complete discussion in Chapter 7 and see Figs. 7.8 and 7.9).

Look for shoulder pain that starts 3 to 5 minutes after the start of activity, including shoulder pain with isolated lower extremity motion (e.g., shoulder pain starts after the client climbs a flight of stairs or rides a stationary bicycle). If the client has known angina and takes nitroglycerin, ask about the influence of the nitroglycerin on shoulder pain.

Shoulder pain associated with MI is unaffected by position, breathing, or movement. Because of the well-known association between shoulder pain and angina, cardiac-related shoulder pain may be medically diagnosed without ruling out other causes, such as adhesive capsulitis or supraspinatus tendinitis, when, in fact, the client may have both a cardiac and a musculoskeletal problem (Case Example 19.6).

CASE EXAMPLE 19.6
Strange Case of the Flu

Referral: A 53-year-old butcher at the local grocery store stopped by the physical therapy clinic located in the same shopping complex with a complaint of unusual shoulder pain. He had been seen at this same clinic several years ago for shoulder bursitis and tendinitis from repetitive overuse (cutting and wrapping meat).

Clinical Presentation: His clinical presentation for this new episode of care was exactly as it had been during the last episode of shoulder impairment. The therapist reinstituted a program of soft tissue mobilization and stretching, joint mobilization, and postural alignment. Modalities were used during the first two sessions to help gain pain control.

At the third appointment, the client mentioned feeling "dizzy and sweaty" all day. His shoulder pain was described as a constant, deep ache that had increased in intensity from a 6 to a 10 on a scale of 0 to 10. He attributed these symptoms to having the flu.

It was not until this point that the therapist conducted a screening examination and found the following red flags:
- Age
- Recent history (past 3 weeks) of middle ear infection on the same side as the involved shoulder
- Constant, intense pain (escalating over time)
- Constitutional symptoms (dizziness, perspiration)
- Symptoms unrelieved by physical therapy treatment

Result: The therapist suggested the client get a medical checkup before continuing with physical therapy. Even though the clinical presentation supported shoulder impairment, there were enough red flags and soft signs of systemic distress to warrant further evaluation.

Taking vital signs would have been ideal.

It turns out the client was having myocardial ischemia masquerading as shoulder pain, the flu, and an ear infection. He had an angioplasty with complete resolution of all his symptoms and even reported feeling energetic for the first time in years.

This is a good example of how shoulder pain and dysfunction can exactly mimic a true musculoskeletal problem—even to the extent of reproducing symptoms from a previous condition.

This case highlights the fact that we must be careful to fully assess our clients with each episode of care.

Using a review of symptoms approach and a specific musculoskeletal shoulder examination, the physical therapist can screen to differentiate between a medical pathologic condition and mechanical dysfunction[9] (Case Example 19.7).

Complex Regional Pain Syndrome

CRPS (types I and II) characterized by chronic extremity pain following trauma is sometimes still referred to by the outdated term *shoulder-hand syndrome* (see Case Example 1.5). CRPS-I was formerly known as *reflex sympathetic dystrophy* (RSD). CRPS-II was formerly referred to as *causalgia*.

CRPS was first recognized in the 1800s as causalgia or burning pain in wounded soldiers. Similar presentations after lesser injuries were labeled as RSD.[32] Shoulder-hand syndrome

was a condition that occurred after MI (heart attack), usually after prolonged bed rest. This condition (as it was known then) has been significantly reduced in incidence by more up-to-date and aggressive cardiac rehabilitation programs.

Today, CRPS-I, primarily affecting the limbs, develops after bone fracture or other injury (even slight or minor trauma, venipuncture, or an insect bite) or surgery to the upper extremity (including shoulder arthroplasty) or lower extremity. CRPS-I is characterized by nociceptive pain, whereas CRPS-II is characterized by neuropathic pain.[33] Type I is not associated with a nerve lesion, whereas type II develops after trauma with a nerve lesion.[34,35]

In 2010, authors established diagnostic criteria for CRPS referred to as the Budapest Criteria as the previous established diagnostic criteria led to poor specificity and overdiagnosis by health care professionals.

Table 19.1 The Budapest Criteria. Diagnostic criteria for CRPS as defined by an international consensus meeting held in Budapest

Budapest Criteria: clinical diagnostic criteria for CRPS

Continuing pain, which is disproportionate to any inciting event.

Must report at least one symptom in three of the four following categories:
- Sensory: reports of hyperalgesia and/or allodynia
- Vasomotor: reports of temperature asymmetry and/or skin color changes and/or skin color asymmetry
- Sudomotor/edema: reports of edema and/or sweating changes and/or sweating asymmetry
- Motor/trophic: reports of decreased range of motion and/or motor dysfunction (weakness, tremor, dystonia) and/or trophic changes (hair, nails, skin)

Must display at least one sign at time of evaluation in two or more of the following categories:
- Sensory: evidence of hyperalgesia (to pinprick) and/or allodynia (to light touch and/or deep somatic pressure and/or joint movement)
- Vasomotor: evidence of temperature asymmetry and/or skin color changes and/or asymmetry
- Sudomotor/edema: evidence of edema and/or sweating changes and/or sweating asymmetry
- Motor/trophic: evidence of decreased range of motion and/or motor dysfunction (weakness, tremor, dystonia) and/or trophic changes (hair, nails, skin)

There is no other diagnosis that better explains the signs and symptoms.
- A sign is counted only if it is observed at the time of diagnosis.
- Research criteria for CRPS are recommended that are more specific, but less sensitive than the clinical criteria; they require that four of the symptom categories and at least two sign categories be present.[36]

CRPS-I is associated with extremity fracture,[33] cerebrovascular accident, heart attack, or diseases of the thoracic or abdominal viscera that can refer pain to the shoulder and arm, which is why it is included here instead of in a section on neurologic conditions. CRPS secondary to deep venous

CASE EXAMPLE 19.7

Angina Versus Shoulder Pathology

Referral: A 54-year-old man was referred to physical therapy for preprosthetic training after a left transtibial (TT) amputation.

Past Medical History

A right transtibial amputation was done 4 years ago

Coronary artery disease (CAD) with coronary artery bypass graft (CABG), myocardial infarction (MI) (heart attack), and angina

Peripheral vascular disease (PVD)

Long-standing diabetes mellitus (insulin-dependent ×47 years)

Gastroesophageal reflux disease (GERD)

Clinical Presentation: At the time of the initial evaluation for the left TT amputation, the client reported substernal chest pain and left upper extremity pain with activity. A typical anginal pain pattern was described as substernal chest pain. The pain occurs with exertion and is relieved by rest.

Arm pain has never been a part of his usual anginal pain pattern. He reports his arm pain began 10 months ago with intermittent pain starting in the left shoulder and radiating down the anterior-medial aspect of the arm, halfway between the shoulder and the elbow.

The pain is made worse by raising his left arm overhead, pushing his wheelchair, and using a walker. He was not sure if the shoulder pain was caused by repetitive motion needed for mobility or by his angina. The shoulder pain is relieved by avoiding painful motion. He has not received any treatment for the shoulder problem.

Neurologic screen was negative.

Vital signs

Heart rate:	88 bpm
Blood pressure:	120/66 mm Hg (position and extremity, not recorded)
Respirations:	WNL

Vital signs (after transfer and pregait activities)

Heart rate:	92 bpm
Blood pressure:	152/76 mm Hg
Respirations:	"Minimal shortness of breath" recorded

Special tests

Yergason's sign:	Positive
Apprehension test:	Positive
Relocation test:	Positive
Speed's test:	Positive

Palpation of the biceps and supraspinatus tendons increased the client's shoulder pain.

Active range of motion (AROM): left shoulder

Flexion:	100 degrees
Abduction:	70 degrees
Internal/external rotation:	60 degrees

There is a capsular pattern in the left glenohumeral joint with limitations in rotation and adduction. Significant capsular tightness is demonstrated with passive or physiologic motion (joint play) of the humerus on the glenoid.

Manual muscle test (gross)

Bilateral upper extremity:	4/5 (throughout available active range of motion [AROM])

Review of Systems: Dyspnea, fatigue, sweats with pain; when grouped together, these three symptoms fall under the cardiovascular category; these do not occur at the same time as the shoulder pain.

- **How can you differentiate between medical pathology and mechanical dysfunction as the cause of this client's shoulder pain?**
- **Is a medical referral advised?**
  1. Complete special tests for shoulder impingement, tendinitis, and capsulitis as demonstrated.
  2. Assess for trigger points (TrPs); eliminate TrPs and reassess symptoms.
  3. Carry out a Review of Systems to identify clusters of systemic signs and symptoms. In this case, a small cluster of cardiovascular symptoms was identified.
  4. Correlate symptoms from Review of Systems with shoulder pain (i.e., Do the associated signs and symptoms reported occur along with the shoulder pain or do these two sets of symptoms occur separately from each other?).
  5. Assess the effect of using just the lower extremities on shoulder pain; this was difficult to assess given this client's status as a bilateral amputee without a prosthetic device on the left side.

Result: Test results point to an untreated biceps and supraspinatus tendinitis. This tendinitis combined with adhesive capsulitis most likely accounted for the left shoulder pain. This assessment was based on the decreased left glenohumeral AROM and decreased joint mobility.

With objective clinical findings to support a musculoskeletal dysfunction, medical referral was not required. There were no indications that the shoulder pain was a signal of a change in the client's anginal pattern.

Left shoulder impairments were limiting factors in his mobility and rehabilitation process. Shoulder intervention to alleviate pain and to improve upper extremity strength were included in the plan of care. The desired outcome was to improve transfer and gait activity.

Left shoulder pain resolved within the first week of physical therapy intervention. This gain made it possible to improve ambulation from 3 feet to 50 feet with a walker while wearing a right lower extremity prosthesis.

The client gained independence with bed mobility and supine-to-sit transfers. The client continued to make improvements in ambulation, ROM, and functional mobility.

Physical therapy intervention for the shoulder impairment had a significant effect on the outcomes of this client's rehabilitation program. By differentiating and treating the shoulder movement dysfunction, the intervention enabled the client to progress faster in the transfer and gait training program than he would have had his left shoulder pain been attributed to angina.[9]

Data from Smith ML: Differentiating angina and shoulder pathology pain, *Phys Ther Case Rep* 1(4):210–212, 1998.

thrombosis (DVT) has also been reported. Individuals developing limb pain and edema after DVT will need further diagnostic investigation to differentiate the cause of symptoms.[37]

Shoulder, arm, or hand pain and ischemia (usually acute) associated with CRPS that develop without a history of trauma may be attributed to cardiac embolism.[38] Structural cardiac causes of upper limb ischemia include a wide variety of conditions (e.g., atrial fibrillation, cardiomyopathy, prosthetic valve, endocarditis, atrial septal defects, aortic dissection).[39]

This syndrome occurs with equal frequency in either or both shoulders, and, except when caused by coronary occlusion, is most common in women.[40] The shoulder is generally involved first, but the painful hand may precede the painful shoulder.

When this condition occurs after MI, the shoulder may initially demonstrate pericapsulitis. Tenderness around the shoulder is diffuse and not localized to a specific tendon or bursal area. The duration of the initial shoulder stage before the hand component begins is extremely variable. The shoulder may be "stiff" for several months before the hand becomes involved or both may become stiff simultaneously. Other accompanying signs and symptoms are usually present, such as edema, skin (trophic) changes, and vasomotor (temperature, hidrosis) changes.

Thoracic Outlet Syndrome

Compression of the neurovascular bundle consisting of the brachial plexus and subclavian artery and vein (see Fig. 17.10) can cause a variety of symptoms affecting the arm, hand,

---

CLINICAL SIGNS AND SYMPTOMS

Complex Regional Pain Syndrome (Type I)

Stage I (acute, lasting several weeks)
- Pain described as burning, aching, throbbing
- Sensitivity to touch
- Swelling
- Muscle spasm
- Stiffness, loss of motion and function
- Skin changes (warm, red, dry skin changes to cold [cyanotic], sweaty skin)
- Accelerated hair growth (usually dark hair in patches)

Stage II (subacute, lasting 3 to 6 months)
- Severity of pain increases
- Swelling may spread; tissue goes from soft to boggy to firm
- Muscle atrophy
- Skin becomes cool, pale, bluish, sweaty
- Change in nail beds (cracked, grooved, ridges)
- Bone demineralization (early onset of osteoporosis)

Stage III (chronic, lasting more than 6 months)
- Pain may remain the same, improve, or get worse; variable
- Irreversible tissue damage
- Muscle atrophy and contracture
- Skin becomes thin and shiny
- Nails are brittle
- Osteoporosis

---

shoulder girdle, neck, and chest (Case Example 19.8). Risk factors and clinical presentation are discussed more completely in Chapter 17.

Bacterial Endocarditis

The most common musculoskeletal symptom in clients with bacterial endocarditis is arthralgia, generally in the proximal joints.[41] The shoulder is affected most often, followed (in declining incidence) by the knee, hip, wrist, ankle, metatarsophalangeal and metacarpophalangeal joints, and by acromioclavicular involvement.

Most clients with endocarditis-related arthralgia have only one or two painful joints, although some may have pain in several joints.[41] Painful symptoms begin suddenly in one or two joints, accompanied by warmth, tenderness, and redness. One helpful clue: As a rule, morning stiffness is not as prevalent in clients with endocarditis as it is in those with RA or polymyalgia rheumatica.

Pericarditis

The inflammatory process accompanying pericarditis may result in an accumulation of fluid in the pericardial sac, preventing the heart from expanding fully. The subsequent chest pain of pericarditis (see Fig. 7.10) closely mimics that of MI because it is substernal, is associated with cough, and may radiate to the shoulder.[42] Pericarditis chest pain can be differentiated from an MI by the pattern of relieving and aggravating factors.

For example, pericarditis pain is sharp and relieved by leaning over when seated. If there is irritation of the diaphragm, it can cause shoulder pain. The pain of MI is unaffected by position, breathing, or movement, whereas the chest and shoulder pain associated with pericarditis may be relieved by kneeling with hands on the floor, leaning forward, or sitting upright. Pericardial pain is often made worse by deep breathing, swallowing, or belching.

Aortic Aneurysm

Aortic aneurysm appears as sudden, severe chest pain with a tearing sensation (see Fig. 7.11), and the pain may extend to the neck, shoulders, low back, or abdomen but rarely to the joints and arms, which distinguishes it from MI.

Isolated shoulder pain is not associated with aortic aneurysm; shoulder pain (usually left shoulder) occurs when the primary pain pattern radiates up and over the trapezius and upper arm(s) (see Fig. 7.11).[43] The client may report a bounding or throbbing pulse (heartbeat) in the abdomen. Risk factors and other associated signs and symptoms help distinguish this condition.

Deep Venous Thrombosis of the Upper Extremity

DVT of the upper extremity is not as common as in the lower extremity, but incidence may be on the rise because

CASE EXAMPLE 19.8

House Painter

Referral: A 44-year-old female referred herself to physical therapy for a 2-month-long history of right upper trapezius and right shoulder pain. She works as a house painter and thinks the symptoms came on after a difficult job with high ceilings.

She reports new symptoms of dizziness when getting up too fast from bed or a chair. She is seeing a chiropractor and a naturopathic physician for a previous back injury 2 years ago when she fell off a ladder.

She wants to try physical therapy because she has reached a "plateau" with her chiropractic care.

Past Medical History: Other significant past medical history includes a total hysterectomy 4 years ago for unexplained heavy menstrual bleeding. She does not smoke or use tobacco products but admits smoking marijuana occasionally and being a "social drinker" (wine coolers and beer on the weekends or at barbeques).

She is nulliparous (never pregnant). She is not taking any medication, except ibuprofen as needed for headaches. She takes a variety of nutritional supplements given to her by the naturopath. No recent history of infection or illness.

Clinical Presentation: There is no numbness or tingling anywhere in her body. No change in vision, balance, or hearing. The client reports normal bowel and bladder function. Neurologic screen was within normal limits (WNL).

Postural screen:	Moderate forward head position, rounded shoulders, arms held in a position of shoulder internal rotation, minimal lumbar lordosis
Temporomandibular joint (TMJ) screen:	Negative
Vertebral artery tests:	Negative
Upper extremity (UE) range of motion (ROM):	Limited right shoulder internal rotation; all other motions in both UEs were full and pain-free
Spurling's test:	Negative
Cervical spine mobility test:	Restriction of the left C4-C5; no apparent cervical instabilities; tenderness along the entire right cervical spine with mild hypertonus
Trigger points (TrPs):	Positive for right sternocleidomastoid, right upper trapezius, and right levator scapula TrPs

Are there any red flags to suggest the need to screen for medical disease? What other tests (if any) would you like to do before making this decision?

- Age
- Unexplained dizziness
- Failure to progress with chiropractic care
- Surgical menopause and nulliparity (both increase her risk for breast cancer; early menopause puts her at risk for osteoporosis and accelerated atherosclerosis/heart disease)

Assessment: It is likely the client's symptoms are directly related to postural overuse. Long hours with her arms overhead may be contributing factors. A more complete examination for thoracic outlet syndrome (TOS) is warranted. Physical therapy intervention can be initiated, but must be reevaluated on an ongoing basis. Eliminating the TrPs, improving her posture, and restoring full shoulder and neck motion will aid in the differential diagnosis.

The therapist should assess vital signs, including blood pressure measurements in both arms (looking for a vascular component of TOS) and from supine to sit to stand to assess for postural orthostatic hypotension. True postural hypotension must be accompanied by both blood pressure and pulse rate changes.

Depending on the results, medical evaluation may be warranted, especially if no underlying cause can be found for the dizziness. Although there is no reported change in her vision or loss of balance with the dizziness, a vestibular screening examination is warranted.

Given her age and risk factors, she should be asked when her last physical examination was done. If she has not been seen since her hysterectomy or within the last 12 months, she should be advised to see her physician for follow-up.

She should be encouraged to exercise regularly (more education can be provided depending on her level of knowledge and the therapist's level of expertise in this area).

If baseline bone density studies have not been done, then she should pursue this now. Likewise, she should ask her doctor about baseline testing for thyroid, glucose, and lipid values if these are not already available.

In a primary care practice, risk factor assessment is a key factor in knowing when to carry out a screening evaluation. Patient education about personal health choices is also essential.

In any practice, we must know what effect a medical condition can have on the neuromuscular and musculoskeletal systems and watch for any links between the visceral and somatic systems.

---

of the increasing use of peripherally inserted central catheters (PICC lines) or central venous catheters (CVCs).[44,45] Thrombosis affects the subclavian vein, axillary vein, or both most often with less common sites being the internal jugular and brachial veins.[46]

CVCs are frequently used in individuals with hematologic/oncologic disorders to administer drugs, stem cell infusions, blood products, parenteral alimentation, and blood sampling. Other risk factors include a blood clotting disorder,[47] clavicle fracture,[48] insertion of pacemaker wires, and arthroscopy of the shoulder or reconstructive shoulder arthroplasty.[49,50] Thrombosis is the second leading cause of death in cancer patients, and cancer is a major risk factor of venous thromboembolism, as a result of activation of coagulation, use of long-term CVC, and the thrombogenic effects of chemotherapy and antiangiogenic drugs.[51]

Symptoms (when present) are similar to those of the lower extremity (see discussion in Chapter 7). The therapist should be aware of the presence of any risk factors and watch for pain and pitting edema or swelling of the entire (usually upper) limb and/or an area of the limb that is 2 cm or more larger than the surrounding area indicating swelling requiring further investigation.

Other symptoms include redness or warmth of the arm, dilated veins, or low-grade fever possibly accompanied by chills and malaise. Bruising or discoloration of the area or proximal to the thrombosis has been observed in some cases.[52] Swelling can contribute to decreased neck or shoulder motion. Severe thromboses can cause superior vena cava syndrome; symptoms include edema of the face and arm, vertigo, and dyspnea.[53]

Unfortunately, the first clinical manifestation of *deep* thrombosis may be pulmonary embolism (PE; see also Box 6.2 for overall risk factors for DVT and PE). Superficial venous thrombosis is usually self-limiting and does not cause PE because the blood flow to deeper veins occurs through small perforating venous channels.[54]

PE as a consequence of upper extremity DVT can be fatal.[50] Chronic venous insufficiency or postthrombotic syndrome are possible sequelae to upper extremity DVT, similar to lower extremity.[52,55]

To our knowledge, at this time, a validated screening tool, such as the Wells' Clinical Decision Rule for DVT, has not been investigated for the upper extremity. A simple model to predict upper extremity DVT has also been proposed and remains under investigation (Table 19.3).[56,57] The best available test for the diagnosis of upper extremity DVT is contrast venography; color Doppler ultrasonography may be preferred for some people because it is noninvasive.[58]

CLINICAL SIGNS AND SYMPTOMS

Upper Extremity Deep Venous Thrombosis

- Numbness or heaviness of the extremity
- Itching, burning, coldness of the extremity
- Swelling, discoloration, warmth, or redness of the extremity; pitting edema
- Limited range of motion (ROM) of neck, shoulder
- Low-grade fever, chills, malaise
- For individuals with a PICC line (in addition to any of the signs and symptoms just listed):
- Pain or tenderness at or above the insertion site

SCREENING FOR RENAL CAUSES OF UPPER QUADRANT/SHOULDER PAIN

The anatomic position of the kidneys (and ureters) is in front of and on both sides of the vertebral column at the level of T11 to L3. The right kidney is usually lower than the left.[59] The lower portions of the kidneys and the ureters extend below the ribs and are separated from the abdominal cavity by the peritoneal membrane. Due to its location in the posterior upper abdominal cavity in the retroperitoneal space and touching the diaphragm, the upper urinary tract can refer pain to the (ipsilateral) shoulder on the same side as the involved kidney.

Renal sensory innervation is not completely understood; the capsule (covering of the kidney) and the lower portions of the collecting system seem to cause pain with stretching (distention) or puncture. Information transmitted by renal

TABLE 19.3	Possible Predictors of Upper Extremity Deep Venous Thrombosis*		
Independent Variable		**Absent**	**Present**
Venous material (catheter or access device in subclavian or jugular vein; pacemaker)		0	1.0
Localized pain		0	1.0
Unilateral pitting edema		0	1.0
Other diagnosis at least as plausible (negative association)		0	–1.0

*Concepts presented here are based on one preliminary study validated in a second sample but with a limited patient population; diagnosis was confirmed with ultrasound study.[56]

NOTE: As with lower extremity deep venous thrombosis (DVT), a low clinical probability does not exclude the diagnosis of upper extremity DVT. The scoring provides a tool to use in determining the need for additional testing (e.g., ultrasonography, venography).

Key: Total score of:
–1.0 or 0: Low probability of upper extremity DVT
1: Intermediate probability
2–3: High probability

and ureteral pain receptors is relayed by sympathetic nerves that enter the spinal cord at T10 to L1; therefore, renal and ureteral pain is typically felt in the posterior subcostal and costovertebral regions (flank).[60–62]

Renal pain is aching and dull but can occasionally be a severe, boring type of pain. The distention or stretching of the renal capsule, pelvis, or collecting system from intrarenal fluid accumulation (e.g., inflammatory edema, an inflamed or bleeding cyst, and a bleeding or neoplastic growth) accounts for the constant, dull, and aching quality of reported pain. Ischemia of renal tissue caused by blockage of blood flow to the kidneys can produce either a *constant dull* or *sharp* pain. True renal pain is seldom affected by change in position or movements of the shoulder or spine.

If the diaphragm becomes irritated because of pressure from a renal lesion, ipsilateral shoulder pain can be the only symptom or may occur in conjunction with other pain and associated signs and symptoms. For example, generalized abdominal pain may develop accompanied by nausea, vomiting, and impaired intestinal motility (progressing to intestinal paralysis) when pain is acute and severe. Nerve fibers from the renal plexus are also in direct communication with the spermatic plexus, and because of this close relationship, testicular pain may also accompany renal pain in males.[63]

Elevation in temperature or a change in color, odor, or amount of urine (flow, frequency, nocturia) presenting with shoulder pain should be reported to a physician. Shoulder pain that is not affected by movement or provocation tests requires a closer look.

The presence of constitutional symptoms, constant pain (even if dull), and failure to change the symptoms with a position change will also alert the therapist to the need for a more thorough screening examination. A past medical history of cancer is always an important risk factor requiring careful assessment. This is true even when patients/clients have a known or traumatic cause for their symptoms.

Flank pain combined with unexplained weight loss, fever, pain, and hematuria should be reported to the physician. The presence of any amount of blood in the urine always requires referral to a physician for further diagnostic evaluation because this is a primary symptom of urinary tract neoplasm.

Additionally, therapists need to be cognizant that those at high risk for chronic renal disease with an associated neuropathy include anyone with diabetes mellitus and those with history of significant nonsteroidal antiinflammatory drug (NSAID) or acetaminophen use.[64]

SCREENING FOR GASTROINTESTINAL CAUSES OF SHOULDER PAIN

Upper abdominal or GI problems with diaphragmatic irritation can refer pain to the ipsilateral shoulder. A perforated gastric or duodenal ulcer, gallbladder disease, and hiatal hernia are the most likely GI causes of shoulder pain seen in the physical therapy clinic. Usually there are associated signs and symptoms, such as nausea, vomiting, anorexia, melena, or early satiety, but the client may not connect the shoulder pain with a GI disorder. A few screening questions may be all that is needed to uncover any coincident GI symptoms.

The therapist should look for a history of previous ulcer, especially in association with the use of NSAIDs. Shoulder pain that is worse 2 to 4 hours after taking the NSAID can be suggestive of GI bleeding and is considered a yellow (caution) flag. With a true musculoskeletal problem, peak NSAID dosage (usually 2 to 4 hours after ingestion; variable with each drug) should reduce or alleviate painful shoulder symptoms. Any pain increase instead of decrease may be a symptom of GI bleeding.

The therapist must also ask about the effect of eating on shoulder pain. If eating makes shoulder pain better or worse (anywhere from 30 minutes to 2 hours after eating), there may be a GI problem. The client may not be aware of the link between these two events until the therapist asks. If the client is not sure, the therapist needs to follow-up with questioning at a future appointment if the client has noticed any unusual symptoms or connection between eating and shoulder pain.

SCREENING FOR LIVER AND BILIARY CAUSES OF SHOULDER/UPPER QUADRANT SYMPTOMS

As with many of the organ systems in the human body, the hepatic and biliary organs (liver, gallbladder, and common bile duct) can develop diseases that mimic primary musculoskeletal lesions.

The musculoskeletal symptoms associated with hepatic and biliary pathologic conditions are generally confined to the midback, scapular, and right shoulder regions. These musculoskeletal symptoms can occur alone (as the only presenting symptom) or in combination with other systemic signs and symptoms. Fortunately, in most cases of shoulder pain referred from visceral processes, shoulder motion is not compromised and local tenderness is not a prominent feature.

Diagnostic interviewing is especially helpful when clients have avoided medical treatment for so long that shoulder pain caused by a hepatic and/or biliary disease may in turn create a biomechanical change in muscular contraction and shoulder movement. These changes eventually create pain of a biomechanical nature.[65]

Referred shoulder pain may be the only presenting symptom of a hepatic or biliary disease. Sympathetic fibers from the biliary system are connected through the celiac and splanchnic plexuses to the hepatic fibers in the region of the dorsal spine. These connections account for the intercostal and radiating interscapular pain that accompanies gallbladder disease (see Fig. 10.11). Although the innervation is bilateral, most of the biliary fibers reach the cord through the right splanchnic nerves, producing pain in the right shoulder.

Carpal Tunnel Syndrome

There are many potential causes of carpal tunnel syndrome (CTS), both musculoskeletal and systemic (see Table 12.2). Careful evaluation is required (see Box 10.1). The presence of bilateral CTS warrants a closer look. For example, liver dysfunction resulting in increased serum ammonia and urea levels can result in impaired peripheral nerve function.

Ammonia from the intestine (produced by protein breakdown) is normally transformed by the liver to urea, glutamine, and asparagine, which are then excreted by the renal system. When the liver does not detoxify ammonia, ammonia is transported to the brain, where it reacts with glutamate (excitatory neurotransmitter), producing glutamine.

The reduction of brain glutamate impairs neurotransmission, leading to altered central nervous system metabolism and function. Asterixis and numbness/tingling (misinterpreted as CTS) can occur as a result of this ammonia abnormality, causing an intrinsic pathologic nerve condition (see Case Example 9.1).

- For any client presenting with bilateral CTS:
- Ask about the presence of similar symptoms in the feet
- Ask about a personal history of liver or hepatic disease (e.g., cirrhosis, cancer, hepatitis)
- Look for a history of hepatotoxic drugs (see Box 10.3)
- Look for a history of alcoholism
- Ask about current or previous use of statins (cholesterol-lowering drugs such as Crestor, Lipitor, Lovastatin, or Zocor)
- Look for other signs and symptoms associated with liver impairment (see Clinical Signs and Symptoms of Liver Disease in Chapter 10)
- Test for signs of liver disease:
  - Change in skin color
  - Spider angioma (see Fig. 10.5)
  - Palmar erythema (live palms; see Fig. 10.6)
  - Change in nail beds (e.g., white nails of Terry, white bands, clubbing; see Fig. 10.7)
  - Asterixis (liver flap; see Fig. 10.8)

SCREENING FOR RHEUMATIC CAUSES OF SHOULDER PAIN

Some systemic rheumatic diseases can appear as shoulder pain, even as unilateral shoulder pain. The HLA-B27–associated spondyloarthropathies (diseases of the joints of the spine), such as ankylosing spondylitis, most frequently involve the SI joints and spine. Involvement of large central joints, such as the hip and shoulder, is common, however.

RA and its variants, likewise, frequently involve the shoulder girdle. These systemic rheumatic diseases are suggested by the details of the shoulder examination, by coincident systemic complaints of malaise and easy fatigability, and by complaints of discomfort in other joints either coincidental with the presenting shoulder complaint or in the past.

Other systemic rheumatic diseases with major shoulder involvement include polymyalgia rheumatica and polymyositis (inflammatory disease of the muscles). Both may be somewhat asymmetric but almost always appear with bilateral involvement and impressive systemic symptoms.

SCREENING FOR INFECTIOUS CAUSES OF SHOULDER PAIN

The most likely infectious causes of shoulder pain in a physical therapy practice include infectious (septic) arthritis (see discussion in Chapter 3 and also Box 3.6), osteomyelitis, and infectious mononucleosis (mono). Immunosuppression for any reason puts people of all ages at risk for infection (Case Example 19.9).

CASE EXAMPLE 19.9
Osteomyelitis

Referral: SC, an active 62-year-old cardiac nurse, was referred by her orthopedic surgeon for "PT [for] possible rotator cuff tear (RCT), three times a week for 4 weeks." SC reported an "open" magnetic resonance imaging (MRI) was negative for RCT and plain films were also negative. She noted that laboratory testing was not done.

Past Medical History
Medications: Current medications included Motrin 800 mg tid for pain; Decadron 0.75 mg qid for atypical dermatitis and asthma (45-year use of corticosteroids); Avapro 75 mg qid to control hypertension; HydroDIURIL 25 mg qid to counteract fluid retention from corticosteroids; and Chlor-Trimeton 12 mg qid to suppress the high level of blood histamine resulting from the long-term comorbid condition of atypical dermatitis and asthma.

Social History: The client consumes one glass of wine per day, quit smoking 20 years ago, and has never done illicit drugs.

Clinical Presentation
Pain Pattern: The client presented with primary complaints of severe and limiting pain of nearly 4 weeks' duration with any active movement at her left shoulder and at rest. Her pain was rated on the visual analog scale (VAS) as 7/10 at rest and 9/10 to 10/10 with motion at the glenohumeral (GH) joint. Pain onset was gradual over 3 days; she was not aware of injury or trauma.

She reported an inability to (1) use her left upper extremity (UE); (2) lie on or bear weight on left side; (3) perform activities of daily living (ADLs); (4) sleep uninterrupted because of pain, awakening four or five times nightly; or (5) participate in regular weekly yoga classes.

Vital Signs: Temperature: 37° C (98.6° F.); blood pressure: 120/98 mm Hg. SC reported that her medication combination of Decadron and Chlor-Trimeton had been implicated in the past by her physician as acting to suppress low-grade fevers.

Observation: Slight puffiness, minimal swelling observed in the left supraclavicular area. SC holds left UE at her side with the elbow flexed to 90 degrees and the shoulder held in internal rotation.

Standing Posture: Forward head position with increased cervical spine lordosis and thoracic spine kyphosis; inability to attain neutral or reverse either spinal curve.

Palpation revealed exquisite tenderness at distal clavicle and both anterior and posterior aspects of proximal humerus.

Cervical Spine Screen: Spurling's compression, distraction, and Cervical Quadrant testing were all negative; deep tendon reflexes (DTRs) at C5, C6, and C7 were symmetrically increased bilaterally; dermatomal testing was within normal limits (WNL); myotomes could not be reliably tested because of pain.

Special tests at the shoulder could not be performed or were unreliable because of pain limitation.

Range of motion (ROM): Left glenohumeral (GH) joint active ROM (AROM) and passive ROM (PROM) were severely limited. AROM: unable to actively perform flexion or abduction at left shoulder. PROM left shoulder (measured in supine with arm at side and elbow flexed to 90 degrees):

Flexion:	35 degrees
Abduction:	35 degrees
Internal rotation:	50 degrees
External rotation:	−10 degrees

All ranges were pain limited with an "empty" end feel.

Evaluation/Assessment: SC's signs, symptoms, and examination findings were consistent with those of a severe, full-thickness RCT, including severity of pain and functional loss with empty end feel at GH joint ROM. However, the inability to perform special tests limited the certainty of the RCT diagnosis.

Red flags included age over 50 years, severe loss of motion with empty end feel, constancy and severity of pain, inability to relieve pain or obtain a comfortable position, bony tenderness, and insidious onset of the condition. Additional risk factors included long-term use of corticosteroids to treat atypical dermatitis with asthma.

Based on the objective examination findings, including swelling, bone tenderness, along with the severity and unrelenting nature of her pain, the presence of a more serious underlying systemic medical condition was considered (in addition to a possible unconfirmed RCT).

Associated Signs and Symptoms: SC denied fever, chills, night sweats, pain in other joints or bones, weight loss, abdominal pain, nausea or vomiting.

Outcomes: The client made very little progress after the prescribed physical therapy intervention. The severity of pain and functional loss remained unchanged. Numerous attempts were made by the client and the therapist to discuss this case with the referring physician. The client eventually referred herself to a second physician.

Result: The client was diagnosed with osteomyelitis as a result of repeat MRI, a triple-phase bone scan, and laboratory test results of elevated levels of erythrocyte sedimentation rate (ESR) and C-reactive protein (CRP) values. A surgical biopsy confirmed the diagnosis. She underwent three different surgical procedures culminating in a total shoulder arthroplasty (TSA) along with repair of the full-thickness RCT.

From West PR: Case report presented in fulfillment of DPT 910, Institute for Physical Therapy Education, Widener University, Chester, PA, 2005. Used with permission.

Septic arthritis of the acromioclavicular joint or hand can present as insidious onset of shoulder pain. Likewise, septic arthritis of the sternoclavicular joint can present as chest pain. Usually, there is local tenderness at the affected joint. A possible history of intravenous drug use, diabetes mellitus, trauma (puncture wound, surgery, human or animal bite), and infection is usually present. Punching someone in the mouth (hand coming in contact with teeth resulting in a puncture wound) has been reported as a potential cause of septic arthritis. With infection of this type, there may or may not be constitutional symptoms.[66,67]

Osteomyelitis (bone or bone marrow infection) is caused most commonly by *Staphylococcus aureus*. Children under 6 months of age are most likely to be affected by *Haemophilus influenzae* or *Streptococcus*. Hematogenous spread from a wound, abscess, or systemic infection (e.g., fracture, TB, urinary tract infection, upper respiratory infection, finger felons) occurs most often. Osteomyelitis of the spine is associated with injection drug use.

Onset of clinical signs and symptoms is usually gradual in adults but may be more sudden in children with high fever, chills, and inability to bear weight through the affected joint. In all ages, there is marked tenderness over the site of the infection when the affected bone is superficial (e.g., spinous process, distal femur, proximal tibia). The most reliable way to recognize infection is the presence of both local and systemic symptoms.[68]

Mononucleosis is a viral infection that affects the respiratory tract, liver, and spleen. Splenomegaly with subsequent rupture is a rare but serious cause of left shoulder pain (Kehr's sign).[69] There is usually left upper abdominal pain and, in many cases, trauma to the enlarged spleen (e.g., sports injury) is the precipitating cause in an athlete with an unknown or undiagnosed case of mono. Palpation of the upper left abdomen may reveal an enlarged and tender spleen (see Fig. 4.53).

The virus can be present 4 to 10 weeks before any symptoms develop, so the person may not know mono is present. Acute symptoms can include sore throat, headache, fatigue, lymphadenopathy, fever, myalgia, and sometimes, skin rash. Enlarged tonsils can cause noisy or difficult breathing. When asking about the presence of other associated signs and symptoms (current or recent past), the therapist may hear a report of some or all of these signs and symptoms.

SCREENING FOR ONCOLOGIC CAUSES OF SHOULDER PAIN

A past medical history of cancer anywhere in the body with new onset of back or shoulder pain (or impairment) is a red-flag finding. Brachial plexus radiculopathy can occur in either or both arms with cancer metastasized to the lymphatics (Case Example 19.10).

Questions about visceral function are relevant when the pattern for malignant invasion at the shoulder emerges. Invasion of the upper humerus and glenoid area by secondary

---

CASE EXAMPLE 19.10
Upper Extremity Radiculopathy

Referral: A 72-year-old woman was referred to physical therapy by her neurologist with a diagnosis of "nerve entrapment" for a postural exercise program and home traction. She was experiencing symptoms of left shoulder pain with numbness and tingling in the ulnar nerve distribution. She had a moderate forward head posture with slumped shoulders and loss of height from known osteoporosis.

Past Medical History: The woman's past medical history was significant for right breast cancer treated with a radical mastectomy and chemotherapy 20 years ago. She had a second cancer (uterine) 10 years ago that was considered separate from her previous breast cancer.

Clinical Presentation: The physical therapy examination was consistent with the physician's diagnosis of nerve entrapment in a classic presentation. There were significant postural components to account for the development of symptoms. However, the therapist palpated several large masses in the axillary and supraclavicular fossa on both the right and left sides. There was no local warmth, redness, or tenderness associated with these lesions. The therapist requested permission to palpate the client's groin and popliteal spaces for any other suspicious lymph nodes. The rest of the examination findings were within normal limits.

Associated Signs and Symptoms: Further questioning about the presence of associated signs and symptoms revealed a significant disturbance in sleep pattern over the last 6 months with unrelenting shoulder and neck pain. There were no other reported constitutional symptoms, skin changes, or noted lumps anywhere. Vital signs were unremarkable at the time of the physical therapy evaluation.

Result: Returning this client to her referring physician was a difficult decision to make because the therapist did not have the benefit of the medical records or results of the neurologic examination and testing. Given the significant past medical history for cancer, the woman's age, presence of progressive night pain, and palpable masses, no other reasonable choice remained. When asked if the physician had seen or felt the masses, the client responded with a definite "no."

There are several ways to approach handling a situation like this one, depending on the physical therapist's relationship with the physician. In this case, the therapist had never communicated with this physician before. A telephone call was made to ask the clerical staff to check the physician's office notes (the client had provided written permission for disclosure of medical records to the therapist).

It is possible that the physician was aware of the masses, knew from medical testing that there was extensive cancer, and chose to treat the client palliatively. Because there was no indication of such, the therapist notified the physician's staff of the decision to return the client to the physician. A brief (one-page) written report summarizing the findings was given to the client to hand-carry to the physician's office.

Further medical testing was performed, and a medical diagnosis of lymphoma was made.

malignant deposits affects the joint and the adjacent muscles (Case Example 19.11).

Muscle wasting is greater than expected with arthritis and follows a bizarre pattern that does not conform to any one neurologic lesion or any one muscle. Localized warmth felt at any part of the scapular area may prove to be the first sign of a malignant deposit eroding bone. Within 1 or 2 weeks after this observation, a palpable tumor will have appeared, and erosion of bone will be visible on x-ray films.[70]

Primary Bone Neoplasm

Bone cancer occurs chiefly in young people, in whom a cause-less limitation of movement of the shoulder leads the physician to order radiographs. If the tumor originates from the shaft of the humerus, the first symptoms may be a feeling of "pins and needles" in the hand, associated with guarding and leading to limitation of movement at the elbow (Case Example 19.12).

CASE EXAMPLE 19.11
Shoulder and Leg Pain

Referral: A 33-year-old woman came to a physical therapy clinic located inside a large health club. She reported right shoulder and right lower leg pain that is keeping her from exercising. She could walk but had an antalgic gait secondary to pain during weight-bearing.

She linked these symptoms with heavy household chores. She could think of no other trauma or injury. She was screened for the possibility of domestic violence with negative results.

Past Medical History: There was no past history of disease, illness, trauma, or surgery. There were no other symptoms reported (e.g., no fever, nausea, fatigue, bowel or bladder changes, sleep disturbance).

Clinical Presentation: The right shoulder and right leg were visibly and palpably swollen. Any and all (global) motions of either the arm or the leg were painful. The skin was tender to light touch in a wide band of distribution around the painful sites. No redness or skin changes of any kind were noted.

Pain prevented strength testing or assessment of muscle weakness. There was no sign of scoliosis. Trendelenburg test was negative, bilaterally. Functionally, she was able to climb stairs and walk, but these and other activities (e.g., exercising, biking, household chores) were limited by pain.

How do you screen this client for systemic or medical disease?

You may have done as much screening as is possible. Pain is limiting any further testing. Assessing vital signs may provide some helpful information.

She has denied any past medical history to link with these symptoms. Her age may be a red flag in that she is young. Bone pain with these symptoms in a 33-year-old is a red flag for bone pathology and needs to be investigated medically.

Immediate medical referral is advised.

Result: X-ray films of the right shoulder showed destruction of the right humeral head consistent with a diagnosis of metastatic disease. X-ray films of the right leg showed two lytic lesions. There was no sign of fracture or dislocation. Computed tomography (CT) scans showed destructive lytic lesions in the ribs and ilium.

Additional testing was performed, including laboratory values, bone biopsy, mammography, and pelvic ultrasonography. The client was diagnosed with bone tumors secondary to hyperparathyroidism.

A large adenoma was found and removed from the left inferior parathyroid gland. Medical treatment resulted in decreased pain and increased motion and function over 3 to 4 months. Physical therapy intervention was prescribed for residual muscle weakness.

Data from Insler H: Shoulder and leg pain in a 33-year-old woman, *J Musculoskel Med* 14(6)36–37, 1997.

CASE EXAMPLE 19.12
Osteosarcoma

Referral: A 14-year-old boy presented to a physical therapist at a sports medicine clinic with a complaint of left shoulder pain that had been present off and on for the last 4 months. There was no reported history of injury or trauma despite active play on the regional soccer team.

Past Medical History: He has seen his pediatrician for this on several occasions. It was diagnosed as "tendinitis" with the suggestion to see a physical therapist of the family's choice. No x rays or other diagnostic imaging was performed to date. The client could not remember if any laboratory work (blood or urinalysis) had been done.

The client reports that his arm feels "heavy." Movement has become more difficult just in the last week. The only other symptom present was intermittent tingling in the left hand. There is no other pertinent medical history.

Clinical Presentation: Physical examination of the shoulder revealed moderate loss of active motion in shoulder flexion, abduction, and external rotation with an empty end feel and pain during passive range of motion (ROM). There was no pain with palpation or isometric resistance of the rotator cuff tendons. Gross strength of the upper extremity was 4/5 for all motions.

There was a palpable firm, soft, but fixed mass along the lateral proximal humerus. The client reported it was "tender" when the therapist applied moderate palpatory pressure. The client was not previously aware of this lump.

Upper extremity pulses, deep tendon reflexes, and sensation were all intact. There were no observed skin changes or palpable temperature changes. Because this was an active athlete with left shoulder pain, screening for Kehr's sign was carried out but was negative.

What are the red flags?
- Age
- Suspicious palpable lesion (likely not present at previous medical evaluation)
- Lack of medical diagnostics
- Unusual clinical presentation for tendinitis with loss of motion and empty end feel but intact rotator cuff

Result: The therapist telephoned the physician's office to report possible changes since the physician's last examination. The family was advised by the doctor's office staff to bring him to the clinic as a walk-in the same day. X-ray studies showed an irregular bony mass of the humeral head and surrounding soft tissues. The biopsy confirmed a diagnosis of osteogenic sarcoma. The cancer had already metastasized to the lungs and liver.

Pulmonary (Secondary) Neoplasm

Occasionally, the client requires medical referral because shoulder pain is referred from metastatic lung cancer. When the shoulder is examined, the client is unable to lift the arm beyond the horizontal position. Muscles respond with spasm that limits joint movement.

If the neoplasm interferes with the diaphragm, diaphragmatic pain (remember the saying "C3, 4, 5: stay alive!") is often felt at the shoulder with each breath (at the fourth cervical dermatome [i.e., at the deltoid area]), in correspondence with the main embryologic derivation of the diaphragm.[71] Pain arising from the part of the pleura that is not in contact with the diaphragm is also brought on by respiration but is felt in the chest.

Although the lung is insensitive, large tumors invading the chest wall set up local pain and cause spasm of the pectoralis major muscle, with consequent shoulder pain and/or limitation of elevation of the arm.[72] If the neoplasm encroaches on the ribs, stretching the muscle attached to the ribs leads to sympathetic spasm of the pectoralis major. By contrast, the scapula is mobile, and a full range of passive movement is present at the shoulder joint.

Pancoast's Tumor

Pancoast's tumors of the lung apex usually do not cause symptoms if confined to the pulmonary parenchyma. Shoulder pain occurs if they extend into the surrounding structures, infiltrating the chest wall into the axilla. Occasionally, brachial plexus involvement (eighth cervical and first thoracic nerve) presents with radiculopathy.[73] See Fig. 19.3 for Pancoast's tumor.

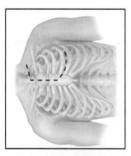

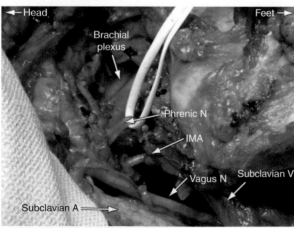

Fig. 19.3 Pancoast's tumors are often found in the apical portion of the lung. Depending on the size, one can appreciate the disruption of the brachial plexus as well as vascular supply to the upper extremity. (From Zwischenberger JB. *Atlas of Thoracic Surgical Techniques*, ed 1, 2010, Saunders.)

This nerve involvement produces sharp neuritic pain in the axilla, shoulder, and subscapular area on the affected side, with eventual atrophy of the upper extremity muscles. Bone pain is aching, exacerbated at night, and a cause of restlessness and musculoskeletal movement.[74]

Usually, general associated systemic signs and symptoms are present (e.g., sore throat, fever, hoarseness, unexplained weight loss, productive cough with blood in the sputum). These features are not found in any regional musculoskeletal disorder, including such disorders of the shoulder.

For example, a similar pain pattern caused by trigger points (TrPs) of the serratus anterior can be differentiated from a neoplasm by a lack of true neurologic findings (indicating TrP) or by lack of improvement after treatment to eliminate the TrP (indicating neoplasm).

Breast Cancer

Breast cancer or breast cancer recurrence is always a consideration with upper quadrant pain or shoulder dysfunction (Case Example 19.13). The therapist must know what to look for when it comes to red flags associated with cancer recurrence versus delayed effects of cancer treatment. See Chapter 13 for a complete discussion of cancer screening and prevention. Breast cancer is discussed in Chapter 17.

CASE EXAMPLE 19.13

Breast Cancer

Referral: A 53-year-old woman with severe adhesive capsulitis was referred to a physical therapist by an orthopedic surgeon. A physical therapy program was initiated. When the client's shoulder flexion and abduction allowed for sufficient movement to place the client's hand under her head in the supine position, ultrasound to the area of capsular redundancy before joint mobilization was added to the treatment protocol.

During the treatment procedure, the client was dressed in a hospital gown wrapped under the axilla on the involved side. With the client in the supine position, the upper outer quadrant of breast tissue was visible and the physical therapist observed skin puckering (peau d'orange) accompanied by a reddened area.

Result: It is always necessary to approach situations like this one carefully to avoid embarrassing or alarming the client. In this case the therapist casually observed, "I noticed when we raised your arm for the ultrasound that there is an area of your skin here that puckers a little. Have you noticed any change in your armpit, chest, or breast areas?"

Depending on the client's response, follow-up questions should include asking about distended veins, discharge from the nipple, itching of the skin or nipple, and the approximate time of the client's last breast examination (self-examination and physician examination). Although not all therapists are trained to perform a clinical breast examination (CBE), palpation of lymph nodes and muscles, such as the pectoral muscle groups, can be performed.

There was no previous history of cancer, and further palpation did not elicit any other suspicious findings. The physical therapist recommended a physician evaluation and a diagnosis of breast cancer was made.

Magnetic resonance imaging (MRI) studies have shown radiation-induced muscle morbidity in cervical, prostate, and breast cancer. Axillary radiation is a predictive factor for the development of shoulder morbidity.[75] Soft tissue changes from radiotherapy is dose-dependent and may develop immediately or several years later.

Primary muscle shortening and secondary loss of muscle activity may produce movement disorders of the shoulder and/or upper quadrant. Radiation-induced changes in vascular networks resulting in ischemia may affect muscle contractility.[76]

SCREENING FOR GYNECOLOGIC CAUSES OF SHOULDER PAIN

Shoulder pain as a result of gynecologic conditions is uncommon, but still very possible. Occasionally a client may present with breast pain as the primary complaint, but most often the description is of shoulder or arm, neck, or upper back pain. When asked if the client has any symptoms anywhere else in the body, breast pain may be mentioned.

Pain patterns associated with breast disease along with a discussion of various breast pathologies are included in Chapter 18. Many of the breast conditions discussed (e.g., tumor, infection, myalgia, implants, lymph disease, trauma) can refer pain to the shoulder either alone or in conjunction with chest and/or breast pain. Shoulder pain or dysfunction in the presence of any of these conditions as a part of the client's current or past medical history raises a red flag.

Ectopic Pregnancy

The therapist must be aware of one other gynecologic condition commonly associated with shoulder pain: ectopic (extrauterine [i.e., outside the uterus]) pregnancy. This type of pregnancy occurs when the fertilized egg implants in some other part of the body other than the inside of the uterus. It may be inside of the fallopian tube, inside of the ovary, outside of the uterus, or even within the lining of the peritoneum (see Fig. 16.6).[27-29]

If the condition goes undetected, the embryo grows too large for the confined space. A tear or rupture of the tissue around the fertilized egg will occur. An ectopic pregnancy is not a viable pregnancy and cannot result in a live birth. This condition is life-threatening and requires immediate medical referral.

The most common symptom of ectopic pregnancy is a sudden, sharp or constant one-sided pain in the lower abdomen or pelvis lasting more than a few hours. The pain may be accompanied by irregular bleeding or spotting after a light or late menstrual period.

Shoulder pain does not usually occur alone without preceding or accompanying abdominal pain, but shoulder pain can be the only presenting symptom with an ectopic pregnancy. When these two symptoms occur together (either alternating or simultaneously), the woman may not realize the abdominal and shoulder pain are connected. She may think these are two separate problems. She may not see the need to tell the therapist about the pelvic or abdominal pain, especially if she thinks it is menstrual cramps or gas. Also ask about the presence of light-headedness, dizziness, or fainting.

The most likely candidate for an ectopic pregnancy is a woman in her childbearing years who is sexually active. Pregnancy can occur when using any form of birth control, so do not be swayed into thinking the woman cannot be pregnant because she is on the pill or some other form of contraception. Factors that put a woman at increased risk for an ectopic pregnancy include:

- History of endometriosis[77]
- Pelvic inflammatory disease
- Previous ectopic pregnancy
- Ruptured ovarian cyst(s) or a ruptured appendix
- Tubal surgery

Many of these conditions can also cause pelvic pain and are discussed in greater detail in Chapter 16. If the therapist suspects a gynecologic basis for the client's symptoms, some additional questions about history, missed menses, shoulder pain, and spotting or bleeding may be helpful.

PHYSICIAN REFERRAL

Here in the last chapter of the text there are no new guidelines for physician referral that have not been discussed in the previous chapters. The therapist must remain alert to yellow (caution) or red (warning) flags in the history and clinical presentation, and ask about associated signs and symptoms.

When symptoms seem out of proportion to the injury or persist beyond the expected time of healing, medical referral may be needed.[78] Likewise, pain that is unrelieved by rest or change in position or pain/symptoms that do not fit the expected mechanical or NMS pattern should serve as red-flag warnings. A past medical history of cancer in the presence of any of these clinical presentation scenarios may warrant consultation with the client's physician.

Guidelines for Immediate Medical Attention

- Presence of suspicious or aberrant lymph nodes, especially hard, fixed nodes in a client with a previous history of cancer
- Clinical presentation and history suggestive of an ectopic pregnancy
- Trauma followed by failure of symptoms to resolve with treatment; pain out of proportion to the injury (**Fracture, acute compartment syndrome**)

Clues to Screening Shoulder/Upper Extremity Pain

- See also Clues to Screening Chest, Breast, or Rib Pain in Chapter 18
- Simultaneous or alternating pain in other joints, especially in the presence of associated signs and symptoms such as easy fatigue, malaise, fever

- Urologic signs and symptoms
- Presence of hepatic symptoms, especially when accompanied by risk factors for jaundice
- Lack of improvement after treatment, including TrP therapy
- Shoulder pain in a woman of childbearing age of unknown cause associated with missed menses (**Rupture of ectopic pregnancy**)
- Left shoulder pain within 24 hours of abdominal surgery, injury, or trauma (**Kehr's sign, ruptured spleen**)

Past Medical History

- History of rheumatic disease
- History of diabetes mellitus (**Adhesive capsulitis**)
- "Frozen" shoulder of unknown cause in anyone with coronary artery disease, recent history of hospitalization in CCU or **ICU/s/p CABG**
- Recent history (past 1 to 3 months) of MI (**CRPS;** formerly RSD)
- History of cancer, especially breast or lung cancer (**Metastasis**)
- Recent history of pneumonia, recurrent upper respiratory infection, or influenza (**Diaphragmatic pleurisy**)
- History of endometriosis

Cancer

- Pectoralis major muscle spasm with no known cause; limited active shoulder flexion but with full passive shoulder motion and mobile scapula (**Neoplasm**)
- Presence of localized warmth felt over the scapular area (**Neoplasm**)
- Marked limitation of movement at the shoulder joint
- Severe muscular weakness and pain with resisted movement

Cardiac

- Exacerbation by exertion unrelated to shoulder movement (e.g., using only the lower extremities to climb stairs or ride a stationary bicycle)
- Excessive, unexplained coincident diaphoresis
- Shoulder pain relieved by leaning forward, kneeling with hands on the floor, sitting upright (**Pericarditis**)
- Shoulder pain accompanied by dyspnea, toothache, belching, nausea, or pressure behind the sternum (**Angina**)
- Shoulder pain relieved by nitroglycerin (men) or antacids/acid-relieving drugs (women) (**Angina**)
- Difference of 10 mm Hg or more in blood pressure in the affected arm compared with the uninvolved or a symptomatic arm (**Dissecting aortic aneurysm, vascular component of thoracic outlet syndrome [TOS]**)

Pulmonary

- Presence of a pleuritic component such as a persistent, dry, hacking, or productive cough; blood-tinged sputum; chest pain; musculoskeletal symptoms are aggravated by respiratory movement
- Exacerbation by recumbency despite proper positioning of the arm in neutral alignment (**Diaphragmatic or pulmonary component**)
- Presence of associated signs and symptoms (e.g., tachypnea, dyspnea, wheezing, hyperventilation)
- Shoulder pain of unknown cause in older adults with accompanying signs of confusion or increased confusion (**Pneumonia**)
- Shoulder pain aggravated by the supine position may be an indication of mediastinal or pleural involvement. Shoulder or back pain alleviated by lying on the painful side may indicate autosplinting (**Pleural**)

Renal

- Shoulder pain accompanied by elevation in temperature or change in color, odor, or amount of urine (flow, frequency, nocturia); pain is not affected by movement or provocation tests
- Shoulder pain accompanied by, or alternating with, flank pain, abdominal pain, or pelvic pain or, in men, testicular pain

Gastrointestinal

- Coincident nausea, vomiting, dysphagia; presence of other GI complaints such as anorexia, early satiety, epigastric pain or discomfort and fullness, melena
- Shoulder pain relieved by belching or antacids and made worse by eating
- History of previous ulcer, especially in association with the use of NSAIDs

Gynecologic

- Shoulder pain preceded or accompanied by one-sided lower abdominal or pelvic pain in a sexually active woman of reproductive age may be a symptom of **ectopic pregnancy;** there may be irregular bleeding or spotting after a light or late menstrual period
- Shoulder pain with reports of light-headedness, dizziness, or fainting in a sexually active woman of reproductive age (**Ectopic pregnancy**)
- Presence of endometrial cyst(s) and/or scar tissue impinging diaphragm, nerve plexus, or the shoulder itself

REFERRED SHOULDER AND UPPER EXTREMITY PAIN PATTERNS

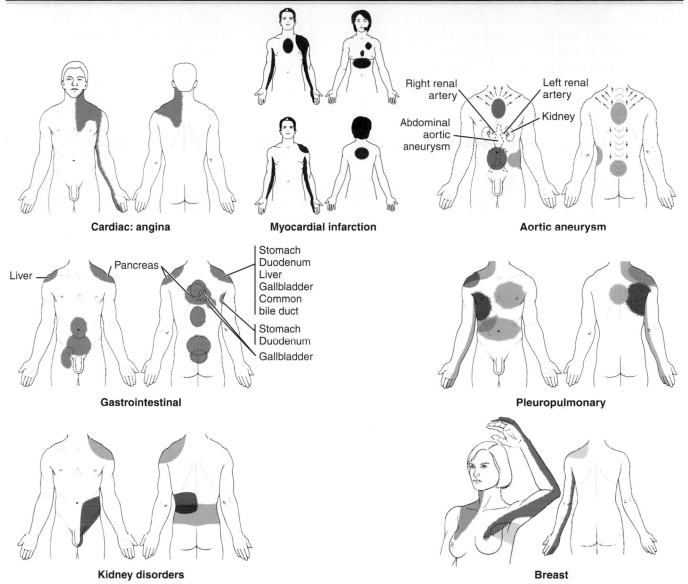

Composite picture of referred shoulder and upper extremity pain patterns. Not pictured: TrP referred pain (see Fig. 17.7).

Key Points to Remember

1. Shoulder dysfunction can look like a true neuromuscular or musculoskeletal problem and still be viscerogenic or systemic in origin.

2. Any adult over the age of 65 years presenting with shoulder pain and/or dysfunction must be screened for a systemic or viscerogenic origin of symptoms, even when there is a known (or attributed) cause or injury.

3. Knowing the key red flags associated with cancer, vascular disease, pulmonary, GI, and gynecologic causes of

shoulder pain and/or dysfunction will help the therapist screen quickly, efficiently, and accurately.

4. Painless weakness of insidious onset is most likely a neurologic problem; painful, insidious weakness may be caused by cervical radiculopathy, a chronic rotator cuff problem, tumor, or arthritis. A medical differential diagnosis is required.[79,80]

5. As mentioned throughout this text, the therapist can collaborate with colleagues in asking questions and

■ **Key Points to Remember—cont'd**

reviewing findings before making a medical referral. Perhaps someone else will see the answer or a solution to the client's unusual presentation, or perhaps another opinion will confirm the findings and give you the confidence you need to guide your professional decision making.

6. Postoperative infection of any kind may not appear with any clinical signs/symptoms for weeks or months,

especially in a client who is taking corticosteroids or is immunocompromised.

7. Consider unreported trauma or assault as a possible etiologic cause of shoulder pain.

8. Palpate the diaphragm and assess breathing patterns; shoulder pain reproduced by diaphragmatic palpation may point to a primary diaphragmatic (muscular) problem.

CLIENT HISTORY AND INTERVIEW

SPECIAL QUESTIONS TO ASK: SHOULDER AND UPPER EXTREMITY

General Systemic

- Does your pain ever wake you at night from a sound sleep? **(Cancer)**
  - Can you find any way to relieve the pain and get back to sleep?
  - *If yes,* how? (Cancer: pain is usually intense and constant; nothing relieves it or if relief is obtained in any way, over time pain gets progressively worse)
- Since your shoulder problem began, have you had any unusual perspiration for no apparent reason, sweats, or fever?
- Have you had any unusual fatigue (more than usual with no change in lifestyle), joint pain in other joints, or general malaise? **(Rheumatic disease)**
- Have you sustained any injuries in the last week during a sports activity, car accident, etc.?
  - (Ruptured spleen associated with pain in the left shoulder: positive Kehr's sign)
  - *For the therapist:* Has the client had a laparoscopy in the last 24 to 48 hours? **(Left shoulder pain: positive Kehr's sign)**

Cardiac

- Have you recently (ever) had a heart attack? **(Referred pain via viscerosomatic zones,** see explanation Chapter 3)
- Do you ever notice sweating, nausea, or chest pain when the pain in your shoulder occurs?
- Have you noticed your shoulder pain increasing with exertion that does not necessarily cause you to use your shoulder (e.g., climbing stairs, stationary bicycle)?
- Do(es) your mouth, jaw, or teeth ever hurt when your shoulder is bothering you? **(Angina)**
- For the client with known angina: Does your shoulder pain go away when you take nitroglycerin? (Ask about the effect of taking antacids/acid-relieving drugs for women.)

Pulmonary

- Have you been treated recently for a lung problem (or think you have any lung or respiratory problems)?

- Do you currently have a cough?
  - *If yes,* is this a smoker's cough?
  - *If no,* how long has this been present?
  - Is this a productive cough (can you bring up sputum), and is the sputum yellow, green, black, or tinged with blood?
- Does coughing bring on your shoulder pain (or make it worse)?
- Do you ever have shortness of breath, have trouble catching your breath, or feel breathless?
- Does your shoulder pain increase when you cough, laugh, or take a deep breath?
- Do you have any chest pain?
- What effect does lying down or resting have on your shoulder pain? (In the supine or recumbent position, a pulmonary problem may be made worse, whereas a musculoskeletal problem may be relieved; on the other hand, pulmonary pain may be relieved when the client lies on the affected side, which diminishes the movement of that side of the chest.)

Gastrointestinal

- Have you ever had an ulcer?
  - *If yes,* when? Do you still have any pain from your ulcer?
  - Have you noticed any association between when you eat and when your symptoms increase or decrease?
- Does eating relieve your pain? **(Duodenal or pyloric ulcer)**
- How soon is the pain relieved after eating?
  - Does eating aggravate your pain? **(Gastric ulcer, gallbladder inflammation)**
- Does your pain occur 1 to 3 hours after eating or between meals? (Duodenal or pyloric ulcers, gallstones)
- For the client taking NSAIDs: Does your shoulder pain increase 2 to 4 hours after taking your NSAIDs? If the client does not know, ask him or her to pay attention for the next few days to the response of their shoulder symptoms after taking the medication.
- Have you ever had gallstones?
- Do you have a feeling of fullness after only one or two bites of food? **(Early satiety: stomach and duodenum or gallbladder)**

CLIENT HISTORY AND INTERVIEW—cont'd

- Have you had any nausea, vomiting, difficulty with swallowing, loss of appetite, or heartburn since the shoulder started bothering you?

Gynecologic

- Have you ever had a breast implant, mastectomy, or other breast surgery? (**Altered lymph drainage, scar tissue**)
- Have you ever had a tubal or ectopic pregnancy?
- Have you ever been diagnosed with endometriosis?
- Have you missed your last period? (**Ectopic pregnancy, endometriosis; blood in the peritoneum irritates diaphragm causing referred pain**)
- Are you having any spotting or irregular bleeding?
- Have you had any spontaneous or induced abortions recently? (**Blood in peritoneum irritating diaphragm**)
- Have you recently had a baby? (**Excessive muscle tension during birth**)
- *If yes:* Are you breastfeeding with the infant supported on pillows?

- Do you have a breast discharge, or have you had mastitis?

Urologic

- Have you recently been diagnosed with a kidney infection, tumor, or kidney stones? (**Pressure from kidney on diaphragm referred to shoulder**)

Trauma

- Have you been in a fight or been assaulted?
- Have you ever been pulled by the arm, pushed against the wall, or thrown by the arm?

If the answer is "Yes" and the history relates to the current episode of symptoms, then the therapist may need to conduct a more complete screening interview related to domestic violence and assault. Specific questions for this section have been discussed in Chapter 2; see also Appendix B-3 in the accompanying enhanced eBook version included with print purchase of this textbook.

CASE STUDY

Steps in the Screening Process

If a client comes to you with shoulder pain with any of the red-flag histories and/or red-flag clinical findings to suggest screening, start by asking yourself these questions:

- Which shoulder is it?
- Which organs could it be? (Use Fig. 3.4 showing the viscera in relation to the diaphragm and Tables 19.1 and 19.2 to help you.)
- What are the associated signs and symptoms of that organ? Are any of these signs or symptoms present?
- What is the history? Does anything in the history correlate with the particular shoulder involved and/or with the associated signs and symptoms? Conduct a Review of Systems as discussed in Chapter 4 (see Box 4.19).
- Can you palpate it, make it better or worse, or reproduce it in any way?

Could it be Cancer?

Remember, the therapist does not determine whether a client has cancer. The therapist's assessment determines whether the client has a true neuromuscular or musculoskeletal problem that is within the scope of our practice. However, knowing red flags for the possibility of cancer helps the therapist know what questions to ask and what red flags to look for. Watch for:

- Previous history of cancer (any kind, but especially breast or lung cancer)
- Pectoralis major muscle spasm with no known cause, but full passive ROM and a mobile scapula. Be sure to assess for TrPs and reassess after TrP therapy.

- Were the symptoms alleviated? Did the movement pattern change?
- Conduct a neurologic screening examination.
- Shoulder flexion and abduction limited to 90 degrees with empty end feel.
- Presence of localized warmth over scapular area. Look for other trophic changes.

Could it be Vascular?

Watch for:

- Exacerbation by exertion unrelated to shoulder movement
- Does the shoulder pain and/or symptoms become worse when the client is just using the lower extremities? What is the effect of riding a stationary bike or climbing stairs without using the arms?
- Excessive, unexplained coincident diaphoresis (i.e., the client breaks out in a cold sweat just before or during an episode of shoulder pain; this may occur at rest but is more likely with mild physical activity).
- Shoulder pain relieved by leaning forward, kneeling with hands on the floor, sitting upright (pericarditis).
- Shoulder pain accompanied by dyspnea, temporomandibular joint (TMJ) pain, toothache, belching, nausea, or pressure behind the sternum.
- Bilateral shoulder pain that comes on after using the arms overhead for 3 to 5 minutes.
- Shoulder pain relieved by nitroglycerin (men) or antacids/acid-relieving drugs (women) [angina]

CASE STUDY—cont'd

- Difference of 10 mm Hg or more (at rest) in diastolic blood pressure in the affected arm (aortic aneurysm; vascular component of thoracic outlet syndrome)
  Remember to correlate any of these symptoms with:
- Client's past medical history (e.g., personal and/or family history of heart disease)
- Age (over 50 years, especially postmenopausal women)
- Characteristics of pain pattern (see Table 7.5; these characteristics of cardiac-related chest pain can also apply to cardiac-related shoulder pain)

Could it be Pulmonary?

- Ask about the presence of a pleuritic component
  - Persistent cough (dry or productive)
  - Blood-tinged sputum; rust, green, or yellow exudate
  - Chest pain
  - Musculoskeletal symptoms are aggravated by respiratory movement; ask the client to take a deep breath. Does this reproduce or increase the pain/symptoms?
- Watch for the exacerbation of symptoms by recumbence even with proper positioning of the arm. Lying down in the supine position can put the shoulder in a position of slight extension.
- This can put pressure on soft tissue structures in and around the shoulder, causing pain in the presence of a true neuromuscular or musculoskeletal problem.
- For this reason, when assessing the effect of recumbence, make sure the shoulder is in a neutral position. You may have to support the upper arm with a towel roll under the elbow and/or put a pillow on the client's abdomen to give the forearms a place to rest.
- Pain is relieved or made better by sidelying on the involved side. This is called autosplinting.
- Pressure on the rib cage prevents respiratory movement on that side, thereby reducing symptoms induced by respiratory movement. This is quite the opposite of a musculoskeletal or neuromuscular cause of shoulder pain; the client often cannot lie on the involved side without increased pain.
- Ask about the presence of associated signs and symptoms. Remember to ask our final question:
- Are there any symptoms of any kind anywhere else in your body?

In the older adult, listen for a self-report or family report of unknown cause of shoulder pain/dysfunction and/or any signs of confusion (confusion or increased confusion is a common first symptom of pneumonia in the older adult).

Could it be Gastrointestinal or Hepatic?

- Ask about a history of chronic (more than 6 months) NSAID use and history of previous ulcer, especially in association with NSAID use. This is the most common cause of medication-induced shoulder pain in all ages, but especially in adults over the age of 65 years.
- History of other GI disease that can refer pain to the shoulder such as:

- Gallbladder
- Acute pancreatitis
- Reflex esophagitis
- Watch for coincident (or alternating) nausea
- Ask if the shoulder pain is relieved by belching
- Look for shoulder pain that is changed by eating

Watch for coincident (or alternating) nausea, vomiting, dysphagia, anorexia, early satiety, or other GI symptoms. Clients often think they have two separate problems. The client may not think the therapist treating the shoulder needs or wants to know about their GI problems. The therapist who is not trained to screen for medical disease may not think to ask.

Ask if shoulder pain is relieved by belching or antacids. This could signal an underlying GI problem, or, for women, cardiac ischemia.

Look for shoulder pain that is changed by eating (better or worse within 30 minutes or worse 1 to 3 hours after eating).

The therapist does not have to identify the specific area of the GI tract that is involved or the specific pathology present. It is important to know that true NMS shoulder pain is not relieved or exacerbated by eating.

If there is a peptic ulcer in the upper GI tract causing referred pain to the shoulder, there is often a history of NSAID use. This client will have that red-flag history along with shoulder pain that gets better after eating. There may also be other GI symptoms present, such as nausea, loss of appetite, or melena from oxidized blood in the upper GI tract.

If there is liver impairment as well, there can be symptoms of CTS. For a list of possible NMS and systemic causes of CTS, see Table 12.2. Again, CTS in the presence of any of these systemic conditions should be assessed carefully. Likewise, CTS may be the first symptom of some of these pathologies.

The client with shoulder pain (GI bleed) and symptoms of CTS (liver impairment) may demonstrate other signs of liver impairment such as:
- Liver flap (asterixis; see Fig. 10.8)
- Liver palms (palmar erythema; see Fig. 10.6)
- Change in nail beds (white nails of Terry; see Fig. 10.7)
- Spider angioma (over the abdomen; see Fig. 10.5)
- These tests along with photos and illustrations are discussed in detail in Chapter 10.

Could it be Breast Pathology?

Remember that men can have breast disease too, although not as often as women. Red-flag clinical presentation and associated signs and symptoms of breast disease referred to the shoulder may include:
- Jarring or squeezing the breast refers pain to the shoulder
- Resisted shoulder motion does not reproduce shoulder pain but does cause breast pain or discomfort
- Obvious change in breast tissue (e.g., lump[s], dimpling or peau d'orange, distended veins, nipple discharge or ulceration, erythema, change in size or shape of the breast)
- Suspicious or aberrant axillary or supraclavicular lymph nodes

PRACTICE QUESTIONS

1. A 66-year-old woman has been referred to you by her physiatrist for preprosthetic training after an above-knee amputation. Her past medical history is significant for chronic diabetes mellitus (insulin dependent), coronary artery disease (CAD) with recent angioplasty and stent placement, and peripheral vascular disease. During the physical therapy evaluation, the client experienced anterior neck pain radiating down the left arm. Name (and/or describe) three tests you can do to differentiate a musculoskeletal cause from a cardiac cause of shoulder pain.

2. Which of the following would be useful information when evaluating a 57-year-old woman with shoulder pain?
   a. Influence of antacids on symptoms
   b. History of chronic NSAID use
   c. Effect of food on symptoms
   d. All of the above

3. Referred pain patterns associated with impairment of the spleen can produce musculoskeletal symptoms in:
   a. The left shoulder
   b. The right shoulder
   c. The mid- or upper back, scapular, and right shoulder areas
   d. The thorax, scapulae, right or left shoulder

4. Referred pain patterns associated with hepatic and biliary pathology can produce musculoskeletal symptoms in:
   a. The left shoulder
   b. The right shoulder
   c. The mid or upper back, scapular, and right shoulder areas
   d. The thorax, scapulae, right or left shoulder

5. The most common sites of referred pain from systemic disease are:
   a. Neck and hip
   b. Shoulder and back
   c. Chest and back
   d. None of the above

6. A 28-year-old mechanic reports bilateral shoulder pain (right more than left) whenever he has to work on a car on a lift overhead. It goes away as soon as he puts his arms down. Sometimes, he has numbness and tingling in his right elbow going down the inside of his forearm to his thumb. The most likely explanation for this pattern of symptoms is:
   a. Angina
   b. Myocardial ischemia
   c. Thoracic outlet syndrome
   d. Peptic ulcer

7. A client reports shoulder and upper trapezius pain on the right that increases with deep breathing. How can you tell if this results from a pulmonary or musculoskeletal cause?
   a. Symptoms become worse when lying supine, but better when right sidelying if the cause is pulmonary
   b. Symptoms become worse when lying supine, but better when right sidelying if the cause is musculoskeletal

8. Organ systems that can cause simultaneous bilateral shoulder pain include:
   a. Spleen
   b. Heart
   c. Gallbladder
   d. None of the above

9. A 23-year-old woman was a walk-in to your clinic with sudden onset of left shoulder pain. She denies any history of trauma and has only a past history of a ruptured appendix 3 years ago. She is not having any abdominal pain or pain anywhere else in her body. How do you know if she is at risk for ectopic pregnancy?
   a. She is sexually active, and her period is late.
   b. She has a history of uterine cancer.
   c. She has a history of peptic ulcer.
   d. None of the above

10. The most significant red flag for shoulder pain secondary to cancer is:
    a. Previous history of coronary artery disease
    b. Subscapularis TrP alleviated with TrP therapy
    c. Negative neurologic screening examination
    d. Previous history of breast or lung cancer

REFERENCES

1. Lollino N, Brunocilla PR, Poglio F, Vannini E, Lollino S, Lancia M. Non-orthopaedic causes of shoulder pain: what the shoulder expert must remember. *Musculoskelet Surg*. 2012;296(Suppl 1):S63–S68.
2. Walter FM, Rubin G, Bankhead C, et al. Symptoms and other factors associated with time to diagnosis and stage of lung cancer: a prospective cohort study. *BJC*. 2015;112:S6–S13.
3. Martin TJ, Moseley JM. Mechanisms in the skeletal complications of breast cancer. *Endocr Relat Cancer*. 2000;7:271–284.
4. Berg J. Symptoms of a first acute myocardial infarction in men and women. *Gend Med*. 2009;6(3):454–462.
5. Logline M. Early warning signs of an acute myocardial infarction and their influence on symptoms during the acute phase, with comparisons by gender. *Gend Med*. 2009;6(3):444–453.
6. Hwang SY. Comparison of factors associated with atypical symptoms in younger and older patients with acute coronary syndromes. *J Korean Med Sci*. 2009;24(5):789–794.
7. Rubba F. Vascular preventive measures: the progression from asymptomatic to symptomatic atherosclerosis management. Evidence on usefulness of early diagnosis in women and children. *Future Cardiol*. 2010;6(2):211–220.
8. Vercoza AM. Cardiovascular risk factors and carotid intima-media thickness in asymptomatic children. *Pediatr Cardiol*. 2009;30(8):1055–1060.
9. Smith ML. Differentiating angina and shoulder pathology pain. *Phys Ther Case Rep*. 1998;1(4):210–212.
10. Ogawa K. Advanced shoulder joint tuberculosis treated with debridement and closed continuous irrigation and suction. *Am J Orthop*. 2010;39(2):E15–E18..
11. Ba-Fall K. Shoulder pain revealing tuberculosis of the humerus. *Rev Pneumonol*. 2009;65(1):13–15.
12. Nagaraj C. Tuberculosis of the shoulder joint with impingement syndrome as initial presentation. *J Microbiol Immunol Infect*. 2008;41(3):275–278.
13. Wohlgethan JR. Frozen shoulder in hyperthyroidism. *Arthritis Rheum*. 1987;Aug;30(8):936–939.
14. Roy A. Adhesive capsulitis in physical medicine and rehabilitation. eMedicine Specialties. Updated Oct. 15, 2009. http://emedicine.medscape.com/article/326828-overview. Accessed March 21, 2011.
15. Lebiedz-Odrobina D. Rheumatic manifestations of diabetes mellitus. *Rheum Dis Clin North Am*. 2010;36(4):681–699.
16. Garcilazo C. Shoulder manifestations of diabetes mellitus. *Curr Diabetes Rev*. 2010;6(5):334–340.

17. Saha NC. Painful shoulder in patients with chronic bronchitis and emphysema. *Am Rev Respir Dis*. 1966;94:455–456.

18. Okada M, Suzuki K, Hidaka T, et al. Complex regional pain syndrome type I induced by pacemaker implantation, with a good response to steroids and neurotrophin. *Intern Med*. 2002;41:498–501.

19. Leff D. Ruptured spleen following laparoscopic cholecystectomy. *JSLS*. 2007;11(1):157–160.

20. Sharami SH. Randomised clinical trial of the influence of pulmonary recruitment manoeuvre on reducing shoulder pain after laparoscopy. *J Obstet Gynaecol*. 2010;30(5):505–510.

21. Shin HY. The effect of mechanical ventilation tidal volume during pneumoperitoneum on shoulder pain after a laparoscopic appendectomy. *Surg Endosc*. 2010;24(8):2002–2007.

22. Wada S, Fukushi Y, Nishimura M, et al. Analysis of risk factors of postlaparoscopic shoulder pain. *J Obstet Gynaecol Res*. 2020;46(2):310–313. https://doi.org/10.1111/jog.14156. Epub 2020 Jan 20. PMID: 31958892.

23. Giles LGF, Singer KP. *The Clinical Anatomy and Management of Thoracic Spine Pain*. Oxford: Butterworth Heinemann; 2000.

24. Kandil TS. Shoulder pain following laparoscopic cholecystectomy: factors affecting the incidence and severity. *J Laparoendosc Adv Surg Tech A*. 2010;20(8):677–682.

25. Chang SH. An evaluation of perioperative pregabalin for prevention and attenuation of postoperative shoulder pain after laparoscopic cholecystectomy. *Anesth Analg*. 2009;109(4):1284–1286.

26. Hadler NM. The patient with low back pain. *Hosp Pract*. 1987;22(10A):17–22.

27. Biolchini F. Emergency laparoscopic splenectomy for haemoperitoneum because of ruptured primary splenic pregnancy: a case report and review of literature. *ANZ J Surg*. 2010;80(102):55–57.

28. Dennert IM. Ectopic pregnancy. *J Minim Invasive Gynecol*. 2008;15(3):377–379.

29. Bildik F. Heterotopic pregnancy presenting with acute left chest pain. *Am J Emerg Med*. 2008;26(7):835.e1–835.e2.

30. Trail CE, Watson A, Schofield AM. Case of hepatic flexure ectopic pregnancy medically managed with methotrexate. *BMJ Case Rep*. 2018 2018:bcr2017220480. https://doi.org/10.1136/bcr-2017-220480. PMID: 29550756.

31. Rossi P, Gargne O, Ayme K, Gavarry O, Boussuges A. Inter-limb changes in arterial function after intense cycling exercise. *Int J Sports Med*. 2014;35(11):889–893.

32. Oaklander AL, Rissmiller JG, Gelman LB, Zheng L, Chang Y, Gott R. Evidence of focal small-fiber axonal degeneration in complex regional pain syndrome-I (reflex sympathetic dystrophy). *Pain*. 2006;120(3):235–243.

33. Urits I, Shen AH, Jones MR, Viswanath O, Kaye AD. Complex regional pain syndrome, current concepts and treatment options. *Curr Pain Headache Rep*. 2018;22(2):10 https://doi.org/10.1007/s11916-018-0667-7. PMID: 29404787.

34. Jänig W, Baron R. Is CRPS: I a neuropathic pain syndrome? *Pain*. 2006;120(3):227–229.

35. Jänig W. The fascination of complex regional pain syndrome. *Exp Neurol*. 2010;221(1):1–4.

36. Harden RN, Bruehl S, Perez RSGM, et al. Validation of proposed diagnostic criteria (the "Budapest Criteria") for complex regional pain syndrome. *Pain*. 2010;150(2):268–274.

37. Duman I. Reflex sympathetic dystrophy secondary to deep venous thrombosis mimicking post-thrombotic syndrome. *Rheumatol Int*. 2009;30(2):249–252.

38. Eyers P, Earnshaw JJ. Acute non-traumatic arm ischemia. *Br J Surg*. 1998;85:1340–1346.

39. Brinkley DM, Hepper CT. Heart in hand: structural cardiac abnormalities that manifest as acute dysvascularity of the hand. *J Hand Surg*. 2010;35A(12):2101–2103.

40. Shenker N, Goebel A, Rockett M, et al. Establishing the characteristics for patients with chronic Complex Regional Pain Syndrome: the value of the CPRS-UK Registry. *British J Pain*. 2015;9(2):122–128.

41. Alozie A, Zimpfer A, Koller K, et al. Arthralgia and blood culture-negative endocarditis in middle age men suggest tropheryma whipplei infection: a report of two cases and review of the literature. *BMC Infect Dis*. 2015;15:339.

42. American Heart Association: Pericardium and Pericarditis. http://www.americanheart.org/presenter.jhtml?identifier=4683. Accessed March 22, 2011.

43. Texas Heart Institute: Aneurysms and Dissections. http://www.texasheartinstitute.org/hic/topics/cond/aneurysm.cfm. Accessed March 22, 2011.

44. Tran H. Deep venous thromboses in patients with hematological malignancies after peripherally inserted central venous catheters. *Leuk Lymphoma*. 2010;51(8):1473–1477.

45. Jones MA. Characterizing resolution of catheter-associated upper extremity deep venous thrombosis. *J Vasc Surg*. 2010;51(1):108–113.

46. Shah MK. Upper extremity deep vein thrombosis. *South Med J*. 2003;96(7):669–672.

47. Linneman B. Hereditary and acquired thrombophilia in patients with upper extremity deep-vein thrombosis. *Thromb Haemost*. 2008;100(3):440–446.

48. Jones RE. Upper limb deep vein thrombosis: a potentially fatal complication of clavicle fracture. *Ann R Coll Surg Engl*. 2010;92(5):W36–W38.

49. Garofalo R. Deep vein thromboembolism after arthroscopy of the shoulder: two case reports and review of the literature. *BMC Musculoskel Disord*. 2010;11:65.

50. Willis AA. Deep vein thrombosis after reconstructive shoulder arthroplasty: a prospective observational study. *J Shoulder Elbow Surg*. 2009;18(1):100–106.

51. Farge D. Lessons from French National Guidelines on the treatment of venous thrombosis and central venous catheter thrombosis in cancer patients. *Thromb Res*. 2010;125(Suppl 2):S108–S116.

52. Lancaster SL. Upper-extremity deep vein thrombosis. *AJN*. 2010;110(5):48–52.

53. Gaitini D. Prevalence of upper extremity deep venous thrombosis diagnosed by color Doppler duplex sonography in cancer patients with central venous catheters. *J Ultrasound Med*. 2006;25(10):1297–1303.

54. Joffe HV. Upper extremity deep vein thrombosis: a prospective registry of 592 patients. *Circulation*. 2004;110:1605–1611.

55. Otten TR. Thromboembolic disease involving the superior vena cava and brachiocephalic veins. *Chest*. 2003;123(3):809–812.

56. Constans J. A clinical prediction score for upper extremity deep venous thrombosis. *Thromb Haemost*. 2008;99:202–207.

57. Rosa-Salazar V, Trujillo-Santos J, Diaz Peromingo JA, et al. A prognostic score to identify low-risk outpatients with acute deep vein thrombosis in the upper extremity. *J Thromb Haemost*. 2015;13(7):1274–1278.

58. Di Nisio M. Accuracy of diagnostic tests for clinically suspected upper extremity deep vein thrombosis: a systematic review. *J Thromb Haemost*. 2010;8(4):684–692.

59. Netter FH. *Atlas of Human Anatomy*. 5 ed. Philadelphia: WB Saunders; 2010.

60. Moore KL. *Clinically Oriented Anatomy*. 6 ed. Baltimore: Lippincott Williams & Wilkins; 2009.

61. Pedersen KV. Flank pain in renal and ureteral calculus. *Ugeskr Laeger*. 2011;173(7):503–505.

62. Pedersen KV. Visceral pain originating from the upper urinary tract. *Urol Res*. 2010;38(5):345–355.

63. Delavierre D. Symptomatic approach to referred chronic pelvic and perineal pain and posterior ramus syndrome. *Prog Urol*. 2010;20(12):990–994.

64. Myslinski MJ. *NSAIDs: The Good, The Bad, and The Ugly*. Las Vegas, NV: Lecture presented at the APTA Combined Sections Meeting; February 11, 2009.

65. Rose SJ, Rothstein JM. Muscle mutability: general concepts and adaptations to altered patterns of use. *Phys Ther.* 1982;62:1773.

66. Yung E. Screening for head, neck, and shoulder pathology in patients with upper extremity signs and symptoms. *J Hand Ther.* 2010;23:173–186.

67. McKay P. Osteomyelitis and septic arthritis of the hand and wrist. *Curr Ortho Pract.* 2010;21(6):542–550.

68. Heick JD, Boissonnault WG, King PM. Physical therapist recognition of signs and symptoms of infection after shoulder reconstruction: a patient case report. *Physiother Theo Pract.* 2013;29(2):166–173.

69. Bonsignore A. Occult rupture of the spleen in a patient with infectious mononucleosis. *G Chir.* 2010;31(3):86–90.

70. Cyriax J. *Textbook of Orthopaedic Medicine.* 8 ed. Baltimore: Williams and Wilkins; 1982.

71. Schumpelick V. Surgical embryology and anatomy of the diaphragm with surgical applications. *Surg Clin North Am.* 2000;80(1):213–239.

72. Tateishi U. Chest wall tumors: radiologic findings and pathologic correlation. *RadioGraphics.* 2003;23:1491–1508. http://radiographics.rsna.org/content/23/6/1491.full. Accessed March 22, 2011.

73. Bhimji S. Pancoast tumor. eMedicine Specialties—Thoracic Surgery (Tumors). http://emedicine.medscape.com/article/428469-overview, August 3, 2010. Accessed March 2, 2011.

74. Cailliet R. *Shoulder Pain.* 3 ed. Philadelphia: FA Davis; 1991.

75. Reitman J. Late morbidity after treatment of breast cancer in relation to daily activities and quality of life: a systematic review. *Eur J Surg Oncol.* 2003;29:229–238.

76. Shamley DR. Changes in shoulder muscle size and activity following treatment for breast cancer. *Breast Cancer Res Treat.* 2007;106(1):19–27.

77. Seoud AA. Endometriosis: a possible cause of right shoulder pain. *Clin Exp Obstet Gynecol.* 2010;37(1):19–20.

78. Prasarn ML, Ouellette EA. Acute compartment syndrome of the upper extremity. *JAAOS.* 2011;19(1):49–58.

79. McFarland EG, Sanguanjit P, Tasaki A, et al. Shoulder examination: established and evolving concepts. *J Musculoskel Med.* 2006;23(1):57–64.

80. McFarland EG. Clinical and diagnostic tests for shoulder disorders: a critical review. *Br J Sports Med.* 2010;44(5):328–332.

81. Neer CS. Anterior acromioplasty for the chronic impingement syndrome in the shoulder: a preliminary report. *J Bone Joint Surg.* 1972;54(1):41–50.

82. Labidi M. Pleural effusions following cardiac surgery: prevalence, risk factors, and clinical features. *Chest.* 2009;136(6):1604–1611.

83. Ashikhmina EA. Pericardial effusion after cardiac surgery: risk factors, patient profiles, and contemporary management. *Ann Thorac Surg.* 2010;89(1):112–118.

84. Ahmed WA. Survival after isolated coronary artery bypass grafting in patients with severe left ventricular dysfunction. *Ann Thorac Surg.* 2009;87(4):1106–1112.

85. Jensen L. Risk factors for postoperative pulmonary complications in coronary artery bypass graft surgery patients. *Eur J Cardiovasc.* 2007;6(3):241–246.

86. Mennell JM. *The Musculoskeletal System: Differential Diagnosis from Symptoms and Physical Signs.* Sudbury, MA: Jones and Bartlett; 1992.

Note: Page numbers followed by *b*, *t*, and *f* indicate boxes, tables, and figures, respectively.